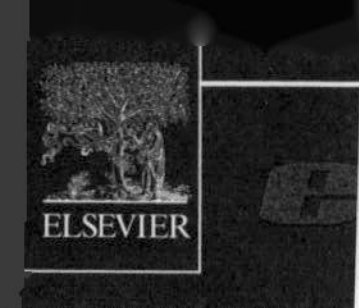

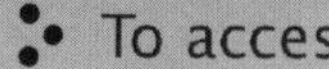

To acces[...]
Web address below.

http://evolve.elsevier.com/DrugConsult/pediatric/

Evolve Resources for *Mosby's Pediatric Drug Consult* offers the following features:

- **Quarterly Drug Updates and Alerts**
  Abbreviated monographs on new drugs and updated information on new indications and new dosages for existing drugs. Important information about drugs recently withdrawn from the market, new drug safety information, and other news to help you provide the best possible care.

- **"Do Not Confuse" Table**
  A complete listing of pediatric drug names that sound alike and are often confused.

- **JCAHO Abbreviations List**
  Up-to-date listing of potentially dangerous abbreviations and the JCAHO recommendations for proper use of abbreviations for medication administration and documentation.

Mosby's PEDIATRIC DRUG CONSULT

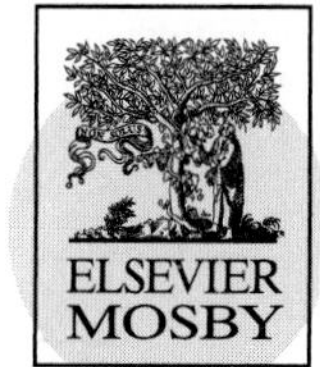

ELSEVIER
MOSBY

11830 Westline Industrial Drive
St. Louis, Missouri 63146

MOSBY'S PEDIATRIC DRUG CONSULT ISBN 0-323-03174-9

Notice

Pharmacology is an ever-changing field. Standard safety precautions must be followed, but as new research and clinical experience broaden our knowledge, changes in treatment and drug therapy may become necessary or appropriate. Readers are advised to check the most current product information provided by the manufacturer of each drug to be administered to verify the recommended dose, the method and duration of administration, and contraindications. It is the responsibility of the licensed prescriber, relying on experience and knowledge of the patient, to determine dosages and the best treatment for each individual patient. Neither the publisher nor the author assumes any liability for any injury and/or damage to persons or property arising from this publication.

International Standard Book Number 0-323-03174-9

Editor: Catherine Jackson
Managing Editor: Michele D. Hayden
Editorial Assistant: Heather Bays
Publishing Services Manager: Julie Eddy
Production Manager: Kelly E.M. Steinmann
Designer: Jyotika Shroff

Printed in the United States

Last digit is the print number: 9 8 7 6 5 4 3 2 1

SPECIAL CONTRIBUTORS

Kelley Ward, PhD, RN, C
Faculty Member
Langston University School of Nursing
Tulsa, Oklahoma

Tracy M. Hagemann, PharmD
Associate Professor
Clinical Pediatric Specialist
University of Oklahoma Health Sciences Center
College of Pharmacy
Oklahoma City, Oklahoma

REVIEWERS

Rebecca Gesler, MSN, RN
Assistant Professor of Nursing
Spalding University
Louisville, Kentucky

Raeann LeBlanc, MSN, RN, BA, CNP
Assistant Professor
Mount Wachusett Community College
Gardner, Massachusetts

Angela S. Wilson, PhD, RN, BC
Associate Professor and Department Chair
The University of Virginia College at Wise
Wise, Virginia

FOREWORD

Nurses are the front-line care providers for patients in pediatric settings. As a pediatric nurse, your actions—including drug administration—directly affect patient outcomes. In today's fast-paced, high-tech world, drug administration errors pose a constant threat and are a leading cause of morbidity, mortality, and litigation. To help prevent life-threatening errors, you need a drug reference that gives you the vital information you need in the most useful way possible. *Mosby's Pediatric Drug Consult* provides you with a resource to help you provide optimal patient care related to drug therapy.

This portable drug handbook includes all the essential information you need to administer hundreds of generic and trade drugs, but it also does much more. Its organization of drugs by therapeutic class, listing drugs alphabetically by generic name in each class, allows you to scan related drugs easily and compare factors that may affect their use in certain patients.

Mosby's Pediatric Drug Consult is edited by Kelley Ward, PhD, RN, C and reviewed by Tracy Hagemann, PharmD. These individuals, in collaboration with our reviewers, ensure that this new pediatric reference meets the highest standards for reliability and accuracy.

Whether you're a student, novice, or seasoned pediatric nurse, you'll find that the book's convenient organization and accurate, comprehensive drug information make it an essential tool for daily use on the job.

WHAT MAKES THIS BOOK SPECIAL

In addition to providing detailed information in each drug entry, *Mosby's Pediatric Drug Consult* offers many special features designed to help make drug administration easier, faster, and more efficient.

KEY FEATURES

Organized by therapeutic class. By grouping drug entries within therapeutic classes, the book helps you identify drugs by clinical application and compare information about alternate drugs used for the same purpose. Each class includes an overview with key information about the drugs' therapeutic uses and mechanisms of action.

Specific to pediatric patients. This drug consult identifies drugs with a clinical application to pediatric patients. This information can be used by a variety of health care providers. Specific information regarding assessment, administration, intervention, and evaluation of drugs is provided, highlighting the importance of pediatric considerations specific to each drug.

Diagnostic test effects. This book identifies diagnostic test effects that specific drugs can have on pediatric patients.

Practice-oriented nursing considerations. In every drug entry this reference provides extensive, practice-oriented nursing considerations, putting essential drug facts directly into the context of your care.

Comprehensive appendixes. Handy time-saving tables, summaries, and charts are included in the appendixes to ensure safe and effective medication administration. Additional drug-related information, such as an English-Spanish translator and Patient/Family Teaching appendix, help you provide appropriate drug therapy and teaching.

UNIQUE FEATURES

Insightful illustrations. Detailed, two-color illustrations help enhance your understanding of the mechanism or site of action for selected drugs and drug classes.

Color plates. More than 20 full-color images are included in a special insert to assist in identifying various pediatric medications by sight.

Prioritized side effects. Side effects for each drug entry are ranked by frequency of occurrence from most common to least common. The percentage of frequency is also included, when known. This information helps you focus your care by knowing which effects to monitor more closely.

Highlights on serious reactions. In each drug entry, the book calls attention to dangerous or life-threatening reactions so you can identify them easily and act on them promptly.

Alert icons. An *Alert* icon is used throughout the drug monographs to spotlight critical nursing considerations that require special attention.

Free updates. The companion website, *http://evolve.elsevier.com/DrugConsult/pediatric/*, provides free late-breaking drug information, to keep you up-to-date on new drugs and indications, recent warnings, withdrawals from the market, and more.

HOW TO USE THE BOOK

Mosby's Pediatric Drug Consult is divided into major sections, such as anti-infective agents, which are then divided into chapters of drugs in the same therapeutic classification, such as antifungal agents. The chapter introduction explains the drugs' general uses and actions, lists generic drugs in the class, and identifies combination products by trade name with generic components and their strengths.

Within each chapter, detailed entries provide all the information you need about the generic drugs in the class. For each drug entry, you'll find:

Generic name, pronunciation, and trade names. Each generic drug name is listed alphabetically—and spelled phonetically—for quick identification.

Do not confuse with. This unique feature identifies generic and trade names that resemble the featured drug to help you avoid drug errors.

Category and schedule. This section lists the drug's pregnancy risk category and, when appropriate, its controlled substance schedule or over-the-counter (OTC) status.

Mechanism of action. Expanding on the chapter overview information, this section clearly and concisely details the drug's mechanism of action and therapeutic effects.

Pharmacokinetics. A quick-reference chart outlines the drug's route, onset, peak, and duration, when known, followed by a discussion of the drug's absorption, distribution, metabolism, excretion, and half-life.

Availability. This section identifies the forms that the drug comes in, for example, in tablets, sustained-release capsules, or an injectable solution. It also lists the available doses and concentrations.

Indications and dosages. Here, you'll find the approved indications and routes, along with the dosage information for children, including neonates and those with pre-existing conditions, such as liver or kidney disease.

Unlabeled uses. This section brings you up-to-date on the unlabeled uses commonly seen in practice.

Contraindications. Here, conditions that prohibit the use of the drug are listed.

Interactions. For drugs, herbal supplements, and food, this section supplies vital information about interactions with the topic drug.

Diagnostic test effects. Brief descriptions of the drug's effects on laboratory and diagnostic test results, such as liver enzyme levels and electrocardiogram tracings, are included in this section.

IV incompatibilities and IV compatibilities. These sections let you know which IV drugs can and cannot be given with the featured drug, whether by IV push, Y-site, or IV piggyback administration.

Side effects. Unlike other handbooks that mix common, deadly effects with rare, minor ones in a lengthy list, this book ranks side effects by frequency of occurrence as expected, frequent, occasional, and rare, and includes the percentage of occurrence, when known.

Serious reactions. Because serious reactions are life-threatening responses that require prompt intervention, this section highlights them, apart from other side effects, for easy identification.

Pediatric considerations. This section presents pediatric considerations in a practice-oriented format in the following categories:

- *Baseline assessment* tells you what to assess before giving the first dose of a drug.
- *Precautions* alerts you to specific conditions or circumstances that call for caution when administering the drug.
- *Administration and handling* features the do's and don'ts of drug administration, with guidelines for PO, IV, IM, and other forms of the drug. Additionally, it provides clear-cut instructions about how to store, prepare, and administer the drug.
- *Intervention and evaluation* describes ongoing interventions and ways to monitor the drug's therapeutic and adverse effects.
- *Patient/family teaching* explains exactly what to teach your patients and their caregivers to help them achieve the maximum therapeutic response to drugs while minimizing possible adverse effects.

ACKNOWLEDGMENTS

A specialized book of this nature requires the commitment of many people. All individuals directly involved in this book appreciate the enduring commitment to excellence and accuracy in those who contributed to the material found in this book. I would like to give a special thank you to Tracy Hagemann for her commitment to excellence in providing valued support and evaluation of the material in this book. She worked diligently to ensure that the information contained in this book is accurate and up-to-date, which is a difficult task in the ever-changing world of drug administration. I also offer acknowledgement to Robert (Bob) Kizior and Barbara Hodgson, who created the basis for this book through *Mosby's 2005 Drug Consult for Nurses*. I would also like to thank Elsevier, who trusted my best efforts and contributed valuable supplies, information, ideas, and presentation. A special thanks to my family who supported me through this eventful process, especially my newborn baby boy, Levin, who slept for 1-hour sessions so I could work on this book.

Kelley Ward, PhD, RN, C

CONTENTS

Unit 4 Central Nervous System Agents

Unit 5 Gastrointestinal Agents

Unit 6 Hematologic Agents

Unit 7 Hormonal Agents

1 Aminoglycosides

Amikacin Sulfate
Gentamicin Sulfate
Kanamycin Sulfate
Neomycin Sulfate
Streptomycin Sulfate
Tobramycin Sulfate

Uses: Aminoglycosides are used to treat serious infections when other, less toxic, agents aren't effective, are contraindicated, or require adjunctive therapy (such as penicillins or cephalosporins). Aminoglycosides primarily treat infections caused by gram-negative microorganisms, such as *Proteus mirabilis, Klebsiella pneumoniae, Pseudomonas aeruginosa, Escherichia coli, Serratia marcescens,* and *Enterobacter* species. They're inactive against most gram-positive microorganisms. These agents aren't well absorbed systemically from the GI tract and must be administered parenterally for systemic infections. Oral agents are given to suppress intestinal bacteria.

Action: Aminoglycosides are transported across bacterial cell membranes and are bactericidal. These drugs irreversibly bind to specific receptor proteins on bacterial ribosomes, thereby interfering with protein synthesis, preventing cell reproduction, and eventually causing cell death. (See illustration, *Sites and Mechanisms of Action: Anti-Infective Agents*, page 2.)

COMBINATION PRODUCTS

NEOSPORIN GU IRRIGANT: neomycin/polymyxin B (an anti-infective) 40 mg/200,000 units/mL. This is a topical product only.
NEOSPORIN OINTMENT, TRIPLE ANTIBIOTIC: neomycin/polymyxin B (an anti-infective)/bacitracin (an anti-infective) 3.5 mg/5,000 units/400 units/g; 3.5 mg/10,000 units/400 units/g.
TOBRADEX: tobramycin/dexamethasone (a steroid) 0.3%/0.1% per mL or per g. This is a ophthalmic product only.

Amikacin Sulfate

am-ih-**kay**-sin
(Amikin)
Do not confuse with Amicar.

CATEGORY AND SCHEDULE

Pregnancy Risk Category: D

MECHANISM OF ACTION

An aminoglycoside antibiotic agent that irreversibly binds to protein on bacterial ribosomes. ***Therapeutic Effect:*** Interferes with protein synthesis of susceptible microorganisms.

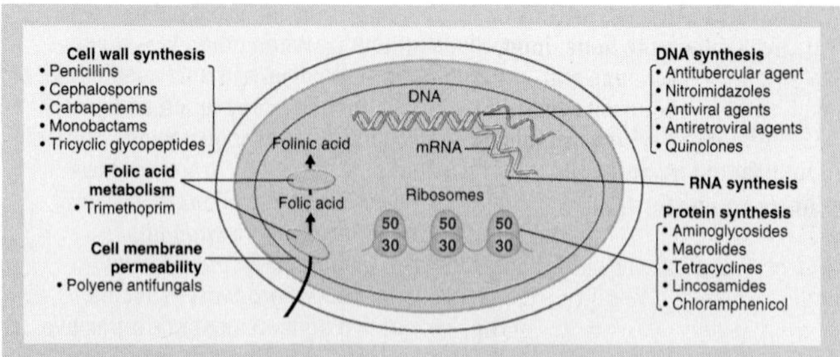

Sites and Mechanisms of Action: Anti-Infective Agents

The goal of anti-infective therapy is to kill or inhibit the growth of microorganisms, such as bacteria, viruses, and fungi. To achieve this goal, anti-infective agents must reach their targets, which usually occurs through absorption and distribution by the circulatory system. When the target is reached, a drug can kill or suppress microorganisms by:

- Inhibiting cell wall synthesis or activating enzymes that disrupt the cell wall, which leads to cellular weakening, lysis, and death. Penicillins (ampicillin), cephalosporins (cefazolin), carbapenems (imipenem), monobactams (aztreonam), and tricyclic glycopeptides (vancomycin) act in this way.
- Altering cell membrane permeability through direct action on the cell wall, which allows intracellular substances to leak out and destabilizes the cell. Polyene antifungals (amphotericin) work by this mechanism.
- Altering protein synthesis by binding to bacterial ribosomes (50/30) or affecting ribosomal function, which leads to cell death or slowed growth, respectively. Aminoglycosides (gentamicin), macrolides (erythromycin), tetracyclines (doxycycline), lincosamides (clindamycin), and the miscellaneous anti-infective chloramphenicol use this action.
- Inhibiting deoxyribonucleic acid (DNA) or ribonucleic acid (RNA), including messenger RNA (mRNA), synthesis by binding to nucleic acids or interacting with enzymes required for their synthesis. Antitubercular agents (rifampin), nitroimidazoles (metronidazole), antiviral agents (acyclovir), antiretroviral agents (stavudine), and quinolones (ciprofloxacin) act like this.
- Inhibiting the metabolism of folic acid and folinic acid or other cellular components that are essential for bacterial cell growth. The miscellaneous anti-infective trimethoprim uses this mechanism of action.

PHARMACOKINETICS

Rapid, complete absorption after IM administration. Protein binding: 0%–10%. Widely distributed (does not cross blood-brain barrier, low concentrations in cerebrospinal fluid). Excreted unchanged in urine. Removed by hemodialysis.

Half-Life: 2–4 hrs (increased in reduced renal function, neonates; decreased in cystic fibrosis, burn, or febrile pts).

AVAILABILITY

Injection: 50 mg/mL, 250 mg/mL. Contains sulfites.

INDICATIONS AND DOSAGES

▸ Serious bacteremia, bone, joint, CNS, and lung infections and complicated or recurrent urinary tract infections in which organisms are resistant to other aminoglycosides:

IM/IV

Children. 15–22.5 mg/kg/day in divided doses q8h. Do not exceed 1.5 g/day. Loading dose: 10 mg/kg, then 7.5 mg/kg q12h.

▸ Dosage in renal impairment

Dosage and frequency are modified based on degree of renal impairment and serum concentration of the drug. After a loading dose of 5–7.5 mg/kg, the maintenance dose and frequency are based on serum creatinine, creatinine clearance, and serum concentrations.

CONTRAINDICATIONS

Sensitivity to amikacin or any component.

INTERACTIONS

Drug

Nephrotoxic medications, other aminoglycosides, ototoxic-producing medications: May increase risk of amikacin toxicity. May increase effects of neuromuscular blocking agents.

Herbal

None known.

Food

None known.

DIAGNOSTIC TEST EFFECTS

May increase serum bilirubin, BUN, serum creatinine, lactate dehydrogenase, SGOT (AST), and SGPT (ALT) levels. May decrease serum calcium, magnesium, potassium, and sodium concentrations. Therapeutic blood serum level: Peak: 20–30 mcg/mL; toxic serum level: greater than 30 mcg/mL; Trough: 1–9 mcg/mL; toxic serum level: greater than 10 mcg/mL.

IV INCOMPATIBILITIES

Amphotericin, ampicillin, cefazolin (Ancef), heparin, propofol (Diprivan)

IV COMPATIBILITIES

Amiodarone (Cordarone), aztreonam (Azactam), calcium gluconate, cefepime (Maxipime), cimetidine (Tagamet), ciprofloxacin (Cipro), clindamycin (Cleocin), diltiazem (Cardizem), enalapril (Vasotec), esmolol (Brevibloc), fluconazole (Diflucan), furosemide (Lasix), levofloxacin (Levaquin), lorazepam (Ativan), magnesium sulfate, midazolam (Versed), morphine, ondansetron (Zofran), potassium chloride, ranitidine (Zantac), vancomycin

SIDE EFFECTS

Frequent

Pain, induration at IM injection site, phlebitis, thrombophlebitis with IV administration

Occasional

Hypersensitivity reactions manifested as rash, fever, urticaria, pruritus

Rare

Neuromuscular blockade manifested as difficulty breathing, drowsiness, weakness

SERIOUS REACTIONS

! Nephrotoxicity as evidenced by increased thirst, decreased appetite, nausea, vomiting, increased BUN and serum creatinine, and decreased creatinine clearance; neurotoxicity manifested as muscle twitching, visual disturbances, seizures, and tingling; ototoxicity as evidenced by tinnitus, dizziness, or loss of hearing may occur.

PEDIATRIC CONSIDERATIONS

Baseline Assessment

• Determine the patient's history of allergies, especially to aminoglycosides and sulfite.
• Expect to correct dehydration before beginning aminoglycoside therapy.
• Establish the patient's baseline hearing acuity before beginning therapy.
• Expect to obtain a specimen for culture and sensitivity testing before giving the first dose.
• Therapy may begin before test results are known.
• Be aware that amikacin readily crosses the placenta and small amounts are distributed in breast milk. Amikacin may produce fetal nephrotoxicity.
• Be aware that neonates and premature infants may be more susceptible to amikacin toxicity because of immature renal function.

Precautions

• Use cautiously in neonates and small infants (because of renal immaturity), in children who have impaired renal function and dehydration, in pts with eighth cranial nerve impairment (vestibulocochlear nerve), myasthenia gravis, and Parkinson's disease.

Administration and Handling

◂ALERT▸ Space amikacin doses evenly around the clock. The drug dosage is based on the patient's ideal body weight. Peak, trough blood serum levels are determined periodically to maintain desired serum concentrations to minimize the risk of amikacin toxicity. Therapeutic blood serum level: Peak: 20–30 mcg/mL; toxic serum level: greater than 30 mcg/mL; Trough: 1–9 mcg/mL; toxic serum level: greater than 10 mcg/mL.

IM

• Give deep IM injections slowly to minimize patient discomfort. Injections administered into the gluteus maximus are less painful than injections into the lateral aspect of the thigh.

IV

• Store vials at room temperature.
• Solutions appear clear but may become pale yellow. The pale yellow color does not affect the drug's potency. Discard if precipitate forms or dark discoloration occurs.
• Intermittent IV infusion (piggyback) is stable for 24 hrs at room temperature.
• Dilute each 500 mg with 100 mL 0.9% NaCl or D_5W.
• Infuse over 30–60 min for older children. Infuse over 60–120 min for infants and young children (30-min infusions should be appropriate for most children).

Intervention and Evaluation

• Monitor the patient's intake and output to maintain hydration.
• Expect to monitor urinalysis results to detect casts, red blood cells, white blood cells, a decrease in specific gravity, and the results of peak and trough amikacin serum levels.
• Be alert to ototoxic and neurotoxic symptoms.
• Check the IM injection site for pain and induration.
• Evaluate the IV site for phlebitis as evidenced by heat, pain, and red streaking over the vein.

- Assess the patient's skin for a rash.
- Assess the patient for superinfection, particularly changes in the oral mucosa, diarrhea, and genital or anal pruritus.
- In pts with neuromuscular disorders, assess the respiratory response carefully.

Patient/Family Teaching

- Explain to the patient/family the importance of receiving the full course of amikacin treatment.
- Warn the patient/family that IM injection may cause discomfort.
- Instruct the patient/family to notify the physician in the event of any hearing, visual, balance, or urinary problems that occur, even if they start after therapy is completed.
- Caution the patient/family not to take any other medications without first notifying the physician.
- Advise the patient/family that lab tests are an essential part of therapy.

Gentamicin Sulfate

jen-tah-**my**-sin
(Alcomicin [CAN], Cidomycin [CAN], Garamycin, Genoptic, Gentacidin)

CATEGORY AND SCHEDULE

Pregnancy Risk Category: D

MECHANISM OF ACTION

An aminoglycoside that irreversibly binds to the protein of bacterial ribosomes. ***Therapeutic Effect:*** Interferes in protein synthesis of susceptible microorganisms. Bactericidal.

PHARMACOKINETICS

Rapid, complete absorption after IM administration. Protein binding: less than 30%. Widely distributed. Does not cross the blood-brain barrier and appears in low concentrations in cerebrospinal fluid (CSF). Excreted unchanged in urine. Removed by hemodialysis. ***Half-Life:*** 2–4 hrs (half-life is increased with impaired renal function as is found in neonates; half-life is decreased in cystic fibrosis, burn, or febrile pts).

AVAILABILITY

Injection: 10 mg/mL 40 mg/mL, 2 mg/mL (intrathecal). May contain sulfites.
Ophthalmic Solution: 3 mg/mL (0.3%).
Ophthalmic Ointment: 3 mg/g (0.3%).
Cream: 0.5%.
Ointment: 0.1%.

INDICATIONS AND DOSAGES

▸ **Treatment of acute pelvic, bone, complicated urinary tract, intra-abdominal, joint, respiratory tract, and skin/skin structure infections, burns, septicemia, meningitis and for postoperative patients**

IM/IV
Children 5–12 years. Usual dosage 2–2.5 mg/kg/dose q8h.
Children younger than 5 years. Usual dosage 2.5 mg/kg/dose q8h.
Neonates. Usual dosage 2.5–3.5 mg/kg/dose q8–12h.

▸ **Hemodialysis**

IM/IV
Children. 2–2.5 mg/kg/dose q8h.
Full-term neonates or infants older than 7 days old. 2.5 mg/kg/dose q8h.
Full-term neonates younger than 7 days old. 2.5 mg/kg/dose q12h.

Premature infants older than 7 days, gestation 28–34 wks. 2.5 mg/kg/dose q12h.
Premature infants older than 7 days, gestation less than 28 wks. 2.5 mg/kg/dose q18h.
Premature infants younger than 7 days, gestation 28–34 wks. 2.5 mg/kg/dose q18h. Premature infants younger than 7 days, gestation less than 28 wks. 2.5 mg/kg/dose q24h.

▸ **Intrathecal**
1–2 mg/day (Note: use preservative-free product).
1 mg/day (Note: use preservative-free product).

▸ **Superficial eye infections**
OPHTHALMIC SOLUTION
Usual dosage 1–2 drops q2–4h up to 2 drops qh into conjunctival sac.

▸ **Superficial skin infections**
TOPICAL
Apply to affected area 3–4 times/day.

UNLABELED USES

Topical: Prophylaxis of minor bacterial skin infections, treatment of dermal ulcer

CONTRAINDICATIONS

Hypersensitivity to gentamicin or other aminoglycosides (cross-sensitivity). Sulfite sensitivity may result in anaphylaxis, especially in asthmatics.

INTERACTIONS

Drug

Other aminoglycosides, nephrotoxic or ototoxic-producing medications: May increase risk of gentamicin toxicity.
Neuromuscular blocking agents: May increase effects of neuromuscular blocking agents.

Herbal

None known.

Food

None known.

DIAGNOSTIC TEST EFFECTS

May increase serum creatinine, serum bilirubin, BUN, serum lactate dehydrogenase, SGOT (AST), and SGPT (ALT) levels. May decrease serum calcium, magnesium, potassium, and sodium concentrations. Therapeutic peak serum level is 5–10 mcg/mL and trough is less than 2 mcg/mL. Toxic peak serum level is greater than 10 mcg/mL and trough is greater than 2 mcg/mL. If you use once daily, dosing peaks are not measured.

IV INCOMPATIBILITIES

Allopurinol (Aloprim), amphotericin B complex (Abelcet, AmBisome, Amphotec), furosemide (Lasix), heparin, hetastarch (Hespan), idarubicin (Idamycin), indomethacin (Indocin), propofol (Diprivan)

IV COMPATIBILITIES

Amiodarone (Cordarone), diltiazem (Cardizem), enalapril (Vasotec), filgrastim (Neupogen), hydromorphone (Dilaudid), insulin, lorazepam (Ativan), magnesium sulfate, midazolam (Versed), morphine, multivitamins

SIDE EFFECTS

Occasional

IM: Pain, induration at IM injection site
IV: Phlebitis, thrombophlebitis with IV administration; hypersensitivity reactions such as fever, pruritus, rash, and urticaria
Ophthalmic: Burning, tearing, itching, blurred vision

Topical: Redness, itching
Rare
Alopecia, hypertension, weakness

SERIOUS REACTIONS

! Nephrotoxicity, as evidenced by increased BUN and serum creatinine and decreased creatinine clearance, may be reversible if the drug is stopped at the first sign of symptoms.
! Irreversible ototoxicity manifested as tinnitus, dizziness, ringing or roaring in the ears, and impaired hearing, and neurotoxicity as evidenced by headache, dizziness, lethargy, tremors, and visual disturbances occur occasionally. The risk of irreversible ototoxicity and neurotoxicity is greater with higher dosages or prolonged therapy or if the solution is applied directly to the mucosa.
! Superinfections, particularly with fungi, may result from bacterial imbalance via any route of administration.
! Ophthalmic application may cause paresthesia of conjunctiva or mydriasis.

PEDIATRIC CONSIDERATIONS

Baseline Assessment

- Expect to correct dehydration before beginning parenteral therapy.
- Establish the patient's baseline hearing acuity.
- Be aware that gentamicin readily crosses the placenta and that it is unknown whether gentamicin is distributed in breast milk.
- Use cautiously in neonates because their immature renal function increases gentamicin half-life and risk of toxicity.
- Use cautiously in children receiving neuromuscular blocking or anesthetic agents.
- Be cautious in observing and assessing treatment of children with neuromuscular disorders.
- The medication is eliminated more quickly in pts with burns, neutropenia, and cystic fibrosis.
- Observe caution in those neonates, infants, and children who have renal immaturity, impaired renal function, eighth cranial nerve impairment, myasthenia gravis, and hypocalcemia.
- It is important to monitor peak and trough levels with this medication. Samples for peak levels should be drawn 30–60 min after the administration of the third successive dose. Samples for troughs should be drawn 30 min before the third successive dose.

◂ALERT▸ Determine whether the patient has a history of allergies, especially to aminoglycosides and sulfites, as well as parabens for topical and ophthalmic routes before giving drug.

Precautions

◂ALERT▸ Cumulative effects may occur with concurrent systemic administration and topical application to large areas.
Use cautiously in neonate pts because of age-related renal insufficiency or immaturity.
Use cautiously in pts with neuromuscular disorders because there is a potential for respiratory depression.
Use cautiously in pts with prior hearing loss, renal impairment, or vertigo.

Administration and Handling

◂ALERT▸ Space parenteral doses evenly around the clock.
Gentamicin dosage is based on ideal body weight. As ordered, monitor serum peak and trough levels periodically to maintain the

desired serum concentrations and to minimize the risk of toxicity. Be aware that the recommended peak serum level is 5–10 mcg/mL, and the recommended trough level is less than 2 mcg/mL. Also, the toxic peak serum level is greater than 10 mcg/mL, and the toxic trough serum level is greater than 2 mcg/mL.

IM

• To minimize discomfort, give deep IM injection slowly.
• To minimize injection-site pain, administer the IM injection in the gluteus maximus rather than lateral aspect of thigh.

IV

• Store vials at room temperature.
• The solution normally appears clear or slightly yellow.
• Intermittent IV infusion or IV piggyback solution is stable for 24 hrs at room temperature.
• Discard the IV solution if precipitate forms.
• Dilute with 50–200 mL D_5W or 0.9% NaCl. The amount of diluent for infants and children depends on individual needs.
• Infuse over 30–60 min for older children. Infuse over 60–120 min for infants and young children (30 min should be adequate for most children).

INTRATHECAL

• Use only 2 mg/mL intrathecal preparation without preservative.
• Mix with 10% estimated CSF volume or NaCl.
• Use intrathecal forms immediately after preparation. Discard unused portion.
• Give over 3–5 min.

OPHTHALMIC

• Place a gloved finger on the patient's lower eyelid and pull it out until a pocket is formed between the eye and lower lid.
• Hold the dropper above the pocket and place the correct number of drops (or ¼ to ½ inch of ointment) into the pocket. Close the eye gently.
• For ophthalmic solution apply digital pressure to the lacrimal sac for 1–2 min to minimize drainage into the nose and throat, thereby reducing the risk of systemic effects.
• For ophthalmic ointment close the patient's eye for 1–2 min. Instruct the patient to roll the eyeball to increase the contact area of the drug to the eye.
• Remove excess solution or ointment around eye with tissue.

Intervention and Evaluation

• Monitor the patient's intake and output and urinalysis results as appropriate. Urge the patient to drink fluids to maintain adequate hydration. Monitor the urinalysis results for casts, RBCs, and WBCs or a decrease in specific gravity.
• Be alert to ototoxic and neurotoxic signs and symptoms.
• Check the IM injection site for induration.
• Evaluate the IV infusion site for signs and symptoms of phlebitis such as heat, pain, and red streaking over the vein.
• Assess the patient's skin for rash. If giving gentamicin for ophthalmic use, monitor the patient's eye for burning, itching, redness, and tearing. If giving gentamicin for topical use, monitor the patient for signs of itching and redness.
• Be alert for signs and symptoms of superinfection, particularly changes in the oral mucosa, diarrhea, and genital or anal pruritus.
• When treating pts with neuromuscular disorders, assess the

patient's respiratory response carefully.
• Be aware that the therapeutic peak serum level is 5–10 mcg/mL and the therapeutic trough serum level is less than 2 mcg/mL. Also, know that the toxic peak serum level is greater than 10 mcg/mL, and the toxic trough serum level is greater than 2 mcg/mL.

Patient/Family Teaching

• Explain to the patient/family that discomfort may occur with IM injection.
• Advise the patient/family that blurred vision or tearing may occur briefly after each ophthalmic dose.
• Instruct the patient/family receiving topical gentamicin to cleanse the area gently before applying the ointment.
• Warn the patient/family to notify the physician of any balance, hearing, urinary, or vision problems that develop, even after gentamicin therapy is completed.
• Warn the patient/family taking ophthalmic gentamicin to notify the physician if irritation, redness, or tearing continues.
• Warn the patient/family receiving topical gentamicin to notify the physician if itching or redness occurs.

Kanamycin Sulfate

can-ah-**my**-sin
(Kantrex)

CATEGORY AND SCHEDULE

Pregnancy Risk Category: Unavailable for irrigating solution.

MECHANISM OF ACTION

• An aminoglycoside antibiotic that irreversibly binds to protein on bacterial ribosomes.
Therapeutic Effect: Interferes with protein synthesis of susceptible microorganisms.

AVAILABILITY

Injection: 1 g/3 mL.

INDICATIONS AND DOSAGES

▸ **Wound and surgical site irrigation**

Infants older than 4 wks and children. 15–30 mg/kg/24 hrs q8–12h (maximum dose 1.5 g/24 hrs).
Birthweight 2 kg or greater, older than 7 days. 30 mg/kg/24 hrs q8h.
Birthweight 2 kg or greater, younger than 7 days. 20 mg/kg/24 hrs q12h.
Birthweight greater than 2 kg, older than 7 days. 22.5 mg/kg/24 hrs q8h.
Birthweight less than 2 kg, younger than 7 days. 15 mg/kg/24 hrs q12h.

CONTRAINDICATIONS

Hypersensitivity to aminoglycosides, kanamycin.

INTERACTIONS

Drug

None significant.

Herbal

None significant.

Food

None significant.

DIAGNOSTIC TEST EFFECTS

None known.

SIDE EFFECTS

Occasional

Hypersensitivity reactions: fever, pruritus, rash, urticaria

Rare

Headache

SERIOUS REACTIONS

None known.

PEDIATRIC CONSIDERATIONS

Baseline Assessment

- Assess the patient for hypersensitivity to aminoglycosides or kanamycin.
- Infuse over 30 min using a volumetric constant infusion devise.
- Do not administer IV push or by continuous infusion.
- Use cautiously in neonates and infants (because of renal immaturity) and in children with dehydration, eighth cranial nerve impairment, myasthenia gravis, hypocalcemia, and impaired renal function or who are pregnant or lactating.
- Infuse separately and flush the line with 0.9% NaCl or D_5W.
- Keep the patient well hydrated to avoid renal toxicity.
- Therapeutic peak levels are 15–30 mg/L, and therapeutic trough levels are less than 5–10 mg/L. Obtain trough within 30 min before the third successive dose and peak 30–60 min after the third successive administration.

Neomycin Sulfate

nee-oh-**my**-sin
(Mycifradin, Myciguent, Neosulf [AUS])

CATEGORY AND SCHEDULE

Pregnancy Risk Category: C
OTC (topical ointment 0.5% only)

MECHANISM OF ACTION

An aminoglycoside antibiotic that binds to bacterial microorganisms. ***Therapeutic Effect:*** Interferes with bacterial protein synthesis.

AVAILABILITY

Topical Ointment (OTC): 0.5%.
Tablets (Rx): 500 mg.

INDICATIONS AND DOSAGES

▸ **Preop bowel antisepsis**

PO

Children. 50–90 mg/kg/day in divided doses q4h for 2 days or 25 mg/kg at 1 P.M., 2 P.M., and 10 P.M. on day before surgery. The doses can also be divided q6h.
Premature infants and neonates. 50 mg/kg/24 hrs q6h.

▸ **Liver encephalopathy**

PO

Children. acute dose—2.5–7 g/m^2/day in divided doses q4–6h for 5–7 days (maximum 12 g/24 hrs). *chronic* dose—2.5 g/m^2/day in divided doses q4–6h or 50–100 mg/kg/day divided q4–6h.

▸ **Diarrhea caused by Escherichia coli**

PO

Preterm and newborns. 50 mg/kg/day in divided doses q6h.

▸ **Minor skin infections**

TOPICAL

Children. Usual dosage, apply to affected area 1–3 times/day.

▸ **Otitis externa**

OTIC

Children. Instill 2–5 drops into auditory canal 3–4 times/day.

CONTRAINDICATIONS

Hypersensitivity to aminoglycosides.

INTERACTIONS

Drug

Other aminoglycosides, other nephrotoxic or ototoxic medications: If significant systemic absorption occurs, neomycin may increase nephrotoxicity and ototoxicity of these drugs.

Herbal
None known.
Food
None known.

DIAGNOSTIC TEST EFFECTS
None known.

SIDE EFFECTS
Frequent
Systemic: Nausea, vomiting, diarrhea, irritation of mouth or rectal area
Topical: Itching, redness, swelling, rash
Rare
Systemic: Malabsorption syndrome, neuromuscular blockade as evidenced by difficulty breathing, drowsiness, or weakness.

SERIOUS REACTIONS
! Nephrotoxicity, as evidenced by increased BUN and serum creatinine and decreased creatinine clearance, may be reversible if the drug is stopped at the first sign of nephrotoxic symptoms.
! Irreversible ototoxicity manifested as tinnitus, dizziness, ringing or roaring in the ears, and impaired hearing, and neurotoxicity as evidenced by headache, dizziness, lethargy, tremors, and visual disturbances, occur occasionally.
! Severe respiratory depression and anaphylaxis occur rarely.
! Superinfections, particularly fungal infections, may occur.

PEDIATRIC CONSIDERATIONS
Baseline Assessment
- Expect to correct dehydration before beginning aminoglycoside therapy.
- Establish the patient's baseline hearing acuity before beginning therapy.
- Use cautiously in infants and children with renal insufficiency or immaturity, neuromuscular disorders, history of hearing loss, renal impairment, vertigo, eighth cranial nerve impairment, myasthenia gravis, hypocalcemia, and impaired renal function or who are pregnant or lactating.

Intervention and Evaluation
- Assess for signs and symptoms of ototoxicity and neurotoxicity.
- Evaluate signs and symptoms of a hypersensitivity reaction. With topical application a hypersensitivity reaction may appear as a rash, redness, or itching.
- Watch the patient for signs and symptoms of superinfection, particularly changes in the oral mucosa, diarrhea, or genital or anal pruritus.

Patient/Family Teaching
- Advise the patient/family to continue the antibiotic for the full length of treatment and to evenly space doses around the clock.
- Instruct pts/family receiving topical neomycin to cleanse the affected area gently before applying the drug.
- Warn pts/family receiving topical neomycin to notify the physician if any itching or redness occurs.
- Warn the patient/family to notify the physician if the patient experiences dizziness, impaired hearing, or ringing in the ears.

Streptomycin
strep-toe-**mye**-sin

CATEGORY AND SCHEDULE
Pregnancy Risk Category: D

MECHANISM OF ACTION

An aminoglycoside that binds directly to the 30S ribosomal subunits causing a faulty peptide sequence to form in the protein chain. ***Therapeutic Effect:*** Inhibits bacterial protein synthesis.

AVAILABILITY

Injection: 1 g.

INDICATIONS AND DOSAGES

▸ Tuberculosis

IM

Children. 20–40 mg/kg/day q6–12h (maximum 1 g in 24 hrs).
Infants. 20–30 mg/kg/24 hrs q12h.
Neonates. 10–20 mg/kg/24 hrs once daily.

▸ Dosage in renal impairment

Creatinine Clearance	Dosage Interval
10–50 ml/min	every 24–72 hrs
less than 10 ml/min	every 72–96 hrs

▸ Tuberculosis

IM

Children. 20–40 mg/kg/24 hrs q12–24h for 7–10 days (maximum of 1 g/24 hrs).
Infants. 20–30 mg/kg/24 hrs q12h for 7–10 days (maximum of 1 g/24 hrs).

CONTRAINDICATIONS

Pregnancy.

INTERACTIONS

Drug

Amphotericin, loop diuretics: May increase the nephrotoxicity of streptomycin.
Neuromuscular blocking agents: May increase the effects of streptomycin.

Herbal

None known.

Food

None known.

DIAGNOSTIC TEST EFFECTS

None known.

SIDE EFFECTS

Occasional

Hypotension, drowsiness, headache, drug fever, paresthesia, skin rash, nausea, vomiting, anemia, arthralgia, weakness, tremor

SERIOUS REACTIONS

! Symptoms of ototoxicity, nephrotoxicity, and neuromuscular toxicity may occur

PEDIATRIC CONSIDERATIONS

Baseline Assessment

- Determine whether the patient is hypersensitive to aminoglycosides, pregnant, or being treated for other medical conditions.
- Therapeutic peak levels are 15–40 mg/L, and therapeutic trough levels are less than 5 mg/L.
- Obtain trough within 30 min before the third successive dose.
- Obtain peak 30–60 min after the third successive dose.

Precautions

- Use cautiously in pts with hearing loss, neuromuscular disorders, preexisting vertigo, renal impairment, and tinnitus.

Administration and Handling

IM/IV

- Give IM injection deeply into a large muscle mass.
- May be given IV over 30–60 min.

Intervention and Evaluation

- Monitor the patient's hearing, renal function, and serum concentrations of streptomycin.

Patient/Family Teaching

- Warn the patient/family to notify the physician if the patient experiences any unusual symptoms of hearing loss, dizziness, fullness in the ears, or roaring noises.

Tobramycin Sulfate

tow-bra-**my**-sin
(Nebcin, Tobi, Tobrex)

CATEGORY AND SCHEDULE

Pregnancy Risk Category: D. (B, Ophthalmic form)

MECHANISM OF ACTION

An aminoglycoside antibiotic that irreversibly binds to protein on bacterial ribosomes. ***Therapeutic Effect:*** Interferes in protein synthesis of susceptible microorganisms.

PHARMACOKINETICS

Rapid, complete absorption after IM administration. Protein binding: less than 30%. Widely distributed but does not cross the blood-brain barrier and is in low concentrations in cerebrospinal fluid. Excreted unchanged in urine. Removed by hemodialysis. ***Half-Life:*** 2–4 hrs. Half-life is increased with impaired renal function and in neonates. Half-life is decreased in cystic fibrosis, burn, or febrile pts.

AVAILABILITY

Injection: 10 mg/mL, 40 mg/mL. May contain sulfites.
Powder for Injection: 1.2 g.
Ophthalmic Solution: 0.3%.
Ophthalmic Ointment: 3 mg/g (0.3%).
Inhalation Solution: 300 mg/ 5 mL.

INDICATIONS AND DOSAGES

▸ Skin/skin structure, bone, joint, respiratory tract infections, postoperative, burn, intra-abdominal infections, complicated urinary tract infections, septicemia, meningitis

IM/IV

Postconceptional age older than 37 wks; postnatal age older than 7 days. 2.5 mg/kg/dose q8h.
Postconceptional age older than 37 wks; postnatal age 0–7 days. 2.5 mg/kg/dose q12h.
Postconceptional age 30–36 wks; postnatal age older than 14 days. 2.5 mg/kg/dose q12h.
Postconceptional age 30–36 wks; postnatal age 0–14 days. 3 mg/kg/dose q24h.
Postconceptional age 29 wks or younger; postnatal age older than 28 days. 3 mg/kg/dose q24h.
Postconceptional age 29 wks or younger; postnatal 0–28 days. 2.5 mg/kg/dose q24h.
Infants and children. 2.5 mg/kg/dose q8h.

▸ Cystic fibrosis

IV

Children. 2.5–3.5 mg/kg/dose q6–8h.

OINTMENT

Children. Usual dosage, a thin strip to conjunctiva q8–12h (q3–4h for severe infections).

SOLUTION

Children. Usual dosage, 1–2 drops q4h (2 drops every hour for severe infections) to the affected eye.

▸ Bronchopulmonary infections in patients with cystic fibrosis

INHALATION

Children. 40–80 mg 2–3 times/day.

▸ Dosage in renal impairment

Dosage and frequency are modified based on degree of renal impairment and the serum concentration of the drug. After a loading dose of 1–2 mg/kg, the maintenance dose and frequency are based on serum creatinine levels, creatinine clearance, and serum concentrations.

CONTRAINDICATIONS

Hypersensitivity to aminoglycosides (cross-sensitivity).

INTERACTIONS

Drug

Other aminoglycosides, nephrotoxic and ototoxic-producing medications: May increase the risk of tobramycin toxicity.
Neuromuscular blocking agents: May increase the effects of neuromuscular blocking agents.

Herbal

None known.

Food

None known.

DIAGNOSTIC TEST EFFECTS

May increase serum bilirubin, BUN, serum creatinine, serum lactate dehydrogenase, SGOT (AST), and SGPT (ALT) levels. May decrease serum calcium, magnesium, potassium, and sodium concentrations.
Therapeutic blood level: Peak is 5–10 mcg/mL; trough is 0.5–2 mcg/mL. Toxic blood level: Peak is greater than 10 mcg/mL; trough is greater than 2 mcg/mL.

IV INCOMPATIBILITIES

Amphotericin B complex (Abelcet, AmBisome, Amphotec), heparin, hetastarch (Hespan), indomethacin (Indocin), propofol (Diprivan), sargramostim (Leukine, Prokine)

IV COMPATIBILITIES

Amiodarone (Cordarone), calcium gluconate, diltiazem (Cardizem), furosemide (Lasix), hydromorphone (Dilaudid), insulin, magnesium sulfate, midazolam (Versed), morphine, theophylline

SIDE EFFECTS

Occasional
IM: Pain, induration at IM injection site
IV: Phlebitis, thrombophlebitis
Topical: Hypersensitivity reaction such as fever, pruritus, rash, and urticaria
Ophthalmic: Tearing, itching, redness, swelling of eyelid
Rare
Hypotension, nausea, vomiting

SERIOUS REACTIONS

! Nephrotoxicity, as evidenced by increased BUN and serum creatinine and decreased creatinine clearance, may be reversible if the drug is stopped at the first sign of nephrotoxic symptoms.
! Irreversible ototoxicity, manifested as tinnitus, dizziness, ringing or roaring in ears, impaired hearing and neurotoxicity, as evidenced by headache, dizziness, lethargy, tremors, and visual disturbances occur occasionally. The risk of irreversible neurotoxicity and ototoxicity is greater with higher dosages, prolonged therapy, or if the solution is applied directly to the mucosa.
! Superinfections, particularly with fungi, may result from bacterial imbalance with any route of administration.
Anaphylaxis may occur.

PEDIATRIC CONSIDERATIONS

Baseline Assessment

- Expect to correct dehydration before beginning parenteral therapy.
- Be aware that tobramycin readily crosses the placenta and is distributed in breast milk.

• Be aware that tobramycin may cause fetal nephrotoxicity. The ophthalmic form should not be used in breastfeeding mothers and only when specifically indicated in pregnancy.
• Be aware that immature renal function in neonates and premature infants may increase the risk of toxicity.
• Therapeutic peak levels are 6–10 mg/L in general and 8–10 mg/L in pulmonary infections, severe sepsis, and neutropenia. Therapeutic trough levels are less than 2 mg/L. Obtain trough within 30 min before the third successive dose and peak 30–60 min after administering the third successive dose.
◂ALERT▸ Determine the patient's history of allergies, especially to aminoglycosides, sulfites, and parabens (for topical and ophthalmic routes) before giving the drug. Establish a baseline for the patient's hearing acuity.

Precautions

• Use cautiously in pts who also use neuromuscular blocking agents or who have impaired renal function or preexisting auditory or vestibular impairment.

Administration and Handling

◂ALERT▸ Be sure to carefully coordinate the drawing of peak and trough blood levels with the drug's administration times.
◂ALERT▸ Evenly space parenteral doses around the clock. Be aware that dosages are based on ideal body weight. Monitor blood peak and trough levels to ensure that the desired blood concentrations are maintained and to minimize the risk of toxicity.

IM

• To minimize injection site discomfort, give deep IM injection slowly. Also, to reduce pain, administer the injection into the gluteus maximus rather than the lateral aspect of the thigh.

IV

• Store vials at room temperature. Solutions may be discolored by light or air, but discoloration does not affect drug potency.
• Dilute with 50–200 mL D_5W or 0.9% NaCl. The amount of diluent for infant and children dosages depends on individual needs.
• Infuse over 20–60 min.

OPHTHALMIC

• Place a gloved finger on the patient's lower eyelid and pull it out until a pocket is formed between the eye and lower lid.
• Hold the dropper above the pocket and place the correct number of drops (or ¼–½ inch of ointment) into the pocket. Have patient close the eye gently.
• To administer ophthalmic solution, apply digital pressure to the lacrimal sac for 1–2 min to minimize drainage into the patient's nose and throat, thereby reducing the risk of systemic effects.
• To administer ophthalmic ointment, close the patient's eye for 1–2 min. Have the patient roll the eyeball to increase the contact area of the drug to the eye.
• Remove excess solution or ointment around the eye with a tissue.

Intervention and Evaluation

• Monitor the patient's intake and output and urinalysis results, as appropriate. To maintain adequate hydration, encourage the patient to drink fluids. Monitor urinalysis results for casts, RBCs, and WBCs or a decrease in specific gravity.
• Expect to monitor the results of peak and trough blood tests. Keep in mind that the therapeutic peak blood level is 5–10 mcg/mL and

the therapeutic trough blood level is 0.5–2 mcg/mL. Also, know that the toxic peak blood level is greater than 10 mcg/mL and the toxic trough level is greater than 2 mcg/mL.

◂ **ALERT** ▸ Assess the patient for ototoxic and neurotoxic symptoms.

• Evaluate the IV site for signs and symptoms of phlebitis such as heat, pain, and red streaking over the vein.

• Assess the patient's skin for rash.

• Be alert for signs and symptoms of superinfection, particularly changes in the oral mucosa, diarrhea, or genital or anal pruritus.

• When treating pts with neuromuscular disorders, assess the patient's respiratory response frequently.

• Assess pts receiving ophthalmic tobramycin for itching, redness, swelling, and tearing.

Patient/Family Teaching

• Warn the patient/family to notify the physician if any balance, hearing, urinary, or vision problems develop, even after therapy is completed.

• Advise pts/families receiving ophthalmic tobramycin that blurred vision and tearing may occur briefly after application.

• Warn pts/families receiving ophthalmic tobramycin to notify the physician if irritation, redness, or tearing continues.

REFERENCES

Gunn, V. L. & Nechyba, C. (2002). The Harriet Lane handbook (16th ed.). St. Louis: Mosby.

Miller, S. & Fioravanti, J. (1997). Pediatric medications: a handbook for nurses. St. Louis: Mosby.

2 Antifungal Agents

Amphotericin B
Fluconazole
Griseofulvin
Ketoconazole
Nystatin
Terbinafine Hydrochloride

Uses: Antifungal agents are used to treat systemic and superficial fungal infections. They are effective against opportunistic and nonopportunistic *systemic* fungal infections. Opportunistic infections, which include candidiasis, aspergillosis, and cryptococcosis, occur primarily in debilitated or immunocompromised pts. Nonopportunistic infections, which include blastomycosis, histoplasmosis, and coccidioidomycosis, are less common.

Antifungal agents are especially effective against *superficial* fungal infections caused by *Candida* species and dermatophytes (ringworm). Candidiasis usually affects the mucous membranes and moist skin areas; in chronic infection, organisms may invade the scalp, skin, and nails. Dermatophytosis typically affects only the skin, hair, and nails.

Action: The three types of antifungal agents act in different ways. *Polyene antifungals,* such as amphotericin and nystatin, bind to sterols in fungal cell walls, forming pores or channels that increase cell wall permeability and allow the leakage of small molecules. *Imidazole antifungals,* such as ketoconazole, inhibit cytochrome P-450 in fungal cells, which impairs ergosterol synthesis and fungal growth. Antimetabolite antifungals, such as flucytosine, disrupt the synthesis of DNA and RNA in fungal cells. (See illustration, *Sites and Mechanism of Action: Antifungal Agents,* page 18.)

COMBINATION PRODUCTS

MYCOLOG: nystatin/triamcinolone (a steroid) 100,000 units/0.1%.
MYCO-TRIACET: nystatin/triamcinolone (a steroid) 100,000 units/0.1%.

Amphotericin B

am-foe-**tear**-ih-sin
(Abelcet, AmBisome, Amphotec, Fungizone)
(See Color Plate)

CATEGORY AND SCHEDULE

Pregnancy Risk Category: B

MECHANISM OF ACTION

This antifungal and antiprotozoal drug is generally fungistatic but

ANTI-INFECTIVE AGENTS

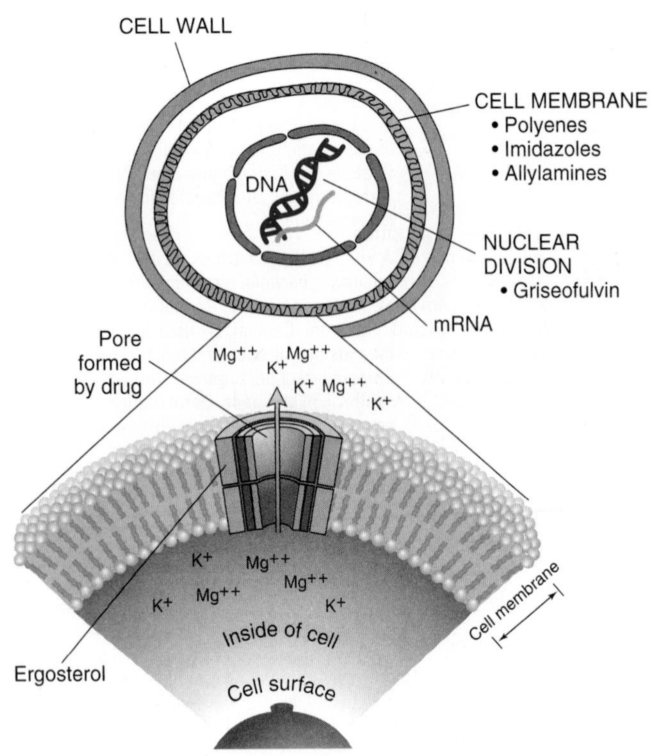

Sites and Mechanism of Action: Antifungal Agents

Antifungal agents primarily affect fungi at one of two sites: the cell membrane or the cell nucleus. Most of these agents, such as polyene, imidazole, and allylamine antifungals, act on the fungal cell membrane. Polyene antifungals, such as amphotericin B, bind to ergosterol and increase cell membrane permeability. Imidazole antifungals, such as fluconazole and ketoconazole, interfere with ergosterol synthesis by inhibiting the cytochrome P_{450} enzyme system, altering the cell membrane, and inhibiting fungal growth. Allylamine antifungals, such as terbinafine, inhibit the enzyme squalene epoxidase, which disrupts ergosterol production and cell membrane integrity. When cell membrane permeability increases, cellular components, including potassium (K^+) and magnesium (Mg^{++}), leak out. Loss of these cellular components leads to cell death.

Another antifungal agent, griseofulvin directly affects the fungal nucleus, interfering with mitosis. By binding to structures in the mitotic spindle, it prevents cells from dividing, which eventually leads to their death.

may become fungicidal with high dosages or very susceptible microorganisms. This drug binds to sterols in the fungal cell membrane. ***Therapeutic Effect:*** Increases fungal cell-membrane permeability, allowing loss of potassium and other cellular components.

PHARMACOKINETICS

Protein binding: 90%. Widely distributed with poor penetration into CNS. Metabolic fate unknown. Cleared by nonrenal pathways. Minimal removal by hemodialysis. Amphotec and Abelcet are not dialyzable. ***Half-Life:*** 24 hrs (half-life increased in neonates, children). Amphotec half-life is 26–28 hrs. Abelcet half-life is 7.2 days. AmBisome half-life is 100–153 hrs.

AVAILABILITY

Injection: 50 mg, 50 mg (Fungizone), 100 mg (Amphotec), 50 mg (AmBisone).
Suspension for Injection: 5 mg/mL (Amphotericin B lipid complex, Abelcet).
Cream, Lotion, Ointment: 3%.

INDICATIONS AND DOSAGES

▸ **Fungizone**
IV INFUSION
Older infants and children weighing less than 30 kg. Test dose: 0.1 mg/kg/dose (maximum of 1 mg) over 30–60 min and if tolerated follow with the remaining first daily dose. Initial dose: 0.25–0.5 mg/kg/dose once daily. May increase dose 0.125–0.25 mg/kg/24 hrs every 1–2 days as tolerated. Typical daily dose: 0.5–1 mg/kg/24 hrs.
Neonates. 1 mg/kg/24 hrs once daily.
INTRATHECAL
Children. 25–100 mcg q48–72h. May increase to 500 mcg as tolerated.

▸ **Amphotec**
IV INFUSION
Children. Initial dose: 3–4 mg/kg/day once daily. Dose may be increased to 6 mg/kg/day as tolerated. Test dose: 10 mL of the solution diluted and given over 15–30 min.

▸ **Abelcet**
IV INFUSION
Children. 2.5–5 mg/kg/day once daily. Infusion rate is 2.5 mg/kg/day.

▸ **AmBisome**
IV INFUSION
Children. 3–5 mg/kg/day once daily. Infusion rate should be over 2 hrs. Can be decreased to over 1 hr as tolerated.
TOPICAL
Children. Apply liberally to the affected area and rub in 2–4 times/day.

CONTRAINDICATIONS

Hypersensitivity to amphotericin B, sulfite.

INTERACTIONS

Drug

Bone marrow depressants: May increase risk for anemia.
Digoxin: May increase risk of digoxin toxicity from hypokalemia.
Nephrotoxic medications: May increase risk of nephrotoxicity.
Steroids: May cause severe hypokalemia.

Herbal

None known.

Food

None known.

DIAGNOSTIC TEST EFFECTS

May increase BUN, serum alkaline phosphatase, serum creatinine, SGOT (AST), and SGPT (ALT) levels. May decrease serum calcium, magnesium, and potassium levels.

IV INCOMPATIBILITIES

Abelcet/Amphotec/AmBisome: Do not mix with any other drug, diluent, or solution. Fungizone: Allopurinol (Aloprim), amifostine (Ethyol), aztreonam (Azactam), calcium gluconate, cefepime (Maxipime), cimetidine (Tagamet), ciprofloxacin (Cipro), docetaxel (Taxotere), dopamine (Intropin), doxorubicin (Adriamycin), enalapril (Vasotec), etoposide (VP-16), filgrastim (Neupogen), fluconazole (Diflucan), fludarabine (Fludara), foscarnet (Foscavir), gemcitabine (Gemzar), magnesium sulfate, meropenem (Merrem IV), ondansetron (Zofran), paclitaxel (Taxol), piperacillin/tazobactam (Zosyn), potassium chloride, propofol (Diprivan), vinorelbine (Navelbine)

IV COMPATIBILITIES

None known; do not mix with other medications or electrolytes.

SIDE EFFECTS

Frequent (greater than 10%)

Abelcet: Chills, fever, increased serum creatinine, multiple organ failure

AmBisome: Hypokalemia, hypomagnesemia, hyperglycemia, hypocalcemia, edema, abdominal pain, back pain, chills, chest pain, hypotension, diarrhea, nausea, vomiting, headache, fever, rigors, insomnia, dyspnea, epistaxis, increased liver/renal function test results

Amphotec: Chills, fever, hypotension, tachycardia, increased creatinine, hypokalemia, bilirubinemia

Fungizone: Fever, chills, headache, anemia, hypokalemia, hypomagnesemia, anorexia, malaise, generalized pain, nephrotoxicity

Topical: Local irritation, dry skin

Rare

Topical: Skin rash

SERIOUS REACTIONS

! Cardiovascular toxicity as evidenced by hypotension and ventricular fibrillation and anaphylaxis occur rarely.

! Vision and hearing alterations, seizures, liver failure, coagulation defects, multiple organ failure, and sepsis may be noted.

PEDIATRIC CONSIDERATIONS

Baseline Assessment

• Determine the patient's history of allergies, especially to amphotericin B and sulfites, before giving the drug.

• Be aware that other nephrotoxic medications should be avoided, if possible.

• Check for or obtain orders for drugs to reduce the risk or severity of adverse reactions during IV therapy. Antiemetics, antihistamines, antipyretics, or small doses of corticosteroids may be given before or during amphotericin administration to help control adverse reactions.

• Be aware that amphotericin B crosses the placenta and that it is unknown whether amphotericin B is distributed in breast milk.

• The safety and efficacy of amphotericin B have not been established in children. Therefore, expect to use the smallest dose necessary to achieve optimal results.

• In infants, use cautiously with other nephrotoxic drugs (because of elimination difficulties).

Precautions

• Use cautiously in pts with renal impairment and in combination

with antineoplastic therapy. Drug is prescribed only for progressive, potentially fatal, fungal infection.
• Keep in mind that conventional amphotericin, Fungizone, is more nephrotoxic than the alternative formulations of amphotericin B, including Abelcet, AmBisome, and Amphotec.

Administration and Handling

IV

• Observe strict aseptic technique because no bacteriostatic agent or preservative is present in the diluent.
• Refrigerate Abelcet as unreconstituted solution. Abelcet reconstituted solution is stable for 48 hrs if refrigerated and 6 hrs at room temperature.
• Refrigerate AmBisome as unreconstituted solution. AmBisone reconstituted solution of 4 mg/mL is stable for 24 hrs. AmBisone reconstituted solution concentration of 1–2 mg/mL is stable for 6 hrs.
• Store Amphotec as unreconstituted solution at room temperature. Amphotec reconstituted solution is stable for 24 hrs.
• Refrigerate Fungizone as unreconstituted solution. Fungizone reconstituted solution is stable for 24 hrs at room temperature or 7 days if refrigerated. Diluted solution less than or equal to 0.1 mg/mL should be used promptly. Do not use the solution if it is cloudy or contains a precipitate.
• Shake Abelcet 20-mL (100-mg) vial gently until contents are dissolved. Withdraw required Abelcet dose using a 5-µ filter needle supplied by the manufacturer.
• Inject Abelcet dose into D_5W; 4 mL D_5W is required for each 1 mL (5 mg) to a final concentration of 1 mg/mL. Reduce dose by half for pediatric or fluid-restricted pts (2 mg/mL).
• Reconstitute each 50-mg AmBisome vial with 12 mL Sterile Water for Injection to provide concentration of 4 mg/mL.
• Shake AmBisome vial vigorously for 30 sec. Then, withdraw the required AmBisone dose and empty the syringe contents through a 5-µ filter into an infusion of D_5W to provide final concentration of 1–2 mg/mL.
• Add 10 mL Sterile Water for Injection to each 50-mg Amphotec vial to provide a concentration of 5 mg/mL. Shake the Amphotec vial gently.
• Further dilute Amphotec vial with D_5W only using the specific amount recommended by manufacturer to provide concentration of 0.16–0.83 mg/mL.
• Rapidly inject 10 mL Sterile Water for Injection to each 50-mg Fungizone vial to provide concentration of 5 mg/mL. Immediately shake Fungizone vial until the solution is clear.
• Further dilute each 1 mg Fungizone in at least 10 mL D_5W to provide a concentration of 0.1 mg/mL.
• Be aware that the potential for thrombophlebitis may be lessened by adding dilute heparin solution, as prescribed.
• Infuse conventional amphotericin, Fungizone, over 2–6 hrs by slow IV infusion.
• Infuse Abelcet over 2 hrs by slow IV infusion. Shake the contents if the infusion time is greater than 2 hrs.
• Infuse Amphotec over 2–4 hrs by slow IV infusion.
• Infuse AmBisome over 1–2 hrs by slow IV infusion.

Intervention and Evaluation

• Monitor the patient's blood pressure, pulse, respirations, and temperature twice every 15 min, then every 30 min for the initial 4 hrs of the infusion to assess for adverse reactions. Adverse reactions include abdominal pain, anorexia, chills, fever, nausea, shaking, and vomiting. If signs and symptoms of adverse reactions occur, slow the infusion and give prescribed drugs to provide symptomatic relief. For a severe reaction or for pts without orders for symptomatic relief, stop the infusion and notify the physician.

• Evaluate the IV site for signs of phlebitis as evidenced by heat, pain, and red streaking over the vein.

• Monitor the patient's intake and output and renal function test results to assess for nephrotoxicity.

• Check the patient's serum potassium and magnesium levels, as well as hematologic and liver function test results.

• Assess the patient's skin for burning, irritation, or itching.

Patient/Family Teaching

• Explain to the patient/family that prolonged amphotericin B therapy over weeks or months is usually necessary to achieve a therapeutic effect.

• Tell the patient/family that the fever reaction may decrease with continued therapy.

• Advise the patient/family that muscle weakness may be noted during therapy from hypokalemia.

• Teach the patient/family to thoroughly rub in the topical cream or lotion because this may prevent staining of the skin or nails. Assure the patient/family that soap and water or dry cleaning will remove fabric stains caused by topical applications.

• Warn the patient/family not to use other preparations or occlusive coverings without consulting the physician.

• Urge the patient/family to keep affected areas clean and dry, to wear light clothing, and to separate out personal items with direct contact to the affected area.

Fluconazole

flu-**con**-ah-zole

(Apo-Fluconazole [CAN], Diflucan)

Do not confuse with diclofenac.

CATEGORY AND SCHEDULE

Pregnancy Risk Category: C

MECHANISM OF ACTION

A fungistatic antifungal that interferes with cytochrome P_{450}, an enzyme necessary for ergosterol formation. ***Therapeutic Effect:*** Directly damages fungal membrane, altering membrane function.

PHARMACOKINETICS

Well absorbed from GI tract. Widely distributed, including cerebrospinal fluid. Protein binding: 11%. Partially metabolized in liver. Primarily excreted unchanged in urine. Partially removed by hemodialysis. ***Half-Life:*** 20–30 hrs (half-life is increased with impaired renal function).

AVAILABILITY

Tablets: 50 mg, 100 mg, 150 mg, 200 mg.

Powder for Oral Suspension: 10 mg/mL, 40 mg/mL.
Injection: 2 mg/mL (in 100- or 200-mL containers).

INDICATIONS AND DOSAGES

▸ Oropharyngeal candidiasis
PO/IV
Children. Initially, 6 mg/kg/day once, then 3 mg/kg/day (maximum: 12 mg/kg/24 hr) for 14 days.
Neonates. Loading dose: 6–12 mg/kg.
Maintenance dose: Postconceptional age 29 wks or younger, 0–14 days postnatally give 5–6 mg/kg/dose beginning 72 hrs after loading dose.
Age 29 wks or younger, older than 14 days. Postnatally give 5–6 mg/kg/dose beginning 48 hrs after loading dose.
Age 30–36 wks, 0–14 days. Postnatally give 3–6 mg/kg/dose beginning 48 hrs after loading dose.
Age 30–36 wks, older than 14 days. Postnatally give 3–6 mg/kg/dose beginning 24 hrs after loading dose.
Age 37–44 wks, 0–7 days. Postnatally give 3–6 mg/kg/dose beginning 48 hrs after loading dose.
Age 37–44 wks, older than 7 days. Postnatally give 3–6 mg/kg/dose beginning 24 hrs after loading dose.
Age 45 wks or older. Give 3–6 mg/kg/dose beginning 24 hrs after loading dose.

▸ Esophageal candidiasis
PO/IV
Children. 10 mg/kg/day once, then 24 hrs after loading dose administer 3 mg/kg/day (up to 12 mg/kg/day) for 21 days.

▸ Systemic candidiasis
PO/IV
Children. 6–12 mg/kg/day for 28 days.

▸ Cryptococcal meningitis
PO/IV
Children. 12 mg/kg/day once, then 6–12 mg/kg/day; 6 mg/kg/day for suppression.

UNLABELED USES

Treatment of coccidioidomycosis, cryptococcosis, fungal pneumonia, onychomycosis, ringworm of the hand, septicemia.

CONTRAINDICATIONS

None known.

INTERACTIONS

Drug

Cyclosporine: High fluconazole doses increase cyclosporine blood concentration.
Oral hypoglycemics: May increase blood concentration and effects of oral hypoglycemics.
Phenytoin, warfarin: May decrease the metabolism of these drugs.
Rifampin: May increase fluconazole metabolism.

Herbal

None known.

Food

None known.

DIAGNOSTIC TEST EFFECTS

May increase serum alkaline phosphatase, serum bilirubin, SGOT (AST), and SGPT (ALT) levels.

IV INCOMPATIBILITIES

Amphotericin (Fungizone), amphotericin B complex (Abelcet, Amphotec, AmBisome), ampicillin (Polycillin), calcium gluconate, cefotaxime (Claforan), ceftazidime (Fortaz), ceftriaxone (Rocephin), cefuroxime (Zinacef), chloramphenicol (Chloromycetin), clindamycin (Cleocin), diazepam (Valium), digoxin (Lanoxin), erythromycin (Erythrocin), furosemide (Lasix), haloperidol (Haldol), hydroxyzine (Vistaril), imipenem/cilastatin (Primaxin), sulfamethoxazole-trimethoprim (Bactrim)

IV COMPATIBILITIES

Diltiazem (Cardizem), dobutamine (Dobutrex), dopamine (Intropin), heparin, lorazepam (Ativan), midazolam (Versed), propofol (Diprivan)

SIDE EFFECTS

Occasional (4%–1%)
Hypersensitivity reaction including chills, fever, pruritus, and rash; dizziness, drowsiness, headache, constipation, diarrhea, nausea, vomiting, abdominal pain

SERIOUS REACTIONS

! Exfoliative skin disorders, serious liver effects, and blood dyscrasias such as eosinophilia, thrombocytopenia, anemia, and leukopenia have been reported rarely.

PEDIATRIC CONSIDERATIONS

Baseline Assessment

- Expect to obtain baseline tests for complete blood count, liver function, and serum potassium.
- Be aware that it is unknown whether fluconazole is excreted in breast milk.
- There are no age-related precautions noted in children.
- Do not administer IV push.
- Use distal veins for IV administration.
- Adjust dosages in pts with renal failure. For creatinine clearance (CrCl) 20–50 mL/min give 50% of recommended dose. For CrCl less than 20 mL/min give 25% of recommended dose.

Precautions

- Use cautiously in pts with liver or renal impairment, hypersensitivity to other triazoles, such as itraconazole or terconazole, or hypersensitivity to imidazoles, such as butoconazole and ketoconazole.

Administration and Handling

PO
- Give without regard to meals.
- Be aware that PO and IV therapy are equally effective and that IV therapy is for pts intolerant of the drug or unable to take it orally.

IV
- Store at room temperature.
- Do not remove from outer wrap until ready to use.
- Squeeze inner bag to check for leaks.
- Do not use parenteral form if the solution is cloudy, a precipitate forms, the seal is not intact, or it is discolored.
- Do not add another medication to the solution.
- Do not exceed maximum flow rate 200 mg/hr.

Intervention and Evaluation

- Assess the patient for signs and symptoms of a hypersensitivity reaction, including chills or fever.
- Expect to monitor the patient's complete blood count, liver and renal function test results, platelet count, and serum potassium levels.
- Warn the patient to report any itching or rash promptly.
- Monitor the patient's temperature daily.
- Assess the patient's daily pattern of bowel activity and stool consistency.
- Evaluate the patient for dizziness and provide assistance as needed.

Patient/Family Teaching

- Caution the patient/family not to drive or use machinery until the

patient's response to the drug is established.
• Warn the patient/family to notify the physician if dark urine, pale stool, rash with or without itching, or yellow skin or eyes develop.
• Teach pts/families with oropharyngeal infections about good oral hygiene.
• Advise the patient/family to consult the physician before taking any other medications.

Griseofulvin

griz-ee-oh-**full**-vin
(Fulvicin P/G, Fulvicin U/F, Grifulvin V, Gris-PEG, Grisovin [AUS])

CATEGORY AND SCHEDULE

Pregnancy Risk Category: C

MECHANISM OF ACTION

An antifungal that inhibits fungal cell mitosis by disrupting mitotic spindle structure. ***Therapeutic Effect:*** Fungistatic.

AVAILABILITY

Tablets (microsize): 250 mg, 500 mg.
Tablets (ultramicrosize): 125 mg, 250 mg, 330 mg.
Oral Suspension: 125 mg/5 mL.
Tablets (ultramicrosize–film coated): Gris-PEG 125 mg, 250 mg.

INDICATIONS AND DOSAGES

▸ Treatment of tinea infections (ringworm): Tinea capitis, tinea corporis, tinea cruris, tinea pedis, tinea unguium

MICROSIZE TABLETS
Children older than 2 yrs. Usual dosage 10–20 mg/kg/day in single or divided doses.

ULTRAMICROSIZE TABLETS
Children older than 2 yrs. 5–10 mg/kg/day as single or divided doses.

CONTRAINDICATIONS

Porphyria, hepatocellular failure, hypersensitivity to griseofulvin or any component.

INTERACTIONS

Drug

Oral contraceptives, warfarin: May decrease the effects of these drugs.
Phenobarbital: May decrease effectiveness of griseofulvin.
Cyclosporine: May decrease the serum concentrations of this drug.

Herbal

None known.

Food

Fatty meals will increase absorption of griseofulvin.

DIAGNOSTIC TEST EFFECTS

None known.

SIDE EFFECTS

Occasional

Hypersensitivity reaction, such as pruritus, rash, and urticaria; headache, nausea, diarrhea, excessive thirst, flatulence, oral thrush, dizziness, insomnia

Rare

Paresthesia of hands or feet, proteinuria, photosensitivity reaction

SERIOUS REACTIONS

! Granulocytopenia occurs rarely.

PEDIATRIC CONSIDERATIONS

Baseline Assessment

• Determine the patient's history of allergies, especially to griseofulvin and penicillins, before giving the drug.

• Safety in children younger than 2 yrs old has not been recognized.
• It is important to ensure appropriate fluid intake.

Precautions

• Use cautiously in pts with hypersensitivity to penicillins or in those who are exposed to sun or ultraviolet light because photosensitivity may develop.

Intervention and Evaluation

◀ **ALERT** ▶ The duration of treatment depends on the site of infection.
• Evaluate the patient's skin for rash and therapeutic response to the drug.
• Assess the patient's daily pattern of bowel activity and stool consistency.
◀ **ALERT** ▶ Monitor the patient's granulocyte count as appropriate. If the patient develops granulocytopenia, notify the physician and expect to discontinue the drug.
• In pts experiencing headache, establish and document the headache's location, onset, and type.
• Assess the patient for dizziness.

Patient/Family Teaching

• Explain to the patient/family that prolonged therapy over weeks or months is usually necessary.
• Advise the patient/family not to miss a dose and to continue therapy as long as it is ordered.
• Warn the patient/family to avoid consuming alcohol because this may produce flushing or tachycardia.
• Advise the patient/family that griseofulvin may cause a photosensitivity reaction, so the patient should avoid exposure to sunlight and wear broad-spectrum sunscreens.
• Urge the patient/family to maintain good hygiene to help prevent superinfection.
• Encourage the patient/family to separate personal items that come in direct contact with affected areas.
• Teach the patient/family to keep affected areas dry and to wear light clothing for ventilation.
• Advise the patient/family to take griseofulvin with foods high in fat, such as milk or ice cream, to reduce GI upset and assist in drug absorption.

Ketoconazole

keet-oh-**con**-ah-zol
(Apo-Ketoconazole [CAN], Nizoral, Nizoral AD, Sebizole [AUS])
Do not confuse with Nasarel.

CATEGORY AND SCHEDULE

Pregnancy Risk Category: C
OTC (1% shampoo only)

MECHANISM OF ACTION

An imidazole derivative that changes the permeability of the fungal cell wall. ***Therapeutic Effect:*** Inhibits fungal biosynthesis of triglycerides, phospholipids. Fungistatic.

AVAILABILITY

Tablets: 200 mg.
Cream: 2%.
Shampoo: 2%, 1% (OTC).

INDICATIONS AND DOSAGES

▸ **Treatment of histoplasmosis, blastomycosis, candidiasis, chronic mucocutaneous candidiasis, coccidioidomycosis, paracoccidioidomycosis, chromomycosis, seborrheic dermatitis, tinea infections (ringworm): tinea corporis, tinea**

capitis, tinea manus, tinea cruris, tinea pedis, tinea unguium (onychomycosis), oral thrush, candiduria

PO

Children 2 yrs or older. 3.3–6.6 mg/kg/day. Maximum: 800 mg/day in 2 divided doses.

TOPICAL

Children. Apply 1–2 times/day to affected area for 2–4 wks.

DANDRUFF SHAMPOO

Children. Twice weekly for 4 wks, allowing at least 3 days between shampooing. Intermittent use to maintain control.

UNLABELED USES

Systemic: Treatment of fungal pneumonia, prostate cancer, septicemia.

CONTRAINDICATIONS

Hypersensitivity to ketoconazole or any component. Not to be used as a single agent for CNS fungal infections because of poor penetration.

INTERACTIONS

Drug

Alcohol, hepatotoxic medications: May increase hepatotoxicity of ketoconazole.

Antacids, anticholinergics, H_2 antagonists, omeprazole, didanosine: May decrease ketoconazole absorption.

Cyclosporine, lovastatin, simvastatin, phenytoin, digoxin, tacrolimus, triazolam, midazolam, corticosteroids, indinavir, warfarin: May increase blood concentration and risk of toxicity of these drugs.

Isoniazid, rifampin, phenytoin: May decrease blood ketoconazole concentration.

Herbal

Echinacea: May have additive hepatotoxic effects.

Food

Food increases ketoconazole absorption. Taking ketoconazole with acidic beverages increases the medication's absorption.

DIAGNOSTIC TEST EFFECTS

May increase serum alkaline phosphatase, serum bilirubin, SGOT (AST), and SGPT (ALT) levels. May decrease serum corticosteroid and testosterone concentrations.

SIDE EFFECTS

Occasional (10%–3%)

Nausea, vomiting

Rare (less than 2%)

Abdominal pain, diarrhea, headache, dizziness, photophobia, pruritus

Topical: itching, burning, irritation

SERIOUS REACTIONS

! Hematologic toxicity as evidenced by thrombocytopenia, hemolytic anemia, and leukopenia occurs occasionally.

! Hepatotoxicity may occur within the first week to several months of therapy.

! Anaphylaxis occurs rarely.

PEDIATRIC CONSIDERATIONS

Baseline Assessment

- Confirm that a culture or histologic test was done for accurate diagnosis; therapy may begin before results are known.
- Oral dose for children: 3.3–6.6 mg/kg/day once daily. Can also be used for prophylaxis of recurrent mucocutaneous candidiasis in HIV infected children: 5–10 mg/kg/day

divided q12–24h. Maximum: 800 mg/day.

Precautions

• Use cautiously in pts with liver impairment.

Administration and Handling

PO

• Give with food to minimize GI irritation.

• Tablets may be crushed.

• Ketoconazole requires acidity; give antacids, anticholinergics, H_2 blockers, and omeprazole at least 2 hrs after dosing.

SHAMPOO

• Apply to wet hair, massage for 1 min, rinse thoroughly, reapply for 3 min, and then rinse.

TOPICAL

• Apply and rub gently into the affected and surrounding area.

Intervention and Evaluation

• Expect to monitor the patient's liver function test results. Be alert for signs and symptoms of hepatotoxicity, including anorexia, dark urine, fatigue, nausea, pale stools, and vomiting, that are unrelieved by giving the medication with food.

• Monitor the patient's complete blood count for evidence of hematologic toxicity.

• Assess the patient's daily pattern of bowel activity and stool consistency.

• Assess the patient for dizziness, provide assistance as needed, and institute safety precautions.

• Evaluate the patient's skin for itching, rash, and urticaria.

• If the patient is receiving topical ketoconazole, check the patient's skin for local burning, itching, and irritation.

Patient/Family Teaching

• Explain to the patient/family that prolonged therapy over weeks or months is usually necessary.

• Instruct the patient/family not to miss a dose and to continue therapy as long as directed.

• Advise the patient to avoid alcohol to avoid potential liver toxicity.

• Warn the patient/family to avoid tasks that require mental alertness or motor skills until the patient's response to the drug is established.

• Encourage the patient/family to take antacids or antiulcer medications at least 2 hrs after taking ketoconazole.

• Warn the patient/family to notify the physician if dark urine, increased irritation with topical use, onset of other new symptoms, pale stool, or yellow skin or eyes develop.

• Teach the patient/family receiving topical ketoconazole to avoid drug contact with the eyes, keep the skin clean and dry, rub the drug well into affected areas, and wear light clothing for ventilation.

• Encourage the patient/family to separate personal items that come in direct contact with the affected area.

• Instruct the patient/family to use the ketoconazole shampoo initially twice weekly for 4 wks with at least 3 days between shampooing. Also explain that further shampooing will be based upon the patient's response to the initial treatment.

Nystatin

nigh-**stat**-in

(Mycostatin, Nilstat, Nyaderm, Nystop)

Do not confuse with Nitrostat.

CATEGORY AND SCHEDULE

Pregnancy Risk Category: C

MECHANISM OF ACTION
An antifungal that binds to sterols in fungal cell membranes, increasing permeability, permitting loss of potassium and other cell components. ***Therapeutic Effect:*** Fungistatic.

PHARMACOKINETICS
PO: Poorly absorbed from the GI tract. Eliminated unchanged in feces.
Topical: Not absorbed systemically from intact skin.

AVAILABILITY
Tablets: 500,000 units.
Oral Suspension: 100,000 units/mL.
Troches: 200,000 units.
Vaginal Tablets: 100,000 units.
Cream: 100,000 units/g.
Ointment: 100,000 units/g.
Powder: 100,000 units/g.

INDICATIONS AND DOSAGES
▸ Intestinal candidiasis
PO
Children. 500,000 units 4 times/day.
▸ Oral candidiasis
PO
Children. Oral suspension: 400,000–600,000 units 4 times/day. Troches: 200,000–400,000 units 4–5 times/day for up to 14 days.
Term infants. 100,000 units to each side of mouth 4 times/day.
Preterm infants. 50,000 units to each side of mouth 4 times/day.
▸ Vulvovaginal candidiasis
INTRAVAGINAL
Children. 1 tablet high in vagina 1 time/day at bedtime for 14 days.
▸ Topical fungal infections
TOPICAL
Children. Apply to affected area 2–4 times/day.

UNLABELED USES
Prophylaxis and treatment of oropharyngeal candidiasis, tinea barbae, tinea capitis.

CONTRAINDICATIONS
Hypersensitivity to nystatin or any component.

INTERACTIONS
Drug
None known.
Herbal
None known.
Food
None known.

DIAGNOSTIC TEST EFFECTS
None known.

SIDE EFFECTS
Occasional
PO: None known
Topical: Skin irritation
Vaginal: Vaginal irritation

SERIOUS REACTIONS
! High dosage with oral form may produce nausea, vomiting, diarrhea, and GI distress.

PEDIATRIC CONSIDERATIONS
Baseline Assessment
- Confirm that cultures or histologic tests were done for accurate diagnosis before giving the drug.
- Be aware that it is unknown whether nystatin is distributed in breast milk.
- During pregnancy, vaginal applicators may be contraindicated, requiring manual insertion of tablets.
- There are no age-related precautions noted for suspension or topical use in children.
- Be aware that lozenges are not recommended for use in children 5 years old or younger.

• Have older children swish suspension and hold in mouth before swallowing.
• For neonates and infants, be aware that you may have to paint nystatin into the recesses of the mouth to ensure effective application.

Precautions

• None known.

Administration and Handling

PO

• Have the patient dissolve lozenges (troches) slowly and completely in the mouth for optimal therapeutic effect. Lozenges should not be chewed or swallowed whole.
• Shake suspension well before administration.
• Instruct the patient to place and hold the suspension in the mouth or swish throughout the mouth as long as possible before swallowing.

Intervention and Evaluation

• Assess the patient for increased irritation with topical application or increased vaginal discharge with vaginal application.

Patient/Family Teaching

• Advise the patient/family not to miss a dose and to complete the full length of treatment.
• Explain that vaginal use should be continued during menses.
• Teach the patient/family to insert the vaginal form high into the vagina.
• Warn the patient/family that the topical form must not come in contact with the eyes.
• Instruct the patient/family to continue use for at least 2 days after symptoms subside.
• Explain that nystatin cream or powder should be used sparingly on erythematous areas.
• Teach the patient/family to rub the topical form well into affected areas, to keep affected areas clean and dry, and to wear light clothing for ventilation.
• Encourage the patient/family to separate personal items that come in contact with affected areas.
• Warn the patient/family to notify the physician if diarrhea, nausea, stomach pain, or vomiting develops.

Terbinafine Hydrochloride

tur-**bin**-ah-feen

(Lamisil, Lamisil Derma Gel)

Do not confuse with Lamictal, terbutaline.

CATEGORY AND SCHEDULE

Pregnancy Risk Category: B

MECHANISM OF ACTION

An antifungal that inhibits the enzyme squalene epoxidase, thereby interfering with biosynthesis in fungi. ***Therapeutic Effect:*** Results in fungal cell death.

AVAILABILITY

Tablets: 250 mg.
Cream: 1%.
Topical Solution: 1%.

INDICATIONS AND DOSAGES

▸ **Tinea pedis**

TOPICAL

Children 12 yrs and older. Apply 2 times/day until signs and symptoms significantly improve.

▸ **Tinea cruris, tinea corporis**

TOPICAL

Children 12 yrs and older. Apply 1–2 times/day until signs and symptoms significantly improve.

▸ **Onychomycosis**

PO

Children 12 yrs and older. 250 mg/day for 6 wks (fingernails), 12 wks (toenails).

CONTRAINDICATIONS

Oral: Preexisting liver disease or renal impairment (creatinine clearance of 50 mL/min or less) and in children younger than 12 years of age.

INTERACTIONS

Drug

Alcohol, other hepatotoxic medications: May increase risk of hepatotoxicity.
Liver enzyme inducers, including rifampin: May increase terbinafine clearance.
Liver enzyme inhibitors, including cimetidine: May decrease terbinafine clearance.
Cyclosporin: May increase cyclosporine clearance.
Dextromethorphan: May increase serum concentrations of dextromethorphan leading to adverse effects and toxicity.

Herbal

None known.

Food

None known.

DIAGNOSTIC TEST EFFECTS

May increase SGOT (AST) and SGPT (ALT) levels.

SIDE EFFECTS

Frequent (13%)
Oral: Headache
Occasional (6%-3%)
Oral: Diarrhea, rash, dyspepsia, pruritus, taste disturbance, nausea
Rare
Oral: Abdominal pain, flatulence, urticaria, visual disturbance
Topical: Irritation, burning, itching, dryness

SERIOUS REACTIONS

! Hepatobiliary dysfunction, including cholestatic hepatitis, serious skin reactions, and severe neutropenia occur rarely.
! Ocular lens and retinal changes have been noted.

PEDIATRIC CONSIDERATIONS

Baseline Assessment

- As appropriate, monitor liver function in pts receiving treatment for longer than 6 wks.
- This medication has not been approved for use in children younger than 12 years of age.

Precautions

- None known.

Intervention and Evaluation

◂ALERT▸ Topical therapy may be used for a minimum of 1 wk and is not to exceed 4 wks.
- Assess the patient for signs of a therapeutic response.
- Discontinue the medication and notify the physician if a local reaction occurs. Signs and symptoms of a local reaction include blistering, burning, irritation, itching, oozing, redness, and swelling.

Patient/Family Teaching

- Teach the patient/family to keep affected areas clean and dry and to wear light clothing to promote ventilation.
- Encourage the patient/family to separate personal items that come in contact with affected areas.
- Warn the patient/family to avoid topical cream contact with eyes, mouth, nose, or other mucous membranes.
- Instruct the patient/family to rub the topical form well into the affected and surrounding area. Reinforce that the treated area should not be covered with an occlusive dressing.
- Warn the patient/family to notify the physician if diarrhea or skin irritation occurs.

REFERENCES

Benitz, W. E. & Tatro, D. S. (1995). The pediatric drug handbook (3rd ed.). St. Louis: Mosby.

Gunn, V. L. & Nechyba, C. (2002). The Harriet Lane handbook (16th ed.). St. Louis: Mosby.

Miller, S. & Fioravanti, J. (1997). Pediatric medications: a handbook for nurses. St. Louis: Mosby.

3 Antiretroviral Agents

Abacavir
Amprenavir
Didanosine
Efavirenz
Enfuvirtide
Lamivudine
Lopinavir/ritonavir
Nelfinavir
Nevirapine
Ritonavir
Saquinavir
Stavudine (dT4)
Zalcitabine
Zidovudine

Uses: Antiretroviral agents are used to treat human immunodeficiency virus (HIV) infection. HIV treatment aims to greatly reduce the viral load, which allows the CD4 cell count to remain at a level that is adequate to fight infections. Antiretroviral therapy typically includes more than one antiretroviral agent, each with a different mechanism of action. When the virus is attacked through different mechanisms of action, the risk of resistance is reduced.

Action: The five classes of antiretroviral agents act in different ways. *Nucleoside reverse transcriptase inhibitors (NRTIs),* such as stavudine and zalcitabine, compete with natural substrates for formation of proviral DNA by reverse transcriptase inhibiting viral replication. *Fusion inhibitors,* such as enfuvirtide, inhibit fusion of viral and cellular membranes. *Nonnucleoside reverse transcriptase inhibitors (NNRTIs),* such as efavirenz, directly bind to reverse transcriptase and block RNA-dependent and DNA-dependent DNA polymerase activities by disrupting the enzyme's catalytic site. *Protease inhibitors (PIs),* such as nelfinavir, bind to the active site of HIV-1 protease and therefore prevent the binding of the enzyme protease. This action prevents protease from processing HIV polyproteins, which renders the structural proteins and enzymes of HIV unable to function. Therefore, the virus remains immature and noninfectious. (See illustration, *Mechanisms and Sites of Action: Antiretroviral Agents,* page 34.)

COMBINATION PRODUCTS

COMBIVIR: lamivudine/zidovudine (an antiretroviral) 150 mg/300 mg.
TRIZIVIR: abacavir/lamivudine (an antiretroviral)/zidovudine (an antiretroviral) 300 mg/150 mg/300 mg.

Abacavir

ah-bah-**kay**-veer
(Ziagen)

CATEGORY AND SCHEDULE

Pregnancy Risk Category: C

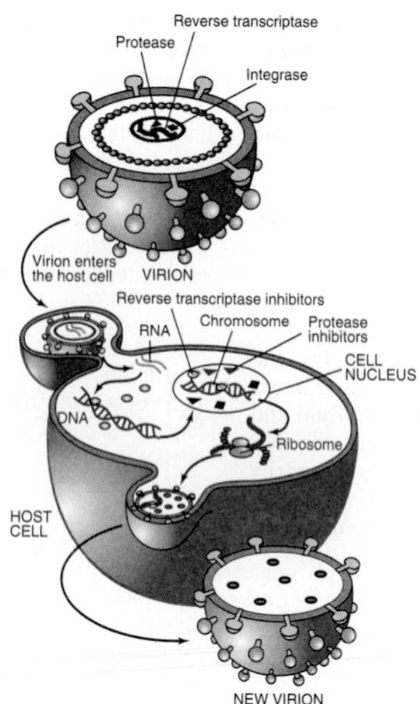

Mechanisms and Sites of Action: Antiretroviral Agents

To understand how antiretroviral agents work, you need to know how viruses reproduce. First, the infectious viral particle or virion (A) enters the host cell. The virion attaches to the cell's surface and then inserts itself into the host cell (B). Once inside, the virion uncoats, and the enzyme reverse transcriptase makes two copies of the viral RNA: one copy is identical; the other is a mirror image. These two copies merge to form double-stranded viral DNA. This newly formed viral DNA enters the host cell's nucleus, where it inserts itself into the host cell's DNA with the help of the enzyme integrase. Then viral DNA reprograms the host cell to produce additional viral RNA, which begins the process of forming new viruses. Specifically, messenger RNA (mRNA) instructs ribosomal RNA (rRNA) to produce a new chain of proteins and enzymes that are used to form new viruses. Protease, another enzyme, cuts the chains of proteins, creating individual proteins. These individual proteins combine with new RNA to create new virions, which bud and are then released from the host cell (C).

Antiretroviral agents target specific enzymes during viral reproduction. Many of them work to inhibit reverse transcriptase. Nucleoside reverse transcriptase inhibitors, such as stavudine, interfere with the action of reverse transcriptase by mimicking naturally occurring nucleosides. Nucleotide reverse transcriptase inhibitors, such as tenofovir, block reverse transcriptase by competing with the natural substrate deoxyadenosine triphosphate and by causing DNA chain termination. Nonnucleoside reverse transcriptase inhibitors, such as delavirdine, work by directly binding to reverse transcriptase. All of these actions block the conversion of single-stranded viral RNA into double-stranded DNA. As a result, no viral DNA is available to insert itself into the host cell's DNA. Protease inhibitors, such as indinavir, bind to and interfere with the action of protease. Because the protease is blocked, the new chain of proteins formed by rRNA cannot be cut into individual proteins to make new viruses.

MECHANISM OF ACTION

This antiretroviral agent inhibits the activity of HIV-1 reverse transcriptase by competing with natural substrate deoxyguanosine triphosphate and by its incorporation into viral DNA. ***Therapeutic Effect:*** Inhibits viral DNA growth.

PHARMACOKINETICS

Rapidly, extensively absorbed after PO administration. Protein binding: 50%. Widely distributed, including cerebrospinal fluid and erythrocytes. Metabolized in liver to inactive metabolites. Primarily excreted in urine. Unknown whether removed by hemodialysis. ***Half-Life:*** 1–1.5 hrs.

AVAILABILITY

Tablets: 300 mg.
Oral Solution: 20 mg/mL.

INDICATIONS AND DOSAGES

▸ HIV (in combination)

PO

Children (3 mos–16 yrs). 8 mg/kg 2 times/day. Maximum: 300 mg 2 times/day.

CONTRAINDICATIONS

Hypersensitivity to any component.

INTERACTIONS

Drug

Alcohol: May increase abacavir blood concentration and half-life.
Methadone: Increases methadone clearance, which may necessitate a larger dose of methadone.

Herbal

St. John's wort: May decrease abacavir blood concentration and effect.

Food

None known.

DIAGNOSTIC TEST EFFECTS

May increase blood glucose, γ-glutamyl transferase, SGOT (AST), SGPT (ALT), and triglycerides.

SIDE EFFECTS

Frequent

Nausea with vomiting (39%), fever (19%), headache, diarrhea (16%), rash (11%)

Occasional

Decreased appetite (9%)

SERIOUS REACTIONS

! Hypersensitivity reaction (may be life-threatening) may occur. Signs and symptoms include fever, rash, fatigue, intractable nausea and vomiting, severe diarrhea, abdominal pain, cough, pharyngitis, and dyspnea.
! Life-threatening hypotension may occur.
! Lactic acidosis and severe hepatomegaly may occur.

PEDIATRIC CONSIDERATIONS

Baseline Assessment

- Determine if the patient is pregnant.
- Expect to obtain baseline laboratory testing, especially liver function tests, before beginning therapy and at periodic intervals during therapy.
- Offer emotional support to the patient and family.
- Be aware that it is unknown whether abacavir is excreted in breast milk. Pts taking abacavir should not breast-feed because this may increase the potential for adverse effects in the infant as well as the risk of HIV transmission.
- Abacavir may be used safely in children aged 3 mos–13 yrs.

Precautions

• Use cautiously in pts with impaired liver function.

Administration and Handling

PO

• May give without regard to food.

• Oral solution may be refrigerated. Do not freeze.

Intervention and Evaluation

• Assess the patient for nausea and vomiting.

• Determine the patient's pattern of bowel activity and stool consistency.

• Assess the patient's eating pattern.

• Monitor the patient for weight loss.

• Monitor laboratory values carefully, particularly liver function.

Patient/Family Teaching

• Explain to the patient/family that the patient should not take any medications, including OTC drugs, without consulting the physician.

• Encourage the patient/family to ingest small, frequent meals to help offset anorexia and nausea.

• Instruct the patient/family that abacavir is not a cure for HIV infection nor does it reduce the risk of transmission to others.

Amprenavir

am-**prenn**-ah-veer
(Agenerase)

CATEGORY AND SCHEDULE

Pregnancy Risk Category: C

MECHANISM OF ACTION

This antiviral inhibits HIV-1 protease by binding to the active site of HIV-1 protease, preventing processing of viral precursors and forming immature noninfectious viral particles. ***Therapeutic Effect:*** Produces impairment of HIV viral replication and proliferation.

PHARMACOKINETICS

Rapidly absorbed after PO administration. Protein binding: 90%. Metabolized in the liver. Primarily excreted in feces. ***Half-Life:*** 7.1–10.6 hrs for adults.

AVAILABILITY

Capsules: 50 mg, 150 mg.
Oral Solution: 15 mg/mL.

INDICATIONS AND DOSAGES

▸ **HIV-1 infection**

PO (CAPSULES)

Children 4–12 yrs, 13–16 yrs weighing less than 50 kg. 20 mg/kg 2 times/day or 15 mg/kg 3 times/day. Maximum: 2,400 mg/day.

Children 13–16 yrs weighing more than 50 kg. 1,200 mg 2 times/day.

PO (ORAL SOLUTION)

Adolescents weighing more than 50 kg. 1,400 mg 2 times/day.

Children 4–12, 13–16 yrs weighing less than 50 kg. 22.5 mg/kg/day (1.5 mL/kg) 2 times/day or 17 mg/kg/day (1.1 mL/kg) 3 times/day. Maximum: 2,800 mg/day.

▸ **Dosage in liver impairment**

Child-Pugh Score	Capsules	Oral Solution
5–8	450 mg bid	513 mg bid
9–12	300 mg bid	342 mg bid

CONTRAINDICATIONS

Hypersensitivity to amprenavir or any component. Solution is contraindicated in infants and children younger than 4 yrs, in pregnancy and hepatic or renal failure, and in pts receiving disulfiram or metronidazole (because of the high amount of propylene glycol in the solution).

INTERACTIONS

Drug

Amiodarone, bepridil, ergotamine, lidocaine, midazolam, oral contraceptives, quinidine, triazolam, tricyclic antidepressants: May interfere with the metabolism of these drugs.
Antacids, didanosine: May decrease amprenavir absorption.
Carbamazepine, phenobarbital, phenytoin, rifampin: May decrease amprenavir blood concentration.
Clozapine, hydroxymethylglutaryl-CoA reductase inhibitors, including statins, warfarin, cyclosporine, tacrolimus, amiodarone: May increase the blood concentration of these drugs.
Flecainide, propafenone: Should not be used if the patient is receiving amprenavir with ritonavir.

Herbal

St. John's wort: May decrease amprenavir blood concentration.

Food

High-fat meals: May decrease amprenavir absorption.

DIAGNOSTIC TEST EFFECTS

May increase blood cholesterol, glucose, and triglyceride levels.

SIDE EFFECTS

Frequent

Diarrhea or loose stools (56%), nausea (38%), oral paresthesia (30%), rash (25%), vomiting (20%)

Occasional

Rash (18%), peripheral paresthesia (12%), depression (4%)

SERIOUS REACTIONS

! Severe hypersensitivity reactions or Stevens-Johnson syndrome as evidenced by blisters, peeling of the skin, loosening of skin and mucous membranes, and fever may occur.

PEDIATRIC CONSIDERATIONS

Baseline Assessment

- Expect to obtain baseline laboratory testing before beginning therapy and at periodic intervals during therapy.
- Offer the patient/family emotional support.
- Be aware that it is unknown whether amprenavir crosses the placenta or is distributed in breast milk.
- Be aware that the safety and efficacy of amprenavir have not established in children younger than 4 yrs.
- Pts in early puberty (Tanner I–II stages) should be given pediatric dosages, and those in late puberty (Tanner V stage) should be given adult dosages.
- Adolescents in the middle of a growth spurt can be given pediatric or adult dosages with close monitoring.

Precautions

- Use cautiously in pts with diabetes mellitus, hemophilia, hypersensitivity to sulfa drugs, liver function impairment, or vitamin K deficiency from anticoagulant malabsorption.

Administration and Handling

PO

- May give without regard to food.

Intervention and Evaluation

- Observe the patient for any nausea or vomiting.
- Determine the patient's pattern of bowel activity and stool consistency.

• Evaluate the patient's eating pattern and monitor the patient for weight loss.
• Examine the patient for tingling or numbness of the peripheral extremities and skin rash.

Patient/Family Teaching

• Urge the patient/family to avoid high-fat meals because they may decrease drug absorption.
• Encourage the patient/family to consume small, frequent meals to help offset anorexia and nausea.
• Advise the patient/family that amprenavir is not a cure for HIV infection nor does it reduce risk of transmission to others.

Didanosine

dye-**dan**-oh-sin
(Videx, Videx-EC)

CATEGORY AND SCHEDULE

Pregnancy Risk Category: B

MECHANISM OF ACTION

A purine nucleoside analogue that is intracellularly converted into a triphosphate, interfering with RNA-directed DNA polymerase (reverse transcriptase). ***Therapeutic Effect:*** Virustatic, inhibiting replication of retroviruses, including HIV.

PHARMACOKINETICS

Variably absorbed from the GI tract. Protein binding: less than 5%. Rapidly metabolized intracellularly to active form. Primarily excreted in urine. Partially (20%) removed by hemodialysis. ***Half-Life:*** 0.8–1.5 hrs; metabolite: 8–24 hrs.

AVAILABILITY

Tablets (chewable): 25 mg, 50 mg, 100 mg, 150 mg, 200 mg.
Capsules (delayed-release): 125 mg, 200 mg, 250 mg, 400 mg.
Powder for Oral Solution (single-dose packet): 100 mg, 250 mg.
Pediatric Solution: 10 mg/mL.

INDICATIONS AND DOSAGES

▸ HIV infection

Children 13 yrs and older, weighing 60 kg or more. 200 mg q12h or 400 mg once daily.
ORAL SOLUTION
Children 13 yrs and older, weighing 60 kg or more. 250 mg q12h.
DELAYED-RELEASE CAPSULE
Children 13 yrs and older, weighing 60 kg or more. 400 mg once daily.
Children 13 yrs and older, weighing less than 60 kg. 125 mg q12h or 250 mg once daily.
ORAL SOLUTION
Children 13 yrs and older, weighing less than 60 kg. 167 mg q12h.
DELAYED-RELEASE CAPSULES
Children 13 yrs and older, weighing less than 60 kg. 250 mg once daily.
Children 3 mos to younger than 13 yrs. 180–300 mg/m²/day in divided doses q12h.
Children younger than 3 mos. 50 mg/m²/day in divided doses q12h.

▸ Dosage in renal impairment

Pts weighing less than 60 kg:

Creatinine Clearance	Tablets	Oral Solution	Delayed-Release Capsules
30–59 mL/min	75 mg 2 times/day	100 mg 2 times daily	125 mg once daily
10–29 mL/min	100 mg once daily	100 mg once daily	125 mg once daily
Less than 10 mL/min	75 mg once daily	100 mg once daily	N/A

Pts weighing 60 kg or more:

Creatinine Clearance	Tablets	Oral Solution	Delayed-Release Capsules
30–59 mL/min	100 mg 2 times/day	100 mg 2 times daily	200 mg once daily
10–29 mL/min	150 mg once daily	167 mg once daily	125 mg once daily
Less than 10 mL/min	100 mg once daily	100 mg once daily	125 mg once daily

CONTRAINDICATIONS

Hypersensitivity to the drug or any component of preparation.

INTERACTIONS

Drug

Dapsone, fluoroquinolones, itraconazole, ketoconazole, tetracyclines: May decrease absorption of these drugs.
Medications producing pancreatitis or peripheral neuropathy such as cisplatin, isoniazid, metronidazole, phenytoin, vincristine, stavudine, zalcitabine, dapsone, ethambutol, ethionamide, hydralazine, nitrofurantoin: May increase risk of pancreatitis or peripheral neuropathy with these drugs.
Stavudine: May increase risk of fatal lactic acidosis in pregnancy.
Antacids, allopurinol, omeprazole, ganciclovir, cimetidine, ranitidine: May increase absorption of didanosine.
Methadone: Decreases didanosine concentrations.

Herbal

None known.

Food

Decreases absorption of didanosine.
Do not mix with acidic beverages.

DIAGNOSTIC TEST EFFECTS

May increase serum alkaline phosphatase, amylase, bilirubin, lipase, triglycerides, uric acid SGOT (AST), and SGPT (ALT) levels. May decrease serum potassium levels.

SIDE EFFECTS

Frequent
Children (greater than 25%): Chills, fever, decreased appetite, pain, malaise, nausea, diarrhea, vomiting, abdominal pain, headache, nervousness, cough, rhinitis, dyspnea, asthenia, rash, itching
Occasional
Children (25%–10%): Failure to thrive, decreased weight, stomatitis, oral thrush, ecchymosis, arthritis, myalgia, insomnia, epistaxis, pharyngitis

SERIOUS REACTIONS

! Pneumonia and opportunistic infection occur occasionally. Peripheral neuropathy and potentially fatal pancreatitis are the major toxicities.

PEDIATRIC CONSIDERATIONS

Baseline Assessment

- Expect to obtain the patient's baseline values for complete blood count (CBC), renal and liver function tests, vital signs, and weight.
- Be aware that didanosine should be used during pregnancy only if clearly needed and that breast-feeding should be discontinued during didanosine therapy.

• Be aware that didanosine is well tolerated in children older than 3 mos.
• Pts in early puberty (Tanner I–II stages) should be given pediatric dosages, and those in late puberty (Tanner V stage) should be given adult dosages.
• Adolescents in the middle of a growth spurt can be given pediatric or adult dosages with close monitoring.

Precautions

• Use cautiously in pts with alcoholism, elevated triglyceride levels, renal or liver dysfunction, or T-cell counts less than 100 cells/mm^3.
• Use didanosine with extreme caution in pts with a history of pancreatitis.
• Use cautiously in pts consuming phenylketonuria and sodium-restricted diets because didanosine contains phenylalanine and sodium.

Administration and Handling

PO

• Store at room temperature.
• Tablets dispersed in water are stable for 1 hr at room temperature; after reconstitution of buffered powder, oral solution is stable for 4 hrs at room temperature.
• Pediatric powder for oral solution after reconstitution, as directed, is stable for 30 days refrigerated.
• Give 1 hr before or 2 hrs after meals because food decreases the rate and extent of didanosine absorption.
• Thoroughly crush and disperse chewable tablets in at least 30 mL water before having the patient swallow it. Stir the mixture well (up to 2–3 min) and have the patient immediately swallow it.
• Reconstitute buffered powder for oral solution before giving it by pouring the contents of the packet into 4 oz of water; stir until completely dissolved (up to 2–3 min). Do not mix with fruit juice or other acidic liquids because didanosine is unstable with an acidic pH.
• Add 100–200 mL water to 2 or 4 g of the unbuffered pediatric powder, respectively, to provide a concentration of 20 mg/mL. Immediately mix with an equal amount of an antacid to provide a concentration of 10 mg/mL. Shake thoroughly before removing each dose.
• Have the patient swallow enteric-coated capsules whole and take them on an empty stomach.

Intervention and Evaluation

◂ **ALERT** ▸ Contact the physician if the patient experiences abdominal pain, elevated serum amylase or triglyceride levels, nausea, and vomiting before administering the medication because these symptoms may indicate pancreatitis.
• Assess the patient for signs and symptoms of peripheral neuropathy, including burning feet, "restless leg syndrome" (unable to find comfortable position for legs and feet), and lack of coordination.
• Monitor the consistency and frequency of the patient's stools. Check the patient's skin for eruptions and rash.
• As appropriate, monitor the patient's blood chemistry values and CBC.
• Assess the patient for signs and symptoms of opportunistic infections, including cough or other respiratory symptoms, fever, or oral mucosa changes.

• Check the patient's weight at least twice a week.
• Assess the patient for visual or hearing difficulty and provide protection from light if photophobia develops.

Patient/Family Teaching

• Advise the patient/family to avoid the intake of alcohol.
• Warn the patient/family to notify the physician if the patient experiences nausea, numbness, persistent severe abdominal pain, or vomiting.
• Teach the patient/family to shake the oral suspension well before using it, to keep it refrigerated, and to discard the solution after 30 days and obtain a new supply.

Efavirenz

eh-fah-vir-enz
(Stocrin [AUS], Sustiva)

CATEGORY AND SCHEDULE

Pregnancy Risk Category: C

MECHANISM OF ACTION

A nonnucleoside reverse transcriptase inhibitor that inhibits the activity of reverse transcriptase of HIV-1. ***Therapeutic Effect:*** Interrupts HIV replication, slowing progression of HIV infection.

PHARMACOKINETICS

Rapidly absorbed after PO administration. Protein binding: 99%. Metabolized to major isoenzymes in liver. Eliminated in urine and feces. ***Half-Life:*** 40–55 hrs.

AVAILABILITY

Capsules: 50 mg, 100 mg, 200 mg.
Tablets: 600 mg.

INDICATIONS AND DOSAGES

▸ HIV infection

PO

Children 3 yrs and older weighing 40 kg or more. 600 mg once daily.
Children older than 3 yrs weighing 32.5 kg to less than 40 KG. 400 mg once daily.
Children older than 3 yrs weighing 25 kg to less than 32.5 kg. 350 mg once daily.
Children older than 3 yrs weighing 20 kg to less than 25 kg. 300 mg once daily.
Children older than 3 yrs weighing 15 kg to less than 20 kg. 250 mg once daily.
Children older than 3 yrs weighing 10 kg to less than 15 kg. 200 mg once daily.

CONTRAINDICATIONS

Concurrent administration with ergot derivatives, midazolam, or triazolam; a history of hypersensitivity to efavirenz; monotherapy.

INTERACTIONS

Drug

Alcohol, psychoactive drugs: May produce additive CNS effects.
Clarithromycin: Decreases clarithromycin plasma levels.
Ergot derivatives, midazolam, triazolam: May cause serious or life-threatening events, such as arrhythmias, prolonged sedation, or respiratory depression.
Indinavir, saquinavir: Decreases the plasma concentrations of these drugs.
Nelfinavir, ritonavir: Increases the plasma concentrations of these drugs.

Rifabutin, rifampin: Lowers efavirenz plasma concentration.
Warfarin: Alters warfarin plasma concentrations.
Phenobarbital, phenytoin, carbamazepine, itraconazole, ketoconazole: Decreases the plasma concentration of these drugs.

Herbal

St. John's wort: May decrease concentrations of efavirenz

Food

None known.

DIAGNOSTIC TEST EFFECTS

May produce false-positive urine test results for cannabinoid and increase liver enzyme, total cholesterol, SGOT (AST), SGPT (ALT), and serum triglyceride levels.

SIDE EFFECTS

Frequent (52%)

Mild to severe symptoms: Dizziness, vivid dreams, insomnia, confusion, impaired concentration, amnesia, agitatio, depersonalization, hallucinations, euphoria

Occasional

Mild to moderate degree maculopapular rash (27%); nausea, fatigue, headache, diarrhea, fever, cough (less than 26%)

SERIOUS REACTIONS

None known.

PEDIATRIC CONSIDERATIONS

Baseline Assessment

- Offer emotional support to the patient and family.
- Expect to obtain the baseline SGOT (AST) and SGPT (ALT) levels in pts with a history of hepatitis B or C before giving the drug.
- Expect to obtain the patient's baseline serum cholesterol and triglyceride levels before giving the drug and at regular intervals during therapy.
- Obtain the patient's history of use of all prescription and nonprescription medications before giving the drug, because efavirenz interacts with several drugs.
- Be aware that breast-feeding is not recommended for pts taking efavirenz.
- Be aware that the safety and efficacy of efavirenz have not been established in children younger than 3 yrs.
- In children, there may be an increased incidence of rash. Discontinue therapy in children who develop a severe rash that has evidence of blistering, fever, mucosal association, or desquamation.
- Use this therapy in combination with at least one other antiretroviral agent.

Precautions

- Use cautiously in pts with a history of liver impairment, mental illness, or substance abuse.

Administration and Handling

PO

- Give without regard to meals.
- High-fat meals may increase drug absorption and should be avoided.

Intervention and Evaluation

- Monitor the patient for signs and symptoms of adverse CNS psychologic side effects, such as abnormal dreams, dizziness, impaired concentration, insomnia, severe acute depression, including suicidal ideation or attempts, and somnolence. Be aware that insomnia may begin during the first or second day of therapy and generally resolves in 2–4 wks.

• Assess the patient for evidence of a rash, a common side effect.
• As appropriate, monitor the patient's liver enzyme studies for abnormalities.
• Assess the patient for diarrhea, headache, and nausea.

Patient/Family Teaching

• Advise the patient/family to avoid high-fat meals during therapy.
• Warn the patient/family to notify the physician immediately if a rash appears.
• Explain to the patient/family that CNS psychologic symptoms occur in more than half of pts and may cause delusions, depression, dizziness, and impaired concentration. Advise the patient to notify the physician if these continue or become problematic.
• Advise the patient/family to take the medication every day as prescribed. Warn the patient/family not to alter the dose or discontinue the medication without first notifying the physician.
• Warn the patient/family to avoid tasks that require mental alertness or motor skills until the patient's response to the drug is established.
• Explain that efavirenz is not a cure for HIV infection nor does it reduce risk of transmission to others.

Enfuvirtide

en-**few**-vir-tide
(Fuzeon)

CATEGORY AND SCHEDULE

Pregnancy Risk Category: B

MECHANISM OF ACTION

A fusion inhibitor that interferes with the entry of HIV-1 into $CD4^+$ cells by inhibiting fusion of viral and cellular membranes.
Therapeutic Effect: Slows HIV replication, reducing progression of HIV infection.

PHARMACOKINETICS

Comparable absorption when injected into subcutaneous tissue of abdomen, arm, or thigh. Protein binding: 92%. Undergoes catabolism to amino acids.
Half-Life: 3.8 hrs.

AVAILABILITY

Powder for Injection: 108 mg (approximately 90 mg/mL when reconstituted) vials.

INDICATIONS AND DOSAGES

▸ **HIV infection**

SUBCUTANEOUS

Children 6–16 yrs. 2 mg/kg 2 times/day up to a maximum dose of 90 mg 2 times/day.

▸ **Pediatric dosing guidelines**

Weight: kg (lbs)	Dose: mg (mL)
11–15.5 (24–34)	27 (0.3)
15.6–20 (more than 34–44)	36 (0.4)
20.1–24.5 (more than 44–54)	45 (0.5)
24.6–29 (more than 54–64)	54 (0.6)
29.1–33.5 (more than 64–74)	63 (0.7)
33.6–38 (more than 74–84)	72 (0.8)
38.1–42.5 (more than 84–94)	81 (0.9)
More than 42.5 (more than 94)	90 (1)

CONTRAINDICATIONS

Those with a known hypersensitivity to enfuvirtide or any component.

INTERACTIONS

Drug
None known.

Herbal
None known.

Food
None known.

DIAGNOSTIC TEST EFFECTS

May elevate blood glucose, serum amylase, serum creatine phosphokinase, serum lipase, serum triglyceride, SGOT (AST), and SGPT (ALT) levels. May decrease blood hemoglobin levels and WBC counts.

SIDE EFFECTS

Expected (98%)
Local injection site reactions (pain, discomfort, induration, erythema, nodules, cysts, pruritus, ecchymosis)
Frequent (26%–16%)
Diarrhea, nausea, fatigue.
Occasional (11%–4%)
Insomnia, peripheral neuropathy, depression, cough, weight or appetite decrease, sinusitis, anxiety, asthenia (loss of energy, strength), myalgia, cold sores.
Rare (3%–2%)
Constipation, influenza, upper abdominal pain, anorexia, conjunctivitis.

SERIOUS REACTIONS

! Enfuvirtide use may potentiate bacterial pneumonia development.
! Hypersensitivity (rash, fever, chills, rigors, hypotension), thrombocytopenia, neutropenia, and renal insufficiency or failure may occur rarely.

PEDIATRIC CONSIDERATIONS

Baseline Assessment

• Expect to obtain baseline laboratory testing, especially liver function tests and serum triglyceride levels, before beginning enfuvirtide therapy and at periodic intervals during therapy.
• Offer the patient/family emotional support.
• Breast-feeding is not recommended in this patient population because of the possibility of HIV transmission.
• Be aware that the safety and efficacy of enfuvirtide have not been established in children younger than 6 yrs of age.

Administration and Handling

• Store at room temperature. Refrigerate reconstituted solution; use within 24 hrs.
• Bring reconstituted solution to room temperature before injection.
• Reconstitute with 1.1 mL Sterile Water for Injection. Visually inspect vial for particulate matter. Solution normally appears clear, colorless. Discard unused portion.
• Administer subcutaneously into the upper abdomen, anterior thigh, or arm. Administer each injection at a different site than the preceding injection site.

Intervention and Evaluation

• Assess the patient's skin for hypersensitivity reaction and local injection site reaction.
• Observe the patient for evidence of fatigue or nausea.
• Evaluate the patient's sleep patterns.
• Monitor the patient for signs and symptoms of depression and insomnia.
• Monitor the patient's blood chemistry test results for marked abnormalities.

Patient/Family Teaching

• Warn the patient/family that an increased rate of bacterial pneumonia has occurred in pts taking enfuvirtide and to seek medical attention if cough with fever, rapid breathing, or shortness of breath occurs.
• Advise the patient/family to continue taking enfuvirtide for the full length of treatment.
• Instruct the patient/family that enfuvirtide is not a cure for HIV

infection nor does it reduce the risk of transmission to others. Explain to the patient/family that he or she still needs to continue practices to prevent transmission of HIV.

Lamivudine

lah-**mih**-view-deen
(Epivir, Epivir-HBV Heptovir [CAN], Zeffix [AUS])
Do not confuse with lamotrigine.

CATEGORY AND SCHEDULE

Pregnancy Risk Category: C

MECHANISM OF ACTION

An antiviral that inhibits HIV reverse transcriptase via viral DNA chain termination. Also inhibits RNA- and DNA-dependent DNA polymerase, an enzyme necessary for viral HIV and hepatitis B virus replication. ***Therapeutic Effect:*** Slows virus replication, reduces progression of viral infection.

PHARMACOKINETICS

Rapidly, completely absorbed from the GI tract. Protein binding: less than 36%. Widely distributed (crosses the blood-brain barrier). Primarily excreted unchanged in urine. Not removed by hemodialysis or peritoneal dialysis. ***Half-Life:*** 11–15 hrs (intracellular); serum (adults) 2–11 hrs, (children) 1.7–2 hrs. Half-life is increased with impaired renal function.

PHARMACOKINETICS

Tablets: 100 mg (Epivir-HBV), 150 mg (Epivir), 300 mg (Epivir).
Oral Solution: 5 mg/mL (Epivir-HBV), 10 mg/mL (Epivir).

INDICATIONS AND DOSAGES

▸ HIV infection

PO

Children 12–16 yrs, weighing less than 50 kg. 2 mg/kg/dose 2 times/day.
Children 12–16 yrs, weighing more than 50 kg. 150 mg 2 times/day or 300 mg once daily.
Children 3 mo-12 yrs. 4 mg/kg/dose 2 times/day. Maximum: 150 mg/dose.
Neonate (younger than 30 days). 2 mg/kg/dose 2 times/day.

▸ Chronic hepatitis B

PO

Children 17 yrs or older. 100 mg daily.
Children younger than 17 yrs. 3 mg/kg/day. Maximum: 100 mg/day.

▸ Dosage in renal impairment for HIV

Dosage and frequency are modified based on creatinine clearance.

Creatinine Clearance	Dosage
50 mL/min or greater	150 mg 2 times/day
30–49 mL/min	150 mg once daily
15–29 mL/min	150 mg first dose, then 100 mg once daily
5–14 mL/min	150 mg first dose, then 50 mg once daily
Less than 5 mL/min	50 mg first dose, then 25 mg once daily

▸ Dosage in renal impairment for chronic hepatitis B

Dosage and frequency are modified based on creatinine clearance.

Creatinine Clearance	Dosage
50 mL/min or greater	100 mg 2 times/day
30–49 mL/min	100 mg first dose, then 50 mg once daily
15–29 mL/min	100 mg first dose, then 25 mg once daily
5–14 mL/min	35 mg first dose, then 15 mg once daily
Less than 5 mL/min	35 mg first dose, then 10 mg once daily

UNLABELED USES

Prophylaxis in health care workers at risk of acquiring HIV after occupational exposure to virus.

CONTRAINDICATIONS

Hypersensitivity to lamivudine or any component.

INTERACTIONS

Drug

Trimethoprim-sulfamethoxazole: Increases lamivudine blood concentration.
Zalcitabine: Concurrent use is not recommended due to inactivation of both drugs.

Herbal

St. John's wort: May decrease lamivudine blood concentration and effect.

Food

None known.

DIAGNOSTIC TEST EFFECTS

May increase blood Hgb values, neutrophil count, and serum amylase, SGOT (AST), and SGPT (ALT) levels.

SIDE EFFECTS

Frequent

Headache (35%), nausea (33%), malaise and fatigue (27%), nasal disturbances (20%), diarrhea, cough (18%), musculoskeletal pain, neuropathy (12%), insomnia (11%), anorexia, dizziness, fever or chills (10%)

Occasional

Depression (9%); myalgia (8%); abdominal cramps (6%); dyspepsia, arthralgia (5%)

SERIOUS REACTIONS

! Pancreatitis occurs in 13% of pediatric pts.
! Anemia, neutropenia, and thrombocytopenia occur rarely.

PEDIATRIC CONSIDERATIONS

Baseline Assessment

• Before starting drug therapy, check the patient's baseline laboratory values, especially renal function.
• Be aware that lamivudine crosses the placenta and it is unknown whether lamivudine is distributed in breast milk. Breast-feeding is not recommended in this patient population because of the possibility of HIV transmission.
• Be aware that the safety and efficacy of this drug have not been established in children younger than 3 mos.
• Pts in early puberty (Tanner I–II stages) should be given pediatric dosages, and those in late puberty (Tanner V stage) should be given adult dosages.
• Adolescents in the middle of a growth spurt can be given pediatric or adult dosages with close monitoring.

Precautions

• Use cautiously in pts with impaired renal function, a history of pancreatitis, or a history of peripheral neuropathy.
• Use cautiously in young children.

Administration and Handling
PO
Give without regard to meals.

Intervention and Evaluation

- Expect to monitor the patient's serum amylase, BUN, and serum creatinine levels.
- Evaluate the patient for altered sleep patterns, cough, dizziness, headache, and nausea.
- Assess the patient's pattern of daily bowel activity and stool consistency.
- Modify the patient's diet or administer a laxative, if ordered, as needed.
- If pancreatitis occurs in a pediatric patient, help the patient to sit up or flex at the waist to relieve abdominal pain aggravated by movement.

Patient/Family Teaching

- Advise the patient/family to continue taking lamivudine for the full length of treatment and to evenly space drug doses around the clock.
- Explain to the patient/family that lamivudine is not a cure for HIV and that the patient may continue to experience illnesses, including opportunistic infections.
- Advise the parents of pediatric pts to closely monitor the patient for symptoms of pancreatitis, manifested as clammy skin, hypotension, nausea, severe and steady abdominal pain often radiating to the back, and vomiting accompanying abdominal pain.
- Warn the patient/family not to engage in activities that require mental acuity if the patient is experiencing dizziness.
- Teach the patient/family that GI discomforts usually subside after 3–4 wks of therapy.

Lopinavir/ritonavir

low-**pin**-ah-veer/rih-**ton**-ah-veer
(Kaletra)
Do not confuse with Keppra.

CATEGORY AND SCHEDULE

Pregnancy Risk Category: C

MECHANISM OF ACTION

A protease inhibitor combination. Lopinavir acts on protease enzyme late in the HIV replication process and inhibits its activity.
Therapeutic Effect: Formation of immature, noninfectious viral particles. Ritonavir inhibits the metabolism of lopinavir. Increases plasma concentrations of lopinavir.

PHARMACOKINETICS

Readily absorbed after PO administration (increased when taken with food). Protein binding: 98%–99%. Metabolized in liver. Primarily eliminated in feces. Not removed by hemodialysis.
Half-Life: 5–6 hrs.

AVAILABILITY

Capsules: 133.3 mg lopinavir/33.3 mg ritonavir.
Oral Solution: 80 mg lopinavir/20 mg ritonavir per mL.

INDICATIONS AND DOSAGES

▸ HIV infection
PO (DOSAGE BASED ON LOPINAVIR COMPONENT)
Children 6 mos and older receiving concomitant antiretroviral treatment without efavirenz or nevirapine:

- More than 40 kg: 400 mg 2 times/day
- 15–40 kg: 10 mg/kg 2 times/day

• 7–15 kg: 12 mg/kg 2 times/day
Children 6 mos and older receiving concomitant antiretroviral treatment with efavirenz or nevirapine:
• More than 45 kg: 533 mg 2 times/day
• 15–45 kg: 11 mg/kg 2 times/day
• 7–15 kg: 13 mg/kg 2 times/day

CONTRAINDICATIONS

Hypersensitivity to lopinavir or ritonavir; concomitant use of ergot derivatives (causes peripheral ischemia of extremities and vasospasm), flecainide, midazolam, pimozide, propafenone (increases the risk of serous cardiac arrhythmias), and triazolam (increases sedation or respiratory depression).

INTERACTIONS

Drug

Atorvastatin: May increase lopinavir/ritonavir blood concentration and risk of myopathy with this drug.
Atovaquone, methadone, oral contraceptives: May decrease blood concentration and effects of these drugs.
Carbamazepine, corticosteroids, efavirenz, nevirapine, phenobarbital, phenytoin, rifampin: May decrease lopinavir/ritonavir blood concentration and effect.
Clarithromycin, felodipine, immunosuppressants, nicardipine, nifedipine, rifabutin: May increase the blood concentration and effects of these drugs.

Herbal

St. John's wort: May decrease lopinavir/ritonavir blood concentration and effect.

Food

None known.

DIAGNOSTIC TEST EFFECTS

May increase blood glucose, γ-glutamyl transferase, serum uric acid, SGOT (AST), SGPT (ALT), total cholesterol, and triglyceride levels.

SIDE EFFECTS

Frequent (14%)
Diarrhea, mild to moderate severity
Occasional (6%–2%)
Nausea, asthenia (loss of strength, energy), abdominal pain, headache, vomiting
Rare (less than 2%)
Insomnia, rash

SERIOUS REACTIONS

! Anemia, leukopenia, lymphadenopathy, deep vein thrombosis, Cushing's syndrome, pancreatitis, and hemorrhagic colitis occur rarely.

PEDIATRIC CONSIDERATIONS

Baseline Assessment

• Expect to establish the patient's baseline values for complete blood count (CBC), renal and liver function tests, and weight.
• Be aware that it is unknown whether lopinavir/ritonavir is excreted in breast milk. Breastfeeding is not recommended in this patient population because of the possibility of HIV transmission.
• Be aware that the safety and efficacy of lopinavir/ritonavir have not been established in children younger than 6 mos.
• Pts in early puberty (Tanner I–II stages) should be given pediatric dosages, and those in late puberty (Tanner V stage) should be given adult dosages.
• Adolescents in the middle of a growth spurt can be given pediatric

or adult dosages with close monitoring.

Precautions

• Use cautiously in pts with hepatitis B or C or impaired liver function.

◂ **ALERT** ▸ High doses of itraconazole or ketoconazole are not recommended in pts taking lopinavir/ritonavir. Lopinavir/ritonavir oral solution contains alcohol and should not be given to pts receiving metronidazole because this combination may cause a disulfiram-type reaction.

Administration and Handling

PO

• Refrigerate until dispensed and avoid exposure to excessive heat.

• If stored at room temperature, use within 2 mos.

• Give all doses with food.

Intervention and Evaluation

• Assess the patient's pattern of daily bowel activity and stool consistency.

• Evaluate the patient for signs and symptoms of opportunistic infections as evidenced by cough, onset of fever, oral mucosa changes, or other respiratory symptoms.

• Check the patient's weight at least twice a week.

• Evaluate the patient for nausea and vomiting.

• Monitor the patient for signs and symptoms of pancreatitis as evidenced by abdominal pain, nausea, and vomiting.

• Monitor the patient's blood glucose, CBC with differential, CD4 cell count, serum cholesterol level, HIV RNA levels (viral load), serum electrolytes, and liver function tests.

Patient/Family Teaching

• Teach the patient/family how to properly take the medication.

• Encourage the patient/family to eat small, frequent meals to offset nausea or vomiting.

• Explain to the patient/family that lopinavir/ritonavir is not a cure for HIV infection nor does it reduce risk of transmission to others.

Nelfinavir

nell-**fine**-ah-veer

(Viracept)

CATEGORY AND SCHEDULE

Pregnancy Risk Category: B

MECHANISM OF ACTION

Inhibits the activity of HIV-1 protease, the enzyme necessary for the formation of infectious HIV. ***Therapeutic Effect:*** Formation of immature noninfectious viral particles rather than HIV replication.

PHARMACOKINETICS

Well absorbed after PO administration. Protein binding: greater than 98%. Absorption increased with food. Metabolized by the liver. Highly bound to plasma proteins. Eliminated primarily in feces. Unknown whether removed by hemodialysis. ***Half-Life:*** 3.5–5 hrs.

AVAILABILITY

Tablets: 250 mg, 625 mg.
Powder: 50 mg/g.

INDICATIONS AND DOSAGES

▸ **HIV infection**

PO

Adolescents. 750 mg (three 250-mg tablets) 3 times/day, or 1,250 mg 2 times/day in combination with

nucleoside analogues (enhances antiviral activity).
Children 2–13 yrs. 20–30 mg/kg/dose, 3 times/day. Maximum: 750 mg q8h.

CONTRAINDICATIONS

Concurrent administration with lovastatin, simvastatin, midazolam, rifampin, or triazolam. Hypersensitivity to nelfinavir or any component.

INTERACTIONS

Drug

Alcohol, psychoactive drugs: May produce additive CNS effects
Anticonvulsants, rifabutin, rifampin: Lower nelfinavir plasma concentration (concurrent use of rifampin and nelfinavir are not recommended: Reduce rifabutin dose by 50% if used with nelfinavir).
Indinavir, saquinavir: Increases plasma concentration of these drugs.
Oral contraceptives: Decreases the effects of these drugs.
Ritonavir: Increases nelfinavir plasma concentration.
Phenobarbital, phenytoin, carbamazepine: Decreases nelfinavir concentrations.

Herbal

St. John's wort: May decrease nelfinavir plasma concentration and effect.

Food

Increases nelfinavir plasma concentration.
Avoid administration with acidic food or juice—increases bitter taste of medication.

DIAGNOSTIC TEST EFFECTS

May decrease Hgb values, neutrophils, and WBCs. May increase serum creatine kinase, SGOT (AST), and SGPT (ALT) levels.

SIDE EFFECTS

Frequent (20%)
Diarrhea
Occasional (7%–3%)
Nausea, rash
Rare (2%–1%)
Flatulence, asthenia

SERIOUS REACTIONS

None known.

PEDIATRIC CONSIDERATIONS

Baseline Assessment

- Expect to check the patient's hematology and liver function tests to establish an accurate baseline before beginning drug therapy.
- Be aware that it is unknown whether nelfinavir is distributed in breast milk.
- There are no age-related precautions noted in children over 2 yrs old.
- Pts in early puberty (Tanner I–II stages) should be given pediatric dosages, and those in late puberty (Tanner V stage) should be given adult dosages.
- Adolescents in the middle of a growth spurt can be given pediatric or adult dosages with close monitoring.

Precautions

- Use cautiously in pts with liver function impairment.

Administration and Handling

PO

- Give with food, a light meal, or snack.
- Mix oral powder with a small amount of dietary supplement, formula, milk, soy formula, soy milk, or water. The entire contents must be consumed to ingest a full dose.

• Do not mix with acidic food such as apple juice, applesauce, or orange juice or with water in its original container.

Intervention and Evaluation

• Assess the patient's pattern of daily bowel activity and stool consistency.

• Monitor the patient's liver enzyme studies for abnormalities.

◀ **ALERT** ▶ Monitor the patient for signs and symptoms of opportunistic infections as evidenced by chills, cough, fever, and myalgia.

Patient/Family Teaching

• Instruct the patient/family to take nelfinavir with food to optimize the drug's absorption.

• Advise the patient/family to take the medication every day as prescribed and to evenly space drug doses around the clock.

• Caution the patient/family not to alter the dose or discontinue the medication without first notifying the physician.

• Explain to the patient/family that this medication is not a cure for HIV infection nor does it reduce the risk of transmitting HIV to others, and that the patient may continue to experience illnesses associated with advanced HIV infection, including opportunistic infections.

• Explain to the patient/family that noncompliance can result in resistant HIV strains.

Nevirapine

neh-vear-ah-peen

(Viramune)

CATEGORY AND SCHEDULE

Pregnancy Risk Category: C

MECHANISM OF ACTION

A nonnucleoside reverse transcriptase inhibitor that binds directly to HIV-1 reverse transcriptase (RT), blocking RNA and DNA-dependent DNA polymerase activity by changing the shape of the RT enzyme. ***Therapeutic Effect:*** Slows HIV replication, reducing progression of HIV infection.

PHARMACOKINETICS

Readily absorbed after PO administration. Protein binding: 60%. Widely distributed. Extensively metabolized in liver; primarily excreted in urine. ***Half-Life:*** 45 hrs (single dose); 25–30 hrs (multiple doses).

AVAILABILITY

Tablets: 200 mg.
Oral Suspension: 50 mg/5 mL.

INDICATIONS AND DOSAGES

▶ **HIV infection**

PO

Children older than 8 yrs. 4 mg/kg once daily for 14 days; then 4 mg/kg 2 times/day. Maximum: 400 mg/day.

Children 2 mos–8 yrs. 4 mg/kg once daily for 14 days; then 7 mg/kg 2 times/day. Maximum: 400 mg/day.

UNLABELED USES

Reduces the risk of transmitting HIV from infected mother to newborn.

CONTRAINDICATIONS

None known.

INTERACTIONS

Drug

Ketoconazole, oral contraceptives, protease inhibitors: May decrease

the plasma concentrations of these drugs.
Rifabutin, rifampin: May decrease nevirapine blood concentration.
Herbal
St. John's wort: May decrease nevirapine blood concentration and effects.
Food
None known.

DIAGNOSTIC TEST EFFECTS

May significantly increase serum bilirubin, GGT, SGOT (AST), and SGPT (ALT) levels. May significantly decrease Hgb level and neutrophil and platelet count.

SIDE EFFECTS

Frequent (8%–3%)
Rash, fever, headache, nausea
Occasional (3%–1%)
Stomatitis, a burning or erythema of the oral mucosa, mucosal ulceration, dysphagia
Rare (less than 1%)
Paresthesia, myalgia, abdominal pain

SERIOUS REACTIONS

! The rash may become severe and life-threatening.
! Hepatitis occurs rarely.

PEDIATRIC CONSIDERATIONS

Baseline Assessment
• Check the patient's baseline diagnostic test results and laboratory values, especially liver function tests, before starting therapy and at intervals during therapy.
• Obtain the patient's medication history, especially regarding the use of oral contraceptives.
• Be aware that nevirapine crosses the placenta and is distributed in breast milk. Breast-feeding is not recommended in this patient population because of the possibility of HIV transmission.
• Granulocytopenia occurs more frequently in children.
• Pts in early puberty (Tanner I–II stages) should be given pediatric dosages and those in late puberty (Tanner V stage) should be given adult dosages.
• Adolescents in the middle of a growth spurt can be given pediatric or adult dosages with close monitoring.
Precautions
• Use cautiously in pts with elevated SGOT (AST) or SGPT (ALT) levels, a history of chronic hepatitis (B or C), or renal or liver dysfunction.
Administration and Handling
◀ **ALERT** ▶ Be aware that nevirapine is always prescribed in combination with at least one additional antiretroviral agent because a resistant HIV virus appears rapidly when nevirapine is given as monotherapy.
PO
• Give without regard to meals.
Intervention and Evaluation
• Closely monitor the patient for evidence of rash, which usually appears on the extremities, face, or trunk, within the first 6 wks of drug therapy.
• Evaluate the patient for rash accompanied by blistering, conjunctivitis, fever, general malaise, muscle or joint aches, oral lesions, and swelling.
Patient/Family Teaching
• Instruct the patient/family that if nevirapine therapy is missed for more than 7 days, to restart therapy by using one 200-mg tablet each day for the first 14 days, followed by one 200-mg tablet 2 times/day.

• Instruct the patient/family that noncompliance can result in resistant HIV strains.
• Advise the patient/family to continue nevirapine therapy for the full length of treatment and to evenly space drug doses around the clock.
• Explain to the patient/family that nevirapine is not a cure for HIV infection nor does it reduce the risk of transmission to others.
• Warn the patient/family to notify the physician before continuing therapy if the patient experiences a rash.

Ritonavir

rih-tone-ah-vir
(Norvir)
Do not confuse with Retrovir.

CATEGORY AND SCHEDULE

Pregnancy Risk Category: B

MECHANISM OF ACTION

Inhibits HIV-1 and HIV-2 proteases, rendering the enzymes incapable of processing the polypeptide precursor that leads to production of immature HIV particles. ***Therapeutic Effect:*** Slows HIV replication, reducing progression of HIV infection.

PHARMACOKINETICS

Well absorbed after PO administration (extent of absorption increased with food). Protein binding: 98%–99%. Extensively metabolized by liver to active and inactive metabolites. Primarily eliminated in feces. Unknown whether removed by hemodialysis. ***Half-Life:*** 2.7–5 hrs.

AVAILABILITY

Soft Gelatin Capsules:
100 mg (contains alcohol and castor oil).
Oral Solution: 80 mg/mL (contains alcohol, castor oil and propylene glycol).

INDICATIONS AND DOSAGES

▸ HIV infection

PO

Children 12 yrs or older: Begin at 300 mg/dose 2 times/day. If nausea becomes apparent, increase by 100 mg up to 600 mg/dose 2 times/day over 5 days as tolerated.

Children younger than 12 yrs. Initially, 250 mg/m^2/dose 2 times/day. Increase by 50 mg/m^2/dose up to 400 mg/m^2/dose. Maximum: 600 mg/dose 2 times/day.

CONTRAINDICATIONS

Hypersensitivity to ritonavir or any component.
Breast-feeding is contraindicated while taking ritonavir.
Because of the potential for serious or life-threatening drug interactions, the following medications should not be given concomitantly with ritonavir: amiodarone, astemizole, bepridil, bupropion, cisapride, clozapine, encainide, flecainide, meperidine, piroxicam, propafenone, propoxyphene, quinidine, rifabutin, terfenadine (increases risk of arrhythmias, hematologic abnormalities, seizures). Alprazolam, clorazepate, diazepam, estazolam, flurazepam, midazolam, triazolam, and zolpidem may produce extreme sedation and respiratory depression.

INTERACTIONS

Drug

Desipramine, fluoxetine, other antidepressants: May increase the blood concentration of these drugs.
Disulfiram or drugs causing disulfiram-like reaction, such as metronidazole: May produce disulfiram-like reaction if taken with these drugs.
Enzyme inducers, including carbamazepine, dexamethasone, nevirapine, phenobarbital, phenytoin, rifabutin, rifampin: May increase ritonavir metabolism and decrease the efficacy of ritonavir.
Oral contraceptives, theophylline: May decrease the effectiveness of these drugs.

Herbal

St. John's wort: May decrease ritonavir blood concentration and effect.

Food

None known.

DIAGNOSTIC TEST EFFECTS

May alter serum creatinine phosphokinase, GGT, triglyceride, uric acid, SGOT (AST), and SGPT (ALT) levels and creatinine clearance.

SIDE EFFECTS

Frequent

GI disturbances (abdominal pain, anorexia, diarrhea, nausea, and vomiting), neurologic disturbances (circumoral and peripheral paresthesias, especially around the feet, hands, or lips, change in sense of taste), headache, dizziness, fatigue, weakness

Occasional

Allergic reaction, flu syndrome, hypotension

SERIOUS REACTIONS

None known.

PEDIATRIC CONSIDERATIONS

Baseline Assessment

- Pts beginning combination therapy with ritonavir and nucleosides may promote GI tolerance by first beginning ritonavir alone and then by adding nucleosides before completing 2 wks of ritonavir monotherapy.
- Check the patient's baseline laboratory test results, if ordered, especially liver function tests and serum triglycerides, before beginning ritonavir therapy and at periodic intervals during therapy.
- Offer the patient/family emotional support.
- Be aware that breast-feeding is not recommended in this patient population because of the possibility of HIV transmission.
- There are no age-related precautions noted in children older than 2 yrs.
- Pts in early puberty (Tanner I–II stages) should be given pediatric dosages, and those in late puberty (Tanner V stage) should be given adult dosages.
- Adolescents in the middle of a growth spurt can be given pediatric or adult dosages with close monitoring.

Precautions

- Use cautiously in pts with impaired hepatic function.

Administration and Handling

PO

- Store capsules or solution in the refrigerator.
- Protect the drug from light.
- Refrigerate the oral solution unless it is used within 30 days and stored below 77°F.
- May give without regard to meals, but preferably give with food.
- May improve the taste of the oral solution by mixing it with

Advera, chocolate milk, or Ensure within 1 hr of dosing.

Intervention and Evaluation

• Closely monitor the patient for signs and symptoms of GI disturbances or neurologic abnormalities, particularly paresthesias.
• Monitor the patient's blood glucose level, CD4 cell count, liver function tests, and plasma levels of HIV RNA.

Patient/Family Teaching

• Advise the patient/family to continue therapy for the full length of treatment and to evenly space drug doses around the clock.
• Explain to the patient/family that ritonavir is not a cure for HIV infection nor does it reduce risk of transmission to others. Also explain that the patient may continue to develop illnesses associated with advanced HIV infection.
• Instruct the patient/family that, if possible, the patient should take ritonavir with food.
• Suggest to the patient/family that the patient mask the taste of the solution by mixing it with Advera, chocolate milk, or Ensure.
• Warn the patient/family to notify the physician if the patient experiences abdominal pain, frequent urination, increased thirst, nausea, or vomiting.
• Instruct the patient/family that noncompliance can result in resistant HIV strains.

Saquinavir

sah-quin-ah-vir
(Fortovase, Invirase)
Do not confuse with Sinequan.

CATEGORY AND SCHEDULE

Pregnancy Risk Category: B

MECHANISM OF ACTION

Inhibits HIV protease, rendering the enzyme incapable of processing the polyprotein precursor to generate functional proteins in HIV-infected cells. ***Therapeutic Effect:*** Slows HIV replication, reducing progression of HIV infection.

PHARMACOKINETICS

Poorly absorbed after PO administration (high-calorie and high-fat meal increases absorption). Protein binding: 99%. Metabolized in liver to inactive metabolite. Primarily eliminated in feces. Unknown whether removed by hemodialysis. ***Half-Life:*** 13 hrs in adults.

AVAILABILITY

Capsules (Invirase): 200 mg.
Capsules (gelatin) (Fortovase): 200 mg.

INDICATIONS AND DOSAGES

▸ HIV infection in combination with other antiretroviral agents

PO

Adolescents 16 yrs and older. Fortovase: 1,200 mg 3 times/day. Invirase: Three 200-mg capsules given 3 times/day within 2 hrs after a full meal. Do not give less than 600 mg/day (does not produce antiviral activity). Recommended daily doses of other antiretroviral agents are zalcitabine (ddC) 0.75 mg 3 times/day or zidovudine (AZT) 200 mg 3 times/day.

CONTRAINDICATIONS

Clinically significant hypersensitivity to drug; concurrent use with ergot medications, lovastatin, midazolam, simvastatin, and triazolam.

INTERACTIONS

Drug

Calcium channel blockers, clindamycin, dapsone, quinidine, triazolam: May increase the plasma concentrations of these drugs.
Carbamazepine, dexamethasone, phenobarbital, phenytoin, rifampin: May reduce saquinavir plasma concentration.
Ketoconazole: Increases saquinavir plasma concentration.

Herbal

Garlic, St. John's wort: May decrease saquinavir plasma concentration and effect.

Food

Grapefruit juice: May increase saquinavir plasma concentration.

DIAGNOSTIC TEST EFFECTS

May alter serum creatinine phosphokinase levels, elevate serum transaminase levels, and lower blood glucose levels.

SIDE EFFECTS

Occasional

Diarrhea, abdominal discomfort and pain, nausea, photosensitivity, buccal mucosa ulceration

Rare

Confusion, ataxia, weakness, headache, rash

SERIOUS REACTIONS

None known.

PEDIATRIC CONSIDERATIONS

Baseline Assessment

• Check the patient's baseline laboratory and diagnostic test results, especially liver function test results, if ordered, before beginning saquinavir therapy and at periodic intervals during therapy.
• Offer emotional support to the patient and family.
• Expect to obtain the patient's medication history.
• Breast-feeding is not recommended in this patient population because of the possibility of HIV transmission.
• Be aware that the safety and efficacy of saquinavir have not been established in children.

Precautions

• Use cautiously in pts with diabetes mellitus or liver impairment.

Administration and Handling

PO
• Give within 2 hrs after a full meal. Keep in mind that if saquinavir is taken on an empty stomach, the drug may not produce antiviral activity.

Intervention and Evaluation

• Monitor the patient's liver function test results, CD4 cell count, blood glucose, HIV RNA levels, and serum triglyceride levels.
• Closely monitor the patient for signs and symptoms of GI discomfort.
• Assess the patient's pattern of daily bowel activity and stool consistency.
• Inspect the patient's mouth for signs of mucosal ulceration.
• Monitor the patient's blood chemistry test results for marked abnormalities.
• If serious or severe toxicities occur, withhold the drug and notify the physician.
• Fortovase and Invirase are not bioequivalent products and should not be interchanged.

Patient/Family Teaching

• Warn the patient/family to notify the physician if the patient experiences nausea, numbness, persistent abdominal pain, tingling, or vomiting.

• Encourage the patient/family to avoid exposure to artificial light sources and sunlight.
• Advise the patient/family to continue therapy for the full length of treatment and to evenly space drug doses around the clock.
• Explain to the patient/family that saquinavir is not a cure for HIV infection nor does it reduce the risk of transmission to others. Also explain that the patient may continue to develop illnesses associated with advanced HIV infection.
• Instruct the patient/family to take saquinavir within 2 hrs after a full meal.
• Warn the patient/family to avoid grapefruit products while taking saquinavir.
• Pts in early puberty (Tanner I–II stages) should be given pediatric dosages, and those in late puberty (Tanner V stage) should be given adult dosages.
• Adolescents in the middle of a growth spurt can be given pediatric or adult dosages with close monitoring.

Stavudine (d4T)

stay-view-deen
(Zerit)

CATEGORY AND SCHEDULE

Pregnancy Risk Category: C

MECHANISM OF ACTION

Inhibits HIV reverse transcriptase via viral DNA chain termination. Also inhibits RNA- and DNA-dependent DNA polymerase, an enzyme necessary for viral HIV replication. ***Therapeutic Effect:*** Slows HIV replication, reducing progression of HIV infection.

PHARMACOKINETICS

Rapidly, completely absorbed after PO administration. Undergoes minimal metabolism. Excreted unchanged in urine. ***Half-Life:*** 1–1.5 hrs (half-life is increased with impaired renal function).

AVAILABILITY

Capsules: 15 mg, 20 mg, 30 mg, 40 mg.
Oral Solution: 1 mg/mL.

INDICATIONS AND DOSAGES

▸ HIV infection

PO
Children weighing more than 60 kg: 40 mg 2 times/day.
Children weighing 30–60 kg: 30 mg 2 times/day.
Children weighing less than 30 kg: 1 mg/kg/dose every 12 hrs.
Newborns birth to 13 days of age: 0.5 mg/kg/dose every 12 hrs.

▸ Dosage in renal impairment

Dosage and frequency are modified based on creatinine clearance and patient weight.

Creatinine Clearance (mL/min)	Weight 60 kg or more	Weight less than 60 kg
Greater than 50	40 mg q12h	30 mg q12h
26–50	20 mg q12h	15 mg q12h
10–25	20 mg q24h	15 mg q24h

CONTRAINDICATIONS

Hypersensitivity to stavudine or any component.

INTERACTIONS

Drug

Drugs associated with peripheral neuropathy (chloramphenicol,

cisplatin, dapsone, ethionamide, gold, hydralazine, isoniazid, lithium, metronidazole, nitrofurantoin, pentamidine, phenytoin, ribavirin, vincristine): May increase risk of stavudine peripheral neuropathy.
Zidovudine: Decreases antiretroviral effect.
Didanosine and hydroxyurea: May increase risk of pancreatitis, lactic acidosis, and hepatomegaly.
Methadone: May decrease stavudine serum concentrations.
Herbal
None known.
Food
None known.

DIAGNOSTIC TEST EFFECTS

Commonly increases SGOT (AST) and SGPT (ALT) levels. May decrease blood neutrophil count.

SIDE EFFECTS

Frequent
Headache (55%), diarrhea (50%), chills and fever (38%), nausea or vomiting, myalgia (35%), rash (33%), asthenia (loss of strength, energy) (28%), insomnia, abdominal pain (26%), anxiety (22%), arthralgia (18%), back pain (20%), sweating (19%), malaise (17%), depression (14%)
Occasional
Anorexia, weight loss, nervousness, dizziness, conjunctivitis, dyspepsia, dyspnea
Rare
Constipation, vasodilation, confusion, migraine, urticaria, abnormal vision

SERIOUS REACTIONS

! Peripheral neuropathy, characterized by numbness, tingling, or pain in the hands and feet occurs frequently (15%–21%).
! Ulcerative stomatitis (erythema or ulcers of oral mucosa, glossitis, and gingivitis), pneumonia, and benign skin neoplasms occur occasionally.
! Pancreatitis and lactic acidosis occur rarely.

PEDIATRIC CONSIDERATIONS

Baseline Assessment
- Check patient's baseline laboratory test results, if ordered, especially liver function and renal function test results, before beginning stavudine therapy and at periodic intervals during therapy.
- Offer the patient/family emotional support.
- Determine the patient's history of peripheral neuropathy.
- Breast-feeding is not recommended in this patient population because of the possibility of HIV transmission.
- There are no age-related precautions noted in children.
- Pts in early puberty (Tanner I–II stages) should be given pediatric dosages, and those in late puberty (Tanner V stage) should be given adult dosages.
- Adolescents in the middle of a growth spurt can be given pediatric or adult dosages with close monitoring.

Precautions
- Use cautiously in pts with a history of peripheral neuropathy or liver or renal impairment.

Administration and Handling
PO
- Give without regard to meals.

Intervention and Evaluation
- Monitor the patient for signs and symptoms of peripheral neuropathy, which is characterized by numbness, pain, or tingling in the feet or hands. Be aware that

peripheral neuropathy symptoms resolve promptly if stavudine therapy is discontinued. Also, know that symptoms may worsen temporarily after the drug is withdrawn. If symptoms resolve completely, expect to resume drug therapy at a reduced dosage.
• Assess the patient for dizziness, headache, muscle or joint aches, myalgia, nausea, and vomiting.
• Monitor the patient for evidence of a rash and signs of chills or a fever.
• Determine the patient's pattern of daily bowel activity and stool consistency.
• Assess the patient for a change in sleep pattern.
• Assess the patient's eating pattern and monitor the patient for weight loss.
• Examine the patient's eyes for signs of conjunctivitis.
• Monitor the patient's CD4 cell count, complete blood count, Hgb, and HIV RNA levels and renal and liver function test results.

Patient/Family Teaching

• Advise the patient/family to continue stavudine therapy for the full length of treatment and to space doses evenly around the clock.
• Caution the patient/family not to take any medications, including OTC drugs, without first notifying the physician.
• Explain to the patient/family that stavudine is not a cure for HIV infection nor does it reduce risk of transmission to others and that the patient may continue to develop illnesses, including opportunistic infections.
• Warn the patient/family to report abdominal discomfort, burning, dyspnea, fatigue, nausea, numbness, pain, tingling, vomiting, and weakness to the physician.

Zalcitabine

zal-**site**-ah-bean
(Hivid)

CATEGORY AND SCHEDULE

Pregnancy Risk Category: C

MECHANISM OF ACTION

A nucleoside reverse transcriptase inhibitor that is intracellularly converted to active metabolite. Inhibits viral DNA synthesis. ***Therapeutic Effect:*** Prevents replication of HIV-1.

PHARMACOKINETICS

Readily absorbed from the GI tract. Food decreases the drug's absorption. Protein binding: less than 4%. Undergoes phosphorylation intracellularly to the active metabolite. Primarily excreted in urine. Removed 50% by hemodialysis. ***Half-Life:*** 1–3 hrs; metabolite: 2.6–10 hrs (half-life is increased with impaired renal function).

AVAILABILITY

Tablets: 0.375 mg, 0.75 mg.

INDICATIONS AND DOSAGES

▸ **HIV infection**

PO

Children 13 yrs and older. 0.75 mg q8h (may be given with zidovudine).
Children younger than 13 yrs. 0.01 mg/kg q8h. Range: 0.005–0.01 mg/kg q8h.

▸ **Dosage in renal impairment**

Based on creatinine clearance.

Creatinine Clearance	Dose
10–40 mL/min	0.75 mg q12h
less than 10 mL/min	0.75 mg q24h

CONTRAINDICATIONS

Pts with moderate or severe peripheral neuropathy.
Pts with hypersensitivity to zalcitabine or any component.

INTERACTIONS

Drug

Medications associated with peripheral neuropathy, including cisplatin, disulfiram, metronidazole, phenytoin, vincristine: May increase the risk of neuropathy.
Medications causing pancreatitis, including IV pentamidine: May increase the risk of pancreatitis.
Didanosine: May increase risk of peripheral neuropathy.

Herbal

None known.

Food

Food decreases absorption of zalcitabine.

DIAGNOSTIC TEST EFFECTS

May increase serum alkaline phosphatase, amylase, bilirubin, lipase, SGOT (AST), SGPT (ALT), and triglyceride levels. May decrease serum calcium, magnesium, and phosphate levels. May alter blood glucose and sodium levels.

SIDE EFFECTS

Frequent (28%–11%)
Peripheral neuropathy, fever, fatigue, headache, rash
Occasional (10%–5%)
Diarrhea, abdominal pain, oral ulcers, cough, pruritus, myalgia, weight loss, nausea, vomiting
Rare (4%–1%)
Fatigue, nasal discharge, dysphagia, depression, night sweats, confusion

SERIOUS REACTIONS

! Peripheral neuropathy occurs commonly (17%–31%) and is characterized by numbness, tingling, burning, and pain of the lower extremities. This situation may be followed by sharp, shooting pain which progresses to a severe, continuous, burning pain that may be irreversible if the drug is not discontinued in time.
! Pancreatitis, leukopenia, neutropenia, eosinophilia, and thrombocytopenia occur rarely.

PEDIATRIC CONSIDERATIONS

Baseline Assessment

- Offer emotional support to the patient and the patient's family.
- Expect to monitor the patient's complete blood count (CBC), serum amylase, and serum triglyceride levels before and during therapy.
- Be aware that it is unknown whether zalcitabine crosses the placenta or is distributed in breast milk. Breast-feeding is not recommended in this patient population because of the possibility of HIV transmission.
- There are no age-related precautions in children younger than 6 mos.
- In children, dosages are not established.
- Pts in early puberty (Tanner I–II stages) should be given pediatric dosages, and those in late puberty (Tanner V stage) should be given adult dosages.
- Adolescents in the middle of a growth spurt can be given pediatric

or adult dosages with close monitoring.

◀ **ALERT** ▶ Use extremely cautiously in pts with preexisting neuropathy and low CD4 cell counts because of an increased risk of development of peripheral neuropathy. Use cautiously in pts with a history of alcohol abuse, diabetes, liver disease, peripheral neuropathy, renal impairment, or weight loss.

Administration and Handling

PO

- Zalcitabine is best taken on an empty stomach because food decreases drug absorption.
- May take with food to decrease GI distress.
- Space doses evenly around the clock.

Intervention and Evaluation

- Withhold the drug and notify the physician immediately if signs and symptoms of peripheral neuropathy develop, including burning, numbness, or shooting or tingling pains of the extremities and loss of the ankle reflex or vibratory sense.

◀ **ALERT** ▶ Although rare, assess the patient for impending, potentially fatal pancreatitis as evidenced by abdominal pain, increasing serum amylase levels, nausea, rising triglyceride levels, and vomiting. If the patient develops any of these signs or symptoms, particularly abdominal pain, withhold the drug and immediately notify the physician.

- Assess the patient for signs and symptoms of a therapeutic response to drug therapy, including decreased fatigue, increased energy, and weight gain.
- Evaluate the patient's CBC for evidence of blood dyscrasias.

Patient/Family Teaching

- Explain to the patient/family that zalcitabine is not a cure for HIV nor does it reduce transmission of the disease and that the patient may continue to contract opportunistic illnesses associated with advanced HIV infection.
- Warn the patient/family to notify the physician if the patient experiences any signs or symptoms of pancreatitis or peripheral neuropathy.
- Caution women of childbearing age to avoid pregnancy. Teach female pts of childbearing age about contraception use.

Zidovudine

zye-**dough**-view-deen

(Apo-Zidovudine [CAN], AZT, Novo-AZT [CAN], Retrovir)

Do not confuse with Combivent or ritonavir.

CATEGORY AND SCHEDULE

Pregnancy Risk Category: C

MECHANISM OF ACTION

A nucleoside reverse transcriptase inhibitor that interferes with viral RNA-dependent DNA polymerase, an enzyme necessary for viral HIV replication. ***Therapeutic Effect:*** Slows HIV replication, reducing progression of HIV infection.

PHARMACOKINETICS

Rapidly, well absorbed from the GI tract. Protein binding: 25%–38%. Undergoes first-pass metabolism in liver to inactive metabolites. Widely distributed. Crosses blood-brain barrier, cerebrospinal fluid. Primarily excreted in urine. Minimal removal by hemodialysis. ***Half-Life:***

0.8–1.2 hrs (half-life is increased with impaired renal function and may be prolonged in premature infants and neonates).

AVAILABILITY

Capsules: 100 mg.
Tablets: 300 mg.
Syrup: 50 mg/5 mL.
Injection: 10 mg/mL.

INDICATIONS AND DOSAGES

▸ HIV infection

IV

Children older than 12 yrs.
1–2 mg/kg/dose q4h.
Children 12 yrs and younger.
120 mg/m²/dose q6h.
Neonates.
1.5 mg/kg/dose q6h.

PO

Children older than 12 yrs.
200 mg q8h or 300 mg q12h.
Children 12 yrs and younger.
160 mg/m²/dose q8h. Range: 90–180 mg/m²/dose q6–8h.
Neonates.
2 mg/kg/dose q6h.

UNLABELED USES

Prophylaxis in pts at risk of acquiring HIV after occupational exposure.

CONTRAINDICATIONS

Life-threatening allergies to zidovudine or components of preparation.

INTERACTIONS

Drug

Bone marrow depressants, ganciclovir: May increase myelosuppression.
Flucytosine, pentamidine, sulfamethoxazole, trimethoprim: May increase hematologic side effects.
Clarithromycin: May decrease zidovudine blood concentration.
Acetaminophen, atovaquone, methadone, valproic acid, cimetidine, indomethacin, lorazepam, fluconazole, probenecid: May increase zidovudine blood concentration and the risk of zidovudine toxicity.

Herbal

None known.

Food

Folate or vitamin B_{12} deficiency may increase zidovudine-associated myelosuppression.

DIAGNOSTIC TEST EFFECTS

May increase mean corpuscular volume.

IV INCOMPATIBILITIES

None known.

IV COMPATIBILITIES

Dexamethasone (Decadron), dobutamine (Dobutrex), dopamine (Intropin), heparin, lorazepam (Ativan), morphine, potassium chloride

SIDE EFFECTS

Expected (46%–42%)
Nausea, headache
Frequent (20%–16%)
GI pain, asthenia (loss of energy, strength), rash, fever
Occasional (12%–8%)
Diarrhea, anorexia, malaise, myalgia, somnolence
Rare (6%–5%)
Dizziness, paresthesia, vomiting, insomnia, dyspnea, altered taste

SERIOUS REACTIONS

! Anemia, occurring most commonly after 4–6 weeks of therapy, and granulocytopenia, particularly significant in those who have low levels before therapy begins, occur rarely.

! Neurotoxicity as evidenced by ataxia, fatigue, lethargy, and nystagmus, as well as seizures, may occur.

PEDIATRIC CONSIDERATIONS

Baseline Assessment

• Be aware that the patient should not receive drugs that are cytotoxic, myelosuppressive, or nephrotoxic, because these drugs may increase the risk of zidovudine toxicity.
• Expect to obtain patient specimens for viral diagnostic tests before starting therapy. Therapy may begin before results are obtained.
• Check the patient's hematology reports to establish an accurate baseline.
• Dosages may differ depending on protocol implemented.
• Be aware that it is unknown whether zidovudine crosses the placenta or is distributed in breast milk.
• Be aware that it is unknown whether fetal harm or effects on fertility can occur from use of this drug.
• There are no age-related precautions noted in children.
• Pts in early puberty (Tanner I–II stages) should be given pediatric dosages, and those in late puberty (Tanner V stage) should be given adult dosages.
• Adolescents in the middle of a growth spurt can be given pediatric or adult dosages with close monitoring.

Precautions

• Use cautiously in pts with bone marrow compromise, decreased liver blood flow, and renal and liver dysfunction.

Administration and Handling

PO

• Keep capsules in a cool, dry place. Protect from light.
• Food or milk does not affect GI absorption of zidovudine.
• Space doses evenly around the clock.
• The patient should be in an upright position when taking the medication to prevent esophageal ulceration.

IV

• After dilution, IV solution is stable for 24 hrs at room temperature; 48 hrs if refrigerated.
• Use within 8 hrs if stored at room temperature; 24 hrs if refrigerated.
• Do not use if particulate matter is present or discoloration occurs.
• Must dilute before administration. Remove calculated dose from vial and add to D_5W to provide a concentration no greater than 4 mg/mL.
• Infuse over 1 hr.
• Do not administer IM.

Intervention and Evaluation

• Monitor the patient's CD4 cell count, complete blood count, Hgb levels, HIV RNA plasma levels, mean corpuscular volume, and reticulocyte count.
• Assess the patient for bleeding, dizziness, headache, and insomnia.
• Assess the patient's pattern of daily bowel activity and stool consistency.
• Evaluate the patient's skin for acne or rash.
• Assess the patient for signs and symptoms of opportunistic infections, such as chills, cough, fever, and myalgia.

• Monitor the patient's intake and output, as well as his or her renal and liver function test results.

Patient/Family Teaching

• Advise the patient/family that zidovudine doses should be evenly spaced around the clock and that blood tests are an essential part of therapy because of the potential for bleeding.
• Explain to the patient/family that zidovudine does not cure HIV or AIDS but acts to reduce symptoms and slow or arrest disease progression.
• Caution the patient/family not to take any medications without the physician's prior approval.
• Warn the patient/family to report bleeding from gums, nose, or rectum to the physician immediately.
• Suggest to the patient/family that dental work be done before therapy or after blood counts return to normal, which is often weeks after therapy has stopped.
• Warn the patient/family to notify the physician if the patient experiences difficulty breathing, headache, inability to sleep, muscle weakness, rash, signs of infection, or unusual bleeding.

REFERENCES

Gunn, V. L. & Nechyba, C. (2002). The Harriet Lane handbook (16th ed.). St. Louis: Mosby.

Ethambutol
Isoniazid
Pyrazinamide
Rifabutin
Rifampin

Uses: Antitubercular agents are used to treat tuberculosis, an infectious disease usually caused by *Mycobacterium tuberculosis* or *Mycobacterium bovis*. Treatment, which aims to eliminate symptoms and prevent relapse, typically consists of combination drug therapy. By using more than one drug, the risk of drug resistance is minimized. Treatment may require three or more drugs and may continue for 6–24 mos.

Action: First-line agents act in different ways, combining the greatest efficacy with an acceptable degree of toxicity. For example, *ethambutol* blocks enzymes in mycobacteria, preventing cell wall synthesis. *Isoniazid* inhibits the synthesis of mycolic acids, which are important to mycobacterial cell walls. *Pyrazinamide* affects enzymes involved in mycolic acid synthesis. *Rifabutin, rifampin,* and *rifapentine* inhibit DNA-dependent RNA polymerase in mycobacteria. (See illustration, *Sites and Mechanisms of Action: Anti-Infective Agents,* page 2.)

COMBINATION PRODUCTS

RIFAMATE: isoniazid/rifampin (an antitubercular) 150 mg/300 mg. **RIFATER:** isoniazid/pyrazinamide (an antitubercular)/rifampin (an antitubercular) 50 mg/300 mg/ 120 mg.

Ethambutol

eth-**am**-byoo-toll
(Etibi [CAN], Myambutol)
Do not confuse with Nembutal.

CATEGORY AND SCHEDULE

Pregnancy Risk Category: B

MECHANISM OF ACTION

An isonicotinic acid derivative that interferes with RNA synthesis. ***Therapeutic Effect:*** Suppresses mycobacterial multiplication.

PHARMACOKINETICS

Rapidly, well absorbed from the GI tract. Widely distributed. Protein binding: 20%–30%. Metabolized in liver to inactive metabolites. Primarily excreted in urine. Removed by hemodialysis slightly (5%–20%). ***Half-Life:*** 3–4 hrs (half-life is increased with impaired renal function).

AVAILABILITY

Tablets: 100 mg, 400 mg.

INDICATIONS AND DOSAGES

▸ **Tuberculosis**

PO

Children. 15–25 mg/kg/day as a single dose or 50 mg/kg 2 times/wk. Maximum: 2.5 g/dose.

▸ **Nontuberculosis mycobacteria**
PO
Children. 15 mg/kg/day. Maximum: 1 g/day.
▸ **Dosage in renal impairment**

Creatinine Clearance	Dosage Interval
10–50 mL/min	q24–36h
less than 10 mL/min	q48h

UNLABELED USES

Treatment of atypical mycobacterial infections.

CONTRAINDICATIONS

Optic neuritis; hypersensitivity to ethambutol or any component.

INTERACTIONS

Drug

Neurotoxic medications: May increase the risk of neurotoxicity.
Aluminum salts: May reduce the absorption of ethambutol—space dosing by 2 hrs.

Herbal

None known.

Food

None known.

DIAGNOSTIC TEST EFFECTS

May increase serum uric acid levels.

SIDE EFFECTS

Occasional

Acute gouty arthritis (as evidenced by chills, pain, swelling of joints with hot skin), confusion, abdominal pain, nausea, vomiting, anorexia, headache

Rare

Rash, fever, blurred vision, eye pain, red-green color blindness

SERIOUS REACTIONS

! Optic neuritis (occurs more often with high ethambutol dosage or long-term ethambutol therapy), peripheral neuritis, thrombocytopenia, and anaphylactoid reaction occur rarely.

PEDIATRIC CONSIDERATIONS

Baseline Assessment

- Evaluate the patient's initial complete blood count and renal and liver function test results.
- Be aware that ethambutol crosses the placenta and is excreted in breast milk.
- Be aware that the safety and efficacy of ethambutol have not been established in children younger than 13 yrs of age.
- Do not use in children whose visual acuity cannot be monitored or evaluated.
- Discontinue use if visual changes occur.
- Maintain age-appropriate fluid and electrolyte balance.

Precautions

- Use cautiously in pts with cataracts, diabetic retinopathy, gout, recurrent ocular inflammatory conditions, and renal dysfunction.

Administration and Handling

PO
- Give with food to decrease GI upset.

Intervention and Evaluation

- Assess the patient for the first signs of vision changes, including altered color perception and decreased visual acuity. If vision changes occur, discontinue the drug and notify the physician immediately.
- Give ethambutol to the patient with food if GI distress occurs.
- Monitor the patient's serum uric acid levels. Also, assess the patient for signs and symptoms of gout,

including hot, painful, or swollen joints, especially in the ankle, big toe, or knee.

• Assess the patient for signs and symptoms of peripheral neuritis as evidenced by burning, numbness, or tingling of the extremities. Notify the physician if peripheral neuritis occurs.

Patient/Family Teaching

• Advise the patient/family not to skip drug doses and to take ethambutol for the full length of therapy, which may be months or years.

• Warn the patient/family to notify the physician immediately of any visual problems. Explain to the patient that visual effects are generally reversible after ethambutol is discontinued and that in rare cases visual problems may take up to a year to disappear or may become permanent.

• Warn the patient/family to promptly report burning, numbness, or tingling of the feet or hands and pain and swelling of joints.

Isoniazid

eye-sew-**nye**-ah-zid
(INH, Isotamine [CAN], Nydrazid, PMS Isoniazid [CAN])

CATEGORY AND SCHEDULE

Pregnancy Risk Category: C

MECHANISM OF ACTION

An isonicotinic acid derivative that inhibits mycolic acid synthesis. Active only during bacterial cell division. ***Therapeutic Effect:*** Causes disruption of bacterial cell wall and loss of acid-fast properties in susceptible mycobacteria. Bactericidal.

PHARMACOKINETICS

Readily absorbed from the GI tract. Protein binding: 10%–15%. Widely distributed (including cerebrospinal fluid). Metabolized in liver. Primarily excreted in urine. Removed by hemodialysis. ***Half-Life:*** 0.5–5 hrs, may be delayed with hepatic dysfunction and renal impairment.

AVAILABILITY

Tablets: 100 mg, 300 mg.
Syrup: 50 mg/5 mL.
Injection: 100 mg/mL.

INDICATIONS AND DOSAGES

▸ Prophylaxis

PO

Infants and children. 10 mg/kg (maximum: 300 mg) PO once daily. After 1 mo of therapy or if daily compliance cannot be achieved may change dosage to 20–40 mg/kg (maximum: 900 mg) PO 2 times/wk.

▸ To treat tuberculosis

PO/IM

Children. 10–15 mg/kg/day as a single dose. Maximum: 300 mg/day.

CONTRAINDICATIONS

Acute liver disease, history of hypersensitivity reactions or liver injury with previous isoniazid therapy.

INTERACTIONS

Drug

Alcohol: May increase hepatotoxicity and isoniazid metabolism.

Carbamazepine, phenytoin, diazepam: May increase the toxicity of these drugs.

Disulfiram: May increase CNS effects.

Hepatotoxic medications: May increase hepatotoxicity.
Ketoconazole: May decrease blood concentration of this drug.
Aluminum salts: May decrease isoniazid absorption.
Meperidine: May lead to serotonin syndrome.
Acetaminophen: May lead to hepatotoxicity and toxic acetaminophen concentrations.
Theophylline: May increase theophylline serum concentrations.

Herbal
None known.

Food
Reduced absorption of isoniazid when administered with food. Avoid foods with histamine or tyramine (cheese, broad beans, dry sausage, salami, liver paté, soya beans, liquid/powder protein supplements, wine).

DIAGNOSTIC TEST EFFECTS
May increase serum bilirubin, SGOT (AST), and SGPT (ALT) levels. May cause false-positive results for urinary glucose with Clinitest.

SIDE EFFECTS
Frequent
Nausea, vomiting, diarrhea, abdominal pain
Rare
Pain at injection site, hypersensitivity reaction

SERIOUS REACTIONS
! Neurotoxicity, as evidenced by clumsiness or unsteadiness and numbness, tingling, burning, or pain in the hands and feet, optic neuritis, and liver toxicity occur rarely.

PEDIATRIC CONSIDERATIONS
Baseline Assessment
- Be aware that prophylactic use of isoniazid is usually postponed until after childbirth.
- Be aware that isoniazid crosses the placenta and is distributed in breast milk.
- May need to increase dietary intake of folate, niacin, magnesium, and pyridoxine.
- The American Academy of Pediatrics recommends that pyridoxine 1–2 mg/kg/day be supplemented in children with nutritional deficiencies taking isoniazid to prevent peripheral neuropathy. These may include symptomatic human immunodeficiency virus (HIV)-infected pts, children or adolescents consuming vegetarian or milk-deficient diets, breast-feeding infants/mothers, and pregnant adolescents/women.

◂ **ALERT** ▸ Determine the patient's history of hypersensitivity reactions or liver injury from isoniazid, as well as his or her sensitivity to nicotinic acid or chemically related medications before starting drug therapy.

- Before beginning therapy, be sure that appropriate specimens are obtained from the patient for culture and sensitivity testing.
- Evaluate the patient's initial liver function test results.

Precautions
- Use cautiously in pts who are alcoholics or have chronic liver disease or severe renal impairment because these pts may be cross-sensitive to nicotinic acid or other chemically related medications.

Administration and Handling
PO
- Give 1 hr before or 2 hrs after meals. May give with food to

decrease GI upset, but this will delay isoniazid absorption.
• Administer at least 1 hr before antacids, especially those containing aluminum.

Intervention and Evaluation

◂ **ALERT** ▸ Monitor the patient's liver function test results. Also assess the patient for signs and symptoms of hepatitis as evidenced by anorexia, dark urine, fatigue, jaundice, nausea, vomiting, and weakness. If you suspect hepatitis, withhold the drug and notify the physician promptly.
• Assess the patient for burning, numbness, and tingling of the extremities. Be aware that pts at risk for neuropathy, such as alcoholics, those with chronic liver disease, diabetics, and malnourished individuals, may receive pyridoxine prophylactically.
• Be alert for signs and symptoms of hypersensitivity reaction, including fever and skin eruptions.

Patient/Family Teaching

• Advise the patient/family not to skip doses and to continue taking isoniazid for the full length of therapy (6–24 mos).
• Instruct the patient/family to take the drug preferably 1 hr before or 2 hrs after meals. Explain that the medication may be taken with food if GI upset occurs.
• Urge the patient/family to avoid consuming alcohol during treatment.
• Caution the patient/family not to take any other medications without first notifying the physician, including antacids. Explain to the patient/family that the patient must take isoniazid at least 1 hr before taking an antacid.
• Warn the patient/family to avoid foods containing tyramine, including aged cheeses, sauerkraut, smoked fish, and tuna because these foods may cause a reaction such as headache, a hot or clammy feeling, lightheadedness, pounding heartbeat, and red or itching skin. Warn the patient/family to notify the physician if any of these reactions occur. Also, provide the patient/family with a list of tyramine-containing foods.
• Warn the patient/family to notify the physician immediately of any new symptoms, such as dark urine, fatigue, nausea, numbness or tingling of the feet or hands, vision difficulties, vomiting, and yellowing of the skin and eyes.

Pyrazinamide

peer-a-**zin**-a-mide
(Pyrazinamide, Tebrazid [CAN], Zinamide [AUS])

CATEGORY AND SCHEDULE

Pregnancy Risk Category: C

MECHANISM OF ACTION

An antitubercular drug whose exact mechanism is unknown. Converted to pyrazinoic acid, which lowers the pH of the environment in susceptible strains of *Mycobacterium*. ***Therapeutic Effect:*** Pyrazinamide is either bacteriostatic or bactericidal, depending on its concentration at the infection site and the susceptibility of the infecting bacteria.

AVAILABILITY

Tablets: 500 mg.

INDICATIONS AND DOSAGES

▸ Tuberculosis

PO

Children. 20–40 mg/kg/day in 1 or 2 doses. Maximum: 2 g/day. May give 50 mg/kg/dose PO twice weekly.

CONTRAINDICATIONS

Severe liver dysfunction; hypersensitivity to pyrazinamide.

INTERACTIONS

Drug

Allopurinol, colchicine, probenecid, sulfinpyrazone: May decrease the effects of these drugs.
Rifampin: Concurrent use has been associated with severe/fatal hepatotoxic reactions.

Herbal

None known.

Food

None known.

DIAGNOSTIC TEST EFFECTS

May increase SGOT (AST), SGPT (ALT), and serum uric acid levels.

SIDE EFFECTS

Frequent

Arthralgia, myalgia (usually mild and self-limiting)

Rare

Hypersensitivity (rash, pruritus, urticaria), photosensitivity

SERIOUS REACTIONS

! Hepatotoxicity, thrombocytopenia, and anemia occur rarely.

PEDIATRIC CONSIDERATIONS

Baseline Assessment

- Determine the patient's hypersensitivity to ethionamide, isoniazid, niacin, and pyrazinamide.
- Ensure the collection of patient specimens for culture and sensitivity tests before beginning drug therapy.
- Evaluate the results of the patient's initial complete blood count (CBC), liver function tests, and serum uric acid levels.
- Maintain age appropriate fluid intake.

Precautions

- Use cautiously in pts with diabetes mellitus, a history of gout, and renal impairment.
- Use cautiously in pts with a possible cross-sensitivity to ethionamide, isoniazid, and niacin.
- Be aware that the safety and efficacy of pyrazinamide have not been established in children.

Intervention and Evaluation

- Monitor the patient's liver function test results and be alert for liver reactions such as anorexia, fever, jaundice, liver tenderness, malaise, nausea, and vomiting. If any liver reactions occur, stop the drug and notify the physician promptly.
- Check the patient's serum uric acid levels, and assess for signs and symptoms of gout, such as hot, painful, swollen joints, especially the ankle, big toe, or knee.
- Evaluate the patient's blood glucose levels, especially in pts with diabetes mellitus, because pyrazinamide administration may make management of diabetes difficult.
- Assess the patient's skin for rash or skin eruptions.
- Monitor the patient's CBC for anemia and development of thrombocytopenia.

Patient/Family Teaching

- Advise the patient/family not to skip drug doses and to complete the full length of therapy, which may be months or years.
- Explain to the patient/family that follow-up physician office visits

and laboratory tests are essential parts of treatment.
• Instruct the patient/family to take pyrazinamide with food to reduce GI upset.
• Encourage the patient/family to avoid overexposure to sun or ultraviolet light to prevent photosensitivity reactions. The patient should use broad-spectrum sunscreens and protective clothing when outdoors.
• Warn the patient/family to immediately notify the physician of any new symptoms, especially fever; hot, painful, swollen joints; unusual tiredness; or yellow eyes or skin.

Rifabutin

rye-fah-**byew**-tin
(Mycobutin)
Do not confuse with rifampin.

CATEGORY AND SCHEDULE

Pregnancy Risk Category: B

MECHANISM OF ACTION

An antitubercular that inhibits DNA-dependent RNA polymerase, an enzyme in susceptible strains of *Escherichia coli* and *Bacillus subtilis*. ***Therapeutic Effect:*** Prevents *Mycobacterium avium* complex (MAC) disease in pts with advanced human immunodeficiency virus (HIV) infection.

PHARMACOKINETICS

Readily absorbed from the GI tract. High-fat meals slow absorption. Protein binding: 85%. Widely distributed. Crosses blood-brain barrier. Extensive intracellular tissue uptake. Metabolized in liver to active metabolite. Excreted in urine; eliminated in feces. Unknown whether removed by hemodialysis. ***Half-Life:*** 16–69 hrs in adults.

AVAILABILITY

Capsules: 150 mg.

INDICATIONS AND DOSAGES

▸ **Prophylaxis (first episode MAC)**
PO
Adolescents. 300 mg/day or 150 mg 2 times/day.
Children older than 6 yrs. 300 mg/day once daily.
Children younger than 6 yrs. 5 mg/kg/day. Maximum: 300 mg/day.
▸ **Prophylaxis (for recurrence of MAC)**
PO
Adolescents. 300 mg/day or 150 mg 2 times/day.
Infants and children. 5 mg/kg/day. Maximum: 300 mg/day.
▸ **MAC treatment**
PO
Children. 5–10 mg/kg/day. Maximum: 300 mg/day.

CONTRAINDICATIONS

Active tuberculosis, hypersensitivity to other rifamycins, including rifampin. Do not give to pts with a WBC less than 1,000/mm^3 or platelet count of less than 50,000 mm^3. Do not use in pts with total bilirubin level more than 3 mg/dL.

INTERACTIONS

Drug

Oral contraceptives: May decrease the effects of these drugs.
Zidovudine: May decrease blood concentration of zidovudine, but does not affect the inhibition of HIV by zidovudine.

Dapsone, methadone, digoxin, theophylline, itraconazole, corticosteroids, barbiturates: May decrease the effects of these drugs.

Herbal

None known.

Food

None known.

DIAGNOSTIC TEST EFFECTS

May increase serum alkaline phosphatase, SGOT (AST), and SGPT (ALT) levels. May cause anemia, leukopenia, neutropenia, or thrombocytopenia.

SIDE EFFECTS

Frequent (30%)

Red-orange or red-brown discoloration of urine, feces, saliva, skin, sputum, sweat, or tears

Occasional (11%–3%)

Rash, nausea, abdominal pain, diarrhea, dyspepsia (heartburn, indigestion, epigastric pain), belching, headache, altered taste, uveitis, corneal deposits

Rare (2% or less)

Anorexia, flatulence, fever, myalgia, vomiting, insomnia

SERIOUS REACTIONS

! Hepatitis and thrombocytopenia occur rarely.

PEDIATRIC CONSIDERATIONS

Baseline Assessment

- Expect the patient to undergo a biopsy of suspicious nodes, if present. Also, expect to obtain blood or sputum cultures and a chest radiograph to rule out active tuberculosis.
- If ordered, obtain the patient's baseline complete blood count (CBC) and liver function test results.
- Be aware that it is unknown if rifabutin crosses the placenta or is excreted in breast milk.

Precautions

- Use cautiously in pts with liver or renal impairment.
- The safety of this drug for use in children is not established.

Administration and Handling

PO

- Give without regard to food. Give with food if GI irritation occurs.
- May mix with applesauce if the patient is unable to swallow capsules whole.

Intervention and Evaluation

- Monitor the patient's CBC and platelet count and Hgb, Hct, and liver function test results.
- Avoid giving the patient IM injections, taking the patient's rectal temperature, and any other trauma that may induce bleeding.
- Check the patient's body temperature and notify the physician of flu-like syndrome, GI intolerance, or rash.

Patient/Family Teaching

- Inform the patient/family that the patient's feces, perspiration, saliva, skin, sputum, tears, and urine may be discolored brown-orange during drug therapy. Also warn the patient/family that soft contact lenses may be permanently discolored.
- Caution the patient/family that rifabutin may decrease the effectiveness of oral contraceptives. Teach the patient about alternative methods of contraception.
- Warn the patient/family to avoid crowds and those with known infection.
- Warn the patient/family to notify the physician if the patient experiences dark urine, flu-like symptoms, nausea, unusual bleeding or bruising, any visual disturbances, or vomiting.

Rifampin

rif-**am**-pin
(Rifadin, Rimactane, Rimycin [AUS], Rofact [CAN])
Do not confuse with rifabutin, Rifamate, rifapentine, or Ritalin.

CATEGORY AND SCHEDULE

Pregnancy Risk Category: C

MECHANISM OF ACTION

This antitubercular interferes with bacterial RNA synthesis by binding to DNA-dependent RNA polymerase, preventing attachment of the enzyme to DNA and thereby blocking RNA transcription. ***Therapeutic Effect:*** Bactericidal activity occurs in susceptible microorganisms. Can be used in combination with other antimicrobials to treat staphylococcal infections.

PHARMACOKINETICS

Well absorbed from the GI tract (food delays absorption). Protein binding: 80%. Widely distributed. Metabolized in liver to active metabolite. Primarily eliminated via biliary system. Not removed by hemodialysis. ***Half-Life:*** 3–5 hrs (increased in liver impairment).

AVAILABILITY

Capsules: 150 mg, 300 mg.
Powder for Injection: 600 mg.

INDICATIONS AND DOSAGES

▸ **Meningococcal prophylaxis**
IV/PO
Infants younger than 1 mo. 10 mg/kg/day in divided doses q12h for 2 days.
Infants older than 1 mo and children. 20 mg/kg/day in divided doses q12–24h. Maximum: 600 mg/dose.

▸ **Treatment**
IV/PO
Children. 10–20 mg/kg/day or twice weekly. Maximum: 600 mg/day.

▸ **Staphylococcal infections**
IV/PO
Children. 15 mg/kg/day in divided doses q12h.

▸ **Synergy for *Staphylococcus aureus* infections**
PO
Neonates. 5–20 mg/kg/day in divided doses q12h (in combination).

▸ ***Haemophilus influenzae* prophylaxis**
PO
Children 1 mo and older. 20 mg/kg/day q24h for 4 days. Maximum: 600 mg.
Children younger than 1 mo. 10 mg/kg/day q24h for 4 days.

UNLABELED USES

Prophylaxis of *H. influenzae* type b infection; treatment of atypical mycobacterial infection, serious infections caused by *Staphylococcus* species.

CONTRAINDICATIONS

Concomitant therapy with amprenavir, hypersensitivity to rifampin or any rifamycins.

INTERACTIONS

Drug

Alcohol, liver-toxic medications: May increase risk of liver toxicity.
Aminophylline, theophylline: May increase creatinine clearance of these drugs.

Chloramphenicol, digoxin, disopyramide, fluconazole, methadone, mexiletine, oral anticoagulants, oral hypoglycemics, phenytoin, quinidine, tacrolimus, cyclosporine, benzodiazepines, tocainide, verapamil: May decrease the effects of these drugs.

Herbal

None known.

Food

None known.

DIAGNOSTIC TEST EFFECTS

May increase serum alkaline phosphatase, bilirubin, uric acid, SGOT (AST), and SGPT (ALT) levels.

IV INCOMPATIBILITIES

Diltiazem (Cardizem)

SIDE EFFECTS

Expected

Red-orange or red-brown discoloration of feces, saliva, skin, sputum, sweat, tears, or urine

Occasional (5%–2%)

Hypersensitivity reaction, such as flushing, pruritus, or rash

Rare (2%–1%)

Diarrhea, dyspepsia, nausea, fungal overgrowth as evidenced by sore mouth or tongue

SERIOUS REACTIONS

! Liver toxicity (risk is increased when rifampin is taken with isoniazid), hepatitis, blood dyscrasias, Stevens-Johnson syndrome, and antibiotic-associated colitis occur rarely.

PEDIATRIC CONSIDERATIONS

Baseline Assessment

- Determine the patient's hypersensitivity to rifampin and rifamycins before beginning drug therapy.
- Ensure the collection of patient specimens for culture and sensitivity tests before beginning drug therapy.
- Evaluate the patient's initial complete blood count (CBC) and liver function test results.
- Be aware that rifampin crosses the placenta and is distributed in breast milk.

Precautions

- Use cautiously in pts with active alcoholism, a history of alcohol abuse, or liver dysfunction.

Administration and Handling

PO

- Preferably give rifampin 1 hr before or 2 hrs after meals with 8 oz of water. Rifampin may be given with food to decrease GI upset; but this will delay the drug's absorption.
- For those pts unable to swallow capsules, the capsule's rifampin may be mixed with applesauce or jelly.
- Give rifampin at least 1 hr before administering antacids, especially antacids containing aluminum.

IV

◂ALERT▸ Administer rifampin by IV infusion only. Avoid IM and SC administration.

- Reconstituted vial is stable for 24 hrs.
- Once the reconstituted vial is further diluted, it is stable for 4 hrs in D_5W or 24 hrs in 0.9% NaCl.
- Reconstitute 600-mg vial with 10 mL Sterile Water for Injection to provide a concentration of 60 mg/mL.
- Withdraw the desired dose and further dilute with 500 mL D_5W.
- Evaluate the patient periodically for extravasation as evidenced by local inflammation and irritation.
- Infuse over 3 hrs (may dilute with 100 mL D_5W and infuse over 30 min).

Intervention and Evaluation

• Assess the patient's IV site at least hourly during infusion. At the first sign of extravasation, restart the IV infusion at another site. Extravasation may cause irritation and inflammation.

• Monitor the patient's liver function test results, and assess the patient for signs and symptoms of hepatitis as evidenced by anorexia, fatigue, nausea, jaundice, vomiting, and weakness. If any signs or symptoms of hepatitis occur, withhold rifampin and inform the physician immediately.

• Report hypersensitivity reactions such as flu-like syndromes and skin eruptions promptly.

• Assess the patient's pattern of daily bowel activity and stool consistency.

• Monitor CBC results for blood dyscrasias and observe the patient for bleeding, bruising, infection manifested as a fever or sore throat, and unusual tiredness and weakness.

Patient/Family Teaching

• Instruct the patient/family to take rifampin on an empty stomach with 8 oz of water 1 hr before or 2 hrs after a meal. If GI upset occurs, tell the patient to take rifampin with food.

• Warn the patient/family to avoid consuming alcohol while taking this drug.

• Explain to the patient/family not to take any other medications, including antacids while taking rifampin without first consulting the physician. Teach the patient/family to take rifampin at least 1 hr before taking an antacid.

• Inform the patient/family that feces, sputum, sweat, tears, or urine may become red-orange colored and that soft contact lenses may be permanently stained.

• Warn the patient/family to notify the physician of any new symptoms and to notify the physician immediately if the patient experiences fatigue, fever, flu, nausea, unusual bleeding or bruising, vomiting, weakness, or yellow eyes and skin.

• Caution women taking oral contraceptives to check with the physician. Explain that the reliability of oral contraceptives may be affected by rifampin. Teach the female patient about barrier contraception.

REFERENCES

Benitz, W. E. & Tatro, D. S. (1995). The pediatric drug handbook (3rd ed.). St. Louis: Mosby.

Gunn, V. L. & Nechyba, C. (2002). The Harriet Lane handbook (16th ed.). St. Louis: Mosby.

5 Antiviral Agents

- Acyclovir
- Amantadine Hydrochloride
- Foscarnet sodium
- Ganciclovir sodium
- Oseltamivir
- Ribavirin
- Rimantadine Hydrochloride
- Valganciclovir Hydrochloride
- Zanamivir

Uses: Antiviral agents are used to treat cytomegalovirus (CMV) retinitis in pts with acquired immunodeficiency syndrome (AIDS), acute herpes zoster infection (shingles), recurrent genital herpes infection, chickenpox, influenza A viral illness, and mucosal and cutaneous infections with herpes simplex virus.

Action: To be effective, antiviral agents must inhibit virus-specific nucleic acid and protein synthesis. They may act by interfering with viral DNA synthesis and viral replication, inactivating viral DNA polymerases, incorporating into and halting the growth of viral DNA chains, preventing the release of viral nucleic acid into host cells, or blocking viral penetration into cells. (See illustration, *Sites and Mechanisms of Action: Anti-Infective Agents,* page 2.)

COMBINATION PRODUCTS

REBETRON: ribavirin/interferon alfa-2b (an immunologic agent). Packaged as ribavirin (Rebetol) 200-mg capsules together with recombinant interferon alfa-2b (Intron A) injection as 3 million IU/0.5 mL or 3 million IU/0.2 mL.

Acyclovir

aye-**sigh**-klo-veer
(Aciclovir-BC IV [AUS], Acihexal [AUS], Acyclo-V [AUS], Avirax [CAN], Lovir [AUS], Zovirax, Zyclir [AUS])
Do not confuse with Zostrix.

CATEGORY AND SCHEDULE

Pregnancy Risk Category: B

MECHANISM OF ACTION

A synthetic nucleoside that converts to acyclovir triphosphate, becoming part of the DNA chain. ***Therapeutic Effect:*** Interferes with DNA synthesis and viral replication. Virustatic.

PHARMACOKINETICS

Poorly absorbed from the GI tract; minimal absorption after topical application. Protein binding: 9%–36%. Widely distributed. Partially metabolized in liver. Excreted primarily in urine. Removed by hemodialysis. ***Half-Life:*** 2.5 hrs (increased in impaired renal function).

AVAILABILITY

Tablets: 400 mg, 800 mg.
Capsules: 200 mg.
Oral Suspension: 200 mg/5 mL.
Powder for Injection: 500 mg, 1,000 mg (50 mg/mL).
Ointment: 5%/50 mg.
Cream: 5%.

INDICATIONS AND DOSAGES

▸ **Herpes simplex**

IV

Children older than 12 yrs. 5 mg/kg/dose q8h for 5–10 days.
Premature neonates. 10 mg/kg/dose q12h for 14–21 days.
Neonates. 10 mg/kg/dose q8h for 14–21 days.

▸ **Genital herpes**

PO

Children older than 12 yrs. 200 mg q4h (5 times/day) for 10 days (initial episode) or 5 days (recurrent episode).

▸ **Varicella zoster (chickenpox)**

IV

Children older than 12 yrs. 30 mg/kg/day divided q8h for 7 days.

PO

Children. 20 mg/kg/dose (maximum: 800 mg/day) 4 times/day for 5 days. Maximum: 3,200 mg/day. Treatment should be initiated within 24 hrs of onset of rash.

▸ **Herpes zoster (shingles)**

IV

Children younger than 12 yrs. 20 mg/kg/dose q8h for 7 days. Maximum: 800 mg/day.

PO

Children (immunocompromised). 250–600 mg/m^2/dose 4–5 times/day for 7–10 days.
Children (nonimmunocompromised). 20 mg/kg/dose 5 times daily for 5–7 days.

TOPICAL

Apply 0.5-inch ribbon of 5% ointment 6 times/day for 7 days.

▸ **Dosage in renal impairment**

Dosage and frequency are modified based on severity of infection and degree of renal impairment.

PO

Creatinine clearance of 10 mL/1.73 m^2 or less: 200 mg q12h.

IV

Creatinine Clearance (mL/min)	Dosage Percent	Dosage Interval
greater than 50	100	8 hrs
25–50	100	12 hrs
10–25	100	24 hrs
less than 10	50	24 hrs

UNLABELED USES

Herpes simplex ocular infections, infectious mononucleosis.

CONTRAINDICATIONS

Acyclovir reconstituted with bacteriostatic water containing benzyl alcohol should not be used in neonates.

INTERACTIONS

Drug

Nephrotoxic medications (e.g., aminoglycosides): May increase nephrotoxicity of acyclovir.
Probenecid: May increase half-life of acyclovir.

Herbal

None known.

Food

None known.

DIAGNOSTIC TEST EFFECTS

May increase BUN and serum creatinine concentrations.

IV INCOMPATIBILITIES

Aztreonam, cefepime (Maxipime), diltiazem (Cardizem), dobutamine (Dobutrex), dopamine (Intropin), levofloxacin (Levaquin), meropenem (Merrem IV), ondansetron (Zofran), piperacillin-tazobactam (Zosyn).

IV COMPATIBILITIES

Allopurinol (Aloprim), amikacin (Amikin), ampicillin, cefazolin (Ancef), cefotaxime (Claforan), ceftazidime (Fortaz), ceftriaxone (Rocephin), cimetidine (Tagamet), clindamycin (Cleocin), famotidine (Pepcid), fluconazole (Diflucan), gentamicin, heparin, hydromorphone (Dilaudid), imipenem (Primaxin), lorazepam (Ativan), magnesium sulfate, methylprednisolone (Solu-Medrol), metoclopramide (Reglan), metronidazole (Flagyl), morphine, multivitamins, potassium chloride, propofol (Diprivan), ranitidine (Zantac), trimethoprim-sulfamethoxazole (Bactrim, Septa), vancomycin

SIDE EFFECTS

Frequent

Parenteral (9%–7%): Phlebitis or inflammation at IV site, nausea, vomiting

Topical (28%): Burning, stinging

Occasional

Parenteral (3%): Itching, rash, hives

Oral (12%–6%): Malaise, nausea, headache

Topical (4%): Itching

Rare

Parenteral (2%–1%): Confusion, hallucinations, seizures, tremors

Topical (less than 1%): Skin rash

Oral (3%–1%): Vomiting, rash, diarrhea, headache

SERIOUS REACTIONS

! Rapid parenteral administration, excessively high doses, or fluid and electrolyte imbalance may produce renal failure exhibited by signs and symptoms such as abdominal pain, decreased urination, decreased appetite, increased thirst, nausea, and vomiting.

! Toxicity not reported with oral or topical use.

PEDIATRIC CONSIDERATIONS

Baseline Assessment

- Determine whether the patient has a history of allergies, particularly to acyclovir.
- Assess herpes simplex lesions before treatment to compare baseline with treatment effect.
- Acyclovir crosses the placenta and is distributed in breast milk.
- Be aware that safety and efficacy have not been established in children younger than 2 yrs of age or younger than 1 yr of age for IV use.
- Do not administer by IV push.
- Maintain age appropriate fluid intake.
- Inform social services if a healthy child is infected with genital herpes.
- Check IV site for phlebitis.

Precautions

- Use cautiously in pts with concurrent use of nephrotoxic agents, dehydration, fluid and electrolyte imbalance, neurologic abnormalities, or renal or hepatic impairment.

Administration and Handling

PO

- May give without regard to food.
- Do not crush or break capsules.
- Store capsules at room temperature.

TOPICAL

- Avoid eye contact.
- Use finger cot or rubber glove to prevent autoinoculation.

IV

- Store vials at room temperature. Solutions of 50 mg/mL will remain stable for 12 hrs at room temperature; may form precipitate when refrigerated. Potency not affected by precipitate and redissolution.

• IV infusion (piggyback) stable for 24 hrs at room temperature. Yellow discoloration does not affect potency.
• Add 10 mL sterile water for injection to each 500-mg vial (50 mg/mL). Do not use bacteriostatic water containing benzyl alcohol or parabens for injection because this will cause a precipitate to form.
• Shake well until solution is clear.
• Further dilute with at least 100 mL D_5W or 0.9% NaCl. Final concentration should be 7 mg/mL or less.
• Infuse over at least 1 hr because renal tubular damage may occur with too rapid administration.
• Maintain adequate hydration during infusion and for 2 hrs after IV administration.

Intervention and Evaluation

• Assess IV site for signs and symptoms of phlebitis, including heat, pain, or red streaking over the vein.
• Evaluate cutaneous lesions for signs of effective drug treatment.
• Ensure adequate ventilation.
• Be sure to maintain appropriate isolation precautions in pts with chickenpox and disseminated herpes zoster.
• Provide analgesics and comfort measures.
• Encourage the patient to drink water.

Patient/Family Teaching

• Encourage the patient to drink adequate fluids.
• Advise the patient/family to avoid touching lesions with fingers to prevent spreading infection to new sites.
• Urge the patient with genital herpes to continue therapy for the full length of treatment and to space doses evenly around the clock.
• Instruct the patient/family to use a finger cot or rubber glove to apply topical ointment.
• Caution the patient to avoid sexual intercourse while visible lesions are present to prevent infecting his or her partner.
• Warn the patient that acyclovir does not cure herpes.
• Encourage the female patient/family to have a Pap smear at least annually because of the increased risk of cervical cancer in women with genital herpes.

Amantadine Hydrochloride

ah-**man**-tih-deen
(Endantadine [CAN], PMS-Amantadine [CAN], Symmetrel)

CATEGORY AND SCHEDULE

Pregnancy Risk Category: C

MECHANISM OF ACTION

A dopaminergic agonist that blocks the uncoating of influenza A virus, preventing penetration into the host and inhibiting M2 protein in the assembly of progeny virions. Amantadine locks the reuptake of dopamine into presynaptic neurons and causes direct stimulation of postsynaptic receptors. ***Therapeutic Effect:*** Antiviral, antiparkinson activity.

PHARMACOKINETICS

Rapidly, completely absorbed from GI tract. Protein binding: 67%. Widely distributed. Primarily excreted in urine. Minimally removed by hemodialysis. ***Half-Life:*** 11–15 hrs (half-life decreased in impaired renal function).

AVAILABILITY
Liquid: 50 mg/5 mL.
Syrup: 50 mg/5 mL.
Tablets: 100 mg.
Capsules: 100 mg.

INDICATIONS AND DOSAGES
▸ Prophylaxis, symptomatic treatment of respiratory illness due to influenza A virus
PO
Children older than 12 yrs. 200 mg/day once daily.
Children 9–12 yrs. 100 mg 2 times/day.
Children 1–8 yrs. 5 mg/kg/day (up to 150 mg/day) once daily or divided q12h.
▸ Dosage in renal impairment
Dosage and frequency are modified based on creatinine clearance.

Creatinine Clearance	Dosage
30–50 mL/min	200 mg first day; 100 mg/day thereafter
15–29 mL/min	200 mg first day; 100 mg on alternate days
less than 15 mL/min	200 mg every 7 days

UNLABELED USES
Treatment of attention-deficit hyperactivity disorder and of fatigue associated with multiple sclerosis.

CONTRAINDICATIONS
Hypersensitivity to amantadine or any component.

INTERACTIONS
Drug
Anticholinergics, antihistamines, phenothiazine, tricyclic antidepressants: May increase anticholinergic effects of amantadine.
Hydrochlorothiazide, triamterene: May increase amantadine blood concentration and risk for toxicity.
Herbal
None known.
Food
None known.

DIAGNOSTIC TEST EFFECTS
None known.

SIDE EFFECTS
Frequent (10%–5%)
Nausea, dizziness, poor concentration, insomnia, nervousness
Occasional (5%–1%)
Orthostatic hypotension, anorexia, headache, livedo reticularis evidenced by reddish blue, netlike blotching of skin, blurred vision, urinary retention, dry mouth or nose
Rare
Vomiting, depression, irritation or swelling of eyes, rash

SERIOUS REACTIONS
! Congestive heart failure (CHF), leukopenia, and neutropenia occur rarely.
! Hyperexcitability, convulsions, and ventricular arrhythmias may occur.

PEDIATRIC CONSIDERATIONS
Baseline Assessment
- When treating infections caused by influenza A virus, expect to obtain specimens for viral diagnostic tests before giving the first dose. Therapy may begin before test results are known.
- Be aware that it is unknown whether amantadine crosses the placenta, but it is distributed in breast milk and is not recommended for use in nursing mothers

• There is no recognized dosing available or recommended in children younger than 1 yr.

Precautions

• Use cautiously in pts with cerebrovascular disease, CHF, history of seizures, liver disease, orthostatic hypotension, peripheral edema, recurrent eczematoid dermatitis, and renal dysfunction and those receiving CNS stimulants.

Administration and Handling

PO

◂ **ALERT** ▸ Give as a single dose or in 2 divided doses.

• May give without regard to food.

• Administer nighttime dose several hours before bedtime to prevent insomnia.

Intervention and Evaluation

• Expect to monitor the patient's intake and output and renal function tests, if ordered.

• Check for peripheral edema.

• Assess the patient's skin for blotching or rash.

• Evaluate the patient's food tolerance and episodes of nausea or vomiting.

• Assess the patient for dizziness.

Patient/Family Teaching

• Advise the patient/family to continue therapy for the full length of treatment and to space drug doses evenly around the clock.

• Explain to the patient/family that the patient should not take any medications, including OTC drugs, without first consulting the physician.

• Warn the patient/family to avoid alcoholic beverages.

• Caution the patient/family not to drive, use machinery, or engage in other activities that require mental acuity if the patient is experiencing dizziness or blurred vision.

• Teach the patient/family to get up slowly from a sitting or lying position.

• Stress to the patient/family to notify the physician of new symptoms, especially any blurred vision, dizziness, nausea or vomiting, and skin blotching or rash.

• Tell the patient/family to take the nighttime dose several hours before bedtime to prevent insomnia.

• Tell the patient/family that amantadine may cause dry mouth.

Foscarnet Sodium

fos-**car**-net
(Foscavir)

CATEGORY AND SCHEDULE

Pregnancy Risk Category: C

MECHANISM OF ACTION

An antiviral that selectively inhibits binding sites on virus-specific DNA polymerases and reverse transcriptases. ***Therapeutic Effect:*** Inhibits replication of herpes virus.

PHARMACOKINETICS

Sequestered into bone and cartilage. Protein binding: 14%–17%. Primarily excreted unchanged in urine. Removed by hemodialysis. ***Half-Life:*** 3.3–6.8 hrs in adults (half-life is increased with impaired renal function).

AVAILABILITY

Injection: 24 mg/mL.

INDICATIONS AND DOSAGES

▸ **CMV retinitis**

IV

Adolescents. Initially, 180 mg/kg/day divided every 8 hours (may dose as 100 mg q12h) for 2–3 wks. Maintenance: 90–120 mg/kg/day as a single IV infusion.

▸ **Herpes simplex (resistant)**

IV

Adolescents. 40 mg/kg q8–12h for 2–3 wks or until healed.

▸ **Dosage in renal impairment**

Dosages are individualized according to the patient's creatinine clearance. Refer to the dosing guide provided by the manufacturer.

CONTRAINDICATIONS

Hypersensitivity to foscarnet. Pts with creatinine clearance less than 0.4 mL/min/kg.

INTERACTIONS

Drug

Nephrotoxic medications: May increase the risk of renal toxicity.
Pentamidine (IV): May cause reversible hypocalcemia, hypomagnesemia, and nephrotoxicity.
Zidovudine (AZT): May increase anemia.
Ciprofloxacin: May increase seizure potential.

Herbal

None known.

Food

None known.

DIAGNOSTIC TEST EFFECTS

May increase serum alkaline phosphatase, bilirubin, creatinine, SGOT (AST), and SGPT (ALT) levels. May decrease serum magnesium and potassium levels. May alter serum calcium and phosphate concentrations.

IV INCOMPATIBILITIES

Acyclovir (Zovirax), amphotericin (Fungizone), diazepam (Valium), digoxin (Lanoxin), diphenhydramine (Benadryl), dobutamine (Dobutrex), droperidol (Inapsine), ganciclovir (Cytovene), haloperidol (Haldol), leucovorin, midazolam (Versed), pentamidine (Pentam IV), prochlorperazine (Compazine), trimethoprim-sulfamethoxazole (Bactrim), vancomycin (Vancocin)

IV COMPATIBILITIES

Dopamine (Intropin), heparin, hydromorphone (Dilaudid), lorazepam (Ativan), morphine, potassium chloride

SIDE EFFECTS

Frequent

Fever (65%); nausea (47%); vomiting, diarrhea (30%)

Occasional (5% or greater)

Anorexia, pain and inflammation at injection site, fever, rigors, malaise, hypertension or hypotension, headache, paresthesia, dizziness, rash, diaphoresis, nausea, vomiting, abdominal pain

Rare (5%–1%)

Back or chest pain, edema, hypertension or hypotension, flushing, pruritus, constipation, dry mouth

SERIOUS REACTIONS

! Renal impairment is a major toxicity that occurs to some extent in most pts.

! Seizures and mineral or electrolyte imbalances may occur and be life-threatening.

PEDIATRIC CONSIDERATIONS

Baseline Assessment

• Expect to obtain the patient's baseline complete blood count values, mineral and electrolyte

levels, renal function, and vital signs.
• Know that the risk of renal impairment is reduced by ensuring sufficient fluid intake to promote diuresis before and during dosing.
• Be aware that it is unknown whether foscarnet is distributed in breast milk.
• Be aware that the safety and efficacy of foscarnet have not been established in young children and infants.
• Ensure adequate fluid intake.
• Stop the medication if signs of electrolyte imbalance occur.

Precautions

• Use cautiously in pts with altered serum calcium or other serum electrolyte levels, a history of renal impairment, or cardiac or neurologic abnormalities.

Administration and Handling

IV

Store parenteral vials at room temperature.
• After dilution, foscarnet is stable for 24 hr at room temperature.
• Do not use if foscarnet solution is discolored or contains particulate material.
• Use the standard 24 mg/mL solution without dilution when a central venous catheter is used for infusion; the 24 mg/mL solution *must* be diluted to 12 mg/mL when the drug is given through a peripheral vein catheter. Use only D_5W or 0.9% NaCl solution for dilution for injection.
• Because foscarnet dosage is calculated on body weight, remove the unneeded quantity before the start of infusion to avoid overdosage. Use an IV infusion pump to administer foscarnet and prevent accidental overdose.
• Use aseptic technique and administer the solution within 24 hrs of the first entry into the sealed bottle.
• Avoid contact with skin.
• Do not administer as IV bolus or IV push.

◀ ALERT ▶ Do not give foscarnet as an IV injection or by rapid infusion because these routes increase the drug's toxicity. Administer foscarnet by IV infusion at a rate not faster than 1 hr for doses up to 60 mg/kg and 2 hrs for doses greater than 60 mg/kg.
• To minimize the risk of phlebitis and toxicity, use central venous lines or veins with an adequate blood flow to permit rapid dilution and dissemination of foscarnet.

Intervention and Evaluation

• Monitor the patient's blood Hct and Hgb levels, renal function test results, and serum calcium, creatinine, magnesium, phosphorus, and potassium levels. Also monitor the results of ophthalmic examinations, as appropriate.
• Assess the patient for signs and symptoms of electrolyte imbalances, especially hypocalcemia as evidenced by numbness or paresthesia of the extremities and perioral tingling, and hypokalemia manifested as irritability, muscle cramps, numbness or tingling of the extremities, and weakness.
• Evaluate the patient for signs and symptoms of anemia, bleeding, superinfections, and tremors. Institute safety measures for potential seizures.

Patient/Family Teaching

• Warn the patient/family to report numbness in the extremities, paresthesias, or perioral tingling, during or after infusion because this may indicate electrolyte abnormalities.
• Warn the patient/family to report tremors promptly because the drug may cause seizures.

Ganciclovir Sodium

gan-sye-klo-vir
(Cymevene [AUS], Cytovene, Vitrasert)
Do not confuse with Cytosar.

CATEGORY AND SCHEDULE
Pregnancy Risk Category: C

MECHANISM OF ACTION
This synthetic nucleoside is converted intracellularly, competes with viral DNA polymerases, and directly incorporates into growing viral DNA chains. ***Therapeutic Effect:*** Interferes with DNA synthesis and viral replication.

PHARMACOKINETICS
Poor oral absorption. Widely distributed. Protein binding: 1%–2%. Undergoes minimal metabolism. Primarily excreted unchanged in urine. Removed 50% by hemodialysis. ***Half-Life:*** 2.5–3.6 hrs (half-life is increased with impaired renal function).

AVAILABILITY
Capsules: 250 mg, 500 mg.
Powder for Injection: 500 mg.
Implant: 4.5 mg.

INDICATIONS AND DOSAGES
▸ **CMV retinitis**
IV
Children older than 3 mos. Initially administer 10 mg/kg/day in divided doses q12h for 14–21 days, then 5 mg/kg/day as a single daily dose.
▸ **Prevention of CMV infection in transplant patients**
IV
Children. Initially administer 10 mg/kg/day in divided doses q12h for 7–14 days, then 5 mg/kg/day as a single daily dose.
▸ **Other CMV infections**
IV
Children. Initially, 10 mg/kg/day in divided doses q12h for 14–21 days, then 5 mg/kg/day as a single daily dose. Maintenance dose: 30 mg/kg q8h.
▸ **Prevention of CMV in HIV-Infected Individuals**
IV
Adolescents. 5–6 mg/kg/dose daily for 7 days.
Infants and children. 5 mg/kg/day.
PO
Adolescents. 1,000 mg 3 times/day with food.
▸ **Intravitreal implant**
Children older than 9 yrs. 1 implant q6–9mos plus ganciclovir orally (30 mg q8h).

UNLABELED USES
Treatment of other CMV infections, such as gastroenteritis, hepatitis, pneumonitis.

CONTRAINDICATIONS
Absolute neutrophil count less than 500/mm^3, platelet count less than 25,000/mm^3, hypersensitivity to acyclovir or ganciclovir. Not for use in nonimmunocompromised persons or those with congenital or neonatal CMV disease.

INTERACTIONS
Drug
Bone marrow depressants: May increase bone marrow depression.
Imipenem-cilastatin: May increase the risk of seizures.
Zidovudine (AZT): May increase the risk of liver toxicity.
Amphotericin B, cyclosporine, tacrolimus: May increase nephrotoxicity.
Herbal
None known.

Food
None known.

DIAGNOSTIC TEST EFFECTS

May increase serum alkaline phosphatase, bilirubin, SGOT (AST), and SGPT (ALT) levels.

IV INCOMPATIBILITIES

Aldesleukin (Proleukin), amifostine (Ethyol), aztreonam (Azactam), cefepime (Maxipime), cytarabine (ARA-C), doxorubicin (Adriamycin), fludarabine (Fludara), foscarnet (Foscavir), gemcitabine (Gemzar), ondansetron (Zofran), piperacillin/tazobactam (Zosyn), sargramostim (Leukine), vinorelbine (Navelbine)

IV COMPATIBILITIES

Amphotericin, enalapril (Vasotec), filgrastim (Neupogen), fluconazole (Diflucan), propofol (Diprivan)

SIDE EFFECTS

Frequent
Diarrhea (41%), fever (40%), nausea (25%), abdominal pain (17%), vomiting (13%)
Occasional (11%–6%)
Diaphoresis, infection, paresthesia, flatulence, pruritus
Rare (4%–2%)
Headache, stomatitis, dyspepsia, vomiting, phlebitis

SERIOUS REACTIONS

! Hematologic toxicity occurs commonly: leukopenia (29%–41%) and anemia (19%–25%).
! Intraocular insertion produces visual acuity loss, vitreous hemorrhage, and retinal detachment occasionally.
! GI hemorrhage occurs rarely.

PEDIATRIC CONSIDERATIONS

Baseline Assessment
- Evaluate the patient's hematologic baseline.
- Obtain specimens (blood, feces, throat culture, and urine) from the patient for culture and sensitivity testing, as ordered, before giving the drug. Keep in mind that test results are needed to support the differential diagnosis and rule out retinal infection as the result of hematogenous dissemination.
- Be aware that ganciclovir should not be used during pregnancy, and breast-feeding should be discontinued during ganciclovir use. Breast-feeding may be resumed no sooner than 72 hrs after the last dose of ganciclovir.
- Be aware that effective contraception should be used during ganciclovir therapy.
- Be aware that the safety and efficacy of ganciclovir have not been established in children younger than 12 yrs of age.

Precautions
- Use cautiously in pediatric pts. The long-term safety of this drug has not been determined because of the potential for long-term adverse reproductive and carcinogenic effects.
- Use cautiously in pts with impaired renal function, neutropenia, and thrombocytopenia.

Administration and Handling
PO
- Do not open or crush contents of capsules.
- Give ganciclovir with food.

IV
- Store vials at room temperature. Do not refrigerate.
- Reconstituted solution in vial is stable for 12 hrs at room temperature.

• After dilution, refrigerate and use within 24 hrs.
• Discard the solution if precipitate forms or discoloration occurs.
• Avoid inhaling the solution. Also avoid solution exposure to the eyes, mucous membranes, or skin. Use latex gloves and safety glasses during preparation and handling of ganciclovir solution. If the solution comes in contact with mucous membranes or the skin, wash the affected area thoroughly with soap and water; rinse eyes thoroughly with plain water.
• Reconstitute 500-mg vial with 10 mL Sterile Water for Injection to provide a concentration of 50 mg/mL; do not use bacteriostatic water that contains parabens and is therefore incompatible with ganciclovir.
• Further dilute with 100 mL D_5W, 0.9% NaCl, lactated Ringer's solution, or any combination thereof to provide a concentration of 5 mg/mL.
◂ **ALERT** ▸ Do not give by IV push or rapid IV infusion because these routes increase the risk of ganciclovir toxicity. Administer only by IV infusion over 1 hr.
• Protect the patient from infiltration because the high pH of this drug causes severe tissue irritation.
• Avoid contact with skin and other mucous membranes. Do not administer IM or SC.
• Use large veins to permit rapid dilution and dissemination of ganciclovir and to minimize the risk of phlebitis. Keep in mind that central venous ports tunneled under SC tissue may reduce catheter-associated infection.

Intervention and Evaluation

• Monitor the patient's intake and output, and ensure that the patient is adequately hydrated. (minimum 1,500 mL/24 hrs).
• Diligently evaluate the patient's hematology reports for decreased platelet count, neutropenia, and thrombocytopenia.
• Evaluate the patient for altered vision, complications, and therapeutic improvement.
• Assess the patient for signs and symptoms of infiltration, phlebitis, pruritus, and rash.

Patient/Family Teaching

• Instruct the patient/family that ganciclovir provides suppression but is not a cure for CMV retinitis.
• Explain to the patient/family that frequent blood tests and eye examinations are necessary during therapy because of the toxic nature of the drug.
• Stress to the patient/family that it is essential to report any new symptom promptly to the physician.
• Tell male pts that ganciclovir use may temporarily or permanently inhibit sperm production.
• Tell female pts that ganciclovir use may suppress fertility.
• Urge pts to use barrier contraception during ganciclovir administration and for 90 days after therapy because of its mutagenic potential.

Oseltamivir

oh-sell-**tam**-ih-veer
(Tamiflu)

CATEGORY AND SCHEDULE
Pregnancy Risk Category: C

MECHANISM OF ACTION

A selective inhibitor of influenza virus neuraminidase, an enzyme essential for viral replication. Acts against both influenza A and B viruses. ***Therapeutic Effect:*** Suppresses spread of infection within respiratory system and reduces duration of clinical symptoms.

PHARMACOKINETICS

Readily absorbed. Protein binding: 3% for active metabolite. Extensively converted to active drug in the liver. Primarily excreted in urine. ***Half-Life:*** 6–10 hrs.

AVAILABILITY

Capsules: 75 mg.
Oral Suspension: 12 mg/mL.

INDICATIONS AND DOSAGES

▸ Influenza (should be started within 2 days of symptom onset)

PO

Children 12 yrs or older. 75 mg 2 times/day for 5 days.
Children weighing more than 40 kg. 75 mg 2 times/day for 5 days.
Children weighing 23–40 kg. 60 mg 2 times/day for 5 days.
Children weighing 15–23 kg. 45 mg 2 times/day for 5 days.
Children weighing less than 15 kg. 30 mg 2 times/day for 5 days.

▸ Prophylaxis against influenza

PO

Children 13 yrs or older. 75 mg once daily for 7 days.

▸ Renal impairment

CREATININE CLEARANCE 10–30 ML/MIN

Treatment. Give dose once daily.
Prophylaxis. Give dose every other day.

CREATININE CLEARANCE LESS THAN 10 ML/MIN

Not recommended.

CONTRAINDICATIONS

Hypersensitivity to oseltamivir or any component.

INTERACTIONS

Drug

None known.

Herbal

None known.

Food

None known.

DIAGNOSTIC TEST EFFECTS

None known.

SIDE EFFECTS

Frequent (greater than 5%)

Nausea, vomiting, diarrhea

Occasional (5%–1%)

Abdominal pain, bronchitis, dizziness, headache, cough, insomnia, fatigue, vertigo

SERIOUS REACTIONS

! Colitis, pneumonia, and pyrexia occur rarely.

PEDIATRIC CONSIDERATIONS

• Be aware that it is unknown whether oseltamivir is excreted in breast milk.
• Be aware that the safety and efficacy of this drug have not been established in children younger than 1 yr of age.
• The safety of repeated treatment or prophylaxis regimens has not been assessed.
• Oral solution contains a metabolite of benzyl alcohol, which in large doses is associated with fatal toxicity in neonates. Oseltamivir is not recommended for use in neonates.

Precautions

• Use cautiously in pts with renal function impairment.

Administration and Handling

PO

• Give oseltamivir without regard to food.

Intervention and Evaluation

• Monitor the patient's renal function.

• In diabetic pts, monitor blood glucose levels.

Patient/Family Teaching

• Instruct the patient/family to begin taking oseltamivir as soon as possible from first appearance of flu symptoms.
• Warn the patient/family to avoid contact with those who are at high risk for influenza.
• Advise the patient/family that oseltamivir is not a substitute for a flu shot.

Ribavirin

rye-bah-**vi**-rin
(Copegus, Rebetol, Virazole)
Do not confuse with riboflavin.

CATEGORY AND SCHEDULE

Pregnancy Risk Category: X

MECHANISM OF ACTION

A synthetic nucleoside that inhibits replication of RNA and DNA viruses. Inhibits influenza virus RNA polymerase activity and interferes with expression of messenger RNA. ***Therapeutic Effect:*** Inhibits viral protein synthesis. ***Half-Life:*** Adults: 24hrs; children: 6.5–11 hrs.

AVAILABILITY

Powder for Reconstitution (aerosol): 6 g/100 mL.
Capsules: 200 mg.
Tablets: 200 mg.

INDICATIONS AND DOSAGES

▸ Severe lower respiratory tract infection caused by respiratory syncytial virus (RSV)

INHALATION

Children and infants. Use with Viratek small-particle aerosol generator at a concentration of 20 mg/mL (6 g reconstituted with 300 mL sterile water) continuously for 12–18 hrs/day for 3 days or up to 7 days.

Oral therapy is for adults older than 18 years of age with chronic hepatitis C.

UNLABELED USES

Treatment of influenza A or B, adenovirus, and west Nile virus.

CONTRAINDICATIONS

Pregnancy, women of childbearing age who will not use contraception reliably.

INTERACTIONS

Drug

Didanosine: May increase the risk of pancreatitis and peripheral neuropathy. May decrease the effects of this drug.

Nucleoside analogues, including adefovir, didanosine, lamivudine, stavudine, zalcitabine, zidovudine: May increase the risk of lactic acidosis.

Herbal

None known.

Food

None known.

DIAGNOSTIC TEST EFFECTS

None known.

SIDE EFFECTS

Frequent (greater than 10%)

Dizziness, headache, fatigue, fever, insomnia, irritability, depression, emotional lability, impaired concentration, alopecia, rash, pruritus, nausea, anorexia, dyspepsia, vomiting, decreased hemoglobin, hemolysis, arthralgia, musculoskeletal pain, dyspnea, sinusitis, flu-like symptoms

Occasional (1%–10%)
Nervousness, altered taste, weakness

SERIOUS REACTIONS

! Cardiac arrest, apnea and ventilator dependence, bacterial pneumonia, pneumonia, and pneumothorax occur rarely.
! If ribavirin therapy exceeds 7 days, anemia may occur.

PEDIATRIC CONSIDERATIONS

Baseline Assessment

- Expect to obtain respiratory tract secretions for diagnostic testing before giving the first dose of ribavirin or at least during the first 24 hrs of therapy.
- Assess the patient's respiratory status and establish a baseline.
- In pts taking oral ribavirin, expect to obtain the patient's complete blood count with differential and to pretreat and test the female patient of childbearing age monthly for pregnancy.
- May be used in infants or young children who are at high risk for serious complications related to RSV disease.
- Do not administer other aerosol medications with this medication.
- Assess for proper respiratory status and age-appropriate fluid intake.
- If aerosolized ribavirin is administered to mechanically ventilated pts, be aware that it may adhere to the ventilatory circuit and compromise ventilation. Frequent (q2h) suctioning is recommended as well as frequent ventilatory monitoring.

Precautions

- Use inhaled ribavirin cautiously in pts with asthma and chronic obstructive pulmonary disease.
- Use inhaled ribavirin cautiously in pts requiring mechanical ventilation.
- Use oral ribavirin cautiously in pts with cardiac or pulmonary disease.
- Use oral ribavirin cautiously in pts with a history of psychiatric disorders.

Administration and Handling

INHALATION

- Ribavirin is teratogenic, and any female of childbearing years should be aware of this potential. This includes health-care workers and close contacts of the patient.
- Ribavirin may adsorb to contact lenses.

◂ **ALERT** ▸ Ribavirin may be given via nasal or oral inhalation.

- Solution normally appears clear and colorless and is stable for 24 hrs at room temperature. Discard solution for nebulization after 24 hrs. Discard solution if discolored or cloudy.
- Add 50–100 mL Sterile Water for Injection or inhalation to 6-g vial.
- Transfer to a flask, serving as reservoir for aerosol generator.
- Further dilute to final volume of 300 mL, giving a solution concentration of 20 mg/mL.
- Use only an aerosol generator available from the manufacturer of the drug.
- Do not give at the same time with other drug solutions for nebulization.
- Discard reservoir solution when fluid levels are low and at least every 24 hrs.

◂ **ALERT** ▸ Be aware that there is controversy over the safety of administering ribavirin to ventilator-dependent pts; only experienced personnel should administer the drug.

ORAL
- Capsules may be taken without regard to food.
- Tablets should be given with food.

Intervention and Evaluation
- Monitor the patient's intake and output and fluid balance carefully.
- Check the patient's hematology reports for anemia resulting from reticulocytosis when therapy exceeds 7 days.
- For ventilator-assisted pts, watch for "rainout" in tubing and empty frequently.
- Be alert to impaired ventilation and gas exchange as a result of drug precipitate.
- Periodically assess the patient's lung sounds and assess the patient's skin for rash.
- Monitor the patient's blood pressure and respirations.

Patient/Family Teaching
- Instruct patient/family to immediately report any difficulty breathing or itching, redness, or swelling of the eyes.
- Educate female pts about prevention of pregnancy and the need for regular pregnancy testing.
- Educate male pts about protection of female partners from pregnancy.

Rimantadine Hydrochloride

rye-**man**-tah-deen
(Flumadine)
Do not confuse with flunisolide, flutamide, or ranitidine.

CATEGORY AND SCHEDULE
Pregnancy Risk Category: C

MECHANISM OF ACTION
An antiviral that appears to exert an inhibitory effect early in the viral replication cycle. May inhibit uncoating of virus. ***Therapeutic Effect:*** Prevents replication of influenza A virus. ***Half-Life:*** Adults: 24–36 hrs; children: 13–38 hrs.

AVAILABILITY
Tablets: 100 mg.
Syrup: 50 mg/5 mL.

INDICATIONS AND DOSAGES
▸ Prophylaxis against influenza A virus
PO
Children 10 yrs and older. 100 mg 2 times/day for at least 10 days after known exposure (usually 6–8 wks).
Children younger than 10 yrs. 5 mg/kg once a day. Maximum: 150 mg/day.

▸ Treatment of influenza A virus
PO
Children 10 yrs and older. 100 mg 2 times/day for 5–7 days.
Children younger than 10 yrs. 5 mg/kg/day 2 times/day for 5–7 days.

CONTRAINDICATIONS.
Hypersensitivity to amantadine or rimantadine

INTERACTIONS
Drug
Acetaminophen, aspirin: May decrease rimantadine blood concentration.
Anticholinergics, CNS stimulants: May increase side effects of rimantadine.
Cimetidine: May increase rimantadine blood concentration.
Herbal
None known.
Food
None known.

DIAGNOSTIC TEST EFFECTS
None known.

SIDE EFFECTS

Occasional (3%–2%)
Insomnia, nausea, nervousness, impaired concentration, dizziness
Rare (less than 2%)
Vomiting, anorexia, dry mouth, abdominal pain, asthenia (loss of energy, strength), fatigue

SERIOUS REACTIONS

None known.

PEDIATRIC CONSIDERATIONS

There are no specific pediatric considerations because of the infrequent use of this medication in pediatric pts.

Precautions

• Use cautiously in pts with a history of recurrent eczematoid dermatitis, liver disease, renal impairment, seizures, and uncontrolled psychosis.
• Use cautiously in pts who also receive CNS stimulants.

Administration and Handling

PO
• Give rimantadine without regard to food.

Intervention and Evaluation

• Assess the patient for nervousness and evaluate the patient's sleep pattern for insomnia.
• Provide assistance to the patient if he or she experiences dizziness.

Patient/Family Teaching

• Stress to the patient/family that the patient should avoid contact with those who are at high risk for developing influenza A (rimantadine-resistant virus may be shed during therapy).
• Warn the patient not to drive or perform tasks that require mental alertness if he or she experiences decreased concentration or dizziness.
• Caution the patient/family against taking acetaminophen, aspirin, or compounds containing these drugs.
• Advise the patient/family that rimantadine may cause dry mouth.

Valacyclovir

val-ah-**sigh**-klo-veer
(Valtrex)

CATEGORY AND SCHEDULE

Pregnancy Risk Category: B

MECHANISM OF ACTION

An antiviral that is converted to acyclovir triphosphate, becoming part of viral DNA chain. Virustatic. ***Therapeutic Effect:*** Interferes with DNA synthesis and viral replication of herpes simplex and varicella zoster virus.

PHARMACOKINETICS

Rapidly absorbed after PO administration. Protein binding: 13%–18%. Rapidly converted by hydrolysis to active compound, acyclovir. Widely distributed to tissues and body fluids (including cerebrospinal fluid). Primarily eliminated in urine. Removed by hemodialysis. ***Half-Life:*** 2.5–3.3 hrs (half-life is increased with impaired renal function).

AVAILABILITY

Tablets: 500 mg, 1,000 mg.

INDICATIONS AND DOSAGES

▸ **Herpes zoster (shingles)**
PO
Adolescents. 1 g 3 times/day for 7 days. Should be started within 48 hrs of onset of rash.

▸ **Genital herpes**
PO
Adolescents. Initial episode give 1 g 2 times/day for 10 days.
Adolescents. Recurrent episodes give 500 mg 2 times/day for 3 days.
Adolescents. Suppressive therapy give 500–1,000 mg/day for 1 year.

UNLABELED USES

Reduce heterosexual transmission of genital herpes.

CONTRAINDICATIONS

Hypersensitivity or intolerance to acyclovir, components of formulation, or valacyclovir.

INTERACTIONS

Drug
Cimetidine, probenecid: May increase acyclovir blood concentration.
Herbal
None known.
Food
None known.

DIAGNOSTIC TEST EFFECTS

None known.

SIDE EFFECTS

Frequent
Herpes zoster (17%–10%): Nausea, headache
Genital herpes (17%): Headache
Occasional
Herpes zoster (7%–3%): Vomiting, diarrhea, constipation (50 yrs or older), asthenia, dizziness (50 yrs or older)
Genital herpes (8%–3%): Nausea, diarrhea, dizziness
Rare
Herpes zoster (3%–1%): Abdominal pain, anorexia
Genital herpes (3%–1%): Asthenia, abdominal pain

SERIOUS REACTIONS

None known.

PEDIATRIC CONSIDERATIONS

Baseline Assessment
• Determine the patient's history of allergies, particularly to acyclovir and valacyclovir, before beginning drug therapy.
• Expect to obtain tissue cultures from herpes simplex and herpes zoster pts before giving the first dose of valacyclovir. Therapy may proceed before test results are known.
• Assess the patient's medical history, especially in those with advanced HIV infection, bone marrow or renal transplantation, and impaired liver or renal function.
• Be aware that valacyclovir may cross the placenta and be distributed in breast milk.
• The safety and efficacy of this drug have not been established in children.
Precautions
• Use cautiously in pts with advanced HIV infection, bone marrow or renal transplantation, concurrent use of nephrotoxic agents, dehydration, fluid or electrolyte imbalance, neurologic abnormalities, and renal or liver impairment.
Administration and Handling
◂ **ALERT** ▸ Be aware that therapy should be initiated at the first sign of shingles and that valacyclovir is most effective within 48 hrs of the onset of zoster rash.
PO
• Give valacyclovir without regard to meals.
• Do not crush or break tablets.

Intervention and Evaluation
- Evaluate the patient for cutaneous lesions.
- Monitor the patient's complete blood count, liver or renal function tests, and urinalysis.
- Manage herpes zoster pts with strict isolation, according to the institution's policies and procedures.
- For herpes zoster pts, provide analgesics, if ordered, and comfort measures.
- Provide the patient with adequate fluids.
- Keep the patient's fingernails short and hands clean.

Patient/Family Teaching
- Encourage the patient to drink adequate fluids.
- Stress to the patient/family that the patient should not touch lesions with fingers to avoid spreading infection to new sites.
- Advise genital herpes pts/families to continue therapy for the full length of treatment and to space doses evenly around the clock.
- Warn genital herpes pts to avoid sexual intercourse during the duration of lesions to prevent infecting partner.
- Instruct the patient that valacyclovir does not cure herpes.
- Warn the patient/family to notify the physician if lesions do not improve or recur.
- Explain to the female genital herpes patient that Pap smears should be done at least annually because of increased risk of cervical cancer in women with genital herpes.
- Teach the patient/family to initiate valacyclovir treatment at the first sign of a recurrent episode of genital herpes or herpes zoster. Explain to the patient that early treatment, that is, within first 24–48 hrs, is imperative for therapeutic results.

Zanamivir

zah-**nam**-ih-vur
(Relenza)

CATEGORY AND SCHEDULE

Pregnancy Risk Category: C

MECHANISM OF ACTION

An antiviral that appears to inhibit the influenza virus enzyme neuraminidase, which is essential for viral replication. ***Therapeutic Effect:*** Prevents viral release from infected cells.

AVAILABILITY

Blisters of Powder for Inhalation: 5 mg.

INDICATIONS AND DOSAGES

▸ Treatment of influenza virus

INHALATION

Children 7 yrs and older. 2 inhalations (one 5-mg blister per inhalation for a total dose of 10 mg) 2 times/day (approximately 12 hrs apart) for 5 days.

CONTRAINDICATIONS

Hypersensitivity to zanamivir or any component

INTERACTIONS

Drug

None known.

Herbal

None known.

Food

None known.

DIAGNOSTIC TEST EFFECTS

May increase serum creatinine phosphokinase and liver enzyme levels.

SIDE EFFECTS

Occasional (3%–2%)
Diarrhea, sinusitis, nausea, bronchitis, cough, dizziness, headache

Rare (less than 1.5%)
Malaise, fatigue, fever, abdominal pain, myalgia, arthralgia, urticaria

SERIOUS REACTIONS

! Neutropenia may occur.
! Bronchospasm may occur in those with history of chronic obstructive pulmonary disease or bronchial asthma.

PEDIATRIC CONSIDERATIONS

Baseline Assessment

- Be aware that pts requiring an inhaled bronchodilator at the same time as zanamivir should receive the bronchodilator before zanamivir.
- Not recommended in pts with asthma and other respiratory diseases.

Precautions

- This medication is not recommended for patients with underlying airway disease (asthma, COPD) because of the risk of fatal bronchospasm.

Administration and Handling

INHALATION

- Using the Diskhaler device provided, instruct the patient to exhale completely; then, holding the mouthpiece 1 inch away from the patient's lips, instruct the patient to inhale and hold his or her breath as long as possible before exhaling.
- Have the patient rinse his or her mouth with water immediately after inhalation to prevent mouth and throat dryness.
- Store at room temperature.

Intervention and Evaluation

- Provide assistance to the patient if he or she experiences dizziness.
- Assess the patient's pattern of daily bowel activity and stool consistency.

Patient/Family Teaching

- Instruct the patient/family on how to use the delivery device.
- Stress to the patient/family that the patient should avoid contact with those who are at high risk for influenza.
- Advise the patient/family to continue treatment for the full 5-day course and to space doses evenly around the clock.
- Teach pts/families with respiratory disease to be sure an inhaled bronchodilator is always readily available.

REFERENCES

Benitz, W. E. & Tatro, D. S. (1995). The pediatric drug handbook (3rd ed.). St. Louis: Mosby.
Gunn, V. L. & Nechyba, C. (2002). The Harriet Lane handbook (16th ed.). St. Louis: Mosby.

Imipenem/Cilastatin Sodium
Meropenem

Uses: Carbapenems are used to treat a wide variety of infections caused by aerobic and anaerobic organisms, including streptococci, *enterococci, staphylococci, Pseudomonas* species, *Acinetobacter* species, and *Bacteroides fragilis*. They have a broader spectrum of activity than most other β-lactam antibiotics.

Action: Carbapenems bind to penicillin-binding proteins, disrupting bacterial cell wall synthesis. Through this action, they are bactericidal. (See illustration, *Sites and Mechanisms of Action: Anti-Infective Agents*, page 2.)

Imipenem/Cilastatin Sodium

im-ih-**peh**-nem/sill-as-**tah**-tin
(Primaxin)

CATEGORY AND SCHEDULE

Pregnancy Risk Category: C

MECHANISM OF ACTION

A fixed-combination carbapenem. Imipenem binds to bacterial cell membrane. ***Therapeutic Effect:*** Inhibits cell wall synthesis. Bactericidal. Cilastatin competitively inhibits the enzyme dehydropeptidase. Prevents renal metabolism of imipenem.

PHARMACOKINETICS

Readily absorbed after IM administration. Widely distributed. Protein binding: 13%–21%. Metabolized in kidney. Primarily excreted in urine. Removed by hemodialysis. ***Half-Life:*** 1.5–3 hrs in neonates,1–1.5 hrs in children (half-life is increased in those with impaired renal function)

AVAILABILITY

IM Injection: 500 mg, 750 mg.
IV Injection: 250 mg, 500 mg.

INDICATIONS AND DOSAGES

▸ **IV***

Children 3 mos and older.
60–100 mg/kg/day in divided doses q6h. Maximum: 4 g/day.
Children 1–3 mos.
100 mg/kg/day in divided doses q6h.
Children younger than 1 month weighing more than 1500 g.
More than 1 week old:
25 mg/kg q12hr.
1–4 weeks old: 25 mg/kg q8h.

CONTRAINDICATIONS

Hypersensitivity to imipenem/cilastatin or any component.

INTERACTIONS

Drug

Ganciclovir: Increased risk of seizures: Do not use concurrently.
Cyclosporin: Increased CNS effects.

*Dosing is based on the imipenem component.

Probenecid: Decreases serum concentrations of imipenem/cilastatin. Do not use concurrently.

Herbal

None known.

Food

None known.

DIAGNOSTIC TEST EFFECTS

May increase BUN, serum alkaline phosphatase, bilirubin, creatinine, lactate dehydrogenase, SGOT (AST), and SGPT (ALT) levels. May decrease blood Hct and Hgb.

IV INCOMPATIBILITIES

Allopurinol (Aloprim), amphotericin B complex (Abelcet, AmBisome, Amphotec), fluconazole (Diflucan)

IV COMPATIBILITIES

Diltiazem (Cardizem), insulin, propofol (Diprivan)

SIDE EFFECTS

Occasional (3%–2%)

Diarrhea, nausea, vomiting

Rare (2%–1%)

Rash

SERIOUS REACTIONS

! Antibiotic-associated colitis and other superinfections may occur.

! Seizures have been reported in pts with CNS infections. Not recommended for use in meningitis.

! Anaphylactic reactions in those concurrently receiving β-lactams have occurred.

PEDIATRIC CONSIDERATIONS

Baseline Assessment

- Be aware that imipenem crosses the placenta and is distributed in amniotic fluid, breast milk, and cord blood.
- This drug may be used safely in children younger than 12 yrs.
- Give slowly through IV over 30–60 min.
- Higher doses of 90 mg/kg/day have been given to children with cystic fibrosis.
- Seizures have been reported in children with imipenem treatment for meningitis. Not recommended for use in pediatric CNS infections.

ALERT Determine the patient's history of allergies, particularly to β-lactams, cephalosporins, and penicillins before beginning drug therapy.

- Determine the patient's history of seizures.

Precautions

- Use cautiously in pts with a history of seizures, renal impairment, and sensitivity to penicillins.

Administration and Handling

IM

- Prepare with 1% lidocaine without epinephrine, as prescribed; 500-mg vial with 2 mL, 750-mg vial with 3 mL lidocaine HCl.
- Administer suspension within 1 hr of preparation.
- Do not mix the suspension with any other medications.
- Give deep IM injections slowly into a large muscle to minimize patient discomfort. To further minimize discomfort, administer IM injections into the gluteus maximus instead of the lateral aspect of the thigh. Be sure to aspirate with the syringe before injecting the drug to decrease risk of injection into a blood vessel.

IV

- Solution normally appears colorless to yellow; discard if solution turns brown.
- IV infusion (piggyback) is stable for 4 hrs at room temperature, 24 hrs if refrigerated.

• Discard if precipitate forms.
• Dilute each 250- or 500-mg vial with 100 mL D_5W or 0.9% NaCl.
• Give by intermittent IV infusion (piggyback). Do not give IV push.
• Infuse over 20–30 min (1-g dose longer than 40–60 min).
• Observe the patient during the first 30 min of the infusion for a possible hypersensitivity reaction.

Intervention and Evaluation

• Monitor the patient's hematologic, liver, and renal function tests.
• Evaluate the patient for phlebitis as evidenced by heat, pain, and red streaking over vein.
• Evaluate that patient for pain at the IV injection site.
• Assess the patient for GI discomfort, nausea, and vomiting.
• Assess the patient's pattern of daily bowel activity and stool consistency.
• Assess the patient's skin for rash.
• Observe the patient for possible seizures and tremors.

Patient/Family Teaching

• Warn the patient/family to immediately notify the physician if the patient experiences severe diarrhea and to avoid taking antidiarrheals until directed to do so by the physician.
• Explain to the patient/family to notify the physician of the onset of troublesome or serious adverse reactions, including infusion site pain, redness, or swelling, nausea or vomiting, or skin rash or itching.

Meropenem

murr-**oh**-pen-em
(Merrem IV)

CATEGORY AND SCHEDULE

Pregnancy Risk Category: B

MECHANISM OF ACTION

A carbapenem that binds to penicillin-binding proteins. ***Therapeutic Effect:*** Inhibits bacterial cell wall synthesis. Bactericidal.

PHARMACOKINETICS

After IV administration, widely distributed into tissues and body fluids, including cerebrospinal fluid. Protein binding: 2%. Primarily excreted unchanged in urine. Removed by hemodialysis. ***Half-Life:*** 2–3 hrs in newborns, 1–1.5 hrs in children.

AVAILABILITY

Powder for Injection: 500 mg, 1 g.

INDICATIONS AND DOSAGES

▸ Mild to moderate infections

IV

Children 3 mos and older.
20 mg/kg/dose q8h.
Children younger than 3 mos.
20 mg/kg/dose q8–12h.

▸ Meningitis

IV

Children weighing 50 kg or more.
2 g q8h.
Children 3 mos and older, weighing less than 50 kg.
40 mg/kg q8h. Maximum: 2 g/dose.

▸ Dosage in renal impairment

Reduce dosage in pts with creatinine clearance less than 50 mL/min.

Creatinine Clearance	Dosage	Interval
26–49 mL/min	Recommended dose	q12h
10–25 mL/min	½ recommended dose	q12h
less than 10 mL/min	½ recommended dose	q24h

UNLABELED USES
Lowers respiratory tract infections, febrile neutropenia, gynecologic and obstetric infections, sepsis.

CONTRAINDICATIONS
Hypersensitivity to meropenem, other carbapenems, or in pts with a previous anaphylactic reaction to β-lactams.

INTERACTIONS
Drug
Probenecid: Inhibits renal excretion of meropenem (do not use concurrently).
Herbal
None known.
Food
None known.

DIAGNOSTIC TEST EFFECTS
May increase BUN, serum alkaline phosphatase, serum bilirubin, serum creatinine, serum lactate dehydrogenase, SGOT (AST), and SGPT (ALT) levels. May decrease blood Hct and Hgb and serum potassium levels.

IV INCOMPATIBILITIES
Acyclovir (Zovirax), amphotericin B (Fungizone), diazepam (Valium), doxycycline (Vibramycin), metronidazole (Flagyl), ondansetron (Zofran)

IV COMPATIBILITIES
Dobutamine (Dobutrex), dopamine (Intropin), heparin, magnesium

SIDE EFFECTS
Frequent (5%–3%)
Diarrhea, nausea, vomiting, headache, inflammation at injection site
Occasional (2%)
Oral moniliasis, rash, pruritus
Rare (less than 2%)
Constipation, glossitis

SERIOUS REACTIONS
! Antibiotic-associated colitis and other superinfections may occur.
! Anaphylactic reactions in those concurrently receiving β-lactams have occurred.
! Seizures may occur in those with bacterial meningitis, CNS disorders (including brain lesions and a history of seizures), and impaired renal function.

PEDIATRIC CONSIDERATIONS
Baseline Assessment
• Determine the patient's history of seizures.
• Be aware that it is unknown whether meropenem is distributed in breast milk.
• Be aware that the safety and efficacy of meropenem have not been established in children younger than 3 mos.
Precautions
• Use cautiously in pts with CNS disorders (particularly a history of seizures), hypersensitivity to cephalosporins, penicillins, or other allergens, and renal function impairment.
Administration and Handling
◂ALERT▸ Space drug doses evenly around the clock.
IV
• Store vials at room temperature.
• After reconstitution with 0.9% NaCl, solution is stable for 2 hrs at room temperature, 18 hrs if refrigerated (with D_5W, stable for 1 hr at room temperature, 8 hrs if refrigerated).
• Reconstitute each 500 mg with 10 mL Sterile Water for Injection to provide a concentration of 50 mg/mL.

- Shake to dissolve until clear.
- May further dilute with 100 mL 0.9% NaCl or D_5W. Final concentration should not exceed 50 mg/mL.
- May give by IV push or IV intermittent infusion (piggyback).
- If administering as IV intermittent infusion (piggyback), give over 15–30 min; if administered by IV push (5–20 mL), give over 3–5 min.

Intervention and Evaluation

- Assess the patient's pattern of daily bowel activity and stool consistency.
- Evaluate the patient for hydration status, nausea, and vomiting.
- Check the patient's IV injection site for inflammation.
- Assess the patient's skin for rash.
- Monitor the patient's electrolytes (especially potassium), intake and output, and renal function test results.
- Observe the patient's mental status and be alert to possible seizure or tremor development.
- Assess the patient's blood pressure and temperature 2 times/day, more often if necessary.

Patient/Family Teaching

- Warn the patient/family to immediately notify the physician if the patient experiences severe diarrhea and to avoid taking antidiarrheals until directed to do so by the physician.
- Explain to the patient/family to notify the physician of the onset of troublesome or serious adverse reactions, including infusion site pain, redness, or swelling, nausea or vomiting, or skin rash or itching.

REFERENCES

Gunn, V. L. & Nechyba, C. (2002). The Harriet Lane handbook (16th ed.). St. Louis: Mosby.

7 Cephalosporins

Cefaclor
Cefadroxil
Cefazolin Sodium
Cefdinir
Cefepime
Cefotaxime Sodium
Cefotetan Disodium
Cefoxitin Sodium
Cefpodoxime Proxetil
Cefprozil
Ceftazidime
Ceftibuten
Ceftizoxime Sodium
Ceftriaxone Sodium
Cefuroxime Axetil, Cefuroxime Sodium
Cephalexin
Loracarbef

Uses: Cephalosporins are used to treat a number of diseases, including respiratory diseases, skin and soft tissue infections, bone and joint infections, and GU infections. These broad-spectrum antibiotics also are used prophylactically in some surgical procedures. First-generation cephalosporins have good activity against gram-positive organisms and moderate activity against gram-negative organisms, including *Proteus mirabilis.* Second-generation cephalosporins have increased activity against gram-negative organisms. Third-generation cephalosporins are less active against gram-positive organisms but more active against the Enterobacteriaceae with some activity against *Pseudomonas aeruginosa.* Fourth-generation cephalosporins have good activity against gram-positive organisms, such as *Staphylococcus aureus,* and gram-negative organisms, such as *Pseudomonas aeruginosa.*

Action: Cephalosporins inhibit bacterial cell wall synthesis or activate enzymes that disrupt the cell wall, causing a weakening in the cell wall, cell lysis, and cell death. (See illustration, *Sites and Mechanisms of Action: Anti-Infective Agents,* page 2.) Cephalosporins may be bacteriostatic or bactericidal and are most effective against rapidly dividing cells.

Cefaclor

sef-ah-klor
(Apo-Cefaclor [CAN], Ceclor, Ceclor CD, Cefkor [AUS], Cefkor CD [AUS], Keflor [AUS])

CATEGORY AND SCHEDULE

Pregnancy Risk Category: B

MECHANISM OF ACTION

A second-generation cephalosporin that binds to bacterial cell membranes. ***Therapeutic Effect:*** Inhibits synthesis of bacterial cell wall. Bactericidal.

PHARMACOKINETICS

Well absorbed from the GI tract. Protein binding: 25%. Widely distributed. Primarily excreted unchanged in urine. Moderately removed by hemodialysis. ***Half-Life:*** 0.6–0.9 hrs (half-life is increased with impaired renal function).

AVAILABILITY

Capsules: 250 mg, 500 mg.
Tablets (extended-release): 375 mg, 500 mg.
Oral Suspension: 125 mg/5 mL, 187 mg/5 mL, 250 mg/5 mL, 375 mg/5 mL.

INDICATIONS AND DOSAGES

▸ **Mild to moderate infections**

PO

Children older than 1 mo.
20 mg/kg/day in divided doses q8h. Maximum: 2 g/day.

▸ **Severe infections**

PO

Children older than 1 mo. 40 mg/kg/day in divided doses q8h. Maximum: 2 g/day.

PO (EXTENDED-RELEASE TABLETS)

Children older than 16 yrs.
375–500 mg q12h.

▸ **Otitis media**

PO

Children older than 1 mo. 40 mg/kg/day in divided doses q8h. Maximum: 1 g/day. May divide q12h for otitis media and pharyngitis.

▸ **Dosage in renal impairment**

Reduced dosage may be necessary in those with creatinine clearance less than 40 mL/min.

CONTRAINDICATIONS

History of anaphylactic reaction to penicillins or hypersensitivity to cephalosporins.

INTERACTIONS

Drug

Probenecid: May increase cefaclor blood concentration.

Herbal

None known.

Food

None known.

DIAGNOSTIC TEST EFFECTS

Positive direct or indirect Coombs' test results may occur. May increase BUN, serum alkaline phosphatase, bilirubin, creatinine, lactate dehydrogenase, SGOT (AST), and SGPT (ALT) levels.

SIDE EFFECTS

Frequent

Oral candidiasis (sore mouth or tongue), mild diarrhea, mild abdominal cramping, vaginal candidiasis (discharge, itching)

Occasional

Nausea, serum sickness reaction (fever, joint pain)

Serum sickness reaction usually occurs after the second course of therapy and resolves after the drug is discontinued.

Rare

Allergic reaction as evidenced by pruritus, rash, and urticaria

SERIOUS REACTIONS

! Antibiotic-associated colitis manifested as severe abdominal pain and tenderness, fever, and watery and severe diarrhea, and other superinfections, may result from altered bacterial balance.

! Nephrotoxicity may occur, especially in pts with preexisting renal disease.

! Severe hypersensitivity reaction including severe pruritus, angioedema, bronchospasm, and anaphylaxis, particularly in pts with a history of allergies, especially to penicillin, may occur.

PEDIATRIC CONSIDERATIONS

Baseline Assessment

◂**ALERT**▸ Determine the patient's history of allergies, particularly to cephalosporins and penicillins, before beginning drug therapy.

- Be aware that cefaclor readily crosses the placenta and is distributed in breast milk.
- There are no age-related precautions noted in children older than 1 mo.
- Extended-release tablets are not currently recommended for children.

• Assure age-appropriate fluid intake.
• Diarrhea may indicate drug toxicity.

Precautions
• Use cautiously in pts with a history of GI disease (especially antibiotic-associated colitis or ulcerative colitis) and renal impairment.
• Use cautiously in pts concurrently using nephrotoxic medications.

Administration and Handling
PO
• After reconstitution, oral solution is stable for 14 days if refrigerated.
• Shake oral suspension well before using.
• Give without regard to meals; if GI upset occurs, give with food or milk.
• Do not cut, crush, or chew extended-release tablets.

Intervention and Evaluation
• Assess the patient's mouth for white patches on the mucous membranes and tongue.
• Assess the patient's pattern of daily bowel activity and stool consistency. Although mild GI effects may be tolerable, an increase in their severity may indicate the onset of antibiotic-associated colitis.
• Monitor the patient's intake and output and renal function reports for nephrotoxicity.
• Be alert for signs and symptoms of superinfection including abdominal pain, moderate to severe diarrhea, severe anal or genital pruritus, and severe mouth soreness.

Patient/Family Teaching
• Advise the patient/family to continue therapy for the full length of treatment and to evenly space doses around the clock.
• Explain to the patient/family that cefaclor may cause GI upset. Instruct the patient to take the drug with food or milk if GI upset occurs.
• Teach the patient/family to refrigerate cefaclor oral suspension.

Cefadroxil

sef-ah-**drocks**-ill
(Duricef)

CATEGORY AND SCHEDULE
Pregnancy Risk Category: B

MECHANISM OF ACTION

A first-generation cephalosporin that binds to bacterial cell membranes. ***Therapeutic Effect:*** Inhibits synthesis of bacterial cell wall. Bactericidal.

PHARMACOKINETICS

Well absorbed from the GI tract. Protein binding: 15%–20%. Widely distributed. Primarily excreted unchanged in urine. Removed by hemodialysis. ***Half-Life:*** 1.2–1.5 hrs (half-life is increased with impaired renal function).

AVAILABILITY

Capsules: 500 mg.
Tablets: 1,000 mg.
Oral Suspension: 125 mg/5 mL, 250 mg/5 mL, 500 mg/5 mL.

INDICATIONS AND DOSAGES

▸ **Skin/skin-structure infections, group A β-hemolytic streptococcal pharyngitis, tonsillitis**
PO
Children. 30 mg/kg/day in 2 divided doses. Maximum: 2 g/day.
Adolescents. 1–2 g/day in 1–2 divided doses. Maximum: 4 g/day

Dosage in renal impairment
Dosage and frequency are based on the degree of renal impairment and the severity of infection. After initial 1-g dose:

Creatinine Clearance	Dosage Interval
25–50 mL/min	q12h
10–25 mL/min	q24h
0–10 mL/min	q36h

CONTRAINDICATIONS

Anaphylactic reaction to penicillins, history of hypersensitivity to cephalosporins.

INTERACTIONS

Drug
Probenecid: Increases cefadroxil blood concentration.
Herbal
None known.
Food
None known.

DIAGNOSTIC TEST EFFECTS

Positive direct or indirect Coombs' test results may occur. May increase BUN, serum alkaline phosphatase, bilirubin, creatinine, lactate dehydrogenase, SGOT (AST), and SGPT (ALT) levels.

SIDE EFFECTS

Frequent
Oral candidiasis (sore mouth or tongue), mild diarrhea, mild abdominal cramping, vaginal candidiasis (discharge, itching)
Occasional
Nausea, unusual bruising or bleeding, serum sickness reaction (fever, joint pain)
Serum sickness reaction usually occurs after the second course of therapy and resolves after the drug is discontinued.
Rare
Allergic reaction (rash, pruritus, urticaria), thrombophlebitis (pain, redness, swelling at injection site)

SERIOUS REACTIONS

! Antibiotic-associated colitis as evidenced by severe abdominal pain and tenderness, fever, and watery and severe diarrhea, and other superinfections may result from altered bacterial balance.
! Nephrotoxicity may occur, especially in pts with preexisting renal disease.
! Severe hypersensitivity reaction including severe pruritus, angioedema, bronchospasm, and anaphylaxis, particularly in pts with history of allergies, especially penicillin, may occur.

PEDIATRIC CONSIDERATIONS

Baseline Assessment
◂ALERT▸ Determine the patient's history of allergies, particularly to cephalosporins and penicillins, before beginning drug therapy.
- Assess for age-appropriate fluid intake.
- Diarrhea may indicate drug toxicity.
- Be aware that cefadroxil readily crosses the placenta and is distributed in breast milk.
- There are no age-related precautions noted in children.

Precautions
- Use cautiously in pts with a history of allergies or GI disease (especially antibiotic-associated colitis or ulcerative-colitis) and renal impairment.
- Use cautiously in pts concurrently using nephrotoxic medications.

Administration and Handling
PO
• After reconstitution, oral solution is stable for 14 days if refrigerated.
• Shake oral suspension well before using.
• Give without regard to meals; if GI upset occurs, give with food or milk.

Intervention and Evaluation
• Assess the patient's mouth for white patches on the mucous membranes and tongue.
• Assess the patient's pattern of daily bowel activity and stool consistency. Although mild GI effects may be tolerable, an increase in their severity may indicate the onset of antibiotic-associated colitis.
• Monitor the patient's intake and output and renal function reports for nephrotoxicity.
• Be alert for signs and symptoms of superinfection as evidenced by abdominal pain, anal or genital pruritus, moderate to severe diarrhea, moniliasis, and sore mouth or tongue.

Patient/Family Teaching
• Advise the patient/family to continue therapy for the full length of treatment and to space doses evenly around the clock.
• Explain that cefadroxil may cause GI upset. Instruct the patient/family to take the drug with food or milk if GI upset occurs.
• Teach the patient/family to refrigerate cefadroxil oral suspension.

Cefazolin Sodium

cef-ah-**zoe**-lin
(Ancef)
Do not confuse with cefprozil or Cefzil.

CATEGORY AND SCHEDULE
Pregnancy Risk Category: B

MECHANISM OF ACTION
A first-generation cephalosporin that binds to bacterial cell membranes. ***Therapeutic Effect:*** Inhibits synthesis of bacterial cell wall. Bactericidal.

PHARMACOKINETICS
Widely distributed. Poor penetration into cerebrospinal fluid. Protein binding: 85%. Primarily excreted unchanged in urine. Moderately removed by hemodialysis. ***Half-Life:*** Neonates: 3–5 hrs. Adults: 1.4–1.8 hrs (half-life is increased with impaired renal function).

AVAILABILITY
Injection: 500 mg, 1 g, 5 g, 10 g, 20 g.
Ready-to-Hang Infusion: 500 mg/50 mL, 1 g/50 mL.

INDICATIONS AND DOSAGES
Neonates 7 days and younger. 40 mg/kg/day in divided doses q12h.
Neonates older than 7 days. 40–60 mg/kg/day in divided doses q8–12h.
Infants older than 1 month and children. 50–100 mg/kg/day in divided doses q8h. Maximum: 6 g/day.

▸ **Dosage in renal impairment**

Creatinine Clearance	Dosing Interval
10–30 mL/min	q12h
less than 10 mL/min	q24h

CONTRAINDICATIONS
Anaphylactic reaction to penicillins, history of hypersensitivity to cephalosporins.

INTERACTIONS

Drug

Probenecid: Increases cefazolin blood concentration.
Nephrotoxic drugs: Increase risk of nephrotoxicity.

Herbal

None known.

Food

None known.

DIAGNOSTIC TEST EFFECTS

Positive direct or indirect Coombs' test results may occur. May increase BUN, serum alkaline phosphatase, bilirubin, creatinine, lactate dehydrogenase, SGOT (AST), and SGPT (ALT) levels.

IV INCOMPATIBILITIES

Amikacin (Amikin), amiodarone (Cordarone), hydromorphone (Dilaudid)

IV COMPATIBILITIES

Calcium gluconate, diltiazem (Cardizem), famotidine (Pepcid), heparin, insulin (regular), lidocaine, magnesium sulfate, midazolam (Versed), morphine, multivitamins, potassium chloride, propofol (Diprivan), vecuronium (Norcuron)

SIDE EFFECTS

Frequent
Discomfort with IM administration, oral candidiasis (sore mouth or tongue), mild diarrhea, mild abdominal cramping, vaginal candidiasis (discharge, itching)
Occasional
Nausea, serum sickness reaction (fever, joint pain)
Serum sickness reaction usually occurs after the second course of therapy and resolves after the drug is discontinued.
Rare
Allergic reaction (rash, pruritus, urticaria), thrombophlebitis (pain, redness, swelling at injection site)

SERIOUS REACTIONS

! Antibiotic-associated colitis manifested as severe abdominal pain and tenderness, fever, and watery and severe diarrhea and other superinfections may result from altered bacterial balance.
! Nephrotoxicity may occur, especially in pts with preexisting renal disease.
! Severe hypersensitivity reaction including severe pruritus, angioedema, bronchospasm, and anaphylaxis, particularly in pts with a history of allergies, especially to penicillin, may occur.

PEDIATRIC CONSIDERATIONS

Baseline Assessment

◂ALERT▸ Determine the patient's history of allergies, particularly to cephalosporins and penicillins, before beginning drug therapy.
• Be aware that cefazolin readily crosses the placenta and is distributed in breast milk.
• Maintain age-appropriate fluid intake.
• Diarrhea could indicate drug toxicity.
• IM injection is less painful than for other cephalosporins.
• Monitor for signs of prolonged bleeding.

Precautions

• Use cautiously in pts with a history GI disease (especially antibiotic-associated colitis or ulcerative colitis) and renal impairment.
• Use cautiously in pts concurrently using nephrotoxic medications.

Administration and Handling

IM

• To minimize discomfort, give IM injection deep and slowly. To minimize injection site discomfort, give the IM injection in the gluteus maximus rather than the lateral aspect of the thigh.

IV

• Solution normally appears light yellow to yellow.
• IV infusion (piggyback) is stable for 24 hrs at room temperature and 96 hrs if refrigerated.
• Discard solution if precipitate forms.
• Reconstitute each 1 g with at least 10 mL Sterile Water for Injection.
• May further dilute in 50–100 mL D_5W or 0.9% NaCl to decrease the incidence of thrombophlebitis.
• For IV push, administer over 3–5 min.
• For intermittent IV infusion (piggyback), infuse over 20–30 min.

Intervention and Evaluation

• Evaluate the patient's IM site for induration and tenderness.
• Assess the patient's mouth for white patches on the mucous membranes or tongue.
• Assess the patient's pattern of daily bowel activity and stool consistency carefully. Although mild GI effects may be tolerable, an increase in their severity may indicate the onset of antibiotic-associated colitis.
• Monitor the patient's intake and output and renal function reports for nephrotoxicity.
• Be alert for signs and symptoms of superinfection including abdominal pain, moderate to severe diarrhea, severe anal or genital pruritus, and severe mouth soreness.

Patient/Family Teaching

• Explain to the patient/family that discomfort may occur with IM injection.
• Advise the patient/family to continue the antibiotic therapy for the full length of treatment and to space drug doses evenly around the clock.

Cefdinir

cef-din-ur
(Omnicef)

CATEGORY AND SCHEDULE

Pregnancy Risk Category: B

MECHANISM OF ACTION

A third-generation cephalosporin that binds to bacterial cell membranes. ***Therapeutic Effect:*** Inhibits synthesis of bacterial cell wall. Bactericidal.

PHARMACOKINETICS

Moderately absorbed from the GI tract. Protein binding: 60%–70%. Widely distributed. Not appreciably metabolized. Primarily excreted unchanged in urine. Minimally removed by hemodialysis. ***Half-Life:*** 1–2 hrs (half-life is increased in those with impaired renal function).

AVAILABILITY

Capsules: 300 mg.
Oral Suspension: 125 mg/5 mL.

INDICATIONS AND DOSAGES

▸ **Community-acquired pneumonia**

PO

Children 13 yrs and older. 300 mg q12h for 10 days.

▸ **Acute exacerbation of chronic bronchitis**
PO
Children 13 yrs and older. 300 mg q12h for 5 days.
▸ **Acute maxillary sinusitis**
PO
Children 13 yrs and older. 300 mg q12h or 600 mg q24h for 10 days.
Children 6 mos–12 yrs. 7 mg/kg q12h or 14 mg/kg q24h for 10 days. Maximum: 600 mg/day.
▸ **Pharyngitis or tonsillitis**
PO
Children 13 yrs and older. 300 mg q12h for 5–10 days or 600 mg q24h for 10 days.
Children 6 mos-12 yrs. 7 mg/kg q12h for 5–10 days or 14 mg/kg q24h for 10 days. Maximum: 600 mg/day.
▸ **Uncomplicated skin/skin-structure infections**
PO
Children 13 yrs and older. 300 mg q12h for 10 days.
Children 6 mos–12 yrs. 7 mg/kg q12h for 10 days. Maximum 600 mg/day.
▸ **Acute bacterial otitis media**
PO
Children 6 mos–12 yrs. 7 mg/kg q12h or 14 mg/kg q24h for 10 days.
▸ **Dosage in renal impairment**
Creatinine clearance less than 30 ml/min. 300 mg/day as single daily dose or 7 mg/kg once daily.
Hemodialysis pts. 300 mg or 7 mg/kg dose every other day.

CONTRAINDICATIONS

Hypersensitivity to cephalosporins.

INTERACTIONS

Drug

Antacids: Decreases cefdinir blood concentration.
Probenecid: Increases cefdinir blood concentration.
Iron: Increases cefdinir blood concentrations.

Herbal

None known.

Food

None known.

DIAGNOSTIC TEST EFFECTS

May produce a false-positive reaction for ketones in urine. May increase serum alkaline phosphatase, bilirubin, lactate dehydrogenase, SGOT (ALT), and SGPT (AST) levels.

SIDE EFFECTS

Frequent
Oral candidiasis (sore mouth or tongue), mild diarrhea, mild abdominal cramping, vaginal candidiasis (discharge, itching)
Occasional
Nausea, serum sickness reaction (fever, joint pain)
Serum sickness reaction usually occurs after the second course of therapy and resolves after the drug is discontinued.
Rare
Allergic reaction (rash, pruritus, urticaria)

SERIOUS REACTIONS

! Antibiotic-associated colitis manifested as severe abdominal pain and tenderness, fever, and watery and severe diarrhea and other superinfections may result from altered bacterial balance.
! Nephrotoxicity may occur, especially in pts with preexisting renal disease.
! Severe hypersensitivity reaction including severe pruritus,

angioedema, bronchospasm, and anaphylaxis, particularly in pts with a history of allergies, especially to penicillins, may occur.

PEDIATRIC CONSIDERATIONS

Baseline Assessment

◂ **ALERT** ▸ Determine the patient's hypersensitivity to cefdinir and other cephalosporins and penicillins before beginning drug therapy.
- Be aware that cefdinir crosses the placenta but is not detected in breast milk.
- Be aware that infants and newborns may have lower renal clearance of cefdinir.
- Assess for age-appropriate fluid intake.
- Diarrhea could indicate drug toxicity.

Precautions
- Use cautiously in pts with hypersensitivity to penicillins or other drugs, a history of GI disease (e.g., colitis), impaired liver function, and renal impairment.

Administration and Handling

PO

Give without regard to meals.
- To reconstitute oral suspension, for the 60-mL bottle, add 39 mL water; for the 120-mL bottle, add 65 mL water.
- Shake oral suspension well before administering.
- Store mixed suspension at room temperature. Discard unused portion after 10 days.

Intervention and Evaluation
- Assess the patient's pattern of daily bowel activity and stool consistency. Although mild GI effects may be tolerable, an increase in their severity may indicate the onset of antibiotic-associated colitis.
- Be alert for signs and symptoms of superinfection including anal or genital pruritus, changes or ulceration of the oral mucosa, moderate to severe diarrhea, and new or increased fever.
- Monitor the patient's hematology reports.

Patient/Family Teaching
- Instruct the patient/family to take antacids 2 hrs before or after taking this medication.
- Advise the patient/family to continue therapy for the full length of treatment and to space doses evenly around the clock.
- Warn the patient/family to notify the nurse or physician of any persistent diarrhea.

Cefepime

sef-eh-**peem**
(Maxipime)

CATEGORY AND SCHEDULE

Pregnancy Risk Category: B

MECHANISM OF ACTION

A fourth-generation cephalosporin that binds to bacterial cell membranes. ***Therapeutic Effect:*** Inhibits synthesis of bacterial cell wall. Bactericidal.

PHARMACOKINETICS

Well absorbed after IM administration. Protein binding: 20%. Minimal metabolism. Widely distributed. Primarily excreted unchanged in urine. Moderately removed by hemodialysis. ***Half-Life:*** 2–2.3 hrs (half-life is increased with impaired renal function).

AVAILABILITY

Powder for Injection: 500 mg, 1 g, 2 g.

INDICATIONS AND DOSAGES

IV/IM

Children 2 mos–16 yrs weighing less than 40 kg. Usual dosage 50 mg/kg q12h.

▸ **Meningitis, neutropenia, serious infections, and fever**

Children 2 mos–16 yrs weighing less than 40 kg. Usual dosage 50 mg/kg q8h. Maximum: 6 g/day.

▸ **Cystic fibrosis**

Children 2 mos–16 yrs weighing less than 40 kg. Usual dosage 50 mg/kg q8h. Maximum: 6 g/day.

CONTRAINDICATIONS

Anaphylactic reaction to penicillins, history of hypersensitivity to cephalosporins.

INTERACTIONS

Drug

Probenecid: May increase cefepime blood concentration.
Aminoglycosides: May increase risk for nephrotoxicity.

Herbal

None known.

Food

None known.

DIAGNOSTIC TEST EFFECTS

Positive direct or indirect Coombs' test results may occur. May increase serum alkaline phosphatase, bilirubin, lactate dehydrogenase, SGOT (AST), and SGPT (ALT) levels.

IV INCOMPATIBILITIES

Acyclovir (Zovirax), amphotericin (Fungizone), cimetidine (Tagamet), ciprofloxacin (Cipro), cisplatin (Platinol), dacarbazine (DTIC), daunorubicin (Cerubidine), diazepam (Valium), diphenhydramine (Benadryl), dobutamine (Dobutrex), dopamine (Intropin), doxorubicin (Adriamycin), etoposide (VePesid), droperidol (Inapsine), famotidine (Pepcid), ganciclovir (Cytovene), haloperidol (Haldol), magnesium, magnesium sulfate, mannitol, meperidine (Demerol), metoclopramide (Reglan), morphine, ofloxacin (Floxin), ondansetron (Zofran), vancomycin (Vancocin)

IV COMPATIBILITIES

Bumetanide (Bumex), calcium gluconate, furosemide (Lasix), hydromorphone (Dilaudid), lorazepam (Ativan), propofol (Diprivan)

SIDE EFFECTS

Frequent

Discomfort with IM administration, oral candidiasis (sore mouth or tongue), mild diarrhea, mild abdominal cramping, vaginal candidiasis (discharge, itching)

Occasional

Nausea, serum sickness reaction (fever, joint pain)
Serum sickness reaction usually occurs after the second course of therapy and resolves after the drug is discontinued.

Rare

Allergic reaction (rash, pruritus, urticaria), thrombophlebitis (pain, redness, swelling at injection site)

SERIOUS REACTIONS

! Antibiotic-associated colitis manifested as severe abdominal pain and tenderness, fever, and watery and severe diarrhea, and other superinfections may result from altered bacterial balance.
! Nephrotoxicity may occur, especially in pts with preexisting renal disease.

! Severe hypersensitivity reaction including severe pruritus, angioedema, bronchospasm, and anaphylaxis, particularly in pts with a history of allergies, especially to penicillins, may occur.

PEDIATRIC CONSIDERATIONS

Baseline Assessment

◂ALERT▸ Determine the patient's history of allergies, particularly to cephalosporins and penicillins, before beginning drug therapy.
- Be aware that it is unknown whether cefepime is distributed in breast milk.
- Assess for age-appropriate fluid intake.
- Diarrhea may indicate drug toxicity.
- There are no age-related precautions noted in children older than 2 mos.

Precautions
- Use cautiously in pts with renal impairment.

Administration and Handling

IM
- Add 1.3 mL Sterile Water for Injection, 0.9% NaCl, or D_5W to 500-mg vial (2.4 mL for 1- and 2-g vials).
- To minimize the pain experienced by the patient, give IM injection slowly and deeply into a large muscle mass (e.g., upper gluteus maximus) instead of the lateral aspect of the thigh.

IV
- Solution is stable for 24 hrs at room temperature or 7 days if refrigerated.
- Add 5 mL to 500-mg vial (10 mL for 1- and 2-g vials).
- Further dilute with 50–100 mL 0.9% NaCl or D_5W.
- For IV push, administer over 3–5 min.
- For intermittent IV infusion (piggyback), infuse over 30 min.

Intervention and Evaluation
- Evaluate the patient's IM site for induration and tenderness.
- Check the patient's mouth for white patches on the mucous membranes and tongue.
- Assess the patient's pattern of daily bowel activity and stool consistency. Although mild GI effects may be tolerable, an increase in their severity may indicate the onset of antibiotic-associated colitis.
- Monitor the patient's intake and output and renal function reports for nephrotoxicity.
- Be alert for signs and symptoms of superinfection including abdominal pain, moderate to severe diarrhea, severe anal or genital pruritus, and severe mouth soreness.

Patient/Family Teaching
- Explain to the patient/family that discomfort may occur with IM injection.
- Advise the patient/family to continue the antibiotic therapy for the full length of treatment and to evenly space drug doses around the clock.

Cefotaxime Sodium

seh-fo-**tax**-eem

(Claforan)

Do not confuse with cefoxitin, ceftizoxime, or cefuroxime.

(See Color Plates)

CATEGORY AND SCHEDULE

Pregnancy Risk Category: B

MECHANISM OF ACTION

A third-generation cephalosporin that binds to bacterial cell membranes. ***Therapeutic Effect:*** Inhibits synthesis of bacterial cell wall. Bactericidal.

PHARMACOKINETICS

Widely distributed, including cerebrospinal fluid. Protein binding: 30%–50%. Partially metabolized in the liver to the active metabolite. Primarily excreted in urine. Moderately removed by hemodialysis. ***Half-Life:*** Neonates 2–6 hrs; Children 1.5 hrs, Adults 1 hr (half-life is increased with impaired renal function).

AVAILABILITY

Powder for Injection: 500 mg, 1 g, 2 g, 10 g
Ready to Hang Piggyback: 1 g, 2 g.

INDICATIONS AND DOSAGES

IM/IV
Infants and children 1 mo–12 yrs. Weighing less than 50 kg give 100–200 mg/kg/day divided q6–8h. Weighing more than 50 kg give 1–2 g q6–8h. Maximum: 12 g/day.
Neonates older than 7 days. 150–200 mg/kg/day divided q6–8h.
Neonates younger than 7 days. 100–150 mg/kg/day divided q8–12h.
Adolescents. 1–2 g q6–8h. Maximum: 12 g/day.

▸ **Meningitis**
Infants and children weighing less than 50 kg. 200 mg/kg/day in divided doses q6h.
Children weighing 50 kg or more. 1–2 g q6–8h. Maximum: 12 g/day.

▸ **Dosage in renal impairment**
Creatinine clearance less than 20 ml/min. Give half dose at usual dosing intervals.

UNLABELED USES

Treatment of Lyme disease.

CONTRAINDICATIONS

Anaphylactic reaction to penicillins, history of hypersensitivity to cephalosporins.

INTERACTIONS

Drug
Probenecid: May increase cefotaxime blood concentration.
Herbal
None known.
Food
None known.

DIAGNOSTIC TEST EFFECTS

Positive direct or indirect Coombs' test results may occur. May increase liver function test results.

IV INCOMPATIBILITIES

Allopurinol (Aloprim), filgrastim (Neupogen), fluconazole (Diflucan), hetastarch (Hespan), pentamidine (Pentam IV), vancomycin (Vancocin)

IV COMPATIBILITIES

Diltiazem (Cardizem), famotidine (Pepcid), hydromorphone (Dilaudid), lorazepam (Ativan), magnesium sulfate, midazolam (Versed), morphine, propofol (Diprivan)

SIDE EFFECTS

Frequent
Discomfort with IM administration, oral candidiasis (sore mouth or tongue), mild diarrhea, mild abdominal cramping, vaginal candidiasis (discharge, itching)
Occasional
Nausea, serum sickness reaction (fever, joint pain)

Serum sickness reaction usually occurs after the second course of therapy and resolves after the drug is discontinued.

Rare

Allergic reaction (rash, pruritus, urticaria), thrombophlebitis (pain, redness, swelling at injection site)

SERIOUS REACTIONS

! Antibiotic-associated colitis manifested as severe abdominal pain and tenderness, fever, and watery and severe diarrhea and other superinfections may result from altered bacterial balance.

! Nephrotoxicity may occur, especially in pts with preexisting renal disease.

! Severe hypersensitivity reaction including severe pruritus, angioedema, bronchospasm, and anaphylaxis, particularly in pts with a history of allergies, especially to penicillins, may occur.

PEDIATRIC CONSIDERATIONS

Baseline Assessment

◂ALERT▸ Determine the patient's history of allergies, particularly to cephalosporins and penicillins, before beginning drug therapy.

• Be aware that cefotaxime readily crosses the placenta and is distributed in breast milk.

• Monitor age-appropriate fluid intake.

• Diarrhea may indicate drug toxicity.

Precautions

• Use cautiously in pts concurrently using nephrotoxic medications.

• Use cautiously in pts with a history of GI disease (especially antibiotic-associated colitis and ulcerative colitis).

• Use cautiously in pts with renal impairment with a creatinine clearance less than 20 mL/min.

Administration and Handling

◂ALERT▸ Space drug doses evenly around the clock.

IM

• Reconstitute with Sterile Water for Injection or Bacteriostatic Water for Injection.

• Add 2, 3, or 5 mL to 500-mg, 1-g, or 2-g vial, respectively, providing a concentration of 230, 300, or 330 mg/mL, respectively.

• To minimize discomfort, give IM injection deeply and slowly into the gluteus maximus rather than the lateral aspect of the thigh.

• For 2-g IM dose, give at 2 separate sites.

IV

• Solution normally appears light yellow to amber. IV infusion (piggyback) may darken in color (does not indicate loss of potency).

• IV infusion (piggyback) is stable for 24 hrs at room temperature, 5 days if refrigerated.

• Discard the solution if a precipitate forms.

• Reconstitute with 10 mL Sterile Water for Injection to provide a concentration of 50, 95, or 180 mg/mL for 500-mg, 1-g, or 2-g vials, respectively.

• May further dilute with 50–100 mL 0.9% NaCl or D_5W.

• For IV push, administer over 3–5 min.

• For intermittent IV infusion (piggyback), infuse over 20–30 min.

Intervention and Evaluation

• Evaluate the patient's IM injection sites for induration and tenderness.

• Assess the patient's mouth for white patches on the

mucous membranes and tongue.

• Assess the patient's pattern of daily bowel activity and stool consistency. Although mild GI effects may be tolerable, an increase in their severity may indicate the onset of antibiotic-associated colitis.

• Monitor the patient's intake and output and renal function reports for nephrotoxicity.

• Be alert for signs and symptoms of superinfection including abdominal pain, moderate to severe diarrhea, severe anal or genital pruritus, and severe mouth soreness.

Patient/Family Teaching

• Explain to the patient/family that discomfort may occur with IM injection.

• Advise the patient/family to continue the antibiotic therapy for the full length of treatment and to space drug doses evenly around the clock.

Cefotetan Disodium

seh-fo-**teh**-tan

(Cefotan)

Do not confuse with cefoxitin or Ceftin.

CATEGORY AND SCHEDULE

Pregnancy Risk Category: B

MECHANISM OF ACTION

A second-generation cephalosporin that binds to bacterial cell membranes. ***Therapeutic Effect:*** Inhibits synthesis of bacterial cell wall. Bactericidal.

PHARMACOKINETICS

Widely distributed. Protein binding: 78%–91%. Primarily excreted unchanged in urine. Minimally removed by hemodialysis. ***Half-Life:*** 3–4.6 hrs (half-life is increased with impaired renal function).

AVAILABILITY

Powder for Injection: 1 g, 2 g, 10 g. *Premixed Infusion, Ready to Hang:* 1 g/50 mL, 2 g/50 mL.

INDICATIONS AND DOSAGES

Infants and children.
40–80 mg/kg/day in divided doses q12h. Maximum: 6 g/day.
Adolescents. 2–4 g/day divided q12h. Maximum: 6 g/day.

▸ **Dosage in renal impairment**

Dosage and frequency are modified on the basis of creatinine clearance and the severity of infection.

Creatinine Clearance	Dosage Interval
10–30 mL/min	Usual dose q24h
less than 10 mL/min	Usual dose q48h

CONTRAINDICATIONS

Anaphylactic reaction to penicillins, history of hypersensitivity to cephalosporins.

INTERACTIONS

Drug

Alcohol: A disulfiram reaction (facial flushing, headache, nausea, sweating, or tachycardia) may occur when alcohol is ingested during cefotetan therapy.

Anticoagulants, heparin, thrombolytics: May increase the risk of bleeding with these drugs.

Herbal

None known.

Food

None known.

DIAGNOSTIC TEST EFFECTS

Positive direct or indirect Coombs' test results may occur. Drug interferes with crossmatching procedures and hematologic tests. Prothrombin times may be prolonged. May increase BUN, serum alkaline phosphatase, serum creatinine, SGOT (AST), and SGPT (ALT) levels.

IV INCOMPATIBILITIES

Vancomycin (Vancocin)

IV COMPATIBILITIES

Diltiazem (Cardizem), famotidine (Pepcid), heparin, insulin (regular), morphine, propofol (Diprivan)

SIDE EFFECTS

Frequent

Discomfort with IM administration, oral candidiasis (sore mouth or tongue), mild diarrhea, mild abdominal cramping, vaginal candidiasis (discharge, itching)

Occasional

Nausea, unusual bleeding or bruising, serum sickness reaction (fever, joint pain)

Serum sickness reaction usually occurs after the second course of therapy and resolves after the drug is discontinued.

Rare

Allergic reaction (rash, pruritus, urticaria), thrombophlebitis (pain, redness, swelling at injection site)

SERIOUS REACTIONS

! Antibiotic-associated colitis manifested as severe abdominal pain and tenderness, fever, and watery and severe diarrhea and other superinfections may result from altered bacterial balance.

! Nephrotoxicity may occur, especially in pts with preexisting renal disease.

! Severe hypersensitivity reaction including severe pruritus, angioedema, bronchospasm, and anaphylaxis, particularly in pts with a history of allergies, especially to penicillins, may occur.

PEDIATRIC CONSIDERATIONS

Baseline Assessment

◂ALERT▸ Determine the patient's history of allergies, particularly to cephalosporins and penicillins, before beginning drug therapy.

- Be aware that cefotetan readily crosses the placenta and is distributed in breast milk.
- The safety and efficacy of this drug have not been established in children.
- Diarrhea may indicate drug toxicity.
- Monitor for age-appropriate fluid intake.

Precautions

- Use cautiously in pts with a history of GI disease (especially antibiotic-associated colitis or ulcerative colitis) and renal impairment.
- Use cautiously in pts concurrently using nephrotoxic medications.

Administration and Handling

◂ALERT▸ Give by IM injection, IV push, or intermittent IV infusion (piggyback) only.

IM

- Add 2, 3 mL Sterile Water for Injection or other appropriate diluent to 1 g, 2 g, providing a concentration of 400 mg/mL, 500 mg/mL, respectively.
- To minimize injection site discomfort, give the IM injection deeply and slowly into the gluteus

maximus rather than the lateral aspect of the thigh.

IV

- Solution normally appears colorless to light yellow. Color change to deep yellow does not indicate loss of potency.
- IV infusion (piggyback) is stable for 24 hrs at room temperature, 96 hrs if refrigerated.
- Discard solution if precipitate forms.
- Reconstitute each 1 g with 10 mL Sterile Water for Injection to provide a concentration of 95 mg/mL.
- May further dilute with 50–100 mL 0.9% NaCl or D_5W.
- For IV push, administer over 3–5 min.
- For intermittent IV infusion (piggyback), infuse over 20–30 min.

Intervention and Evaluation

- Evaluate the patient's IV site for signs and symptoms of phlebitis as evidenced by heat, pain, and red streaking over the vein.
- Evaluate the patient's IM injection sites for induration and tenderness.
- Assess the patient's mouth for white patches on the mucous membranes and tongue.
- Assess the patient's pattern of daily bowel activity and stool consistency. Although mild GI effects may be tolerable, an increase in their severity may indicate the onset of antibiotic-associated colitis.
- Monitor renal function reports for nephrotoxicity.
- Be alert for signs and symptoms of superinfection including abdominal pain, moderate to severe diarrhea, severe anal or genital pruritus, and severe mouth soreness.

Patient/Family Teaching

- Explain to the patient/family that discomfort may occur with IM injection.
- Advise the patient/family to continue the antibiotic therapy for the full length of treatment and to space drug doses evenly around the clock.
- Warn the patient/family to avoid consuming alcohol and alcohol-containing preparations, such as cough syrups, salad dressings, and sauces, during treatment and for 72 hrs after the last dose of cefotetan.

Cefoxitin Sodium 

seh-**fox**-ih-tin

(Mefoxin)

Do not confuse with cefotaxime, cefotetan, or Cytoxan.

CATEGORY AND SCHEDULE

Pregnancy Risk Category: B

MECHANISM OF ACTION

A second-generation cephalosporin that binds to bacterial cell membranes. ***Therapeutic Effect:*** Inhibits synthesis of bacterial cell wall. Bactericidal.

AVAILABILITY

Powder for Injection: 1 g, 2 g, 10 g. *Premixed Infusion, Ready to Hang*: 1 g/50mL, 2 g/50mL.

INDICATIONS AND DOSAGES

▸ **Surgical prophylaxis**

IM/IV

Children older than 3 mos.

30–40 mg/kg 30–60 min before surgery and q6h postop for no more than 24 hrs.

▸ **Usual treatment**
IM/IV
Adolescents. 1–2 g q6–8h. Maximum: 12 g/day.
Children older than 3 mos. 80–160 mg/kg/day divided q6–8h. Maximum: 12 g/day.
Neonates. 90–100 mg/kg/day in divided doses q8h.

▸ **Dosage in renal impairment**
After a loading dose of 1–2 g, dosage and frequency are modified on the basis of creatinine clearance and the severity of infection.

Creatinine Clearance	Interval
30–50 mL/min	q8–12h
10–29 mL/min	q12–24h
less than 10 mL/min	q24–48h

CONTRAINDICATIONS
Anaphylactic reaction to penicillins, history of hypersensitivity to cephalosporins.

INTERACTIONS
Drug
Probenecid: Increases serum concentrations of cefoxitin.
Herbal
None known.
Food
None known.

DIAGNOSTIC TEST EFFECTS
Positive direct or indirect Coombs' test results may occur. Drug interferes with crossmatching procedures and hematologic tests. May increase BUN, serum alkaline phosphatase, serum creatinine, SGOT (AST), and SGPT (ALT) levels.

IV INCOMPATIBILITIES
Filgrastim (Neupogen), pentamidine (Pentam IV), vancomycin (Vancocin)

IV COMPATIBILITIES
Diltiazem (Cardizem), famotidine (Pepcid), heparin, hydromorphone (Dilaudid), magnesium sulfate, morphine, multivitamins, propofol (Diprivan)

SIDE EFFECTS
Frequent
Discomfort with IM administration, oral candidiasis (sore mouth or tongue), mild diarrhea, mild abdominal cramping, vaginal candidiasis (discharge, itching)
Occasional
Nausea, serum sickness reaction (fever, joint pain). Serum sickness reaction usually occurs after the second course of therapy and resolves after the drug is discontinued.
Rare
Allergic reaction (pruritus, rash, urticaria), thrombophlebitis (pain, redness, swelling at injection site)

SERIOUS REACTIONS
! Antibiotic-associated colitis manifested as severe abdominal pain and tenderness, fever, and watery and severe diarrhea and other superinfections may result from altered bacterial balance.
! Nephrotoxicity may occur, especially in pts with preexisting renal disease.
! Severe hypersensitivity reaction including severe pruritus, angioedema, bronchospasm, and anaphylaxis, particularly in those with history of allergies, especially to penicillins, may occur.

PEDIATRIC CONSIDERATIONS
Baseline Assessment
◂**ALERT**▸ Determine the patient's history of allergies, particularly to

cephalosporins and penicillins, before beginning drug therapy.
• Monitor age-appropriate fluid intake.
• Diarrhea may indicate drug toxicity.
• Monitor for increased bleeding time.

Precautions

• Use cautiously in pts with a history of GI disease, especially antibiotic-associated colitis or ulcerative colitis, and renal impairment.
• Use cautiously in pts concurrently using nephrotoxic medications.

Administration and Handling

◀ **ALERT** ▶ Give by IM, intermittent IV infusion (piggyback), or IV push.
◀ **ALERT** ▶ Space doses evenly around the clock.

IM

• Reconstitute each 1 g with 2 mL Sterile Water for Injection or 0.5% or 1% lidocaine to provide concentration of 400 mg/mL.
• Give deep IM injections slowly to minimize patient discomfort. To further minimize discomfort, administer IM injections into the gluteus maximus instead of the lateral aspect of the thigh.

IV

• Solution normally appears colorless to light amber but may darken (does not indicate loss of potency).
• IV infusion (piggyback) is stable for 24 hrs at room temperature, 48 hrs if refrigerated.
• Discard if precipitate forms.
• Reconstitute each 1 g with 10 mL Sterile Water for Injection to provide a concentration of 95 mg/mL.
• May further dilute with 50–100 mL Sterile Water for Injection, 0.9% NaCl, or D_5W.
• For IV push, administer over 3–5 min.
• For intermittent IV infusion (piggyback), infuse over 15–30 min.

Intervention and Evaluation

• Evaluate the patient's IV site for phlebitis as evidenced by heat, pain, and red streaking over the vein.
• Assess the patient's IM injection sites for induration and tenderness.
• Assess the patient's mouth for white patches on the mucous membranes and tongue.
• Assess the patient's pattern of daily bowel activity and stool consistency. Mild GI effects may be tolerable, but increasing severity may indicate the onset of antibiotic-associated colitis.
• Monitor the patient's intake and output and renal function reports for signs of nephrotoxicity.
• Be alert for signs and symptoms of superinfection including abdominal pain, moderate to severe diarrhea, severe anal or genital pruritus, and severe mouth soreness.

Patient/Family Teaching

• Explain to the patient/family that discomfort may occur with IM injection.
• Advise the patient/family to continue the antibiotic therapy for the full length of treatment and to space drug doses evenly around the clock.

Cefpodoxime Proxetil

sef-poe-**docks**-em
(Vantin)
Do not confuse with Ventolin.

CATEGORY AND SCHEDULE

Pregnancy Risk Category: B

MECHANISM OF ACTION

A third-generation cephalosporin that binds to bacterial cell membranes. ***Therapeutic Effect:*** Inhibits synthesis of bacterial cell wall. Bactericidal.

PHARMACOKINETICS

Well absorbed from the GI tract (food increases absorption). Protein binding: 21%–40%. Widely distributed. Primarily excreted unchanged in urine. Partially removed by hemodialysis. ***Half-Life:*** 2.3 hrs (half-life is increased in those with impaired renal function).

AVAILABILITY

Tablets: 100 mg, 200 mg.
Oral Suspension: 50 mg/5 mL, 100 mg/5 mL.

INDICATIONS AND DOSAGES

▸ Chronic bronchitis, pneumonia
PO
Children older than 13 yrs. 200 mg q12h for 10–14 days.

▸ Gonorrhea, rectal gonococcal infection (female patients only)
PO
Children older than 13 yrs. 200 mg as single dose.

▸ Skin and skin-structure infections
PO
Children older than 13 yrs. 400 mg q12h for 7–14 days.

▸ Pharyngitis, tonsillitis
PO
Children older than 13 yrs. 100 mg q12h for 5–10 days.
Children 6 mos–13 yrs. 5 mg/kg q12h for 5–10 days. Maximum: 100 mg/dose.

▸ Acute maxillary sinusitis
PO
Children older than 13 yrs. 200 mg 2 times/day for 10 days.
Children 2 mos–13 yrs. 5 mg/kg q12h for 10 days. Maximum: 400 mg/day.

▸ Urinary tract infection
PO
Children older than 13 yrs. 100 mg q12h for 7 days.

▸ Acute otitis media
PO
Children 6 mos–13 yrs. 5 mg/kg q12h for 5 days. Maximum: 400 mg/dose.

▸ Dosage in renal impairment
Dosage and frequency are based on the degree of renal impairment and creatinine clearance.
Creatinine clearance less than 30 mL/min. Dose q24h.
Pts on hemodialysis. 3 times/wk after dialysis.

CONTRAINDICATIONS

History of anaphylactic reaction to penicillins, hypersensitivity to cephalosporins.

INTERACTIONS

Drug

Antacids, H_2 antagonists: May decrease cefpodoxime absorption.
Probenecid: May increase cefpodoxime blood concentration.

Herbal

None known.

Food

None known.

DIAGNOSTIC TEST EFFECTS

Positive direct or indirect Coombs' test results. May increase BUN, serum alkaline phosphatase, serum bilirubin, serum creatinine, serum lactate dehydrogenase, SGOT (AST), and SGPT (ALT) levels.

SIDE EFFECTS

Frequent

Oral candidiasis (sore mouth or tongue), mild diarrhea, mild abdominal cramping, vaginal candidiasis (discharge, itching)

Occasional

Nausea, serum sickness reaction (fever, joint pain)

Serum sickness reaction usually occurs after the second course of therapy and resolves after the drug is discontinued.

Rare

Allergic reaction (pruritus, rash, urticaria)

SERIOUS REACTIONS

! Antibiotic-associated colitis manifested as severe abdominal pain and tenderness, fever, and watery and severe diarrhea and other superinfections may result from altered bacterial balance.

! Nephrotoxicity may occur, especially in pts with preexisting renal disease.

! Severe hypersensitivity reaction including severe pruritus, angioedema, bronchospasm, and anaphylaxis, particularly in pts with a history of allergies, especially to penicillins, may occur.

PEDIATRIC CONSIDERATIONS

Baseline Assessment

◀ALERT▶ Determine the patient's history of allergies, particularly to cephalosporins and penicillins, before beginning drug therapy.

- Be aware that cefpodoxime readily crosses the placenta and is distributed in breast milk.
- Be aware that the safety and efficacy of cefpodoxime have not been established in children younger than 6 mos.
- Assess for age-appropriate fluid intake.
- Monitor for increased bleeding time.
- Diarrhea may indicate drug toxicity.

Precautions

- Use cautiously in pts with a history of allergies or GI disease, especially antibiotic-associated colitis or ulcerative colitis, and renal impairment.
- Use cautiously in pts concurrently using nephrotoxic medications.

Administration and Handling

PO

- Administer with food to enhance drug absorption.
- After reconstitution, oral suspension is stable for 14 days if refrigerated.

Intervention and Evaluation

- Assess the patient's mouth for white patches on the mucous membranes and tongue.
- Assess the patient's pattern of daily bowel activity and stool consistency. Mild GI effects may be tolerable, but increasing severity may indicate the onset of antibiotic-associated colitis.
- Monitor the patient's intake and output and renal function reports for signs of nephrotoxicity.
- Be alert for signs and symptoms of superinfection including abdominal pain, moderate to severe diarrhea, severe anal or genital pruritus, and severe mouth soreness.

Patient/Family Teaching

- Advise the patient/family to continue cefpodoxime therapy for the full length of treatment and to space drug doses evenly around the clock.
- Instruct the patient/family to refrigerate the oral suspension, to shake the oral suspension well before using, and to take the oral suspension with food.

Cefprozil

sef-**proz**-ill
(Cefzil)
Do not confuse with Cefazolin or Ceftin.

CATEGORY AND SCHEDULE

Pregnancy Risk Category: B

MECHANISM OF ACTION

A second-generation cephalosporin that binds to bacterial cell membranes. ***Therapeutic Effect:*** Inhibits synthesis of bacterial cell wall. Bactericidal.

PHARMACOKINETICS

Well absorbed from the GI tract. Protein binding: 36%–45%. Widely distributed. Primarily excreted unchanged in urine. Moderately removed by hemodialysis. ***Half-Life:*** 1.3 hrs (half-life is increased in those with impaired renal function).

AVAILABILITY

Tablets: 250 mg, 500 mg.
Oral Suspension: 125 mg/5 mL, 250 mg/5 mL.

INDICATIONS AND DOSAGES

▸ Pharyngitis, tonsillitis
PO
Children 2–12 yrs. 7.5 mg/kg q12h for 10 days.

▸ Skin and skin-structure infections
PO
Children. 20 mg/kg q24h for 10 days.

Acute sinusitis
▸ PO
Children 6 mos–12 yrs. 7.5–15 mg/kg q12h for 10 days.

▸ Otitis media
PO
Children 6 mos–12 yrs.
15 mg/kg q12h for 10 days.
Maximum: 1 g/day.

▸ Dosage in renal impairment
Dosage and frequency are based on the degree of renal impairment and creatinine clearance.
Creatinine clearance less than 30 mL/min. 50% dosage at usual interval.

CONTRAINDICATIONS

History of anaphylactic reaction to penicillins, hypersensitivity to cephalosporins.

INTERACTIONS

Drug
Probenecid: Increases serum concentrations of cefprozil.
Herbal
None known.
Food
None known.

DIAGNOSTIC TEST EFFECTS

Positive direct or indirect Coombs' test results may occur. Drug interferes with crossmatching procedures and hematologic tests. May increase liver function test results.

SIDE EFFECTS

Frequent
Oral candidiasis (sore mouth or tongue), mild diarrhea, mild abdominal cramping, vaginal candidiasis (discharge, itching)
Occasional
Nausea, serum sickness reaction (fever, joint pain)
Serum sickness reaction usually occurs after the second course of therapy and resolves after the drug is discontinued.

Rare
Allergic reaction (pruritus, rash, urticaria)

SERIOUS REACTIONS

! Antibiotic-associated colitis manifested as severe abdominal pain and tenderness, fever, and watery and severe diarrhea and other superinfections may result from altered bacterial balance.
! Nephrotoxicity may occur, especially in pts with preexisting renal disease.
! Severe hypersensitivity reaction including severe pruritus, angioedema, bronchospasm, and anaphylaxis, particularly in pts with a history of allergies, especially to penicillins, may occur.

PEDIATRIC CONSIDERATIONS

Baseline Assessment
◀ ALERT ▶ Determine the patient's history of allergies, particularly to cephalosporins and penicillins before beginning drug therapy.
• Be aware that cefprozil readily crosses the placenta and is distributed in breast milk.
• Be aware that the safety and efficacy of cefprozil have not been established in children younger than 6 mos.
• Diarrhea may indicate drug toxicity.
• Monitor and assess for increased bleeding time.
• Maintain age-appropriate fluid intake.

Precautions
• Use cautiously in pts with a history of GI disease, especially antibiotic-associated colitis or ulcerative colitis, and renal impairment.
• Use cautiously in pts concurrently using nephrotoxic medications.

Administration and Handling
PO
• After reconstitution, oral suspension is stable for 14 days if refrigerated.
• Shake oral suspension well before using.
• Give without regard to meals; if GI upset occurs, give with food or milk.

Intervention and Evaluation
• Assess the patient's mouth for white patches on the mucous membranes and tongue.
• Assess the patient's pattern of daily bowel activity and stool consistency. Mild GI effects may be tolerable, but increasing severity may indicate the onset of antibiotic-associated colitis.
• Monitor the patient's intake and output and renal function reports for signs of nephrotoxicity.
• Be alert for signs and symptoms of superinfection including abdominal pain, moderate to severe diarrhea, severe anal or genital pruritus, and severe mouth soreness.

Patient/Family Teaching
• Advise the patient/family to continue cefprozil therapy for the full length of treatment and to evenly space drug doses around the clock.
• Explain to the patient/family that cefprozil may cause GI upset. Instruct the patient to take the drug with food or milk if GI upset occurs.

Ceftazidime

sef-**taz**-ih-deem
(Ceptaz, Fortaz, Fortum [AUS], Tazicef, Tazidime)
Do not confuse with ceftizoxime.

CATEGORY AND SCHEDULE

Pregnancy Risk Category: B

MECHANISM OF ACTION

A third-generation cephalosporin that binds to bacterial cell membranes. ***Therapeutic Effect:*** Inhibits synthesis of bacterial cell wall. Bactericidal.

PHARMACOKINETICS

Widely distributed (including cerebrospinal fluid). Protein binding: 5%–17%. Primarily excreted unchanged in urine. Removed by hemodialysis. ***Half-Life:*** 2 hrs (half-life is increased in those with impaired renal function).

AVAILABILITY

Powder for Injection: 500 mg, 1 g, 2 g, 6 g.
Premixed, Ready to Hang Infusion: 1 g/50 mL, 2 g/50 mL.

INDICATIONS AND DOSAGES

Children 1 mo–12 yrs. 100–150 mg/kg/day in divided doses q8h. Maximum: 6 g/day.
Neonates 7 days or older. 1,200 g or greater usual dose: 150 mg/kg/day divided q8h. Less than 1,200 g usual dose: 100 mg/kg/day divided q12h.
Neonates younger than 7 days old. 100 mg/kg/day divided q12h.

▸ **Meningitis**

IV/IM
Infants and children. 150 mg/kg/day divided q8h.

▸ **Cystic fibrosis**

IV/IM
Infants and children. 50 mg/kg/day divided q8h. Maximum dose: 6 g/day.

▸ **Dosage in renal impairment**

After initial 1-g dose, dosage and frequency are modified on the basis of creatinine clearance and the severity of infection.

Creatinine Clearance	Dosage Interval
30–50 mL/min	q12h
10–30 mL/min	q24h
less than 10 mL/min	q24–48h

CONTRAINDICATIONS

History of anaphylactic reaction to penicillins, hypersensitivity to cephalosporins.

INTERACTIONS

Drug

Probenecid: Increases blood concentrations of ceftazidime
Aminoglycosides: Increases risk of nephrotoxicity.

Herbal

None known.

Food

None known.

DIAGNOSTIC TEST EFFECTS

Positive direct or indirect Coombs' test results. Drug interfere with crossmatching procedures and hematologic tests. May increase BUN, serum alkaline phosphatase, serum creatinine, serum lactate dehydrogenase, SGOT (AST), and SGPT (ALT) levels.

IV INCOMPATIBILITIES

Amphotericin B complex (AmBisome, Amphotec, Abelcet), doxorubicin liposome (Doxil), fluconazole (Diflucan), idarubicin (Idamycin), midazolam (Versed), pentamidine (Pentam IV), vancomycin (Vancocin)

IV COMPATIBILITIES

Diltiazem (Cardizem), famotidine (Pepcid), heparin, hydromorphone (Dilaudid), morphine, propofol (Diprivan)

SIDE EFFECTS

Frequent

Discomfort with IM administration, oral candidiasis (sore mouth or tongue), mild diarrhea, mild abdominal cramping, vaginal candidiasis (discharge, itching)

Occasional

Nausea, serum sickness reaction (fever, joint pain)

Serum sickness reaction usually occurs after the second course of therapy and resolves after the drug is discontinued.

Rare

Allergic reaction (pruritus, rash, urticaria), thrombophlebitis (pain, redness, swelling at injection site)

SERIOUS REACTIONS

! Antibiotic-associated colitis manifested as severe abdominal pain and tenderness, fever, and watery and severe diarrhea and other superinfections may result from altered bacterial balance.

! Nephrotoxicity may occur, especially in pts with preexisting renal disease.

! Severe hypersensitivity reaction including severe pruritus, angioedema, bronchospasm, and anaphylaxis, particularly in pts with a history of allergies, especially to penicillins, may occur.

PEDIATRIC CONSIDERATIONS

Baseline Assessment

◂ALERT▸ Determine the patient's history of allergies, particularly to cephalosporins and penicillins, before beginning drug therapy.

• Be aware that ceftazidime readily crosses the placenta and is distributed in breast milk.

• There are no age-related precautions noted in children.

• Diarrhea may indicate drug toxicity.

• Assess for age-appropriate fluid intake.

• Monitor for increased bleeding time.

Precautions

• Use cautiously in pts with a history of GI disease, especially antibiotic-associated colitis or ulcerative colitis, and renal impairment.

• Use cautiously in pts concurrently using nephrotoxic medications.

Administration and Handling

◂ALERT▸ Give by IM injection, direct IV injection, or intermittent IV infusion (piggyback).

IM

• For reconstitution, add 1.5 mL Sterile Water for Injection or lidocaine 1% to 500 mg, if prescribed, or 3 mL to 1-g vial to provide a concentration of 280 mg/mL.

• Give deep IM injections slowly to minimize patient discomfort. To further minimize discomfort, administer IM injections into the gluteus maximus instead of the lateral aspect of the thigh.

IV

• Solution normally appears light yellow to amber, tends to darken (color change does not indicate loss of potency).

• IV infusion (piggyback) stable for 18 hrs at room temperature, 7 days if refrigerated.

• Discard if precipitate forms.

• Add 10 mL Sterile Water for Injection to each 1 g to provide concentration of 90 mg/mL.

• May further dilute with 50–100 mL 0.9% NaCl, D_5W, or other compatible diluent.

• For IV push, administer over 3–5 min.

• For intermittent IV infusion (piggyback), infuse over 15–30 min.

Intervention and Evaluation

• Evaluate the patient's IV site for phlebitis as evidenced by heat, pain, and red streaking over the vein.
• Assess the patient's IM injection site for induration and tenderness.
• Assess the patient's mouth for white patches on the mucous membranes or tongue.
• Assess the patient's pattern of daily bowel activity and stool consistency. Mild GI effects may be tolerable, but increasing severity may indicate the onset of antibiotic-associated colitis.
• Monitor the patient's intake and output and renal function reports for signs of nephrotoxicity.
• Be alert for signs and symptoms of superinfection including abdominal pain, moderate to severe diarrhea, severe anal or genital pruritus, and severe mouth soreness.

Patient/Family Teaching

• Explain to the patient/family that discomfort may occur with IM injection.
• Advise the patient/family to continue ceftazidime therapy for the full length of treatment and explain that doses will be evenly spaced around the clock.

Ceftibuten

sef-tih-**byew**-ten
(Cedax)

CATEGORY AND SCHEDULE

Pregnancy Risk Category: B

MECHANISM OF ACTION

A third-generation cephalosporin that binds to bacterial cell membranes. ***Therapeutic Effect:*** Inhibits bacterial cell wall synthesis. Bactericidal.

AVAILABILITY

Capsules: 400 mg.
Oral Suspension: 90 mg/5 mL.

INDICATIONS AND DOSAGES

▸ **Chronic bronchitis, acute bacterial otitis media, pharyngitis, tonsillitis**
PO
Children 12 yrs and older. 400 mg/day as single daily dose for 10 days.
Children younger than 12 yrs. 9 mg/kg/day as single daily dose for 10 days. Maximum: 400 mg/day.

▸ **Dosage in renal impairment**
Based on creatinine clearance.

Creatinine Clearance	Dosage
greater than 50 mL/min	400 mg or 9 mg/kg q24h
30–49 mL/min	200 mg or 4.5 mg/kg q24h
less than 30 mL/min	100 mg or 2.25 mg/kg q24h

CONTRAINDICATIONS

Hypersensitivity to cephalosporins

INTERACTIONS

Drug

Aminoglycosides: Increased risk of nephrotoxicity with concurrent use of drugs in this class.
Probenecid: Increases serum levels of cephalosporins.

Herbal

None known.

Food

None known.

DIAGNOSTIC TEST EFFECTS

Positive direct or indirect Coombs' test results. May increase BUN, serum alkaline phosphatase, serum bilirubin, serum creatinine, serum lactate dehydrogenase, SGOT (AST), and SGPT (ALT) levels.

SIDE EFFECTS

Frequent
Oral candidiasis (sore mouth or tongue), mild diarrhea, mild abdominal cramping, vaginal candidiasis (discharge, itching)

Occasional
Nausea, serum sickness reaction (fever, joint pain)
Serum sickness reaction usually occurs after the second course of therapy and resolves after the drug is discontinued.

Rare
Allergic reaction (rash, pruritus, urticaria)

SERIOUS REACTIONS

! Antibiotic-associated colitis manifested as severe abdominal pain and tenderness, fever, and watery and severe diarrhea and other superinfections may result from altered bacterial balance.
! Nephrotoxicity may occur, especially in pts with preexisting renal disease.
! Severe hypersensitivity reaction including severe pruritus, angioedema, bronchospasm, and anaphylaxis, particularly in pts with a history of allergies, especially to penicillins, may occur.

PEDIATRIC CONSIDERATIONS

Baseline Assessment
◂ALERT▸ Determine the patient's history of allergies, particularly to cephalosporins and penicillins, before beginning drug therapy.

Precautions
• Use cautiously in pts with a history of allergies or GI disease (especially antibiotic-associated colitis or ulcerative colitis), hypersensitivity to penicillins or other drugs, and renal impairment.

Administration and Handling
◂ALERT▸ Use this drug's oral suspension to treat otitis media to achieve higher peak blood levels.

Intervention and Evaluation
• Assess the patient's mouth for white patches on the mucous membranes and tongue.
• Assess the patient's pattern of daily bowel activity and stool consistency. Mild GI effects may be tolerable, but increasing severity may indicate the onset of antibiotic-associated colitis.
• Monitor the patient's intake and output and renal function reports for signs of nephrotoxicity.
• Be alert for signs and symptoms of superinfection including abdominal pain, moderate to severe diarrhea, severe anal or genital pruritus, and severe mouth soreness.

Patient/Family Teaching
• Advise the patient/family to continue ceftibuten therapy for the full length of treatment and to space drug doses evenly around the clock.
• Explain to the patient/family that ceftibuten may cause GI upset. Instruct the patient to take the drug with food or milk if GI upset occurs.

Ceftizoxime Sodium

cef-tih-**zox**-eem
(Cefizox)
Do not confuse with cefotaxime or ceftazidime.

CATEGORY AND SCHEDULE

Pregnancy Risk Category: B

MECHANISM OF ACTION

A third-generation cephalosporin that binds to bacterial cell membranes. ***Therapeutic Effect:*** Inhibits synthesis of bacterial cell wall. Bactericidal.

PHARMACOKINETICS

Widely distributed (including cerebrospinal fluid). Protein binding: 30%. Primarily excreted unchanged in urine. Moderately removed by hemodialysis. ***Half-Life:*** 1.7 hrs (half-life is increased in those with impaired renal function).

AVAILABILITY

Powder for Injection: 1 g, 2 g, 10 g.
Premixed, Ready to Hang Infusion: 1 g/50 mL, 2 g/50 mL.

INDICATIONS AND DOSAGES

Children older than 6 mos. 50 mg/kg q6–8h. Maximum: 12 g/day.

▸ **Dosage in renal impairment**

After a loading dose of 0.5–1 g, dosage and frequency are modified on the basis of creatinine clearance and the severity of infection.

Creatinine Clearance	Dosage Interval
50–80 mL/min	q8–12h
10–50 mL/min	q36–48h
less than 10 mL/min	q48–72h

CONTRAINDICATIONS

History of anaphylactic reaction to penicillins, hypersensitivity to cephalosporins.

INTERACTIONS

Drug

Probenecid: Increases serum concentration of ceftizoxime.

Herbal

None known.

Food

None known.

DIAGNOSTIC TEST EFFECTS

Positive direct or indirect Coombs' test results may occur. May increase BUN, serum alkaline serum phosphatase, serum creatinine, SGOT (AST), and SGPT (ALT) levels.

IV INCOMPATIBILITIES

Filgrastim (Neupogen)

IV COMPATIBILITIES

Hydromorphone (Dilaudid), morphine, propofol (Diprivan)

SIDE EFFECTS

Frequent

Discomfort with IM administration, oral candidiasis (sore mouth or tongue), mild diarrhea, mild abdominal cramping, vaginal candidiasis (discharge, itching)

Occasional

Nausea, serum sickness reaction (fever, joint pain)
Serum sickness reaction usually occurs after the second course of therapy and resolves after the drug is discontinued.

Rare

Allergic reaction (rash, pruritus, urticaria), thrombophlebitis (pain, redness, swelling at injection site)

SERIOUS REACTIONS

! Antibiotic-associated colitis manifested as severe abdominal pain and tenderness, fever, and watery and severe diarrhea and other superinfections may result from altered bacterial balance.

! Nephrotoxicity may occur, especially in pts with preexisting renal disease.

! Severe hypersensitivity reaction including severe pruritus, angioedema, bronchospasm, and anaphylaxis, particularly in pts with a history of allergies, especially to penicillins, may occur.

PEDIATRIC CONSIDERATIONS

Baseline Assessment

◀ALERT▶ Determine the patient's history of allergies, particularly to cephalosporins and penicillins, before beginning drug therapy.

- Be aware that ceftizoxime readily crosses the placenta and is distributed in breast milk.
- Be aware that ceftizoxime use in children is associated with transient elevations of blood eosinophil and serum creatine kinase, SGOT (AST), and SGPT (ALT) levels.
- Assess for age-appropriate fluid intake.
- Diarrhea may indicate drug toxicity.

Precautions

- Use cautiously in pts with a history of GI disease, especially antibiotic-associated colitis or ulcerative colitis, and liver or renal impairment.

Administration and Handling

IM

- Add 1.5 mL Sterile Water for Injection to each 0.5 g to provide concentration of 270 mg/mL.
- Give deep IM injections slowly to minimize patient discomfort.
- When giving 2-g dose, divide dose and give in different large muscle masses.

IV

- Solution normally appears clear to pale yellow. Color change from yellow to amber does not indicate loss of potency.
- IV infusion (piggyback) is stable for 24 hrs at room temperature, 96 hrs if refrigerated.
- Discard if precipitate forms.
- Add 5 mL Sterile Water for Injection to each 0.5 g to provide concentration of 95 mg/mL.
- May further dilute with 50–100 mL 0.9% NaCl, D_5W, or other compatible fluid.
- For IV push, administer over 3–5 min.
- For intermittent IV infusion (piggyback), infuse over 15–30 min.

Intervention and Evaluation

- Assess the patient's mouth for white patches on the mucous membranes and tongue.
- Assess the patient's pattern of daily bowel activity and stool consistency. Mild GI effects may be tolerable, but increasing severity may indicate the onset of antibiotic-associated colitis.
- Monitor the patient's intake and output and renal function reports for signs of nephrotoxicity.
- Be alert for signs and symptoms of superinfection including abdominal pain, moderate to severe diarrhea, severe anal or genital pruritus, and severe mouth soreness.

Patient/Family Teaching

- Advise the patient/family to continue ceftizoxime therapy for the full length of treatment and explain that the doses will be evenly spaced around the clock.
- Explain to the patient/family that discomfort may occur with IM injection.

Ceftriaxone Sodium

cef-try-**ax**-zone
(Rocephin)

CATEGORY AND SCHEDULE

Pregnancy Risk Category: B

MECHANISM OF ACTION

A third-generation cephalosporin that binds to bacterial cell membranes. ***Therapeutic Effect:*** Inhibits synthesis of bacterial cell wall. Bactericidal.

PHARMACOKINETICS

Widely distributed (including cerebrospinal fluid). Protein binding: 83%–96%. Primarily excreted unchanged in urine. Not removed by hemodialysis. ***Half-Life:*** 4.3–4.6 hrs IV; 5.8–8.7 hrs IM (half-life is increased in those with impaired renal function).

AVAILABILITY

Powder for Injection: 250 mg, 500 mg, 1 g, 2 g.
Premixed, Ready-to-Hang Infusion: 1 g/50 mL, 2 g/50 mL.

INDICATIONS AND DOSAGES

▸ Serious respiratory and GU tract, bone, intra-abdominal, and biliary tract infections and septicemia

IM/IV

Children. 50–75 mg/kg/day in divided doses q12h. Maximum: 2 g/day.

▸ Skin and skin-structure infections

IM/IV

Children. 50–75 mg/kg/day as single or 2 divided doses. Maximum: 2 g/day.

▸ Meningitis

IV

Children. Initially, 75 mg/kg loading dose, then 100 mg/kg/day as single or in divided doses q12h. Maximum: 4 g/day.

▸ Acute bacterial otitis media

IM

Children. 50 mg/kg/day as single dose. Maximum: 1 g/day.

▸ Relapsing acute otitis media

Children. 50 mg/kg as a single dose for 3 days. Maximum: 1 g/day.

▸ Gonococcal Infections

IM

Conjunctivitis. 50 mg/kg once (max dose 1 g)

Uncomplicated. 125 mg once

IM/IV

Complicated—Neonates. 25–50 mg/kg/day p24h for 7 days (max 125 mg)

Complicated—Children. 50 mg/kg/day once daily for 7 days (max 1 g)

Meningitis—Neonates. 25–50 mg/kg/day p24h for 14 days (max 125 mg)

Meningitis—Children. 50 mg/kg/day divided q12h for 14 days (max 2 g)

▸ Dosage in renal impairment

Dosage modification is usually unnecessary.

CONTRAINDICATIONS

History of anaphylactic reaction to penicillins, hypersensitivity to cephalosporins.
Do not use in neonates with hyperbilirubinemia because ceftriaxone can displace bilirubin from albumin binding sites and increase the risk for kernicterus.

INTERACTIONS

Drug

Probenecid: May increase blood concentration of ceftriaxone.
Aminoglycosides: May increase the risk for nephrotoxicity.

Herbal

None known.

Food

None known.

DIAGNOSTIC TEST EFFECTS

Positive direct or indirect Coombs' test results may occur. Drug interferes with crossmatching procedures and hematologic tests. May increase BUN, serum alkaline phosphatase, bilirubin, creatinine, SGOT (AST), and SGPT (ALT) levels.

IV INCOMPATIBILITIES

Aminophylline, amphotericin B complex (AmBisome, Amphotec, Abelcet), filgrastim (Neupogen), fluconazole (Diflucan), labetalol (Normodyne), pentamidine (Pentam IV), vancomycin (Vancocin)

IV COMPATIBILITIES

Diltiazem (Cardizem), heparin, lidocaine, morphine, propofol (Diprivan)

SIDE EFFECTS

Frequent

Discomfort with IM administration, oral candidiasis (sore mouth or tongue), mild diarrhea, mild abdominal cramping, vaginal candidiasis (discharge, itching)

Occasional

Nausea, serum sickness reaction (fever, joint pain)

Serum sickness reaction usually occurs after the second course of therapy and resolves after the drug is discontinued.

Rare

Allergic reaction (rash, pruritus, urticaria), thrombophlebitis (pain, redness, swelling at injection site)

SERIOUS REACTIONS

! Antibiotic-associated colitis manifested as severe abdominal pain and tenderness, fever, and watery and severe diarrhea and other superinfections may result from altered bacterial balance.

! Nephrotoxicity may occur, especially in pts with preexisting renal disease.

! Severe hypersensitivity reaction including severe pruritus, angioedema, bronchospasm, and anaphylaxis, particularly in pts with a history of allergies, especially to penicillins, may occur.

PEDIATRIC CONSIDERATIONS

Baseline Assessment

◂ALERT▸ Determine the patient's history of allergies, particularly to cephalosporins and penicillins, before beginning drug therapy.

- Be aware that ceftriaxone readily crosses the placenta and is distributed in breast milk.
- Be aware that ceftriaxone use in children may displace serum bilirubin from serum albumin.
- Use ceftriaxone with caution in neonates, who may become hyperbilirubinemic.
- Be aware that ceftriaxone use can lead to false increases in liver function tests.
- Diarrhea may indicate drug toxicity.
- Monitor for increased bleeding time.

Precautions

- Use cautiously in pts with a history of allergies or GI disease, especially antibiotic-associated colitis or ulcerative colitis, and liver or renal impairment.
- Use cautiously in pts concurrently using nephrotoxic medications.

Administration and Handling

IM

- Add 0.9 mL Sterile Water for Injection, 0.9% NaCl, D_5W,

Bacteriostatic Water and 0.9% Benzyl Alcohol or lidocaine to each 250 mg to provide concentration of 250 mg/mL.
• Give deep IM injections slowly to minimize patient discomfort. To further minimize discomfort, administer IM injections into the gluteus maximus instead of the lateral aspect of the thigh.

IV

• Solution normally appears light yellow to amber.
• IV infusion (piggyback) is stable for 3 days at room temperature, 10 days if refrigerated.
• Discard if precipitate forms.
• Add 2.4 mL Sterile Water for Injection to each 250 mg to provide concentration of 100 mg/mL.
• May further dilute with 50–100 mL 0.9% NaCl or D_5W.
• For intermittent IV infusion (piggyback), infuse over 15–30 min for adults or 10–30 min in children and neonates.
• Alternate IV sites and use large veins to reduce the potential for phlebitis development.

Intervention and Evaluation

• Assess the patient's mouth for white patches on the mucous membranes and tongue.
• Assess the patient's pattern of daily bowel activity and stool consistency. Mild GI effects may be tolerable, but increasing severity may indicate the onset of antibiotic-associated colitis.
• Monitor the patient's intake and output and renal function reports for nephrotoxicity.
• Be alert for signs and symptoms of superinfection including abdominal pain, moderate to severe diarrhea, severe anal or genital pruritus, and severe mouth soreness.

Patient/Family Teaching

• Advise the patient/family to continue ceftriaxone therapy for the full length of treatment and explain that doses will be evenly spaced around the clock.
• Explain to the patient/family that discomfort may occur with IM injection.

Cefuroxime Axetil

sef-yur-**ox**-ime
(Ceftin, Zinnat [AUS])
Do not confuse with cefotaxime or Cefzil.
cefuroxime sodium
(Kefurox, Zinacef)
(See Color Plates)

CATEGORY AND SCHEDULE

Pregnancy Risk Category: B

MECHANISM OF ACTION

A second-generation cephalosporin that binds to bacterial cell membranes. ***Therapeutic Effect:*** Inhibits synthesis of bacterial cell wall. Bactericidal.

PHARMACOKINETICS

Rapidly absorbed from the GI tract. Protein binding: 33%–50%. Widely distributed (including cerebrospinal fluid). Primarily excreted unchanged in urine. Moderately removed by hemodialysis. ***Half-Life:*** 1.3 hrs (half-life is increased in those with impaired renal function).

AVAILABILITY

Tablets: 250 mg, 500 mg.
Oral Suspension: 125 mg/5 mL, 250 mg/5 mL.
Powder for Injection: 750 mg, 1.5 g.

Premixed, Ready-to-Hang Infusion: 750 mg/50 mL, 1.5 g/50 mL

INDICATIONS AND DOSAGES

▸ **Ampicillin-resistant influenza; bacterial meningitis; early Lyme disease; GU tract, gynecologic, skin, and bone infections; septicemia; gonorrhea and other gonococcal infections**

IM/IV

Children. 75–150 mg/kg/day divided q8h. Maximum: 6 g/day.
Neonates. 50–100 mg/kg/day divided q12h.

▸ **Pharyngitis, tonsillitis**

PO

Children 3 mos–12 yrs. Tablets: 125 mg q12h. Suspension: 20 mg/kg/day in 2 divided doses. Maximum: 500 mg/day.

▸ **Acute otitis media, acute bacterial maxillary sinusitis, impetigo**

PO

Children 3 mos–12 yrs. Tablets: 250 mg q12h. Suspension: 30 mg/kg/day in 2 divided doses. Maximum: 1 g/day.

▸ **Bacterial meningitis**

IV

Children 3 mos–12 yrs. 200–240 mg/kg/day in divided doses q6–8h. Maximum: 9 g/day.

▸ **Usual neonate dosage**

IM/IV

Neonates. 50–100 mg/kg/day in divided doses q12h.

▸ **Dosage in renal impairment**

Adult dosage is modified on the basis of creatinine clearance and the severity of infection.

Creatinine Clearance	Dosage Interval
10–20 mL/min	q12h
less than 10 mL/min	q24h

CONTRAINDICATIONS

History of anaphylactic reaction to penicillins, hypersensitivity to cephalosporins.

INTERACTIONS

Drug

Probenecid: Increases serum concentration of cefuroxime.

Herbal

None known.

Food

None known.

DIAGNOSTIC TEST EFFECTS

Positive direct or indirect Coombs' test results may occur. Drug interferes with crossmatching procedures and hematologic tests. May increase serum alkaline phosphatase, serum bilirubin, serum lactate dehydrogenase, SGOT (AST), and SGPT (ALT) levels.

IV INCOMPATIBILITIES

Filgrastim (Neupogen), fluconazole (Diflucan), midazolam (Versed), vancomycin (Vancocin)

IV COMPATIBILITIES

Diltiazem (Cardizem), hydromorphone (Dilaudid), morphine, propofol (Diprivan)

SIDE EFFECTS

Frequent

Discomfort with IM administration, oral candidiasis (sore mouth or tongue), mild diarrhea, mild abdominal cramping, vaginal candidiasis (discharge, itching)

Occasional

Nausea, serum sickness reaction (fever, joint pain)

Serum sickness reaction usually occurs after the second course of therapy and resolves after the drug is discontinued.

Rare

Allergic reaction (rash, pruritus, urticaria), thrombophlebitis (pain, redness, swelling at injection site)

SERIOUS REACTIONS

! Antibiotic-associated colitis manifested as severe abdominal pain and tenderness, fever, and watery and severe diarrhea and other superinfections may result from altered bacterial balance.

! Nephrotoxicity may occur, especially in pts with preexisting renal disease.

! Severe hypersensitivity reaction including severe pruritus, angioedema, bronchospasm, and anaphylaxis, particularly in pts with a history of allergies, especially to penicillins, may occur.

PEDIATRIC CONSIDERATIONS

Baseline Assessment

◂ALERT▸ Determine the patient's history of allergies, particularly to cephalosporins and penicillins, before beginning drug therapy.

• Be aware that cefuroxime readily crosses the placenta and is distributed in breast milk.

• If a child has difficulty swallowing the tablet whole, provide fluids before/after administration.

• Assess for age-appropriate fluid intake.

• Diarrhea may indicate drug toxicity.

• Assess for prolonged bleeding time.

Precautions

• Use cautiously in pts with a history of GI disease, especially antibiotic-associated colitis or ulcerative colitis, and renal impairment.

• Use cautiously in pts concurrently using nephrotoxic medications.

Administration and Handling

PO

• Give without regard to meals. If GI upset occurs, give with food or milk.

• Avoid crushing tablets because of a bitter taste.

• Suspension must be given with food.

IM

• Give deep IM injections slowly to minimize patient discomfort. To further minimize discomfort, administer IM injections into the gluteus maximus instead of the lateral aspect of the thigh.

IV

• Solution normally appears light yellow to amber; may darken, but color change does not indicate loss of potency

• IV infusion (piggyback) is stable for 24 hrs at room temperature, 7 days if refrigerated.

• Discard if precipitate forms.

• Reconstitute 750 mg in 8 mL (1.5 g in 14 mL) Sterile Water for Injection to provide a concentration of 100 mg/mL.

• For intermittent IV infusion (piggyback), further dilute with 50–100 mL 0.9% NaCl or D_5W.

• For IV push, administer over 3–5 min.

• For intermittent IV infusion (piggyback), infuse over 15–60 min.

Intervention and Evaluation

• Assess the patient's mouth for white patches on the mucous membranes and tongue.

• Assess the patient's pattern of daily bowel activity and stool consistency. Mild GI effects may be tolerable, but increasing severity may indicate the onset of antibiotic-associated colitis.

• Monitor the patient's intake and output and renal function reports for signs of nephrotoxicity.
• Be alert for signs and symptoms of superinfection including abdominal pain, moderate to severe diarrhea, severe anal or genital pruritus, and severe mouth soreness.

Patient/Family Teaching

• Advise the patient/family to continue cefuroxime therapy for the full length of treatment and to space drug doses evenly around the clock.
• Explain to the patient/family that cefuroxime may cause GI upset. Instruct the patient to take the drug with food or milk if GI upset occurs.
• Explain to the patient/family that discomfort may occur with IM injection.

Cephalexin

cef-ah-**lex**-in
(Apo-Cephalex [CAN], Ceporex [AUS], Ibilex [AUS], Keflex, Keftab, Novo-Lexin [CAN])

CATEGORY AND SCHEDULE

Pregnancy Risk Category: B

MECHANISM OF ACTION

A first-generation cephalosporin that binds to bacterial cell membranes. ***Therapeutic Effect:*** Inhibits synthesis of bacterial cell wall. Bactericidal.

PHARMACOKINETICS

Rapidly absorbed from the GI tract. Absorption may be delayed in young children and neonates. Protein binding: 10%–15%. Widely distributed. Primarily excreted unchanged in urine. Moderately removed by hemodialysis.

Half-Life: Young children, 2.5 hrs; Adults, 0.9–1.2 hrs (half-life is increased in those with impaired renal function).

AVAILABILITY

Capsules: 250 mg, 500 mg.
Tablets: 250 mg, 500 mg, 1 g.
Oral Suspension: 125 mg/5 mL, 250 mg/5 mL.

INDICATIONS AND DOSAGES

Children. 25–100 mg/kg/day in 2–4 divided doses. Maximum: 4 g/day.

▸ Otitis media

PO

Children. 75–100 mg/kg/day in 4 divided doses.

▸ Dosage in renal impairment

After usual initial dose, dosage and frequency are modified on the basis of creatinine clearance and the severity of infection.

Creatinine Clearance	Dosage Interval
10–40 mL/min	q8–12h
less than 10 mL/min	q12–24h

CONTRAINDICATIONS

History of anaphylactic reaction to penicillins, hypersensitivity to cephalosporins.

INTERACTIONS

Drug

Probenecid: Increases serum concentration of cephalexin.

Herbal

None known.

Food

None known.

DIAGNOSTIC TEST EFFECTS

Positive direct or indirect Coombs' test results may occur. Drug interferes with crossmatching procedures and hematologic tests. May increase serum alkaline phosphatase, SGOT (AST), and SGPT (ALT) levels.

SIDE EFFECTS

Frequent

Oral candidiasis (sore mouth or tongue), mild diarrhea, mild abdominal cramping, vaginal candidiasis (discharge, itching)

Occasional

Nausea, serum sickness reaction (fever, joint pain)

Serum sickness reaction usually occurs after the second course of therapy and resolves after the drug is discontinued.

Rare

Allergic reaction (rash, pruritus, urticaria)

SERIOUS REACTIONS

! Antibiotic-associated colitis manifested as severe abdominal pain and tenderness, fever, and watery and severe diarrhea and other superinfections may result from altered bacterial balance.

! Nephrotoxicity may occur, especially in pts with preexisting renal disease.

! Severe hypersensitivity reaction including severe pruritus, angioedema, bronchospasm, and anaphylaxis, particularly in pts with a history of allergies, especially to penicillin, may occur.

PEDIATRIC CONSIDERATIONS

Baseline Assessment

◂ALERT▸ Determine the patient's history of allergies, particularly to cephalosporins and penicillins, before beginning drug therapy.

- Be aware that cephalexin readily crosses the placenta and is distributed in breast milk.
- May cause false readings on certain urine tests (e.g., Coombs' and Clinitest).
- Assess for age-appropriate fluid intake.
- Diarrhea may indicate drug toxicity.
- Monitor for signs of prolonged bleeding time (e.g., ecchymosis, hematuria, and bleeding gums).

Precautions

- Use cautiously in pts with a history of GI disease, especially antibiotic-associated colitis or ulcerative colitis, and renal impairment.
- Use cautiously in pts concurrently using nephrotoxic medications.

Administration and Handling

◂ALERT▸ Space drug doses evenly around the clock.

PO

- After reconstitution, oral suspension is stable for 14 days if refrigerated.
- Shake oral suspension well before using.
- Give without regard to meals. If GI upset occurs, give with food or milk.

Intervention and Evaluation

- Assess the patient's mouth for white patches on the mucous membranes and tongue.
- Assess the patient's pattern of daily bowel activity and stool consistency. Mild GI effects may be tolerable, but increasing severity may indicate the onset of antibiotic-associated colitis.
- Monitor the patient's intake and output and renal function reports for signs of nephrotoxicity.

• Be alert for signs and symptoms of superinfection including abdominal pain, moderate to severe diarrhea, severe anal or genital pruritus, and severe mouth soreness.

Patient/Family Teaching

• Advise the patient/family to continue cephalexin therapy for the full length of treatment and to evenly space drug doses around the clock.
• Explain to the patient/family that cephalexin may cause GI upset. Instruct the patient to take the drug with food or milk if GI upset occurs.
• Teach the patient/family to refrigerate an oral suspension of cephalexin.

Loracarbef

laur-ah-**car**-bef
(Lorabid)
Do not confuse with Lortab.

CATEGORY AND SCHEDULE

Pregnancy Risk Category: B

MECHANISM OF ACTION

A cephalosporin that acts as a bactericidal by binding to bacterial cell membranes. ***Therapeutic Effect:*** Inhibits bacterial cell wall synthesis.

AVAILABILITY

Capsules: 200 mg, 400 mg.
Powder for PO Suspension: 100 mg/5 mL, 200 mg/5 mL.

INDICATIONS AND DOSAGES

▸ Bronchitis

PO

Children older than 12 yrs. 200–400 mg q12h for 7 days.

▸ Pharyngitis

PO

Children older than 12 yrs. 200 mg q12h for 10 days.
Children 6 mos–12 yrs. 7.5 mg/kg q12h for 10 days.

▸ Pneumonia

PO

Children older than 12 yrs. 400 mg q12h for 14 days.

▸ Sinusitis

PO

Children older than 12 yrs. 400 mg q12h for 10 days.
Children 6 mos–12 yrs. 15 mg/kg q12h for 10 days.

▸ Skin, soft tissue infections

PO

Children older than 12 yrs. 200 mg q12h for 7 days.
Children 6 mos–12 yrs. 7.5 mg/kg q12h for 7 days.

▸ Urinary tract infections

PO

Children older than 12 yrs. 200–400 mg q12h for 7–14 days.

▸ Otitis media

PO

Children 6 mos–12 yrs. 15 mg/kg q12h for 10 days (use suspension for better plasma concentrations).

CONTRAINDICATIONS

History of anaphylactic reaction to penicillins, hypersensitivity to cephalosporins.

INTERACTIONS

Drug

Probenecid: Increases serum concentrations and half-life of loracarbef.

Herbal

None known.

Food

None known.

DIAGNOSTIC TEST EFFECTS

May increase BUN, serum alkaline phosphatase, serum creatinine, SGOT (AST), and SGPT (ALT) levels. May decrease blood leukocyte and platelet counts.

SIDE EFFECTS

Frequent
Abdominal pain, anorexia, nausea, vomiting, diarrhea

Occasional
Skin rash, itching

Rare
Dizziness, headache, vaginitis

SERIOUS REACTIONS

! Antibiotic-associated colitis and other superinfections may result from altered bacterial balance.

! Hypersensitivity reactions (ranging from rash, urticaria, and fever to anaphylaxis) occur in less than 5% of pts. Generally, hypersensitivity reactions develop in pts with a history of allergies, especially to penicillins.

PEDIATRIC CONSIDERATIONS

Baseline Assessment

◂ALERT▸ Determine the patient's history of allergies, particularly to cephalosporins and penicillins, before beginning drug therapy.

- Can cause false increases in certain urine tests (e.g., Coombs' and Jaffe's reaction).
- Diarrhea may be a sign of drug toxicity.
- Assess for age-appropriate fluid intake.

Precautions

- Use cautiously in pts with a history of colitis or renal impairment.

Administration and Handling

PO

- Give 1 hr before or 2 hrs after meals.
- After reconstitution, powder for suspension may be kept at room temperature for 14 days.
- Discard unused portion after 14 days.
- Shake oral suspension well before using.

Intervention and Evaluation

- Assess the patient for nausea or vomiting.
- Assess the patient's pattern of daily bowel activity and stool consistency.
- Evaluate the patient's skin for rash, especially in the diaper area in children.
- Monitor the patient's intake and output, renal function reports, and urinalysis results for signs of nephrotoxicity.
- Be alert for signs and symptoms of superinfection including abdominal pain, anal or genital pruritus, moderate to severe diarrhea, moniliasis, and sore mouth or tongue.

Patient/Family Teaching

- Advise the patient/family to continue loracarbef therapy for the full length of treatment and to evenly space drug doses around the clock, giving the drug 1 hr before or 2 hrs after a meal.

REFERENCES

Gunn, V. L. & Nechyba, C. (2002). The Harriet Lane handbook (16th ed.). St. Louis: Mosby.

Miller, S. & Fioravanti, J. (1997). Pediatric medications: a handbook for nurses. St. Louis: Mosby.

Azithromycin
Clarithromycin
Erythromycin

Uses: Macrolides are used to treat pharyngitis, tonsillitis, sinusitis, chronic bronchitis, pneumonia, and uncomplicated skin and skin-structure infections.

Action: Macrolides can be bacteriostatic or bactericidal and act primarily against gram-positive microorganisms and gram-negative cocci by reversibly binding to the P site of the 50S ribosomal subunit of susceptible organisms. This action inhibits RNA-dependent protein synthesis and causes bacterial cell death. (See illustration, *Sites and Mechanisms of Action: Anti-Infective Agents,* page 2.) Azithromycin and clarithromycin appear to be more potent than erythromycin.

COMBINATION PRODUCTS

ERYZOLE: erythromycin/sulfisoxazole (a sulfonamide) 200 mg/600 mg/5 mL.
PEDIAZOLE: erythromycin/sulfisoxazole (a sulfonamide) 200 mg/600 mg per 5 mL.

Azithromycin

aye-**zith**-row-my-sin
(Zithromax)
Do not confuse with erythromycin.
(See Color Plate)

CATEGORY AND SCHEDULE

Pregnancy Risk Category: B

MECHANISM OF ACTION

A macrolide antibiotic that binds to ribosomal receptor sites of susceptible organisms. ***Therapeutic Effect:*** Inhibits RNA-dependent protein synthesis.

PHARMACOKINETICS

Rapidly absorbed from the GI tract. Protein binding: 7%–50%. Widely distributed. Eliminated primarily unchanged via biliary excretion. ***Half-Life:*** 68 hrs.

AVAILABILITY

Tablets: 250 mg, 500 mg, 600 mg.
Injection: 500 mg.
Oral Suspension: 100 mg/5 mL, 200 mg/5 mL.

INDICATIONS AND DOSAGES

▸ **Respiratory tract, skin, soft tissue infection**

PO

Adolescents. 500 mg on day 1, then 250 mg/day on days 2–5.
Children older than 6 mos. 10 mg/kg on day 1 (maximum 500), then 5 mg/kg/day on days 2–5 (maximum 250).

▸ **Otitis media**

PO

Children older than 6 mos. 5-day regimen. 10 mg/kg once (maximum 500 mg), then 5 mg/kg/day for 4 days (maximum 250 mg).
3-day regimen. 10 mg/kg/day for 3 days (maximum 500 mg/day).
1-day regimen. 30 mg/kg in a single dose (maximum 1500 mg).

▸ **Pharyngitis, tonsillitis**
PO
Children 2 yrs and older.
12 mg/kg/day (maximum 500 mg) for 5 days.

▸ **Treatment of *Mycobacterium avium* complex (MAC)**
PO
Adolescents. 600 mg qd in combination with ethambutol.
Children. 5 mg/kg/day (maximum 250 mg) in combination with ethambutol.

▸ **MAC prevention**
PO
Adolescents. 1,200 mg once weekly, alone or with rifabutin.
Children. 5 mg/kg/day (maximum 250 mg) or 20 mg/kg/wk (maximum 1200 mg) alone or with rifabutin.

▸ **Usual pediatric dosage**
Children older than 6 mos. 10 mg/kg once (maximum 500 mg), then 5 mg/kg/day for 4 days (maximum 250 mg).

UNLABELED USES

Chlamydial infections, gonococcal pharyngitis, uncomplicated gonococcal infections of cervix, urethra, and rectum, *Helicobacter pylori* infections, Lyme disease, toxoplasmosis.

CONTRAINDICATIONS

Hypersensitivity to azithromycin, erythromycins, or any macrolide antibiotic.

INTERACTIONS

Drug

Aluminum- or magnesium-containing antacids: May decrease azithromycin blood concentration. Give azithromycin 1 hr before or 2 hrs after antacids.
Carbamazepine, cyclosporine, theophylline, warfarin, tacrolimus, phenytoin, digoxin: May increase the serum concentrations of these drugs.

Herbal

None known.

Food

None known.

DIAGNOSTIC TEST EFFECTS

May increase serum creatinine phosphokinase, SGOT (AST), and SGPT (ALT) levels.

IV INCOMPATIBILITIES

Information is not available.

IV COMPATIBILITIES

None known; do not mix with other medications.

SIDE EFFECTS

Occasional
Nausea, vomiting, diarrhea, abdominal pain
Rare
Headache, dizziness, allergic reaction

SERIOUS REACTIONS

! Superinfections, especially antibiotic-associated colitis as evidenced by abdominal cramps, severe and watery diarrhea, and fever, may result from altered bacterial balance.
! Acute interstitial nephritis occurs rarely.

PEDIATRIC CONSIDERATIONS

Baseline Assessment

- Determine the patient's history of hepatitis or allergies to azithromycin and erythromycin.
- Be aware that it is unknown whether azithromycin is distributed in breast milk.
- Be aware that the safety and efficacy of azithromycin have not been established in children younger than 16 yrs for IV use or

for children younger than 6 mos for oral use.
• Assess for age-appropriate fluid intake.

Precautions

• Use cautiously in pts with liver or renal dysfunction.

Administration and Handling

PO

• May give tablets without regard to food.
• Store the suspension at room temperature. The suspension is stable for 10 days after reconstitution.
• Do not administer oral suspension with food. Give at least 1 hr before or 2 hrs after meals.

IV

• Store vials at room temperature.
• After reconstitution, the solution is stable for 24 hrs at room temperature or 7 days if refrigerated.
• Reconstitute each 500-mg vial with 4.8 mL Sterile Water for Injection to provide concentration of 100 mg/mL.
• Shake well to ensure dissolution.
• Further dilute with 250 or 500 mL 0.9% NaCl or D_5W to provide final concentration of 2 mg/mL with 250 mL diluent or 1 mg/mL with 500 mL diluent.
• Infuse over 60 min. Never give IV push.

Intervention and Evaluation

• Assess the patient for GI discomfort, nausea, or vomiting.
• Assess the patient's pattern of daily bowel activity and stool consistency.
• Monitor the patient's liver function test results.
• Assess the patient for signs and symptoms of hepatotoxicity manifested as abdominal pain, fever, GI disturbances, and malaise.
• Evaluate the patient for signs and symptoms of superinfection including genital or anal pruritus, sore mouth or tongue, and moderate to severe diarrhea.

Patient/Family Teaching

• Advise the patient/family to continue therapy for the full length of treatment and to space drug doses evenly around the clock.
• Teach the patient/family to take oral medication with 8 oz of water at least 1 hr before or 2 hrs after consuming any food or beverages.

Clarithromycin

clair-**rith**-row-my-sin
(Biaxin, Biaxin XL, Klacid [AUS])

CATEGORY AND SCHEDULE

Pregnancy Risk Category: C

MECHANISM OF ACTION

A macrolide that is bacteriostatic and binds to ribosomal receptor sites. May be bactericidal with high dosage or very susceptible microorganisms. ***Therapeutic Effect:*** Inhibits protein synthesis of bacterial cell wall.

PHARMACOKINETICS

Well absorbed from the GI tract. Protein binding: 65%–75%. Widely distributed. Metabolized in liver to active metabolite. Primarily excreted in urine. Not removed by hemodialysis. ***Half-Life:*** 3–7 hrs; metabolite: 5–7 hrs (half-life is increased in those with impaired renal function).

AVAILABILITY

Tablets: 250 mg, 500 mg.
Tablets (extended-release): 500 mg.
Oral Suspension: 125 mg/5 mL, 250 mg/5mL.

INDICATIONS AND DOSAGES

▸ **Usual treatment**

Adolescents. 250 mg in 2 divided doses for 7–14 days.

▸ **Sinusitis and chronic bronchitis due to *Haemophilus influenzae***

Adolescents. 500 mg in 2 divided doses for 7–14 days.

▸ **Acute otitis media**

Children. 15 mg/kg/day in 2 divided doses for 10 days.

▸ **Respiratory, skin, and skin-structure infections**

PO

Children. 15 mg/kg/day in 2 divided doses for 7–14 days.

▸ **Prophylaxis for bacterial endocarditis**

Children. 15 mg/kg 1 hr before procedure

▸ **Dosage in renal impairment**

Creatinine clearance less than 30 mL/min: Reduce dose by 50% and administer once or twice daily.

CONTRAINDICATIONS

Hypersensitivity to clarithromycin, erythromycins, or any macrolide antibiotic.

INTERACTIONS

Drug

Carbamazepine, digoxin, theophylline, tacrolimus, cyclosporine, omeprazole, lovastatin: May increase blood concentration and toxicity of these drugs.

Rifampin: May decrease clarithromycin blood concentration.

Warfarin: May increase warfarin effects.

Zidovudine: May decrease blood concentration of zidovudine.

Herbal

None known.

Food

None known.

DIAGNOSTIC TEST EFFECTS

May rarely increase BUN, SGOT (AST), and SGPT (ALT) levels.

SIDE EFFECTS

Occasional (6%–3%)

Diarrhea, nausea, altered taste, abdominal pain

Rare (2%–1%)

Headache, dyspepsia

SERIOUS REACTIONS

! Antibiotic-associated colitis as evidenced by severe abdominal pain and tenderness, fever, and watery and severe diarrhea and other superinfections may result from altered bacterial balance.

! Hepatotoxicity and thrombocytopenia occur rarely.

PEDIATRIC CONSIDERATIONS

Baseline Assessment

◂ **ALERT** ▸ Determine the patient's allergies, especially to clarithromycin and erythromycins and history of hepatitis before beginning drug therapy.

- Be aware that it is unknown whether clarithromycin is distributed in breast milk.
- Be aware that the safety and efficacy of this drug have not been established in children younger than 6 mos.
- May lead to false increases in liver function test results.
- Assess for age-appropriate fluid intake.

Precautions

- Use cautiously in pts with liver and renal dysfunction and in pts with severe renal impairment.

Administration and Handling

PO

- Give without regard to food.
- Do not crush or break tablets.

• Shake suspension well before administration.

Intervention and Evaluation

• Assess the patient's pattern of daily bowel activity and stool consistency. Mild GI effects may be tolerable, but increasing severity may indicate the onset of antibiotic-associated colitis.
• Be alert for signs and symptoms of superinfection, including abdominal pain, anal or genital pruritus, moderate to severe diarrhea, and mouth soreness.

Patient/Family Teaching

• Advise the patient/family to continue clarithromycin therapy for the full length of treatment and to space drug doses evenly around the clock.
• Instruct the patient/family to take this medication with 8 oz of water. Explain that the drug may be taken without regard to food.

Erythromycin

eh-rith-row-**my**-sin
(Akne-Mycin, Apo-Erythro Base [CAN], EES, Eryacne [AUS], Erybid [CAN], Eryc, Eryc LD [AUS], EryDerm, EryPed, Ery-Tab, Erythrocin, Erythromid [CAN], PCE)
(See Color Plate)

CATEGORY AND SCHEDULE

Pregnancy Risk Category: B

MECHANISM OF ACTION

A macrolide that is bacteriostatic, penetrates bacterial cell membranes, and reversibly binds to bacterial ribosomes. ***Therapeutic Effect:*** Inhibits bacterial protein synthesis.

PHARMACOKINETICS

Variably absorbed from the GI tract (affected by dosage form used). Widely distributed. Protein binding: 70%–90%. Metabolized in liver. Primarily eliminated in feces via bile. Not removed by hemodialysis. ***Half-Life:*** 1.4–2 hrs (half-life is increased in those with impaired renal function).

AVAILABILITY

Powder for Injection: 500 mg, 1 g.
Tablets (base): 250 mg, 333 mg, 500 mg.
Tablets (delayed-release [base]): 250 mg, 333 mg, 500 mg.
Capsules (delayed-release): 250 mg.
Tablets (estolate): 500 mg.
Capsules (estolate): 250 mg.
Oral Suspension (estolate): 125 mg/5 mL, 250 mg/5 mL.
Tablets (chewable [ethylsuccinate]): 200 mg.
Tablets (ethylsuccinate): 400 mg.
Oral Suspension (ethylsuccinate): 200 mg/5 mL, 400 mg/5 mL.
Oral Drops (ethylsuccinate): 100 mg/2.5 mL.
Tablets (stearate): 250 mg, 500 mg.
Ophthalmic Ointment (stearate): 5%.
Topical Solution (stearate): 1.5%, 2%.
Topical Gel (stearate): 2%.
Topical Ointment (stearate): 2%.

INDICATIONS AND DOSAGES

▸ **Respiratory infections, otitis media, pertussis, diphtheria (adjunctive therapy), Legionnaires' disease, intestinal amebiasis**

IV

Children. 15–50 mg/kg/day in divided doses. Maximum: 4 g/day.

PO

Children. 30–50 mg/kg/day in divided doses up to 60–100 mg/kg/day for severe infections.

Maximum: 2 g/day (base, estolate, or stearate) or 3.2 g/day (ethylsuccinate).
PO
Neonates 1–7 days. 20 mg/kg/day divided q12h (ethylsuccinate).
Neonates older than 7 days and weighing less than 1,200 g. 20 mg/kg/day divided q12h (ethylsuccinate).
Neonates older than 7 days and weighing more than 1,200 g. 30–40 mg/kg/day divided q8h (ethylsuccinate).

▸ Preop intestinal antisepsis
PO
Children. 20 mg/kg of base at 1, 2, and 11 PM the day before the surgery.

▸ Acne vulgaris
TOPICAL
Children. Apply to affected area 2 times/day to clean dry skin.

▸ Gonococcal ophthalmia neonatorum
OPHTHALMIC
Neonates. 0.5–2 cm no later than 1 hr after delivery.

UNLABELED USES

Systemic: Treatment of acne vulgaris, chancroid, *Campylobacter* enteritis, gastroparesis, Lyme disease.
Topical: Treatment of minor bacterial skin infections.
Ophthalmic: Treatment of blepharitis, conjunctivitis, keratitis, chlamydial trachoma.

CONTRAINDICATIONS

Do not administer the fixed-combination, Pediazole (erythromycin and sulfisoxazole), to infants younger than 2 mos. Pediazole is contraindicated in those with a history of hepatitis, resulting in difficulty in metabolizing the medications, erythromycins, hypersensitivity to erythromycins, preexisting liver disease, and hypersensitivity to erythromycin or any component.

INTERACTIONS

Drug

Buspirone, cyclosporine, felodipine, lovastatin, simvastatin: May increase the blood concentration and toxicity of these drugs.
Carbamazepine: May inhibit the metabolism of carbamazepine.
Chloramphenicol, clindamycin: May decrease the effects of chloramphenicol and clindamycin.
Hepatotoxic medications: May increase the risk of liver toxicity.
Theophylline: May increase the risk of theophylline toxicity.
Warfarin: May increase the effects of this drug.

Herbal

None known.

Food

None known.

DIAGNOSTIC TEST EFFECTS

May increase serum alkaline phosphatase, serum bilirubin, SGOT (AST), and SGPT (ALT) levels.

IV INCOMPATIBILITIES

Fluconazole (Diflucan)

IV COMPATIBILITIES

Aminophylline, amiodarone (Cordarone), diltiazem (Cardizem), heparin, hydromorphone (Dilaudid), lidocaine, lorazepam (Ativan), magnesium sulfate, midazolam (Versed), morphine, multivitamins, potassium chloride

SIDE EFFECTS

Frequent
IV: Abdominal cramping or discomfort, phlebitis or thrombophlebitis
Topical: Dry skin (50%)

Occasional
Nausea, vomiting, diarrhea, rash, urticaria

Rare
Ophthalmic: Sensitivity reaction with increased irritation, burning, itching, inflammation
Topical: Urticaria

SERIOUS REACTIONS

! Superinfections, especially antibiotic-associated colitis as evidenced by genital and anal pruritus, sore mouth or tongue, and moderate to severe diarrhea, and reversible cholestatic hepatitis may occur.
! High dosages in pts with renal impairment may lead to reversible hearing loss.
! Anaphylaxis occurs rarely.

PEDIATRIC CONSIDERATIONS

Baseline Assessment

◂ALERT▸ Determine the patient's history of allergies, particularly to erythromycins, and hepatitis before beginning drug therapy.

- Be aware that erythromycin crosses the placenta and is distributed in breast milk.
- Be aware that erythromycin estolate may increase liver function enzymes in pregnant women.
- There are no age-related precautions noted in children.
- Be aware that high dosages in pts with decreased liver or renal function increase the risk of hearing loss.
- Do not administer IV push.
- Assess for age-appropriate fluid intake.

Precautions

- Use cautiously in pts with liver dysfunction.
- Consider the precautions for sulfonamides if erythromycin is used in combination therapy (Pediazole).
- IV erythromycin contains benzyl alcohol; use with caution in neonates.
- IV erythromycin may cause tachycardia and a prolonged QT interval.

Administration and Handling

PO

- Store capsules and tablets at room temperature.
- Oral suspension is stable for 14 days at room temperature.
- Administer erythromycin base, stearate, 1 hr before or 2 hrs after food. Erythromycin estolate or ethylsuccinate may be given without regard to meals, but optimal absorption occurs when it is given on an empty stomach.
- Give with 8 oz of water.
- If the patient has difficulty swallowing, sprinkle capsule contents on teaspoon of applesauce and follow with water.
- Be sure the patient does not swallow chewable tablets whole.

IV

- Store parenteral form at room temperature.
- Initial reconstituted solution in vial is stable for 2 wks if refrigerated or 24 hrs at room temperature.
- Diluted IV solutions are stable for 8 hrs at room temperature, 24 hrs if refrigerated.
- Discard if precipitate forms.
- Reconstitute each 500 mg with 10 mL Sterile Water for Injection without preservative to provide a concentration of 50 mg/mL.

• Further dilute with 100–250 mL D_5W or 0.9% NaCl.
• For intermittent IV infusion (piggyback), infuse over 20–60 min.
• For continuous infusion, infuse over 6–24 hrs.

OPHTHALMIC

• Place a gloved finger on the patient's lower eyelid and pull the lower eyelid out until a pocket is formed between eye and lower lid. Place ¼–½ inch ointment into pocket.
• Have the patient close the eye gently for 1–2 min and roll the eyeball to increase the contact area of drug to eye.
• Remove excess ointment around the eye with a tissue.

Intervention and Evaluation

• Assess the patient's pattern of daily bowel activity and stool consistency.
• Assess the patient's skin for rash.
• Evaluate the patient for signs and symptoms of liver toxicity, including abdominal pain, fever, GI disturbances, and malaise.
• Evaluate the patient for signs and symptoms of superinfection.
• Check the patient's injection site for signs and symptoms of phlebitis as evidenced by heat, pain, and red streaking over the vein.
• Monitor the patient for signs of high-dose hearing loss.

Patient/Family Teaching

• Advise the patient/family to continue erythromycin therapy for the full length of treatment and to evenly space drug doses around the clock.
• Instruct the patient/family to take the oral form of erythromycin with 8 oz of water 1 hr before or 2 hrs after food or beverage. Teach the patient/family not to swallow chewable tablets whole.
• Warn the patient/family receiving the ophthalmic form of erythromycin to notify the physician if the patient experiences burning, inflammation, and itching.
• Advise the patient/family receiving the topical form of erythromycin to notify the physician if the patient experiences burning, excessive dryness, and itching.
• Explain to the patient/family that acne improvement may not occur for 1–2 mos and that the maximum benefit of the drug may take 3 mos to appear. Also inform the patient that erythromycin therapy may last for months or years.
• Warn the patient/family taking erythromycin for acne vulgaris to use caution if using other topical acne preparations containing abrasive or peeling agents, abrasive or medicated soaps, and cosmetics containing alcohol (e.g., astringents or aftershave lotion).

REFERENCES

Gunn V. L. & Nechyba, C. (2002). The Harriet Lane handbook (16th ed.). St. Louis: Mosby.
Miller, S. & Fioravanti, J. (1997). Pediatric medications: A handbook for nurses. St. Louis: Mosby.
Taketomo, C. K., Hodding, J. H. & Kraus, D. M. (2003–2004). Pediatric dosage handbook (10th ed.). Hudson, OH: Lexi-Comp.

9 Penicillins

Amoxicillin
Amoxicillin/ Clavulanate Potassium
Ampicillin Sodium
Ampicillin/ Sulbactam Sodium
Oxacillin
Penicillin G Benzathine
Penicillin G Potassium
Penicillin V Potassium
Piperacillin Sodium/ Tazobactam Sodium
Ticarcillin Disodium/ Clavulanate Potassium

Uses: Penicillins may be used to treat a large number of infections, including pneumonia and other respiratory diseases, urinary tract infections, septicemia, meningitis, intra-abdominal infections, gonorrhea, syphilis, and bone and joint infections.

These agents are classified by antimicrobial spectrum:

Natural penicillins, such as penicillin G benzathine and penicillin V potassium, are very active against gram-positive cocci but are ineffective against most strains of *Staphylococcus aureus* because the drugs are inactivated by the enzyme penicillinase, which is produced by these organisms.

Penicillinase-resistant penicillins, such as oxacillin, are effective against penicillinase-producing *S. aureus* but are less effective against gram-positive cocci than the natural penicillins.

Broad-spectrum penicillins, such as amoxicillin and ampicillin sodium, are effective against gram-positive cocci and some gram-negative bacteria, such as *Haemophilus influenzae, Escherichia coli,* and *Proteus mirabilis.*

Extended-spectrum penicillins, such as piperacillin sodium/tazobactam sodium and ticarcillin disodium/clavulanate potassium, are effective against *Pseudomonas aeruginosa, Enterobacter* species, *Proteus* species, *Klebsiella* species, and some other gram-negative organisms.

Action: Penicillins inhibit cell wall synthesis or activate enzymes that disrupt bacterial cell walls, weakening the walls and causing cell lysis and death. They may be bacteriostatic or bactericidal and are most effective against bacteria undergoing active growth and division. (See illustration, *Mechanisms of Action: Penicillins*, page 147.)

COMBINATION PRODUCTS

BICILLIN CR: penicillin G benzathine/penicillin procaine 600,000 units/600,000 units.

Amoxicillin

ah-**mocks**-ih-sill-in

(Alphamox [AUS], Amohexal [AUS], Amoxil, Apo-Amoxi [CAN], Cilamox [AUS], Clamoxyl [AUS], DisperMox, Fisamox [AUS], Moxacin [AUS], Moxamox [AUS], Novamoxin [CAN], Polymox, Trimox, Wymox)

Do not confuse with amoxapine or Tylox.

CATEGORY AND SCHEDULE

Pregnancy Risk Category: B

MECHANISM OF ACTION

A penicillin that acts as a bactericidal in susceptible microorganisms. ***Therapeutic Effect:*** Inhibits bacterial cell wall synthesis.

PHARMACOKINETICS

Well absorbed from GI tract. Protein binding: 20%. Partially metabolized in liver. Primarily excreted in urine. Moderately removed by hemodialysis. ***Half-Life:*** Children: 1–2 hrs; adolescents: 1–1.3 hrs (half-life increased in reduced renal function).

AVAILABILITY

Tablets (chewable): 125 mg, 200 mg, 250 mg, 400 mg.
Tablets: 500 mg, 875 mg.
Tablets for Oral Suspension: 200 mg, 400 mg.
Capsules: 250 mg, 500 mg.
Powder for Oral Suspension: 50 mg/mL, 125 mg/5 mL, 200 mg/mL, 250 mg/5 mL, 400 mg/5 mL.

INDICATIONS AND DOSAGES

▸ **Usual pediatric dosage**

Neonates and children younger than 3 mos. 20–30 mg/kg/day in divided doses q12h.

▸ **Ear, nose, throat, GU, skin/skin-structure infections**

PO

Children older than 3 mos weighing less than 40 kg. 25–45 mg/kg/day divided q12h or 20–40 mg/kg/day divided q8h.

Children weighing more than 40 kg. 500–875 mg q8h or 250–500 mg q8h.

▸ **Lower respiratory tract infections**

PO

Children weighing more than 40 kg. 500 mg q8h or 875 mg q12h.

Children weighing less than 40 kg. 45 mg/kg/day in divided doses q12h or 40 mg/kg/day divided q8h.

▸ **Acute, uncomplicated gonorrhea**

PO

Children 2 yrs and older. 50 mg/kg plus probenecid 25 mg/kg as a single dose.

Adolescents. 3 g as a single dose.

▸ **Acute otitis media due to highly resistant strains of *Streptococcus pneumoniae***

PO

Children. 80–90 mg/kg/day in divided doses q12h.

▸ **Endocarditis**

PO

Children. 50 mg/kg 1 hr before procedure. Do not exceed adult dose.

▸ **Dosage in renal impairment**

Creatinine clearance 10–30 mL/min. Administer q12h.

Creatinine clearance less than 10 mL/min. Administer q24h.

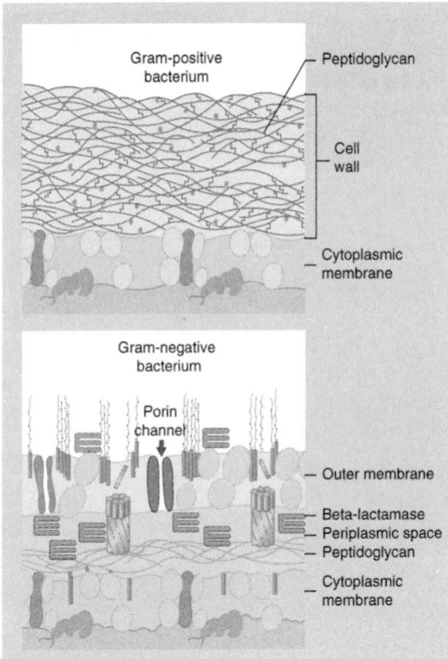

Mechanisms of Action: Penicillins

Generally, penicillins act by weakening the normally rigid cell walls of bacteria. A weakened wall causes the cell to absorb excess water, leading to cellular swelling and rupture. However, the effectiveness of penicillins is determined by the bacterial cell wall, which differs in gram-positive and gram-negative bacteria.

Gram-positive bacteria (A) have a rigid cell wall composed of long strands of peptidoglycan. This peptidoglycan is held together by cross-bridges, which are formed by transpeptidase and give the cell wall its strength. In addition, autolysins (bacterial enzymes that adhere to cellular bonds in the wall) are present in the cell wall. Bacteria use these enzymes to break down portions of the cell wall to permit growth and cell division. Penicillins inhibit transpeptidases, thereby interfering with the creation of cross-bridges and weakening the cell wall. These drugs also activate autolysins, which then leads to cell wall breakdown and cell destruction.

Gram-negative bacteria (B) have a different cell wall structure. Unlike gram-positive bacteria, which have two layers (a cell wall and a cytoplasmic membrane), gram-negative bacteria have three layers (an outer membrane, a thin cell wall, and a cytoplasmic membrane). Although penicillins can penetrate the cell wall, they must first penetrate the outer membrane. Only a few penicillins are small enough to pass through the tiny openings (porin channels) in the outer member to be effective against gram-negative bacteria.

In addition, gram-positive and gram-negative bacteria produce enzymes called β-lactamases, which can render penicillins ineffective. β-Lactamases that act specifically on penicillins are known as penicillinases. Gram-positive bacteria produce large amount of penicillinases, but release them into the environment around the cell. In contrast, gram-negative bacteria produce smaller amounts of these enzymes, but release them into the periplasmic space. So even if a penicillin can pass through the porin channel, it must also be resistant to penicillinase to achieve its therapeutic effect.

UNLABELED USES

Treatment of Lyme disease and typhoid fever.

CONTRAINDICATIONS

Hypersensitivity to any penicillin, infectious mononucleosis.

INTERACTIONS

Drug

Allopurinol: May increase incidence of rash.
Oral contraceptives: May decrease effects of oral contraceptives.
Probenecid: May increase amoxicillin blood concentration and risk for amoxicillin toxicity.

Herbal

None known.

Food

None known.

DIAGNOSTIC TEST EFFECTS

May increase BUN, lactate dehydrogenase, serum bilirubin, serum creatinine, SGOT (AST), and SGPT (ALT) levels. May cause positive Coombs' test results.

SIDE EFFECTS

Frequent
GI disturbances (mild diarrhea, nausea, or vomiting), headache, oral or vaginal candidiasis
Occasional
Generalized rash, urticaria

SERIOUS REACTIONS

! Altered bacterial balance may result in potentially fatal superinfections and antibiotic-associated colitis as evidenced by abdominal cramps, watery or severe diarrhea, and fever.
! Severe hypersensitivity reactions, including anaphylaxis and acute interstitial nephritis, occur rarely.

PEDIATRIC CONSIDERATIONS

Baseline Assessment

- Determine the patient's history of allergies, especially to cephalosporins or penicillins, before giving the drug.
- Be aware that amoxicillin crosses the placenta, appears in cord blood and amniotic fluid, and is distributed in breast milk in low concentrations.
- Be aware that amoxicillin use may lead to allergic sensitization, candidiasis, diarrhea, and skin rash in infants.
- Be aware that immature renal function in neonates and young infants may delay renal excretion of amoxicillin.

Precautions

- Use cautiously in pts with antibiotic-associated colitis or a history of allergies, especially to cephalosporins.

Administration and Handling

PO
- Store capsules or tablets at room temperature.
- After reconstitution, the oral solution is stable for 14 days, whether at room temperature or refrigerated.
- Give without regard to meals.
- May mix the suspension with milk, formula, or juice.
- Instruct the patient to chew or crush chewable tablets thoroughly before swallowing.

Intervention and Evaluation

- Withhold amoxicillin and promptly notify the physician if the patient experiences a rash or diarrhea. Severe diarrhea with abdominal pain, blood or mucus in stools, and fever may indicate antibiotic-associated colitis.
- Monitor the patient for signs and symptoms of superinfection,

including anal or genital pruritus, black, hairy tongue, diarrhea, increased fever, sore throat, ulceration or changes of oral mucosa, and vomiting.

Patient/Family Teaching

• Urge the patient/family to continue taking the antibiotic for the full length of treatment and to space doses evenly around the clock.
• Instruct the patient/family to take amoxicillin with meals if GI upset occurs.
• Stress to the patient/family that he or she must thoroughly chew or crush the chewable tablets before swallowing.
• Warn the patient/family to notify the physician if diarrhea, a rash, or other new symptoms occur.

Amoxicillin/ Clavulanate Potassium

a-**mocks**-ih-sill-in/klah-view-**lan**-ate
(Augmentin, Augmentin ES 600, Augmentin XR, Ausclav [AUS], Ausclav Duo 400 [AUS], Ausclav Duo Forte [AUS], Clamoxyl [AUS], Clamoxyl Duo Forte [AUS], Clavulin [CAN], Clavulin Duo Forte [AUS])
(See Color Plates)

CATEGORY AND SCHEDULE

Pregnancy Risk Category: B

MECHANISM OF ACTION

An antibiotic, amoxicillin, is bactericidal in susceptible microorganisms whereas clavulanate inhibits bacterial β-lactamase.
Therapeutic Effect: Amoxicillin inhibits cell wall synthesis. Clavulanate protects amoxicillin from enzymatic degradation.

PHARMACOKINETICS

Well absorbed from the GI tract. Protein binding: 20%. Partially metabolized in liver. Primarily excreted in urine. Moderately removed by hemodialysis.
Half-Life: Children: 1–2 hrs; adolescents: 1–1.3 hrs (half-life increased in reduced renal function).

AVAILABILITY

Tablets (chewable): 125 mg, 200 mg, 250 mg, 400 mg.
Tablets: 250 mg, 500 mg, 875 mg, 1000 mg (extended release).
Powder for PO Suspension: 125 mg/5 mL, 200 mg/5 mL, 250 mg/5 mL, 400 mg/5 mL, 600 mg/5 mL.

INDICATIONS AND DOSAGES (DOSES BASED ON AMOXICILLIN COMPONENT)

▸ **Mild to moderate infections**

PO

Children weighing more than 40 kg. 250 mg q8h or 500 mg q12h.
Children weighing less than 40 kg. 20 mg/kg/day in divided doses q8h or 25 mg/kg/day in divided doses q12h (because of different amoxicillin to clavulanic acid ratios, use only 200 or 400 mg/5 mL suspension or 200- or 400-mg chewable tablets).

▸ **Respiratory tract infections, severe infections**

PO

Children weighing more than 40 kg. 500 mg q8h or 875 mg q12h.
Children weighing less than 40 kg. 40 mg/kg/day in divided doses q8h or 45 mg/kg/day in divided doses q12h (because of different amoxicillin to clavulanic acid ratios, use only 200 mg or 400 mg/5 mL suspension or 200 or 400 mg chewable tablets).

▸ **Otitis media with multidrug resistance**
PO
Children. 80–90 mg/kg/day in divided doses q12h for 10 days.

▸ **Sinusitis, lower respiratory tract infections**
PO
Children. 40 mg/kg/day in divided doses q8h or 45 mg/kg/day in divided doses q12h.

▸ **Usual neonate dosage**
PO
Neonates or children younger than 3 mos. 30 mg/kg/day in divided doses q12h.

▸ **Intervals in renal impairment**
Creatinine clearance 10–30 ml/min. q12h.
Creatinine crearance less than 10 ml/min. q24h.

OFF-LABEL USES
Treatment of bronchitis and chancroid.

CONTRAINDICATIONS
Hypersensitivity to any penicillins, infectious mononucleosis.

INTERACTIONS
Drug
Allopurinol: May increase incidence of rash.
Oral contraceptives: May decrease effects of oral contraceptives.
Probenecid: May increase amoxicillin and clavulanate blood concentration and risk of toxicity.
Herbal
None known.
Food
None known.

DIAGNOSTIC TEST EFFECTS
May increase SGOT (AST) and SGPT (ALT) levels. May cause positive Coombs' test results.

SIDE EFFECTS
Frequent
GI disturbances (mild diarrhea, nausea, vomiting), headache, oral or vaginal candidiasis
Occasional
Generalized rash, urticaria

SERIOUS REACTIONS
! Altered bacterial balance may result in potentially fatal superinfections and antibiotic-associated colitis as evidenced by abdominal cramps, watery or severe diarrhea, and fever.
! Severe hypersensitivity reactions, including anaphylaxis and acute interstitial nephritis, occur rarely.

PEDIATRIC CONSIDERATIONS
Baseline Assessment
◂ **ALERT** ▸ Determine the patient's history of allergies, especially to cephalosporins and penicillins, before giving the drug.
• Be aware that amoxicillin/clavulanate crosses the placenta, appears in cord blood and amniotic fluid, and is distributed in breast milk in low concentrations.
• Be aware that amoxicillin/clavulanate use may lead to allergic sensitization, candidiasis, diarrhea, and skin rash in infants.
• Be aware that immature renal function in neonates and young infants may delay renal excretion of amoxicillin/clavulanate.
• Giving the medication 2 times/day instead of 3 times/day is often associated with less diarrhea in children.
• Assess for age-appropriate fluid intake.
Precautions
• Use cautiously in pts with antibiotic-associated colitis or a history of allergies, especially to cephalosporins.

Administration and Handling

◀ **ALERT** ▶ Drug dosage is expressed in terms of amoxicillin. Be aware that an alternative dosing for adults is 500–875 mg 2 times/day and for children is 200–400 mg 2 times/day.

PO

- Store tablets at room temperature.
- After reconstitution, oral solution is stable for 14 days whether at room temperature or refrigerated.
- Give without regard to meals.
- Instruct the patient to chew or crush chewable tablets thoroughly before swallowing.

Intervention and Evaluation

- Withhold amoxicillin and promptly notify the physician if the patient experiences a rash or diarrhea. Immediately notify the physician if the patient develops severe diarrhea with abdominal pain, blood or mucus in stools, and fever. These symptoms may indicate antibiotic-associated colitis.
- Be alert for signs and symptoms of superinfection, including anal or genital pruritus, black hairy tongue, diarrhea, increased fever, sore throat, ulceration or changes of oral mucosa, and vomiting.
- Be aware that because of the amount of clavulanic acid in each formulation, two 250 mg tablets are not equivalent to one 500 mg tablet and that four 250 mg tablets or two 500 mg tablets are not equivalent to one 1,000 mg extended-release tablet.

Patient/Family Teaching

- Advise the patient/family to continue taking the antibiotic for the full length of treatment and to space drug doses evenly around the clock.
- Instruct the patient/family to take the drug with meals if GI upset occurs.
- Stress that the patient should thoroughly chew or crush the chewable tablets before swallowing.
- Warn the patient/family to notify the physician if diarrhea, rash, or other new symptoms occur.

Ampicillin Sodium

amp-ih-**sill**-in

(Alphacin [AUS], Apo-Ampi [CAN], Novo-Ampicillin [CAN], Nu-Ampi [CAN], Polycillin, Principen)

Do not confuse with aminophylline, Imipenem, or Unipen.

(See Color Plate)

CATEGORY AND SCHEDULE

Pregnancy Risk Category: B

MECHANISM OF ACTION

A penicillin that inhibits cell wall synthesis in susceptible microorganisms. ***Therapeutic Effect:*** Produces a bactericidal effect.

PHARMACOKINETICS

Moderately absorbed from the GI tract. Protein binding: 10%–28%. Widely distributed. Partially metabolized in liver. Primarily excreted in urine. Moderately removed by hemodialysis. ***Half-Life:*** 1–1.5 hrs (half-life increased in impaired renal function).

AVAILABILITY

Capsules: 250 mg, 500 mg.
Powder for PO Suspension: 125 mg/5 mL, 250 mg/5 mL, 500 mg/5 mL.
Powder for Injection: 125 mg, 250 mg, 500 mg, 1 g, 2 g.

INDICATIONS AND DOSAGES

▸ Respiratory tract, skin/skin-structure infections

PO

Children weighing more than 20 kg. 250–500 mg q6h.

Children weighing less than 20 kg. 50 mg/kg/day in divided doses q6–8h.

IM/IV

Children weighing more than 40 kg. 250–500 mg q6h.

Children weighing less than 40 kg. 25–50 mg/kg/day in divided doses q6–8h.

▸ Bacterial meningitis, septicemia

IM/IV

Children. 200–400 mg/kg/day in divided doses q4h. Maximum: 12 g/day.

▸ Perioperative prophylaxis

IM/IV

Children. 50 mg/kg using same dosage regimen.

▸ Usual neonate dosage

IM/IV

Neonates 7–28 days old. 50–100 mg/ kg/day in divided doses q6–12h up to 200 mg/kg/day in divided doses q6h.

Neonates 0–7 days old. 50–75 mg/kg/day in divided doses q8–12h up to 150 mg/kg/day in divided doses q8h.

CONTRAINDICATIONS

Hypersensitivity to any penicillin, infectious mononucleosis.

INTERACTIONS

Drug

Allopurinol: May increase incidence of rash.

Oral contraceptives: May decrease effectiveness of oral contraceptives.

Probenecid: May increase ampicillin blood concentration and risk of ampicillin toxicity.

Herbal

None known.

Food

None known.

DIAGNOSTIC TEST EFFECTS

May increase SGOT (AST) and SGPT (ALT) levels. May cause positive Coombs' test results.

IV INCOMPATIBILITIES

Amikacin (Amikin), gentamicin, diltiazem (Cardizem), midazolam (Versed)

IV COMPATIBILITIES

Calcium gluconate, cefepime (Maxipime), dopamine (Inotropin), famotidine (Pepcid), furosemide (Lasix), heparin, hydromorphone (Dilaudid), insulin (regular), levofloxacin (Levaquin), magnesium sulfate, morphine, multivitamins, potassium chloride, propofol (Diprivan)

SIDE EFFECTS

Frequent

Pain at IM injection site, GI disturbances, including mild diarrhea, nausea, or vomiting, oral or vaginal candidiasis

Occasional

Generalized rash, urticaria, phlebitis, thrombophlebitis with IV administration, headache

Rare

Dizziness, seizures, especially with IV therapy

SERIOUS REACTIONS

! Altered bacterial balance may result in potentially fatal superinfections and antibiotic-associated colitis as evidenced by abdominal cramps, watery or severe diarrhea, and fever.

! Severe hypersensitivity reactions, including anaphylaxis and acute interstitial nephritis, occur rarely.

PEDIATRIC CONSIDERATIONS

Baseline Assessment

◀ **ALERT** ▶ Determine the patient's history of allergies, especially to cephalosporins and penicillins, before giving the drug.

• Be aware that ampicillin readily crosses the placenta, appears in cord blood and amniotic fluid, and is distributed in breast milk in low concentrations.

• Ampicillin use may lead to allergic sensitization, candidiasis, diarrhea, and skin rash in infants.

• Immature renal function in neonates and young infants may delay renal excretion of ampicillin.

• May cause false-positive Coombs' test or urine protein test results and false levels of serum aminoglycosides.

• Maintain age-appropriate fluid intake.

• A rash occurs in 5%–10% of children receiving ampicillin. This rash is characterized as dull red, beginning 3–14 days after the first dose.

◀ **ALERT** ▶ Keep in mind that higher dosages may be needed for neonatal meningitis.

Precautions

• Use cautiously in pts with antibiotic-associated colitis or a history of allergies, particularly to cephalosporins.

Administration and Handling

PO

• Store capsules at room temperature.

• Oral suspension, after reconstituted, is stable for 7 days at room temperature, 14 days if refrigerated.

• Give orally 1 hr before or 2 hrs after meals for maximum absorption.

IM

• Reconstitute each vial with Sterile Water for Injection or Bacteriostatic Water for Injection. Consult individual ampicillin vials for specific volumes of diluent. Reconstituted solution is stable for 1 hr.

• Give injection deeply in a large muscle mass.

IV

• An IV solution, diluted with 0.9% NaCl, is stable for 2–8 hrs at room temperature or 3 days if refrigerated.

• An IV solution diluted with D_5W is stable for 2 hrs at room temperature or 3 hrs if refrigerated.

• Discard the IV solution if a precipitate forms.

• For IV injection, dilute each vial with 5 or 10 mL Sterile Water for Injection for 1- or 2-g vials.

• For intermittent IV infusion or piggyback, further dilute with 50–100 mL 0.9% NaCl or D_5W.

• For IV injection, give over 3–5 min or 10–15 min for a 1- to 2-g dose.

• For intermittent IV infusion or piggyback, infuse over 20–30 min.

• Because of the potential for hypersensitivity and anaphylaxis, start the initial dose at a few drops per minute, increase the dosage slowly to the prescribed rate; and stay with the patient for the first 10–15 min. Then assess the patient every 10 min for signs and symptoms of hypersensitivity or anaphylaxis.

• Expect to switch to the PO route as soon as possible.

Intervention and Evaluation

• Withhold ampicillin and promptly notify the physician if the patient experiences a rash or diarrhea. Although a rash is common with ampicillin, it also may indicate hypersensitivity. Severe diarrhea with abdominal pain, blood or mucus in stools, and fever

may indicate antibiotic-associated colitis.
• Evaluate the IV site for phlebitis as evidenced by heat, pain, and red streaking over the vein.
• Check the IM injection site for pain and swelling.
• Monitor the patient's intake and output, renal function tests, and urinalysis results.
• Assess the patient for signs and symptoms of superinfection such as anal or genital pruritus, black hairy tongue, oral ulcerations or pain, diarrhea, increased fever, sore throat, and vomiting.

Patient/Family Teaching

• Advise the patient/family to take the antibiotic for the full length of treatment and to space doses evenly around the clock.
• Explain that the antibiotic is more effective if taken 1 hr before or 2 hrs after the patient consumes food or beverages.
• Instruct the patient/family that discomfort may occur with IM injection.
• Warn the patient/family to notify the physician if diarrhea, rash, or other new symptoms occur.

Ampicillin/Sulbactam Sodium

amp-ih-**sill**-in/sull-**bak**-tam
(Unasyn)

CATEGORY AND SCHEDULE

Pregnancy Risk Category: B

MECHANISM OF ACTION

A penicillin that is bactericidal in susceptible microorganisms and inhibits bacterial β-lactamase. ***Therapeutic Effect:*** Ampicillin inhibits cell wall synthesis. Sulbactam protects ampicillin from enzymatic degradation.

PHARMACOKINETICS

Protein binding: 28%–38%. Widely distributed. Partially metabolized in liver. Primarily excreted in urine. Removed by hemodialysis. ***Half-Life:*** 1–1.8 hrs (half-life increased in impaired renal function).

AVAILABILITY

Powder for Injection: 1.5 g (1 g ampicillin and 0.5 g sulbactam), 3 g (2 g ampicillin and 1 g sulbactam).

INDICATIONS AND DOSAGES (DOSES BASED ON AMPICILLIN COMPONENT)

▸ **Skin/skin-structure infections**

IV

Children 1–12 yrs. 150–300 mg/kg/day in divided doses q6h.

▸ **Mild/moderate infections**

IM/IV

Children. 100–200 mg/kg/day divided q6h.

Infants younger than 1 mo. 100–150 mg/kg/day divided q6h.

▸ **Meningitis/severe infections**

IM/IV

Children. 200–400 mg/kg/day divided q4–6h. Maximum: 8 g ampicillin/day.

Infants younger than 1 mo. 200–300 mg/kg/day divided q6h.

▸ **Dosage in renal impairment**

Modifications of dosage and frequency are based on creatinine clearance and the severity of infection.

Creatinine Clearance	Dosage
Greater than 30 mL/min	0.5–3 g q6–8h
15–29 mL/min	1.5–3 g q12h
5–14 mL/min	1.5–3 g q24h
Less than 5 mL/min	Not recommended

CONTRAINDICATIONS
Hypersensitivity to any penicillin, infectious mononucleosis.

INTERACTIONS
Drug
Allopurinol: May increase incidence of rash.
Oral contraceptives: May decrease effectiveness of oral contraceptives.
Probenecid: May increase ampicillin blood concentration and risk of ampicillin toxicity.
Herbal
None known.
Food
None known.

DIAGNOSTIC TEST EFFECTS
May increase serum lactate dehydrogenase, alkaline phosphatase, creatinine, SGOT (AST), and SGPT (ALT) levels. May cause positive Coombs' test results.

IV INCOMPATIBILITIES
Diltiazem (Cardizem), idarubicin (Idamycin), ondansetron (Zofran), sargramostim (Leukine)

IV COMPATIBILITIES
Famotidine (Pepcid), heparin, insulin (regular), morphine

SIDE EFFECTS
Frequent
Diarrhea and rash (most common), urticaria, pain at IM injection site; thrombophlebitis with IV administration; oral or vaginal candidiasis
Occasional
Nausea, vomiting, headache, malaise, urinary retention

SERIOUS REACTIONS
! Severe hypersensitivity reactions, including anaphylaxis, acute interstitial nephritis, and blood dyscrasias may be noted.
! Altered bacterial balance may result in potentially fatal superinfections and antibiotic-associated colitis as evidenced by abdominal cramps, watery or severe diarrhea, and fever.
! Overdose may produce seizures.

PEDIATRIC CONSIDERATIONS
Baseline Assessment
• Determine the patient's history of allergies, especially to cephalosporins and penicillins, before giving the drug.
• Be aware that ampicillin readily crosses the placenta, appears in cord blood and amniotic fluid, and is distributed in breast milk in low concentrations.
• Be aware that ampicillin use may lead to allergic sensitization, candidiasis, diarrhea, and skin rash in infants.
• Be aware that the safety and efficacy of ampicillin have not been established in children younger than 1 yr.
• Be aware that ampicillin use may lead to false-positive readings for urine protein and Coombs' tests.
• Assess for age-appropriate fluid intake.
Precautions
• Use cautiously in pts with antibiotic-associated colitis or a history of allergies, particularly to cephalosporins.
Administration and Handling
IM
• Reconstitute each 1.5-g vial with 3.2 mL Sterile Water for Injection to provide concentration of 250 mg ampicillin and 125 mg sulbactam/mL.
• Give injection deeply into a large muscle mass within 1 hr of preparation.

IV

• When reconstituted with 0.9% NaCl, IV solution is stable for 8 hrs at room temperature or 48 hrs if refrigerated. Stability may be different with other diluents.
• Discard IV solution if precipitate forms.
• For IV injection, dilute with 10–20 mL Sterile Water for Injection.
• For intermittent IV infusion or piggyback, further dilute with 50–100 mL D_5W or 0.9% NaCl.
• For IV injection, give slowly over a minimum of 10–15 min.
• For intermittent IV infusion or piggyback, infuse over 15–30 min.
• Because of the potential for hypersensitivity and anaphylaxis, start the initial dose at a few drops per minute, then increase the dose slowly to the ordered rate. Stay with the patient for the first 10–15 min and assess for signs and symptoms of hypersensitivity or anaphylaxis, and then check the patient every 10 min during the infusion.
• Expect to switch to a PO antibiotic as soon as possible.

Intervention and Evaluation

• Withhold ampicillin and promptly notify the physician if the patient experiences a rash or diarrhea. Although a rash is common with ampicillin, it also may indicate hypersensitivity. Severe diarrhea with abdominal pain, blood or mucus in stools, and fever may indicate antibiotic-associated colitis.
• Evaluate the IV site for phlebitis as evidenced by heat, pain, and red streaking over vein.
• Check the IM injection site for pain and swelling.
• Monitor the patient's intake and output, renal function tests, and urinalysis results.
• Assess the patient for signs and symptoms of superinfection such as anal or genital pruritus, black hairy tongue, changes in oral mucosa, diarrhea, increased fever, onset of sore throat, and vomiting.

Patient/Family Teaching

• Advise the patient/family to take the antibiotic for the full length of therapy and to space drug doses evenly around the clock.
• Instruct the patient/family that discomfort may occur at the IM injection site.
• Warn the patient/family to notify the physician if diarrhea, rash, or other new symptoms occur.

Oxacillin

ox-ah-**sill**-inn

CATEGORY AND SCHEDULE

Pregnancy Risk Category: B

MECHANISM OF ACTION

A penicillin that binds to bacterial membranes. ***Therapeutic Effect:*** Inhibits bacterial cell wall synthesis. Bactericidal.

AVAILABILITY

Powder for Injection: 1-g vials, 2-g vials.
Premixed infusion: 1 g, 2 g.

INDICATIONS AND DOSAGES

▸ **Upper respiratory tract, skin/skin-structure infections**

IM/IV

Children weighing more than 40 kg. 250–500 mg q4–6h.
Children weighing less than 40 kg. 50 mg/kg/day in divided doses q6h. Maximum: 12 g/day.

▸ **Lower respiratory tract, serious infections**
IM/IV
Children weighing more than 40 kg. 1 g q4–6h. Maximum: 12 g/day.
Children weighing less than 40 kg. 100 mg/kg/day in divided doses q4–6h.
▸ **Mild to moderate infections**
PO
Infants and children. 100–150 mg/kg/day divided q6h.
▸ **Severe infections**
PO
Infants and children. 150–200 mg/kg/day divided q4–6h. Maximum: 12 g/day.
▸ **Usual dosage for neonates**
IM/IV
Postnatal age older than 7 days. Weighing less than 1,200 g: 50 mg/kg/day divided q12h.
Weighing 1,200–2,000 g: 75 mg/kg/day divided q8h.
Weighing more than 2,000 g: 100 mg/kg/day divided q6h.
Postnatal age 7 days or younger. Weighing less than 2,000 g: 50 mg/kg/day divided q12h.
Weighing more than 2,000 g: 75 mg/kg/day divided q8h.

CONTRAINDICATIONS

Hypersensitivity to penicillin.

INTERACTIONS

Drug
Probenecid: May increase oxacillin blood concentration and risk of toxicity.
Herbal
None known.
Food
None known.

DIAGNOSTIC TEST EFFECTS

May increase SGOT (AST) levels. May cause positive Coombs' test results.

SIDE EFFECTS

Frequent
Mild hypersensitivity reaction including fever, rash, and pruritus, GI effects including nausea, vomiting, and diarrhea
Occasional
Phlebitis, thrombophlebitis (more common in pts with liver toxicity with high IV oxacillin dosage)

SERIOUS REACTIONS

! Superinfections and antibiotic-associated colitis may result from altered bacteria balance and a hypersensitivity reaction ranging from mild to severe may occur in those allergic to penicillin.

PEDIATRIC CONSIDERATIONS

Baseline Assessment
- Determine whether the patient has a history of allergies, especially to cephalosporins and penicillin.

Precautions
- Use cautiously in pts with a history of allergies, especially to cephalosporins, and in those with impaired renal function.
- High doses in infants and neonates have been associated with hematuria and azotemia.
- Use with care in neonates with impaired hepatic or renal function.
- Be aware that use of this medication may lead to false-positive urine protein and increased liver function test results.
- Never infuse by IV push. This could lead to seizures.
- Assure age-appropriate fluid intake.

Administration and Handling
IV
- Store at room temperature.
- Once reconstituted, vials are stable for 3 days at room temperature or 7 days if refrigerated.

• Remember that the solution is stable for 24 hrs when further diluted with D_5W or 0.9% NaCl.
• To each 1-g vial, add 10 mL Sterile Water for Injection to provide a concentration of 100 mg/mL.
• For piggyback administration, further dilute with 50–100 mg D_5W or 0.9% NaCl.
• Administer IV push over 10 min, IV piggyback over 30 min.

Intervention and Evaluation

• Withhold the medication and promptly report to the physician if the patient experiences diarrhea with abdominal pain, blood or mucus in stools, and fever or rash.
• Evaluate the patient's IV site frequently for phlebitis as evidenced by heat, pain, and red streaking over the vein.
• Monitor the patient's intake and output, renal function tests, and urinalysis results.
• Be alert for development of anal or genital pruritus, black hairy tongue, diarrhea, changes or ulcerations of the oral mucosa, signs and symptoms of superinfection, and vomiting.

Patient/Family Teaching

• Tell the patient/family to immediately report burning or pain at the IV site.
• Tell the patient/family to immediately report shortness of breath, chest tightness, or hives, signs of an allergic reaction.
• Encourage the patient/family to use good oral hygiene.

Penicillin G Benzathine

pen-ih-**sil**-lin G **benz**-ah-thene
(Bicillin LA, Permapen)

CATEGORY AND SCHEDULE

Pregnancy Risk Category: B

MECHANISM OF ACTION

A penicillin that binds to one or more of the penicillin-binding proteins of bacteria. ***Therapeutic Effect:*** Inhibits bacterial cell wall synthesis. Bactericidal.

AVAILABILITY

Injection (prefilled syringe): 600,000 units/mL.

INDICATIONS AND DOSAGES

▸ Group A streptococcal infection

IM

Infants and children. 25,000–50,000 units/kg as a single dose. Maximum: 1.2 million units/dose.

▸ Prophylaxis for rheumatic fever

IM

Infants and children. 25,000–50,000 units/kg q3–4wks. Maximum: 1.2 million units/dose.

▸ Congenital syphilis

IM

Children. 50,000 units/kg/wk for 3 wks. Maximum: 2.4 million units/dose.

▸ Syphilis duration longer than 1 yr

IM

Children. 50,000 units/kg qwk for 3 doses. Maximum: 2.4 million units/dose.

CONTRAINDICATIONS

Hypersensitivity to any penicillin.

INTERACTIONS

Drug

Erythromycin, chloramphenicol, tetracyclines: May antagonize effects of penicillin.
Probenecid: Increases serum concentration of penicillin.

Herbal

None known.

Food

None known.

DIAGNOSTIC TEST EFFECTS
May cause positive Coombs' test results.

SIDE EFFECTS
Occasional
Lethargy, fever, dizziness, rash, pain at injection site
Rare
Seizures, interstitial nephritis

SERIOUS REACTIONS
! Hypersensitivity reactions ranging from chills, fever, and rash to anaphylaxis occur.

PEDIATRIC CONSIDERATIONS

Baseline Assessment
• Determine the patient's history of allergies, particularly to aspirin, cephalosporins, and penicillins, before beginning drug therapy.
• Cardiac arrest and death can occur from IV administration.
• Do not administer repeated IM injections into the anterolateral thigh in neonates and infants because atrophy of the quadriceps femoris can occur.
• May lead to false-positive Coombs' and urine protein test results.
• Assess for age-appropriate fluid intake.
• Administer into the largest muscle mass to prevent painful administration.
Precautions
• Use cautiously in pts with a hypersensitivity to cephalosporins, impaired cardiac or renal function, and seizure disorders.
Administration and Handling
IM
• Store in refrigerator. Do not freeze.
• Administer undiluted by deep IM injection in the upper outer quadrant of the buttock for adolescents and adults and the midlateral muscle of the thigh for infants and children.
◂ **ALERT** ▸ Do not give IV, intra-arterially, or subcutaneously because giving penicillin G via these routes may cause death, heart attack, severe neurovascular damage, and thrombosis.
Intervention and Evaluation
• Monitor the patient's complete blood count, renal function tests, and urinalysis results.
Patient/Family Teaching
• Warn the patient/family to immediately report if the patient experiences, chills, fever, rash, or any other unusual sign or symptom.
• Explain to the patient/family that the patient may experience temporary pain at the injection site.

Penicillin G Potassium
pen-ih-**sil**-lin G
(Megacillin [CAN], Novepen-G [CAN], Pfizerpen)

CATEGORY AND SCHEDULE
Pregnancy Risk Category: B

MECHANISM OF ACTION
A penicillin that binds to one or more of the penicillin-binding proteins of bacteria. ***Therapeutic Effect:*** Inhibits bacterial cell wall synthesis. Bactericidal.

AVAILABILITY
Injection: 1 million units, 5 million units, 20 million units.
Premixed Dextrose Solution:
1 million units, 2 million units, 3 million units.

INDICATIONS AND DOSAGES

▸ Treatment of sepsis, meningitis, pericarditis, endocarditis, pneumonia due to susceptible gram-positive organisms (not *Staphylococcus aureus*), some gram-negative organisms

IM/IV

Children. 100,000–400,000 units/kg/day in divided doses q4–6h. Maximum: 24 million units/day.

▸ Dosage in renal impairment

Creatinine Clearance	Dosage Interval
10–30 mL/min	q8–12h
Less than 10 mL/min	q12–18h

CONTRAINDICATIONS

Hypersensitivity to any penicillin.

INTERACTIONS

Drug

Erythromycin, chloramphenicol, tetracyclines: May antagonize effects of penicillin.

Probenecid: Increases serum concentration of penicillin.

Herbal

None known.

Food

None known.

DIAGNOSTIC TEST EFFECTS

May cause positive Coombs' test results.

IV INCOMPATIBILITIES

Amikacin (Amikin), aminophylline, amphotericin, dopamine (Intropin)

IV COMPATIBILITIES

Amiodarone (Cordarone), calcium gluconate, diltiazem (Cardizem), diphenhydramine (Benadryl), furosemide (Lasix), heparin, hydromorphone (Dilaudid), lidocaine, magnesium sulfate, methylprednisolone (Solu-Medrol), morphine, potassium chloride

SIDE EFFECTS

Occasional

Lethargy, fever, dizziness, rash, electrolyte imbalance, diarrhea, thrombophlebitis

Rare

Seizures, interstitial nephritis

SERIOUS REACTIONS

! Hypersensitivity reactions ranging from rash, fever, and chills to anaphylaxis occur.

PEDIATRIC CONSIDERATIONS

Baseline Assessment

◂ **ALERT** ▸ Determine the patient's history of allergies, particularly to aspirin, cephalosporins, and penicillins, before beginning drug therapy.

- Rapid IV administration may lead to electrolyte imbalances or seizures.
- Administer into the infant or child's largest muscle to decrease pain.
- Assess for age-appropriate fluid intake.

Precautions

- Use cautiously in pts with a hypersensitivity to cephalosporins, impaired liver or renal function, and seizure disorders.

Administration and Handling

IV

- Reconstituted solution is stable for 7 days if refrigerated.
- Follow dilution guide per manufacturer.
- After reconstitution, further dilute with 50–100 mL D_5W or 0.9% NaCl for a final concentration of 100–500,000 units/mL (50,000 units/mL for infants and neonates).
- Infuse over 15–60 min.

Intervention and Evaluation
- Monitor the patient's complete blood count, electrolytes, renal function tests, and urinalysis results.

Patient/Family Teaching
- Advise the patient/family to continue to take the drug for the full course of treatment.
- Explain to the patient/family that drug doses should be spaced evenly around the clock.
- Warn the patient/family to immediately notify the physician if the patient experiences diarrhea, a rash, fever, or chills, or any other unusual sign or symptoms.

Penicillin V Potassium

pen-ih-**sil**-lin V
(Abbocillin VK [AUS], Apo-Pen-VK [CAN], Cilicaine VK [AUS], L.P.V. [AUS], Novo-Pen-VK [CAN], Pen-Vee K, V-Cillin-K, Veetids)
(See Color Plate)

CATEGORY AND SCHEDULE
Pregnancy Risk Category: B

MECHANISM OF ACTION
A penicillin that binds to bacterial cell membranes. ***Therapeutic Effect:*** Inhibits cell wall synthesis. Bactericidal.

PHARMACOKINETICS
Moderately absorbed from the GI tract. Protein binding: 80%. Widely distributed. Metabolized in liver. Primarily excreted in urine. ***Half-Life:*** 1 hr (half-life is increased in those with impaired renal function).

AVAILABILITY
Tablets: 250 mg, 500 mg.
Powder for Oral Solution: 125 mg/5 mL, 250 mg/5 mL.

INDICATIONS AND DOSAGES
▸ **Mild to moderate respiratory tract or skin or skin-structure infections; otitis media; or necrotizing ulcerative gingivitis**
PO
Children 12 yrs and older. 125–500 mg q6–8h.
Children younger than 12 yrs. 25–50 mg/kg/day in divided doses q6–8h. Maximum: 3 g/day.
▸ **Primary prevention of rheumatic fever**
PO
Children older than 5 yrs. 250–500 mg 2–3 times/day for 10 days.
Children younger than 5 yrs. 125 mg 2–3 times/day for 10 days.
▸ **Prophylaxis for recurrent rheumatic fever**
PO
Children older than 5 yrs. 250 mg 2 times/day.
Children between the ages of 2 mos. and 3 yrs. 125 mg 2 times/day.
▸ **Systemic infections**
PO
Children younger than 12 yrs. 25–50 mg/kg/day divided q6–8h. Maximum: 3 g/day.
Children older than 12 yrs. 125–500 mg divided q6–8h.

CONTRAINDICATIONS
Hypersensitivity to any penicillin.

INTERACTIONS
Drug
Probenecid: May increase penicillin V blood concentration and risk of toxicity.
Herbal
None known.
Food
Food or milk may decrease absorption.

DIAGNOSTIC TEST EFFECTS

May cause positive Coombs' test results.

SIDE EFFECTS

Frequent
Mild hypersensitivity reaction (chills, fever, rash), nausea, vomiting, diarrhea
Rare
Bleeding, allergic reaction

SERIOUS REACTIONS

! Severe hypersensitivity reaction, including anaphylaxis, may occur.
! Nephrotoxicity, antibiotic-associated colitis (severe abdominal pain and tenderness, fever, and watery and severe diarrhea), and other superinfections may result from high dosages or prolonged therapy.

PEDIATRIC CONSIDERATIONS

Baseline Assessment
◂ALERT▸ Determine the patient's history of allergies, particularly to aspirin, cephalosporins and penicillins before beginning drug therapy.
• Be aware that penicillin V readily crosses the placenta, appears in amniotic fluid and cord blood, and is distributed in breast milk in low concentrations.
• Be aware that penicillin V use may lead to allergic sensitization, candidiasis, diarrhea, and skin rash in infants.
• Use caution when giving penicillin V to neonates and young infants because these pts may have delayed renal elimination of the drug.
• Assess for age-appropriate fluid intake.
Precautions
• Use cautiously in pts with a history of allergies, particularly to aspirin or cephalosporins, a history of seizures, and renal impairment.
Administration and Handling
PO
• Store tablets at room temperature. Oral solution, after reconstitution, is stable for 14 days if refrigerated.
• Space drug doses evenly around the clock.
• Give without regard to meals.
Intervention and Evaluation
• Withhold penicillin V potassium and promptly notify the physician if the patient experiences any diarrhea (may indicate antibiotic-associated colitis if abdominal pain, fever, and mucus and blood in stools are also seen) or rash (may indicate hypersensitivity).
• Monitor the patient's intake and output, renal function tests, and urinalysis results for signs of nephrotoxicity.
• Be alert for signs and symptoms of superinfection including anal or genital pruritus, diarrhea, increased fever, nausea, sore throat, ulceration or changes of oral mucosa, vaginal discharge, and vomiting.
• Review the patient's blood Hgb levels.
• Check the patient for signs of bleeding including bruising, overt bleeding, and swelling of tissue.
Patient/Family Teaching
• Advise the patient/family to continue penicillin V potassium for the full length of treatment and to space drug doses evenly around the clock.
• Warn the patient/family to immediately notify the physician if the patient experiences bleeding, bruising, diarrhea, rash, or any other new symptom.

Piperacillin Sodium/Tazobactam Sodium

pip-ur-ah-**sill**-in/tay-zoe-**back**-tam
(Tazocin [CAN], Zosyn)
Do not confuse with Zofran or Zyvox.

CATEGORY AND SCHEDULE
Pregnancy Risk Category: B

MECHANISM OF ACTION
A penicillin antibiotic.
Piperacillin: binds to bacterial cell membranes. ***Therapeutic Effect:*** Inhibits cell wall synthesis. Bactericidal.
Tazobactam: inactivates bacterial β-lactamase enzymes. ***Therapeutic Effect:*** Protects piperacillin from inactivation by β-lactamase–producing organisms, extends spectrum of activity, and prevents bacterial overgrowth.

PHARMACOKINETICS
Protein binding: 16%–30%. Widely distributed. Primarily excreted unchanged in urine. Moderately removed by hemodialysis. ***Half-Life:*** 0.7–1.2 hrs (half-life is increased in those with hepatic cirrhosis or impaired renal function).

AVAILABILITY
Powder for Injection: 2.25 g, 3.375 g, 4.5 g.
Premix Ready to Use: 2.25 g, 3.375 g, 4.5 g.

INDICATIONS AND DOSAGES (DOSES ARE BASED ON THE PIPERACILLIN COMPONENT)
▸ **Severe infections**
IV
Children older than 12 yrs. 4 g divided q6h. Maximum: 18 g/day.

▸ **Moderate infections**
IV
Infants and children older than 6 mos. 240 mg/kg/day (piperacillin component) divided q8h. Maximum: 18 g piperacillin component/day.
Children older than 12 yrs. 3.375 g q6h. Maximum: 18 g piperacillin component/day.

▸ **Dosage in renal impairment for adolescents/adults**
Dosage and frequency are based on creatinine clearance.

Creatinine Clearance	Interval
20–40 mL/min	2.25 g q6h
Less than 20 mL/min	2.25 g q8h

CONTRAINDICATIONS
Hypersensitivity to any penicillin.

INTERACTIONS
Drug
Hepatotoxic medications: May increase the risk of liver toxicity.
Probenecid: May increase piperacillin blood concentration and the risk of toxicity.
Methotrexate: May decrease clearance of methotrexate.
Herbal
None known.
Food
None known.

DIAGNOSTIC TEST EFFECTS
May increase serum alkaline phosphatase, serum bilirubin, serum lactate dehydrogenase, SGOT (AST), SGPT (ALT), and serum sodium levels. May cause positive Coombs' test results. May decrease serum potassium level.

IV INCOMPATIBILITIES
Amphotericin (Fungizone), amphotericin B complex (Abelcet, AmBisome, Amphotec),

chlorpromazine (Thorazine), dacarbazine (DTIC), daunorubicin (Cerubidine), dobutamine (Dobutrex), doxorubicin (Adriamycin), doxorubicin liposome (Doxil), droperidol (Inapsine), famotidine (Pepcid), haloperidol (Haldol), hydroxyzine (Vistaril), idarubicin (Idamycin), minocycline (Minocin), nalbuphine (Nubain), prochlorperazine (Compazine), promethazine (Phenergan), vancomycin (Vancocin)

IV COMPATIBILITIES

Aminophylline, bumetanide (Bumex), calcium gluconate, diphenhydramine (Benadryl), dopamine (Intropin), enalapril (Vasotec), furosemide (Lasix), granisetron (Kytril), heparin, hydrocortisone (Solu-Cortef), hydromorphone (Dilaudid), lorazepam (Ativan), magnesium sulfate, methylprednisolone (Solu-Medrol), metoclopramide (Reglan), morphine, ondansetron (Zofran), potassium chloride

SIDE EFFECTS

Frequent
Diarrhea, headache, constipation, nausea, insomnia, rash
Occasional
Vomiting, dyspepsia, pruritus, fever, agitation, pain, moniliasis, dizziness, abdominal pain, edema, anxiety, dyspnea, rhinitis

SERIOUS REACTIONS

! Antibiotic-associated colitis as evidenced by severe abdominal pain and tenderness, fever, and watery and severe diarrhea may result from altered bacterial balance.
! Overdosage, more often with renal impairment, may produce seizures and neurologic reactions.
! Severe hypersensitivity reactions, including anaphylaxis, occur rarely.

PEDIATRIC CONSIDERATIONS

Baseline Assessment

◂ALERT▸ Determine the patient's history of allergies, especially to cephalosporins and penicillins, before beginning drug therapy.
• Be aware that piperacillin readily crosses the placenta, appears in amniotic fluid and cord blood, and is distributed in breast milk in low concentrations.
• Piperacillin use in infants may lead to allergic sensitization, candidiasis, diarrhea, and skin rash.
• Be aware that piperacillin dosage has not been established for children younger than 12 yrs of age.
• Assure age-appropriate fluid intake.
• Seizures can occur with rapid IV administration.

Precautions

• Use cautiously in pts with a history of allergies, especially to cephalosporins, preexisting seizure disorder, and renal impairment.

Administration and Handling

IV

• Reconstituted vial is stable for 24 hrs at room temperature or 48 hrs if refrigerated.
• After further dilution, the solution is stable for 24 hrs at room temperature or 7 days if refrigerated.
• Reconstitute each 1 g with 5 mL D_5W or 0.9% NaCl. Shake vigorously to dissolve.
• Further dilute with at least 50 mL D_5W, 0.9% NaCl, or lactated Ringer's solution.
• Infuse over 30 min.

Intervention and Evaluation

• Assess the patient's pattern of daily bowel activity and stool consistency. Mild GI effects may be tolerable, but increasing severity may indicate onset of antibiotic-associated colitis.

- Be alert for signs and symptoms of superinfection including abdominal pain, moderate to severe diarrhea, severe anal or genital pruritus, and severe mouth soreness.
- Monitor the patient's electrolytes, especially potassium, intake and output, renal function tests, and urinalysis results.

Patient/Family Teaching

- Advise the patient/family to immediately notify the physician if the patient experiences severe diarrhea and to avoid taking antidiarrheals until directed to do so by the physician.
- Warn the patient/family to notify the physician if the patient experiences pain, redness, or swelling at the infusion site.
- Explain to the patient/family that piperacillin contains 1.85 mEq of sodium and that the patient should discuss a reduction in salt intake with the physician.

Ticarcillin Disodium/Clavulanate Potassium

tie-car-**sill**-in/klah-view-**lan**-ate (Timentin)

CATEGORY AND SCHEDULE

Pregnancy Risk Category: B

MECHANISM OF ACTION

A penicillin antibiotic.
Ticarcillin: Binds to bacterial cell wall, inhibiting bacterial cell wall synthesis. ***Therapeutic Effect:*** Causes cell lysis, death. Bactericidal.
Clavulanate: Inhibits action of bacterial beta-lactamase. ***Therapeutic Effect:*** Protects ticarcillin from enzymatic degradation.

PHARMACOKINETICS

Widely distributed. Protein binding: ticarcillin: 45%–60%; clavulanate: 9%–30%. Minimal metabolism in liver. Primarily excreted unchanged in urine. Removed by hemodialysis. ***Half-Life:*** 1–1.2 hrs (half-life is increased in those with impaired renal function).

AVAILABILITY

Powder for Injection: 3.1 g (ticarcillin 3 g/clavulanic acid 0.1 g).
Solution for Infusion: 3.1 g/100 mL. (ticarcillin 3 g/clavulanic acid 0.1 g).

INDICATIONS AND DOSAGES (DOSES ARE BASED ON THE TICARCILLIN COMPONENT)

▸ **Septicemia; skin and skin-structure, bone, joint, and lower respiratory tract infections; endometriosis**

IV

Infants and children older than 3 mos. 200–300 mg/kg/day (as ticarcillin) divided q4–6h. Maximum: 24 g/day.
Infants younger than 3 mos and term neonates. 200–300 mg/kg/day of ticarcillin component divided q6–8h.

▸ **Cystic fibrosis**

IM/IV

Children. 300–600 mg/kg/day of ticarcillin component divided q4–6h. Maximum: 24 g/day.

▸ **Dosage in renal impairment**

Creatinine Clearance	Dosage Interval
10–30 mL/min	q8h
Less than 10 mL/min	q12h

CONTRAINDICATIONS

Hypersensitivity to any penicillin or clavulanate.

INTERACTIONS

Drug

Probenecid: May increase ticarcillin blood concentration and risk of toxicity.

Herbal

None known.

Food

None known.

DIAGNOSTIC TEST EFFECTS

May cause positive Coombs' test results. May increase bleeding time, serum alkaline phosphatase, serum bilirubin, serum creatinine, serum lactate dehydrogenase, SGOT (AST), and SGPT (ALT) levels. May decrease serum potassium, sodium, and uric acid levels.

IV INCOMPATIBILITIES

Amphotericin B complex (Abelcet, AmBisome, Amphotec), vancomycin (Vancocin)

IV COMPATIBILITIES

Diltiazem (Cardizem), heparin, insulin, morphine, propofol (Diprivan)

SIDE EFFECTS

Frequent

Phlebitis, thrombophlebitis with IV dose, rash, urticaria, pruritus, smell or taste disturbances

Occasional

Nausea, diarrhea, vomiting

Rare

Headache, fatigue, hallucinations, bleeding or bruising

SERIOUS REACTIONS

! Overdosage may produce seizures and neurologic reactions.

! Superinfections, including potentially fatal antibiotic-associated colitis, may result from bacterial imbalance.

! Severe hypersensitivity reactions, including anaphylaxis, occur rarely.

PEDIATRIC CONSIDERATIONS

Baseline Assessment

◂ALERT▸ Determine the patient's history of allergies, especially to cephalosporins and penicillins, before beginning drug therapy.

- Be aware that ticarcillin readily crosses the placenta, appears in amniotic fluid and cord blood, and is distributed in breast milk in low concentrations.
- Ticarcillin use in infants may lead to allergic sensitization, candidiasis, diarrhea, and skin rash.
- Be aware that the safety and efficacy of this drug have not been established in children younger than 3 mos.
- Assess for age-appropriate fluid intake.
- Rapid IV infusion may cause seizures.

Precautions

- Use cautiously in pts with a history of allergies, especially to cephalosporins, and renal impairment.

Administration and Handling

IV

- Solution normally appears colorless to pale yellow (if solution darkens, this indicates loss of potency).
- Reconstituted IV infusion (piggyback) is stable for 24 hrs at room temperature, 3 days if refrigerated.
- Discard if precipitate forms.
- Available in ready-to-use containers.
- For IV infusion (piggyback), reconstitute each 3.1-g vial with

13 mL Sterile Water for Injection or 0.9% NaCl to provide concentration of 200 mg ticarcillin and 6.7 mg clavulanic acid per mL.
• Shake vial to assist reconstitution.
• Further dilute with 50–100 mL D_5W or 0.9% NaCl.
• Infuse over 30 min.
• Because of the potential for hypersensitivity reactions such as anaphylaxis, start the initial dose at a few drops per minute and increase slowly to the ordered rate. Monitor the patient for the first 10–15 min, and then check the patient every 10 min.

Intervention and Evaluation

• Withhold the drug and promptly notify the physician if the patient experiences diarrhea (with fever, abdominal pain, and mucus and blood in stools may indicate antibiotic-associated colitis) or rash (may indicate hypersensitivity).
• Assess the patient's food tolerance.
• Provide the patient with mouth care, sugarless gum, or hard candy to offset the drug's taste and smell effects.
• Evaluate the patient's IV site for signs and symptoms of phlebitis as evidenced by heat, pain, and red streaking over the vein.
• Monitor the patient's intake and output, renal function tests, and urinalysis results.
• Assess the patient for signs and symptoms of bruising or tissue swelling and overt bleeding.
• Monitor the patient's hematology reports and serum electrolytes, particularly potassium.
• Be alert for signs and symptoms of superinfection including anal or genital pruritus, diarrhea, increased fever, sore throat, ulceration or other oral changes, and vomiting.

Patient/Family Teaching

• Advise the patient/family to immediately notify the physician if the patient experiences pain, redness, or swelling at the infusion site.
• Warn the patient/family to immediately notify the physician if the patient experiences severe diarrhea, a rash or itching, or any other unusual sign or symptom.

REFERENCES

Gunn, V. L. & Nechyba, C. (2002). The Harriet Lane handbook (16th ed.). St. Louis: Mosby.
Miller, S. & Fioravanti, J. (1997). Pediatric medications: A handbook for nurses. St. Louis: Mosby.
Taketomo, C. K., Hodding, J. H. & Kraus, D. M. (2003–2004). Pediatric dosage handbook (10th ed.). Hudson, OH: Lexi-Comp.

10 Quinolones

Ciprofloxacin Hydrochloride
Ofloxacin

Uses: Quinolones are used primarily to treat lower respiratory tract infections, skin and skin-structure infections, urinary tract infections, and sexually transmitted diseases.

Action: Quinolones are bactericidal and act against a wide range of gram-negative and gram-positive organisms. In susceptible microorganisms, they inhibit DNA gyrase, the enzyme responsible for unwinding and supercoiling DNA before it replicates. By inhibiting DNA gyrase, quinolones interfere with bacterial cell replication and repair and cause cell death. (See illustration, *Sites and Mechanisms of Action: Anti-Infective Agents,* page 2.)

COMBINATION PRODUCTS

CIPRODEX OTIC: ciprofloxacin/dexamethasone (a steroid) 0.3%/0.1%.

CIPRO HC OTIC: ciprofloxacin/hydrocortisone (a steroid) 0.2%/1%.

Ciprofloxacin Hydrochloride

sip-row-**flocks**-ah-sin
(C-Flox [AUS], Ciloquin [AUS], Ciloxan (ophthalmic), Cipro, Ciproxin [AUS])
Do not confuse with cinoxacin or Cytoxan.
(See Color Plate)

CATEGORY AND SCHEDULE

Pregnancy Risk Category: C

MECHANISM OF ACTION

A fluoroquinolone that inhibits DNA enzyme in susceptible bacteria. ***Therapeutic Effect:*** Interferes with bacterial DNA replication. Bactericidal.

PHARMACOKINETICS

Well absorbed from the GI tract (absorption is delayed by food). Protein binding: 20%–40%. Widely distributed (including cerebrospinal fluid). Metabolized in liver to active metabolite. Primarily excreted in urine. Minimal removal by hemodialysis. ***Half-Life:*** 2–3 hrs in children.

AVAILABILITY

Tablets: 100 mg, 250 mg, 500 mg, 750 mg.
Tablets (extended-release): 500 mg.
Oral Suspension: 50 mg/mL, 100 mg/mL.
Injection: 200 mg, 400 mg.
Ophthalmic Solution: 3.33 mg/mL (0.3% base).
Ophthalmic Ointment: 3.33 mg/mL (0.3% base).

INDICATIONS AND DOSAGES

▸ **Usual pediatric dosage**

PO

Children. 20–30 mg/kg/day in 2 divided doses. Maximum: 1.5 g/day.

IV
Children. 10–20 mg/kg/day in 2 divided doses q12h. Maximum: 800 mg/day.

▸ **Cystic fibrosis**
PO
Children. 40 mg/kg/day in 2 divided doses q12h. Maximum: 2 g/day.
IV
Children. 30 mg/kg/day in 2 divided doses q12. Maximum: 1.2 g/day.
OPHTHALMIC DROPS
Children. 1–2 drops q2h when awake for 2 days, then 1–2 drops q4h when awake for 5 days.
OINTMENT
Children. Apply 0.5-in ribbon of ointment 3 times/day for 2 days, then 2 times/day for 5 days.

▸ **Dosage in renal impairment**
The dosage and frequency are modified in pts based on the severity of infection and the degree of renal impairment.

Creatinine Clearance	Dosage Interval
Less than 30 mL/min	q18–24h

Hemodialysis, peritoneal dialysis 250–500 mg q24h (after dialysis).

UNLABELED USES
Treatment of chancroid.

CONTRAINDICATIONS
Hypersensitivity to ciprofloxacin, quinolones.
Ophthalmic: Vaccinia, varicella, epithelial herpes simplex, keratitis, mycobacterial infection, fungal disease of ocular structure. Not for use after uncomplicated removal of foreign body.

INTERACTIONS
Drug
Antacids, iron preparations, sucralfate: May decrease ciprofloxacin absorption. Separate administration by 2 hrs.
Oral anticoagulants: May increase the effects of oral anticoagulants.
Theophylline: Decreases clearance and may increase blood concentration and risk of toxicity of this drug.
Cyclosporin: Decreases clearance and may increase blood concentration and risk of toxicity of this drug.
Herbal
None known.
Food
None known.

DIAGNOSTIC TEST EFFECTS
May increase BUN, serum alkaline phosphatase, serum bilirubin, serum creatinine, lactate dehydrogenase, SGOT (AST), and SGPT (ALT) levels.

IV INCOMPATIBILITIES
Aminophylline, ampicillin/sulbactam (Unasyn), cefepime (Maxipime), dexamethasone (Decadron), furosemide (Lasix), heparin, hydrocortisone (Solu-Cortef), methylprednisolone (Solu-Medrol), phenytoin (Dilantin), sodium bicarbonate

IV COMPATIBILITIES
Calcium gluconate, diltiazem (Cardizem), dobutamine (Dobutrex), dopamine (Intropin), lidocaine, lorazepam (Ativan), magnesium, midazolam (Versed), potassium chloride

SIDE EFFECTS
Frequent (5%–2%)
Nausea, diarrhea, dyspepsia, vomiting, constipation, flatulence, confusion, crystalluria
Ophthalmic: Burning, crusting in corner of eye

Occasional (less than 2%)
Abdominal pain or discomfort, headache, rash
Ophthalmic: Bad taste, sense of something in eye, redness of eyelids, eyelid itching
Rare (less than 1%)
Dizziness, confusion, tremors, hallucinations, hypersensitivity reaction, insomnia, dry mouth, paresthesia, tendonitis

SERIOUS REACTIONS

! Superinfection (especially enterococcal or fungal), nephropathy, cardiopulmonary arrest, and cerebral thrombosis may occur.
! Arthropathy may occur if the drug is given to children younger than 18 yrs.
! Sensitization to the ophthalmic form of the drug may contraindicate later systemic use of ciprofloxacin.

PEDIATRIC CONSIDERATIONS

Baseline Assessment

◂ALERT▸ Determine the patient's history of hypersensitivity to ciprofloxacin and quinolones before beginning drug therapy.
• Be aware that it is unknown whether ciprofloxacin is distributed in breast milk. If possible, do not use during pregnancy or breast-feeding because of the risk of arthropathy to the fetus or infant.
• The safety and efficacy of ciprofloxacin have not been established in children younger than 18 yrs of age.
• Never give the medication by IV push.
• Assure age-appropriate fluid intake.

Precautions

• Use cautiously in pts with CNS disorders, renal impairment, and seizures and those taking caffeine or theophylline.
• Do not use the suspension in a nasogastric tube.

Administration and Handling

PO
• May be given without regard to meals (preferred dosing time: 2 hrs after meals).
• Do not administer antacids (aluminum or magnesium) within 2 hrs of ciprofloxacin.
• Provide the patient with sufficient amounts of citrus fruits and cranberry juice to acidify urine.
• Suspension may be stored for 14 days at room temperature.
• Shake suspension well before administration.

IV
• Store at room temperature.
• Solution normally appears clear and colorless to slightly yellow.
• Available prediluted in infusion container ready for use.
• Infuse over 60 min.

OPHTHALMIC
• Tilt the patient's head back and place the solution in the conjunctival sac of the affected eye.
• Have the patient close his or her eye, then press gently on the lacrimal sac for 1 min.
• Do not use ophthalmic solutions for injection.
• Unless the infection is very superficial, systemic administration generally accompanies ophthalmic use.

Intervention and Evaluation

• Evaluate the patient's food tolerance.
• Assess the patient's pattern of daily bowel activity and stool consistency.
• Evaluate the patient for dizziness, headache, tremors, and visual difficulties.

• Assess the patient for chest and joint pain.
• Observe pts receiving the ophthalmic form for therapeutic response.

Patient/Family Teaching

• Advise the patient/family not to skip drug doses and to take ciprofloxacin for the full length of therapy.
• Instruct the patient/family to take ciprofloxacin during meals with 8 oz of water and to drink several glasses of water between meals.
• Encourage the patient/family to eat foods and drink liquids that are high in ascorbic acid (e.g., citrus fruits and cranberry juice) to prevent crystalluria.
• Warn the patient/family not to take antacids while taking this drug because antacids reduce or destroy the effectiveness of ciprofloxacin.
• Teach the patient/family to shake the suspension well before using and not to chew the microcapsules in suspension.
• Explain to the patient/family that sugarless gum or hard candy may relieve the bad taste of ciprofloxacin.
• For pts receiving the ophthalmic form of ciprofloxacin, explain to the patient/family that a crystal precipitate may form, which usually resolves in 1–7 days.
• Advise the patient/family to notify a health care provider if tendon pain or swelling is evident.
• Because ciprofloxacin may cause photosensitivity; caution the patient/family against exposure to sunlight and tanning beds and advise the patient/family to wear protective clothing and use a broad-spectrum sunscreen when outdoors.
• Instruct the patient/family to remove contact lenses before administration of the ophthalmic solution or ointment.

Ofloxacin

oh-**flocks**-ah-sin
(Apo-Oflox [CAN], Floxin, Floxin Otic, Ocuflox)
Do not confuse with Flexeril, Flexon, or Ocufen.

CATEGORY AND SCHEDULE

Pregnancy Risk Category: C

MECHANISM OF ACTION

A fluoroquinolone that inhibits DNA gyrase in susceptible microorganisms. ***Therapeutic Effect:*** Interferes with bacterial DNA replication and repair. Bactericidal.

PHARMACOKINETICS

Rapidly, well absorbed from the GI tract. Protein binding: 20%–25%. Widely distributed (penetrates cerebrospinal fluid). Metabolized in liver. Primarily excreted in urine. Removed by hemodialysis. ***Half-Life:*** 4.7–7 hrs (half-life is increased with impaired renal function and cirrhosis).

AVAILABILITY

Tablets: 200 mg, 300 mg, 400 mg.
Premix Injection: 400 mg/100 mL D_5W.
Ophthalmic Solution: 0.3%.
Otic Solution: 0.3%.

INDICATIONS AND DOSAGES

OTIC

▸ **Otitis media**

Children 1–12 yrs. 5 drops 2 times/day for 10 days. Eardrops

should be at body temperature (wrap hand around bottle).
Children older than 12 yrs. 10 drops 2 times/day for 10 days.

▸ **Chronic suppurative otitis media**
Children older than 12 yrs. 10 drops 2 times/day for 14 days.

▸ **Acute otitis media with tympanostomy tubes**
Children 1–12 yrs. 5 drops 2 times/day for 10 days.
OPHTHALMIC
Children older than 1 yr. 1 drop q2–4h for 2 days, then 4 times/day for 5 extra days.

CONTRAINDICATIONS

For children younger than 18 yrs of age, hypersensitivity to any quinolones.

INTERACTIONS

Drug

Antacids, sucralfate: May decrease absorption and effects of ofloxacin.
Theophylline: May increase blood concentrations and risk of theophylline toxicity.
Cyclosporin: May increase blood concentrations and risk of cyclosporine toxicity

Herbal

None known.

Food

None known.

DIAGNOSTIC TEST EFFECTS

None known.

IV INCOMPATIBILITIES

Amphotericin B complex (Abelcet, AmBisome, Amphotec), cefepime (Maxipime), doxorubicin liposome (Doxil)

IV COMPATIBILITIES

Propofol (Diprivan)

SIDE EFFECTS

Frequent (10%–7%)
Nausea, headache, insomnia
Occasional (5%–3%)
Abdominal pain, diarrhea, vomiting, dry mouth, flatulence, dizziness, fatigue, drowsiness, rash, pruritus, fever
Rare (less than 1%)
Constipation, numbness of the feet and hands

SERIOUS REACTIONS

! Superinfection and severe hypersensitivity reaction occur rarely.
! Arthropathy manifested as swelling, pain, clubbing of fingers and toes, and degeneration of stress-bearing portion of a joint may occur if the drug is given to children.

PEDIATRIC CONSIDERATIONS

Baseline Assessment

◂ **ALERT** ▸ Determine the patient's history of hypersensitivity to ofloxacin or any quinolones before beginning drug therapy.
• Be aware that ofloxacin is distributed in breast milk, has potentially serious adverse reactions in nursing infants, and presents a risk of arthropathy development to a fetus.
• Be aware that the safety and efficacy of ofloxacin have not been established in children. The safety and efficacy of the otic form of ofloxacin have not been established in children younger than 1 yr of age.

Precautions

• Use cautiously in pts with CNS disorders, renal impairment, and seizures, and those taking caffeine or theophylline.
• Use cautiously in pts with syphilis because ofloxacin may

mask or delay symptoms of syphilis. A serologic test for syphilis should be done at diagnosis and 3 mos after treatment.

Administration and Handling

PO

• Do not give with food. The preferred dosing time is 1 hr before or 2 hrs after meals.
• Do not administer antacids (aluminum or magnesium) or iron- or zinc-containing products within 2 hrs of administering ofloxacin.
• Provide the patient with citrus fruits and cranberry juice to acidify urine.
• Give with 8 oz of water and encourage fluid intake.

OPHTHALMIC

• Tilt the patient's head back and place the solution in the conjunctival sac.
• Have the patient close his or her eye; then press gently on the lacrimal sac for 1 min.
• Do not use ophthalmic solutions for injection.
• Unless the infection is very superficial, expect to also administer systemic drug therapy.

OTIC

• Instruct the patient to lie down with his or her head turned so the affected ear is upright.
• Instill drops toward the canal wall, not directly on the eardrum.
• Pull the auricle down and posterior in children or up and posterior in adults.

Intervention and Evaluation

• Monitor the patient for signs and symptoms of infection.
• Monitor the patient's mental status and WBC count.
• Assess the patient's skin for rash. Withhold the drug at the first sign of rash or other allergic reaction and promptly notify the physician.
• Assess the patient's pattern of daily bowel activity and stool consistency.
• Observe the patient during the night for insomnia.
• Evaluate the patient for dizziness, headache, tremors, and visual difficulties.
• Evaluate the patient for joint tenderness, swelling.
• Provide ambulation assistance as needed.
• Be alert for signs of superinfection manifested as anal or genital pruritus, discomfort in the mouth, fever, sores, and vaginitis.

Patient/Family Teaching

• Instruct the patient/family not to take antacids within 6 hrs before or 2 hrs after taking ofloxacin. Teach the patient/family that ofloxacin is best taken 1 hr before or 2 hrs after meals.
• Warn the patient/family that ofloxacin may cause dizziness, drowsiness, headache, and insomnia.
• Advise the patient/family to avoid tasks requiring mental alertness or motor skills until the patient's response to ofloxacin is established.

REFERENCES

Gunn, V. L. & Nechyba, C. (2002). The Harriet Lane handbook (16th ed.). St. Louis: Mosby. Louis.

Miller, S. & Fioravanti, J. (1997). Pediatric medications: A handbook for nurses. St. Louis: Mosby.

Taketomo, C. K., Hodding, J. H. & Kraus, D. M. (2003–2004). Pediatric dosage handbook (10th ed.). Hudson, OH: Lexi-Comp.

11 Tetracyclines

Demeclocycline Hydrochloride
Doxycycline
Minocycline Hydrochloride
Tetracycline Hydrochloride

Uses: Tetracyclines are used to treat rickettsial diseases (such as typhus fever and Q fever), *Chlamydia trachomatis* infections, brucellosis, cholera, pneumonia caused by *Mycoplasma pneumoniae,* Lyme disease, *Helicobacter pylori* gastric infections (in combination therapy), and periodontal disease. Topical formulations are used to treat acne.

Action: Tetracyclines are bacteriostatic. They inhibit bacterial protein synthesis by binding to the 30S ribosomal subunit and preventing the binding of transfer RNA to messenger RNA. (See illustration, *Mechanism of Action: Tetracyclines,* page 175.)

Demeclocycline Hydrochloride

deh-meh-clo-**sigh**-clean
(Declomycin, Ledermycin [AUS])

CATEGORY AND SCHEDULE
Pregnancy Risk Category: D

MECHANISM OF ACTION
This tetracycline antibiotic produces bacteriostasis by binding to ribosomal receptor sites; it also inhibits antidiuretic hormone–induced water reabsorption. ***Therapeutic Effect:*** Inhibits bacterial protein synthesis. Produces water diuresis.

AVAILABILITY
Tablets: 150 mg, 300 mg.

INDICATIONS AND DOSAGES
▸ **Mild to moderate infections, including acne, pertussis, chronic bronchitis, and urinary tract infection**

PO

Children older than 8 yrs.
8–12 mg/kg/day in 2–4 divided doses.

CONTRAINDICATIONS
Hypersensitivity to tetracyclines, last half of pregnancy, infants, children up to 8 yrs of age.

INTERACTIONS
Drug

Antacids containing aluminum, calcium, or magnesium; laxatives containing magnesium; oral iron preparations: Impair the absorption of tetracyclines.
Cholestyramine, colestipol: May decrease demeclocycline absorption.
Oral contraceptives: May decrease the effects of these drugs.

Herbal

None known.

Food

Milk, dairy products: May decrease demeclocycline absorption.

DIAGNOSTIC TEST EFFECTS
May increase BUN, serum alkaline phosphatase, serum amylase, serum bilirubin, SGOT (AST), and SGPT (ALT) levels.

SIDE EFFECTS
Frequent

Anorexia, nausea, vomiting, diarrhea, dysphagia

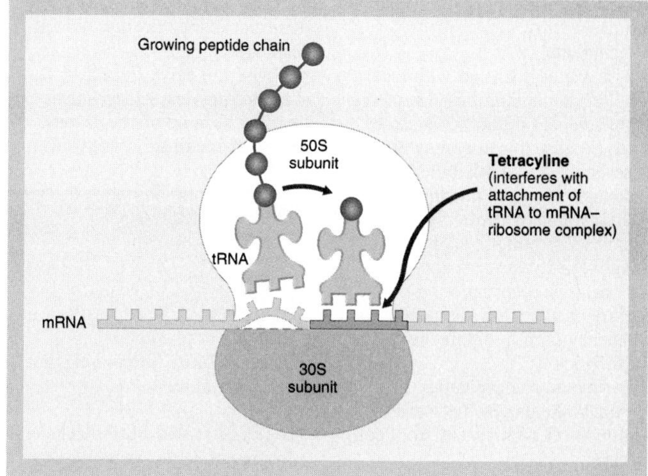

Mechanism of Action: Tetracyclines

Like certain other anti-infectives, tetracyclines work by interfering with bacterial protein synthesis. Protein synthesis normally occurs when the ribosomal subunits 50S and 30S bind to messenger RNA (mRNA), which arranges amino acids into peptide chains that form proteins. Then transfer RNA (tRNA) helps carry out genetic instructions from mRNA to arrange certain amino acids in a specific sequence to form a growing peptide chain. Once the peptide chain is complete, mRNA detaches from the ribosomal subunits, and the new protein is created.

Tetracyclines inhibit bacterial protein synthesis by attaching to the 30S ribosomal subunit. As a result, tRNA cannot bind with the mRNA-ribosome complex, and no new amino acids can be synthesized or added to the growing peptide chain.

Exaggerated sunburn reaction may occur with moderate to high demeclocycline dosage.

Occasional

Urticaria, rash

Long-term therapy may result in diabetes insipidus syndrome: polydipsia, polyuria, and weakness.

SERIOUS REACTIONS

! Superinfection (especially fungal), anaphylaxis, and increased intracranial pressure occur rarely.

! Bulging fontanelles occur rarely in infants.

PEDIATRIC CONSIDERATIONS

Baseline Assessment

◂ **ALERT** ▸ Determine the patient's history of allergies, especially to tetracyclines, before beginning drug therapy.

• May cause permanent discoloration of teeth, retardation of bone growth and development, and defects in enamel in children younger than 8 yrs.

• Assess for age-appropriate fluid intake.

Precautions

• Use cautiously in pts with renal impairment and in those who cannot avoid sun or ultraviolet exposure, because this drug may produce a severe photosensitivity reaction.

Administration and Handling

• Give antacids containing aluminum, calcium, or magnesium, laxatives containing magnesium, or oral iron preparations 1–2 hrs before or after demeclocycline so that they do not impair the drug's absorption.

Intervention and Evaluation

• Assess the patient's pattern of daily bowel activity and stool consistency.
• Evaluate the patient's food intake and tolerance.
• Monitor the patient's intake and output and renal function test results.
• Assess the patient's skin for rash.
• Be alert to signs and symptoms of superinfection as evidenced by anal or genital pruritus, diarrhea, and ulceration or changes of oral mucosa or tongue.
• Monitor the patient's blood pressure and level of consciousness because of the potential for increased intracranial pressure.

Patient/Family Teaching

• Advise the patient/family to continue taking the antibiotic for the full length of treatment and to space drug doses evenly around the clock.
• Instruct the patient/family to take oral doses of demeclocycline on an empty stomach with a full glass of water.
• Encourage the patient/family to avoid overexposure to sun or ultraviolet light to prevent photosensitivity reactions.
• Advise the patient/family that demeclocycline may discolor fingernails.
• Advise the patient/family to avoid taking demeclocycline at bedtime because of the diuretic effects of the drug.

Doxycycline

dock-see-**sigh**-clean
(Adoxa, Apo-Doxy [CAN], Doryx, Doxsig [AUS], Doxycin [CAN], Doxylin [AUS], Periostat, Vibra-Tabs, Vibramycin)
Do not confuse with dicyclomine or doxylamine.

CATEGORY AND SCHEDULE

Pregnancy Risk Category: D

MECHANISM OF ACTION

A tetracycline antibiotic that inhibits bacterial protein synthesis by binding to ribosomes. ***Therapeutic Effect:*** Prevents bacterial cell growth.

AVAILABILITY

Capsules: 50 mg, 100 mg.
Tablets: 50 mg, 100 mg.
Powder for Oral Suspension: 25 mg/5 mL.
Syrup: 50 mg/5 mL.
Powder for Injection: 100 mg, 200 mg.
Capsules (extended release): 75 mg, 100 mg.

INDICATIONS AND DOSAGES

▸ **Treatment of respiratory, skin and soft tissue, and urinary tract infections; pelvic inflammatory disease; brucellosis; trachoma; Rocky Mountain spotted fever; typhus; Q fever; rickettsia; severe acne (Adoxa); smallpox; psittacosis; ornithosis; granuloma inguinale; and lymphogranuloma venereum;**

rheumatic fever prophylaxis; adjunctive treatment of intestinal amebiasis
PO/IV
Adolescents. 100–200 mg/day in 1–2 divided doses.
Children older than 8 yrs. 2–4 mg/kg/day divided q12–24 hrs. Maximum: 200 mg/day.

▸ **Lyme disease**
Children older than 8 yrs. 100 mg/dose q12h for 14–21 days.

▸ **Chlamydial infections**
Children older than 8 yrs. 100 mg/dose q12h for 7–10 days.

UNLABELED USES

Treatment of atypical mycobacterial infections, gonorrhea, malaria, prevention of Lyme disease, prophylaxis or treatment of traveler's diarrhea, rheumatoid arthritis.

CONTRAINDICATIONS

Hypersensitivity to tetracyclines, sulfites, last half of pregnancy, children younger than 8 yrs, severe liver dysfunction.

INTERACTIONS

Drug

Antacids containing aluminum, calcium, or magnesium; laxatives containing magnesium: Decrease doxycycline absorption.
Barbiturates, carbamazepine, phenytoin: May decrease doxycycline blood concentrations.
Cholestyramine, colestipol: May decrease doxycycline absorption.
Oral contraceptives: May decrease the effects of these drugs.
Oral iron preparations: Impair absorption of tetracyclines.

Herbal

None known.

Food

Calcium, milk, or dairy product–containing food/beverages: Decrease doxycycline absorption.

DIAGNOSTIC TEST EFFECTS

May increase serum alkaline phosphatase, serum amylase, serum bilirubin, SGOT (AST), and SGPT (ALT) levels. May alter complete blood count.

IV INCOMPATIBILITIES

Allopurinol (Aloprim), heparin, piperacillin/tazobactam (Zosyn)

IV COMPATIBILITIES

Amiodarone (Cordarone), diltiazem (Cardizem), hydromorphone (Dilaudid), magnesium sulfate, morphine, propofol (Diprivan)

SIDE EFFECTS

Frequent
Anorexia, nausea, vomiting, diarrhea, dysphagia, photosensitivity, which may be severe
Occasional
Rash, urticaria

SERIOUS REACTIONS

! Superinfection (especially fungal) and benign intracranial hypertension (headache, visual changes) may occur.
! Liver toxicity, fatty degeneration of liver, and pancreatitis occur rarely.

PEDIATRIC CONSIDERATIONS

Baseline Assessment

◂ **ALERT** ▸ Determine the patient's history of allergies, especially to sulfites and tetracyclines, before beginning drug therapy.
• May discolor teeth and/or fingernails in children younger than 8 yrs of age.
• Assess for age-appropriate fluid intake.

Precautions

• Use cautiously in pts who cannot avoid sun or ultraviolet light exposure because this drug may produce a severe photosensitivity reaction.

Administration and Handling

◀ **ALERT** ▶ Do not administer IM or SC. Space doses evenly around clock.

• Give doxycycline 1–2 hrs before or after antacids that contain aluminum, calcium, or magnesium, laxatives that contain magnesium, or oral iron preparations because these drugs may impair doxycycline absorption.

PO

Store capsules and tablets at room temperature.

• Store oral suspension for up to 2 wks at room temperature.

• Give with a full glass of fluid. Know that drug may be given with food if GI upset is present, although this can reduce drug absorption.

IV

After reconstitution, store IV piggyback infusion for up to 12 hrs at room temperature, or refrigerate for up to 72 hrs.

• Protect from direct sunlight. Discard if precipitate forms.

• Reconstitute each 100-mg vial with 10 mL Sterile Water for Injection for concentration of 10 mg/mL.

• Further dilute each 100 mg with at least 100 mL D_5W, 0.9% NaCl, or lactated Ringer's solution.

• Give by intermittent IV piggyback infusion.

• Infuse over more than 1–4 hrs.

Intervention and Evaluation

• Assess the patient's pattern of daily bowel activity and stool consistency.

• Assess the patient's skin for rash.

• Monitor the patient's level of consciousness because of the potential for increased intracranial pressure.

• Be alert for signs and symptoms of superinfection as evidenced by anal or genital pruritus, diarrhea, and ulceration or changes of the oral mucosa.

Patient/Family Teaching

• Encourage the patient/family to avoid overexposure to sun or ultraviolet light to prevent photosensitivity reactions.

• Instruct the patient/family not to take doxycycline with antacids, dairy products, or iron products because these substances decrease the absorption of doxycycline.

• Advise the patient/family to continue taking doxycycline for the full course of therapy.

Minocycline Hydrochloride

min-know-**sigh**-clean

(Akamin [AUS], Dynacin, Minocin, Minomycin [AUS], Novo Minocycline [CAN])

Do not confuse with Dynabac or Mithracin.

CATEGORY AND SCHEDULE

Pregnancy Risk Category: D

MECHANISM OF ACTION

A tetracycline antibiotic that binds to ribosomes. ***Therapeutic Effect:*** Inhibits bacterial protein synthesis. Bacteriostatic.

AVAILABILITY

Capsules: 50 mg, 75 mg, 100 mg.
Tablets: 50 mg, 75 mg, 100 mg.
Powder for Injection: 100 mg.

INDICATIONS AND DOSAGES

▶ **Mild to moderate to severe prostate, urinary tract, and CNS infections (excluding meningitis);**

uncomplicated gonorrhea; inflammatory acne; brucellosis; skin granulomas; cholera; trachoma; nocardiosis; yaws; syphilis when penicillins are contraindicated
PO/IV
Adolescents. Initially, 200 mg/dose, then 100 mg q12 hrs.
Children older than 8 yrs. Initially, 4 mg/kg, then 2 mg/kg q12h. Maximum: 200 mg/day.

UNLABELED USES

Treatment of atypical mycobacterial infections, rheumatoid arthritis, scleroderma.

CONTRAINDICATIONS

Hypersensitivity to tetracyclines, last half of pregnancy, children younger than 8 yrs.

INTERACTIONS

Drug
Carbamazepine, phenytoin: May decrease minocycline blood concentration.
Cholestyramine, colestipol: May decrease minocycline absorption.
Oral contraceptives: May decrease the effects of these drugs.
Herbal
St. John's wort: May increase risk of photosensitivity.
Food
Calcium, milk, or dairy product–containing food/beverages: Decrease doxycycline absorption.

DIAGNOSTIC TEST EFFECTS

May increase serum alkaline phosphatase, serum amylase, serum bilirubin, SGOT (AST), and SGPT (ALT) levels.

IV INCOMPATIBILITIES

Adrenocorticotropic hormone, aminophylline, amphotericin B, bicarbonate, calcium gluconate or chloride, carbenicillin, cefazolin, chloramphenicol, heparin, hydrocortisone, iodine, methicillin, penicillin, phenytoin, piperacillin/tazobactam (Zosyn), prochlorperazine, sulfadiazine, sulfisoxazole, vitamin K.

SIDE EFFECTS

Frequent
Dizziness, lightheadedness, diarrhea, nausea, vomiting, stomach cramps, photosensitivity (may be severe)
Occasional
Pigmentation of skin or mucous membranes, itching in rectal and genital area, sore mouth or tongue

SERIOUS REACTIONS

! Superinfection (especially fungal), anaphylaxis, and increased intracranial pressure may occur.
! Bulging fontanelles occur rarely in infants.

PEDIATRIC CONSIDERATIONS

Baseline Assessment
◂ALERT▸ Determine the patient's history of allergies, especially to sulfites and tetracyclines, before beginning drug therapy.
• Assess for age-appropriate fluid intake.
• May cause discoloration of teeth in children younger than 8 yrs of age.
Precautions
• Use cautiously in pts with renal impairment and in those who cannot avoid sun or ultraviolet exposure because this drug may produce a severe photosensitivity reaction.
Administration and Handling
◂ALERT▸ Space drug doses evenly around the clock.

PO
Store at room temperature.
• Give capsules and tablets with a full glass of water.

IV
• Store IV solution for up to 24 hrs at room temperature.
• Use piggyback IV infusion immediately after reconstitution.
• Discard solution if precipitate forms.
• For intermittent piggyback IV infusion, reconstitute each 100-mg vial with 5–10 mL Sterile Water for Injection to provide concentration of 20 or 10 mg/mL, respectively.
• Further dilute with 500–1,000 mL D_5W or 0.9% NaCl.
• Infuse over 6 hrs.

Intervention and Evaluation
• Assess the patient's ability to ambulate. Minocycline may cause dizziness, drowsiness, or vertigo.
• Assess the patient's pattern of daily bowel activity and stool consistency.
• Assess the patient's skin for rash.
• Check the patient's blood pressure and level of consciousness for increased intracranial pressure.
• Be alert for signs and symptoms of superinfection as evidenced by anal or genital pruritus, diarrhea, and ulceration or changes of the oral mucosa.

Patient/Family Teaching
• Advise the patient/family to continue taking the antibiotic for the full length of treatment and to space drug doses evenly around the clock.
• Teach the patient/family to drink a full glass of water with minocycline capsules or tablets and to avoid bedtime doses.
• Warn the patient/family to avoid tasks that require mental alertness or motor skills until the patient's response to the drug is established.
• Instruct the patient/family to notify the physician if diarrhea, rash, or other new symptoms occur.
• Encourage the patient/family to protect the patient's skin from sun exposure.

Tetracycline Hydrochloride

tet-rah-**sigh**-klin
(Achromycin, Apo-Tetra [CAN], Latycin [AUS], Mysteclin [AUS], Novotetra [CAN], Sumycin, Tetrex [AUS])

CATEGORY AND SCHEDULE
Pregnancy Risk Category: D (B with topical)

MECHANISM OF ACTION
A tetracycline antibiotic that inhibits bacterial protein synthesis by binding to ribosomes. ***Therapeutic Effect:*** Prevents bacterial cell growth. Bacteriostatic.

PHARMACOKINETICS
Readily absorbed from the GI tract. Protein binding: 30%–60%. Widely distributed. Excreted in urine; eliminated in feces via the biliary system. Not removed by hemodialysis. ***Half-Life:*** 6–11 hrs (half-life is increased with impaired renal function).

AVAILABILITY
Capsules: 250 mg, 500 mg.
Tablets: 250 mg, 500 mg.
Suspension: 125 mg/5 mL.

INDICATIONS AND DOSAGES
▸ **Treatment of inflammatory acne vulgaris, Lyme disease, *Mycoplasma* disease, *Legionella*, Rocky**

Mountain spotted fever, chlamydial infection in patients with gonorrhea
PO
Adolescents. 250–500 mg/dose q6–12hrs.
Children older than 8 yrs. 25–50 mg/kg/day in 4 divided doses. Maximum: 3 g/day.
OPHTHALMIC OINTMENT
Apply ointment every 2–12 hrs.
SUSPENSION
Instill 1–2 drops into conjunctival sac 2–4 times/day.

▸ **Dosage in renal impairment**

Creatinine Clearance	Dosage Interval
50–80 mL/min	q8–12h
10–50 mL/min	q12–24h
Less than 10 mL/min	q24h

CONTRAINDICATIONS

Hypersensitivity to tetracyclines or sulfites, children 8 yrs and younger.

INTERACTIONS

Drug

Carbamazepine, phenytoin: May decrease tetracycline blood concentration.
Cholestyramine, colestipol: May decrease tetracycline absorption.
Oral contraceptives: May decrease the effects of these drugs.
Calcium, magnesium, and aluminum-containing antacids, iron, zinc, and antidiarrheals: May decrease tetracycline absorption.

Herbal

St. John's wort: May increase risk of photosensitivity.

Food

Dairy products: Inhibit tetracycline absorption.

DIAGNOSTIC TEST EFFECTS

May increase BUN, serum alkaline phosphatase, serum amylase, serum bilirubin, SGOT (AST), and SGPT (ALT) levels.

SIDE EFFECTS

Frequent
Dizziness, lightheadedness, diarrhea, nausea, vomiting, stomach cramps, increased sensitivity of skin to sunlight

Occasional
Pigmentation of skin, mucous membranes, itching in rectal or genital area, sore mouth or tongue

SERIOUS REACTIONS

! Superinfection (especially fungal), anaphylaxis, and increased intracranial pressure may occur.
! Bulging fontanelles occur rarely in infants.

PEDIATRIC CONSIDERATIONS

Baseline Assessment

◂ALERT▸ Determine the patient's history of allergies, especially to sulfites and tetracyclines, before beginning drug therapy.
• Be aware that tetracycline readily crosses the placenta and is distributed in breast milk.
• Avoid tetracycline use in women during the last half of pregnancy.
• Be aware that tetracycline use may produce permanent tooth discoloration or enamel hypoplasia and inhibit skeletal growth in children 8 yrs of age or younger.
• Be aware that tetracycline use is not recommended in children 8 yrs of age and younger.

• Assess for age-appropriate fluid intake.

Precautions

• Use cautiously in pts who cannot avoid sun or ultraviolet light exposure because this drug may produce a severe photosensitivity reaction.

Administration and Handling

◂**ALERT**▸ Space drug doses evenly around the clock.

PO

• Give capsules and tablets with a full glass of water 1 hr before or 2 hrs after meals.

Intervention and Evaluation

• Assess the patient's skin for rash.
• Assess the patient's pattern of daily bowel activity and stool consistency.
• Monitor the patient's food intake and tolerance.
• Be alert for signs and symptoms of superinfection as evidenced by anal or genital pruritus, diarrhea, and ulceration or changes of the oral mucosa.
• Monitor the patient's blood pressure and level of consciousness because of the potential for increased intracranial pressure.

Patient/Family Teaching

• Advise the patient/family to continue taking the antibiotic for the full length of treatment and to space drug doses evenly around the clock.
• Instruct the patient/family to take oral tetracycline doses on an empty stomach 1 hr before or 2 hrs after consuming beverages or food.
• Teach the patient/family to drink a full glass of water with tetracycline capsules and to avoid bedtime tetracycline doses.
• Warn the patient/family to notify the physician if diarrhea, rash, or any other new symptoms occur.
• Encourage the patient/family to protect the patient's skin from sun exposure and to avoid overexposure to sun or ultraviolet light to prevent photosensitivity reactions.
• Explain to the patient/family that the patient should not take any medications, including OTC drugs, without consulting the physician.

REFERENCES

Gunn V. L. & Nechyba, C. (2002). The Harriet Lane handbook (16th ed.). St. Louis: Mosby.
Miller, S. & Fioravanti, J. (1997). Pediatric medications: A handbook for nurses. St. Louis: Mosby.
Taketomo, C. K., Hodding, J. H. & Kraus, D. M. (2003–2004). Pediatric dosage handbook (10th ed.). Hudson, OH: Lexi-Comp.

12 Miscellaneous Anti-Infective Agents

Atovaquone
Aztreonam
Bacitracin
Chloramphenicol
Clindamycin
Co-Trimoxazole (Sulfamethoxazole-Trimethoprim)
Dapsone
Hydroxychloroquine Sulfate
Linezolid
Metronidazole Hydrochloride
Nitrofurantoin Sodium
Pentamidine Isethionate
Sulfasalazine
Trimethoprim
Vancomycin Hydrochloride

Uses: Miscellaneous anti-infective agents have a wide variety of uses because they belong to many different subclasses. Some agents, such as atovaquone, chloramphenicol, and linezolid, are used for serious infections when other, less toxic agents have failed or are not appropriate. Others are prescribed to treat uncommon infections, such as malaria (with hydrochloroquine), leprosy (with dapsone), and trichomoniasis and amebiasis (with metronidazole). Several, including aztreonam, clindamycin, and quinupristin, combat a broad range of systemic infections; yet some are used for just one indication, such as fosfomycin and nitrofurantoin, which are given solely for urinary tract infections. In addition to treatment, some miscellaneous anti-infectives are used prophylactically, such as vancomycin (to prevent bacterial endocarditis) and co-trimoxazole and pentamidine (to prevent *Pneumocystis carinii* pneumonia).

Action: Miscellaneous anti-infective agents may be bacteriostatic or bactericidal and work in many different ways. (See illustration, *Sites and Mechanisms of Action: Anti-Infective Agents,* page 2.) For details, see the specific drug entries.

COMBINATION PRODUCTS

BACTRIM: trimethoprim/sulfamethoxazole (a sulfonamide) 16 mg/80 mg/mL (injection), 40 mg/200 mg/5 mL (suspension), 80 mg/400 mg or 160 mg/800 mg (tablets).

HELIDAC: metronidazole/bismuth (an antisecretory)/tetracycline (an anti-infective) 250 mg/262 mg/500 mg.

MYCITRACIN: bacitracin/polymyxin B (an anti-infective)/neomycin (an aminoglycoside). 400 units/5,000 units/3.5 mg/g, 500 units/5,000 units/3.5 mg/g.

NEOSPORIN OINTMENT, TRIPLE ANTIBIOTIC: bacitracin (an anti-infective)/neomycin/polymyxin B (an anti-infective) 400 units/3.5 mg/5,000 units, 400 units/3.5 mg/10,000 units.

POLYSPORIN: bacitracin/polymyxin B (an anti-infective) 500 units/10,000 units/g.

SEPTRA: trimethoprim/sulfamethoxazole (a sulfonamide) 16 mg/80 mg/mL (injection), 40 mg/200 mg/5 mL (suspension), 80 mg/400 mg or 160 mg/800 mg (tablets).

ZOTRIM: trimethoprim/sulfamethoxazole (a sulfonamide)/phenazopyridine (a urinary analgesic) 160 mg/800 mg/200 mg.

Atovaquone

ah-tow-vah-quon

(Mepron, Wellvone [AUS])

CATEGORY AND SCHEDULE

Pregnancy Risk Category: C

MECHANISM OF ACTION

A systemic anti-infective that inhibits the mitochondrial electron transport system at the cytochrome bc_1 complex (complex III). ***Therapeutic Effect:*** Interrupts nucleic acid and adenosine triphosphate synthesis.

PHARMACOKINETICS

Absorption is enhanced with food. Highly protein bound (99%). ***Half-Life:*** 2–3 days. Mostly excreted unchanged in feces.

AVAILABILITY

Suspension: 750 mg/5 mL (contains benzyl alcohol).

INDICATIONS AND DOSAGES

▸ Usual pediatric dosage

PO

Adolescents. 750 mg/dose q12h for 21 days.

Children. 40 mg/kg/day divided q12h. Maximum: 1,500 mg/day.

▸ Prophylaxis of *P. carinii* pneumonia

Adolescents. 1,500 mg once daily.

Infants 4–24 mos. 45 mg/kg/day once a day. Maximum: 1,500 mg/day.

Infants 1–3 mos and older than 24mos. 30 mg/kg/day once a day. Maximum: 1,500 mg/day

▸ Babesiosis

Adolescents. 750 mg/dose q12h for 7–10 days with azithromycin 1,000 mg once daily for 3 days, then 500 mg once daily for 7 days.

Children. 40 mg/kg/day q12h with azithromycin 12 mg/kg/day once daily for 7–10 days.

CONTRAINDICATIONS

Development or history of potentially life-threatening allergic reaction to the drug.

INTERACTIONS

Drug

Rifampin: May decrease atovaquone blood concentration. Atovaquone may increase rifampin blood concentration.

Herbal

None known.

Food

None known.

DIAGNOSTIC TEST EFFECTS

May elevate serum alkaline phosphatase, serum amylase, SGOT (AST), and SGPT (ALT) levels. May decrease serum sodium levels.

SIDE EFFECTS

Frequent (greater than 10%)

Rash, nausea, diarrhea, headache, vomiting, fever, insomnia, cough

Occasional (less than 10%)

Abdominal discomfort, thrush, asthenia (loss of strength, energy), anemia, neutropenia

SERIOUS REACTIONS

None known.

PEDIATRIC CONSIDERATIONS

◂ ALERT ▸ Suspension contains benzyl alcohol. Large amounts of benzyl alcohol have been linked to potentially fatal toxicity in neonates.

Precautions

- Use cautiously in pts with chronic diarrhea, malabsorption syndromes, or severe *P. carinii* pneumonia.

Intervention and Evaluation

- Assess the patient for GI discomfort, nausea, and vomiting.
- Assess the patient's pattern of daily bowel activity and stool consistency.
- Assess the patient's skin for rash.
- Monitor the patient's Hgb levels, intake and output, and renal function test results.

Patient/Family Teaching

- Advise the patient/family to continue therapy for the full length of treatment.
- Warn the patient/family not to take any other medications without first notifying the physician.
- Urge the patient/family to notify the physician if diarrhea, rash, or other new symptoms develop.
- Shake suspension well before administration.
- Administer with a high-fat meal for increased absorption.

Aztreonam 

az-**tree**-oh-nam
(Azactam)

CATEGORY AND SCHEDULE

Pregnancy Risk Category: B

MECHANISM OF ACTION

A monobactam bactericidal antibiotic that inhibits bacterial cell wall synthesis. ***Therapeutic Effect:*** Produces bacterial cell lysis and death.

PHARMACOKINETICS

Completely absorbed after IM administration. Protein binding: 56%–60%. Partially metabolized by hydrolysis. Primarily excreted unchanged in urine. Moderately removed by hemodialysis. ***Half-Life:*** 1.4–2.2 hrs (half-life increased in reduced renal, liver function).

AVAILABILITY

Injection: 500 mg, 1 g, 2 g.
Premixed Infusion: 1 g, 2 g.

INDICATIONS AND DOSAGES

▸ **Mild to severe infections in children**

IV/IM

Children. 90–120 mg/kg/day divided q6–8h.

Neonates. Younger than 7 days: 30 mg/kg/dose q8–12h.
Older than 7 days: 30 mg/kg/dose q6–12h.

▸ **Dosage in renal impairment**

Dosage and frequency are modified based on creatinine clearance and the severity of infection.

Creatinine Clearance	Dosage
10–30 mL/min	½ the usual dose at usual intervals
Less than 10 mL/min	¼ the usual dose at usual intervals

UNLABELED USES

Treatment of bone and joint infections.

CONTRAINDICATIONS

Hypersensitivity to aztreonam or any related component.

INTERACTIONS

Drug

Probenecid, furosemide: May increase aztreonam serum concentrations.

Herbal

None known.

Food

None known.

DIAGNOSTIC TEST EFFECTS

May cause positive Coombs' test results. May increase serum alkaline phosphatase, serum creatinine, lactate dehydrogenase,

SGOT (AST), and SGPT (ALT) levels.

IV INCOMPATIBILITIES
Acyclovir (Zovirax), amphotericin (Fungizone), daunorubicin (Cerubidine), ganciclovir (Cytovene), lorazepam (Ativan), metronidazole (Flagyl), vancomycin (Vancocin)

IV COMPATIBILITIES
Aminophylline, bumetanide (Bumex), calcium gluconate, cimetidine (Tagamet), diltiazem (Cardizem), dobutamine (Dobutrex), dopamine (Intropin), famotidine (Pepcid), furosemide (Lasix), heparin, hydromorphone (Dilaudid), insulin (regular), magnesium sulfate, morphine, potassium chloride, propofol (Diprivan)

SIDE EFFECTS
Occasional (less than 3%)
Discomfort and swelling at IM injection site, nausea, vomiting, diarrhea, rash
Rare (less than 1%)
Phlebitis or thrombophlebitis at IV injection site, abdominal cramps, headache, hypotension

SERIOUS REACTIONS
! Superinfections and antibiotic-associated colitis manifested as abdominal cramps, severe and watery diarrhea, and fever may result from altered bacterial balance.
! Severe hypersensitivity reactions, including anaphylaxis, occur rarely.

PEDIATRIC CONSIDERATIONS

Baseline Assessment
◂ **ALERT** ▸ Determine the patient's history of allergies, especially to antibiotics, before giving aztreonam.
- Be aware that aztreonam crosses the placenta and is distributed in amniotic fluid as well as in low concentrations in breast milk.
- Be aware that the safety and efficacy of aztreonam have not been established in children younger than 9 mos of age.
- Assess for age-appropriate fluid intake.

Precautions
- Use cautiously in pts with a history of allergy, especially to antibiotics, or liver or renal impairment.

Administration and Handling
IM
- Shake immediately and vigorously after adding diluent.
- Inject deeply into a large muscle mass.
- After reconstitution for IM injection, solution is stable for 48 hrs at room temperature or 7 days if refrigerated.

IV
- Store vials at room temperature.
- Solution normally appears colorless to light yellow.
- After reconstitution, the solution is stable for 48 hrs at room temperature or 7 days if refrigerated.
- Discard the solution if a precipitate forms. Discard unused portions of solution.
- For IV push, dilute each 1 g with 6–10 mL Sterile Water for Injection.
- For intermittent IV infusion, further dilute with 50–100 mL D_5W or 0.9% NaCl.
- For IV push, give over 3–5 min at maximum concentration of 66 mg/mL.
- For IV infusion, administer over 20–60 min; final concentration should not exceed 20 mg/mL.

Intervention and Evaluation
- Evaluate the patient for signs and symptoms of phlebitis, mani-

fested as heat, pain, and red streaking over the vein and pain at the IM injection site.
• Observe the patient for GI discomfort, nausea, or vomiting.
• Assess the patient's pattern of daily bowel activity and stool consistency.
• Assess the patient's skin for rash.
• Be alert for signs and symptoms of superinfection, including anal or genital pruritus, black hairy tongue, diarrhea, increased temperature, sore throat, ulceration or changes of oral mucosa, and vomiting.

Patient/Family Teaching

• Urge the patient/family to report any diarrhea, nausea, rash, or vomiting the patient experiences.

Bacitracin

bah-cih-**tray** -sin
(Baci-IM, Baciguent, Bacitracin)
Do not confuse with Bactrim or Bactroban.

CATEGORY AND SCHEDULE

Pregnancy Risk Category: C
OTC

MECHANISM OF ACTION

An antibiotic that interferes with plasma membrane permeability in susceptible bacteria. ***Therapeutic Effect:*** Inhibits bacterial cell wall synthesis and is bacteriostatic.

AVAILABILITY

Powder for Reconstitution: 50,000 units.
Ophthalmic Ointment: 500 units/g
Topical Ointment: 500 units/g

INDICATIONS AND DOSAGES

OPHTHALMIC OINTMENT
Children. ¼–½ in ribbon in conjunctival sac q3–4h.
TOPICAL OINTMENT
Children. Apply 1–5 times/day to the affected area.
IM (NOT RECOMMENDED)
Children. 800–1,200 units/kg/day divided q8h.
Infants weighing more than 2.5 kg. 1,000 units/kg/day in 2 or 3 divided doses.
Infants weighing less than 2.5 kg. 900 units/kg/day in 2 or 3 divided doses.
IRRIGATION SOLUTION
50–100 units/mL in 0.9% NaCl, lactated Ringer's solution, or Sterile Water for Irrigation. Soak sponges in solution for topical compresses 1–5 times/day or as needed.

CONTRAINDICATIONS

Hypersensitivity to bacitracin or any component. IM use is contraindicated in pts with renal failure/impairment.

INTERACTIONS

Drug

Nephrotoxic drugs: Increase renal toxicity.
Neuromuscular blockers and anesthetics: Increase neuromuscular blockade.

Herbal

None known.

Food

None known.

DIAGNOSTIC TEST EFFECTS

None known.

SIDE EFFECTS

Rare

Topical: Hypersensitivity reaction as evidenced by allergic contact dermatitis, burning, inflammation, and itching
Ophthalmic: Burning, itching, redness, swelling, pain
IM: Renal tubular necrosis, glomerular necrosis, azotemia, renal failure.

SERIOUS REACTIONS

! Severe hypersensitivity reaction, including apnea and hypotension, occurs rarely.

PEDIATRIC CONSIDERATIONS

Precautions

◂ALERT▸ Familiarize yourself with the side effects of each of a drug's components when bacitracin is used in a fixed combination.

- The IM route is not recommended for use in pediatric pts.
- Assess for age-appropriate fluid intake.

Administration and Handling

OPHTHALMIC

- Place a gloved finger on the patient's lower eyelid and pull it out until a pocket is formed between the eye and lower lid. Place ¼–½ in ointment in the pocket.
- Have the patient close the eye gently for 1–2 min, rolling his or her eyeball to increase contact area of drug to eye.
- Remove excess ointment around the eye with a tissue.

Intervention and Evaluation

TOPICAL

- Evaluate the patient for signs and symptoms of hypersensitivity as evidenced by burning, inflammation, and itching.
- With preparations containing corticosteroids, closely monitor the patient for any unusual signs or symptoms, because corticosteroids may mask clinical signs.

OPHTHALMIC

- Assess the patient's eye for the therapeutic response or a hypersensitivity reaction manifested as increased burning, itching, redness, and swelling.

Patient/Family Teaching

- Advise the patient/family to continue therapy for the full length of treatment and to space drug doses evenly around the clock.
- Urge the patient/family to report any burning, increased irritation, itching, and rash the patient experiences.

Chloramphenicol

klor-am-**fen**-ih-call
(Chloromycetin, Chloroptic, Chlorsig [AUS])
Do not confuse with chlorambucil.

CATEGORY AND SCHEDULE

Pregnancy Risk Category: C

MECHANISM OF ACTION

A dichloroacetic acid derivative that acts as a bacteriostatic agent (may be bactericidal in high concentrations) by binding to bacterial ribosomal receptor sites. ***Therapeutic Effect:*** Inhibits bacterial protein synthesis.

AVAILABILITY

Powder for Injection: 100 mg/mL.
Ophthalmic Solution: 5 mg/mL (0.5%).
Ophthalmic Ointment: 10 mg/g.

INDICATIONS AND DOSAGES

▸ Mild to moderate infections from organisms resistant to other, less toxic antibiotics

PO/IV

Children. 50 mg/kg/day in divided doses q6h. Maximum: 4 g/day.
Newborns. 25 mg/kg/day in 4 doses q6h. Maximum: 4 g/day.
Infants older than 2 wks. 50 mg/kg/day in 4 doses q6h.
Neonates weighing less than 2 kg. 25 mg/kg once daily.
Neonates younger than 7 days weighing more than 2 kg. 25 mg/kg once daily.

Neonates 7 days and older weighing more than 2 kg. 50 mg/kg/day in divided doses q12h.
OPHTHALMIC
Children. Apply thin strip of ointment to conjunctiva q3–4h. 1–2 drops of solution 4–6 times/day.
OTIC
Children. 2–3 drops into ear 3 times/day.

▸ Severe infections, infections due to moderately resistant organisms, including meningitis
PO/IV
Children. 75–100 mg/kg/day in divided doses q6h.

▸ Dosage in liver or renal impairment
Dosage is reduced based on the degree of renal impairment and plasma concentration of the drug.

CONTRAINDICATIONS

Hypersensitivity to chloramphenicol.

INTERACTIONS

Drug

Anticonvulsants, bone marrow depressants: May increase bone marrow depression.
Clindamycin, erythromycin: May antagonize the effects of these drugs.
Oral hypoglycemics: May increase the effects of these drugs.
Phenobarbital, phenytoin, warfarin: May increase blood concentrations of these drugs.

Herbal

None known.

Food

May decrease the absorption of vitamin B_{12}.
May increase dietary requirement for riboflavin, pyridoxine, and vitamin B_{12}.

DIAGNOSTIC TEST EFFECTS

None known. Therapeutic peak blood level: 10–20 mcg/mL; therapeutic trough blood level: 5–10 mcg/mL; toxic level: greater than 25 mcg/mL.

SIDE EFFECTS

Occasional
Systemic: Nausea, vomiting, diarrhea
Ophthalmic: Blurred vision, burning, stinging, hypersensitivity reaction
Otic: Hypersensitivity reaction
Rare
"Gray baby" syndrome in neonates (abdominal distention, blue-gray skin color, cardiovascular collapse, unresponsiveness), rash, shortness of breath, confusion, headache, optic neuritis (blurred vision, eye pain), peripheral neuritis (numbness and weakness in feet and hands)

SERIOUS REACTIONS

! Superinfection as a result of bacterial or fungal overgrowth may occur.
! There is a narrow margin between effective therapy and toxic levels producing blood dyscrasias.
! Bone marrow depression with resulting aplastic anemia, hypoplastic anemia, and pancytopenia may occur weeks or months later.

PEDIATRIC CONSIDERATIONS

Baseline Assessment

• Be aware that, if possible, chloramphenicol should not be given concurrently with other drugs that cause bone marrow depression.
• Expect to obtain blood studies to establish the patient's baseline before beginning chloramphenicol therapy.
• Draw blood for peak levels 90 min after the end of a 30-min

infusion; draw blood for trough levels just before the third dose.

Precautions

• Use cautiously in pts with bone marrow depression, liver or renal impairment, previous cytotoxic drug therapy, and radiation therapy.
• Use cautiously in pediatric pts, infants, and children younger than 2 yrs of age.
• Use cautiously in pediatric pts who have impaired renal or hepatic function.
• The three main toxicities seen with chloramphenicol are aplastic anemia (usually 3 wks–12 mos after initial exposure), bone marrow suppression (dose-related and reversible after discontinuation of the drug), and gray baby syndrome.

Intervention and Evaluation

• Assess the patient's nausea and monitor the patient for vomiting.
• Evaluate the patient's mental status.
• Test the patient to determine if he or she is experiencing visual disturbances.
• Assess the patient's skin for rash.
• Assess the patient's pattern of daily bowel activity and stool consistency.
• Be alert for signs and symptoms of superinfection manifested as anal or genital pruritus, a change in the oral mucosa, diarrhea, and increased fever.
• Monitor the patient's drug blood levels and know that the therapeutic peak blood level is 10–20 mcg/mL and the toxic level is greater than 25 mcg/mL.

Patient/Family Teaching

• Advise the patient/family to continue taking chloramphenicol for the full length of treatment and to space drug doses evenly around the clock.
• Instruct the patient/family that ophthalmic treatment should continue at least 48 hrs after the eye returns to normal appearance.
• Warn the family to report signs of gray baby syndrome in newborns (pallor, cyanosis, failure to feed, irregular respiration, or abdominal distention).

Clindamycin

klin-da-**my**-sin
(Cleocin, Dalacin [CAN])

CATEGORY AND SCHEDULE

Pregnancy Risk Category: B

MECHANISM OF ACTION

A lincosamide antibiotic that acts as a bacteriostatic by binding to bacterial ribosomal receptor sites. Topically, decreases fatty acid concentration on skin. ***Therapeutic Effect:*** Inhibits protein synthesis of the bacterial cell wall. Prevents outbreak of acne vulgaris.

PHARMACOKINETICS

Rapidly absorbed from the GI tract. Protein binding: 92%–94%. Widely distributed. Metabolized in liver to some active metabolites. Primarily excreted in urine. Not removed by hemodialysis. ***Half-Life:*** 2.4–3 hrs (half-life is increased with impaired renal function, in premature infants).

AVAILABILITY

Capsules: 75 mg, 150 mg, 300 mg.
Oral Solution: 75 mg/5 mL.
Injection: 150 mg/mL.
Premixed Infusion: 300 mg, 600 mg, 900 mg.
Vaginal Cream: 2%.
Vaginal Suppository: 100 mg.
Lotion: 1%.
Topical Solution: 1%.

INDICATIONS AND DOSAGES

▸ **Treatment of chronic bone and joint, respiratory tract, skin and soft tissue, intra-abdominal, female, and GU infections, endocarditis, septicemia**

IM/IV

Adolescents. 1.2–1.8 g/day divided 2–4 times. Maximum: 4.8 g/day.
Children. 25–40 mg/kg/day in 3–4 divideds. Maximum: 4.8 g/day.
Neonates 7 days or younger weighing 2 kg or less. 5 mg/kg/dose q12h.
Neonates 7 days or younger weighing more than 2 kg. 5 mg/kg/dose q8h.
Neonates older than 7 days weighing 1.2 kg or less. 5 mg/kg/dose q12h.
Neonates older than 7 days weighing 1.2–2 kg. 5 mg/kg/dose q8h.
Neonates older than 7 days weighting more than 2 kg. 5 mg/kg/dose q6h.

PO

Infants and children. 10–30 mg/kg/day in 3–4 divided doses. Maximum: 1.8 g/day.
Adolescents. 150–450 mg/dose q6–8h. Maximum: 1.8 g/day.

▸ **Acne vulgaris**

TOPICAL

Adolescents. Apply thin layer 2 times/day to affected area.

VAGINAL

Adolescents. Insert one full application (100 mg) into vagina once daily before to bedtime for 7 days.

UNLABELED USES

Treatment of malaria, otitis media, *P. carinii* pneumonia, toxoplasmosis

CONTRAINDICATIONS

History of antibiotic-associated colitis, regional enteritis, or ulcerative colitis, hypersensitivity to clindamycin or lincomycin, known allergy to tartrazine dye (oral therapy).

INTERACTIONS

Drug

Adsorbent antidiarrheals: May delay absorption of clindamycin.
Chloramphenicol, erythromycin: May antagonize the effects of clindamycin.
Neuromuscular blockers: May increase the effects of these drugs.

Herbal

None known.

Food

None known.

DIAGNOSTIC TEST EFFECTS

May increase serum alkaline phosphatase, SGOT (AST), and SGPT (ALT) levels.

IV INCOMPATIBILITIES

Allopurinol (Aloprim), filgrastim (Neupogen), fluconazole (Diflucan), idarubicin (Idamycin)

IV COMPATIBILITIES

Amiodarone (Cordarone), diltiazem (Cardizem), heparin, hydromorphone (Dilaudid), magnesium sulfate, midazolam (Versed), morphine, multivitamins, propofol (Diprivan)

SIDE EFFECTS

Frequent

Abdominal pain, nausea, vomiting, diarrhea
Vaginal: Vaginitis, itching
Topical: Dry scaly skin

Occasional

Phlebitis, thrombophlebitis with IV administration, pain, induration at IM injection site, allergic reaction, urticaria, pruritus
Vaginal: Headache, dizziness, nausea, vomiting, abdominal pain
Topical: Contact dermatitis, abdominal pain, mild diarrhea, burning or stinging

Rare
Vaginal: Hypersensitivity reaction

SERIOUS REACTIONS

! Antibiotic-associated colitis as evidenced by severe abdominal pain and tenderness, fever, and watery and severe diarrhea may occur during and several weeks after clindamycin therapy, including the topical form.
! Blood dyscrasias (leukopenia and thrombocytopenia) and nephrotoxicity (proteinuria, azotemia, and oliguria) occur rarely.

PEDIATRIC CONSIDERATIONS

Baseline Assessment

◂ALERT▸ Determine the patient's history of allergies, particularly to aspirin, clindamycin, and lincomycin, before beginning drug therapy.

• Avoid, if possible, concurrent use of neuromuscular blocking agents.
• Be aware that clindamycin readily crosses the placenta and is distributed in breast milk.
• Be aware that it is unknown whether the topical and vaginal forms of clindamycin are distributed in breast milk.
• Use cautiously in children younger than 1 mo of age.
• Assess for age-appropriate fluid intake.

Precautions

• Use cautiously in pts concomitantly using neuromuscular blocking agents.
• Use cautiously in pts with severe renal or liver dysfunction.
• Use cautiously in neonates.
• Use topical preparations cautiously; they should not be applied to abraded areas or near the eyes.

Administration and Handling

PO
• Store capsules at room temperature.
• After reconstitution, oral solution is stable for 2 wks at room temperature.
• Do not refrigerate oral solution to avoid thickening the solution.
• Give with 8 oz of water. May give without regard to food.

IM
• Do not exceed 600 mg/dose.
• Give by deep IM injection.

IV
• IV infusion (piggyback) is stable at room temperature for up to 16 days.
• Dilute 300–600 mg with 50 mL D_5W or 0.9% NaCl (900–1,200 mg with 100 mL). Never exceed concentration of 18 mg/mL.
• Infuse 50 mL (300–600 mg) piggyback over more than 20 min; infuse 100 mL (900 mg–1.2 g) piggyback over more than 40 min. Be aware that severe hypotension or cardiac arrest can occur with too rapid administration.
• Do not administer more than 1.2 g in a single infusion.

Intervention and Evaluation

• Assess the patient's pattern of daily bowel activity and stool consistency. Report diarrhea promptly to the physician because of the potential for development of serious colitis (even with topical or vaginal clindamycin).
• Assess the patient's skin for dryness, irritation, and rash with topical application.
• Be alert for signs and symptoms of superinfection manifested as anal or genital pruritus, a change in oral mucosa, increased fever, and severe diarrhea.

Patient/Family Teaching

• Advise the patient/family to continue taking clindamycin for the full

length of treatment and to space drug doses evenly around the clock.
• Teach the patient/family to take oral doses with 8 oz of water.
• Warn the patient/family to use caution when applying topical clindamycin concurrently with abrasive, peeling acne agents, soaps, or alcohol-containing cosmetics to avoid cumulative effect.
• Instruct the patient/family not to apply topical preparations near the eyes or abraded areas.
• Teach the patient/family that if the vaginal form of clindamycin accidentally comes in contact with the eyes to rinse them with copious amounts of cool tap water.
• Advise the patient not to engage in sexual intercourse during clindamycin treatment.

Co-Trimoxazole (Sulfamethoxazole-Trimethoprim)

koe-try-**mox**-oh-zole
(Apo-Sulfatrim [CAN], Bactrim, Bactrim DS [AUS], Cosig Forte [AUS], Novotrimel [CAN], Resprim [AUS], Resprim Forte [AUS], Septra, Septrin [AUS], Septrin Forte [AUS])
Do not confuse with bacitracin, clotrimazole, Sectral, or Septa.

CATEGORY AND SCHEDULE
Pregnancy Risk Category: C

MECHANISM OF ACTION
A sulfonamide and folate antagonist that blocks bacterial synthesis of essential nucleic acids. ***Therapeutic Effect:*** Produces bactericidal action in susceptible microorganisms.

PHARMACOKINETICS
Rapidly well absorbed from the GI tract. Widely distributed. Protein binding: 45%–60%. Metabolized in liver. Excreted in urine. Minimally removed by hemodialysis. ***Half-Life:*** 6–12 hrs (trimethoprim 8–10 hrs). Half-life is increased with impaired renal function.

AVAILABILITY
Tablets: 80 mg trimethoprim/400 mg sulfamethoxazole; 160 mg/800 mg.
Oral Suspension: 40 mg/200 mg/5 mL.
Injection: 16 mg/80 mg/mL

INDICATIONS AND DOSAGES
▸ Mild to moderate infections
PO/IV (BASE DOSE ON TRIMETHOPRIM [TMP] COMPONENT)
Children older than 2 mos. 6–12 mg TMP/kg/day in divided doses q12h.
▸ Serious infections, *P. carinii* pneumonia
PO/IV
Children older than 2 mos. 15–20 mg TMP/kg/day in divided doses q6–8h.
▸ Prevention of *P. carinii* pneumonia
PO
Children. 150 mg TMP/m^2/day on 3 consecutive days/wk.
▸ Urinary tract infection prophylaxis
PO
Children older than 2 mos. 2 mg TMP/kg/dose once daily.
▸ Dosage in renal impairment
The dosage and frequency are modified based on the severity of infection, degree of renal impairment, and serum concentration of the drug. For those with creatinine clearance of 15–30 mL/min, a reduction in dose of 50% is recommended.

UNLABELED USES

Treatment of bacterial endocarditis, biliary tract, bone or joint, and chancroid infections, chlamydial infection, gonorrhea, intra-abdominal infection, meningitis, septicemia, sinusitis, skin and soft tissue infections.

CONTRAINDICATIONS

Hypersensitivity to trimethoprim or any sulfonamides, megaloblastic anemia as a result of folate deficiency, infants younger than 2 mos of age, porphyria.

INTERACTIONS

Drug

Hemolytics: May increase the risk of toxicity with other hemolytics.
Hydantoin anticonvulsants, oral hypoglycemics, warfarin: May increase or prolong the effects of and increase the risk of toxicity with these drugs.
Liver toxic medications: May increase the risk of liver toxicity.
Methenamine: May form precipitate.
Methotrexate: May increase the effect of methotrexate.
Cyclosporin: May decrease serum concentrations of this drug.

Herbal

None known.

Food

None known.

DIAGNOSTIC TEST EFFECTS

May increase BUN, serum alkaline phosphatase, serum creatinine, serum potassium, SGOT (AST), and SGPT (ALT) levels.

IV INCOMPATIBILITIES

Fluconazole (Diflucan), foscarnet (Foscavir), midazolam (Versed), vinorelbine (Navelbine)

IV COMPATIBILITIES

Diltiazem (Cardizem), heparin, hydromorphone (Dilaudid), lorazepam (Ativan), magnesium sulfate, morphine

SIDE EFFECTS

Frequent
Anorexia, nausea, vomiting, rash (generally 7–14 days after therapy begins), urticaria
Occasional
Diarrhea, abdominal pain, local pain or irritation at IV site
Rare
Headache, vertigo, insomnia, seizures, hallucinations, depression

SERIOUS REACTIONS

! Rash, fever, sore throat, pallor, purpura, cough, and shortness of breath may be early signs of serious adverse reactions.
! Fatalities are rare but have occurred with sulfonamide therapy after Stevens-Johnson syndrome, toxic epidermal necrolysis, fulminant hepatic necrosis, agranulocytosis, aplastic anemia, and other blood dyscrasias.

PEDIATRIC CONSIDERATIONS

Baseline Assessment

◂ALERT▸ Determine the patient's history of bronchial asthma, hypersensitivity to trimethoprim or any sulfonamide, and sulfite sensitivity before beginning drug therapy.
- Expect to establish the patient's hematologic, liver, and renal baselines.
- Be aware that co-trimoxazole use is contraindicated during pregnancy, at term, and during lactation.
- Be aware that co-trimoxazole use is contraindicated in children

younger than 2 mos of age and that co-trimoxazole use in newborns may produce kernicterus.
• Assess for age-appropriate fluid intake.
• Use cautiously in children with AIDS, renal or hepatic impairment, asthma, or urinary problems.
• May cause kernicterus in newborns.

Precautions

• Use cautiously in pts with glucose 6-phosphate dehydrogenase deficiency or hepatic or renal impairment.

Administration and Handling

◂ **ALERT** ▸ Be aware that drug potency is expressed in terms of TMP content.

PO

• Store tablets and suspension at room temperature.
• Give to the patient on an empty stomach with 8 oz of water, and be sure to provide the patient with several extra glasses of water each day.

IV

• Be aware that the piggyback IV infusion solution is stable for 2–6 hrs. Use the solution immediately.
• Discard the solution if it is cloudy or precipitate forms.
• For piggyback IV infusion, dilute each 5 mL with 75–125 mL D_5W.
• Do not mix co-trimoxazole with other drugs or solutions.
• Infuse over 60–90 min and avoid bolus or rapid infusion.
• Do not give IM.
• Ensure that the patient is adequately hydrated.

Intervention and Evaluation

• Monitor the patient's intake and output.
• Assess the patient's pattern of daily bowel activity and stool consistency.
• Assess the patient's skin for pallor, purpura, and rash.
• Check the patient's IV site and flow rate.
• Monitor the patient's hematology, liver, and renal function test reports.
• Evaluate the patient for CNS symptoms such as hallucinations, headache, insomnia, and vertigo.
• Monitor the patient's vital signs at least 2 times/day.
• Evaluate the patient for cough or shortness of breath.
• Assess the patient for signs and symptoms of bruising, overt bleeding, or swelling.

Patient/Family Teaching

• Advise the patient/family to continue taking co-trimoxazole for the full length of treatment and to space drug doses evenly around the clock.
• Instruct the patient/family to take oral co-trimoxazole doses with 8 oz of water and to drink several extra glasses of water each day.
• Warn the patient/family to notify the physician immediately if the patient experiences any new symptoms, especially bleeding, bruising, fever, rash or other skin changes, and sore throat.

Dapsone

dap-sewn
(Dapsone)

CATEGORY AND SCHEDULE

Pregnancy Risk Category: C

MECHANISM OF ACTION

An antibiotic that is a competitive antagonist of *para*-aminobenzoic acid (PABA) and prevents normal bacterial utilization of PABA for synthesis of folic acid. ***Therapeutic Effect:*** Inhibits bacterial growth.

AVAILABILITY

Tablets: 25 mg, 100 mg.

INDICATIONS AND DOSAGES

▸ **Leprosy**

PO

Children. 1–2 mg/kg/24 hrs. Maximum: 100 mg/day.

▸ ***P. carinii*** **pneumonia prophylaxis**

PO

Children older than 1 mo. 2 mg/kg/day. Maximum: 100 mg/day.

UNLABELED USES

Treatment of inflammatory bowel disorder, malaria.

CONTRAINDICATIONS

Hypersensitivity to dapsone or any component, pts with severe anemia.

INTERACTIONS

Drug

Methotrexate, pyrimethamine, nitrofurantoin: May increase hematologic reactions.
Probenecid: May decrease the excretion of dapsone.
Protease inhibitors, including ritonavir: May increase dapsone blood concentration.
Rifampin: May decrease rifampin blood concentration.
Trimethoprim: May increase the risk of toxic effects.

Herbal

St. John's wort: May decrease dapsone blood concentration.

Food

Do not administer with antacids or alkaline foods or drugs: may decrease dapsone absorption.

DIAGNOSTIC TEST EFFECTS

None significant.

SIDE EFFECTS

Frequent (greater than 10%)
Hemolytic anemia, methemoglobinemia, skin rash

Occasional (10%–1%)
Hemolysis, photosensitivity reaction

SERIOUS REACTIONS

! Agranulocytosis and blood dyscrasias may occur.

PEDIATRIC CONSIDERATIONS

Baseline Assessment

- As ordered, obtain the patient's baseline complete blood count (CBC).
- Determine whether the patient has a hypersensitivity to sulfa drugs.
- Assess for age-appropriate fluid intake.

Precautions

- Use cautiously in pts with agranulocytosis, aplastic anemia, glucose 6-phosphate dehydrogenase deficiency, sensitivity to sulfa drugs, and severe anemia.

Administration and Handling

PO

- May give dapsone with or without food.

Intervention and Evaluation

- Assess the patient's skin for a dermatologic reaction.
- Monitor the patient for signs and symptoms of hemolysis and jaundice.
- Monitor the patient's CBC.

Patient/Family Teaching

- Explain to the patient/family that frequent blood tests are necessary, especially during early dapsone therapy.
- Instruct the patient/family to notify the physician and discontinue dapsone use if a rash develops.
- Warn the patient/family to report if the patient experiences persistent fatigue, fever, or sore throat.
- Encourage the patient/family to avoid overexposure to sun or ultraviolet light.

Hydroxychloroquine Sulfate

hi-drocks-ee-**klor**-oh-kwin
(Plaquenil)
Do not confuse with hydrocortisone or hydroxyzine.

CATEGORY AND SCHEDULE

Pregnancy Risk Category: C

MECHANISM OF ACTION

An antimalarial and antirheumatic that concentrates in parasite acid vesicles, interfering with parasite protein synthesis and increasing pH. Its antirheumatic action is unknown but may involve suppressing formation of antigens responsible for hypersensitivity reactions. ***Therapeutic Effect:*** Inhibits parasite growth.

AVAILABILITY

Tablets: 200 mg (155 mg base).

INDICATIONS AND DOSAGES

▸ Prophylaxis of malaria

PO

Children. 5 mg base/kg/wk. Begin 2 wks before exposure; continue 4 wks after leaving endemic area or if therapy is not begun before exposure. Maximum: 310 mg/kg/day.

▸ Treatment of malaria

PO

Children. 10 mg base/kg given in 2 divided doses 6 hrs apart.

▸ Treatment of malaria (acute attack; dose [mg base]):

Dose	Times	Adults	Children
Initial	Day 1	620 mg	10 mg/kg
Second	6 hrs later	310 mg	5 mg/kg
Third	Day 2	310 mg	5 mg/kg
Fourth	Day 3	310 mg	5 mg/kg

UNLABELED USES

Treatment of juvenile arthritis, sarcoid-associated hypercalcemia.

CONTRAINDICATIONS

Hypersensitivity to hydroxychloroquine. Long-term therapy for children, porphyria, psoriasis, retinal or visual field changes.

INTERACTIONS

Drug

Penicillamine: May increase blood concentration of this drug. May increase the risk of hematologic and renal or severe skin reaction when taken concurrently with this drug.
Digoxin: Increases digoxin serum concentrations, which may increase toxicity of digoxin.

Herbal

None known.

Food

None known.

DIAGNOSTIC TEST EFFECTS

None known.

SIDE EFFECTS

Frequent

Mild transient headache, anorexia, nausea, vomiting

Occasional

Visual disturbances, nervousness, fatigue, pruritus (especially of palms, soles, scalp), irritability, personality changes, diarrhea

Rare

Stomatitis dermatitis, impaired hearing

SERIOUS REACTIONS

! Ocular toxicity, especially retinopathy, which may progress even after the drug is discontinued, may occur.

! Prolonged therapy may result in peripheral neuritis, neuromyopathy, hypotension, EKG changes, agranulocytosis, aplastic anemia, thrombocytopenia, seizures, and psychosis.

! Overdosage may result in headache, vomiting, visual disturbance, drowsiness, seizures, and hypokalemia followed by cardiovascular collapse and death.

PEDIATRIC CONSIDERATIONS

Baseline Assessment

- Evaluate the patient's complete blood count and liver function test results.
- Use cautiously in children with retinal or visual field changes, which could indicate hypersensitivity to the medication.
- Death has occurred in children who have ingested 3–4 tablets. Keep out of reach of children to avoid potentially fatal outcomes.

Precautions

- Use cautiously in pts who abuse alcohol or have a history of alcohol abuse.
- Use cautiously in pts with glucose 6-phosphate dehydrogenase deficiency and liver disease.
- Be aware that children are especially susceptible to the fatal effects of hydroxychloroquine.

Administration and Handling

◂ **ALERT** ▸ 200 mg hydroxychloroquine = 155 mg base.

Intervention and Evaluation

- Monitor the patient and promptly report any visual disturbances experienced by the patient to the physician.
- Evaluate the patient for GI distress.
- Give the drug dose with food for treatment of malaria.
- Monitor the patient's liver function test results.
- Assess the patient's buccal mucosa and skin. Evaluate the patient for pruritus.
- Report to the physician immediately if the patient experiences impaired hearing.

Patient/Family Teaching

- Advise the patient/family to continue taking hydroxychloroquine sulfate for the full length of treatment.
- Explain to the patient/family that in long-term therapy, a therapeutic response may not be evident for up to 6 mos.
- Warn the patient/family to immediately notify the physician of any new symptom of decreased hearing, muscular weakness, tinnitus, and visual difficulties.
- Teach the patient/family that hydroxychloroquine sulfate may cause photosensitivity reactions and that pts should avoid exposure to sunlight and wear broad-spectrum sunscreen, sunglasses, and protective clothing.

Linezolid

lyn-eh-**zoe**-lid

(Zyvox)

Do not confuse with Vioxx.

CATEGORY AND SCHEDULE

Pregnancy Risk Category: C

MECHANISM OF ACTION

An oxalodinone that binds to a site on bacterial 23S ribosomal RNA This action prevents the formation of the complex that is an essential component of the bacterial translation process. ***Therapeutic Effect:*** Bacteriostatic against enterococci and staphylococci; bactericidal against streptococci.

PHARMACOKINETICS

Rapidly, extensively absorbed after PO administration. Protein binding: 31%. Metabolized in liver by oxidation. Excreted in urine. ***Half-Life:*** Neonates and infants: 1.5–5 hrs; children: 2–4 hrs; adults: 4–5.4 hrs.

AVAILABILITY

Tablets: 400 mg, 600 mg.
Oral Powder for Suspension: 20 mg/mL.
Injection (premixed): 2 mg/mL in 100 mL or 300-mL bags.

INDICATIONS AND DOSAGES

‣ Treatment of vancomycin-resistant *Enterococcus faecium* infections

PO/IV

Children older than 12 yrs. 600 mg q12h for 14–28 days.

Children younger than 12 yrs. 10 mg/kg/dose q8h.

‣ Uncomplicated skin infections

PO/IV

Children older than 12 yrs. 600 mg q12h.

Children 5–11 yrs. 10 mg/kg/dose q12h.

CONTRAINDICATIONS

Hypersensitivity to linezolid.

INTERACTIONS

Drug

Adrenergic agents (sympathomimetics, dopamine, epinephrine): Increase vasopressor effects.
MAOIs: Decreases the effects of these drugs.
Antidepressants (tricyclic, selective serotonin reuptake inhibitors, venlafaxine, trazodone), meperidine, dextromethorphan: Increased risk of serotonin syndrome.

Herbal

None known.

Food

Ingestion of tyramine-containing foods may lead to hypertensive crisis.

DIAGNOSTIC TEST EFFECTS

May decrease blood Hgb, platelet count, WBC count, and SGPT (ALT) levels.

IV INCOMPATIBILITIES

Amphotericin B complex (Abelcet, AmBisome, Amphotec), chlorpromazine (Thorazine), diazepam (Valium), erythromycin (Erythrocin), pentamidine (Pentam IV), phenytoin (Dilantin), sulfamethoxazole-trimethoprim (Bactrim)

SIDE EFFECTS

Occasional (5%–2%)

Diarrhea, nausea, headache

Rare (less than 2%)

Taste alteration, vaginal candidiasis (discharge, itching), fungal infection, dizziness, tongue discoloration

SERIOUS REACTIONS

! Thrombocytopenia occurs rarely.
! Myelosuppression occurs.
! Antibiotic-associated colitis manifested as severe abdominal pain and tenderness, fever, and watery and severe diarrhea may result from altered bacterial balance.

PEDIATRIC CONSIDERATIONS

- Be aware that it is unknown whether linezolid is distributed in breast milk.
- Be aware that the safety and efficacy of linezolid have not been established in children.
- Children younger than 40 mos of age experience faster clearance. Therefore, q8h dosing interval is recommended.

Precautions

- Use cautiously in pts with carcinoid syndrome, pheochromocytoma, severe renal or liver impairment, uncontrolled hypertension, and untreated hyperthyroidism.

Administration and Handling

PO

- Give without regard to meals.
- Use suspension within 21 days after reconstitution.
- Do not shake suspension; gently invert bottle several times before use.
- Store at room temperature.

IV

◂ALERT▸ Do not mix with other medications. If same line is used, flush with compatible fluid (D_5W, 0.9% NaCl, lactated Ringer's solution).

- Store at room temperature and protect from light.
- Know that yellow color does not affect potency.
- Infuse over 30–120 min.

Intervention and Evaluation

- Assess the patient's pattern of daily bowel activity and stool consistency. Mild GI effects may be tolerable, but increasing severity may indicate the onset of antibiotic-associated colitis.
- Be alert for signs and symptoms of superinfection manifested as abdominal pain, moderate to severe diarrhea, severe anal or genital pruritus, and severe mouth soreness.
- Monitor the patient's complete blood count weekly.

Patient/Family Teaching

- Advise the patient/family to continue linezolid therapy for the full length of treatment and to evenly space drug doses around the clock.
- Explain that linezolid may cause GI upset. Tell the patient/family that the patient may take linezolid with food or milk if GI upset occurs.
- Teach the patient/family to avoid excessive amounts of tyramine-containing foods (e.g., aged cheese, red wine). Give the patient/family a list of tyramine-containing foods.
- Warn the patient/family to notify the physician if symptoms of infection get persistently worse.

Metronidazole Hydrochloride

meh-trow-**nye**-dah-zoll

(Apo-Metronidazole [CAN], Flagyl, MetroCream, MetroGel, Metrogyl [AUS], MetroLotion, Metronide [AUS], NidaGel [CAN], Noritate, Novonidazol [CAN], Rozex [AUS], Satric 500)

CATEGORY AND SCHEDULE

Pregnancy Risk Category: B

MECHANISM OF ACTION

A nitroimidazole derivative that is an antibacterial and antiprotozoal. Disrupts bacterial and protozoal DNA and inhibits nucleic acid synthesis. ***Therapeutic Effect:*** Produces bactericidal, amebicidal, trichomonacidal effects. Produces anti-inflammatory, immunosuppressive effects when applied topically.

PHARMACOKINETICS

Well absorbed from the GI tract, minimal absorption after topical application. Protein binding: less than 20%. Widely distributed, crosses blood-brain barrier. Metabolized in liver to active metabolite. Primarily excreted in urine; partially eliminated in feces. Removed by hemodialysis. ***Half-Life:*** Neonates: 25–75 hrs; children and adults: 8 hrs (half-life is increased in pts with alcoholic liver disease, in neonates).

AVAILABILITY

Tablets: 250 mg, 500 mg.
Tablets (extended release): 750 mg.

Capsules: 375 mg.
Powder for Injection: 500 mg.
Premixed Injection (infusion): 5 mg/mL.
Lotion: 0.75% (60 mL).
Vaginal Gel: 0.75% (70 g).
Topical Gel: 0.75% (30 g, 45 g).
Topical Cream: 0.75% (45 g), 1% (30 g).

INDICATIONS AND DOSAGES

▸ Amebiasis

PO

Children. 35–50 mg/kg/day in divided doses q8h for 10 days.

▸ Parasitic infections

PO

Children. 15–30 mg/kg/day in divided doses q8h.

▸ Anaerobic skin and skin-structure, CNS, lower respiratory tract, bone, joint, intra-abdominal, and gynecologic infections; endocarditis; septicemia

PO/IV

Children. 30 mg/kg/day in divided doses q6h. Maximum: 4 g/day.
Neonates younger than 7 days weighing less than 1.2 kg. 7.5 mg/kg q48h.
Neonates younger than 7 days weighing 1.2–2 kg. 7.5 mg/kg q24h.
Neonates younger than 7 days weighing 2 kg or more. 15 mg/kg/day q12h.
Neonates older than 7 days weighing less than 1.2 kg. 7.5 mg/kg q48h.
Neonates older than 7 days weighing 1.2–2 kg. 15 mg/kg/day q12h.
Neonates older than 7 days weighing 2 kg or more. 30 mg/kg/day q12h.

▸ Antibiotic-associated pseudomembranous colitis

PO

Children. 30 mg/kg/day in divided doses q6h for 7–10 days.

▸ Helicobacter pylori

PO

Children. 15–20 mg/kg/day in 2 divided doses for 4 wks (in combination with amoxicillin and bismuth subsalicylate).

UNLABELED USES

Topical application in treatment of acne rosacea, treatment of bacterial vaginosis, treatment of grade III–IV decubitus ulcers with anaerobic infection, treatment of *H. pylori*–associated gastritis and duodenal ulcer, treatment of inflammatory bowel disease.

CONTRAINDICATIONS

Hypersensitivity to metronidazole or other nitroimidazole derivatives (also parabens with topical application) and first trimester of pregnancy.

INTERACTIONS

Drug

Alcohol: May cause disulfiram-type reaction.
Disulfiram: May increase toxicity with disulfiram.
Oral anticoagulants: May increase the effects of these drugs.
Phenytoin, lithium: May increase the effects of these drugs.

Herbal

None known.

Food

None known.

DIAGNOSTIC TEST EFFECTS

May increase lactate dehydrogenase, SGOT (AST), and SGPT (ALT) levels.

IV INCOMPATIBILITIES

Amphotericin B complex (Abelcet, AmBisome, Amphotec), filgrastim (Neupogen)

IV COMPATIBILITIES

Diltiazem (Cardizem), dopamine (Intropin), heparin, hydromorphone (Dilaudid), lorazepam (Ativan), magnesium sulfate, midazolam (Versed), morphine

SIDE EFFECTS

Frequent

Anorexia, nausea, dry mouth, metallic taste
Vaginal: Symptomatic cervicitis and vaginitis, abdominal cramps, uterine pain

Occasional

Diarrhea or constipation, vomiting, dizziness, erythematous rash, urticaria, reddish brown or dark urine
Topical: Transient redness, mild dryness, burning, irritation, stinging, tearing when applied too close to eyes
Vaginal: Vaginal, perineal, vulvar itching; vulvar swelling

Rare

Mild, transient leukopenia, thrombophlebitis with IV therapy

SERIOUS REACTIONS

! Oral therapy may result in furry tongue, glossitis, cystitis, dysuria, pancreatitis, and flattening of T waves on EKG readings.
! Peripheral neuropathy manifested as numbness, tingling, and paresthesia, which is usually reversible if treatment is stopped immediately after neurologic symptoms appear, occurs.
! Seizures occur occasionally.

PEDIATRIC CONSIDERATIONS

Baseline Assessment

• Determine the patient's history of hypersensitivity to metronidazole or other nitroimidazole derivatives (and parabens with topical application).
• Obtain patient specimens for diagnostic tests before giving the first dose of metronidazole. Therapy may begin before the test results are known.
• Be aware that metronidazole readily crosses the placenta and is distributed in breast milk.
• Be aware that metronidazole use is contraindicated during the first trimester of pregnancy in women with trichomoniasis. Topical use during pregnancy or during breast-feeding is discouraged.
• There are no age-related precautions noted in children.
• Do not administer by IV push.
• Assess for age-appropriate fluid intake.

Precautions

• Use cautiously in pts with blood dyscrasias, CNS disease, a predisposition to edema, and severe liver dysfunction.
• Use cautiously in pts concurrently receiving corticosteroid therapy.
• Be aware that the safety and efficacy of topical administration in those younger than 21 yrs of age have not been established.

Administration and Handling

PO
• Give metronidazole without regard to meals. Give with food to decrease GI irritation.

IV
• Store ready-to-use infusion bags at room temperature.
• Infuse over more than 30–60 min. Do not give as a bolus.

Intervention and Evaluation

• Avoid prolonged use of indwelling catheters.
• Assess the patient's pattern of daily bowel activity and stool consistency.
• Monitor the patient's intake and output and assess the patient for urinary problems.
• Be alert for neurologic symptoms, such as dizziness or numb-

ness, tingling, or paresthesia of the extremities.
• Assess the patient for rash and urticaria.
• Be alert for signs and symptoms of superinfection manifested as anal or genital pruritus, furry tongue, ulceration or change of oral mucosa, and vaginal discharge.

Patient/Family Teaching

• Explain to the patient/family that the patient's urine may be red-brown or dark during drug therapy.
• Urge the patient/family to avoid alcohol and alcohol-containing preparations (e.g., cough syrups, elixirs) while taking metronidazole.
• Warn the patient/family to avoid tasks requiring mental alertness or motor skills until the patient's response to the drug is established. Metronidazole may cause dizziness.
• In pts with amebiasis, check stool specimens frequently.
• Warn the patient/family using the topical version of metronidazole to avoid drug contact with eyes.
• Tell the patient that he or she may apply cosmetics after topical drug application.
• Explain to the patient/family that metronidazole acts on papules, pustules, and redness but has no effect on ocular problems (conjunctivitis, keratitis, blepharitis), rhinophyma (hypertrophy of nose), or telangiectasia.

Nitrofurantoin Sodium

ny-tro-feur-**an**-twon
(Apo-Nitrofurantoin [CAN], Furadantin, Macrobid, Macrodantin, Novo-Furan [CAN], Ralodantin [AUS])

CATEGORY AND SCHEDULE

Pregnancy Risk Category: B

MECHANISM OF ACTION

An antibacterial, urinary tract infection agent. Inhibits bacterial enzyme systems that may alter ribosomal proteins. ***Therapeutic Effect:*** Inhibits protein, DNA, RNA, and cell wall synthesis. Bacteriostatic (bacteriocidal at high concentration).

PHARMACOKINETICS

Microcrystalline: rapidly, completely absorbed; macrocrystalline: more slowly absorbed. Food increases absorption. Protein binding: 40%. Primarily concentrated in urine, kidneys. Metabolized in most body tissues. Primarily excreted in urine. Removed by hemodialysis. ***Half-Life:*** 20–60 min (prolonged with renal impairment).

AVAILABILITY

Capsules (Macrodantin): 25 mg, 50 mg, 100 mg
Capsules (Macrobid): 100 mg.
PO Suspension (Furadantin): 25 mg/5 mL.

INDICATIONS AND DOSAGES

▸ Initial or recurrent urinary tract infection (UTI)

PO

Children older than 1 mo. 5–7 mg/kg in 4 divided doses. Maximum: 400 mg/day.

▸ Long-term prophylactic therapy of UTI

PO

Children. 1–2 mg/kg in 1–2 divided doses. Maximum: 100 mg/day.

UNLABELED USES

Prophylaxis of bacterial UTIs.

CONTRAINDICATIONS

Hypersensitivity to nitrofurantoin. Renal impairment. Infants younger than 1 mo of age because of hemolytic anemia, anuria, oliguria, and substantial renal impairment (creatinine clearance less than 40 mL/min). Pregnant pts at term and during labor.

INTERACTIONS

Drug

Hemolytics: May increase the risk of nitrofurantoin toxicity.
Neurotoxic medications: May increase the risk of neurotoxicity.
Probenecid: May increase blood concentration and toxicity of nitrofurantoin.

Herbal

None known.

Food

None known.

DIAGNOSTIC TEST EFFECTS

None known.

SIDE EFFECTS

Frequent
Anorexia, nausea, vomiting, dark yellow or brown urine
Occasional
Abdominal pain, diarrhea, rash, pruritus, urticaria, hypertension, headache, dizziness, drowsiness
Rare
Photosensitivity, transient alopecia, asthmatic attack in those with history of asthma

SERIOUS REACTIONS

! Superinfection, liver toxicity, peripheral neuropathy (may be irreversible), Stevens-Johnson syndrome, permanent pulmonary function impairment, and anaphylaxis occur rarely.

PEDIATRIC CONSIDERATIONS

Baseline Assessment

• Determine the patient's history of asthma.
• Evaluate the patient's laboratory test results for renal and liver baselines.
• Be aware that nitrofurantoin readily crosses the placenta and is distributed in breast milk.
• Be aware that nitrofurantoin use is contraindicated at term and during breast-feeding when an infant is suspected of having glucose 6-phosphate dehydrogenase (G6PD) deficiency.
• There are no age-related precautions noted in children older than 1 mo of age.
• Assess for age-appropriate fluid intake.

Precautions

• Use cautiously in pts with anemia, diabetes mellitus, electrolyte imbalance, G6PD deficiency (greater risk of hemolytic anemia), renal impairment, and vitamin B deficiency and in debilitated pts (greater risk of peripheral neuropathy).

Administration and Handling

PO
• Give nitrofurantoin with food or milk to enhance absorption and reduce GI upset.

Intervention and Evaluation

• Monitor the patient's intake and output and renal function test results.
• Assess the patient's pattern of daily bowel activity and stool consistency.
• Assess the patient's skin for rash and urticaria.
• Be alert for signs and symptoms of peripheral neuropathy, such as numbness or tingling, especially of the lower extremities.
• Observe the patient for signs and symptoms of liver toxicity manifested as arthralgia, fever, hepatomegaly, and rash.
• Perform a respiratory assessment of the patient. Auscultate the

patient's lungs; check for chest pain, cough, and difficulty breathing.

Patient/Family Teaching

- Explain to the patient/family that the patient's urine may become dark yellow or brown with nitrofurantoin use.
- Teach the patient/family to take nitrofurantoin with food or milk for best results and to reduce GI upset.
- Advise the patient/family to continue taking nitrofurantoin for the full length of therapy.
- Urge the patient/family to avoid sun and ultraviolet light, to use sunscreens, and wear protective clothing.
- Warn the patient/family to notify the physician if chest pain, cough, difficult breathing, fever, or numbness and tingling of fingers or toes occurs.
- Explain to the patient/family that alopecia is a rare occurrence and is only temporary.

Pentamidine Isethionate

pen-**tam**-ih-deen
(NebuPent, Pentacarinat [CAN], Pentam-300)

CATEGORY AND SCHEDULE

Pregnancy Risk Category: C

MECHANISM OF ACTION

An anti-infective, antiprotozoal that interferes with nuclear metabolism and incorporation of nucleotides. ***Therapeutic Effect:*** Inhibits DNA, RNA, phospholipid, and protein synthesis.

PHARMACOKINETICS

Minimal absorption after inhalation, well absorbed after IM administration. Widely distributed. Primarily excreted in urine. Minimally removed by hemodialysis. ***Half-Life:*** 6.5 hrs (half-life is increased with impaired renal function).

AVAILABILITY

Injection (Pentam-300): 300 mg.
Powder for Nebulization (NebuPent): 300 mg.

INDICATIONS AND DOSAGES

▸ *P. carinii* pneumonia (PCP) treatment

IV/IM

Children. 4 mg/kg/day once daily for 14–21 days.

▸ PCP prevention

INHALATION

Children 5 yrs and older. 300 mg q3–4wks.

Children younger than 5 yrs. 8 mg/kg/dose q3–4wks.

IV/IM

4 mg/kg/dose q2–4wks.

▸ Trypanosomiasis

IM

Children. 4 mg/kg/day once daily for 10 days.

UNLABELED USES

Treatment of African trypanosomiasis, cutaneous or visceral leishmaniasis.

CONTRAINDICATIONS

Hypersensitivity to pentamidine or any component. Do not use concurrently with didanosine.

INTERACTIONS

Drug

Blood dyscrasia–producing medication, bone marrow depressants: May increase abnormal hematologic effects of pentamidine.

Didanosine: May increase the risk of pancreatitis.

Foscarnet: May increase the risk of hypocalcemia, hypomagnesemia, and nephrotoxicity of pentamidine.
Nephrotoxic medications: May increase the risk of nephrotoxicity.

Herbal
None known.

Food
None known.

DIAGNOSTIC TEST EFFECTS

May increase BUN, serum alkaline phosphatase, serum bilirubin, serum creatinine, SGOT (AST), and SGPT (ALT) levels. May decrease serum calcium and magnesium levels. May alter blood glucose levels.

IV INCOMPATIBILITIES

Cefazolin (Ancef), cefotaxime (Claforan), ceftazidime (Fortaz), ceftriaxone (Rocephin), fluconazole (Diflucan), foscarnet (Foscavir), interleukin (Proleukin)

IV COMPATIBILITIES

Diltiazem (Cardizem), zidovudine (AZT, Retrovir)

SIDE EFFECTS

Frequent
Injection (greater than 10%): Abscess, pain at injection site
Inhalation (greater than 5%): Fatigue, metallic taste, shortness of breath, decreased appetite, dizziness, rash, cough, nausea, vomiting, chills

Occasional
Injection (10%–1%): Nausea, decreased appetite, hypotension, fever, rash, bad taste, confusion
Inhalation (5%–1%): Diarrhea, headache, anemia, muscle pain

Rare
Injection (less than 1%): Neuralgia, thrombocytopenia, phlebitis, dizziness

SERIOUS REACTIONS

! Life-threatening or fatal hypotension, arrhythmias, hypoglycemia, or leukopenia, nephrotoxicity and renal failure, anaphylactic shock, Stevens-Johnson syndrome, and toxic epidural necrolysis occur rarely.
! Hyperglycemia and insulin-dependent diabetes mellitus (often permanent) may occur even months after therapy.

PEDIATRIC CONSIDERATIONS

Baseline Assessment

- Avoid concurrent use of nephrotoxic drugs.
- Establish the patient's baseline blood glucose and blood pressure (B/P).
- Obtain patient specimens for diagnostic tests before giving the first dose of pentamidine.
- Be aware that it is unknown if pentamidine crosses the placenta or is distributed in breast milk.
- There are no age-related precautions noted in children.
- Be sure to administered IV pentamidine while the patient is lying down to decrease the effects of severe hypotension.
- Assess for age-appropriate fluid intake.

Precautions

- Use cautiously in pts with diabetes mellitus, hypertension, hypotension, and liver or renal impairment.

Administration and Handling

◀ **ALERT** ▶ Patient must be in the supine position during administration, with frequent B/P checks until B/P is stable because of the potential for developing a life-threatening hypotensive reaction. Have resuscitative equipment immediately available.

IM
Reconstitute 300-mg vial with 3 mL Sterile Water for Injection to provide concentration of 100 mg/mL.

IV

- Store vials at room temperature.
- After reconstitution, IV solution is stable at room temperature for 48 hrs.
- Discard unused portion.
- For intermittent IV infusion (piggyback), reconstitute each vial with 3–5 mL D_5W or Sterile Water for Injection.
- Withdraw desired dose and further dilute with 50–250 mL D_5W.
- Infuse over 60 min.
- Do not give by IV injection or rapid IV infusion because this increases the potential for development of severe hypotension.

AEROSOL (NEBULIZER)

- Store aerosol at room temperature for 48 hrs.
- Reconstitute 300-mg vial with 6 mL Sterile Water for Injection. Avoid use of 0.9% NaCl because this may cause precipitate to form.
- Do not mix with other medications in nebulizer reservoir.

Intervention and Evaluation

- Monitor the patient's B/P during pentamidine administration until stable for both IM and IV administration. The patient should remain supine until stable.

◂ALERT▸ Check the patient's blood glucose levels. Also assess the patient for signs and symptoms of hypoglycemia as evidenced by diaphoresis, double vision, headache, incoordination, lightheadedness, nervousness, numbness of lips, palpitation, tachycardia, and tremor, and hyperglycemia manifested as abdominal pain, headache, malaise, nausea, polydipsia, polyphagia, polyuria, visual changes, and vomiting.

- Evaluate the patient's IM sites for induration, pain, and redness.
- Evaluate the patient's IV sites for phlebitis as evidenced by heat, pain, and red streaking over the vein.
- Monitor the patient's hematology, liver, and renal function test results.
- Assess the patient's skin for rash.
- Evaluate the patient's equilibrium during ambulation.
- Be alert for respiratory difficulty when administering pentamidine by the inhalation route.

Patient/Family Teaching

- Teach the patient/family to remain flat in bed during administration of this medication and to get up slowly and with assistance only when B/P becomes stable.
- Warn the patient/family to notify the nurse immediately if the patient experiences lightheadedness, palpitations, shakiness, or sweating.
- Advise the patient/family that even several months after therapy stops, anorexia, drowsiness, and increased thirst and urination may develop.
- Instruct the patient/family to drink plenty of water to maintain adequate fluid intake.
- Warn the patient/family to notify the physician if cough, fever, or shortness of breath occurs.
- Urge the patient to avoid consuming alcohol.

Sulfasalazine

sul-fah-**sal**-ah-zeen
(Azulfidine, EN-tabs, Pyralin EN [AUS], Salazopyrin [CAN], SAS-500 [CAN])
Do not confuse with azathioprine, sulfadiazine, or sulfisoxazole.

CATEGORY AND SCHEDULE

Pregnancy Risk Category: B (D if given near term)

MECHANISM OF ACTION

A sulfonamide that inhibits prostaglandin synthesis. Acts locally in the colon. ***Therapeutic Effect:*** Decreases inflammatory response and interferes with GI secretion. Effect may be the result of antibacterial action with a change in intestinal flora.

PHARMACOKINETICS

Poorly absorbed from the GI tract. Cleaved in the colon by intestinal bacteria forming sulfapyridine and mesalamine (5-ASA). Absorbed in colon. Widely distributed. Metabolized in liver. Primarily excreted in urine. ***Half-Life:*** Sulfapyridine: 6–14 hrs; 5-ASA: 0.6–1.4 hrs.

AVAILABILITY

Tablets (Azulfidine): 500 mg.
Tablets (delayed release) (Azulfidine EN-tabs): 500 mg.

INDICATIONS AND DOSAGES

▸ Ulcerative colitis

PO

Children older than 2 yrs. 40–75 mg/kg/day in divided doses q4–6h. Maximum: 6 g/day. Maintenance: 30–50 mg/kg/day in divided doses q4–8h. Maximum: 2 g/day.

▸ Juvenile rheumatoid arthritis

PO

Children older than 2 yrs. Initially, 10 mg/kg/day. May increase by 10 mg/kg/day at weekly intervals. Range: 30–50 mg/kg/day. Maximum: 2 g/day.

UNLABELED USES

Treatment of ankylosing spondylitis.

CONTRAINDICATIONS

Children younger than 2 yrs of age; hypersensitivity to carbonic anhydrase inhibitors, local anesthetics, salicylates, sulfonamides, sulfonylureas, sunscreens containing para-aminobenzoic acid, thiazide or loop diuretics; intestinal or urinary tract obstruction; porphyria; pregnancy at term; severe liver or renal dysfunction.

INTERACTIONS

Drug

Anticonvulsants, oral anticoagulants, oral hypoglycemics, methotrexate: May increase the effects of these drugs.
Hemolytics: May increase toxicity of sulfasalazine.
Liver toxic medications: May increase the risk of liver toxicity of sulfasalazine.

Herbal

None known.

Food

None known.

DIAGNOSTIC TEST EFFECTS

None known.

SIDE EFFECTS

Frequent (33%)
Anorexia, nausea, vomiting, headache, oligospermia (generally reversed by withdrawal of drug)
Occasional (3%)
Hypersensitivity reaction: rash, urticaria, pruritus, fever, anemia
Rare (less than 1%)
Tinnitus, hypoglycemia, diuresis, photosensitivity

SERIOUS REACTIONS

! Anaphylaxis, Stevens-Johnson syndrome, hematologic toxicity (leukopenia, agranulocytosis), liver toxicity, and nephrotoxicity occur rarely.

PEDIATRIC CONSIDERATIONS

Baseline Assessment

◂ **ALERT** ▸ Determine the patient's hypersensitivity to medications (see Contraindications) before beginning drug therapy.

- Check the patient's initial complete blood count (CBC) and liver and renal function and urinalysis test results.
- Be aware that sulfasalazine may produce infertility and oligospermia in men while taking the medication.
- Be aware that sulfasalazine readily crosses the placenta and is excreted in breast milk. Do not breast-feed premature infants or those with hyperbilirubinemia or glucose 6-phosphate dehydrogenase (G6PD) deficiency.
- Be aware that if sulfasalazine is given near term, it may produce hemolytic anemia, jaundice, and kernicterus in the newborn.
- There are no age-related precautions noted in children older than 2 yrs of age.
- Assess for age-appropriate fluid intake.
- Diaper rash, fever, malaise, or diarrhea can be signs of superinfection.

Precautions

- Use cautiously in pts with bronchial asthma, G6PD deficiency, impaired liver or renal function, and severe allergies.

Administration and Handling

PO

- Space drug doses evenly at intervals not to exceed 8 hrs.
- Administer the drug after meals, if possible, to prolong intestinal passage.
- Have the patient swallow enteric-coated tablets whole; do not chew or crush.
- Give with 8 oz of water; encourage drinking of several glasses of water between meals.

Intervention and Evaluation

- Monitor the patient's intake and output and renal function and urinalysis test results.
- Ensure that the patient drinks plenty of water to maintain adequate hydration (minimum output 1,500 mL/24 hr) to prevent nephrotoxicity.
- Assess the patient's skin for rash. Withhold the drug and notify the physician at the first sign of a rash.
- Assess the patient's pattern of daily bowel activity and stool consistency. Drug dosage may need to be increased if diarrhea continues or recurs.
- Monitor the patient's CBC closely.
- Assess the patient for hematologic effects: bleeding, bruising, fever, jaundice, pallor, purpura, sore throat, and weakness. If hematologic effects occur, notify the physician immediately.

Patient/Family Teaching

- Explain to the patient/family that sulfasalazine may cause orange-yellow discoloration of the skin and urine.
- Advise the patient/family to continue sulfasalazine therapy for the full length of treatment and to space drug doses evenly around the clock. Explain to the patient/family that it may be necessary to continue taking the drug even after symptoms are relieved.
- Instruct the patient/family to take sulfasalazine after food with 8 oz of water and to drink several glasses of water between meals.
- Stress to the patient/family the importance of follow-up and laboratory tests.

• Tell the patient/family that if the patient is to have dental or other surgery, he or she must inform the dentist or surgeon about the sulfasalazine therapy.
• Urge the patient/family to avoid exposure to sun and ultraviolet light until the patient's photosensitivity is determined. Explain to the patient/family that photosensitivity may last for months after the last dose of sulfasalazine.

Trimethoprim

try-**meth**-oh-prim
(Primsol, Proloprim, Trimpex)

CATEGORY AND SCHEDULE

Pregnancy Risk Category: C

MECHANISM OF ACTION

A folate antagonist that blocks bacterial biosynthesis of nucleic acids and proteins by interfering with metabolism of folinic acid. ***Therapeutic Effect:*** Produces antibacterial activity.

PHARMACOKINETICS

Rapidly, completely absorbed from the GI tract. Protein binding: 42%–46%. Widely distributed, including cerebrospinal fluid. Metabolized in liver. Primarily excreted in urine. Moderately removed by hemodialysis. ***Half-Life:*** 8–10 hrs (half-life is increased with impaired renal function in newborns; decreased in children).

AVAILABILITY

Tablets: 100 mg, 200 mg.
Oral Solution: 50 mg/5 mL.

INDICATIONS AND DOSAGES

▸ **Acute, uncomplicated urinary tract infections (UTIs)**

PO

Children 12 yrs and older. 100 mg q12h or 200 mg once daily for 10 days.
Children younger than 12 yrs. 4–6 mg/kg/day in 2 divided doses for 10 days.

▸ **Dosage in renal impairment**

Creatinine Clearance	Dosage Interval
Greater than 30 mL/min	No change
15–30 mL/min	Give 50% of normal dose
Less than 15 mL/min	Avoid use

UNLABELED USES

Prophylaxis of bacterial UTIs, treatment of pneumonia caused by *P. carinii.*

CONTRAINDICATIONS

Infants younger than 2 mos of age, megaloblastic anemia due to folic acid deficiency.

INTERACTIONS

Drug

Folate antagonists, including methotrexate: May increase the risk of myeloblastic anemia.
Phenytoin: Increases phenytoin concentrations.

Herbal

None known.

Food

None known.

DIAGNOSTIC TEST EFFECTS

May increase BUN, serum bilirubin, serum creatinine, SGOT (AST), and SGPT (ALT) levels.

SIDE EFFECTS

Occasional

Nausea, vomiting, diarrhea, decreased appetite, stomach cramps, headache

Rare

Hypersensitivity reaction (pruritus, rash), methemoglobinemia (blue color on fingernails, lips, or skin, fever, pale skin, sore throat, unusual tiredness)

SERIOUS REACTIONS

! Stevens-Johnson syndrome, erythema multiforme, exfoliative dermatitis, and anaphylaxis occur rarely.

! Hematologic toxicity (thrombocytopenia, neutropenia, leukopenia, megaloblastic anemia) is more likely to occur in debilitated pts and pts with impaired renal function or receiving prolonged high dosage.

PEDIATRIC CONSIDERATIONS

Baseline Assessment

- Assess the patient's baseline hematology and renal function test reports.
- Be aware that trimethoprim readily crosses the placenta and is distributed in breast milk.
- Be aware that the safety and efficacy of trimethoprim have not been established in children.
- Assess for age-appropriate fluid intake.

Precautions

- Use cautiously in those with impaired liver or renal function and in pts who have folic acid deficiency.

Administration and Handling

PO

- Space doses evenly around the clock to maintain constant drug level in urine.
- Give without regard to meals (if stomach upset occurs, give with food).

Intervention and Evaluation

- Assess the patient's skin for rash.
- Evaluate the patient's food tolerance.
- Monitor the patient's hematology reports and liver or renal function test results, if ordered.
- Observe the patient for signs and symptoms of hematologic toxicity manifested as bleeding, bruising, fever, malaise, pallor, and sore throat.

Patient/Family Teaching

- Advise pts/families to complete the full course of trimethoprim therapy, usually 10–14 days, and to space drug doses evenly around the clock.
- Instruct the patient/family that trimethoprim may be taken on an empty stomach or with food if stomach upset occurs.
- Urge the patient/family to avoid sun and ultraviolet light, to use sunscreen, and wear protective clothing.
- Warn the patient/family to immediately report any bleeding, bruising, discoloration of the skin, fever, pallor, rash, sore throat, and tiredness the patient experiences to the physician.

Vancomycin Hydrochloride

van-koe-**my**-sin

(Vancocin, Vancoled)

CATEGORY AND SCHEDULE

Pregnancy Risk Category: C

MECHANISM OF ACTION

A tricyclic glycopeptide antibiotic that binds to the bacterial cell wall, altering cell membrane permeability and inhibiting RNA synthesis. ***Therapeutic Effect:***

Inhibits cell wall synthesis and produces bacterial cell death. Bactericidal.

PHARMACOKINETICS

PO: Poorly absorbed from the GI tract. Primarily eliminated in feces.
Parenteral: Widely distributed. Protein binding: 55%. Primarily excreted unchanged in urine. Not removed by hemodialysis.
Half-Life: 4–11 hrs (half-life is increased with impaired renal function).

AVAILABILITY

Capsules: 125 mg, 250 mg.
Powder for Injection: 500 mg, 1 g, 5 g.
Infusion (premix): 500 mg/100 mL, 1 g/200 mL.
Powder for Oral Solution: 250 mg/5 mL.

INDICATIONS AND DOSAGES

▸ Treatment of bone, respiratory tract, skin and soft tissue infections; endocarditis; peritonitis; septicemia

Given prophylactically to those at risk for bacterial endocarditis (if penicillin contraindicated) when undergoing biliary, dental, GI, GU, or respiratory surgery or invasive procedures.

IV

Children older than 1 mo. 40 mg/kg/day in divided doses q6–8h. Maximum: 3–4 g/day.
Neonates. 15 mg/kg q8–12h.

▸ Dosage in renal impairment

Dosages and frequency are modified based on the degree of renal impairment, severity of infection, and serum concentration of drug.

▸ Staphylococcal enterocolitis, antibiotic-associated pseudomembranous colitis caused by *Clostridium difficile*

PO

Children. 40 mg/kg/day in 3–4 divided doses for 7–10 days. Maximum: 2 g/day.

UNLABELED USES

Treatment of brain abscess, perioperative infections, staphylococcal or streptococcal meningitis.

CONTRAINDICATIONS

Hypersensitivity to vancomycin.

INTERACTIONS

Drug

Aminoglycosides, amphotericin, aspirin, bumetanide, carmustine, cisplatin, cyclosporine, ethacrynic acid, furosemide, streptozocin: May increase ototoxicity and nephrotoxicity of parenteral vancomycin.
Cholestyramine, colestipol: May decrease the effects of oral vancomycin.

Herbal

None known.

Food

None known.

DIAGNOSTIC TEST EFFECTS

May increase BUN level. Therapeutic peak blood level is 20–40 mcg/mL; trough level is 5–15 mcg/mL. The toxic peak blood level is greater than 40 mcg/mL; the toxic trough level is greater than 15 mcg/mL.

IV INCOMPATIBILITIES

Albumin, amphotericin B complex (Abelcet, AmBisome, Amphotec), aztreonam (Azactam), cefazolin (Ancef), cefepime (Maxipime), cefotaxime (Claforan), cefotetan (Cefotan), cefoxitin (Mefoxin), ceftazidime (Fortaz), ceftriaxone (Rocephin), cefuroxime (Zinacef), foscarnet (Foscavir), heparin, idarubicin (Idamycin), nafcillin (Nafcil), piperacillin/tazobactam (Zosyn), ticarcillin/clavulanate (Timentin)

IV COMPATIBILITIES

Amiodarone (Cordarone), calcium gluconate, diltiazem (Cardizem), hydromorphone (Dilaudid), insulin, lorazepam (Ativan), magnesium sulfate, midazolam (Versed), morphine, potassium chloride, propofol (Diprivan)

SIDE EFFECTS

Frequent

PO: Bitter or unpleasant taste, nausea, vomiting, mouth irritation (oral solution)

Rare

Systemic: Phlebitis, thrombophlebitis, pain at peripheral IV site; necrosis may occur with extravasation, dizziness, vertigo, tinnitus, chills, fever, rash

PO: Rash.

SERIOUS REACTIONS

! Nephrotoxicity (a change in the amount or frequency of urination, nausea, vomiting, increased thirst, anorexia), ototoxicity (deafness resulting from damage to auditory branch of eighth cranial nerve), and red-neck syndrome (from too rapid injection—redness on face, neck, arms, and back) may occur.

! Chills, fever, tachycardia, nausea, vomiting, itching, rash, and unpleasant taste may occur.

PEDIATRIC CONSIDERATIONS

Baseline Assessment

- Know that, if possible, vancomycin should not be given while administering other ototoxic and nephrotoxic medications.
- Obtain patient culture and sensitivity tests before giving the first dose of vancomycin. Therapy may begin before test results are known.
- Be aware that vancomycin crosses the placenta and that it is unknown whether vancomycin is distributed in breast milk.
- Be aware that close monitoring of drug serum levels is recommended in premature neonates and young infants. Blood for peak levels is drawn 30 min–1 hr after the initial dose of the medication has been infused, and blood for trough levels is drawn before the second dose.
- Be aware that red-neck syndrome (redness on face, neck, arms, and back) can develop in children. Stop the infusion immediately if signs of red-neck syndrome are observed.
- Assess for age-appropriate fluid intake.

Precautions

- Use cautiously in pts with preexisting hearing impairment and renal dysfunction.
- Use cautiously in pts concurrently taking other ototoxic or nephrotoxic medications.

Administration and Handling

PO

- Be aware that vancomycin is usually not given for systemic infections because of poor absorption from GI tract; however, some pts with colitis may effectively absorb the drug.
- Reconstitute powder for oral solution as appropriate and give it PO or via nasogastric tube. Do not use powder for oral solution for IV administration.

• Refrigerated oral solution is stable for 2 wks.

IV

ALERT Give by intermittent IV infusion (piggyback) or continuous IV infusion. Do not give IV push because this may result in exaggerated hypotension.

• After reconstitution, IV solution may be refrigerated; use within 14 days.
• Discard if precipitate forms.
• For intermittent IV infusion (piggyback), reconstitute each 500-mg vial with 10 mL Sterile Water for Injection (20 mL for 1-g vial) to provide concentration of 50 mg/mL.
• Further dilute to a final concentration not to exceed 5 mg/mL.
• Administer over 60 min or more.
• Monitor the patient's blood pressure (B/P) closely during IV infusion.
• ADD-Vantage vials should not be used in neonates, infants, or children requiring less than a 500 mg dose.

Intervention and Evaluation

• Monitor the patient's intake and output and renal function test results.
• Assess the patient's skin for rash.
• Evaluate the patient's balance and hearing acuity.
• Monitor the patient's B/P carefully during infusion.
• Evaluate the patient's IV site for phlebitis as evidenced by heat, pain, and red streaking over the vein.
• Know that the vancomycin therapeutic peak blood level is 20–40 mcg/mL; the trough level is 5–5 mcg/mL. The toxic peak blood level is greater than 40 mcg/mL; the toxic trough level is greater than 15 mcg/mL.

Patient/Family Teaching

• Advise the patient/family to continue vancomycin therapy for the full length of treatment and to space drug doses evenly around the clock.
• Warn the patient/family to notify the physician if the patient experiences rash, signs and symptoms of nephrotoxicity, or tinnitus.
• Stress to the patient/family that laboratory tests are an important part of total therapy.

REFERENCES

Gunn V. L. & Nechyba, C. (2002). The Harriet Lane handbook (16th ed.). St. Louis: Mosby.
Miller, S. & Fioravanti, J. (1997). Pediatric medications: A handbook for nurses. St. Louis: Mosby.
Taketomo, C. K., Hodding, J. H. & Kraus, D. M. (2003–2004). Pediatric dosage handbook (10th ed.). Hudson, OH: Lexi-Comp.

13 Alkylating Agents

Busulfan
Carboplatin
Chlorambucil
Cisplatin
Cyclophosphamide
Ifosfamide
Lomustine
Thiotepa

Uses: Alkylating agents are used to treat many types of cancer, including acute and chronic leukemias, lymphomas, multiple myeloma, and solid tumors in the breasts, uterus, lungs, bladder, and stomach.

Action: Alkylating agents form cross-links on DNA strands, which disturb DNA synthesis and cell division. In this way, these agents interfere with DNA integrity and function in rapidly proliferating tissues. They affect all phases of the cell cycle.

Busulfan

bew-**sull**-fan
(Busulfex, Myleran)
Do not confuse with Alkeran or Leukeran.

CATEGORY AND SCHEDULE

Pregnancy Risk Category: D

MECHANISM OF ACTION

An alkylating agent that interferes with DNA replication and RNA synthesis and is cell cycle–phase nonspecific. ***Therapeutic Effect:*** Disrupts nucleic acid function. Myelosuppressant.

PHARMACOKINETICS

Completely absorbed from the GI tract. Protein binding: 33%. Metabolized in liver. Primarily excreted in urine. Minimal removal by hemodialysis. ***Half-Life:*** 2.5 hrs.

AVAILABILITY

Tablets: 2 mg.
Injection: 60 mg ampule (6 mg/mL).

INDICATIONS AND DOSAGES

Refer to individual protocols. Base dose on ideal body weight.

▸ **Treatment of chronic myelogenous leukemia (CML); remission induction**

PO

Children. 0.06–0.12 mg/kg once daily.

▸ **Conditioning regimen before allogeneic hematopoietic cell transplantation**

IV

Children. 0.8 mg/kg/dose q6h for 16 doses over 4 consecutive days.

UNLABELED USES

Treatment of acute myelocytic leukemia.

CONTRAINDICATIONS

Hypersensitivity to busulfan. Disease resistance to previous therapy with this drug. Do not use during pregnancy and lactation.

INTERACTIONS

Drug

Antigout medications: May decrease the effects of these drugs.

Bone marrow depressants: May increase the risk of bone marrow depression.

Live virus vaccines: May potentiate virus replication, increase vaccine side effects, and decrease the patient's antibody response to the vaccine.

Itraconazole: May increase busulfan toxicity.

Herbal
None known.
Food
None known.

DIAGNOSTIC TEST EFFECTS

May decrease serum magnesium, potassium, phosphate, and sodium levels. May increase blood glucose, BUN, serum calcium, serum alkaline phosphatase, serum bilirubin, serum creatinine, and SGPT (ALT) levels.

IV INCOMPATIBILITIES

Do not mix with any other medications.

SIDE EFFECTS

Expected (98%–72%)
Nausea, stomatitis, vomiting, anorexia, insomnia, diarrhea, fever, abdominal pain, anxiety
Frequent (69%–44%)
Headache, rash, asthenia (loss of energy, strength), infection, chills, tachycardia, dyspepsia
Occasional (38%–16%)
Constipation, dizziness, edema, pruritus, cough, dry mouth, depression, abdominal enlargement, pharyngitis, hiccups, back pain, alopecia, myalgia
Rare (13%–5%)
Injection site pain, arthralgia, confusion, hypotension, lethargy

SERIOUS REACTIONS

! The major adverse reaction with busulfan is bone marrow depression resulting in hematologic toxicity as evidenced by severe leukopenia, anemia, and severe thrombocytopenia.
! Very high busulfan dosages may produce blurred vision, muscle twitching, and tonic-clonic seizures.
! Long-term therapy (more than 4 yrs) may produce pulmonary syndrome or "busulfan lung," which is characterized by persistent cough, congestion, rales, and dyspnea.
! Hyperuricemia may produce uric acid nephropathy, renal stones, and acute renal failure.

PEDIATRIC CONSIDERATIONS

Baseline Assessment
• Expect to perform hematologic studies, including blood Hct and Hgb, WBC count, differential, platelet count, and liver and renal function tests weekly. Know that the dosage of busulfan is based on hematologic values.
• Teach the patient/family about the expected effects of busulfan treatment.
• If possible, busulfan use should be avoided during pregnancy, especially in the first trimester.
• Be aware that busulfan use may cause fetal harm, and it is unknown whether the drug is distributed in breast milk. Breastfeeding is not recommended in this patient population.
• Assess for and maintain age-appropriate fluid intake.
Precautions
• Use extremely cautiously in pts with compromised bone marrow reserve.
• Use cautiously in pts with chicken pox, herpes zoster, a history of gout, or infection.
Administration and Handling
◂**ALERT**▸ Busulfan dosage is individualized based on the patient's clinical response and tolerance of the adverse effects of the drug. When used in combination therapy, consult specific protocols for optimum dosage and sequence of drug administration.
◂**ALERT**▸ Busulfan may be carcinogenic, mutagenic, or teratogenic.

Handle with extreme care during administration. Use of gloves is recommended. If contact with skin or mucosa occurs, wash thoroughly with water.
PO
Give at same time each day.
• Give to the patient on an empty stomach if nausea or vomiting occurs.

IV infusion

◂ALERT▸ Premedicate the patient with phenytoin to decrease the risk of seizures.
• Refrigerate ampules.
• After dilution, the solution is stable for 8 hrs at room temperature, 12 hrs if refrigerated when diluted with 0.9% NaCl.
• Dilute with 0.9% NaCl or D_5W only. The diluent quantity must be 10 times the volume of busulfan (e.g., 9.3 mL busulfan must be diluted with 93 mL diluent).
• Use a filter to withdraw busulfan from the ampule.
• Add busulfan to calculated diluent.
• Lock infusion pump when administering busulfan.
• Infuse over 2 hrs.
• Before and after infusion, flush catheter line with 5 mL 0.9% NaCl or D_5W.

Intervention and Evaluation

• Monitor the patient's laboratory values diligently for evidence of bone marrow depression.
• Assess the patient's mouth for onset of stomatitis as evidenced by difficulty swallowing, gum inflammation, and redness or ulceration of the oral mucous membranes.
• Give the patient antiemetic medications to prevent nausea or vomiting.
• Assess the patient's pattern of daily bowel activity and stool consistency.

Patient/Family Teaching

• Instruct the patient/family to maintain adequate daily fluid intake to protect against renal impairment.
• Warn the patient/family to report congestion, consistent cough, difficulty breathing, easy bruising, fever, signs of local infection, sore throat, or unusual bleeding from any site.
• Stress to the patient/family that the patient should not receive vaccinations without the physician's approval because busulfan lowers the body's resistance and that he or she should avoid contact with anyone who recently received a live virus vaccine.
• Teach the patient/family to take busulfan at the same time each day.
• Caution women of childbearing age to avoid pregnancy. Educate the patient regarding contraception options.
• Teach the patient/family to avoid products containing aspirin because aspirin could cause an increased risk of bleeding.

Carboplatin

car-bow-**play**-tin
(Paraplatin)
Do not confuse with Cisplatin or Platinol.

CATEGORY AND SCHEDULE
Pregnancy Risk Category: D

MECHANISM OF ACTION

A platinum coordination complex that inhibits DNA synthesis by cross-linking with DNA strands. Cell cycle-phase nonspecific. ***Therapeutic Effect:*** Prevents cellular division, interferes with DNA function.

PHARMACOKINETICS

Protein binding: Low. Hydrolyzed in solution to active form. Primarily excreted in urine. ***Half-life:*** 2.6–5.9 hrs.

AVAILABILITY

Powder for Injection: 50 mg, 150 mg, 450 mg.

INDICATIONS AND DOSAGES

Refer to individual protocols.

IV

Children. Solid tumor: 560 mg/m² q4wks.

Brain tumor: 175 mg/m² q4wks.

Sarcoma: 400 mg/m2/day for 2 days

Bone marrow transplant preparative: 500 mg/m2/day for 3 days

DOSAGE IN RENAL IMPAIRMENT

Initial dosage is based on creatinine clearance; subsequent dosages are based on the patient's tolerance and degree of myelosuppression.

UNLABELED USES

Treatment of bony and soft tissue sarcomas; germ cell tumors; neuroblastoma; pediatric brain tumor; small cell lung cancer; solid tumors of the bladder, cervix, and testes; and squamous cell carcinoma of the esophagus.

CONTRAINDICATIONS

History of severe allergic reaction to cisplatin, platinum compounds, and mannitol; severe bleeding; and severe myelosuppression.

INTERACTIONS

Drug

Bone marrow depressants: May increase bone marrow depression.

Live virus vaccines: May potentiate virus replication, increase vaccine side effects, and decrease the patient's antibody response to the vaccine.

Nephrotoxic-, ototoxic-producing agents: May increase the risk of toxicity.

Herbal

None known.

Food

None known.

DIAGNOSTIC TEST EFFECTS

May decrease serum electrolytes, including calcium, magnesium, potassium, and sodium. High dosages (>4 times the recommended dosage) may elevate BUN, serum alkaline phosphatase, serum bilirubin, serum creatinine, and SGOT (AST) levels.

IV INCOMPATIBILITIES

Amphotericin B complex (AmBisome, Amphotec, Abelcet)

IV COMPATIBILITIES

Etoposide (VePesid), granisetron (Kytril), ondansetron (Zofran), paclitaxel (Taxol)

SIDE EFFECTS

Frequent

Nausea (75%-80%), vomiting (65%)

Occasional

Generalized pain (17%), diarrhea or constipation (6%), peripheral neuropathy (4%)

Rare (3%-2%)

Alopecia, asthenia (loss of energy, strength), hypersensitivity reaction (erythema, pruritus, rash, urticaria)

SERIOUS REACTIONS

! Bone marrow suppression may be severe, resulting in anemia, infection, and bleeding (gastrointestinal bleeding, sepsis, pneumonia).

! Prolonged treatment may result in peripheral neurotoxicity.

PEDIATRIC CONSIDERATIONS

Baseline Assessment

• Offer the patient emotional support.

• Be aware that treatment should not be repeated until the patient's white blood cell (WBC) count recovers from previous therapy.

• Expect to administer transfusions in those patients receiving prolonged therapy.

• If possible, carboplatin use should be avoided during pregnancy, especially in the first trimester.

• Be aware that carboplatin use may cause fetal harm and that it is unknown if the drug is distributed in breast milk. Breast-feeding is not recommended in this patient population.

• Be aware that the safety and efficacy of carboplatin have not been established in children.

• Assess for and maintain age-appropriate fluid intake.

• Can cause severe vomiting and bone marrow suppression. Assess for and provide supportive care.

Precautions

• Use cautiously in patients with chickenpox, herpes zoster, infection, and renal function impairment.

Administration and Handling

◂ALERT▸ Be aware that carboplatin dosage is individualized based on the patient's clinical response and tolerance of the drug's adverse effects. Also, know that platelets must be greater than 100,000 mm^3 and neutrophils greater than 2,000 mm^3 before giving any dosage.

◂ALERT▸ Know that carboplatin may be carcinogenic, mutagenic, or teratogenic. Handle with extreme care during preparation and administration.

IV

• Store vials at room temperature.

• After reconstitution, solution is stable for 8 hrs. Discard unused portion after 8 hrs.

• Reconstitute immediately before use.

• Do not use aluminum needles or administration sets that come in contact with drug because this may produce black precipitate and a loss of potency.

• Reconstitute each 50 mg with 5 ml Sterile Water for Injection, D_5W, or 0.9% NaCl to provide concentration of 10 mg/ml.

• Further dilute solution with D_5W or 0.9% NaCl to provide concentration as low as 0.5 mg/ml, if needed.

• Infuse over 15 to 60 min.

• Be aware that rarely, an anaphylactic reaction may occur minutes after administration. Use epinephrine and corticosteroid, as prescribed, to alleviate symptoms.

Intervention and Evaluation

• Monitor the patient's hematologic status, pulmonary function studies, and liver and renal function tests. Be aware that myelosuppression is increased in those who have received previous carboplatin therapy or have impaired renal function.

• Assess the patient for easy bruising, fever, signs of local infection, sore throat, symptoms of anemia (excessive fatigue, weakness), and unusual bleeding from any site.

Patient/Family Teaching

• Advise the patient/family that nausea or vomiting is a side effect

of carboplatin that generally abates in less than 24 hrs.
• Stress to the patient/family that the patient should not receive vaccinations without the physician's approval, because carboplatin lowers the body's resistance. Also advise patient/family to avoid contact with anyone who recently received a live virus vaccine.

Chlorambucil

klor-**am**-bew-sill
(Leukeran)
Do not confuse with Alkeran, Chloromycetin, or Myleran.

CATEGORY AND SCHEDULE

Pregnancy Risk Category: D

MECHANISM OF ACTION

An alkylating agent and nitrogen mustard that inhibits DNA and RNA synthesis by cross-linking with DNA and RNA strands. Cell cycle–phase nonspecific.
Therapeutic Effect: Interferes with nucleic acid function.

PHARMACOKINETICS

Rapidly, completely absorbed from the GI tract. Protein binding: 99%. Rapidly metabolized in liver to active metabolite. Not removed by hemodialysis. Excreted as metabolites in the urine. ***Half-Life:*** 1.5 hrs; metabolite: 2.5 hrs.

AVAILABILITY

Tablets: 2 mg.

INDICATIONS AND DOSAGES

Refer to individual protocols.

▸ **Palliative treatment of advanced Hodgkin disease, advanced malignant (non-Hodgkin) lymphomas, chronic lymphocytic leukemia, giant follicular lymphomas, and lymphosarcoma**

PO

Children. Initial or short-course therapy: 0.1–0.2 mg/kg/day as single or divided dose for 3–6 wks. Average dose is 4–10 mg/day. Maintenance dose: 0.03–0.1 mg/kg/day. Average dose is 2–4 mg/day.
Chronic myelogenous leukemia (CML) use: Single daily dose q2wks is 0.4 mg/kg initially. Increase by 0.1 mg/kg q2wks until response and myelosuppression occur.

UNLABELED USES

Treatment of hairy cell leukemia; nephrotic syndrome; ovarian, testicular carcinoma; polycythemia vera.

CONTRAINDICATIONS

Previous allergic reaction, disease resistance to previous therapy with drug.

INTERACTIONS

Drug

Antigout medications: May decrease the effect of these drugs.
Bone marrow depressants: May increase bone marrow depression.
Live virus vaccines: May potentiate virus replication, increase vaccine side effects, or decrease the patient's antibody response to the vaccine.
Other immunosuppressants, including steroids: May increase the risk of infection or development of neoplasms.
Phenobarbital: May increase chlorambucil toxicity.

Herbal

None known.

Food

Acidic, hot foods and spices: May excessively irritate oral mucosal area and exacerbate mucositis.

DIAGNOSTIC TEST EFFECTS

May increase serum alkaline phosphatase, serum uric acid, and SGOT (AST) levels.

SIDE EFFECTS

Expected

GI effects such as nausea, vomiting, anorexia, diarrhea, and abdominal distress are generally mild, last less than 24 hrs, and occur only if a single dose exceeds 20 mg.

Occasional

Rash or dermatitis, pruritus, cold sores

Rare

Alopecia, urticaria (hives), erythema, hyperuricemia

SERIOUS REACTIONS

! Bone marrow depression manifested as hematologic toxicity, including neutropenia, leukopenia, progressive lymphopenia, anemia, and thrombocytopenia, may occur.

! After discontinuation of therapy, thrombocytopenia and leukopenia usually occur at 1–3 wks and last 1–4 wks.

! Neutrophil count decreases up to 10 days after the last dose.

! Toxicity appears to be less severe with intermittent rather than continuous drug administration.

! Overdosage may produce seizures in children.

! Excessive serum uric acid level and liver toxicity occur rarely.

PEDIATRIC CONSIDERATIONS

Baseline Assessment

- Expect to obtain a complete blood count (CBC) each week during chlorambucil therapy.
- Expect to obtain a WBC count 3–4 days after each weekly CBC during the first 3–6 weeks of chlorambucil therapy or 4–6 weeks if the patient is on an intermittent dosing schedule.
- If possible, chlorambucil use should be avoided during pregnancy, especially in the first trimester.
- Be aware that breast-feeding is not recommended in this patient population.
- Be aware that when chlorambucil is taken for nephritic syndrome, seizures may increase.

Precautions

- Use extremely cautiously in pts within 4 wks after full-course radiation therapy or a myelosuppressive drug regimen.

Administration and Handling

◂ALERT▸ Be aware that chlorambucil may be carcinogenic, mutagenic, or teratogenic. Handle with extreme care during administration. Know that dosage is individualized on the basis of the patient's clinical response and tolerance of the adverse effects of the drug. When using this drug in combination therapy, consult specific protocols for optimum dosage and sequence of drug administration.

PO

Give chlorambucil without regard to food. Avoid acidic, hot, or spicy foods.

Intervention and Evaluation

- Monitor the patient for signs and symptoms of hematologic toxicity as evidenced by easy bruising, fever, signs of local infection, sore throat, symptoms of anemia (excessive fatigue, weakness), or unusual bleeding from any site.
- Assess the patient's skin for rash, pruritus, and urticaria.

Patient/Family Teaching

• Instruct the patient/family to maintain adequate daily fluid intake to protect against hyperuricemia.
• Stress to the patient/family that the patient should not receive vaccinations without the physician's approval because chlorambucil lowers the body's resistance. Also advise the patient to avoid contact with anyone who recently received a live virus vaccine.
• Warn the patient/family to report congestion, consistent cough, difficulty breathing, easy bruising, fever, signs of local infection, sore throat, or unusual bleeding from any site.

Cisplatin

sis-**plah**-tin
(Platinol-AQ)
Do not confuse with carboplatin, Paraplatin, or Patanol.

CATEGORY AND SCHEDULE

Pregnancy Risk Category: D

MECHANISM OF ACTION

A platinum coordination complex that inhibits DNA and, to a lesser extent, RNA and protein synthesis by cross-linking with DNA strands. Cell cycle–phase nonspecific. ***Therapeutic Effect:*** Prevents cellular division.

PHARMACOKINETICS

Widely distributed. Protein binding: greater than 90%. Undergoes rapid nonenzymatic conversion to inactive metabolite. Excreted in urine. Minimally removed by hemodialysis. ***Half-Life:*** 44 hrs (half-life is increased with impaired renal function).

AVAILABILITY

Injection: 1 mg/mL (50-mg vials, 100-mg vials).

INDICATIONS AND DOSAGES

Refer to individual protocols.

▸ **Treatment of advanced bladder carcinoma, metastatic ovarian tumors, metastatic testicular tumors**

IV

Children. Intermittent dosage schedule: 37–75 mg/m^2 once every 2–3 wks or 50–100 mg/m^2 over 4–6 hrs once every 21–28 days.

IV

Children. Daily dosage schedule: 15–20 mg/m^2/day for 5 days every 3–4 wks.

▸ **Osteogenic sarcoma and neuroblastoma**

IV

Children. 60–100 mg/m^2 on day 1 of cycle every 3–4 wks.

▸ **Brain tumor**

IV

Children. 60 mg/m^2 once daily for 2 consecutive days every 3–4 wks.

▸ **Bone marrow or stem cell transplantation**

Children. Continuous infusion: 55 mg/m^2/day for 72 hrs: Total dose: 165 mg/m^2.

▸ **Dosage in renal impairment**

Creatinine Clearance	% of Dose
10–50 mL/min	75%
less than 10 mL/min	50%

UNLABELED USES

Treatment of carcinoma of breast, cervix, endometrium, stomach, head and neck, lung, prostate; germ cell tumors; neuroblastoma; osteosarcoma.

CONTRAINDICATIONS

Hypersensitivity to cisplatin or platinum-containing agents. Hearing impairment, myelosuppression, pregnancy, renal impairment.

INTERACTIONS

Drug

Antigout medications: May decrease the effects of these drugs.
Bone marrow depressants: May increase bone marrow depression.
Live virus vaccines: May potentiate virus replication, increase vaccine side effects, and decrease the patient's antibody response to the vaccine.
Nephrotoxic, ototoxic agents: May increase the risk of respective toxicities.

Herbal

None known.

Food

None known.

DIAGNOSTIC TEST EFFECTS

May cause positive Coombs' test results. May increase BUN, serum creatinine, serum uric acid, and SGOT (AST) levels. May decrease creatinine clearance and serum calcium, magnesium, phosphate, potassium, and sodium levels.

IV INCOMPATIBILITIES

Amifostine (Ethyol), amphotericin B complex (AmBisome, Amphotec, Abelcet), cefepime (Maxipime), piperacillin/tazobactam (Zosyn), thiotepa

IV COMPATIBILITIES

Etoposide (VePesid), granisetron (Kytril), heparin, hydromorphone (Dilaudid), lorazepam (Ativan), magnesium sulfate, mannitol, morphine, ondansetron (Zofran)

SIDE EFFECTS

Frequent

Nausea or vomiting (begins 1–4 hrs after administration, generally lasts up to 24 hrs).
Myelosuppression occurs in 25%–30% of pts. Recovery can generally be expected in 18–23 days.

Occasional

Peripheral neuropathy (numbness, tingling of face, fingers, toes) may occur with prolonged therapy (4–7 mos).
Pain or redness at injection site, loss of taste or appetite

Rare

Hemolytic anemia, blurred vision, stomatitis

SERIOUS REACTIONS

! Anaphylactic reaction manifested as facial edema, wheezing, tachycardia, and hypotension may occur in the first few minutes of IV administration in pts previously exposed to cisplatin.
! Nephrotoxicity occurs in 28%–36% of pts treated with single dose of cisplatin, usually during the second week of therapy.
! Ototoxicity, including tinnitus and hearing loss, occurs in 31% of pts treated with a single dose of cisplatin (more severe in children). Ototoxicity may become more frequent or severe with repeated doses.

PEDIATRIC CONSIDERATIONS

Baseline Assessment

- Keep pts well hydrated before and 24 hrs after receiving this drug to ensure good urinary output and decrease the risk of nephrotoxicity.
- If possible, cisplatin use should be avoided during pregnancy, especially in the first trimester.
- Be aware that breast-feeding is not recommended in this patient population.

• Be aware that the ototoxic effects of this drug may be more severe in children.
• Assess for age-appropriate fluid intake.
• Assess for hearing loss periodically.

Precautions

• Use cautiously in pts who have had previous therapy with other antineoplastic agents or radiation.

Administration and Handling

◂ALERT▸ Verify any cisplatin dose exceeding 120 mg/m² per course. Know that the dosage is individualized based on the patient's clinical response and tolerance of the adverse effects of the drug. When used in combination therapy, consult specific protocols for optimum dosage and sequence of drug administration. Be aware that repeat courses should not be given more frequently than every 3–4 wks. Also, know that the course should not be repeated unless the patient's auditory acuity is within normal limits, serum creatinine level is less than 1.5 mg/dL, BUN level is less than 25 mg/dL, and platelet count and WBC count are within acceptable levels.

◂ALERT▸ Wear protective gloves during handling of cisplatin. Cisplatin may be carcinogenic, mutagenic, or teratogenic. Handle with extreme care during preparation and administration.

IV

• After reconstitution, solution normally appears clear and colorless.
• Protect from direct sunlight; do not refrigerate because the solution may form a precipitate. Discard if precipitate forms.
• Reconstituted solution is stable for up to 20 hrs at room temperature.
• Reconstitute 10-mg vial with 10 mL Sterile Water for Injection (50 mL for 50-mg vial) to provide concentration of 1 mg/mL.
• For IV infusion, dilute desired dose in up to 1,000 mL D_5W or 0.33% or 0.45% NaCl containing 12.5–50 g mannitol/L.
• Infuse over 2–24 hrs.
• Avoid rapid infusion because this increases the risk of nephrotoxicity and ototoxicity.
• Monitor for an anaphylactic reaction during first few minutes of IV infusion.

Intervention and Evaluation

• Measure all of the patient's vomitus. If the patient vomits 750 mL or more over 8 hrs, notify the physician immediately.
• Monitor the patient's intake and output every 1–2 hrs, beginning with pretreatment hydration, and continuing for 48 hrs after cisplatin therapy. If the patient has a urinary output less than 100 mL each hour (or for children less than 1 mL/kg), notify the physician immediately.
• Assess the patient's vital signs every 1–2 hrs during cisplatin infusion.
• Monitor the patient's urinalysis and renal function test results for evidence of nephrotoxicity.

Patient/Family Teaching

• Warn the patient/family to report signs and symptoms of ototoxicity, including hearing loss or ringing or roaring in the ears.
• Stress to the patient/family that the patient should not receive vaccinations without the physician's approval because cisplatin lowers the body's resistance and that he or she should avoid contact with anyone who recently received an oral polio vaccine (oral polio vaccine is no longer available in the United States).

• Warn the patient/family to contact the physician if nausea or vomiting continues at home.
• Teach the patient to recognize signs and symptoms of peripheral neuropathy.

Cyclophosphamide

sigh-klo-**phos** -fah-mide
(Cycloblastin [AUS], Cytoxan, Endoxan Asta [AUS], Endoxon Asta [AUS], Neosar, Procytox [CAN])
Do not confuse with cefoxitin, Ciloxan, or Cytotec.

CATEGORY AND SCHEDULE

Pregnancy Risk Category: D

MECHANISM OF ACTION

An alkylating agent that inhibits DNA and RNA protein synthesis by cross-linking with DNA and RNA strands. ***Therapeutic Effect:*** Inhibits protein synthesis and prevents cell growth. Potent immunosuppressant.

PHARMACOKINETICS

Well absorbed from the GI tract. Crosses the blood-brain barrier. Protein binding: Low. Metabolized in liver to active metabolites. Primarily excreted in urine. Moderately removed by hemodialysis. ***Half-Life:*** 3–12 hrs.

AVAILABILITY

Tablets: 25 mg, 50 mg.
Powder for Injection: 100 mg, 200 mg, 500 mg, 1 g, 2 g.

INDICATIONS AND DOSAGES

Refer to individual protocols.

▸ **Treatment of adenocarcinoma of ovary, carcinoma of breast, disseminated neuroblastoma, Hodgkin disease, multiple myeloma, leukemia (acute lymphoblastic, acute myelogenous, acute monocytic, chronic granulocytic, chronic lymphocytic), mycosis fungoides, non-Hodgkin lymphomas, retinoblastoma**
PO
Children. Initially, 2–8 mg/kg/day. Maintenance: 2–5 mg/kg 2 times/wk.
IV
Children. Initially, 40–50 mg/kg in divided doses over 2–5 days. Maintenance: 10–15 mg/kg q7–10days or 3–5 mg/kg 2 times/wk.

▸ **Biopsy-proven minimal-change nephrotic syndrome**
PO
Children. 2.5–3 mg/kg/day for 60–90 days when corticosteroids are not successful.

▸ **Systemic lupus erythematosus**
IV
Children: 500–750 mg/m^2 every month: Maximum: 1 g/m^2.

▸ **Bone marrow transplant preparatory regimen**
IV
Children. 50 mg/kg/day once daily for 3–4 days.

UNLABELED USES

Treatment of carcinoma of bladder, cervix, endometrium, lung, prostate, testicles; germ cell ovarian tumors; osteosarcoma; rheumatoid arthritis; systemic lupus erythematosus.

CONTRAINDICATIONS

Hypersensitivity to cyclophosphamide or any related component.

INTERACTIONS

Drug

Allopurinol, bone marrow depressants: May increase bone marrow depression.

Antigout medications: May decrease the effects of these drugs.
Cytarabine: May increase risk of cardiomyopathy.
Immunosuppressants: May increase the risk of infection and development of neoplasms.
Live virus vaccines: May potentiate virus replication, increase vaccine side effects, and decrease the patient's antibody response to the vaccine.

Herbal
None known.

Food
None known.

DIAGNOSTIC TEST EFFECTS

May increase serum uric acid levels.

IV INCOMPATIBILITIES

Amphotericin B complex (Abelcet, AmBisome, Amphotec)

IV COMPATIBILITIES

Granisetron (Kytril), heparin, hydromorphone (Dilaudid), lorazepam (Ativan), morphine, ondansetron (Zofran), propofol (Diprivan)

SIDE EFFECTS

Expected
Marked leukopenia 8–15 days after initial therapy

Frequent
Nausea or vomiting beginning about 6 hrs after administration and lasting about 4 hrs, alopecia (33%)

Occasional
Diarrhea, darkening of skin and fingernails, stomatitis (may include oral ulceration), headache, diaphoresis

Rare
Pain or redness at injection site

SERIOUS REACTIONS

! The major toxic effect of cyclophosphamide is bone marrow depression resulting in blood dyscrasias manifested as leukopenia, anemia, thrombocytopenia, and hypoprothrombinemia.
! Thrombocytopenia may occur 10–15 days after drug initiation.
! Anemia generally occurs after large doses of the drug or prolonged therapy.
! Hemorrhagic cystitis occurs commonly in long-term therapy, especially in pediatric pts.
! Pulmonary fibrosis and cardiotoxicity have been noted with high doses.
! Amenorrhea, azoospermia, and hyperkalemia may also occur.

PEDIATRIC CONSIDERATIONS

Baseline Assessment
- Expect to obtain the patient's WBC count weekly during cyclophosphamide therapy or until the drug's maintenance dose is established, then at 2- to 3-wk intervals.

Precautions
- Use cautiously in pts with severe leukopenia, thrombocytopenia, tumor infiltration of bone marrow, or previous therapy with other antineoplastic agents or radiation.
- Know that cyclophosphamide use should be avoided during pregnancy because of the risk of malformations such as cardiac anomalies, hernias, and limb abnormalities.
- Be aware that cyclophosphamide is distributed in breast milk and that breast-feeding is not recommended in this patient population.
- There are no age-related precautions noted in children.

• Assess and maintain age-appropriate fluid intake.

Administration and Handling

◂ **ALERT** ▸ Be aware that cyclophosphamide dosage is individualized based on the patient's clinical response and tolerance of the adverse effects of the drug. When used in combination therapy, consult specific protocols for optimum dosage and sequence of drug administration.

◂ **ALERT** ▸ Because cyclophosphamide may be carcinogenic, mutagenic, or teratogenic, handle the drug with extreme care during drug preparation and administration.

PO

• Give on an empty stomach. If GI upset occurs, give with food.

IV

• Reconstituted solution is stable for up to 24 hrs at room temperature or up to 6 days if refrigerated.
• For IV push, reconstitute each 100 mg with 5 mL Sterile Water for Injection or Bacteriostatic Water for Injection to provide a concentration of 20 mg/mL.
• Shake to dissolve. Allow solution to stand until clear.
• Give by IV push or further dilute with 250 mL D_5W, 0.9% NaCl, 0.45% NaCl, lactated Ringer's solution (LR) or D_5W/LR.
• Infuse each 100 mg or fraction thereof over 15 min or more.
• Be aware that IV administration may produce diaphoresis, facial flushing, faintness, and oropharyngeal sensation.

Intervention and Evaluation

• Monitor the patient's blood chemistry values, complete blood count, and serum uric acid concentration.
• Monitor the patient's WBC count closely during initial therapy.
• Monitor the patient for signs and symptoms of anemia, such as excessive fatigue and weakness, and hematologic toxicity, such as easy bruising, fever, signs of local infection, sore throat, and unusual bleeding from any site.
• Expect recovery from marked leukopenia due to bone marrow depression in 17–28 days.
• Verify that the patient's urine specific gravity is less than 1.010 and urine output is more than 3 mg/kg/hr before initiating cyclophosphamide.

Patient/Family Teaching

• To help prevent cystitis, encourage the patient to drink fluids 24 hrs before, during, and after therapy and to void frequently.
• Stress to the patient/family that the patient should not receive vaccinations without the physician's approval because cyclophosphamide lowers the body's resistance. Also warn the patient to avoid contact with anyone who recently received a live virus vaccine.
• Warn the patient/family to report easy bruising, fever, signs of local infection, sore throat, or unusual bleeding from any site.
• Explain to the patient/family that hair loss (alopecia) is reversible, but new hair growth may have a different color or texture.

Ifosfamide

eye-**fos**-fah-mid
(Holoxan [AUS], Ifex)

CATEGORY AND SCHEDULE

Pregnancy Risk Category: D

MECHANISM OF ACTION

An alkylating agent that is converted to the active metabolite and binds with intracellular structures. Action is primarily due to cross-linking strands of DNA and RNA. ***Therapeutic Effect:*** Inhibits protein synthesis.

PHARMACOKINETICS

Metabolized in liver to the active metabolite. Crosses blood-brain barrier (limited). Primarily excreted in urine. ***Half-Life:*** 4–15 hrs.

AVAILABILITY

Powder for Injection: 1 g, 3 g.

INDICATIONS AND DOSAGES

Refer to individual protocols.

▸ **Hodgkin disease, breast cancer, acute lymphocytic leukemia, ovarian cancer, testicular cancer, sarcomas**

IV

Children. 1,200–1,800 mg/m^2/day for 5 days q21–28days or 5,000 mg/m^2 as a single 24-hr infusion or 3 g/m^2/day for 2 days.

UNLABELED USES

Treatment of Ewing sarcoma; non-Hodgkin lymphomas; lung, pancreatic, and soft tissue carcinoma.

CONTRAINDICATIONS

Hypersensitivity to ifosfamide or any related component. Pregnancy, severely depressed bone marrow function.

INTERACTIONS

Drug

Bone marrow depressants: May increase bone marrow depression.
Live virus vaccines: May potentiate virus replication, increase vaccine side effects, and decrease the patient's antibody response to the vaccine.
Phenytoin, phenobarbital, and chloral hydrate: May increase toxicity of ifosfamide.

Herbal

None known.

Food

None known.

DIAGNOSTIC TEST EFFECTS

May increase BUN, serum bilirubin, serum creatinine, serum uric acid, SGOT (AST), and SGPT (ALT) levels.

IV INCOMPATIBILITIES

Cefepime (Maxipime), methotrexate

IV COMPATIBILITIES

Granisetron (Kytril), ondansetron (Zofran)

SIDE EFFECTS

Frequent

Alopecia (83%); nausea, vomiting (58%)

Occasional (15%–5%)

Confusion, somnolence, hallucinations, infection

Rare (less than 5%)

Dizziness, seizures, disorientation, fever, malaise, stomatitis (mucosal irritation, glossitis, gingivitis)

SERIOUS REACTIONS

! Hemorrhagic cystitis with hematuria or dysuria occurs frequently if a protective agent (mesna) is not used.

! Myelosuppression characterized as leukopenia and, to a lesser extent, thrombocytopenia occurs frequently.

! Pulmonary toxicity, liver toxicity, nephrotoxicity, cardiotoxicity, CNS toxicity manifested as confusion, hallucinations, somnolence, and coma may require discontinuation of therapy.

PEDIATRIC CONSIDERATIONS

Baseline Assessment

• Obtain the patient's urinalysis test results, as appropriate, before each dose. If hematuria occurs, evidenced by greater than 10 RBCs per field, notify the physician because therapy should be withheld until resolution occurs.
• Expect to obtain the patient's WBC count, platelet count, and blood Hgb levels before each dose.

Precautions

• Use cautiously in pts with compromised bone marrow function and impaired liver or renal function.
• If possible, ifosfamide use should be avoided during pregnancy, especially in the first trimester.
• Be aware that ifosfamide may cause fetal harm.
• Be aware that ifosfamide is distributed in breast milk. Breastfeeding is not recommended in this patient population.
• Assess for and maintain age-appropriate fluid intake.

Administration and Handling

◀ **ALERT** ▶ Be aware that ifosfamide dosage is individualized based on the patient's clinical response and tolerance of the adverse effects of the drug. When used in combination therapy, consult specific protocols for optimum dosage and sequence of drug administration.
◀ **ALERT** ▶ Because ifosfamide may be carcinogenic, mutagenic, or teratogenic, handle the drug with extreme care during preparation and administration.
◀ **ALERT** ▶ Hemorrhagic cystitis may occur if mesna is not given concurrently with ifosfamide. Mesna should always be given with ifosfamide.

IV

• Store vial at room temperature.
• After reconstitution with Bacteriostatic Water for Injection, store solution for up to 1 wk at room temperature or refrigerate for up to 3 wks. Refrigerate further diluted solution for up to 6 wks.
• Use solution prepared with other diluents within 6 hrs.
• Reconstitute 1-g vial with 20 mL Sterile Water for Injection or Bacteriostatic Water for Injection to provide a concentration of 50 mg/mL. Shake to dissolve.
• Further dilute with D_5W or 0.9% NaCl to provide concentration of 0.6–20 mg/mL.
• Infuse over a minimum of 30 min.
• Give with at least 2,000 mL PO or IV fluid to prevent bladder toxicity.
• Give with a prescribed protectant against hemorrhagic cystitis, such as mesna. Be aware that mesna should always be given with ifosfamide to prevent other adverse reactions, including chills, fever, jaundice, joint pain, sore throat, stomatitis, or unusual bleeding or bruising.

Intervention and Evaluation

• Monitor the patient's hematologic studies and urinalysis results diligently.
• Assess the patient for easy bruising, fever, signs of local infection, sore throat, symptoms of anemia, such as excessive fatigue, weakness, and unusual bleeding from any site.

Patient/Family Teaching

• Encourage the patient/family to drink fluids to protect against cystitis.
• Stress to the patient/family that the patient should not receive vaccinations without the physician's

approval because ifosfamide lowers the body's resistance. Also warn the patient to avoid contact with anyone who recently received a live virus vaccine. Explain to the patient/family that the patient should avoid crowds and those with known infection.

• Warn the patient/family to notify the physician if the patient experiences chills, fever, joint pain, sores in the mouth or on the lips, sore throat, yellowing of the skin or eyes, unusual bleeding, or bruising.

Lomustine

low-**meuw**-steen
(CeeNU)

CATEGORY AND SCHEDULE

Pregnancy Risk Category: D

MECHANISM OF ACTION

An alkylating agent and nitrosourea that inhibits DNA and RNA synthesis by cross-linking with DNA and RNA strands, preventing cellular division. Cell cycle–phase nonspecific.
Therapeutic Effect: Interferes with DNA and RNA function.

AVAILABILITY

Capsules: 10 mg, 40 mg, 100 mg.

PHARMACOKINETICS

Rapid and complete absorption from oral administration. Distributes into the CNS and breast milk. Rapidly metabolized in the liver to active metabolites. Primarily eliminated in the urine.
Half-Life: 1–2 days.

INDICATIONS AND DOSAGES

Refer to individual protocols.

▸ Treatment of disseminated Hodgkin disease; primary and metastatic brain tumors

PO

Children. 75–150 mg/m^2 as single dose q6wks.

UNLABELED USES

Treatment of breast, GI, lung, and renal carcinoma; malignant melanoma; multiple myeloma

CONTRAINDICATIONS

Hypersensitivity to lomustine or any related component and pregnancy.

INTERACTIONS

Drug

Bone marrow depressants: May increase bone marrow depression.
Live virus vaccines: May potentiate virus replication, increase vaccine side effects, and decrease a patient's antibody response to the vaccine.
Phenobarbital: May reduce activity of lomustine.

Herbal

None known.

Food

None known.

DIAGNOSTIC TEST EFFECTS

May cause elevated liver function test results.

SIDE EFFECTS

Frequent

Nausea or vomiting occurs 45 min–6 hrs after dosing and lasts 12–24 hrs. Anorexia often follows for 2–3 days.

Occasional

Neurotoxicity (confusion, slurred speech), stomatitis, darkening of skin, diarrhea, skin rash, itching, hair loss

SERIOUS REACTIONS

! Bone marrow depression manifested as hematologic toxicity (principally leukopenia, mild anemia, and thrombocytopenia) may occur.

! Leukopenia occurs at about 6 wks. Thrombocytopenia occurs at about 4 wks and persists for 1–2 wks.

! Refractory anemia and thrombocytopenia occur commonly if lomustine therapy is continued for more than 1 yr.

! Liver toxicity occurs infrequently.

! Large cumulative doses of lomustine may result in renal damage.

PEDIATRIC CONSIDERATIONS

Baseline Assessment

• As ordered, obtain weekly blood counts and know that this procedure is recommended by the manufacturer. Be aware that experts recommend that the first blood count be obtained 2–3 wks after initial therapy and that subsequent blood counts should be obtained based on prior hematologic toxicity.

• Give antiemetics, as prescribed, to reduce the duration and frequency of nausea or vomiting.

• Maintain age-appropriate fluid intake.

Precautions

• Use cautiously in pts with depressed erythrocyte, leukocyte, or platelet counts.

Administration and Handling

◂ **ALERT** ▸ Be aware that lomustine dosage is individualized based on the patient's clinical response and tolerance of the adverse effects of the drug. When used in combination therapy, consult specific protocols for optimum dosage and sequence of drug administration.

Intervention and Evaluation

• Monitor the patient's complete blood count with differential; platelet count; and liver, renal, and pulmonary function tests.

• Assess the patient for stomatitis as evidenced by burning or erythema of the oral mucosa at the inner margin of lips, difficulty swallowing, and sore throat.

• Monitor for the patient for signs and symptoms of anemia, including excessive fatigue and weakness, and hematologic toxicity, including easy bruising, fever, signs of local infection, sore throat, and unusual bleeding from any site.

Patient/Family Teaching

• Instruct the patient/family to immediately report exposure to chickenpox.

• Explain that nausea or vomiting usually abates in less than 1 day. Further explain that fasting before therapy can reduce the frequency and duration of GI effects.

• Teach the patient/family to maintain fastidious oral hygiene to prevent stomatitis.

• Stress to the patient/family that the patient should not receive vaccinations without the physician's approval because lomustine lowers the body's resistance. Warn the patient to avoid contact with anyone who recently received a live virus vaccine. Explain to the patient/family that the patient should avoid crowds and those with known illness.

• Warn the patient/family to notify the physician if the patient experiences easy bruising, fever, jaundice, signs of local infection, sore throat, swelling of the legs and feet, or unusual bleeding from any site.

Thiotepa

thigh-oh-**teh**-pah
(Thioplex)

CATEGORY AND SCHEDULE

Pregnancy Risk Category: D

MECHANISM OF ACTION

An alkylating agent that binds with many intracellular structures. Cross-links strands of DNA and RNA. Cell cycle–phase nonspecific. ***Therapeutic Effect:*** Disrupts protein synthesis, producing cell death.

AVAILABILITY

Powder for Injection: 15 mg.

PHARMACOKINETICS

Variable absorption, increased absorption with tissue inflammation. Distributes to CNS. Protein binding: 8%–13%. Metabolized in liver to the active metabolite. ***Half-Life:*** Active metabolite 10–21 hrs.

INDICATIONS AND DOSAGES

Refer to individual protocols.

▸ **Treatment of adenocarcinoma of breast and ovary, Hodgkin disease, lymphomas, lymphosarcoma, superficial papillary carcinoma of urinary bladder, sarcomas**

IV

Children. 25–65 mg/m^2 as a single dose q3–4wks.

UNLABELED USES

Treatment of lung carcinoma.

CONTRAINDICATIONS

Hypersensitivity to thiotepa or related components, pregnancy, severe myelosuppression (WBC count less than 3,000/mm^3 or platelet count less than 150,000 mm^3).

INTERACTIONS

Drug

Antigout medications: May decrease the effects of these drugs.
Bone marrow depressants: May increase bone marrow depression.
Live virus vaccines: May potentiate virus replication, increase vaccine side effects, and decrease the patient's antibody response to vaccine.

Herbal

None known.

Food

None known.

DIAGNOSTIC TEST EFFECTS

May increase serum uric acid levels.

IV INCOMPATIBILITIES

Cisplatin (Platinol AQ), filgrastim (Neupogen)

IV COMPATIBILITIES

Allopurinol (Aloprim), bumetanide (Bumex), calcium gluconate, carboplatin (Paraplatin), cyclophosphamide (Cytoxan), dexamethasone (Decadron), diphenhydramine (Benadryl), doxorubicin (Adriamycin), etoposide (VePesid), fluorouracil, gemcitabine (Gemzar), granisetron (Kytril), heparin, hydromorphone (Dilaudid), leucovorin, lorazepam (Ativan), magnesium sulfate, morphine, ondansetron (Zofran), paclitaxel (Taxol), potassium chloride, vincristine (Oncovin), vinorelbine (Navelbine)

SIDE EFFECTS

Occasional

Pain at injection site, headache, dizziness, hives, rash, nausea, vomiting, anorexia, stomatitis

Rare

Alopecia, cystitis, hematuria after intravesical dosing

SERIOUS REACTIONS

! Hematologic toxicity manifested as leukopenia, anemia, thrombocytopenia, and pancytopenia due to bone marrow depression may occur.

! Although the WBC count falls to its lowest point at 10–14 days after initial therapy, bone marrow effects are not evident for 30 days.

! Stomatitis and ulceration of intestinal mucosa may be noted.

PEDIATRIC CONSIDERATIONS

Baseline Assessment

- Expect the patient to undergo hematologic testing at least weekly during therapy and for 3 wks after therapy is discontinued.
- If the medication comes in contact with the skin, the area should be immediately washed with soap and water.

Precautions

- Use cautiously in pts with bone marrow dysfunction and liver or renal impairment.

Administration and Handling

◂ALERT▸ Know that thiotepa dosage is individualized based on the patient's clinical response and tolerance of the adverse effects of the drug. When used in combination therapy, consult specific protocols for optimum dosage and sequence of drug administration.

◂ALERT▸ Because thiotepa may be carcinogenic, mutagenic, or teratogenic, handle the drug with extreme care during preparation and administration.

◂ALERT▸ Know that the drug may be given by intrapericardial, intraperitoneal, intrapleural, intratumoral, or IV injection and by intravesical instillation.

IV

- Refrigerate unopened vials.
- Reconstituted solution normally appears clear to slightly opaque. Store refrigerated solution for up to 5 days. Discard if solution appears grossly opaque or precipitate forms.
- Reconstitute 15-mg vial with 1.5 mL Sterile Water for Injection to provide concentration of 10 mg/mL. Shake solution gently; let stand to clear.
- Withdraw reconstituted drug through a 0.22-μ filter before administering. For IV push, give over 5 min at concentration of 10 mg/mL. Give IV infusion at concentration of 1 mg/mL.

Intervention and Evaluation

- Interrupt thiotepa therapy if the patient's platelet count falls below 150,000/mm^3 and the WBC count falls below 3,000/mm^3 or if the patient's platelet or WBC count declines rapidly.
- Monitor the patient's hematologic tests and serum uric acid levels.
- Assess the patient for signs and symptoms of stomatitis, such as burning or erythema of the oral mucosa at the inner margin of lips, difficulty swallowing, oral ulceration, and sore throat.
- Monitor the patient for signs and symptoms of symptoms of anemia, including excessive fatigue and weakness, and hematologic toxicity, including easy bruising, fever, signs of local infection, sore throat, or unusual bleeding from any site.
- Assess the patient's skin for hives and rash.

Patient/Family Teaching

- Teach the patient/family to maintain fastidious oral hygiene to guard against development of stomatitis.

• Stress to the patient/family that the patient should not receive vaccinations and should avoid contact with crowds and anyone with known infection or who recently received a live virus vaccine.
• Warn the patient/family to promptly notify the physician if the patient experiences easy bruising, fever, signs of local infection, sore throat, or unusual bleeding from any site.

REFERENCES

Miller, S. & Fioravanti, J. (1997). Pediatric medications: a handbook for nurses. St. Louis: Mosby.
Taketomo, C. K., Hodding, J. H. & Kraus, D. M. (2003–2004). Pediatric dosage handbook (10th ed.). Hudson, OH: Lexi-Comp.

Daunorubicin
Doxorubicin
Idarubicin Hydrochloride
Mitomycin

Uses: Antineoplastic antibiotics are cytotoxic and are therefore only used to treat cancer and not infections. *Daunorubicin* is effective in acute lymphocytic and acute myelogenous leukemias. *Doxorubicin* is used in acute leukemias, malignant lymphomas, and breast cancer. *Idarubicin* is active against acute myelogenous leukemia. *Mitomycin* may be prescribed for carcinoma of cervix, stomach, breasts, bladder, head, or neck.

Action: Originally isolated from cultures of *Streptomyces,* antineoplastic antibiotics act by inhibiting RNA synthesis and binding with DNA. These actions cause fragmentation of DNA molecules.

Daunorubicin

dawn-oh-**rue**-bih-sin
(Cerubidine, DaunoXome)
Do not confuse with dactinomycin or doxorubicin

CATEGORY AND SCHEDULE

Pregnancy Risk Category: D

MECHANISM OF ACTION

An anthracycline antibiotic that is cell cycle–phase nonspecific. Most active in S phase of cell division. Appears to bind to DNA. ***Therapeutic Effect:*** Inhibits DNA and DNA-dependent RNA synthesis.

PHARMACOKINETICS

Widely distributed. Does not cross the blood-brain barrier. Protein binding: High. Metabolized in liver to active metabolite. Excreted in urine, eliminated by biliary excretion. ***Half-Life:*** 18.5 hrs; metabolite: 26.7 hrs.

AVAILABILITY

CERUBIDINE
Powder for Injection: 20 mg.
Solution for Injection: 5 mg/mL.
DAUNOXOME (LYPOSOMAL)
Injection: 2 mg/mL. Equivalent to 50 mg daunorubicin base.

INDICATIONS AND DOSAGES

Refer to individual protocols.

▸ **Acute lymphocytic leukemia**

IV

Children. 25–45 mg/m^2 on days 1 and 8 of cycle.

▸ **Acute myeloid leukemia**

IV

Children. 30–60 mg/m^2 on days 1–3 of cycle.

UNLABELED USES

Treatment of chronic myelocytic leukemia, Ewing sarcoma, neuroblastoma, non-Hodgkin lymphoma, Wilms tumor.

CONTRAINDICATIONS

Hypersensitivity to daunorubicin or any related component.

Arrhythmias, congestive heart failure (CHF), left ventricular ejection fraction less than 40%, preexisting bone marrow suppression.

INTERACTIONS

Drug

Antigout medications: May decrease the effects of these drugs.
Bone marrow depressants: May enhance myelosuppression.
Live virus vaccines: May potentiate virus replication, increase vaccine side effects, and decrease the patient's antibody response to the vaccine.

Herbal

None known.

Food

None known.

DIAGNOSTIC TEST EFFECTS

May increase serum alkaline phosphatase, serum bilirubin, serum uric acid, and SGOT (AST) levels.

IV INCOMPATIBILITIES

Allopurinol (Aloprim), aztreonam (Azactam), cefepime (Maxipime), fludarabine (Fludara), piperacillin/tazobactam (Zosyn)
DaunoXome: Do not mix with any other solution, especially NaCl or bacteriostatic agents (e.g., benzyl alcohol).

IV COMPATIBILITIES

Cytarabine (Cytosar), etoposide (VePesid), filgrastim (Neupogen), granisetron (Kytril), ondansetron (Zofran)

SIDE EFFECTS

Frequent

Complete alopecia (scalp, axillary, pubic hair), nausea or vomiting beginning a few hours after administration and lasting 24–48 hrs
DaunoXome: Mild to moderate nausea, fatigue, fever

Occasional

Diarrhea, abdominal pain, esophagitis, stomatitis (redness or burning of oral mucous membranes, inflammation of gums or tongue), transverse pigmentation of fingernails and toenails

Rare

Transient fever, chills

SERIOUS REACTIONS

! Bone marrow depression manifested as hematologic toxicity (severe leukopenia, anemia, and thrombocytopenia) may occur.
! A decrease in platelet count and WBC count occurs in 10–14 days; counts return to normal levels by the third week of daunorubicin treatment.
! Cardiotoxicity noted as either acute with transient abnormal electrocardiogram (EKG) findings or as chronic with cardiomyopathy manifested as CHF. The risk of cardiotoxicity increases when the cumulative dose exceeds 550 mg/m^2 in adults and 300 mg/m^2 in children older than 2 yrs of age, or the total dosage is greater than 10 mg/kg in children younger than 2 yrs of age.

PEDIATRIC CONSIDERATIONS

Baseline Assessment

- Expect to obtain the patient's RBC, platelet, and WBC counts before beginning daunorubicin therapy and at frequent intervals during therapy.
- Obtain the patient's baseline EKG before beginning daunorubicin therapy.

• Give antiemetics, if ordered, to the patient to prevent and treat nausea.

Precautions

• Use cautiously in pts with biliary, liver, or renal impairment.

• Be aware that daunorubicin use should be avoided during pregnancy, especially in the first trimester because it may cause fetal harm. Know that breast-feeding is not recommended in this patient population.

• Be aware that the safety and efficacy of daunorubicin have not been established in children.

• This medication is contraindicated in children with cardiac disease and infections such as chickenpox.

• This medication is very potent so ensure that the IV line is patent before and during administration.

• Assess and maintain appropriate fluid intake.

Administration and Handling

◂**ALERT**▸ Be aware that daunorubicin dosage is individualized based on the patient's clinical response and tolerance of the adverse effects of the drug. When used in combination therapy, consult specific protocols for optimum dosage and sequence of drug administration. Do not exceed total dosage of 500–600 mg/m^2 in adults, 400–450 mg/m^2 in those who received irradiation of the cardiac region, 300 mg/m^2 in children older than 2 yrs of age, or 10 mg/kg in children younger than 2 yrs of age (increases the risk of cardiotoxicity). Expect to reduce dosage in those with liver or renal impairment. Use body weight to calculate dose in children younger than 2 yrs of age or with a body surface area less than 0.5 m^2.

◂**ALERT**▸ Give daunorubicin by IV push or IV infusion. IV infusion is not recommended because of the risk of thrombophlebitis and vein irritation. Avoid areas overlying joints and tendons, small veins, and swollen or edematous extremities. Because daunorubicin may be carcinogenic, mutagenic, or teratogenic, handle the drug with extreme care during preparation and administration.

IV

Cerubidine. Store reconstituted solution for up to 24 hrs at room temperature or up to 48 hrs if refrigerated.

• Discard the solution if the color changes from red to blue-purple because this indicates decomposition.

• Reconstitute each 20-mg vial with 4 mL Sterile Water for Injection to provide a concentration of 5 mg/mL.

• Gently agitate vial until completely dissolved.

• For IV push, withdraw desired dose into syringe containing 10–15 mL 0.9% NaCl. Inject over 2–3 min into tubing of running IV solution of D_5W or 0.9% NaCl.

• For IV infusion, further dilute with 100 mL D_5W or 0.9% NaCl. Infuse over 30–45 min.

• Know that extravasation produces immediate pain and severe local tissue damage. Aspirate as much infiltrated drug as possible and then infiltrate the area with hydrocortisone sodium succinate injection (50–100 mg hydrocortisone) or isotonic sodium thiosulfate injection or 1 mL of 5% ascorbic acid injection, as ordered. Apply cold compresses.

Daunoxome. Refrigerate unopened vials.

• Be aware that reconstituted solution is stable for 6 hrs if refrigerated.
• Do not use solution if it is opaque.
• Must dilute with an equal part of D_5W to provide a concentration of 1 mg/mL.
• Do not use any other diluent.
• Infuse over 60 min.

Intervention and Evaluation

• Monitor the patient for signs and symptoms of stomatitis, including burning and erythema of oral mucosa. Know that stomatitis may lead to ulceration within 2–3 days.
• Assess the patient's skin and nailbeds for hyperpigmentation.
• Monitor the patient's hematologic status, liver and renal function studies, and serum uric acid level.
• Assess the patient's pattern of daily bowel activity and stool consistency.
• Monitor the patient for signs and symptoms of anemia, including excessive fatigue and weakness, and hematologic toxicity, including easy bruising, fever, signs of local infection, sore throat, or unusual bleeding from any site.

Patient/Family Teaching

• Advise the patient/family that the patient's urine may turn a reddish color for 1–2 days after beginning daunorubicin therapy.
• Explain to the patient/family that alopecia is reversible, but new hair growth may have a different color or texture. Tell the patient/family that new hair growth resumes about 5 wks after the last daunorubicin therapy dose.
• Teach the patient/family to maintain fastidious oral hygiene.
• Stress to the patient/family that the patient should not receive vaccinations and should avoid contact with anyone who recently received a live virus vaccine.
• Warn the patient/family to notify the physician if the patient experiences easy bruising, fever, signs of local infection, sore throat, or unusual bleeding from any site.
• Urge the patient/family to increase the patient's fluid intake to help protect against development of hyperuricemia.
• Caution the patient/family to notify the physician if nausea and vomiting persist at home.

Doxorubicin

dox-o-**roo**-bi-sin
(Adriamycin PFS, Adriamycin RDF, Doxil)
Do not confuse with daunorubicin, Idamycin, or idarubicin.

CATEGORY AND SCHEDULE

Pregnancy Risk Category: D

MECHANISM OF ACTION

An anthracycline antibiotic that inhibits DNA and DNA-dependent RNA synthesis by binding with DNA strands. Liposomal encapsulation increases uptake by tumors, prolongs action, and may decrease toxicity. ***Therapeutic Effect:*** Prevents cellular division.

PHARMACOKINETICS

Widely distributed. Does not cross blood-brain barrier. Protein binding: 74%–76%. Metabolized rapidly in liver to active metabolite. Primarily eliminated via biliary system. Not removed by hemodialysis. ***Half-Life:*** 16 hrs; metabolite: 32 hrs.

AVAILABILITY

Powder for Injection: 10 mg, 20 mg, 50 mg, 200 mg.
Solution for Injection (preservative free): 2 mg/mL.
Lipid Complex (Doxil): 2 mg/mL.

INDICATIONS AND DOSAGES

Refer to individual protocols.

▸ **Treatment of breast, bronchogenic, gastric, ovarian, thyroid, and transitional cell bladder carcinoma; lymphomas of Hodgkin and non-Hodgkin type; neuroblastoma; primary liver cancer; soft tissue and bone sarcomas; Wilms tumor; regression in acute lymphoblastic and myeloblastic leukemia**

IV

Children. 35–75 mg/m² as single dose q3wks or 20–30 mg/m² weekly or 60–90 mg/m² as continuous infusion over 96 hrs q3–4wks.

▸ **Dose adjustment for hyperbilirubinemia:**

BILIRUBIN LEVEL 1–3 MG/DL.
Decrease dose by 50%.
BILIRUBIN LEVEL MORE THAN 3 MG/DL.
Decrease dose by 75%.

UNLABELED USES

Treatment of cervical, head or neck, endometrial, liver, pancreatic, prostatic, and testicular carcinoma; treatment of germ cell tumors, multiple myeloma

CONTRAINDICATIONS

Hypersensitivity to doxorubicin or related components.
Cardiomyopathy; preexisting myelosuppression; previous or concomitant treatment with cyclophosphamide, idarubicin, mitoxantrone, or irradiation of the cardiac region; severe congestive heart failure (CHF) and pregnancy.

INTERACTIONS

Drug

Antigout medications: May decrease the effects of these drugs.
Bone marrow depressants: May increase bone marrow depression.
Daunorubicin: May increase the risk of cardiotoxicity.
Live virus vaccines: May potentiate virus replication, increase vaccine side effects, and decrease the patient's antibody response to vaccine.
Carbamazepine, digoxin, phenytoin: May decrease the serum concentrations of these drugs.

Herbal

None known.

Food

None known.

DIAGNOSTIC TEST EFFECTS

May cause electrocardiogram (EKG) changes. May increase serum uric acid.
Doxil: May reduce neutrophil and RBC count.

IV INCOMPATIBILITIES

Doxil: Do not mix with any other medications.
Doxorubicin: Allopurinol (Aloprim), amphotericin B complex (Abelcet, AmBisome, Amphotec), cefepime (Maxipime), furosemide (Lasix), ganciclovir (Cytovene), heparin, piperacillin/tazobactam (Zosyn), propofol (Diprivan)

IV COMPATIBILITIES

Dexamethasone (Decadron), diphenhydramine (Benadryl), etoposide (VePesid), granisetron (Kytril), hydromorphone (Dilaudid), lorazepam (Ativan), morphine, ondansetron (Zofran), paclitaxel (Taxol), propofol (Diprivan)

SIDE EFFECTS

Frequent

Complete alopecia (scalp, axillary, pubic hair), nausea, vomiting, stomatitis, esophagitis (especially if drug is given each day on several successive days), reddish urine

Doxil: Nausea

Occasional

Anorexia, diarrhea, hyperpigmentation of nailbeds, phalangeal and dermal creases

Rare

Fever, chills, conjunctivitis, lacrimation

SERIOUS REACTIONS

! Bone marrow depression manifested as hematologic toxicity (principally leukopenia and, to a lesser extent, anemia and thrombocytopenia) may occur, generally within 10–15 days and returning to normal levels by the third week.

! Cardiotoxicity noted as either acute, transient abnormal EKG findings and cardiomyopathy manifested as CHF may occur.

PEDIATRIC CONSIDERATIONS

Baseline Assessment

- As ordered, obtain the patient's blood Hct and Hgb and platelet and WBC counts before beginning doxorubicin therapy and at frequent intervals during therapy.
- Obtain a baseline EKG of the patient before doxorubicin therapy.
- As ordered, obtain liver function studies of the patient before administering each doxorubicin dose.
- Give antiemetics, if ordered, to the patient to prevent or treat nausea.
- Know that doxorubicin use should be avoided, if possible, during pregnancy, especially in the first trimester and that breast-feeding is not recommended in this patient population.
- Be aware that cardiotoxicity may be more frequent in children younger than 2 yrs.
- Assess and maintain appropriate fluid intake.
- This medication is contraindicated in children with preexisting cardiac defects and active infections.
- This medication is very potent so be sure and assess and maintain IV patency during drug administration.
- Doxorubicin can lead to potentially fatal cardiomyopathy so assess for resting heart rate and blood pressure routinely.

Precautions

- Use cautiously in pts with impaired liver function.

Administration and Handling

◂ **ALERT** ▸ Know that doxorubicin dosage is individualized based on the patient's clinical response and tolerance of the adverse effects of the drug. When used in combination therapy, consult specific protocols for optimum dosage and sequence of drug administration.

◂ **ALERT** ▸ Wear gloves. If doxorubicin powder or solution comes in contact with skin, wash thoroughly. When accessing a vein for infusion, avoid areas overlying joints and tendons, small veins, and swollen or edematous extremities. For Doxil, do not use with an in-line filter or mix with any diluent except D_5W. Because Doxil may be carcinogenic, mutagenic, or teratogenic, handle the drug with extreme care during preparation and administration.

IV

- Store at room temperature.
- Reconstituted solution is stable for up to 24 hrs at room temperature or up to 48 hrs if refrigerated.

• Protect from prolonged exposure to sunlight; discard unused solution.
• Reconstitute each 10-mg vial with 5 mL preservative-free 0.9% NaCl (10 mL for 20 mg; 25 mL for 50 mg) to provide concentration of 2 mg/mL.
• Shake vial; allow contents to dissolve.
• Withdraw an appropriate volume of air from the vial during reconstitution to avoid excessive pressure build-up.
• Further dilute with 50 mL D_5W or 0.9% NaCl, if necessary, and give as a continuous infusion through a central venous line.
• For IV push, administer into the tubing of a freely running IV infusion of D_5W or 0.9% NaCl, preferably through a butterfly needle. To avoid local erythematous streaking along the vein and facial flushing, administer at a rate no faster than 3–5 min.
• Test for flashback every 30 sec to be certain that the needle remains in the vein during injection.
• Be aware that extravasation produces immediate pain and severe local tissue damage. If extravasation occurs, terminate drug administration immediately; withdraw as much medication as possible, obtain an extravasation kit and follow the protocol.

DOXIL
• Refrigerate unopened vials.
• After solution is diluted, use within 24 hrs.
• Dilute each dose in 250 mL D_5W.
• Give as infusion over more than 30 min.
• Do not use in-line filters.

Intervention and Evaluation
• Monitor the patient for signs and symptoms of stomatitis, including burning or erythema of oral mucosa at inner margin of lips and difficulty swallowing. Be aware that stomatitis may lead to ulceration of mucous membranes within 2–3 days.
• Assess the patient's nailbeds and skin for hyperpigmentation.
• Monitor the patient's hematologic status, liver and renal function studies, and serum uric acid levels.
• Assess the patient's pattern of daily bowel activity and stool consistency.
• Monitor the patient for signs and symptoms of anemia, including excessive fatigue and weakness, and hematologic toxicity, including easy bruising, fever, signs of local infection, sore throat, and unusual bleeding from any site.

Patient/Family Teaching
• Explain to the patient/family that alopecia is reversible, but new hair growth may have a different color or texture. Tell the patient that new hair growth resumes 2–3 mos after the last doxorubicin therapy dose.
• Teach the patient/family to maintain fastidious oral hygiene.
• Stress to the patient/family that the patient should not receive vaccinations and should avoid contact with anyone who recently received a live virus vaccine.
• Warn the patient/family to notify the physician if the patient experiences easy bruising, fever, signs of local infection, sore throat, or unusual bleeding from any site.
• Caution the patient/family to notify the physician if nausea and vomiting persist after discharge.
• Urge the patient to avoid consuming alcohol during doxorubicin therapy.
• Pts should avoid exposure to sunlight or artificial light sources because of the risk of

photosensitivity. Encourage patient/family to wear broad-spectrum sunscreen and protective clothing when sun exposure is unavoidable.

Idarubicin Hydrochloride

eye-dah-**roo**-bi-sin
(Idamycin PFS)
Do not confuse with Adriamycin or doxorubicin.

CATEGORY AND SCHEDULE
Pregnancy Risk Category: D

MECHANISM OF ACTION
An anthracycline antibiotic that inhibits nucleic acid synthesis by interacting with the enzyme topoisomerase II, which promotes DNA strand supercoiling. ***Therapeutic Effect:*** Produces death of rapidly dividing cells.

PHARMACOKINETICS
Widely distributed including in cerebrospinal fluid. Protein binding: 97%. Rapidly metabolized in liver to the active metabolite. Primarily eliminated via biliary excretion. Not removed by hemodialysis. ***Half-Life:*** 4–46 hrs; metabolite: 8–92 hrs.

AVAILABILITY
Injection: 1 mg/mL (5 mL, 10 mL, 20 mL)

INDICATIONS AND DOSAGES
Refer to individual protocols.

▸ Treatment of acute myeloid leukemia

IV

Children (solid tumor). 5 mg/m^2 once daily for 3 days.

Children (leukemia). 10–12 mg/m^2 once daily for 3 days.

▸ Dosage in liver or renal impairment

Serum Level	Dose Reduction
Serum creatinine 2 mg/dL or more	25%
Serum bilirubin greater than 2.5 mg/dL	50%
Serum bilirubin greater than 5 mg/dL	Do not give

CONTRAINDICATIONS
Hypersensitivity to idarubicin or any related component. Preexisting arrhythmias, bone marrow suppression, cardiomyopathy, pregnancy, severe congestive heart failure (CHF).

INTERACTIONS
Drug

Antigout medications: May decrease the effects of these drugs.
Bone marrow depressants: May increase bone marrow depression.
Live virus vaccines: May potentiate virus replication, increase vaccine side effects, and decrease the patient's antibody response to vaccine.

Herbal

None known.

Food

None known.

DIAGNOSTIC TEST EFFECTS
May increase serum alkaline phosphatase, serum bilirubin, SGOT (AST), SGPT (ALT), and serum uric acid levels. May cause EKG changes.

IV INCOMPATIBILITIES
Acyclovir (Zovirax), allopurinol (Aloprim), ampicillin-sulbactam (Unasyn), cefazolin (Ancef,

Kefzol), cefepime (Maxipime), ceftazidime (Fortaz), clindamycin (Cleocin), dexamethasone (Decadron), furosemide (Lasix), hydrocortisone (Solu-Cortef), lorazepam (Ativan), meperidine (Demerol), methotrexate, piperacillin/tazobactam (Zosyn), sodium bicarbonate, teniposide (Vumon), vancomycin (Vancocin), vincristine (Oncovin)

IV COMPATIBILITIES

Diphenhydramine (Benadryl), granisetron (Kytril), magnesium, potassium

SIDE EFFECTS

Frequent
Nausea, vomiting (82%); complete alopecia (scalp, axillary, pubic hair) (77%); abdominal cramping, diarrhea (73%); mucositis (50%)
Occasional
Hyperpigmentation of nailbeds, phalangeal and dermal creases (46%); fever (36%); headache (20%)
Rare
Conjunctivitis, neuropathy

SERIOUS REACTIONS

! Bone marrow depression manifested as hematologic toxicity (principally leukopenia and, to a lesser extent, anemia and thrombocytopenia) generally occurs within 10–15 days, returning to normal levels by the third week.
! Cardiotoxicity noted as either acute, transient abnormal electrocardiogram (EKG) findings and cardiomyopathy manifested as CHF may occur.

PEDIATRIC CONSIDERATIONS

Baseline Assessment
- Evaluate the patient's baseline complete blood count (CBC) results and liver and renal function test results.
- Obtain an EKG of the patient, as ordered, before starting idarubicin therapy.
- Give an antiemetic, if ordered, to the patient before and during idarubicin therapy to prevent or treat nausea and vomiting.
- Inform the patient of the high potential for alopecia development.
- Know that idarubicin use should be avoided during pregnancy because the drug may be embryotoxic.
- Be aware that it is unknown whether idarubicin is distributed in breast milk and the patient should discontinue breast-feeding before starting idarubicin therapy.
- Be aware that the safety and efficacy of idarubicin have not been established in children.
- Assess for and maintain age-appropriate fluid intake.

Precautions
- Use cautiously in pts receiving concurrent radiation therapy or with impaired liver or renal function.

Administration and Handling
◂ALERT▸ Know that idarubicin dosage is individualized based on the patient's clinical response and tolerance of the drug's adverse effects. When used in combination therapy, consult specific protocols for optimum dosage and sequence of drug administration.
◂ALERT▸ Give idarubicin by free-flowing IV infusion and never by the SC or IM route. Use gloves, gowns, and eye goggles during the preparation and administration of this medication. If powder or solution comes in contact with skin, wash thoroughly. Avoid areas overlying joints and tendons, small

veins, and swollen or edematous extremities.

◀ **ALERT** ▶ Be aware that Idamycin prefilled syringe does not require reconstitution and is stored refrigerated.

◀ **ALERT** ▶ Do not administer idarubicin IM or SC.

IV

• Reconstituted solution is stable for up to 72 hrs, or 3 days, at room temperature or up to 168 hrs, or 7 days, if refrigerated.
• Discard unused solution.
• Reconstitute each 10-mg vial with 10 mL or each 5-mg vial with 5 mL of 0.9% NaCl to provide a concentration of 1 mg/mL.
• Administer into the tubing of a freely running IV infusion of D_5W or 0.9% NaCl, preferably through a butterfly needle, slowly over more than 10–15 min.
• Monitor for signs and symptoms of extravasation, such as immediate pain and severe local tissue damage. Terminate the infusion immediately. Apply cold compresses for ½ hr immediately then for ½ hr 4 times/day for 3 days. Keep the affected extremity elevated.

Intervention and Evaluation

• Monitor the patient's CBC with differential, EKG, platelet count, and liver and renal function tests.
• Monitor the patient for signs and symptoms of anemia, including excessive fatigue and weakness, and hematologic toxicity, including easy bruising, fever, signs of local infection, sore throat, or unusual bleeding from any site.
• Avoid giving the patient IM injections or rectal medications and causing other trauma that may precipitate bleeding.
• Check the patient's infusion site frequently for evidence of extravasation, which causes severe local necrosis.
• Assess the patient for potentially fatal CHF (dyspnea, edema, and rales) and life-threatening arrhythmias.

Patient/Family Teaching

• Explain to the patient/family that total body alopecia may occur and that it is reversible. Take measures to help the patient cope with hair loss. Tell the patient that new hair growth resumes 2–3 mos after the last idarubicin dose and that new hair may have a different color or texture than the original.
• Teach the patient/family to maintain fastidious oral hygiene.
• Stress to the patient/family that the patient should avoid crowds and those with known infections.
• Teach the patient and family how to recognize the early signs and symptoms of bleeding and infection.
• Warn the patient/family to notify the physician if the patient experiences easy bruising, bleeding, fever, or sore throat.
• Advise the patient/family that idarubicin use may turn the patient's urine pink or red.
• Explain to the patient that he or she should use contraceptive measures during idarubicin therapy.

Mitomycin

my-toe-**my**-sin
(Mutamycin)

CATEGORY AND SCHEDULE

Pregnancy Risk Category: D

MECHANISM OF ACTION

An antibiotic that acts as an alkylating agent and cross-links the strands of DNA. ***Therapeutic Effect:*** Inhibits DNA and RNA synthesis.

PHARMACOKINETICS

Widely distributed. Does not cross blood-brain barrier. Primarily metabolized in liver and excreted in bile and urine. ***Half-Life:*** 50 min.

AVAILABILITY

Powder for Injection: 5 mg, 20 mg, 40 mg.

INDICATIONS AND DOSAGES

Refer to individual protocols.

▸ **Treatment of disseminated adenocarcinoma of pancreas and stomach**

IV

Children. Initial dosage: 10–20 mg/m² as a single dose. Repeat q6–8wks. Give additional courses only after platelet and WBC counts are within acceptable levels.

▸ **Dosage in renal impairment**

Creatinine Clearance	% Normal Dose
Less than 10 mL/min	75%

Leukocytes/ mm³	Platelets/ mm³	% of Prior Dose to Give
4,000	more than 100,000	100
3,000–3,999	75,000–99,000	100
2,000–2,999	25,000–74,999	70
1,999 or less	less than 25,000	50

UNLABELED USES

Treatment of biliary, bladder, breast, cervical, colorectal, head and neck, and lung carcinoma and chronic myelocytic leukemia

CONTRAINDICATIONS

Hypersensitivity to mitomycin or any related component. Coagulation disorders and bleeding tendencies, platelet count less than 75,000/mm³, serious infection, serum creatinine level greater than 1.7 mg/dL, WBC count less than 3,000/mm³.

INTERACTIONS

Drug

Bone marrow depressants: May increase bone marrow depression.

Live virus vaccines: May potentiate virus replication, increase vaccine side effects, and decrease the patient's antibody response to vaccine.

Anthracyclines: May increase cardiotoxicity.

Herbal

None known.

Food

None known.

DIAGNOSTIC TEST EFFECTS

May increase BUN and serum creatinine levels.

IV INCOMPATIBILITIES

Do not mix with any other medications.

IV COMPATIBILITIES

Cisplatin (Platinol AQ), cyclophosphamide (Cytoxan), doxorubicin (Adriamycin), fluorouracil, granisetron (Kytril), leucovorin, methotrexate, ondansetron (Zofran), vinblastine (Velban), vincristine (Oncovin)

SIDE EFFECTS

Frequent (greater than 10%)

Fever, anorexia, nausea, vomiting

Occasional (10%–2%)

Stomatitis, numbness of fingers and toes, purple color bands on nails, skin rash, alopecia, unusual tiredness

Rare (less than 1%)
Thrombophlebitis, cellulitis, extravasation

SERIOUS REACTIONS

! Marked bone marrow depression results in hematologic toxicity manifested as leukopenia, thrombocytopenia, and to a lesser extent, anemia, which generally occurs within 2–4 wks after initial therapy.
! Renal toxicity evidenced by a rise in BUN and serum creatinine levels may occur.
! Pulmonary toxicity manifested as dyspnea, cough, hemoptysis, and pneumonia may occur.
! Long-term therapy may produce hemolytic uremic syndrome, characterized by hemolytic anemia, thrombocytopenia, renal failure, and hypertension.

PEDIATRIC CONSIDERATIONS

Baseline Assessment

• If ordered, obtain the patient's bleeding time, complete blood count, and prothrombin time before and periodically during mitomycin therapy.
• Give antiemetics, if ordered, to the patient before and during mitomycin therapy to prevent or treat nausea and vomiting.
• Be aware that mitomycin use should be avoided during pregnancy, especially in the first trimester and that breast-feeding is not recommended in this patient population.
• Contraindicated in children who have impaired hepatic or renal function or those with active infections such as chicken pox.
• This medication is a vesicant so it is important to assess and maintain IV patency during drug administration.
• Assess for and maintain age-appropriate fluid intake.
• There are no age-related precautions noted in children.

Precautions

• Use cautiously in pts with impaired liver or renal function and myelosuppression.

Administration and Handling

◀ALERT▶ Be aware that mitomycin dosage is individualized based on the patient's clinical response and tolerance of the adverse effects of the drug. When used in combination therapy, consult specific protocols for optimum dosage and sequence of drug administration.

◀ALERT▶ Because mitomycin may be carcinogenic, mutagenic, or teratogenic, handle the drug with extreme care during preparation and administration. Be aware that this drug is extremely irritating to veins and may produce pain during infusion with induration, paresthesia, and thrombophlebitis.

IV

• Use only clear, blue-gray solutions.
• Concentration of 0.5 mg/mL is stable for up to 7 days at room temperature or up to 2 wks if refrigerated.
• If solution is further diluted with D_5W, solution is stable for up to 3 hrs or if diluted with 0.9% NaCl is stable for up to 24 hrs at room temperature.
• Reconstitute 5-mg vial with 10 mL and a 20-mg vial with 40 mL of Sterile Water for Injection to provide solution containing 0.5 mg/mL.
• Do not shake vial to dissolve. Allow vial to stand at room temperature until complete dissolution occurs.
• For IV infusion, further dilute with 50–100 mL D_5W or 0.9% NaCl.

- Give IV push over 5–10 min.
- Give IV through tubing running IV infusion.
- Monitor for signs and symptoms of extravasation, which may produce cellulitis, tissue sloughing, and ulceration. If extravasation occurs, terminate the infusion immediately and inject the ordered antidote as appropriate. Apply ice intermittently for up to 72 hrs and keep the affected area elevated.

Intervention and Evaluation

- Monitor the patient's BUN and serum creatinine levels and hematologic status.
- Assess the patient's IV site for evidence of extravasation and phlebitis.
- Monitor the patient for signs and symptoms of anemia, including excessive fatigue and weakness, hematologic toxicity, including easy bruising, fever, signs of local infection, sore throat, and unusual bleeding from any site, and renal toxicity, including a rise in BUN and serum creatinine levels.

Patient/Family Teaching

- Teach the patient/family to maintain fastidious oral hygiene.
- Warn the patient/family to immediately report any burning or pain felt at the injection site.
- Stress to the patient/family that the patient should not receive vaccinations and should avoid contact with anyone who recently received a live virus vaccine.
- Warn the patient/family to notify the physician if the patient experiences bleeding, easy bruising, burning or painful urination, increased urinary frequency, fever, nausea, signs of local infection, shortness of breath, sore throat, unusual bleeding from any site, and vomiting.
- Explain to the patient/family that alopecia is reversible, but that new hair growth may have a different color or texture.

REFERENCES

Miller, S. & Fioravanti, J. (1997). Pediatric medications: A handbook for nurses. St. Louis: Mosby.

Taketomo, C. K., Hodding, J. H. & Kraus, D. M. (2003–2004). Pediatric dosage handbook (10th ed.). Hudson, OH: Lexi-Comp.

15 Antimetabolites

Cytarabine
Fludarabine Phosphate
Fluorouracil
Hydroxyurea
Mercaptopurine
Methotrexate Sodium

Uses: Antimetabolites produce the best response in pts with lymphomas, acute leukemias, cancer of the gastrointestinal tract, or breast cancer.

Action: Structurally similar to natural metabolites, antimetabolites act by disrupting critical metabolic processes. Some agents inhibit enzymes that synthesize essential cellular components; others are incorporated into DNA, interfering with DNA replication and function. By altering DNA synthesis and metabolism, antimetabolites affect the S phase of the cell cycle.

Cytarabine

sigh-**tar**-ah-bean
(Ara-C, Cytosar [CAN], Cytosar-U)
Do not confuse with Cytadren, Cytovene, or vidarabine.

CATEGORY AND SCHEDULE

Pregnancy Risk Category: D

MECHANISM OF ACTION

An antimetabolite that is converted intracellularly to a nucleotide. Cell cycle-specific for S phase of cell division. Potent immunosuppressive activity. ***Therapeutic Effect:*** May inhibit DNA synthesis.

PHARMACOKINETICS

Widely distributed; moderate amount crosses the blood-brain barrier. Protein binding: 15%. Primarily excreted in urine. ***Half-Life:*** 1–3 hrs.

AVAILABILITY

Powder for Injection: 100 mg, 500 mg, 1 g, 2 g.

INDICATIONS AND DOSAGES

Refer to individual protocols.

▸ **Treatment of acute lymphocytic leukemia, acute and chronic myelocytic leukemia, meningeal leukemia, non-Hodgkin lymphoma in children; induction remission**

IV

Children. 200 mg/m²/day for 5 days at 2-wk intervals as a single agent. 100–200 mg/m²/day for 5- to 10-day therapy course every 2–4 wks in combination therapy.

INTRATHECAL

Children. 5–7.5 mg/m² q2–7days.

▸ **Treatment of acute lymphocytic leukemia, acute and chronic myelocytic leukemia, meningeal leukemia, non-Hodgkin lymphoma in children; maintenance of remission**

IV

Children. 70–200 mg/m²/day for 2–5 days every month.

IM, SC

Children. 1–1.5 mg/m² as a single dose at 1- to 4-wk intervals.

INTRATHECAL

Children. 5–7.5 mg/m² q2–7days.

UNLABELED USES

Treatment of Hodgkin lymphoma, myelodysplastic syndrome.

CONTRAINDICATIONS
Hypersensitivity to cytarabine or related component.

INTERACTIONS
Drug
Antigout medications: May decrease the effects of these drugs.
Bone marrow depressants: May increase bone marrow depression.
Cyclophosphamide: May increase risk of developing cardiomyopathy.
Live virus vaccines: May potentiate virus replication, increase vaccine side effects, and decrease the patient's antibody response to vaccine.
Herbal
None known.
Food
None known.

DIAGNOSTIC TEST EFFECTS
May increase serum alkaline phosphatase, serum bilirubin, SGOT (AST), and serum uric acid levels.

IV INCOMPATIBILITIES
Amphotericin B complex (AmBisome, Amphotec, Abelcet), ganciclovir (Cytovene), heparin, insulin (regular)

IV COMPATIBILITIES
Dexamethasone (Decadron), diphenhydramine (Benadryl), filgrastim (Neupogen), granisetron (Kytril), heparin, hydromorphone (Dilaudid), lorazepam (Ativan), morphine, ondansetron (Zofran), potassium chloride, propofol (Diprivan)

SIDE EFFECTS
Frequent
SC, IV (33%–16%): Asthenia, fever, pain, change in taste and smell, nausea, vomiting (risk of nausea and vomiting greater with IV push than with continuous IV infusion)
Intrathecal (28%–11%): Headache, asthenia, change in taste and smell, confusion, somnolence, nausea, vomiting
Occasional
SC, IV (11%–7%): Abnormal gait, somnolence, constipation, back pain, urinary incontinence, peripheral edema, headache, confusion
Intrathecal (7%–3%): Peripheral edema, back pain, constipation, abnormal gait, urinary incontinence

SERIOUS REACTIONS
! The major toxic effect of cytarabine use is bone marrow depression resulting in blood dyscrasias, including leukopenia, anemia, thrombocytopenia, megaloblastosis, and reticulocytopenia, occurring minimally after a single IV dose.
! Leukopenia, anemia, and thrombocytopenia should be expected with daily or continuous IV therapy.
! Cytarabine syndrome evidenced by fever, myalgia, rash, conjunctivitis, malaise, or chest pain and hyperuricemia may be noted.
! High-dose cytarabine therapy may produce severe CNS, GI, and pulmonary toxicity.

PEDIATRIC CONSIDERATIONS
Baseline Assessment
• Expect the patient's WBC count to decrease within 24 hrs after the initial cytarabine dose, continue to decrease for 7–9 days, show a brief rise at 12 days, decrease again at 15–24 days, and finally rise rapidly for the next 10 days.
• Expect the patient's platelet count to decrease 5 days after

cytarabine initiation to a low count at 12–15 days and then rise rapidly for the next 10 days.

- Know that cytarabine use should be avoided during pregnancy because the drug may cause fetal malformations.
- Be aware that it is unknown whether cytarabine is distributed in breast milk. Breast-feeding is not recommended in this patient population.
- Assess for and maintain age-appropriate fluid intake.
- Do not use diluents that contain benzyl alcohol for reconstitution in neonatal regimens or high-dose regimens.

PRECAUTIONS

- Use cautiously in pts with impaired liver function.

Administration and Handling

◂ALERT▸ Know that cytarabine dosage is individualized based on the patient's clinical response and tolerance of the adverse effects of the drug. When used in combination therapy, consult specific protocols for optimum dosage and sequence of drug administration. Expect to modify the dosage when serious hematologic depression occurs.

◂ALERT▸ May give cytarabine by SC injection, IV infusion, IV push, or intrathecally. Because cytarabine may be carcinogenic, mutagenic, or teratogenic, causing embryonic deformity, handle the drug with extreme care during preparation and administration.

SC, IV, Intrathecal

- Reconstituted solution is stable for up to 48 hrs at room temperature.
- IV infusion solutions at concentration up to 0.5 mg/mL are stable for up to 7 days at room temperature.
- Discard if a slight haze develops.
- Reconstitute 100-mg vial with 5 mL Bacteriostatic Water for Injection with benzyl alcohol (10 mL for 500-mg vial) to provide concentration of 20 mg/mL and 50 mg/mL, respectively.
- Further dilute the dose, if necessary, with up to 1,000 mL D_5W or 0.9% NaCl for IV infusion.
- For intrathecal use, reconstitute vial with preservative-free 0.9% NaCl or patient's spinal fluid. Be aware that the dose is usually administered in 5–15 mL of solution, after equivalent volume of cerebrospinal fluid is removed.
- For IV push, give over 1–3 min. For IV infusion, give over 30 min–24 hrs.

Intervention and Evaluation

- Monitor the patient's complete blood count for signs of bone marrow depression.
- Monitor the patient for signs and symptoms of anemia, including excessive tiredness and weakness, and blood dyscrasias, including easy bruising, fever, signs of local infection, sore throat, or unusual bleeding from any site.
- Evaluate the patient for neuropathy as evidenced by gait disturbances, handwriting difficulties, and numbness.
- Administer corticosteroid eye drops for prophylaxis of conjunctivitis around-the-clock before, during, and after high-dose cytarabine treatment.

Patient/Family Teaching

- Instruct the patient/family to increase the patient's fluid intake to help protect against hyperuricemia development.
- Stress to the patient/family that the patient should not receive vac-

cinations and should avoid contact with anyone who recently received a live virus vaccine.

• Warn the patient/family to promptly report if the patient experiences easy bruising, fever, signs of local infection, sore throat, or unusual bleeding from any site.

Fludarabine Phosphate

flew-**dare**-ah-bean
(Fludara)
Do not confuse with FUDR.

CATEGORY AND SCHEDULE

Pregnancy Risk Category: D

MECHANISM OF ACTION

An antimetabolite that interferes with DNA polymerase alpha, ribonucleotide reductase, and DNA primase. ***Therapeutic Effect:*** Inhibits DNA synthesis; induces cell death.

PHARMACOKINETICS

Rapidly dephosphorylated in serum, then phosphorylated intracellularly to active triphosphate. Protein binding: 19%–29%. Primarily excreted in urine. ***Half-Life:*** 7–20 hrs.

AVAILABILITY

Injection: 50 mg.

INDICATIONS AND DOSAGES

Refer to individual protocols.

▸ **Acute leukemia**

IV

Children. 10 mg/m^2 bolus (over 15 min), then IV continuous infusion of 30.5 mg/m^2/day over 5 days.

▸ **Solid tumors**

IV

Children. 9 mg/m^2 bolus, then 27 mg/m^2/day for 5 days as continuous infusion.

▸ **Dosage in renal impairment**

Creatinine Clearance	Dosage
30–70 mL/min	Decrease dose by 20%
Less than 30 mL/min	Not recommended

CONTRAINDICATIONS

Hypersensitivity to fludarabine or any related component. Concomitant administration with pentostatin and pregnancy.

INTERACTIONS

Drug

Antigout medications: May decrease the effects of these drugs.

Bone marrow depressants: May increase risk of bone marrow depression.

Live virus vaccines: May potentiate virus replication, increase vaccine side effects, and decrease the patient's antibody response to the vaccine.

Pentostatin: Increases pulmonary toxicity.

Herbal

None known.

Food

None known.

DIAGNOSTIC TEST EFFECTS

May increase serum alkaline phosphatase, SGOT (AST), and uric acid levels.

IV INCOMPATIBILITIES

Acyclovir (Zovirax), amphotericin (Fungizone), hydroxyzine (Vistaril), prochlorperazine (Compazine)

IV COMPATIBILITIES

Heparin, hydromorphone (Dilaudid), lorazepam (Ativan), magnesium sulfate, morphine, multivitamins, potassium chloride

SIDE EFFECTS

Frequent
Fever (60%), nausea and vomiting (36%), chills (11%)
Occasional (20%–10%)
Fatigue, generalized pain, rash, diarrhea, cough, weakness, stomatitis (burning or erythema of oral mucosa, sore throat, difficulty swallowing), dyspnea, weakness, peripheral edema
Rare (7%–3%)
Anorexia, sinusitis, dysuria, myalgia, paresthesia, headaches, visual disturbances

SERIOUS REACTIONS

! Pneumonia occurs frequently.
! Severe bone marrow toxicity as evidenced by anemia, thrombocytopenia, and neutropenia may occur.
! Tumor lysis syndrome may occur with onset of flank pain and hematuria. This syndrome may include hypercalcemia, hyperphosphatemia, hyperuricemia, and result in renal failure.
! GI bleeding may occur.
! High fludarabine dosage may produce acute leukemia, blindness, and coma.

PEDIATRIC CONSIDERATIONS

Baseline Assessment

- Assess the patient's baseline complete blood count and serum creatinine level.
- Expect to discontinue fludarabine if intractable diarrhea, GI bleeding, stomatitis, or vomiting occurs.
- Know that fludarabine use should be avoided during pregnancy, if possible, especially in the first trimester.
- Be aware that fludarabine may cause fetal harm and it is unknown whether it is distributed in breast milk. Breast-feeding is not recommended in this patient population.
- The safety and efficacy of fludarabine have not been established in children.

Precautions

- Use cautiously in pts with preexisting bone marrow suppression, neurologic problems, and renal insufficiency.

Administration and Handling

◂ALERT▸ Be aware that fludarabine dosage is individualized on the basis of the patient's clinical response and tolerance of the drug's adverse effects. When used in combination therapy, consult specific protocols for optimum dosage and sequence of drug administration. Drug dosage is based on the patient's actual weight. Use ideal body weight in edematous or obese pts.
◂ALERT▸ Give fludarabine by IV infusion. Do not add to other IV infusions. Avoid areas overlying joints and tendons, small veins, and swollen or edematous extremities.

IV

- Store in refrigerator.
- Handle with extreme care during preparation and administration.
- If contact with skin or mucous membranes occurs, wash thoroughly with soap and water; rinse eyes profusely with plain water.
- After reconstitution, use within 8 hrs; discard unused portion.

• Reconstitute 50-mg vial with 2 mL Sterile Water for Injection to provide a concentration of 25 mg/mL.
• Further dilute with 100–125 mL 0.9% NaCl or D_5W.
• Infuse over 30 min.

Intervention and Evaluation
• Assess the patient for onset of peripheral edema, pneumonia, visual disturbances, and weakness.
• Monitor the patient for cough, dyspnea, GI bleeding, including bright red or tarry stools, intractable diarrhea, and rapidly falling WBC count.
• Examine the patient for difficulty swallowing, mucosal erythema, sore throat, and ulceration at the inner margin of the lips, which indicate the presence of stomatitis.
• Assess the patient's skin for rash.
• Be alert to signs and symptoms of possible tumor lysis syndrome manifested as hematuria and onset of flank pain.
• Pts with a large tumor burden at risk for tumor lysis syndrome should receive prophylactic allopurinol, good hydration, and urinary alkalinization.

Patient/Family Teaching
• Stress to the patient/family to avoid crowds and exposure to those with known infection.
• Teach the patient/family to maintain fastidious oral hygiene.
• Warn the patient/family to notify the physician if the patient experiences easy bruising, fever, signs of local infection, sore throat, or unusual bleeding from any site.
• Caution the patient/family to contact the physician if nausea and vomiting continue at home.

Fluorouracil

phlur-oh-**your**-ah-sill
(Adrucil, Efudex, Efudix [AUS], Fluoroplex)
Do not confuse with Efidac.

CATEGORY AND SCHEDULE

Pregnancy Risk Category: D

MECHANISM OF ACTION

An antimetabolite that blocks formation of thymidylic acid. ***Therapeutic Effect:*** Inhibits DNA and RNA synthesis.
Topical: Destroys rapidly proliferating cells. Cell cycle–specific for S phase of cell division.

PHARMACOKINETICS

Crosses blood-brain barrier. Widely distributed. Rapidly metabolized in tissues to active metabolite, which is localized intracellularly. Primarily excreted via lungs as CO_2. Removed by hemodialysis. ***Half-Life:*** 20 hrs.

AVAILABILITY

Injection: 50 mg/mL.
Cream: 0.5%, 1%, 5%.
Topical Solution: 1%, 2%, 5%.

INDICATIONS AND DOSAGES

Refer to individual protocols.

▸ **Treatment of carcinoma of breast, colon, pancreas, rectum, and stomach**

IV

Children. Initially, 12 mg/kg/day for 4–5 days. Maximum: 800 mg/day. Maintenance: 6 mg/kg every other day for 4 doses. Repeat in 4 wks. As single weekly dosing: 15 mg/kg as a single bolus dose, then 5–15 mg/kg/wk as a single dose, not to exceed 1 g.

▸ **Colorectal carcinoma/hepatoma**
PO
Children. 15–20 mg/kg/day for 5–8 days or 15 mg/kg/wk.
▸ **Superficial basal cell carcinomas or actinic keratoses**
TOPICAL
Children. Apply twice weekly.

UNLABELED USES

Parenteral: Treatment of bladder, cervical, endometrial, head and neck, liver, lung, ovarian, prostate carcinomas; treatment of pericardial, peritoneal, pleural effusions.
Topical: Treatment of actinic cheilitis, radiodermatitis

CONTRAINDICATIONS

Hypersensitivity to fluorouracil or any related component. Depressed bone marrow function, major surgery within previous month, poor nutritional status, potentially serious infections.

INTERACTIONS

Drug

Bone marrow depressants: May increase risk of bone marrow depression.
Live virus vaccines: May potentiate virus replication, increase vaccine side effects, and decrease the patient's antibody response to vaccine.
Cimetidine: Increases fluorouracil serum concentrations

Herbal

None known.

Food

Use of acidic juices to dilute oral form may result in precipitation and decreased absorption.

DIAGNOSTIC TEST EFFECTS

May decrease serum albumin. May increase excretion of 5-hydroxyindoleacetic acid in urine.
Topical: May cause eosinophilia, leukocytosis, thrombocytopenia, and toxic granulation.

IV INCOMPATIBILITIES

Amphotericin B complex (Abelcet, Amphotec, AmBisome), droperidol (Inapsine), filgrastim (Neupogen), ondansetron (Zofran), vinorelbine (Navelbine)

IV COMPATIBILITIES

Granisetron (Kytril), heparin, hydromorphone (Dilaudid), leucovorin, morphine, ondansetron (Zofran), potassium chloride, propofol (Diprivan)

SIDE EFFECTS

Occasional
Anorexia, diarrhea, minimal alopecia, fever, dry skin, fissuring, scaling, erythema
Topical: Pain, pruritus, hyperpigmentation, irritation, inflammation, burning at application site
Rare
Nausea, vomiting, anemia, esophagitis, proctitis, GI ulcer, confusion, headache, lacrimation, visual disturbances, angina, allergic reactions

SERIOUS REACTIONS

! The earliest sign of toxicity, which may occur 4–8 days after beginning of therapy, is stomatitis as evidenced by dry mouth, burning sensation, mucosal erythema, and ulceration at the inner margin of the lips.
! The most common dermatologic toxicity is a pruritic rash that generally appears on the extremities and less frequently on trunk.
! Leukopenia generally occurs within 9–14 days after drug admin-

istration and may occur as late as the 25th day.

! Thrombocytopenia occasionally occurs within 7–17 days after administration.

! Hematologic toxicity may also manifest itself as pancytopenia or agranulocytosis.

PEDIATRIC CONSIDERATIONS

Baseline Assessment

- Monitor the patient's complete blood count with differential, liver and renal function tests, and platelet count.
- Be aware that fluorouracil use should be avoided during pregnancy, if possible, especially in the first trimester.
- Be aware that fluorouracil may cause fetal harm and it is unknown whether fluorouracil is distributed in breast milk. Breast-feeding is not recommended in this patient population.
- Assess for and maintain age-appropriate fluid intake.
- Be sure to maintain IV patency because fluorouracil is a potent vesicant.
- Do not give medication to children who have been exposed to chicken pox or herpes zoster.

Precautions

- Use cautiously in pts with a history of high-dose pelvic irradiation, impaired liver or renal function, and metastatic cell infiltration of bone marrow.

Administration and Handling

◂ALERT▸ Know that fluorouracil dosage is individualized on the basis of the patient's clinical response and tolerance of the adverse effects of the drug. When used in combination therapy, consult specific protocols for optimum dosage and sequence of drug administration. Be aware that dosage is based on the patient's actual weight. Use ideal body weight in edematous or obese pts.

◂ALERT▸ Give fluorouracil by IV injection or IV infusion. Do not add to other IV infusions. Avoid areas overlying joints and tendons, small veins, and swollen or edematous extremities. Because fluorouracil may be carcinogenic, mutagenic, or teratogenic, handle the drug with extreme care during preparation and administration.

IV

- Solution normally appears colorless to faint yellow. Slight discoloration does not adversely affect potency or safety.
- If precipitate forms, redissolve by heating and shaking vigorously; allow to cool to body temperature.
- Administer IV push as undiluted or unreconstituted, as appropriate. Inject through Y-tube or 3-way stopcock of free-flowing solution.
- For IV infusion, further dilute with D_5W or 0.9% NaCl.
- Give IV push slowly over 1–2 min.
- Administer IV infusion over 30 min–24 hrs.
- Monitor patient for signs and symptoms of extravasation, including immediate pain and severe local tissue damage. If this occurs, follow the protocol of your facility.

TOPICAL

- Apply with a nonmetallic applicator or gloved fingers. Avoid contact with mucous membranes. Do not cover area with occlusive dressings.

Intervention and Evaluation

- Monitor the patient for signs of GI bleeding, including bright red or tarry stool, intractable diarrhea, and rapidly falling WBC count.

• Assess the patient for signs and symptoms of stomatitis, including difficulty swallowing, mucosal erythema, sore throat, and ulceration of inner margin of lips.
• Discontinue fluorouracil if intractable diarrhea, GI bleeding, or stomatitis occurs.
• Assess the patient's skin for rash.

Patient/Family Teaching

• Teach the patient/family to maintain fastidious oral hygiene.
• Warn the patient/family to notify the physician if the patient experiences bleeding, bruising, chest pain, diarrhea, nausea, palpitations, signs and symptoms of infection, or visual changes.
• Encourage the patient/family to avoid overexposure to sun or ultraviolet light and to wear protective clothing, sunglasses, and sunscreen.
• Instruct the patient/family using topical fluorouracil to apply the drug only to the affected area and not to use occlusive coverings. Explain to the patient that he or she needs to be careful when applying topical drug near the eyes, mouth, and nose. Teach the patient to wash hands thoroughly after topical drug application. Explain to the patient/family that treated areas may be unsightly for several weeks after therapy.

Hydroxyurea

high-**drocks**-ee-your-e-ah
(Droxia, Hydrea, Mylocel)

CATEGORY AND SCHEDULE

Pregnancy Risk Category: D

MECHANISM OF ACTION

A synthetic urea analogue that is cell cycle–specific for the S phase. Inhibits DNA synthesis without interfering with RNA synthesis or protein. ***Therapeutic Effect:*** Interferes with the normal repair process of cells damaged by irradiation.

PHARMACOKINETICS

Well absorbed orally. Crosses blood-brain barrier; excreted in breast milk. Metabolized in the liver. Eliminated unchanged in the urine. ***Half-Life:*** 3–4 hrs.

AVAILABILITY

Capsules: 200 mg, 300 mg, 400 mg, 500 mg.
Tablets: 1,000 mg.

INDICATIONS AND DOSAGES

Refer to individual protocols.

▸ Resistant chronic myelocytic leukemia

PO

Children. Initially, 10–20 mg/kg once daily.

▸ Sickle cell anemia

PO

Children. Initially, 15 mg/kg once daily. May increase by 5 mg/kg/day every 12 wks. Maximum: 35 mg/kg/wk.

UNLABELED USES

Treatment of cervical carcinoma, polycythemia vera. Long-term suppression of HIV.

CONTRAINDICATIONS

WBC count less than 2,500/mm^3 or platelet count less than 100,000/mm^3.

INTERACTIONS

Drug

Antigout medications: May decrease the effects of these drugs.
Bone marrow depressants: May increase bone marrow depression.

Live virus vaccines: May potentiate virus replication, increase vaccine side effects, and decrease the patient's antibody response to vaccine.

Herbal

None known.

Food

None known.

DIAGNOSTIC TEST EFFECTS

May increase BUN, serum creatinine, and serum uric acid levels.

SIDE EFFECTS

Frequent

Nausea, vomiting, anorexia, constipation or diarrhea

Occasional

Mild reversible rash, facial flushing, pruritus, fever, chills, malaise

Rare

Alopecia, headache, drowsiness, dizziness, disorientation

SERIOUS REACTIONS

! Bone marrow depression manifested as hematologic toxicity (leukopenia and, to a lesser extent, thrombocytopenia and anemia) may occur.

PEDIATRIC CONSIDERATIONS

Baseline Assessment

- Expect the patient to undergo bone marrow studies and liver and kidney function tests before hydroxyurea therapy begins and periodically thereafter.
- Obtain baseline blood Hgb and serum uric acid levels and platelet and WBC counts weekly during hydroxyurea therapy.
- Know that those pts with marked renal impairment may develop auditory or visual hallucinations and marked hematologic toxicity.
- Assess for and maintain age-appropriate fluid intake.
- Report exposure to chicken pox or herpes zoster.

Precautions

- Use cautiously in pts with impaired liver or renal function, who have had previous radiation therapy or who are using other cytotoxic drugs.
- Hydroxyurea is presumed to be a human carcinogen: it is embryotoxic and can cause fetal malformations. Pts taking hydroxyurea should use appropriate contraceptives if of childbearing age.

Administration and Handling

◀ALERT▶ Be aware that hydroxyurea dosage is individualized based on the patient's clinical response and tolerance of the drug's adverse effects. When used in combination therapy, consult specific protocols for optimum dosage and sequence of drug administration. Know that dosage is based on actual or ideal body weight, whichever is less. Expect therapy to be interrupted when the platelet count falls below 100,000/mm^3 or the WBC count falls below 2,500/mm^3 and to resume when counts rise toward normal.

◀ALERT▶ Store in a tightly sealed container: moisture will degrade this drug.

◀ALERT▶ Hydroxyurea should be handled properly: the Food and Drug Administration recommends that appropriate antineoplastic handling and disposal procedures be used.

Intervention and Evaluation

- Assess the patient's pattern of daily bowel activity and stool consistency.
- Monitor the patient for signs and symptoms of anemia, including

excessive tiredness and weakness, and hematologic toxicity, including easy bruising, fever, signs of local infection, sore throat, or unusual bleeding from any site.

- Assess the patient's skin for erythema or rash.
- Monitor the patient's blood Hgb, complete blood count with differential, liver function test results, platelet count, renal function studies, and serum uric acid levels.

Patient/Family Teaching

- Warn the patient/family to notify the physician if the patient experiences easy bruising, fever, signs of local infection, sore throat, or unusual bleeding from any site.
- Teach the patient/family about the importance of follow-up care to monitor and assess blood counts.

Mercaptopurine 

mur-cap-**tow**-pure-een
(6-MP, Purinethol)

CATEGORY AND SCHEDULE

Pregnancy Risk Category: D

MECHANISM OF ACTION

An antimetabolite that is incorporated into RNA and DNA. Blocks purine synthesis. ***Therapeutic Effect:*** Inhibits DNA and RNA synthesis.

PHARMACOKINETICS

Absorption variable. Widely distributed, including in cerebrospinal fluid. Protein binding: 19%. Metabolized in the liver, excreted unchanged in the urine. ***Half-Life:*** 36–90 min (age dependent).

AVAILABILITY

Tablets: 50 mg.

INDICATIONS AND DOSAGES

Refer to individual protocols.

▸ Acute lymphoblastic leukemia

PO (INDUCTION)

Children. 2.5–5 mg/kg/day once daily.

PO (MAINTENANCE)

Children. 1.5–2.5 mg/kg/day once daily.

▸ Dosage in renal impairment

Creatinine clearance less than 50 mL/min. Administer q48h.

CONTRAINDICATIONS

Hypersensitivity to mercaptopurine or related component. Pregnancy, severe bone marrow suppression, severe liver disease.

INTERACTIONS

Drug

Allopurinol, doxorubicin, liver-toxic drugs: May increase the effects and risk of toxicity of mercaptopurine.

Warfarin: May decrease the effects of this drug.

Herbal

None known.

Food

Decreases bioavailability of mercaptopurine.

DIAGNOSTIC TEST EFFECTS

None known.

SIDE EFFECTS

Frequent (greater than 10%)

Myelosuppression, leukopenia, thrombocytopenia, anemia, intrahepatic cholestasis, focal centrilobular necrosis

Occasional (10%–1%)

Drug fever, hyperpigmentation, rash, hyperuricemia, nausea, vomiting, diarrhea, stomatitis, anorexia, stomach pain, mucositis

SERIOUS REACTIONS

! Nausea, vomiting, bone marrow suppression, liver necrosis, and gastroenteritis may occur.

PEDIATRIC CONSIDERATIONS

Baseline Assessment

• Determine whether the patient is pregnant or breast-feeding (not recommended) and taking other medication, especially allopurinol, other bone marrow suppressants, and other liver-toxic medications, before beginning mercaptopurine therapy.
• Assess for and maintain IV patency. Mercaptopurine is a strong vesicant.
• It is important to assess liver function because the drug is initially metabolized in the liver.
• Assess for and maintain age-appropriate fluid intake.

Precautions

• Use cautiously in pts with a history of gout, infection, liver impairment, prior bone marrow suppression, and renal impairment.

Administration and Handling

PO

• Do not administer with meals.

Intervention and Evaluation

• Monitor the patient's liver function tests, platelet count, renal function, and serum uric acid level.

Patient/Family Teaching

• Urge the patient/family to avoid consuming alcohol during mercaptopurine therapy. Explain to the patient that alcohol may increase the risk of toxicity with this drug.
• Stress to the patient/family that the patient should not receive vaccinations and should avoid contact with anyone with known infection.
• Warn the patient/family to notify the physician if the patient experiences unusual bleeding or bruising.

Methotrexate Sodium

meth-oh-**trex**-ate
(Ledertrexate [AUS], Methoblastin [AUS], Rheumatrex)

CATEGORY AND SCHEDULE

Pregnancy Risk Category: D (X for psoriasis or rheumatoid arthritis pts)

MECHANISM OF ACTION

An antimetabolite that competes with enzymes necessary to reduce folic acid to tetrahydrofolic acid, a component essential to DNA, RNA, and protein synthesis. ***Therapeutic Effect:*** Inhibits DNA, RNA, and protein synthesis.

PHARMACOKINETICS

Variably absorbed from the GI tract. Completely absorbed after IM administration. Protein binding: 50%–60%. Widely distributed. Metabolized in liver, intracellularly. Primarily excreted in urine. Removed by hemodialysis; not removed by peritoneal dialysis. ***Half-Life:*** 8–12 hrs (large doses: 8–15 hrs).

AVAILABILITY

Tablets: 2.5 mg, 5 mg, 7.5 mg, 10 mg, 15 mg.
Powder for Injection: 20 mg, 1 g.
Injection: 25 mg/mL.
Injection (preservative-free): 25 mg/mL.

INDICATIONS AND DOSAGES

Refer to individual protocols.

▸ **Juvenile rheumatoid arthritis**

PO/IM/SC

Children. 5–15 mg/m^2/wk as a single dose or in 3 divided doses given 12 hrs apart.

▸ **Antineoplastic dosage for children**
PO/IM
Children. 7.5–30 mg/m²/wk or q2wks.
IV
Children. 10 to 33,000 mg/m² bolus or continuous infusion over 6–42 hrs.

▸ **Pediatric solid tumors**
Children older than 12 yrs. 8 g/m². Maximum: 18 g.
Children younger than 12 yrs. 12 g/m². Maximum 18 g.

▸ **CNS leukemia**
INTRATHECAL
Children. 10–15 mg/m² at 2- to 5-day intervals until cerebrospinal fluid counts return to normal, then one dose weekly for 2 wks, then monthly doses. Maximum: 15 mg.

▸ **Acute lymphoblastic leukemia high-dose regimen**
IV
Children. Loading dose of 200 mg/m², then 1,200 mg/m²/day as a continuous infusion for 24 hrs.

▸ **Dosing in renal impairment**

Creatinine Clearance	Dosage Interval
61–80 mL/min	Decrease dose by 25%
51–60 mL/min	Decrease dose by 33%
10–50 mL/min	Decrease dose by 50%–70%

UNLABELED USES
Treatment of acute myelocytic leukemia, bladder, cervical, ovarian, prostatic, renal, and testicular carcinoma, psoriatic arthritis, systemic dermatomyositis.

CONTRAINDICATIONS
Hypersensitivity to methotrexate or any related component. Preexisting bone marrow suppression, severe liver or renal impairment.

INTERACTIONS
Drug
Asparaginase: May decrease the effects of methotrexate.
Bone marrow depressants: May increase bone marrow depression.
Live virus vaccines: May potentiate virus replication, increase vaccine side effects, and decrease the patient's antibody response to vaccine.
Liver toxic medications: May increase liver toxicity.
Nonsteroidal anti-inflammatory drugs: May increase risk of methotrexate toxicity.
Parenteral acyclovir: May increase risk of neurotoxicity.
Probenecid, salicylates: May increase blood methotrexate concentration and risk of toxicity.
Herbal
None known.
Food
Alcohol: May increase risk of liver toxicity.
Dairy foods: May decrease absorption.

DIAGNOSTIC TEST EFFECTS
May increase serum uric acid and SGOT (AST) levels.

IV INCOMPATIBILITIES
Chlorpromazine (Thorazine), cytarabine, droperidol (Inapsine), gemcitabine (Gemzar), idarubicin (Idamycin), midazolam (Versed), nalbuphine (Nubain), fluorouracil, prednisolone, sodium phosphate

IV COMPATIBILITIES
Cisplatin (Platinol AQ), cyclophosphamide (Cytoxan), daunorubicin (DaunoXome), doxorubicin (Adriamycin), etoposide (VePesid), fluorouracil, granisetron (Kytril), leucovorin, mitomycin (Mutamycin), ondansetron

(Zofran), paclitaxel (Taxol), vinblastine (Velban), vincristine (Oncovin), vinorelbine (Navelbine)

SIDE EFFECTS

Frequent (10%–3%)
Nausea, vomiting, stomatitis
In pts with psoriasis, burning, erythema at psoriatic site.

Occasional (3%–1%)
Diarrhea, rash, dermatitis, pruritus, alopecia, dizziness, anorexia, malaise, headache, drowsiness, blurred vision

SERIOUS REACTIONS

! There is a high potential for various, severe toxicity development.
! GI toxicity may produce oral ulcers of mouth, gingivitis, glossitis, pharyngitis, stomatitis, enteritis, and hematemesis.
! Liver toxicity occurs more frequently with frequent, small doses than with large, intermittent doses.
! Pulmonary toxicity is characterized as interstitial pneumonitis.
! Hematologic toxicity, which may develop rapidly, resulting from marked bone marrow depression may be manifested as leukopenia, thrombocytopenia, anemia, and hemorrhage.
! Skin toxicity produces rash, pruritus, urticaria, pigmentation, photosensitivity, petechiae, ecchymosis, and pustules.
! Severe nephropathy produces azotemia, hematuria, and renal failure.

PEDIATRIC CONSIDERATIONS

Baseline Assessment

- Determine whether the patient with psoriasis or rheumatoid arthritis is pregnant before initiating methotrexate therapy because the drug has a Pregnancy Category rating of X.
- Evaluate diagnostic test results, including renal and liver function tests, Hgb and Hct levels, and platelet count, before methotrexate therapy and throughout therapy.
- Give antiemetics, if ordered, to prevent and treat nausea and vomiting.
- Know that pts should not try to conceive during methotrexate therapy; male pts should wait for a minimum of 3 mos after therapy is completed and female pts should wait for at least one ovulatory cycle after therapy is completed.
- Be aware that methotrexate may cause congenital anomalies and fetal death.
- Be aware that methotrexate is distributed in breast milk and that breast-feeding is not recommended in this patient population.
- In children, decreased liver and renal function requires caution and may require dosage adjustment.
- Assess for and maintain age-appropriate fluid intake.
- Know that exposure to chicken pox or herpes zoster should be reported immediately.

Precautions

- Use cautiously in pts with ascites, bone marrow suppression, peptic ulcer disease, pleural effusion, and ulcerative colitis.

Administration and Handling

◂ **ALERT** ▸ Because methotrexate may be carcinogenic, mutagenic, or teratogenic, handle the drug with extreme care during preparation and administration. Wear gloves when preparing solution. If powder or solution comes in contact with skin, wash immediately and thoroughly with soap and water.

• Be aware that the drug may be given IM, IV, intra-arterially, or intrathecally.

IV

• Store vials at room temperature.
• Reconstitute each 5 mg with 2 mL Sterile Water for Injection or 0.9% NaCl to provide a concentration of 2.5 mg/mL up to a maximum concentration of 25 mg/mL.
• May further dilute with D_5W or 0.9% NaCl.
• For intrathecal use, dilute with preservative-free 0.9% NaCl to provide a 1 mg/mL concentration.
• Give IV push at rate of 10 mg/min.
• Give IV infusion over 30 min to 4 hrs.

Intervention and Evaluation

• Monitor the patient's blood Hgb and Hct levels, chest radiograph results, liver and renal function tests, platelet count, serum uric acid level, urinalysis, and WBC count with differential.
• Monitor the patient for signs and symptoms of anemia, including excessive fatigue and weakness, and hematologic toxicity, including easy bruising, fever, signs of local infection, sore throat, and unusual bleeding from any site.
• Assess the patient's skin for evidence of dermatologic toxicity.
• As prescribed, administer IV fluids to keep the patient well hydrated and medication, such as bicarbonate, to alkalinize the urine.
• Avoid giving IM injections, taking rectal temperatures, and performing traumatic procedures that induce bleeding.
• Apply 5 full min of pressure to the patient's IV sites after discontinuation.

Patient/Family Teaching

• Teach the patient/family to maintain fastidious oral hygiene.
• Stress to the patient/family that the patient should not receive vaccinations and should avoid contact with crowds and those with known infection.
• Urge the patient/family to avoid alcohol and salicylates during methotrexate therapy.
• Encourage the patient/family to avoid overexposure to sun or ultraviolet light.
• Instruct the male patient in the use of contraceptive measures during therapy and for 3 mos after therapy.
• Instruct the female patient in the use of contraceptive measures during therapy and for one ovulatory cycle after therapy.
• Warn the patient/family to report if the patient experiences easy bruising, fever, signs of local infection, sore throat, and unusual bleeding from any site.
• Explain to the patient/family that alopecia is reversible, but new hair growth may have a different color or texture.
• Caution the patient/family to notify the physician if nausea and vomiting continue at home.

REFERENCES

Miller, S. & Fioravanti, J. (1997). Pediatric medications: A handbook for nurses. St. Louis: Mosby.
Taketomo, C. K., Hodding, J. H. & Kraus, D. M. (2003–2004). Pediatric dosage handbook (10th ed.). Hudson, OH: Lexi-Comp.

16 Antimitotic Agents

Paclitaxel
Vinblastine Sulfate
Vincristine Sulfate

Uses: Antimitotic agents are used to treat lymphoma, lymphosarcomas, neuroblastomas, multiple myeloma, and cancer of testes, breasts, kidneys, lungs, or ovaries.

Action: Antimitotic agents include two groups that act in different ways—vinca alkaloids and taxoids. *Vinca alkaloids,* which include vinblastine and vincristine, block mitosis during metaphase (M phase) by disrupting the assembly of microtubules (filaments that move chromosomes during cell division). This action prevents cell division. *Taxoids,* such as docetaxel and paclitaxel, act during the late G_2 phase to enhance the formation of stable microtubules, which prevents cell division.

Paclitaxel

pass-leh-**tax**-ell
(Anzatax [AUS], Onxol, Taxol)
Do not confuse with Paxil or Taxotere.

CATEGORY AND SCHEDULE

Pregnancy Risk Category: D

MECHANISM OF ACTION

An antimitotic agent in the taxoid family that promotes the assembly of microtubules and stabilizes them by preventing depolymerization. ***Therapeutic Effect:*** Inhibits mitotic cellular functions and cell replication. Blocks cells in late G_2 phase/M phase of the cell cycle.

PHARMACOKINETICS

Does not readily cross blood-brain barrier. Protein binding: 89%–98%. Metabolized in liver (active metabolites); eliminated via bile. Not removed by hemodialysis. ***Half-Life:*** Children: 4.5–17 hrs; adults: 1.3–8.6 hrs.

AVAILABILITY

Injection: 6 mg/mL (5 mL, 17 mL, 25 mL and 50 mL vials)

INDICATIONS AND DOSAGES

Refer to individual protocols.
IV INFUSION
Children. 135–250 mg/m²/dose over 1–24 hrs q3wks.

▸ **Recurrent Wilms tumor**
Children. 250–350 mg/m²/dose over 24 hrs q3wks.

▸ **Dosage in liver impairment**

Total Bilirubin	Total Dose
1.5 mg/dL or less	Less than 135 mg/m²
1.6–3 mg/dL	Less than 75 mg/m²
More than 3 mg/dL	Less than 50 mg/m²

UNLABELED USES

Treatment of adenocarcinoma of upper GI tract, head and neck cancer, hormone-refractory prostate cancer, non-Hodgkin lymphoma, small-cell lung cancer, transitional cell cancer of urothelium.

CONTRAINDICATIONS

Baseline neutropenia less than 1,500 cells/mm³, hypersensitivity to paclitaxel or drugs developed with Cremophor EL (polyoxyethylated castor oil).

INTERACTIONS

Drug

Bone marrow depressants: May increase bone marrow depression.
Live virus vaccines: May potentiate virus replication, increase vaccine side effects, and decrease the patient's antibody response to vaccine virus.

Herbal

None known.

Food

None known.

DIAGNOSTIC TEST EFFECTS

May elevate serum alkaline phosphatase, serum bilirubin, SGOT (AST), and SGPT (ALT) levels. Decreases blood Hgb and Hct levels, and platelet, RBC, and WBC counts.

IV INCOMPATIBILITIES

Amphotericin B complex (Abelcet, AmBisome, Amphotec), chlorpromazine (Thorazine), doxorubicin liposome (Doxil), hydroxyzine (Vistaril), methylprednisolone (Solu-Medrol), mitoxantrone (Novantrone)

IV COMPATIBILITIES

Carboplatin (Paraplatin), cisplatin (Platinol AQ), cyclophosphamide (Cytoxan), cytarabine (Cytosar), dacarbazine (DTIC-Dome), dexamethasone (Decadron), diphenhydramine (Benadryl), doxorubicin (Adriamycin), etoposide (VePesid), gemcitabine (Gemzar), granisetron (Kytril), hydromorphone (Dilaudid), magnesium sulfate, mannitol, methotrexate, morphine, ondansetron (Zofran), potassium chloride, vinblastine (Velban), vincristine (Oncovin)

SIDE EFFECTS

Expected (90%–70%)
Diarrhea, alopecia, nausea, vomiting

Frequent (48%–46%)
Myalgia or arthralgia, peripheral neuropathy

Occasional (20%–13%)
Mucositis, hypotension during infusion, pain or redness at injection site

Rare (3%)
Bradycardia

SERIOUS REACTIONS

! Neutropenic nadir occurs at the median of 11 days.
! Anemia and leukopenia occur commonly.
! Thrombocytopenia occurs occasionally.
! A severe hypersensitivity reaction, including dyspnea, severe hypotension, angioedema, and generalized urticaria, occurs rarely.

PEDIATRIC CONSIDERATIONS

Baseline Assessment

- Offer emotional support to the patient and family.
- Use strict asepsis and protect the patient from infection.
- Assess the patient's blood counts, particularly neutrophil and platelet counts, before each course of paclitaxel therapy or as clinically indicated.
- Be aware that paclitaxel may produce fetal harm, and it is unknown whether paclitaxel is distributed in breast milk. Paclitaxel use should be avoided during pregnancy.
- Be aware that the safety and efficacy of paclitaxel have not been

established in children younger than 8 yrs of age.
• Assess for and maintain age-appropriate fluid intake.

Precautions

• Use cautiously in pts with liver impairment, peripheral neuropathy, and severe neutropenia.

Administration and Handling

◂ **ALERT** ▸ Pretreat the patient with corticosteroids, diphenhydramine, and H_2 antagonists, as prescribed.
◂ **ALERT** ▸ Wear gloves during handling of the drug; if contact with skin occurs, wash hands thoroughly with soap and water. If drug comes in contact with mucous membranes, flush with water.

IV

• Refrigerate unopened vials.
• Reconstituted solution is stable at room temperature for up to 24 hrs.
• Store diluted solutions in bottles or plastic bags and administer through polyethylene-lined administration sets. Avoid storing diluted solutions in plasticized PVC equipment or devices.
• Dilute with 0.9% NaCl or D_5W to final concentration of 0.3–1.2 mg/mL.
• Administer at rate as ordered by physician through in-line filter not greater than 0.22 μ.
• Monitor the patient's vital signs during infusion, especially during the first hour.
• Discontinue paclitaxel administration, and notify the physician if the patient experiences severe hypersensitivity reaction.

Intervention and Evaluation

• Monitor the patient's complete blood count, liver enzyme levels, platelet count, and vital signs.
• Monitor the patient for signs and symptoms of anemia, including excessive fatigue and weakness, and hematologic toxicity, including easy bruising, fever, signs of local infection, sore throat, and unusual bleeding.
• Assess the patient's response to medication. Monitor the patient for and report diarrhea.
• Avoid giving the patient IM injections or rectal medications or causing other trauma that may induce bleeding.
• Put pressure to the patient's injection sites for a full 5 min.

Patient/Family Teaching

• Explain to the patient/family that alopecia is reversible, but new hair may have a different color or texture.
• Stress to the patient/family that the patient should not receive vaccinations and should avoid contact with crowds and those with known infection.
• Warn the patient/family to immediately notify the physician if the patient experiences signs of infection, including fever and flu-like symptoms.
• Caution the patient/family to notify the physician if nausea and vomiting continue at home.
• Teach the patient/family to recognize the signs and symptoms of peripheral neuropathy.
• Warn the patient/family to avoid pregnancy during paclitaxel therapy. Teach the patient about various contraception methods.

Vinblastine Sulfate

vin-**blass**-teen
(Velbe [CAN])
Do not confuse with vincristine or vinorelbine.

CATEGORY AND SCHEDULE

Pregnancy Risk Category: D

MECHANISM OF ACTION

A vinca alkaloid and antineoplastic agent that binds to microtubular protein of the mitotic spindle. ***Therapeutic Effect:*** Causes metaphase arrest. Inhibits cellular division.

PHARMACOKINETICS

Does not cross blood-brain barrier. Protein binding: 75%. Metabolized in liver to the active metabolite. Primarily eliminated in feces via biliary system. ***Half-Life:*** 24.8 hrs.

AVAILABILITY

Powder for Injection: 10 mg.
Injection: 1 mg/mL.

INDICATIONS AND DOSAGES

Refer to individual protocols.

▸ **Advanced carcinoma of testis, advanced stage of mycosis fungoides, breast carcinoma, choriocarcinoma, disseminated Hodgkin disease, Kaposi sarcoma, Letterer-Siwe disease, non-Hodgkin lymphoma**

IV

Children. 2.5–6 mg/mg^2/day one time every 1–2 wks for 3–6 wks. Maximum weekly dose: 12.5 mg/m^2.

▸ **Histiocytosis**

IV

Children. 0.4 mg/kg one time every 7–10 days.

▸ **Germ cell tumor**

IV

Children. 0.2 mg/kg on days 1 and 2 of regimen cycle every 3 wks for 4 cycles.

Dose adjustment for hepatic impairment: Direct serum bilirubin level greater than 3 mg/dL: Decrease dose by 50%.

UNLABELED USES

Treatment of carcinoma of bladder, head and neck, kidneys, lungs, chronic myelocytic leukemia, germ cell ovarian tumors, neuroblastoma.

CONTRAINDICATIONS

Hypersensitivity to vinblastine or related agents. Bacterial infection, severe leukopenia, significant granulocytopenia unless a result of disease being treated.

INTERACTIONS

Drug

Antigout medications: May decrease the effects of these drugs.
Bone marrow depressants: May increase bone marrow depression.
Live virus vaccines: May potentiate virus replication, increase vaccine side effects, and decrease the patient's antibody response to vaccine.
Mitomycin: Severe bronchospasm and shortness of breath.
Phenytoin: May decrease serum phenytoin concentrations.

Herbal

None known.

Food

None known.

DIAGNOSTIC TEST EFFECTS

May increase serum uric acid levels.

IV INCOMPATIBILITIES

Cefepime (Maxipime), furosemide (Lasix)

IV COMPATIBILITIES

Allopurinol (Aloprim), cisplatin (Platinol AQ), cyclophosphamide (Cytoxan), doxorubicin (Adriamycin), etoposide (VePesid), fluorouracil, gemcitabine (Gemzar), granisetron (Kytril), heparin, leucovorin, methotrexate, ondansetron (Zofran), paclitaxel (Taxol), vinorelbine (Navelbine)

SIDE EFFECTS

Frequent

Nausea, vomiting, alopecia

Occasional

Constipation or diarrhea, rectal bleeding, paresthesia, headache, malaise, weakness, dizziness, pain at tumor site, jaw or face pain, mental depression, dry mouth GI distress, headache, paresthesia (occurs 4–6 hrs after administration, persists for 2–10 hrs)

Rare

Dermatitis, stomatitis, phototoxicity, hyperuricemia

SERIOUS REACTIONS

! Hematologic toxicity manifested most commonly as leukopenia and less frequently as anemia may occur. The WBC count falls to its lowest point 4–10 days after initial therapy with recovery within another 7–14 days. High vinblastine dosages may require a 21-day recovery period.

! Thrombocytopenia is usually slight and transient, with rapid recovery within few days.

! Liver insufficiency may increase the risk of toxicity.

! Acute shortness of breath or bronchospasm may occur, particularly when vinblastine is administered concurrently with mitomycin.

PEDIATRIC CONSIDERATIONS

Baseline Assessment

- Give antiemetics, if ordered, to control nausea and vomiting. Be aware that usually these side effects are easily controlled by antiemetics.
- Expect to discontinue therapy if WBC and thrombocyte counts fall abruptly. However, be aware that the physician may continue the drug if it is clearly destroying tumor cells in bone marrow.
- Expect to obtain a complete blood count weekly or before each vinblastine dosing.
- Know that vinblastine use should be avoided during pregnancy, if possible, and especially in the first trimester. Breast-feeding is not recommended in this patient population.
- Do not give vinblastine to children who potentially have active infections such as chicken pox or herpes zoster.
- Assess for and maintain age-appropriate fluid intake.

Precautions

- Use cautiously in pts with liver function impairment, neurotoxicity, and recent exposure to radiation therapy or chemotherapy.

Administration and Handling

◂ **ALERT** ▸ Know that vinblastine dosage is individualized based on the patient's clinical response and tolerance of the drug's adverse effects. When used in combination therapy, consult specific protocols for optimum dosage and sequence of drug administration. Reduce dosage if serum bilirubin is greater than 3 mg/dL. Repeat dosage at intervals of no less than 7 days and if the WBC count is at least 4,000/mm^3.

◂ **ALERT** ▸ Because vinblastine may be carcinogenic, mutagenic, or teratogenic, handle the drug with extreme care during preparation and administration. Give by IV injection. Leakage from IV site into surrounding tissue may produce extreme irritation. Avoid eye contact with solution because severe eye irritation and possible corneal ulceration may result. If eye contact occurs, immediately irrigate eye with water.

◂ **ALERT** ▸ Do not remove protective overwrap from the vial until the moment of injection. Must be protected from light. *Do not* administer intrathecally.

IV

- Refrigerate unopened vials.
- Solutions normally appears clear, colorless.
- After reconstitution, solution is stable for up to 30 days if refrigerated.
- Discard if precipitate forms or discoloration occurs.
- Reconstitute 10-mg vial with 10 mL 0.9% NaCl preserved with phenol or benzyl alcohol to provide concentration of 1 mg/mL.
- Inject into tubing of running IV infusion or directly into vein over 1 min.
- Do not inject into an extremity with impaired or potentially impaired circulation caused by compression or invading neoplasm, phlebitis, or varicosity.
- After completing administration directly into a vein, withdraw a minute amount of venous blood before withdrawing the needle to minimize the possibility of extravasation.
- Be aware that extravasation may result in cellulitis and phlebitis and that a large amount of extravasation may result in tissue sloughing. If extravasation occurs, give a local injection of hyaluronidase, if ordered, and apply warm compresses to the affected area.

Intervention and Evaluation

- Assess the patient diligently for signs and symptoms of infection if his or her WBC count falls below 2,000/mm^3.
- Assess the patient for signs and symptoms of stomatitis, including burning or erythema of the oral mucosa at the inner margin of lips, difficulty swallowing, oral ulceration, and sore throat.
- Monitor the patient for signs and symptoms of anemia, including excessive fatigue and weakness, and hematologic toxicity, including easy bruising, fever, signs of local infection, sore throat, and unusual bleeding from any site.
- Assess the patient's pattern of daily bowel activity and stool consistency. Practice measures to prevent the patient from becoming constipated.
- Maintain adequate hydration.
- Vinblastine may be given with allopurinol to prevent uric acid nephropathy.

Patient/Family Teaching

- Warn the patient/family to immediately notify the physician if the patient experiences any pain or burning at injection site during administration.
- Advise the patient/family that pain at the tumor site may occur during or shortly after vinblastine injection.
- Stress to the patient/family that the patient should not receive vaccinations and should avoid contact with crowds and those with known infection.
- Caution the patient/family to promptly notify the physician if the patient experiences easy bruising, fever, signs of local infection, sore throat, or unusual bleeding from any site.
- Explain to the patient/family that alopecia is reversible, but new hair growth may have a different color or texture.
- Instruct the patient/family to notify the physician if nausea and vomiting continue at home.
- Urge the patient/family increase the patient's fluid intake and bulk in diet, as well as exercise as tolerated, to avoid constipation.

• Caution patient/family to avoid exposure to sunlight. The patient should wear protective clothing and a broad-spectrum sunscreen because this drug may cause photosensitivity reactions.

Vincristine Sulfate

vin-**cris**-teen
(Vincasar PFS)
Do not confuse with Ancobon or vinblastine.

CATEGORY AND SCHEDULE

Pregnancy Risk Category: D

MECHANISM OF ACTION

A vinca alkaloid and antineoplastic agent that binds to microtubular protein of the mitotic spindle. ***Therapeutic Effect:*** Causes metaphase arrest. Inhibits cellular division.

PHARMACOKINETICS

Does not cross blood-brain barrier. Protein binding: 75%. Metabolized in liver. Primarily eliminated in feces via biliary system. ***Half-Life:*** 10–37 hrs.

AVAILABILITY

Injection: 1 mg/mL.

INDICATIONS AND DOSAGES

Refer to individual protocols.

▸ **Treatment of acute leukemia, advanced non-Hodgkin lymphomas, disseminated Hodgkin disease, neuroblastoma, rhabdomyosarcoma, Wilms tumor (administer at weekly intervals)**

IV

Children. 1–2 mg/m^2. Maximum single dose: 2 mg.

Children weighing less than 10 kg or with a body surface area less than 1 m^2. 0.05 mg/kg. Maximum single dose: 2 mg.

▸ **Liver function impairment**

Reduce dosage by 50% in pts with a direct serum bilirubin concentration greater than 3 mg/dL.

UNLABELED USES

Treatment of breast, cervical, colorectal, lung, and ovarian carcinoma, chronic lymphocytic, germ cell ovarian tumors, idiopathic thrombocytopenia purpura, malignant melanoma, multiple myeloma, mycosis fungoides, myelocytic leukemia.

CONTRAINDICATIONS

Hypersensitivity to vincristine. Pts receiving radiation therapy through ports that include the liver.

INTERACTIONS

Drug

Asparaginase, neurotoxic medications: May increase the risk of neurotoxicity.
Antigout medications: May decrease the effects of these drugs.
Doxorubicin: May increase myelosuppression.
Live virus vaccines: May potentiate virus replication, increase vaccine side effects, and decrease the patient's antibody response to vaccine.
Mitomycin C: Acute pulmonary reactions may occur.
Itraconazole: Increased risk of neuromuscular side effects.

Herbal

None known.

Food

None known.

DIAGNOSTIC TEST EFFECTS

May increase serum uric acid levels.

IV INCOMPATIBILITIES

Cefepime (Maxipime), furosemide (Lasix), idarubicin (Idamycin)

IV COMPATIBILITIES

Allopurinol (Aloprim), cisplatin (Platinol AQ), cyclophosphamide (Cytoxan), cytarabine (Ara-C, Cytosar), doxorubicin (Adriamycin), etoposide (VePesid), fluorouracil, gemcitabine (Gemzar), granisetron (Kytril), leucovorin, methotrexate, ondansetron (Zofran), paclitaxel (Taxol), vinorelbine (Navelbine)

SIDE EFFECTS

Expected

Peripheral neuropathy occurs in nearly every patient. Its first clinical sign is depression of the Achilles tendon reflex.

Frequent

Peripheral paresthesia, alopecia, constipation or obstipation (upper colon impaction with empty rectum), abdominal cramps, headache, jaw pain, hoarseness, double vision, ptosis or drooping of eyelid, urinary tract disturbances

Occasional

Nausea, vomiting, diarrhea, abdominal distention, stomatitis, fever

Rare

Mild leukopenia, mild anemia, thrombocytopenia

SERIOUS REACTIONS

! Acute shortness of breath and bronchospasm may occur, especially when vincristine is used in combination with mitomycin.

! Prolonged or high-dose therapy may produce foot or wrist drop, difficulty walking, slapping gait, ataxia, and muscle wasting.

! Acute uric acid nephropathy may be noted.

PEDIATRIC CONSIDERATIONS

Baseline Assessment

- Monitor the patient's hematologic status, liver and renal function tests, and serum uric acid levels.
- Assess the patient's Achilles tendon reflex for evidence of peripheral neuropathy.
- Assess the patient's pattern of daily bowel activity and stool consistency.
- Monitor the patient for development of blurred vision or ptosis.
- Evaluate the patient's urine output for changes.
- Be aware that vincristine use should be avoided during pregnancy, especially in the first trimester because it may cause fetal harm. Breast-feeding is not recommended in this patient population.
- Be sure and maintain IV patency because the medication is a strong vesicant.
- Assess for and maintain age-appropriate fluid intake.

Precautions

- Use cautiously in pts with liver function impairment, neurotoxicity, and preexisting neuromuscular disease.

Administration and Handling

◂ **ALERT** ▸ Know that vincristine dosage is individualized based on the patient's clinical response and tolerance of the drug's adverse effects. When used in combination therapy, consult specific protocols for optimum dosage and sequence of drug administration.

◂ **ALERT** ▸ Because vincristine may be carcinogenic, mutagenic, or teratogenic, handle the drug with extreme care during preparation and administration. Give by IV injection. Use extreme caution in calculating and administering vincristine, and know that overdose may result in serious or fatal outcomes.

◂ **ALERT** ▸ Do not remove protective overwrap until the moment of injection. Vincristine is fatal if given intrathecally.

• Do not administer intrathecally, SC, or IM.

IV

• Refrigerate unopened vials.
• Solutions normally appears clear, colorless.
• Discard if precipitate forms or discoloration occurs.
• May give undiluted.
• Inject dose into tubing of running IV infusion or directly into the vein over more than 1 min.
• Do not inject vincristine into an extremity with impaired or potentially impaired circulation caused by compression or an invading neoplasm, phlebitis, or varicosity.
• Be aware that extravasation produces burning, edema, and stinging at the injection site. If this occurs, terminate injection immediately, notify the physician, locally inject hyaluronidase, if ordered, and apply heat to the affected area to disperse vincristine and minimize cellulitis and discomfort.
• May be administered with allopurinol to prevent uric acid nephropathy.

Patient/Family Teaching

• Warn the patient/family to immediately notify the physician of any pain or burning at the injection site occurs during administration.
• Explain to the patient/family that alopecia is reversible, but new hair growth may have a different color and texture.
• Caution the patient/family to notify the physician if nausea and vomiting continue at home.
• Teach the patient/family to recognize the signs of peripheral neuropathy.
• Warn the patient/family to notify the physician if the patient experiences easy bruising, fever, signs of infection, sore throat, shortness of breath, or unusual bleeding for any site.

REFERENCES

Miller, S. & Fioravanti, J. (1997). Pediatric medications: a handbook for nurses. St. Louis: Mosby.
Taketomo, C. K., Hodding, J. H. & Kraus, D. M. (2003–2004). Pediatric dosage handbook (10th ed.). Hudson, OH: Lexi-Comp.

17 Cytoprotective Agents

Dexrazoxane
Mesna

Uses: During antineoplastic therapy, specific cytoprotective agents are used to help prevent or reduce the severity of specific adverse reactions. *Dexrazoxane* reduces the risk of cardiomyopathy related to doxorubicin therapy. *Mesna* protects against hemorrhagic cystitis, which may result from cyclophosphamide or ifosfamide.

Action: Each cytoprotective agent works by a different action. In myocardial cell membranes, *dexrazoxane* binds with intracellular iron, preventing the generation of free radicals by the anthracycline doxorubicin. *Mesna* binds with and detoxifies the urotoxic metabolites of cyclophosphamide and ifosfamide.

Dexrazoxane

dex-rah-**zox**-ann
(Zinecard)

CATEGORY AND SCHEDULE

Pregnancy Risk Category: C

MECHANISM OF ACTION

A cytoprotective antineoplastic adjunct that rapidly penetrates the myocardial cell membrane. Binds intracellular iron and prevents generation of oxygen free radicals by anthracyclines (doxorubicin and daunorubicin), which may be responsible for anthracycline-induced cardiomyopathy. ***Therapeutic Effect:*** Protects against anthracycline-induced cardiomyopathy.

PHARMACOKINETICS

Rapidly distributed after IV administration. Not bound to plasma proteins. Primarily excreted in urine. Removed by peritoneal dialysis. ***Half-Life:*** 2–3 hrs.

AVAILABILITY

Powder for Injection: 250 mg (10 mg/mL reconstituted in 25 mL single-use vial), 500 mg (10 mg/mL reconstituted in 50-mL single-use vial).

INDICATIONS AND DOSAGES

Refer to individual protocols.

▸ **Reduction of incidence and severity of cardiomyopathy associated with doxorubicin therapy**

IV

Children. Recommended dosage ratio of dexrazoxane to doxorubicin is 10:1 (e.g., 500 mg/m^2 dexrazoxane, 50 mg/m^2 doxorubicin).

CONTRAINDICATIONS

Hypersensitivity to dexrazoxane. Chemotherapy regimens that do not contain an anthracycline.

INTERACTIONS

Drug

Concurrent FAC therapy (fluorouracil, Adriamycin, cyclophosphamide): May produce severe blood dyscrasias.

Herbal
None known.
Food
None known.

DIAGNOSTIC TEST EFFECTS

Concurrent FAC therapy may produce abnormal liver or renal function test results.

IV INCOMPATIBILITIES

Do not mix with other medications.

SIDE EFFECTS

Frequent
Alopecia, nausea, vomiting, fatigue, malaise, anorexia, stomatitis, fever, infection, diarrhea
Occasional
Pain with injection, neurotoxicity, phlebitis, dysphagia, streaking, or erythema
Rare
Urticaria, skin reaction

SERIOUS REACTIONS

! FAC therapy with dexrazoxane may produce more severe leukopenia, granulocytopenia, and thrombocytopenia than FAC therapy without dexrazoxane.
! Dexrazoxane overdosage can be removed with peritoneal dialysis or hemodialysis.

PEDIATRIC CONSIDERATIONS

Baseline Assessment
• Give antiemetics, if ordered, to prevent and treat nausea.
• Be aware that dexrazoxane may be embryotoxic or teratogenic, and it is unknown whether dexrazoxane is distributed in breast milk. Breast-feeding is not recommended in this patient population.
• The safety and efficacy of dexrazoxane have not been established in children.
• Assess for and maintain appropriate age-related fluid intake.
Precautions
• Use cautiously in pts taking chemotherapeutic agents that increase the risk of myelosuppression or those also receiving FAC therapy.
Administration and Handling
◂ **ALERT** ▸ Be aware that dexrazoxane should be used only in those pts who have received a cumulative doxorubicin dose of 300 mg/m^2 and are continuing with doxorubicin therapy.
◂ **ALERT** ▸ Do not mix dexrazoxane with other drugs. Use caution and wear gloves during the handling and preparation of reconstituted solution. If powder or solution comes in contact with skin, wash immediately with soap and water.
◂ **ALERT** ▸ Dexrazoxane should be handled, prepared, and disposed of as an antineoplastic agent.
IV
• Store vials at room temperature.
• Reconstituted solution is stable for up to 6 hrs at room temperature or if refrigerated. Discard unused solution.
• Reconstitute with 0.167 M (M/6) sodium lactate injection to give a concentration of 10 mg dexrazoxane for each mL of sodium lactate.
• May further dilute with 0.9% NaCl or D_5W. Concentration should range from 1.3 to 5 mg/mL.
• Give reconstituted solution by slow IV push or IV infusion over 15–30 min.
• After infusion is completed and before a total elapsed time of 30 min from the beginning of dexrazoxane infusion, give an IV injection of doxorubicin.

Intervention and Evaluation

• Frequently monitor the patient's blood counts for evidence of blood dyscrasias.
• Monitor the patient for signs and symptoms of stomatitis, including burning or erythema of oral mucosa at the inner margin of the lips, difficulty swallowing, and sore throat.
• Monitor the patient's cardiac function, hematologic status, and liver and renal function studies.
• Assess the patient's pattern of daily bowel activity and stool consistency.
• Monitor the patient for signs and symptoms of hematologic toxicity, including easy bruising, fever, signs of local infection, sore throat, and unusual bleeding from any site.

Patient/Family Teaching

• Explain to the patient/family that alopecia is reversible, but new hair growth may have a different color or texture. Tell the patient that new hair growth resumes 2–3 mos after the last dexrazoxane therapy dose.
• Teach the patient/family to maintain fastidious oral hygiene.
• Warn the patient/family to notify the physician if the patient experiences fever, signs of local infection, or sore throat.
• Caution the patient/family to notify the physician if nausea and vomiting persist at home.

Mesna

mess-nah
(Mesnex, Uromitexan [CAN])

CATEGORY AND SCHEDULE

Pregnancy Risk Category: B

MECHANISM OF ACTION

A cytoprotective agent and antineoplastic adjunct that binds with and detoxifies urotoxic metabolites of ifosfamide and cyclophosphamide. ***Therapeutic Effect:*** Inhibits ifosfamide- and cyclophosphamide-induced hemorrhagic cystitis.

PHARMACOKINETICS

Rapidly metabolized after IV administration to mesna disulfide, which is reduced to mesna in kidney. Excreted in urine. ***Half-Life:*** 24 min.

AVAILABILITY

Injection: 100 mg/mL.
Tablets: 400 mg.

INDICATIONS AND DOSAGES

Refer to individual protocols.
IV
Children. IV fractionated dosing of IV bolus infusions equal to the complete dose of ifosfamide. This dose needs to be administered 15 min before administration of ifosfamide, then administered after 2–3 additional doses at given hours.

▸ **To prevent hemorrhagic cystitis in patients receiving ifosfamide**
IV
Children. 20% of ifosfamide dose at time of ifosfamide administration and 4 and 8 hrs after each dose of ifosfamide. Total: 60% of ifosfamide dosage.

▸ **To prevent hemorrhagic cystitis in patients receiving cyclophosphamide**
IV
Children. 20% of cyclophosphamide dose at time of cyclophosphamide administration and q3h for 3–4 doses.
PO
Children. 40% of antineoplastic agent dose in 3 doses at 4-hr intervals.

CONTRAINDICATIONS

Hypersensitivity to mesna or other thiol agents.

INTERACTIONS

Drug

None known.

Herbal

None known.

Food

None known.

DIAGNOSTIC TEST EFFECTS

May produce false-positive test results for urinary ketones.

IV INCOMPATIBILITIES

Amphotericin B complex (Abelcet, AmBisome, Amphotec)

IV COMPATIBILITIES

Allopurinol (Aloprim), docetaxel (Taxotere), doxorubicin (Adriamycin), etoposide (VP-16, VePesid), gemcitabine (Gemzar), granisetron (Kytril), methotrexate, ondansetron (Zofran), paclitaxel (Taxol), vinorelbine (Navelbine)

SIDE EFFECTS

Frequent (more than 17%)

Bad taste in mouth, soft stools
Large doses: Diarrhea, limb pain, headache, fatigue, nausea, hypotension, allergic reaction

SERIOUS REACTIONS

! Hematuria occurs rarely.

PEDIATRIC CONSIDERATIONS

Baseline Assessment

- Administer each mesna dose with ifosfamide, as prescribed.
- Be aware that it is unknown whether mesna crosses placenta or is distributed in breast milk.
- Be aware that the safety and efficacy of mesna have not been established in children.
- Assess for and maintain age-appropriate fluid intake.
- Assess for and monitor ketones and glucose in urine.

Administration and Handling

PO

- Dilute mesna solution before oral administration to decrease sulfur odor. If desired, dilute in carbonated cola drinks, fruit juices, or milk.

IV

- Store parenteral form at room temperature.
- After reconstitution, the solution is stable up to 24 hrs at room temperature. Recommended use is within 6 hrs. Discard unused medication.
- Dilute with D_5W or 0.9% NaCl to concentration of 1–20 mg/mL, as appropriate.
- Add to solutions containing ifosfamide or cyclophosphamide, as appropriate.
- Administer by IV infusion (piggyback) over 15–30 min or by continuous infusion.

Intervention and Evaluation

- Test the patient's morning urine specimen for hematuria. If hematuria occurs, mesna dosage reduction or discontinuation may be necessary.
- Assess the patient's pattern of daily bowel activity and stool consistency. Record time of evacuation.
- Monitor the patient's blood pressure for hypotension.
- It is absolutely important that all ordered doses are given on time as ordered. Failure to do so may lead to prolonged toxicity.

Patient/Family Teaching

- Warn the patient/family to notify the physician or nurse if the patient experiences headache, limb pain, or nausea.

• Encourage the patient/family to be sure to take all doses of mesna and drink adequate fluids before and after chemotherapy.

REFERENCES

Miller, S. & Fioravanti, J. (1997). Pediatric medications: a handbook for nurses. St. Louis: Mosby.

Taketomo, C. K., Hodding, J. H. & Kraus, D. M. (2003–2004). Pediatric dosage handbook (10th ed.). Hudson, OH: Lexi-Comp.

18 Hormones

Leuprolide Acetate	**Uses:** In antineoplastic therapy, hormones are used to treat cancers and precocious puberty. Antineoplastic hormones are less toxic than other antineoplastic agents. **Action:** Antineoplastic hormones may act as agonists that inhibit tumor cell growth or as antagonists that compete with endogenous hormones. These agents include *gonadotropin-releasing hormone analogues,* such as leuprolide. Specifically, antiestrogens compete with endogenous estrogen and estrogen-receptor binding sites. Gonadotropin-releasing hormone analogues stimulate the release of luteinizing hormone (LH) and follicle-stimulating hormone (FSH) from the anterior pituitary gland.

Leuprolide Acetate

leu-pro-lied
(Eligard, Lucrin [AUS], Lupron, Lupron Depot-Ped, Viadur)
Do not confuse with Lopurin or Nuprin.

CATEGORY AND SCHEDULE
Pregnancy Risk Category: X

MECHANISM OF ACTION
A gonadotropin-releasing hormone analogue and antineoplastic agent whose initial or intermittent administration stimulates release of LH and FSH from anterior pituitary, increasing testosterone level in males. Continuous daily administration suppresses secretion of gonadotropin-releasing hormone. ***Therapeutic Effect:*** In central precocious puberty, gonadotropins reduced to prepubertal levels.

PHARMACOKINETICS
Rapidly, well absorbed after subcutaneous administration. Slow absorption after IM administration. Protein binding: 43%–49%. ***Half-Life:*** 3–4 hrs.

AVAILABILITY
Implant: 65 mg (Viadur).
Injection solution: 5 mg/mL (Lupron).
Injection Depot Formulation: 3.75 mg (Lupron Depot), 7.5 mg (Eligard), 7.5 mg (Lupron Depot), 7.5 mg, 22.5 mg, 30 mg, (Lupron Depot-Ped), 11.25 mg (Lupron Depot monthly), 11.25 mg (Lupron Depot-Ped), 15 mg (Lupron Depot-Ped), 22.5 mg (Lupron Depot monthly), 30 mg (Lupron Depot monthly).

INDICATIONS AND DOSAGES
▸ **Central precocious puberty**
SUBCUTANEOUS
Children. Initially, 35–50 mcg/kg/day; if down regulation is not achieved, titrate upward by 10 mcg/kg/day.
IM
Children. Initially, 0.15–0.3 mg/kg/4 wks (minimum: 7.5 mg); if

down regulation is not achieved, titrate upward in 3.75-mg increments q4wks.

CONTRAINDICATIONS

Hypersensitivity to leuprolide, gonadotropin-releasing hormone, or agonist analogs. Pernicious anemia and pregnancy.

INTERACTIONS

Drug

None known.

Herbal

None known.

Food

None known.

DIAGNOSTIC TEST EFFECTS

May increase serum acid phosphatase levels. Initially increases and then decreases testosterone concentration.

SIDE EFFECTS

Frequent

Hot flashes (ranging from mild flushing to diaphoresis)
Females: Amenorrhea, spotting

Occasional

Arrhythmias, palpitations, blurred vision, dizziness, edema, headache, burning or itching, swelling at injection site, nausea, insomnia, increased weight
Females: Deepening voice, increased hair growth, decreased libido, increased breast tenderness, vaginitis, altered mood
Males: Constipation, decreased testicle size, gynecomastia, impotence, decreased appetite, angina

Rare

Males: Thrombophlebitis

SERIOUS REACTIONS

! Increased bone pain and less frequently dysuria or hematuria, weakness, or paresthesia of the lower extremities may be noted.
! Myocardial infarction and pulmonary embolism occur rarely.

PEDIATRIC CONSIDERATIONS

Baseline Assessment

• Determine whether the patient is pregnant before initiating leuprolide therapy.
• Expect to obtain serum testosterone and prostatic acid phosphatase (PAP) levels periodically during leuprolide therapy. Be aware that serum testosterone and PAP levels should increase during the first week of therapy. The testosterone level then should decrease to the baseline level or less within 2 wks, PAP level within 4 wks.
• Be aware that depot use is contraindicated in pregnancy. The depot form may cause spontaneous abortion.
• Be aware that the long-term safety of leuprolide has not been established in children.
• Be aware that during the first several months of therapy, females may experience spotting or menses.

Precautions

• Use cautiously in children for long-term use.

Administration and Handling

◀ALERT▶ Because leuprolide may be carcinogenic, mutagenic, or teratogenic, handle with extreme care during preparation and administration.

SC
• Solution normally appears clear, colorless.
• Refrigerate.
• Store opened vial at room temperature.
• Discard if precipitate forms or solution appears discolored.

- Store Depot vials at room temperature. Reconstitute only with diluent provided; use immediately. Do not use needles less than 22 gauge.
- Use syringes provided by manufacturer or use a 0.5-mL low-dose insulin syringe as an alternative.

Intervention and Evaluation

- Monitor the patient for arrhythmias and palpitations.
- Assess the patient for peripheral edema behind the medial malleolus or in the sacral area in bedridden patients.
- Evaluate the patient's sleep pattern.
- Monitor the patient for visual difficulties.
- Assist the patient with ambulation if dizziness occurs.
- Offer the patient antiemetics, if ordered, to treat any nausea and vomiting he or she experiences.

Patient/Family Teaching

- Advise the patient/family that hot flashes tend to decrease in frequency during continued leuprolide therapy.
- Explain to the patient/family that a temporary exacerbation of signs and symptoms of the disease may occur during the first few weeks of leuprolide therapy.
- Encourage the patient to use contraceptive measures during leuprolide therapy.
- Warn the patient/family to notify the physician if regular menstruation persists or if the patient becomes pregnant.

REFERENCES

Miller, S. & Fioravanti, J. (1997). Pediatric medications: a handbook for nurses. St. Louis: Mosby.

19 Monoclonal Antibodies

Imatinib Mesylate

Uses: Imatinib mesylate monoclonal antibody is used to treat B-cell chronic lymphocytic leukemia.

Action: Although their exact mechanism of action is unknown, monoclonal antibodies may act by binding to specific cell-surface antigens. The agents' cytotoxic effects may be related to T-cell–mediated recognition of the bound antibody and interference with cell proliferation.

Imatinib Mesylate

ih-**mah**-tin-ib
(Gleevec, Glivec [AUS])

CATEGORY AND SCHEDULE

Pregnancy Risk Category: D

MECHANISM OF ACTION

An antineoplastic that inhibits the Bcr-Abl tyrosine kinase, a translocation-created enzyme, created by the Philadelphia chromosome abnormality noted in chronic myeloid leukemia (CML). ***Therapeutic Effect:*** Inhibits proliferation and tumor growth during the three stages of CML, including CML in myeloid blast crisis, CML in accelerated phase, and CML in chronic phase.

PHARMACOKINETICS

Well absorbed after PO administration. Binds to plasma proteins, particularly albumin. Metabolized in the liver. Eliminated mainly in the feces as metabolites. ***Half-Life:*** 18 hrs.

AVAILABILITY

Tablets: 100 mg, 400 mg.

INDICATIONS AND DOSAGES

▸ **CML**

PO

Children. 260 mg/m^2 daily as a single daily dose or 2 divided doses.

CONTRAINDICATIONS

Known hypersensitivity to imatinib.

INTERACTIONS

Drug

Calcium channel blockers, dihydropyridine, simvastatin, triazolobenzodiazepines: Increase the blood concentration of these drugs.
Carbamazepine, dexamethasone, phenobarbital, phenytoin, rifampicin: Decrease imatinib plasma concentration.
Clarithromycin, erythromycin, itraconazole, ketoconazole: Increase imatinib plasma concentration.
Cyclosporine, pimozide: May alter the therapeutic effects of these drugs.
Warfarin: Reduces the effect of warfarin.

Herbal

St. John's wort: Decreases imatinib concentration.

Food

None known.

DIAGNOSTIC TEST EFFECTS

May increase serum bilirubin and transaminase levels. May decrease platelet count, serum potassium level, and WBC count.

SIDE EFFECTS

Frequent (68%–24%)
Nausea, diarrhea, vomiting, headache, fluid retention (periorbital, lower extremities), rash, musculoskeletal pain, muscle cramps, arthralgia
Occasional (23%–10%)
Abdominal pain, cough, myalgia, fatigue, pyrexia, anorexia, dyspepsia (heartburn, gastric upset), constipation, night sweats, pruritus
Rare (less than 10%)
Nasopharyngitis, petechiae, weakness, epistaxis

SERIOUS REACTIONS

! Severe fluid retention manifested as pleural effusion, pericardial effusion, pulmonary edema, and ascites and hepatotoxicity occur rarely.
! Neutropenia and thrombocytopenia are expected responses to the drug.
! Respiratory toxicity, manifested as dyspnea and pneumonia, may occur.

PEDIATRIC CONSIDERATIONS

Baseline Assessment

- Expect to obtain the patient's complete blood count (CBC) weekly for the first month, biweekly for the second month, and periodically thereafter.
- Monitor the patient's liver function tests, including serum alkaline phosphatase, bilirubin, and transaminase, before imatinib treatment begins and monthly thereafter.
- Be aware that imatinib has the potential for severe teratogenic effects. Female pts should avoid breast-feeding while taking this drug.
- Be aware that the safety and efficacy of imatinib have not been established in children.
- Assess and monitor for age-appropriate fluid intake.

Precautions

- Use cautiously in pts with liver or renal impairment.

Administration and Handling

PO

- Give imatinib with a meal and a large glass of water.
- For pediatric pts unable to swallow tablets, the tablets may be dispersed in a glass of water or apple juice. Place the required number of tablets in an appropriate volume of beverage (approximately 50 mL for a 100 mg tablet or 200 mL for a 400 mg tablet) and stir with a spoon. Administer the suspension immediately after complete disintegration of the tablet(s).

Intervention and Evaluation

- Assess the patient's eye area and lower extremities for early evidence of fluid retention.
- Weigh and monitor the patient for unexpected rapid weight gain.
- Administer antiemetics, if ordered, to the patient to control nausea and vomiting.
- Assess the patient's pattern of daily bowel activity and stool consistency.
- Monitor the patient's CBC for evidence of neutropenia and thrombocytopenia and liver function tests for hepatotoxicity. Duration of neutropenia and thrombocytopenia ranges from 2 to 4 wks.

Patient/Family Teaching

- Stress to the patient/family that the patient should not receive vaccinations and should avoid contact with anyone who recently received a live virus vaccine, crowds, and those with known infection.

- Instruct the patient/family to take imatinib with food and a full glass of water.

20 Miscellaneous Antineoplastic Agents

Asparaginase
Dacarbazine
Etoposide, VP-16
Interleukin-2
Mitoxantrone
Pegasparagase
Procarbazine Hydrochloride
Teniposide

Uses: Miscellaneous antineoplastic agents have a wide range of specific uses. The enzyme *asparaginase* and its derivative *pegaspargase* are used to treat acute lymphocytic leukemia; asparaginase is also given with other drugs for lymphoma. *Dacarbazine* is used for metastatic malignant melanoma and, with other drugs, for Hodgkin disease. The podophyllotoxins *etoposide* and *teniposide* are used in acute lymphocytic leukemia; etoposide is also used to treat testicular tumors, small-cell lung carcinoma, and other cancers. *Mitoxantrone* is helpful not only in leukemias and prostate cancer but also in multiple sclerosis. *Procarbazine* is used primarily to treat advanced Hodgkin disease.

Action: Because miscellaneous antineoplastic agents belong to many different subcategories, their mechanisms of action are diverse. For details, see the specific drug entries.

Asparaginase

ah-spa-**raj**-in-ace
(Elspar, Kidrolase [CAN], Leunase [AUS])

CATEGORY AND SCHEDULE

Pregnancy Risk Category: C

MECHANISM OF ACTION

Asparaginase is an enzyme that inhibits protein synthesis by deaminating asparagines, thus depriving tumor cells of this essential amino acid. ***Therapeutic Effect:*** Interferes with DNA, RNA, and protein synthesis in leukemic cells. Cell cycle–specific for the G_1 phase of cell division.

PHARMACOKINETICS

Metabolized via slow sequestration by the reticuloendothelial system. ***Half-Life:*** 39–49 hrs IM; 8–30 hrs IV.

AVAILABILITY

Powder for Injection: 10,000 units.

INDICATIONS AND DOSAGES

Refer to individual protocols

▸ **Acute lymphocytic leukemia**

IV

Children (combination therapy). 1,000 units/kg/day for 10 days.

Children (single drug therapy). 200 units/kg/day for 28 days.

IM

Children (combination therapy). 6,000–10,000 units/m²/dose 3 times/wk for 3 wks.

UNLABELED USES

Treatment of acute myelocytic leukemia, acute myelomonocytic leukemia, chronic lymphocytic leukemia, Hodgkin disease, lymphosarcoma, melanosarcoma, and reticulum cell sarcoma.

CONTRAINDICATIONS
Hypersensitivity to *Escherichia coli.* Pancreatitis.

INTERACTIONS
Drug
Antigout medications: May decrease the effect of antigout medications.
Live virus vaccines: May decrease the patient's antibody response to vaccine, increase vaccine side effects, and potentiate virus replication.
Methotrexate: May block effects of methotrexate.
Steroids, vincristine: May increase disturbances of erythropoiesis, hyperglycemia, and risk of neuropathy.
Prednisone: Increases risk of hyperglycemia.
Herbal
None known.
Food
None known.

DIAGNOSTIC TEST EFFECTS
May increase activated partial thromboplastin time, platelet count, prothrombin time, thrombin time, serum alkaline phosphatase, blood ammonia, serum bilirubin, BUN, blood glucose, serum uric acid, SGOT (AST), and SGPT (ALT) levels. May decrease blood-clotting factors, including antithrombin, plasma fibrinogen, and plasminogen, as well as blood levels of albumin, calcium, and cholesterol.

IV INCOMPATIBILITIES
None known. Consult pharmacy.

SIDE EFFECTS
Frequent
Allergic reaction, manifested as rash, urticaria, arthralgia, facial edema, hypotension, and respiratory distress; pancreatitis as evidenced by severe stomach pain with nausea and vomiting
Occasional
CNS effects, including confusion, drowsiness, depression, nervousness, and tiredness; stomatitis, as evidenced by sores in the mouth and on the lips; hypoalbuminemia or uric acid nephropathy, manifested as swelling of the feet or lower legs; hyperglycemia.
Rare
Hyperthermia, including fever or chills; thrombosis, seizures.

SERIOUS REACTIONS
! Hepatotoxicity usually occurs within 2 wks of the initial treatment.
! There is an increased risk of allergic reaction, including anaphylaxis, after repeated therapy, and severe bone marrow depression.

PEDIATRIC CONSIDERATIONS
Baseline Assessment
◂ALERT▸ Be sure to keep antihistamines, epinephrine, and an IV corticosteroid readily available as well as oxygen equipment, before administering asparaginase. May do a test dose of 2 units of asparaginase intradermally before the first dose and when more than 1 week has elapsed between doses.
• Assess baseline CNS function and expect to obtain blood chemistry analysis, complete blood count, and liver, pancreatic, and renal function tests and results before therapy begins and when longer than 1 week has elapsed between doses.
• Be aware that asparaginase use should be avoided during

pregnancy, especially during the first trimester, and in pts who are breast-feeding.

- Be aware that signs of toxicity include nausea, vomiting, and increased lipase and serum amylase levels.
- Assess for and maintain age-appropriate fluid intake.

Precautions

- Use cautiously in pts with diabetes mellitus, existing or recent chickenpox, gout, herpes zoster infection, liver or renal function impairment, or recent cytotoxic and radiation therapy.

Administration and Handling

◀ALERT▶ This drug's dosage is individualized based on clinical response and the patient's tolerance to adverse effects. When used in combination therapy, consult specific protocols for optimum drug dosage and sequence of drug administration.

◀ALERT▶ Asparaginase may be carcinogenic, mutagenic, or teratogenic. Handle with extreme care during preparation and administration. Urine should be treated as infectious waste. Asparaginase powder or solution may irritate the skin on contact. Wash the affected area for 15 min if contact occurs.

IM

- Add 2 mL 0.9% NaCl to a 10,000-international unit vial to provide a concentration of 5,000 international units/mL.
- Administer no more than 2 mL at any one site. If more than 2 mL is required, use multiple injection sites.

IV

- Refrigerate the powder for the injected form.
- Reconstituted solutions are stable for 8 hrs if refrigerated.
- Gelatinous fiber-like particles may develop in the solution. If this occurs, remove the particles using a 5-μ filter during administration.

◀ALERT▶ Administer an intradermal test dose (2 units) before beginning therapy or when longer than 1 week has elapsed between doses. Observe the patient for any appearance of erythema or of a wheal for 1 hr after drug administration.

- For a test solution reconstitute a 10,000-unit vial with 5 mL Sterile Water for Injection or 0.9% NaCl. Shake to dissolve. Withdraw 0.1 mL, inject into a vial containing 9.9 mL of the same diluent for a concentration of 20 units/mL.
- Reconstitute a 10,000-unit vial with 5 mL Sterile Water for Injection or 0.9% NaCl to provide a concentration of 2,000 units/mL.
- Shake gently to ensure complete dissolution. Vigorous shaking will produce foam and cause some loss of potency.
- For IV injection, administer asparaginase solution into the tubing of a freely running IV solution of D_5W or 0.9% NaCl over at least 30 min.
- For IV infusion, further dilute with up to 1,000 mL D_5W or 0.9% NaCl.

Intervention and Evaluation

- As appropriate, monitor serum amylase levels frequently during therapy.

◀ALERT▶ Expect to discontinue asparaginase use at the first sign or symptom of renal failure (oliguria or anuria) or pancreatitis, as evidenced by abdominal pain, nausea, and vomiting, or elevated serum amylase and lipase levels.

- Monitor the patient for signs and symptoms of hematologic toxicity,

manifested as easy bruising, fever, signs of local infection, sore throat, and unusual bleeding, as well as for signs and symptoms of anemia, including excessive fatigue and weakness.
• Expect to monitor patient closely for an allergic reaction for 1 hr after IM injection, because of delayed onset of hypersensitivity with this route.

Patient/Family Teaching
• Advise the patient/family to increase the patient's fluid intake to protect against any kidney problems.
• Explain to the patient/family that any nausea the patient experiences may decrease during therapy.
• Caution the patient/family to avoid contact with those who have recently received a live virus vaccine and to avoid receiving any immunizations without the physician's approval.
• Advise the patient/family to avoid contact with individuals who have known active infections such as chickenpox.

Dacarbazine

day-**car**-bah-zeen
(DTIC [CAN], DTIC-Dome)
Do not confuse with Dicarbosil or procarbazine.

CATEGORY AND SCHEDULE
Pregnancy Risk Category: C

MECHANISM OF ACTION
An alkylating, antineoplastic agent that forms methyl-diazonium ions, which attack nucleophilic groups in DNA. Cross-links DNA strands.
Therapeutic Effect: Inhibits DNA, RNA, and protein synthesis.

PHARMACOKINETICS
Minimally crosses brain barrier. Protein binding: 5%. Metabolized in liver. Excreted in urine. ***Half-Life:*** 5 hrs (half-life is increased in those with impaired renal function).

AVAILABILITY
Powder for Injection: 100-mg, 200-mg vials.

INDICATIONS AND DOSAGES
Refer to individual protocols.

▸ **Hodgkin disease**
IV
Adolescents. 375 mg/m^2 on days 1 and 15; repeat every 28 days.

▸ **Solid tumors**
IV
Children. 200–470 mg/m^2/day over 5 days every 21–28 days.

▸ **Neuroblastoma**
IV
Children. 800–900 mg/m^2 as single dose on day 1 of therapy every 3–4 wks in combination therapy.

UNLABELED USES
Treatment of islet cell carcinoma, neuroblastoma, soft tissue sarcoma.

CONTRAINDICATIONS
Demonstrated hypersensitivity to dacarbazine.

INTERACTIONS
Drug
Bone marrow depressants: May enhance myelosuppression.
Live virus vaccines: May potentiate virus replication, increase vaccine side effects, and

decrease the patient's antibody response to vaccine.
Phenytoin, phenobarbital: May increase metabolism of dacarbazine.
Herbal
None known.
Food
None known.

DIAGNOSTIC TEST EFFECTS
May increase BUN, serum alkaline phosphatase, SGOT (AST), and SGPT (ALT) levels.

IV INCOMPATIBILITIES
Allopurinol (Aloprim), cefepime (Maxipime), heparin, piperacillin/tazobactam (Zosyn)

IV COMPATIBILITIES
Etoposide (VePesid), granisetron (Kytril), ondansetron (Zofran), paclitaxel (Taxol)

SIDE EFFECTS
Frequent (90%)
Nausea, vomiting, anorexia (occurs within 1 hr of initial dose, may last up to 12 hrs)
Occasional
Facial flushing, paresthesia, alopecia, flu-like syndrome (fever, myalgia, and malaise), dermatologic reactions, CNS symptoms (confusion, blurred vision, headache, lethargy)
Rare
Diarrhea, stomatitis (redness or burning of oral mucous membranes, gum or tongue inflammation), photosensitivity

SERIOUS REACTIONS
! Bone marrow depression resulting in blood dyscrasias, such as leukopenia and thrombocytopenia, generally appears 2–4 wks after last dacarbazine dose.
! Liver toxicity occurs rarely.

PEDIATRIC CONSIDERATIONS
Baseline Assessment
• Hydrate the patient before treatment to avoid dehydration from vomiting.
• Be aware that dacarbazine use should be avoided during pregnancy, if possible, especially during the first trimester, and that breast-feeding is not recommended in this patient population.
Precautions
• Use cautiously in pts with impaired liver function.
Administration and Handling
◀ **ALERT** ▶ Know that dacarbazine dosage is individualized based on the patient's clinical response and tolerance of the drug's adverse effects. When used in combination therapy, consult specific protocols for optimum dosage and sequence of drug administration.
◀ **ALERT** ▶ Give dacarbazine by IV push or IV infusion, as prescribed. Because dacarbazine may be carcinogenic, mutagenic, or teratogenic, handle the drug with extreme care during preparation and administration.
IV
• Protect from light; refrigerate vials.
• Discard if the color changes from ivory to pink because this indicates decomposition.
• Reconstituted solution containing 10 mg/mL is stable for up to 8 hrs at room temperature or up to 72 hrs if refrigerated.
• Store solution diluted with up to 500 mL D_5W or 0.9% NaCl for up

to 8 hrs at room temperature or up to 24 hrs if refrigerated.
- Reconstitute 100-mg vial with 9.9 mL Sterile Water for Injection (19.7 mL for 200-mg vial) to provide concentration of 10 mg/mL.
- Give IV push over 2–3 min.
- For IV infusion, further dilute with up to 250 mL D_5W or 0.9% NaCl. Infuse over 15–30 min.
- Apply hot packs if a burning sensation, irritation, or local pain at the injection site occurs.
- Monitor for signs and symptoms of extravasation, including coolness, slight or no blood return at the injection site, and stinging and swelling at the injection site.

Intervention and Evaluation
- Monitor the patient's erythrocyte, leukocyte, and platelet counts for evidence of bone marrow depression.
- Monitor the patient for signs and symptoms of hematologic toxicity including easy bruising, fever, signs of local infection, sore throat, and unusual bleeding from any site.

Patient/Family Teaching
- Advise the patient/family that the gastrointestinal side effects are usually better tolerated after 1–2 days of treatment.
- Stress to the patient/family that the patient should not receive vaccinations and should avoid contact with anyone who recently received a live virus vaccine.
- Advise the patient/family to notify the physician if the patient experiences easy bruising, fever, signs of local infection, sore throat, and unusual bleeding from any site.
- Explain that the patient/family should notify the physician if nausea and vomiting persist at home.
- Advise the patient/family to avoid excessive exposure to sunlight: Use a broad spectrum sunscreen and protective clothing.

Etoposide, VP-16

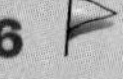

eh-**toe**-poe-side
(Etopophos, Toposar, VePesid)
Do not confuse with Pepcid or Versed.

CATEGORY AND SCHEDULE
Pregnancy Risk Category: D

MECHANISM OF ACTION
An epipodophyllotoxin that induces single- and double-stranded breaks in DNA. Cell cycle–dependent and phase-specific with maximum effect on S and G_2 phases of cell division. ***Therapeutic Effect:*** Inhibits or alters DNA synthesis.

PHARMACOKINETICS
Variably absorbed from the GI tract. Rapidly distributed. Low concentrations in cerebrospinal fluid. Protein binding: 97%. Metabolized in liver. Primarily excreted in urine. Not removed by hemodialysis. ***Half-Life:*** 3–12 hrs.

AVAILABILITY
Capsules: 50 mg.
Injection: 20 mg/mL.
Injection (water soluble): 100 mg/mL (Etopophos).

INDICATIONS AND DOSAGES
Refer to individual protocols.

▸ **Usual pediatric dosage**
Children. 60–150 $mg/m^2/day$ for 2–5 days every 3–6 wks.

UNLABELED USES
Treatment of acute myelocytic leukemia, AIDS-associated Kaposi

sarcoma, bladder carcinoma, Ewing sarcoma, Hodgkin and non-Hodgkin lymphoma

CONTRAINDICATIONS

Hypersensitivity to etoposide or any related component and pregnancy.

INTERACTIONS

Drug

Bone marrow depressants: May increase bone marrow depression.
Live virus vaccines: May potentiate virus replication, increase vaccine side effects, and decrease the patient's antibody response to vaccine.
Cyclosporin: May increase toxicity of etoposide.

Herbal

None known.

Food

None known.

DIAGNOSTIC TEST EFFECTS

None known.

IV INCOMPATIBILITIES

Cefepime (Maxipime), filgrastim (Neupogen), idarubicin (Idamycin).
Etopophos: amphotericin (Fungizone), cefepime (Maxipime), chlorpromazine (Thorazine), methylprednisolone (Solu-Medrol), prochlorperazine (Compazine)

IV COMPATIBILITIES

Carboplatin (Paraplatin), cisplatin (Platinol), cytarabine (Cytosar), daunorubicin (Cerubidine), doxorubicin (Adriamycin), granisetron (Kytril), mitoxantrone (Novantrone), ondansetron (Zofran)
Etopophos: carboplatin (Paraplatin), cisplatin (Platinol), cytarabine (Cytosar), dacarbazine (DTIC-Dome), daunorubicin (Cerubidine), dexamethasone (Decadron), diphenhydramine (Benadryl), doxorubicin (Adriamycin), granisetron (Kytril), magnesium sulfate, mannitol, mitoxantrone (Novantrone), ondansetron (Zofran), potassium chloride

SIDE EFFECTS

Frequent (66%–43%)
Mild to moderate nausea and vomiting, alopecia
Occasional (13%–6%)
Diarrhea, anorexia, stomatitis (redness or burning of oral mucous membranes, gum or tongue inflammation)
Rare (2% or less)
Hypotension, peripheral neuropathy

SERIOUS REACTIONS

! Bone marrow depression manifested as hematologic toxicity, principally anemia, leukopenia, thrombocytopenia and, to a lesser extent, pancytopenia may occur. Leukopenia occurs within 7–14 days after drug administration. Thrombocytopenia occurs within 9–16 days after administration. Bone marrow recovery occurs by day 20.
! Liver toxicity occurs occasionally.

PEDIATRIC CONSIDERATIONS

Baseline Assessment

• Monitor the patient hematology test results before and at frequent intervals during etoposide therapy.
• Administer antiemetics, if ordered, to readily control nausea and vomiting.
• Be aware that etoposide use should be avoided during

pregnancy, especially during the first trimester because of the risk of fetal harm and that breast-feeding is not recommended.
• Be aware that the safety and efficacy of etoposide have not been established in children.
• Assess for and maintain age-appropriate fluid intake.
• Use cautiously in individuals who have renal or hepatic insufficiency.
• Assess for active signs of infection or bleeding.
• Inspect and assess oral mucosa daily for ulcerations or bleeding.

Precautions
• Use cautiously in pts with bone marrow suppression and liver or renal impairment.

Administration and Handling
◀ **ALERT** ▶ Be aware that etoposide dosage is individualized based on the patient's clinical response and tolerance of the drug's adverse effects and that treatment is repeated at 3- to 4-week intervals.
◀ **ALERT** ▶ Administer etoposide by slow IV infusion. Wear gloves when preparing solution. If powder or solution comes in contact with skin, wash immediately and thoroughly with soap and water. Because etoposide may be carcinogenic, mutagenic, or teratogenic, handle the drug with extreme care during preparation and administration.
PO
Refrigerate gelatin capsules.
IV
• Store VePesid injection at room temperature before dilution.
• Know that VePesid concentrate for injection normally is clear and yellow.
• Reconstituted VePesid solution is stable at room temperature for up to 96 hrs at 0.2 mg/mL and 48 hrs at 0.4 mg/mL.
• Discard VePesid solution if crystallization occurs.
• Dilute each 100 mg (5 mL) of VePesid with at least 250 mL D_5W or 0.9% NaCl to provide a concentration of 0.4 mg/mL (500 mL for a concentration of 0.2 mg/mL).
• Infuse VePesid slowly, over 30–60 min. Rapid IV infusion may produce marked hypotension.
• Monitor the patient receiving VePesid for an anaphylactic reaction manifested as back, chest, or throat pain, chills, diaphoresis, dyspnea, fever, lacrimation, and sneezing.
• Refrigerate Etopophos vials.
• Etopophos is stable for up to 24 hrs after reconstitution.
• Reconstitute each 100 mg of Etopophos with 5 or 10 mL Sterile Water for Injection, D_5W, or 0.9% NaCl to provide a concentration of 20 or 10 mg/mL, respectively.
• As desired, give Etopophos without further dilution or further dilute to a concentration as low as 0.1 mg/mL with 0.9% NaCl or D_5W.
• Administer Etopophos over at least 5 min or up to 210 min, as appropriate.

Intervention and Evaluation
• Monitor the patient's blood Hgb and Hct levels and platelet and WBC counts. Monitor bilirubin level and liver and renal function tests.
• Assess the patient's pattern of daily bowel activity and stool consistency.
• Monitor the patient for signs and symptoms of anemia, including excessive fatigue and weakness, and hematologic toxicity, including easy bruising, fever, signs of local infection, sore throat, or unusual bleeding from any site.

• Assess the patient for signs and symptoms of paresthesias and peripheral neuropathy.
• Monitor the patient for signs and symptoms of stomatitis manifested as burning or redness of the oral mucous membranes and gum or tongue inflammation.

Patient/Family Teaching

• Explain to the patient/family that alopecia is reversible, but new hair growth may have a different color or texture.
• Stress to the patient/family that the patient should not receive vaccinations and should avoid contact with anyone who recently received a live virus vaccine.
• Warn the patient/family to notify the physician if the patient experiences easy bruising, fever, signs of local infection, sore throat, or unusual bleeding from any site.

Interleukin-2 (Aldesleukin)

in-tur-**lew**-kin
(IL-2, Proleukin)
Do not confuse with interferon 2.

CATEGORY AND SCHEDULE

Pregnancy Risk Category: C

MECHANISM OF ACTION

A biologic response modifier that acts as an antineoplastic agent and modifies human recombinant interleukin-2. ***Therapeutic Effect:*** Promotes proliferation, differentiation, and recruitment of T and B cells, natural killer cells, and thymocytes. Causes cytolytic activity in lymphocytes.

PHARMACOKINETICS

Primarily distributed into plasma, lymphocytes, lungs, liver, kidney, and spleen. Metabolized to amino acids in the cells lining the kidney. ***Half-Life:*** Children: 14–61 min; adults: 85 min.

AVAILABILITY

Powder for Injection: 22 million units (1.3 mg).

INDICATIONS AND DOSAGES

Refer to individual protocols.

▸ **Metastatic melanoma, metastatic renal cell carcinoma**

IV

Children older than 18 yrs. 600,000 units/kg q8h for 14 doses; rest 9 days, repeat 14 doses. Total: 28 doses. May repeat treatment no sooner than 7 wks from date of hospital discharge.

▸ **Acute myelocytic leukemia (investigational)**

IV

Children. 9 million units daily for 4 days, repeat 4 days later with 1.6 million units daily for 10 days.

UNLABELED USES

Treatment of colorectal cancer, Kaposi sarcoma, non-Hodgkin lymphoma.

CONTRAINDICATIONS

Hypersensitivity to aldesleukin or any related component. Abnormal pulmonary function tests or thallium stress test, bowel ischemia or perforation, coma or toxic psychosis longer than 48 hrs, gastrointestinal bleeding requiring surgery, intubation more than 72 hrs, organ allografts, pericardial tamponade, renal dysfunction requiring dialysis longer than 72 hrs, repetitive or difficult-to-control seizures, retreatment in those who experience the following toxicities: angina, myocardial infarction, recurrent chest pain with EKG changes, sustained ventricular tachycardia, uncontrolled or unresponsive cardiac rhythm disturbances.

INTERACTIONS

Drug

Antihypertensives: May increase hypotensive effect.
Cardiotoxic, liver toxic, nephrotoxic, and myelotoxic medications: May increase the risk of toxicity.
Glucocorticoids: May decrease the effects of interleukin.
Iodinated contrast media: Acute reactions including fever, chills, nausea, vomiting, pruritus, rash, diarrhea, hypotension, edema, oliguria. May occur within 4 wks to several months after aldesleukin administration.

Herbal

None known.

Food

None known.

DIAGNOSTIC TEST EFFECTS

May increase BUN, serum alkaline phosphatase, bilirubin, creatinine, and transaminase levels. May decrease serum calcium, magnesium, phosphorus, potassium, and sodium.

IV INCOMPATIBILITIES

Ganciclovir (Cytovene), pentamidine (Pentam), prochlorperazine (Compazine), promethazine (Phenergan)

IV COMPATIBILITIES

Calcium gluconate, dopamine (Intropin), heparin, lorazepam (Ativan), magnesium, potassium

SIDE EFFECTS

Side effects are generally self-limiting and reversible within 2–3 days after discontinuation of therapy.

Frequent (89%–48%)
Fever, chills, nausea, vomiting, hypotension, diarrhea, oliguria or anuria, mental status changes, irritability, confusion, depression, sinus tachycardia, pain (abdomen, chest, back), fatigue, dyspnea, pruritus

Occasional (47%–17%)
Edema, erythema, rash, stomatitis, anorexia, weight gain, infection (urinary tract, injection site, catheter tip), dizziness

Rare (15%–4%)
Dry skin, sensory disorders (vision, speech, taste), dermatitis, headache, arthralgia, myalgia, weight loss, hematuria, conjunctivitis, proteinuria

SERIOUS REACTIONS

! Anemia, thrombocytopenia, and leukopenia occur commonly.
! GI bleeding and pulmonary edema occur occasionally.
! Capillary leak syndrome results in hypotension (less than 90 mm Hg or a 20 mm Hg drop from baseline systolic pressure) and extravasation of plasma proteins and fluid into extravascular space and loss of vascular tone. May result in cardiac arrhythmias, angina, myocardial infarction, and respiratory insufficiency.
! Fatal malignant hyperthermia, cardiac arrest or stroke, pulmonary emboli and bowel perforation or gangrene, and severe depression leading to suicide have occurred in less than 1% of pts.

PEDIATRIC CONSIDERATIONS

Baseline Assessment

• Treat pts with bacterial infection and those with indwelling central

lines with antibiotic therapy before beginning interleukin therapy.
• Confirm that the patient is neurologically stable with a negative computed tomography scan before beginning interleukin therapy.
• Obtain results of blood chemistry analysis (including electrolyte levels), chest radiograph, complete blood count (CBC), and liver and renal function tests before beginning interleukin therapy and every day thereafter.
• Be aware that interleukin use should be avoided in pts of either sex not practicing effective contraception.
• Be aware that the safety and efficacy of interleukin have not been established in children younger than 18 yrs.
• Assess for and maintain age-appropriate fluid intake.

Precautions
• Use extremely cautiously in pts with normal thallium stress tests and pulmonary function tests who have a history of prior cardiac or pulmonary disease.
• Use cautiously in pts with fixed requirements for large volumes of fluid (e.g., those with hypercalcemia) or a history of seizures.

Administration and Handling
◀ **ALERT** ▶ Withhold the drug in pts who develop moderate to severe lethargy or somnolence (continued administration may result in coma).
◀ **ALERT** ▶ Restrict interleukin therapy to pts with normal cardiac and pulmonary functions as defined by thallium stress testing and pulmonary function testing. Dosage is individualized based on the patient's clinical response and tolerance of the adverse effects of the drug.

IV
• Refrigerate vials; do not freeze.
• Reconstituted solution is stable for 48 hrs refrigerated or at room temperature (refrigeration is preferred).
• Reconstitute 22-million unit vial with 1.2 mL Sterile Water for Injection to provide concentration of 18 million units/mL. Do not use Bacteriostatic Water for Injection or 0.9% NaCl.
• During reconstitution, direct the Sterile Water for Injection at the side of vial. Swirl contents gently to avoid foaming. Do not shake. Bacteriostatic Water for Injection or 0.9% NaCl should not be used for reconstitution because of increased aggregation.
• Further dilute dose in 50 mL D_5W and infuse over 15 min. Do not use an in-line filter.
• Solution should be warmed to room temperature before infusion.
• Monitor diligently for a drop in mean arterial blood pressure, a sign of capillary leak syndrome. Continued treatment may result in edema, pleural effusion, mental status changes, and significant hypotension (less than 90 mm Hg or a 20 mm Hg drop from baseline systolic pressure).

Intervention and Evaluation
• Monitor the patient's CBC, electrolyte levels, liver function tests, platelets, pulse oximetry, renal function, and weight.
• Determine the patient's serum amylase concentration frequently during therapy.
• Discontinue interleukin at the first sign of hypotension and withhold the drug for moderate to severe lethargy (physician must decide whether therapy should continue).
• Assess the patient's mental status changes (irritability, confusion, and depression) and weight gain or loss.

- Maintain strict intake and output protocols.
- Assess the patient for extravascular fluid accumulation evidenced by dependent edema and rales in lungs.

Patient/Family Teaching

- Advise the patient/family that nausea may decrease during continued therapy.
- Instruct the patient/family to increase the patient's fluid intake to protect against renal impairment.
- Warn the patient/family against receiving immunizations without the physician's approval because interleukin lowers the body's resistance.
- Urge the patient/family to avoid contact with those who have recently received a live virus vaccine.

Mitoxantrone

my-toe-**zan**-trone
(Novantrone, Onkotrone [AUS])

CATEGORY AND SCHEDULE

Pregnancy Risk Category: D

MECHANISM OF ACTION

An anthracenedione that inhibits DNA and RNA synthesis. Active throughout the entire cell cycle. ***Therapeutic Effect:*** Inhibits B-cell, T-cell, and macrophage proliferation. Causes cell death.

PHARMACOKINETICS

Protein binding: 78%. Widely distributed. Metabolized in liver. Primarily eliminated in feces via the biliary system. Not removed by hemodialysis. ***Half-Life:*** 2.3–13 days.

AVAILABILITY

Injection: 2 mg/mL.

INDICATIONS AND DOSAGES

Refer to individual protocols.

▸ Leukemias

IV

Children older than 2 yrs. 12 mg/m^2/day once daily for 2–3 days.

Children younger than 2 yrs. 0.4 mg/kg/day once daily for 3–5 days.

▸ Acute leukemia in relapse

Children older than 2 yrs. 8–12 mg/m^2/day once daily for 4–5 days.

▸ Acute, nonlymphocytic leukemia

Children older than 2 yrs. 10 mg/m^2/day once daily for 3–5 days.

▸ Solid tumors

IV

Children. 18–20 mg/m^2 once every 3–4 wks.

UNLABELED USES

Treatment of breast carcinoma, liver carcinoma, non-Hodgkin lymphoma.

CONTRAINDICATIONS

Hypersensitivity to mitoxantrone or any related component. Baseline left ventricular ejection fraction less than 50%, cumulative lifetime mitoxantrone dose 140 mg/m^2 or more, multiple sclerosis with liver impairment.

INTERACTIONS

Drug

Antigout medications: May decrease the effects of these drugs.
Bone marrow depressants: May increase bone marrow depression.
Live virus vaccines: May potentiate virus replication, increase vaccine side effects, and decrease the patient's antibody response to vaccine.

Herbal

None known.

Food

None known.

DIAGNOSTIC TEST EFFECTS

May increase serum bilirubin, uric acid, SGOT (AST), and SGPT (ALT) levels.

IV INCOMPATIBILITIES

Heparin, paclitaxel (Taxol), piperacillin/tazobactam (Zosyn)

IV COMPATIBILITIES

Allopurinol (Aloprim), etoposide (VePesid), gemcitabine (Gemzar), granisetron (Kytril), ondansetron (Zofran), potassium chloride

SIDE EFFECTS

Frequent (greater than 10%)
Nausea, vomiting, diarrhea, cough, headache, stomatitis, abdominal discomfort, fever, alopecia
Occasional (9%–4%)
Easy bruising, fungal infection, conjunctivitis, urinary tract infection
Rare (3%)
Arrhythmias

SERIOUS REACTIONS

! Bone marrow suppression may be severe, resulting in GI bleeding, sepsis, and pneumonia.
! Renal failure, seizures, jaundice, and CHF may occur.

PEDIATRIC CONSIDERATIONS

Baseline Assessment

- Offer the patient and family emotional support.
- Assess the patient's baseline body temperature, complete blood count, as ordered, respiratory status including lung sounds, and pulse quality and rate.
- Know that mitoxantrone use should be avoided during pregnancy, if possible, especially during the first trimester because it can cause fetal harm. Also know that breast-feeding is not recommended in this patient population.
- Be aware that the safety and efficacy of mitoxantrone have not been established in children.
- Caution the family about avoiding others with active infections such as chicken pox or herpes zoster.
- This medication can be toxic to the cardiac system. It is important to monitor heart rate and echocardiograms regularly.
- Assess for and maintain age-appropriate fluid intake.
- Be sure to notify provider of bleeding or infection.

Precautions

- Use cautiously in pts with impaired hepatobiliary function, preexisting bone marrow suppression, and previous treatment with cardiotoxic medications.

Administration and Handling

◂ **ALERT** ▸ Because mitoxantrone may be carcinogenic, mutagenic, or teratogenic, handle the drug with extreme care during preparation and administration. Give by IV injection or IV infusion after dilution.

IV

- Store vials at room temperature.
- Dilute with at least 50 mL D_5W or 0.9% NaCl.
- Do not administer by SC, IM, intrathecal, or intra-arterial injection. Do not give IV push over less than 3 min. Give IV bolus over more than 3 min or intermittent IV infusion over 15–60 min. Administer continuous IV infusion of 0.02–0.5 mg/mL in D_5W or 0.9% NaCl.

Intervention and Evaluation

- Monitor the patient's hematologic status, liver and renal function test results, and pulmonary function studies.

• Monitor the patient for signs and symptoms of hematologic toxicity, including easy bruising, fever, signs of local infection, and unusual bleeding from any site, and stomatitis, including burning or erythema of the oral mucosa, difficulty swallowing, oral ulcerations, and sore throat.
• Evaluate the patient for signs and symptoms of extravasation including blue discoloration of skin, burning, pain, and swelling.

Patient/Family Teaching

• Advise the patient/family that the patient's urine will appear blue or green 24 hrs after mitoxantrone administration. Explain to the patient that a blue tint to the sclera may also appear.
• Urge the patient to drink plenty of fluids to maintain adequate hydration and protect against renal impairment.
• Stress to the patient/family that the patient should not receive vaccinations and should avoid contact with crowds and those with known infection.
• Instruct the patient to use contraceptive measures during mitoxantrone therapy.

Pegasparagase

peg-ah-spa-**raj**-ace
(Oncaspar)

CATEGORY AND SCHEDULE

Pregnancy Risk Category: C

MECHANISM OF ACTION

An enzyme that breaks down extracellular supplies of the amino acid asparagines that are necessary for survival of leukemic cells. Normal cells produce their own asparagines. Binding to polyethylene glycol causes asparaginase to be less antigenic and less likely to cause a hypersensitivity reaction.
Therapeutic Effect: Interferes with DNA, RNA, and protein synthesis in leukemic cells. Cell cycle–specific for the G_1 phase of cell division.

AVAILABILITY

Injection: 7,500 international units/mL vial.

INDICATIONS AND DOSAGES

Refer to individual protocols.
Acute lymphocytic leukemia
IM/IV
Children with a body surface area 0.6 m² or greater. 2,500 international units/m² every 14 days.
Children with a body surface area less than 0.6 m². 82.5 international units/kg every 14 days.

CONTRAINDICATIONS

Previous anaphylactic reaction or significant hemorrhagic event associated with prior L-asparaginase therapy, pancreatitis, history of pancreatitis.

INTERACTIONS

Drug

Antigout medications: May decrease the effects of antigout medications.
Methotrexate: May block the effects of methotrexate.
Live virus vaccine: May potentiate virus replication, increase vaccine side effects, and decrease the patient's antibody response to vaccine.
Steroids, vincristine: May increase hyperglycemia, risk of neuropathy, and disturbance of erythropoiesis.

Warfarin, aspirin, heparin, NSAIDs, or dipyridamole: May increase risk of bleeding.
Herbal
None known.
Food
None known.

DIAGNOSTIC TEST EFFECTS

May increase blood ammonia levels, activated partial thromboplastin time, thrombin time, blood glucose, BUN, uric acid, serum alkaline phosphatase, bilirubin, uric acid, SGOT (AST), and SGPT (ALT) levels. May decrease blood clotting factors, including plasma fibrinogen, antithrombin, and plasminogen, and serum albumin, calcium, and cholesterol levels.

SIDE EFFECTS

Frequent
Allergic reaction, including rash, urticaria, arthralgia, facial edema, hypotension, and respiratory distress
Occasional
CNS effects, including confusion, drowsiness, depression, nervousness, and tiredness; stomatitis or sores to the mouth or lips; hypoalbuminemia; uric acid nephropathy or pedal or lower extremity edema; hyperglycemia
Rare
Hyperthermia (fever or chills)

SERIOUS REACTIONS

! There is a risk of a hypersensitivity reaction including anaphylaxis.
! An increased risk of blood coagulopathies occurs occasionally.
! Seizures occur rarely.
! Pancreatitis, evidenced by severe abdominal pain with nausea and vomiting, occurs frequently.

PEDIATRIC CONSIDERATIONS

Baseline Assessment
- Keep agents for adequate airway and allergic reaction readily available before giving pegaspargase and during administration.
- Closely monitor the patient following drug administration.
- Assess the patient's complete blood count, bone marrow tests, fibrinogen, liver, pancreatic, and renal function tests, prothrombin time, and partial thromboplastin time before beginning the drug and when 1 week or more has elapsed between drug doses.
- Assess for and maintain age-appropriate fluid intake.
- Caution the family to avoid those with active infections such as chicken pox or herpes zoster.
- Pts should be observed for 1 hr after injection. Treatment for hypersensitivity reactions should be readily available (oxygen, corticosteroids, epinephrine, and antihistamines).

Precautions
- Use cautiously in pts concurrently taking aspirin or NSAIDs and those receiving concurrent anticoagulant therapy.

Administration and Handling
◀**ALERT**▶ Avoid inhalation of vapors. Wear gloves when handling pegaspargase and avoid contact with skin or mucous membranes (drug is a contact irritant). If contact occurs, wash the affected area with copious amount of water for at least 15 min. Avoid excessive agitation of the vial; do not shake. The IM route is preferred because of the decreased risk of coagulopathy, GI disorders, liver toxicity, and renal disorders.
- Refrigerate; do not freeze.
- Discard if cloudy, if precipitate is present, if stored at room

temperature for longer than 48 hrs, or if vial has been previously frozen because freezing destroys activity.
• Use one dose per vial, do not re-enter vial. Discard unused portion.
IM
• Administer no more than 2 mL at any one IM site.
• Use multiple injection sites if more than 2 mL is administered.
IV
• Add 100 mL 0.9% NaCl or D_5W and administer through an infusion that is already running.
• Infuse over 1–2 hrs.
Intervention and Evaluation
• Monitor the patient's response and toxicity.
• Monitor the patient's serum amylase and lipase concentrations frequently during and after therapy for evidence of pancreatitis.
• Monitor the patient's BUN and serum creatinine for signs of renal failure.
• Discontinue the drug at the first sign of pancreatitis or renal failure.
• Monitor the patient for signs and symptoms of anemia, such as excessive fatigue and weakness, infection, and hematologic toxicity, including easy bruising, fever, signs of local infection, sore throat, and unusual bleeding.
Patient/Family Teaching
• Urge the patient/family to increase the patient's fluid intake to protect against renal impairment.
• Explain to the patient/family that nausea may decrease during therapy.
• Stress to the patient/family that the patient should not receive vaccinations and should avoid contact with anyone who recently received a live virus vaccine.
• Warn the patient/family to notify the physician if nausea and vomiting continue at home.

Procarbazine Hydrochloride

pro-**car**-bah-zeen
(Matulane, Natulan [CAN])
Do not confuse with dacarbazine.

CATEGORY AND SCHEDULE
Pregnancy Risk Category: D

MECHANISM OF ACTION
A methylhydrazine derivative that inhibits DNA, RNA, and protein synthesis. May also directly damage DNA. Cell cycle–specific for the S phase of cell division. ***Therapeutic Effect:*** Cell death.

PHARMACOKINETICS
Good oral absorption. Widely distributed, including cerebrospinal fluid. Metabolized in liver. Eliminated in urine as metabolites. ***Half-Life:*** 10 min.

AVAILABILITY
Capsules: 50 mg.

INDICATIONS AND DOSAGES
Refer to individual protocols.
▸ **Advanced Hodgkin disease**
PO
Children. 50–100 mg/m^2/day for 10–14 days of a 28-day cycle. Continue until maximum response, leukocyte count falls below 4,000/mm^3, or platelet count falls below 100,000/mm^3. Maintenance: 50 mg/m^2/day.
▸ **Neuroblastoma**
PO
Doses have been reported to be as high as 100–200 mg/m^2/day once daily.

▸ **Conditioning for bone marrow transplantation for aplastic anemia**
PO
Children. 12.5 mg/kg/dose every other day for 4 doses.

UNLABELED USES

Treatment of lung carcinoma, malignant melanoma, multiple myeloma, non-Hodgkin lymphoma, polycythemia vera, primary brain tumors

CONTRAINDICATIONS

Hypersensitivity to procarbazine or any related component. Inadequate bone marrow reserve.

INTERACTIONS

Drug

Alcohol: May cause disulfiram reaction.
Anticholinergics, antihistamines: May increase anticholinergic effects of these drugs.
Bone marrow depressants: May increase bone marrow depression.
Buspirone, caffeine-containing medications: May increase blood pressure with these drugs.
Carbamazepine, cyclobenzaprine, MAOIs, maprotiline: May cause hyperpyretic crisis, seizures, or death with these drugs.
CNS depressants: May increase CNS depression.
Insulin, oral hypoglycemics: May increase the effects of these drugs.
Meperidine: May produce coma, convulsions, immediate excitation, rigidity, severe hypertension or hypotension, severe respiratory distress, sweating, and vascular collapse.
Sympathomimetics: May increase cardiac stimulant and vasopressor effects.
Tricyclic antidepressants: May increase anticholinergic effects and cause convulsions and hyperpyretic crisis.

Herbal

None known.

Food

Tyramine-containing foods (cheese, tea, dark beer, coffee, cola, wine, bananas): May lead to hypertensive crisis, tremor, excitation, cardiac effects, and angina.

DIAGNOSTIC TEST EFFECTS

None known.

SIDE EFFECTS

Frequent

Severe nausea, vomiting, respiratory disorders (cough, effusion), myalgia, arthralgia, drowsiness, nervousness, insomnia, nightmares, sweating, hallucinations, seizures

Occasional

Hoarseness, tachycardia, nystagmus, retinal hemorrhage, photophobia, photosensitivity, urinary frequency, nocturia, hypotension, diarrhea, stomatitis, paresthesia, unsteadiness, confusion, decreased reflexes, foot drop

Rare

Hypersensitivity reaction (dermatitis, pruritus, rash, urticaria), hyperpigmentation, alopecia

SERIOUS REACTIONS

! The major toxic effects of procarbazine are bone marrow depression manifested as hematologic toxicity (mainly leukopenia, thrombocytopenia, or anemia) and liver toxicity manifested as jaundice and ascites.
! Urinary tract infection secondary to leukopenia may occur.
! Therapy should be discontinued if stomatitis, diarrhea, paresthesia,

neuropathies, confusion, or a hypersensitivity reaction occurs.

PEDIATRIC CONSIDERATIONS

Baseline Assessment

• Expect the patient to undergo bone marrow tests. Monitor the patient's leukocyte count, differential, platelet count, and reticulocyte count Also, check the results of the patient's urinalysis, blood Hgb, Hct levels, BUN, serum alkaline phosphatase, and transaminase levels before beginning procarbazine therapy and periodically thereafter.

• Be aware that therapy should be interrupted if the patient's WBC count falls below 4,000/mm^3 or the platelet count falls below 100,000/mm^3.

• Be sure to notify the provider of any signs and symptoms of infection or bleeding.

• Assess for and maintain age-appropriate fluid intake.

Precautions

• Use cautiously in pts with impaired liver or renal function.

Intervention and Evaluation

• Monitor the results of the patient's hematologic tests and liver and renal function studies.

• Assess the patient for signs and symptoms of stomatitis, including burning or erythema of the oral mucosa at the inner margin of the lips, difficulty swallowing, oral ulceration, and sore throat.

• Monitor for the patient for signs and symptoms of anemia, including excessive fatigue and weakness, and hematologic toxicity, including easy bruising, fever, signs of local infection, sore throat, and unusual bleeding from any site.

Patient/Family Teaching

• Warn the patient/family to notify the physician if the patient experiences bleeding, easy bruising, fever, or sore throat.

• Caution the patient/family to avoid consumption of alcohol because it may cause a disulfiram reaction characterized by nausea, sedation, severe headache, visual disturbances, and vomiting.

• Caution the patient/family to avoid foods with a high-tyramine content.

Teniposide

ten-**ih**-poe-side

(Vumon)

CATEGORY AND SCHEDULE

Pregnancy Risk Category: D

MECHANISM OF ACTION

An epipodophyllotoxin that induces single- and double-stranded breaks in DNA, inhibiting or altering DNA synthesis. ***Therapeutic Effect:*** Prevents cells from entering mitosis. Phase-specific acting in late S and early G_2 phases of the cell cycle.

PHARMACOKINETICS

Protein binding: greater than 99%. Eliminated mostly in urine with some minimal excretion in the feces. ***Half-Life:*** 5 hrs.

AVAILABILITY

Injection: 50 mg.

INDICATIONS AND DOSAGES

Refer to individual protocols.

▸ **In combination with other antineoplastic agents, induction therapy in patients with refractory childhood acute lymphoblastic leukemia (ALL)**

Dosage is individualized based on the patient's clinical response and tolerance of the adverse effects of the drug. When used in combination therapy, consult specific protocols for optimum dosage or sequence of drug administration.

▸ **Recurrent ALL**

IV

Children and adolescents.
165 mg/m^2 2 times/wk for 9 doses (combined with cytarabine).

CONTRAINDICATIONS

Hypersensitivity to Cremophor EL (polyoxyethylated castor oil), etoposide, or teniposide. Absolute neutrophil count less than 500/mm^3, platelet count less than 50,000/mm^3.

INTERACTIONS

Drug

Bone marrow depressants: May increase bone marrow depression.
Live virus vaccines: May potentiate virus replication, increase vaccine side effects, and decrease the patient's antibody response to the vaccine.
Methotrexate: May increase intracellular accumulation of this drug.
Vincristine: May increase severity of peripheral neuropathy with this drug.
Sodium salicylate, sulfamethizole, tolbutamide: May increase toxicity of teniposide because of displacement from protein binding sites.

Herbal

None known.

Food

None known.

DIAGNOSTIC TEST EFFECTS

None significant.

SIDE EFFECTS

Frequent (greater than 30%)

Mucositis, nausea, vomiting, diarrhea, anemia

Occasional (5%–3%)

Alopecia, rash

Rare (less than 3%)

Liver dysfunction, fever, renal dysfunction, peripheral neurotoxicity

SERIOUS REACTIONS

! Bone marrow depression manifested as hematologic toxicity (principally leukopenia, neutropenia, and thrombocytopenia) with increased risk of infection or bleeding may occur.

! Hypersensitivity reaction including anaphylaxis (chills, fever, tachycardia, bronchospasm, dyspnea, and facial flushing) may occur.

PEDIATRIC CONSIDERATIONS

Baseline Assessment

- Assess the patient's hematology test results, liver function tests, and renal function tests before beginning and frequently during teniposide therapy.
- Individuals with Down syndrome might be moderately sensitive to the drug so use with caution.
- Assess for and maintain age-appropriate fluid intake.
- The medication needs to be administered slowly to prevent hypotension (over 30–60 min).
- It is important to administer this medication through a central line to avoid extravasation.

Precautions

- Use cautiously in pts with brain tumors, decreased liver function, Down syndrome, and neuroblastoma (increases risk of anaphylaxis).

Administration and Handling

IV

- Refrigerate unopened ampules.
- Protect from light.

- Reconstituted solutions are stable for 24 hrs at room temperature.
- Discard if precipitation occurs.
- Use 1 mg/mL solutions within 4 hrs of preparation to reduce the potential for precipitation.
- Do not refrigerate reconstituted solutions.
- Wear gloves when preparing solution. If solution comes in contact with skin, wash immediately and thoroughly with soap and water.
- Dilute with 0.9% NaCl or D_5W to provide a concentration of 0.1–1 mg/mL.
- Prepare and administer in containers such as glass or polyolefin plastic bags or containers. Avoid use of PVC containers.
- Give over at least 30–60 min. Avoid rapid IV injection.

Intervention and Evaluation

- Have medication and supportive measures readily available for the first dose because life-threatening anaphylaxis characterized by bronchospasm, chills, dyspnea, facial flushing, fever, and tachycardia may occur.
- Monitor the patient for signs and symptoms of myelosuppression, including anemia, infection, and unusual bleeding or bruising.

Patient/Family Teaching

- Stress to the patient/family that the patient should not receive vaccinations without physician approval and should avoid contact with crowds and anyone with known infection.
- Warn the patient/family to notify the physician if the patient experiences easy bruising, difficulty breathing, fever, signs of infection, or unusual bleeding from any site.
- Caution the patient to avoid becoming pregnant during teniposide therapy. Teach the patient about various methods of contraception.
- Explain to the patient/family that hair loss is reversible, but new growth may have a different color or texture.

REFERENCES

Miller, S. & Fioravanti, J. (1997). Pediatric medications: a handbook for nurses. St. Louis: Mosby.
Taketomo, C. K., Hodding, J. H. & Kraus, D. M. (2003–2004). Pediatric dosage handbook (10th ed.). Hudson, OH: Lexi-Comp.

21 Angiotensin-Converting Enzyme (ACE) Inhibitors

Captopril
Enalapril Maleate

Uses: Angiotensin-converting enzyme (ACE) inhibitors are used to treat hypertension and, as adjuncts, to treat CHF.

Action: ACE inhibitors act primarily by suppressing the renin-angiotensin-aldosterone system. (See illustration, *Site of Action: ACE Inhibitors,* page 304.) They reduce peripheral arterial resistance and increase cardiac output, but produce little or no change in the heart rate.

COMBINATION PRODUCTS

ACCURETIC: quinapril/hydrochlorothiazide (a diuretic) 10 mg/12.5 mg; 20 mg/12.5 mg; 20 mg/25 mg.
CAPOZIDE: captopril/hydrochlorothiazide (a diuretic) 25 mg/15 mg; 25 mg/25 mg; 50 mg/15 mg; 50 mg/25 mg.
LEXXEL: enalapril/felodipine (a calcium channel blocker) 5 mg/2.5 mg; 5 mg/5 mg.
LOTENSIN HCT: benazepril/hydrochlorothiazide (a diuretic) 5 mg/6.25 mg; 10 mg/12.5 mg; 20 mg/12.5 mg; 20 mg/25 mg.
LOTREL: benazepril/amlodipine (a calcium channel blocker) 2.5 mg/10 mg; 5 mg/10 mg; 5 mg/20 mg; 10 mg/20 mg.
PRINZIDE: lisinopril/hydrochlorothiazide (a diuretic) 10 mg/12.5 mg; 20 mg/12.5 mg; 20 mg/25 mg.
TARKA: trandolapril/verapamil (a calcium channel blocker) 1 mg/240 mg; 2 mg/180 mg; 2 mg/240 mg; 4 mg/240 mg.
TECZEM: enalapril/diltiazem (a calcium channel blocker) 5 mg/180 mg.
UNIRETIC: moexipril/hydrochlorothiazide (a diuretic) 7.5 mg/12.5 mg; 15 mg/12.5 mg; 15 mg/25 mg.
VASERETIC: enalapril/hydrochlorothiazide (a diuretic) 5 mg/12.5 mg; 10 mg/25 mg.
ZESTORETIC: lisinopril/hydrochlorothiazide (a diuretic) 10 mg/12.5 mg; 20 mg/12.5 mg; 20 mg/25 mg.

Captopril

cap-toe-prill
(Acenorm [AUS], Capoten, Captohexal [AUS], Novo-Captoril [CAN], Topace [AUS])
Do not confuse with Capitrol.

CATEGORY AND SCHEDULE

Pregnancy Risk Category: C (D if used in second or third trimester)

MECHANISM OF ACTION

This ACE inhibitor suppresses the renin-angiotensin-aldosterone system and prevents conversion of angiotensin I to angiotensin II, a potent vasoconstrictor; it may also inhibit angiotensin II at local vascular and renal sites. Decreases plasma angiotensin II, increases plasma renin activity, decreases aldosterone secretion. ***Therapeutic Effect:*** Reduces peripheral arterial

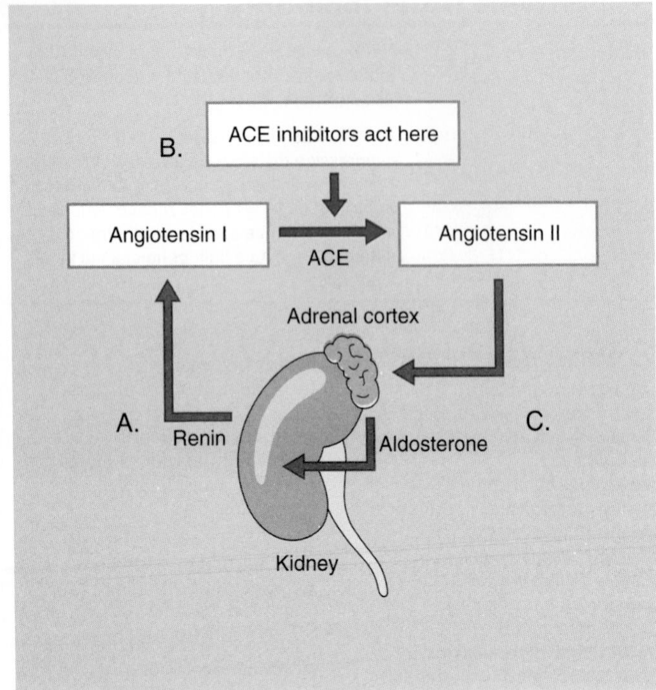

Site of Action: ACE Inhibitors

The renin-angiotensin-aldosterone system plays a major role in regulating blood pressure. Any condition that decreases renal blood flow, reduces blood pressure, or stimulates $beta_1$-adrenergic receptors prompts the kidneys to release renin (A). Renin acts on angiotensinogen, which is converted to angiotensin I, a weak vasoconstrictor. ACE converts angiotensin I to angiotensin II, which causes systemic and renal blood vessels to constrict (B). Systemic vasoconstriction increases peripheral vascular resistance, raising the blood pressure. Renal vasoconstriction decreases glomerular filtration, resulting in sodium and water retention and increasing blood volume and blood pressure. In addition, angiotensin II also acts on the adrenal cortex causing it to release aldosterone (C). This makes the kidneys retain additional sodium and water, which further increases the blood pressure.

ACE inhibitors, such as captopril and enalapril, block the action of ACE. As a result, angiotensin II cannot form, which prevents systemic and renal vasoconstriction and the release of aldosterone.

resistance and pulmonary capillary wedge pressure; improves cardiac output and exercise tolerance.

PHARMACOKINETICS

Rapidly well absorbed from the GI tract (absorption is decreased in the presence of food). Protein binding: 25%–30%. Metabolized in liver. Primarily excreted in urine. Removed by hemodialysis. ***Half-Life:*** Less than 3 hrs (half-life is increased in those with impaired renal function). Infants with CHF: 2–12 hr.

AVAILABILITY

Tablets: 12.5 mg, 25 mg, 50 mg, 100 mg.

INDICATIONS AND DOSAGES

PO

Adolescents. Initially 12.5–25 mg/dose q8–12h; may increase by 25 mg/dose. Maximum: 450 mg/day.
Older children. Initially 6.25–12.5 mg/dose in 1–2 divided doses. Titrate up to maximum of 6 mg/kg/day in 2–4 divided doses.
Children. Initially 0.3–0.5 mg/kg/dose titrated up to a maximum of 6 mg/kg/day in 2–4 divided doses.
Infants. 0.15–0.3 mg/kg/dose in 1–4 divided doses. Maximum: 6 mg/kg/day.
Neonates. Initially, 0.05–0.1 mg/kg/dose q8–24h titrated up to 0.5 mg/kg/dose given q6–24h.

▸ **Dosing in renal impairment**

Creatinine clearance 10–50 mL/min: give 75% of dose
Creatinine clearance less than 10 mL/min: give 50% of dose.

UNLABELED USES

Diagnosis of anatomic renal artery stenosis, hypertensive crisis, rheumatoid arthritis.

CONTRAINDICATIONS

History of angioedema with previous treatment with ACE inhibitors.

INTERACTIONS

Drug

Alcohol, diuretics, hypotensive agents: May increase the effects of captopril.
Lithium: May increase lithium blood concentration and risk of toxicity.
NSAIDs: May decrease the effects of captopril.
Potassium-sparing diuretics, potassium supplements: May cause hyperkalemia.

Herbal

None known.

Food

None known.

DIAGNOSTIC TEST EFFECTS

May increase BUN, serum alkaline phosphatase, serum bilirubin, serum creatinine, serum potassium, SGOT (AST), and SGPT (ALT) levels. May decrease serum sodium levels. May cause positive ANA titer.

SIDE EFFECTS

Frequent (7%–4%)

Rash

Occasional (4%–2%)

Pruritus, dysgeusia (change in sense of taste)

Rare (less than 2%–0.5%)

Headache, cough, insomnia, dizziness, fatigue, paresthesia, malaise, nausea, diarrhea or constipation, dry mouth, tachycardia

SERIOUS REACTIONS

! Excessive hypotension ("first-dose syncope") may occur in those with CHF and those who are severely salt and volume depleted.
! Angioedema (swelling of face and lips) and hyperkalemia occur rarely.

! Agranulocytosis and neutropenia may be noted in those with collagen vascular disease, including scleroderma and systemic lupus erythematosus, and impaired renal function.
! Nephrotic syndrome may be noted in those with history of renal disease.

PEDIATRIC CONSIDERATIONS

Baseline Assessment

• Expect to obtain the patient's blood pressure (B/P) immediately before each captopril dose, in addition to regular monitoring. Be alert to fluctuations in B/P. If an excessive reduction in B/P occurs, place the patient in the supine position with legs elevated and notify the physician.
• Test the patient's first urine of the day for protein by the dipstick method before beginning captopril therapy and periodically thereafter in pts with prior renal disease or those receiving captopril dosages greater than 150 mg/day.
• As ordered, obtain a complete blood count (CBC) and blood chemistry analysis before beginning captopril therapy, then every 2 wks for the next 3 mos, and periodically thereafter in pts with autoimmune disease or renal impairment and in those who are taking drugs that affect immune response or leukocyte count.
• Be aware that captopril crosses the placenta, is distributed in breast milk, and may cause fetal or neonatal morbidity or mortality.
• Be aware that the safety and efficacy of captopril have not been established in children.

Precautions

• Use cautiously in pts with cerebrovascular or coronary insufficiency, hypovolemia, renal impairment, and sodium depletion.
• Use cautiously in pts receiving dialysis or diuretic therapy.

Administration and Handling

PO
• Give captopril 1 hr before meals for maximum absorption because food significantly decreases drug absorption.
• Crush tablets if necessary.

Intervention and Evaluation

• Examine the patient's skin for pruritus and rash.
• Assist the patient with ambulation if he or she experiences dizziness.
• Check the patient's urinalysis test results for proteinuria.
• Assess the patient for anorexia resulting from decreased taste perception.
• Monitor the BUN, CBC, serum creatinine, and serum potassium levels in pts also receiving a diuretic.

Patient/Family Teaching

• Explain that the full therapeutic effect of captopril may not occur for several weeks.
• Warn the patient/family that noncompliance with drug therapy or skipping captopril doses may cause severe rebound hypertension.
• Urge the patient not to consume alcohol while taking captopril.

Enalapril Maleate

en-**al**-ah-prill
(Alphapril [AUS], Amprace [AUS], Apo-Enalapril [CAN], Auspril [AUS], Renitec [AUS], Vasotec)
Do not confuse with Anafranil, Eldepryl, or ramipril.

CATEGORY AND SCHEDULE

Pregnancy Risk Category: D (C if used in first trimester)

MECHANISM OF ACTION

This ACE inhibitor suppresses the renin-angiotensin-aldosterone system and prevents conversion of angiotensin I to angiotensin II, a potent vasoconstrictor; it may inhibit angiotensin II at local vascular, renal sites. Decreases plasma angiotensin II, increases plasma renin activity, and decreases aldosterone secretion. ***Therapeutic Effect:*** In hypertension, reduces peripheral arterial resistance. In CHF, increases cardiac output; decreases peripheral vascular resistance, blood pressure (B/P), pulmonary capillary wedge pressure, and heart size.

PHARMACOKINETICS

Readily absorbed from the GI tract (not affected by food). Protein binding: 50%–60%. Converted to active metabolite (enalaprilat). Primarily excreted in urine. Removed by hemodialysis. ***Half-Life:*** 11 hrs (half-life is increased in those with impaired renal function).

AVAILABILITY

Tablets: 2.5 mg, 5 mg, 10 mg, 20 mg.
Injection: 1.25 mg/mL.

INDICATIONS AND DOSAGES

▸ **Hypertension alone or in combination with other antihypertensives**

PO

Adolescents. 2.5–5 mg/day, may increase as needed. Maximum: 40 mg/day.

Children. 0.1 mg/kg/day in 1–2 divided doses. Maximum: 0.5 mg/kg/day.

Neonates. 0.1 mg/kg/day q24h.

IV

Adolescents. 0.625–1.25 mg q6h up to 5 mg q6h.

Children, neonates. 5–10 mcg/kg/dose q8–24h.

▸ **Dosage in renal impairment**

Creatinine Clearance	% Usual Dose
10–50 mL/min	75–100
Less than 10 mL/min	50

UNLABELED USES

Treatment of diabetic nephropathy or renal crisis in scleroderma.

CONTRAINDICATIONS

History of angioedema with previous treatment with ACE inhibitors.

INTERACTIONS

Drug

Alcohol, diuretics, hypotensive agents: May increase the effects of enalapril.

Indomethacin, NSAIDs: May decrease hypotensive effect of enalapril.

Lithium: Increased risk of lithium toxicity.

Herbal

None known.

Food

Licorice (natural): Leads to sodium and water retention and increases potassium loss.

DIAGNOSTIC TEST EFFECTS

May increase BUN and serum alkaline phosphatase, serum bilirubin, serum creatinine, serum potassium, SGOT (AST), and SGPT (ALT) levels. May decrease serum sodium levels. May cause positive ANA titer.

IV INCOMPATIBILITIES

Amphotericin (Fungizone), amphotericin B complex (Abelcet,

AmBisome, Amphotec), cefepime (Maxipime), phenytoin (Dilantin)

IV COMPATIBILITIES

Calcium gluconate, dobutamine (Dobutrex), dopamine (Inotropin), fentanyl (Sublimaze), heparin, lidocaine, magnesium sulfate, morphine, nitroglycerin, potassium chloride, potassium phosphate, propofol (Diprivan)

Side Effects

Frequent (7%–5%)
Postural hypotension, headache, dizziness

Occasional (3%–2%)
Orthostatic hypotension, fatigue, diarrhea, cough, syncope

Rare (less than 2%)
Angina, abdominal pain, vomiting, nausea, rash, asthenia (loss of strength, energy), syncope

SERIOUS REACTIONS

! Excessive hypotension (first-dose syncope) may occur in those with CHF and those who are severely salt or volume depleted.
! Angioedema (swelling of face, lips) and hyperkalemia occur rarely.
! Agranulocytosis and neutropenia may be noted in pts with collagen vascular diseases, including scleroderma and systemic lupus erythematosus, and impaired renal function.
! Nephrotic syndrome may be noted in those with a history of renal disease.

PEDIATRIC CONSIDERATIONS

Baseline Assessment

- Assess the patient's B/P immediately before each enalapril dose. Be alert to fluctuations in B/P.
- As ordered, obtain a complete blood count and blood chemistry analysis before beginning enalapril therapy, then every 2 wks for 3 mos, and periodically thereafter in pts with autoimmune disease or renal impairment and in those who are taking drugs that affect immune or leukocyte responses.
- Be aware that enalapril crosses the placenta and is distributed in breast milk. Enalapril may cause fetal or neonatal morbidity or mortality.
- Be sure to assess for adequate sodium intake in pediatric pts. Severe hypotension may result in pts who are sodium depleted.
- Assess for and maintain age-appropriate fluid intake.
- Be aware that the safety and efficacy of enalapril have not been established in children.

Precautions

- Use cautiously in pts with cerebrovascular or coronary insufficiency, hypovolemia, renal impairment, and sodium depletion.
- Use cautiously in pts who are receiving dialysis and diuretic therapy.

Administration and Handling

PO

- Give enalapril without regard to food.
- Crush tablets if necessary.

IV

- Store parenteral form at room temperature.
- Use only clear, colorless solution.
- Diluted IV solution is stable for up to 24 hrs at room temperature.
- Give undiluted or dilute with D_5W or 0.9% NaCl.
- For IV push, give undiluted over 5 min.
- For IV piggyback, infuse over 10–15 min.

Intervention and Evaluation

- Assist the patient with ambulation if he or she experiences dizziness.

- Monitor the patient's B/P and BUN, serum creatinine, and potassium levels.
- Assess the patient's pattern of daily bowel activity and stool consistency.

Patient/Family Teaching

- Advise the patient/family to rise slowly from lying to sitting position and to permit the legs to dangle from the bed momentarily before standing to reduce the hypotensive effect of enalapril.
- Explain to the patient/family that the full therapeutic effect of B/P reduction may take several weeks to appear.
- Caution the patient/family against noncompliance with drug therapy or skipping drug doses because this may produce severe rebound hypertension.
- Urge the patient to limit consumption of alcohol while taking enalapril.
- Warn the patient/family to notify the physician if diarrhea, difficulty breathing, excessive perspiration, swelling of the face, lips, or tongue, and vomiting occur.

REFERENCES

Miller, S. & Fioravanti, J. (1997). Pediatric medications: a handbook for nurses. St. Louis: Mosby.

Taketomo, C. K., Hodding, J. H. & Kraus, D. M. (2003–2004). Pediatric dosage handbook (10th ed.). Hudson, OH: Lexi-Comp.

22 Angiotensin II Receptor Antagonists

Irbesartan

Uses: Angiotensin II receptor antagonists (AIIRAs) are used to treat hypertension alone or in combination with other antihypertensive drugs.

Action: AIIRAs block the vasoconstricting and aldosterone-secreting effects of angiotensin II, a potent vasoconstrictor. By selectively blocking the binding of angiotensin II to the angiotensin II type AT_1 receptors in vascular smooth muscle and the adrenal gland, AIIRAs cause vasodilation, decrease aldosterone effects, and reduce blood pressure.

COMBINATION PRODUCTS

AVALIDE: irbesartan/hydrochlorothiazide (a diuretic) 150 mg/12.5 mg; 300 mg/12.5 mg.

Irbesartan

ir-beh-**sar**-tan

(Avapro, Karvea [AUS])

CATEGORY AND SCHEDULE

Pregnancy Risk Category: C (D if used in second or third trimester)

MECHANISM OF ACTION

This type AT_1 AIIRA blocks the vasoconstrictor and aldosterone-secreting effects of angiotensin II, inhibiting the binding of angiotensin II to AT_1 receptors. ***Therapeutic Effect:*** Produces vasodilation, decreases peripheral resistance, and decreases blood pressure (B/P).

PHARMACOKINETICS

Rapidly and completely absorbed after PO administration. Protein binding: 90%. Undergoes hepatic metabolism to inactive metabolite. Recovered primarily in feces and, to a lesser extent, in urine. Not removed by hemodialysis.
Half-Life: 11–15 hrs.

AVAILABILITY

Tablets: 75 mg, 150 mg, 300 mg.

INDICATIONS AND DOSAGES

▸ **Hypertension alone or in combination with other antihypertensives**

PO

Children 13 yrs and older. Initially, 150 mg/day. May increase to 300 mg/day.

Children 6–12 yrs. Initially 75 mg/day. May increase to 150 mg/day.

UNLABELED USES

Treatment of heart failure.

CONTRAINDICATIONS

Hypersensitivity to irbesartan or any related component. Bilateral renal artery stenosis, biliary cirrhosis or obstruction, primary hyperaldosteronism, severe liver insufficiency, and pregnancy.

INTERACTIONS

Drug

Hydrochlorothiazide: Produces further reduction in B/P.

Herbal

None known.

Food

None known.

DIAGNOSTIC TEST EFFECTS

Minor increase in BUN and serum creatinine levels. May decrease blood Hgb levels.

SIDE EFFECTS

Occasional (9%–3%)

Upper respiratory infection, fatigue, diarrhea, cough

Rare (2%–1%)

Heartburn, dizziness, headache, nausea, rash, flushing, sleep disturbances, muscle cramps.

SERIOUS REACTIONS

! Overdosage may manifest as hypotension and tachycardia. Bradycardia occurs less often.

PEDIATRIC CONSIDERATIONS

Baseline Assessment

- Obtain the patient's apical pulse and B/P immediately before each irbesartan dose and monitor regularly throughout therapy. Be alert to fluctuations in apical pulse and B/P. If an excessive reduction in B/P occurs, place the patient in the supine position with feet slightly elevated.
- Determine whether the patient is pregnant before beginning therapy.
- Assess the patient's medication history, especially for diuretics.
- Be aware that it is unknown whether irbesartan is distributed in breast milk. Irbesartan may cause fetal or neonatal morbidity or mortality.
- Be aware that the safety and efficacy of irbesartan have not been established in children.

Precautions

- Use cautiously in pts with CHF, coronary artery disease, mild to moderate liver dysfunction, sodium or water depletion, and unilateral renal artery stenosis.

Administration and Handling

◀ **ALERT** ▶ Know that irbesartan may be given concurrently with other antihypertensives and if the B/P is not controlled by irbesartan alone, a diuretic may also be prescribed.

PO

- Give irbesartan without regard to meals.

Intervention and Evaluation

- Offer the patient fluids frequently to maintain hydration.
- Assess the patient for signs and symptoms of an upper respiratory infection.
- Assist the patient with ambulation if he or she experiences dizziness.
- Monitor the patient's B/P and pulse rate. Also check the results of serum electrolyte tests, liver and renal function tests, and urinalysis.
- Assess the patient for signs and symptoms of hypotension.

Patient/Family Teaching

- Advise female pts of the consequences of second- and third-trimester exposure to irbesartan.
- Stress to the patient/family that the patient should avoid tasks that require mental alertness or motor skills until his or her response to the drug is established.
- Warn the patient/family to report signs or symptoms of infection, including fever and sore throat.
- Encourage the patient to avoid outdoor exercise during hot weather to avoid the risks of dehydration and hypotension.

23 Antiarrhythmic Agents

Adenosine
Amiodarone Hydrochloride
Atropine Sulfate
Disopyramide Phosphate
Lidocaine Hydrochloride
Procainamide Hydrochloride
Quinidine

Uses: Antiarrhythmic agents are used to prevent and treat cardiac arrhythmias, such as premature ventricular contractions, ventricular tachycardia, premature atrial contractions, paroxysmal atrial tachycardia, atrial fibrillation, and atrial flutter.

Action: Antiarrhythmic agents affect certain ion channels and receptors on the myocardial cell membrane. They are divided into four classes; class I drugs are further divided into three subclasses (IA, IB, and IC) based on the electrophysiologic effects of the drugs'.

Class I: Blocks cardiac sodium channels and slows conduction velocity, prolonging refractoriness and decreasing automaticity of sodium-dependent tissue.

Class IA: Blocks sodium and potassium channels.

Class IB: Shortens the repolarization phase.

Class IC: Does not affect the repolarization phase but slows conduction velocity.

Class II: Slows sinoatrial (SA) and atrioventricular (AV) nodal conduction.

Class III: Blocks cardiac potassium channels, prolonging the repolarization phase of electrical cells.

Class IV: Inhibits the influx of calcium through its channels, causing slower conduction through the SA and AV nodes.

COMBINATION PRODUCTS

EMLA: lidocaine/prilocaine (an anesthetic) 2.5%/2.5%.

LIDOCAINE WITH EPINEPHRINE: lidocaine/epinephrine (a vasopressor) 2%/1:50,000; 1%/1:100,000; 1%/1:200,000; 0.5%/1:200,000.

LOMOTIL: atropine/diphenoxylate (an antidiarrheal) 0.025 mg/2.5 mg.

Adenosine

ah-**den**-oh-seen
(Adenocard, Adenocor [AUS])

CATEGORY AND SCHEDULE

Pregnancy Risk Category: C

MECHANISM OF ACTION

A cardiac agent that slows impulse formation in the SA node and conduction time through the AV node. Adenosine also acts as a diagnostic aid in myocardial perfusion imaging or stress echocardiography. ***Therapeutic Effect:*** Depresses left ventricular function and restores normal sinus rhythm.

AVAILABILITY

Injection: 3 mg/mL in 6- and 12-mg syringes.

INDICATIONS AND DOSAGES

▸ **Paroxysmal supraventricular tachycardia (PSVT).**

RAPID IV BOLUS

Adolescents weighing more than 0 kg. 6 mg. If not effective within 1–2 min, may give 12 mg.

Children. Initially 0.1 mg/kg (maximum 6 mg). If not effective, may give 0.2 mg/kg (maximum 12 mg).

Neonates. 0.05 mg/kg. If not effective within 2 min, increase dose by 0.05 mg/kg increments q2min to a maximum dose of 0.25 mg/kg or termination of PSVT.

CONTRAINDICATIONS

Hypersensitivity to adenosine or any related component, atrial fibrillation or flutter, second- or third-degree AV block or sick sinus syndrome (with functioning pacemaker), ventricular tachycardia.

INTERACTIONS

Drug

Carbamazepine: May increase degree of heart block caused by adenosine.

Dipyridamole: May increase effect of adenosine.

Methylxanthines (e.g., caffeine, theophylline): May decrease effect of adenosine.

Digoxin, verapamil: Rare cases of ventricular fibrillation.

Herbal

None known.

Food

None known.

DIAGNOSTIC TEST EFFECTS

None known.

IV INCOMPATIBILITIES

Any drug or solution other than 0.9% NaCl or D_5W.

SIDE EFFECTS

Frequent (18%–12%)

Facial flushing, shortness of breath or dyspnea

Occasional (7%–2%)

Headache, nausea, lightheadedness, chest pressure

Rare (1% or less)

Numbness or tingling in arms, dizziness, sweating, hypotension, palpitations, chest, jaw, or neck pain

SERIOUS REACTIONS

! May produce short-lasting heart block.

PEDIATRIC CONSIDERATIONS

Baseline Assessment

- Identify the arrhythmia on a 12-lead EKG. Also assess the patient's heart rate and rhythm on a continuous cardiac monitor and evaluate the apical pulse rate, rhythm, and quality.
- Be cautious of dyspnea, shortness of breath, and asthma in children.

Precautions

- Use cautiously in pts with arrhythmias at time of conversion, asthma, heart block, or liver or renal failure.

Administration and Handling

IV

• Store at room temperature. Solution normally appears clear.
• Crystallization occurs if refrigerated; if crystallization occurs, dissolve crystals by warming to room temperature. Discard unused portion.
• Administer very rapidly, over 1–2 sec, undiluted, directly into vein, or if using an IV line, use the closest port to the insertion site. If the IV line is being used to infuse any fluid other than 0.9% NaCl, flush the line first before administering adenosine.
• Follow the rapid bolus injection with a rapid 0.9% NaCl flush.

Intervention and Evaluation

• Continue to assess the patient's heart rate and rhythm with continuous cardiac monitoring.
• Monitor the patient's apical pulse rate, rhythm, and strength, blood pressure, and quality of respirations.
• Monitor the patient's intake and output.
• Assess the patient for fluid retention.
• Check serum electrolyte levels.

Patient/Family Teaching

• Advise the patient/family to report unusual signs or symptoms, including chest pain, chest pounding or palpitations, or difficulty breathing or shortness of breath.
• Explain that facial flushing, headache, and nausea may occur and that these symptoms will resolve.

Amiodarone Hydrochloride

ah-me-**oh**-dah-roan
(Aratac [AUS], Cordarone, Cordarone X [AUS], Pacerone)
Do not confuse with amiloride or Cardura.

CATEGORY AND SCHEDULE

Pregnancy Risk Category: D

MECHANISM OF ACTION

A cardiac agent that prolongs myocardial cell action potential duration and refractory period by acting directly on all cardiac tissue. ***Therapeutic Effect:*** Decreases AV conduction and sinus node function.

PHARMACOKINETICS

Slowly, variably absorbed from GI tract. Protein binding: 96%. Extensively metabolized in liver to the active metabolite. Excreted via bile; not removed by hemodialysis. ***Half-Life:*** Adults: 26–107 days; metabolite: 61 days.

AVAILABILITY

Tablets: 200 mg, 400 mg.
Injection: 50 mg/mL.

INDICATIONS AND DOSAGES

▸ **Life-threatening recurrent ventricular fibrillation or hemodynamically unstable ventricular tachycardia.**

PO

Children. Initially, 10–15 mg/kg/day in 1–2 divided doses, for 4–14 days, then 5 mg/kg/day for several wks. Maintenance: 2.5 mg/kg minimal dose for 5 of 7 days/wk.

IV/IO (PALS DOSE)
Children. 5 mg/kg over 20–60 min. May repeat to a maximum dose of 15/kg/day.

UNLABELED USES

Treatment and prophylaxis of supraventricular arrhythmias refractory to conventional treatment and symptomatic atrial flutter.

CONTRAINDICATIONS

Hypersensitivity to amiodarone or any related component. Bradycardia-induced syncope (except in the presence of a pacemaker), second- and third-degree AV block, severe liver disease, severe sinus node dysfunction.

INTERACTIONS

Drug

Antiarrhythmics: May increase cardiac effects.
Beta-blockers, oral anticoagulants: May increase effect of beta-blockers and oral anticoagulants.
Digoxin, phenytoin, cyclosporine, methotrexate, theophylline: May increase drug concentration and risk of toxicity of these drugs.
Fentanyl: May cause bradycardia, hypotension, decreased cardiac output.
Lovastatin, simvastatin: May increase the risk of myopathy or rhabdomyolysis.

Herbal

St. John's wort: Significantly decreases concentrations of amiodarone. Concurrent use is not recommended.

Food

Grapefruit juice: Increases oral absorption of amiodarone.

DIAGNOSTIC TEST EFFECTS

May increase ANA titer, serum alkaline phosphatase, SGOT (AST), and SGPT (ALT) levels. May cause changes in the EKG and thyroid function tests. Therapeutic blood serum level is 0.5–2.5 mcg/mL; toxic serum level has not been established.

IV INCOMPATIBILITIES

Aminophylline (theophylline), cefazolin (Ancef), heparin, sodium bicarbonate

IV COMPATIBILITIES

Dobutamine (Dobutrex), dopamine (Intropin), furosemide (Lasix), insulin (regular), labetalol (Normodyne), lidocaine, midazolam (Versed), morphine, nitroglycerin, norepinephrine (Levophed), phenylephrine (Neo-Synephrine), potassium chloride, vancomycin

SIDE EFFECTS

Expected
Corneal microdeposits are noted in almost all pts treated for more than 6 mos (can lead to blurry vision).

Frequent (greater than 3%)
Parenteral: Hypotension, nausea, fever, bradycardia
Oral: Constipation, headache, decreased appetite, nausea, vomiting, numbness of fingers and toes, photosensitivity, muscular incoordination

Occasional (less than 3%)
Oral: Bitter or metallic taste; decreased sexual ability and interest; dizziness; facial flushing; blue-gray coloring of skin of face, arms, and neck; blurred vision; slow heartbeat; asymptomatic corneal deposits

Rare (less than 1%)
Oral: Skin rash, vision loss, blindness

SERIOUS REACTIONS

! Serious, potentially fatal pulmonary toxicity (alveolitis, pulmonary fibrosis, pneumonitis, and acute respiratory distress syndrome) may begin with progressive dyspnea and cough with rales, decreased breath sounds, pleurisy, CHF or liver toxicity.

! Amiodarone may worsen existing arrhythmias or produce new arrhythmias called proarrhythmias.

PEDIATRIC CONSIDERATIONS

Baseline Assessment

• Expect patient to undergo baseline chest radiograph, EKG, and pulmonary function tests. Also, if ordered, check the results of baseline liver enzyme tests and serum alkaline phosphatase, SGOT (AST), and SGPT (ALT) levels.

• Assess the apical pulse and blood pressure (B/P) immediately before giving the drug. Withhold the medication and notify the physician if the pulse is 60 beats/min or lower or the systolic B/P is less than 90 mm Hg.

• Be aware that amiodarone crosses the placenta and is distributed in breast milk. Know that fetal development is adversely affected by amiodarone.

• The preservative-free IV product should be used with children.

• Be aware that the injectable products contain benzyl alcohol, which can lead to fatal toxicity in neonates who receive large doses.

• Be aware that the safety and efficacy of amiodarone have not been established in children.

Precautions

• Use cautiously in pts with thyroid disease. Amiodarone contains approximately 40% iodine.

Administration and Handling

PO

• Give with meals to reduce GI distress.

• May crush tablets if necessary.

IV

◀ALERT▶ Be aware that solution concentrations greater than 3 mg/mL can cause peripheral vein phlebitis.

• Store at room temperature.

• Use glass or polyolefin containers for dilution. Dilute the loading dose of 150 mg in 100 mL D_5W to yield a solution of 1.5 mg/mL. Dilute the maintenance dose of 900 mg in 500 mL D_5W to yield a solution of 1.8 mg/mL.

• Use solutions held in polyvinyl chloride containers within 2 hrs of dilution. Use solutions in glass or polyolefin containers within 24 hrs of dilution.

• Give the drug through a central venous catheter (CVC) if possible, using an in-line filter. The solution does not need protection from light during administration.

• Give a bolus over 10 min (15 mg/min) not to exceed 30 mg/min; then 1 mg/min over 6 hrs; then 0.5 mg/min over 18 hrs. For infusions lasting longer than 1 hr, drug concentration should not exceed 2 mg/mL, unless a CVC is used.

Intervention and Evaluation

◀ALERT▶ Assess the patient for signs and symptoms of pulmonary toxicity, including progressively worsening cough and dyspnea. Expect to discontinue or reduce the drug dosage if toxicity occurs.

• Monitor the patient's serum alkaline phosphatase, SGOT

(AST), and SGPT (ALT) levels as well as liver and thyroid function tests for evidence of toxicity. Expect to reduce or discontinue the drug if toxicity is evident or liver enzyme levels are elevated.
• Monitor the patient's amiodarone blood level. Know that the therapeutic blood level of amiodarone is 0.5–2.5 mcg/mL and the toxic level has not been established.
• Assess the patient's pulse for bradycardia and an irregular rhythm as well as its quality. Monitor the patient's EKG for changes, particularly widening of the QRS complex and prolonged PR and QT intervals. Notify the physician of any significant interval changes.
• Assess the patient for signs and symptoms of hyperthyroidism, such as breathlessness, bulging eyes (exophthalmos), eyelid edema, frequent urination, hot and dry skin, and weight loss. Also assess the patient for signs and symptoms of hypothyroidism, such as cool and pale skin, lethargy, night cramps, periorbital edema, and pudgy hands and feet.
• Assess the patient for nausea and vomiting.
• Check for bluish discoloration of the skin and cornea in pts receiving therapy for longer than 2 mos.

Patient/Family Teaching

• Urge the patient/family not to abruptly discontinue the medication. Explain that compliance with the prescribed therapy is essential to control arrhythmias.
• Teach the patient/family to monitor the patient's pulse before taking the drug.
• Instruct the patient/family to report shortness of breath, cough, or vision changes.
• Warn the patient/family to limit the patient's exposure to sunlight to protect against photosensitivity.
• Inform the patient/family that the bluish skin and cornea discoloration gradually disappear after the drug is discontinued.
• Encourage the patient/family to restrict the patient's salt and alcohol intake.
• Recommend that the patient/family seek ophthalmic examinations every 6 mos. Advise the patient to report any vision changes to the physician.

Atropine Sulfate

ah-trow-peen
(Atropine Sulfate, Atropisol [CAN], Atropt [AUS])

CATEGORY AND SCHEDULE

Pregnancy Risk Category: C

MECHANISM OF ACTION

An acetylcholine antagonist that competes with acetylcholine for common binding sites on muscarinic receptors, which are located on exocrine glands, cardiac and smooth muscle ganglia, and intramural neurons. This action blocks all muscarinic effects. ***Therapeutic Effect:*** Inhibits the action of acetylcholine, decreases GI motility and secretory activity, GU muscle tone (ureter and bladder); produces ophthalmic cycloplegia and mydriasis.

AVAILABILITY

Injection: 0.05 mg/mL, 0.1 mg/mL, 0.4 mg/0.5 mL, 0.4 mg/mL, 0.5 mg/mL, 1 mg/mL.

INDICATIONS AND DOSAGES

▸ Preanesthetic

IV/IM/SC

Children weighing 5 kg and more. 0.01–0.02 mg/kg/dose 30–60 min preop, to maximum of 0.4 mg/dose. May repeat q4–6h.

Children weighing less than 5 kg. 0.02 mg/kg/dose 30–60 min preop. may repeat q4–6h.

▸ Bradycardia

IV

Children. 0.02 mg/kg with a minimum of 0.1 mg to a maximum of 0.5 mg in children and 1 mg in adolescents. May repeat in 5 min. Maximum total dose: 1 mg in children, 2 mg in adolescents.

CONTRAINDICATIONS

Hypersensitivity to atropine or any related component. Bladder neck obstruction, cardiospasm, intestinal atony, myasthenia gravis in those not treated with neostigmine, narrow-angle glaucoma, obstructive disease of the GI tract, paralytic ileus, severe ulcerative colitis, tachycardia secondary to cardiac insufficiency or thyrotoxicosis, toxic megacolon, unstable cardiovascular status in acute hemorrhage

INTERACTIONS

Drug

Antacids, antidiarrheals: May decrease absorption of atropine.
Anticholinergics: May increase effects of atropine.
Ketoconazole: May decrease absorption of ketoconazole.
Potassium chloride: May increase severity of GI lesions with KCl (wax matrix).

Herbal

None known.

Food

None known.

DIAGNOSTIC TEST EFFECTS

None known.

IV INCOMPATIBILITIES

Thiopental (Pentothal)

IV COMPATIBILITIES

Diphenhydramine (Benadryl), droperidol (Inapsine), fentanyl (Sublimaze), glycopyrrolate (Robinul), heparin, hydromorphone (Dilaudid), midazolam (Versed), morphine, potassium chloride, propofol (Diprivan)

SIDE EFFECTS

Frequent

Dry mouth, nose, and throat that may be severe, decreased sweating, constipation, irritation at SC or IM injection site

Occasional

Swallowing difficulty, blurred vision, bloated feeling, impotence, urinary hesitancy

Rare

Allergic reaction, including rash and urticaria; mental confusion or excitement, particularly in children; fatigue

SERIOUS REACTIONS

! Overdosage may produce tachycardia, palpitations, hot, dry, or flushed skin, absence of bowel sounds, increased respiratory rate, nausea, vomiting, confusion, drowsiness, slurred speech, and CNS stimulation.

! Overdosage may produce psychosis as evidenced by agitation, restlessness, rambling speech, visual hallucinations, paranoid behavior, and delusions, followed by depression.

PEDIATRIC CONSIDERATIONS

Baseline Assessment

• Instruct the patient to urinate before giving this drug to reduce the risk of urinary retention.
• Use with caution in those children who are sensitive to sulfites.

Precautions

◀ **ALERT** ▶ Use extremely cautiously in pts with autonomic neuropathy, diarrhea, known or suspected GI infections, and mild to moderate ulcerative colitis.
• Use cautiously in pts with chronic obstructive pulmonary disease, CHF, coronary artery disease, esophageal reflux or hiatal hernia associated with reflux esophagitis, gastric ulcer, liver or renal disease, hypertension, hyperthyroidism, and tachyarrhythmias.
• Use atropine cautiously in infants.

Administration and Handling

◀ **ALERT** ▶ Notify physician and expect to discontinue this medication immediately if blurred vision, dizziness, or increased pulse occurs.

IM

May be given by SC or IM injection.

IV

• To prevent paradoxical slowing of the heart rate, give the drug rapidly.

Intervention and Evaluation

• Monitor for changes in the patient's blood pressure, pulse, and temperature.
• Monitor the patient with heart disease for signs of tachycardia.
• Assess the patient's skin turgor and mucous membranes to evaluate his or her hydration status.
• Encourage the patient to drink fluids unless the patient is to have nothing by mouth for surgery.
• Assess the patient's bowel sounds for the presence of peristalsis, and be alert for diminished bowel sounds.
• Monitor the patient for fever because pts receiving atropine are at an increased risk of hyperthermia.
• Monitor the patient's intake and output and palpate his or her bladder to assess for urinary retention.
• Assess the patient's stool frequency and consistency.

Patient/Family Teaching

• If atropine is being given preoperatively, explain to the patient that a warm, dry, flushing feeling may occur upon administration.
• Remind the patient/family to remain in bed and not to eat or drink anything before surgery.

Disopyramide Phosphate

dye-so-**peer**-ah-myd
(Norpace, Norpace CR, Rythmodan [CAN])
Do not confuse with desipramine, dipyridamole, or Rythmol.

CATEGORY AND SCHEDULE

Pregnancy Risk Category: C

MECHANISM OF ACTION

An antiarrhythmic that prolongs the refractory period of the cardiac cell by a direct effect, decreasing myocardial excitability and conduction velocity.
Therapeutic Effect: Depresses myocardial contractility. Has anticholinergic and negative inotropic effects.

AVAILABILITY

Capsules: 100 mg, 150 mg.
Capsules (extended release): 100 mg, 150 mg.

INDICATIONS AND DOSAGES

▸ Suppression and prevention of ventricular ectopy, unifocal or multifocal premature ventricular contractions, paired ventricular contractions (couplets), episodes of ventricular tachycardia

PO

Children 12–18 yrs. 6–15 mg/kg/day in divided doses q6h.
Children 5–11 yrs. 10–15 mg/kg/day in divided doses q6h.
Children 1–4 yrs. 10–20 mg/kg/day in divided doses q6h.
Children younger than 1 yr. 10–30 mg/kg/day in divided doses q6h.

▸ Severe refractory arrhythmias

PO

Children 12–18 yrs. 6–15 mg/kg/day.
Children 4–12 yrs. 10–15 mg/kg/day.
Children 1–4 yrs. 10–20 mg/kg/day.
Children younger than 1 yr. 10–30 mg/kg/day.

▸ Dosage in renal impairment

Creatinine Clearance	Dosage Interval
30–40 mL/min	q8h
15–30 mL/min	q12h
Less than 15 mL/min	q24h

UNLABELED USES

Prophylaxis and treatment of supraventricular tachycardia.

CONTRAINDICATIONS

Hypersensitivity to disopyramide or any related component. Cardiogenic shock, narrow-angle glaucoma (unless patient is undergoing cholinergic therapy), preexisting second- or third-degree AV block, preexisting urinary retention. Do not administer to pts receiving erythromycin or clarithromycin.

INTERACTIONS

Drug

Other antiarrhythmics, including diltiazem, propranolol, verapamil: May prolong cardiac conduction, decrease cardiac output.
Pimozide: May increase cardiac arrhythmias.
Phenytoin, phenobarbital, rifampin: May lower serum concentrations of disopyramide.
Clarithromycin and erythromycin: May increase disopyramide concentrations to a toxic, potentially fatal, level. Do not use these drugs concomitantly.

Herbal

None known.

Food

None known.

DIAGNOSTIC TEST EFFECTS

May decrease blood glucose levels. May cause EKG changes. May increase serum cholesterol and triglyceride levels. The therapeutic blood level is 2–8 mcg/mL, and the toxic blood level is greater than 8 mcg/mL.

SIDE EFFECTS

Frequent (greater than 9%)
Dry mouth (32%), urinary hesitancy, constipation
Occasional (9%–3%)
Blurred vision; dry eyes, nose, or throat; urinary retention; headache; dizziness; fatigue nausea
Rare (less than 1%)
Impotence, hypotension, edema, weight gain, shortness of breath, syncope, chest pain, nervousness,

diarrhea, vomiting, decreased appetite, rash, itching

SERIOUS REACTIONS

! May produce or aggravate CHF.
! May produce severe hypotension, shortness of breath, chest pain, syncope (especially in pts with primary cardiomyopathy or CHF).
! Hepatotoxicity occurs rarely.

PEDIATRIC CONSIDERATIONS

Baseline Assessment

- Have the patient empty his or her bladder before administering disopyramide to reduce the risk of urine retention.
- Use cautiously in children who have diabetes mellitus, liver or renal disease, or Wolff-Parkinson White syndrome.

Precautions

- Use cautiously in pts with bundle-branch block, CHF, impaired liver or renal function, myasthenia gravis, prostatic hypertrophy, sick sinus syndrome (sinus bradycardia alternating with tachycardia), and Wolff-Parkinson-White syndrome.

Intervention and Evaluation

- Monitor the patient's EKG for cardiac changes, particularly widening of the QRS complex and prolongation of the PR and QT intervals.
- Monitor the patient's blood glucose, liver enzyme, serum alkaline phosphatase, bilirubin, potassium, SGOT (AST), and SGPT (ALT) levels. Also monitor the patient's blood pressure. Be aware that the therapeutic blood level of disopyramide is 2–8 mcg/mL and the toxic blood level is greater than 8 mcg/mL.
- Monitor the patient's intake and output for signs of urine retention.
- Assess the patient for signs and symptoms of CHF including cough, dyspnea (particularly on exertion), fatigue, and rales at the base of the lungs.
- Assist the patient with ambulation if he or she experiences dizziness.

Patient/Family Teaching

- Warn the patient/family to notify the physician if the patient has a productive cough or shortness of breath.
- Explain to the patient/family that the patient should not take nasal decongestants or OTC cold preparations, especially those containing stimulants, without consulting the physician for approval.
- Encourage the patient/family to restrict the patient's alcohol and salt consumption while he or she is taking disopyramide.

Lidocaine Hydrochloride

lie-doe-cane
(Lidoderm, Lignocaine [AUS], Xylocaine, Xylocard [CAN], Zilactin-L [CAN])

CATEGORY AND SCHEDULE

Pregnancy Risk Category: B

MECHANISM OF ACTION

An amide anesthetic that inhibits conduction of nerve impulses. ***Therapeutic Effect:*** Causes temporary loss of feeling and sensation. Also an antiarrhythmic that decreases depolarization, automaticity, and excitability of the ventricle during diastole by direct action.
Reverses ventricular arrhythmias.

PHARMACOKINETICS

Route	Onset	Peak	Duration
IV	30–90 sec	N/A	10–20 min
Local anesthetic	2.5 min	N/A	30–60 min

Completely absorbed after IM administration. Protein binding: 60%–80%. Widely distributed. Metabolized in liver. Primarily excreted in urine. Minimally removed by hemodialysis.
Half-Life: 1–2 hrs.

AVAILABILITY

IM Injection: 300 mg/3 mL.
Direct IV Injection: 10 mg/mL, 20 mg/mL.
IV Admixture Injection: 40 mg/mL, 100 mg/mL, 200 mg/mL.
IV Infusion: 2 mg/mL, 4 mg/mL, 8 mg/mL.
Injection (anesthesia): 0.5%, 1%, 1.5%, 2%, 4%.
Liquid: 2.5%, 5%.
Ointment: 2.5%, 5%.
Cream: 3%, 4%, 5%.
Gel: 0.5%, 2.5%, 4%
Topical Spray: 0.5%.
Topical Solution: 2%, 4%.
Topical Jelly: 2%.
Dermal Patch: 5%.

INDICATIONS AND DOSAGES

▸ **Rapid control of acute ventricular arrhythmias after a myocardial infarction (MI), cardiac catheterization, cardiac surgery, or digitalis-induced ventricular arrhythmias**
IV
Children and Infants. Initially, 0.5–1 mg/kg IV bolus; may repeat but total dose not to exceed 3–5 mg/kg. Maintenance: 20–50 mcg/kg/min as IV infusion.
ENDOTRACHEAL TUBE
Children and Infants. 2–10 times the bolus IV dose.

▸ **Local skin disorders (minor burns, insect bites, prickly heat, skin manifestations of chickenpox, abrasions), mucous membrane disorders (local anesthesia of oral, nasal, and laryngeal mucous membranes; local anesthesia of respiratory or urinary tract; relief of discomfort of pruritus ani, hemorrhoids, or pruritus vulvae)**
TOPICAL

▸ **Treatment of shingles-related skin pain**
Children. 3 mg/kg/dose no more frequently than q2h.

CONTRAINDICATIONS

Adams-Stokes syndrome, hypersensitivity to amide-type local anesthetics, septicemia (spinal anesthesia), supraventricular arrhythmias, Wolff-Parkinson-White syndrome.

INTERACTIONS

Drug
Anticonvulsants: May increase cardiac depressant effects.
Beta-adrenergic blockers, cimetidine: May increase risk of toxicity.
Other antiarrhythmics: May increase cardiac effects.
Herbal
None known.
Food
None known.

DIAGNOSTIC TEST EFFECTS

IM lidocaine may increase creatinine phosphokinase level (used in diagnostic test for presence of acute MI).
Therapeutic blood level is 1.5–6 mcg/mL; toxic blood level is greater than 6 mcg/mL.

IV INCOMPATIBILITIES

Amphotericin B complex (Abelcet, AmBisome, Amphotec), thiopental

IV COMPATIBILITIES

Aminophylline, amiodarone (Cordarone), calcium gluconate, digoxin (Lanoxin), diltiazem (Cardizem), dobutamine (Dobutrex), dopamine (Intropin), enalapril (Vasotec), furosemide (Lasix), heparin, insulin, nitroglycerin, potassium chloride

SIDE EFFECTS

CNS effects are generally dose related and of short duration.

Occasional

IM: Pain at injection site
Topical: Burning, stinging, tenderness

Rare

Generally with high dose: Drowsiness, dizziness, disorientation, lightheadedness, tremors, apprehension, euphoria, sensation of heat or cold or numbness, blurred or double vision, ringing or roaring in ears (tinnitus), nausea

SERIOUS REACTIONS

! Although serious adverse reactions to lidocaine are uncommon, high dosage by any route may produce cardiovascular depression, bradycardia, somnolence, hypotension, arrhythmias, heart block, cardiovascular collapse, and cardiac arrest.
! There is a potential for malignant hyperthermia.
! CNS toxicity may occur, especially with regional anesthesia use, progressing rapidly from mild side effects to tremors, convulsions, vomiting, and respiratory depression.
! Methemoglobinemia (evidenced by cyanosis) has occurred after topical application of lidocaine for teething discomfort and laryngeal anesthetic spray.
! Overuse of oral lidocaine has caused seizures in children.
! Allergic reactions are rare.

PEDIATRIC CONSIDERATIONS

Baseline Assessment

- Determine whether the patient has a hypersensitivity to amide anesthetics and lidocaine before beginning drug therapy.
- Obtain the patient's baseline blood pressure (B/P), pulse, respirations, EKG, and serum electrolyte levels.
- Be aware that lidocaine crosses the placenta and is distributed in breast milk.
- Keep patches out of the reach of children.
- There are no age-related precautions noted in children.

Precautions

- Use cautiously in pts with atrial fibrillation, bradycardia, heart block, hypovolemia, liver disease, marked hypoxia, and severe respiratory depression.

Administration and Handling

◀ALERT▶ Keep resuscitative equipment and drugs, including O_2, readily available when administering lidocaine by any route.
◀ALERT▶ Know that the therapeutic blood level of lidocaine is 1.5–6 mcg/mL and the toxic blood level is greater than 6 mcg/mL.

IM

- Use 10% solution (100 mg/mL) and clearly identify that the lidocaine preparation is for IM use.
- Give injection in deltoid muscle because the blood level will be significantly higher than if the

injection is given in the gluteus muscle or lateral thigh.

IV

‹ALERT› Use only lidocaine without preservative, clearly marked for IV use.

- Store at room temperature.
- For IV infusion, prepare the solution by adding 1 g to 1 L D_5W to provide a concentration of 1 mg/mL (0.1%).
- Know that commercially available preparations of 0.2%, 0.4%, and 0.8% may be used for IV infusion. Be aware that the maximum concentration is 4 g/250 mL.
- For IV push, use 1% (10 mg/mL) or 2% (20 mg/mL).
- Administer IV push at rate of 25–50 mg/min.
- Administer for IV infusion at rate of 1–4 mg/min (1–4 mL) and use a volume control IV set.

TOPICAL

- Be aware that the topical form is not for ophthalmic use.
- For skin disorders, apply directly to the affected area or put on a gauze pad or bandage, which can then be applied to the skin.
- For mucous membrane use, apply to desired area using the manufacturer's insert.
- Administer the lowest dosage possible that still provides anesthesia.

Intervention and Evaluation

- Monitor the patient's EKG and vital signs closely for cardiac performance during and after lidocaine administration.
- Inform the physician immediately if the patient's EKG shows arrhythmias or prolongation of the PR interval or QRS complex.
- Assess the patient's pulse for its quality and for bradycardia and irregularity.
- Assess the patient's B/P for signs of hypotension.
- Monitor the patient for a therapeutic blood level, which is 1.5–6 mcg/mL.
- For lidocaine given by all routes, monitor the patient's level of consciousness and vital signs. Be aware that drowsiness may signal high lidocaine blood levels.

Patient/Family Teaching

- Ensure that the patient/family receiving lidocaine as a local anesthetic understands that the patient will experience a loss of feeling or sensation and will need protection until the anesthetic wears off.
- Warn the patient/family not to chew gum, drink, or eat for 1 hr after lidocaine application to oral mucous membranes. The swallowing reflex may be impaired, increasing the risk of aspiration; and numbness of tongue or buccal mucosa may lead to biting trauma.

Procainamide Hydrochloride

pro-**cane**-ah-myd
(Apo-Procainamide [CAN], Procanbid, Procan-SR, Pronestyl)
Do not confuse with Ponstel or probenecid.

CATEGORY AND SCHEDULE
Pregnancy Risk Category: C

MECHANISM OF ACTION

An antiarrhythmic that increases the electrical stimulation threshold of the ventricles and His-Purkinje system. Possesses direct cardiac effects. ***Therapeutic Effect:*** Decreases myocardial excitability and conduction velocity and depresses myocardial contractility. Produces an antiarrhythmic effect.

PHARMACOKINETICS
Rapidly, completely absorbed from the GI tract. Protein binding: 15%–20%. Widely distributed. Metabolized in liver to the active metabolite. Primarily excreted in urine. Moderately removed by hemodialysis. ***Half-Life:*** Children: 1.7 hrs; adults: 2.5–4.5 hrs; metabolite: 6 hrs.

AVAILABILITY
Capsules: 250 mg, 375 mg, 500 mg.
Tablets: 250 mg, 375 mg, 500 mg.
Tablets (extended release): 500 mg, 750 mg, 1,000 mg.
Injection: 100 mg/mL, 500 mg/mL.

INDICATIONS AND DOSAGES
▸ **Maintain normal sinus rhythm after conversion of atrial fibrillation or flutter; treat premature ventricular contractions, paroxysmal atrial tachycardia, atrial fibrillation, and ventricular tachycardia**

IV

Children. Loading dose: 3–6 mg/kg/dose over 5 min (maximum: 100 mg). Do not exceed 500 mg in 30 min for a loading dose. May repeat q5–10min to maximum total dose of 15 mg/kg then maintenance dose of 20–80 mcg/kg/min. Maximum: 2 g/day.

PO

Children. 15–50 mg/kg/day of immediate-release tablets in divided doses q3–6h. Maximum: 4 g/day.

▸ **Dosage in renal impairment**

Creatinine Clearance	Dosage Interval
10–50 mL/min	q6–12h
Less than 10 mL/min	q8–24h

UNLABELED USES
Conversion and management of atrial fibrillation.

CONTRAINDICATIONS
Hypersensitivity to procainamide or any related component. Complete heart block, myasthenia gravis, preexisting QT prolongation, second- or third-degree heart block, systemic lupus erythematosus, torsades de pointes.

INTERACTIONS
Drug
Antihypertensives (IV procainamide), neuromuscular blockers: May increase the effects of these drugs. May decrease the antimyasthenic effect on skeletal muscle.

Other antiarrhythmics, pimozide: May increase cardiac effects.

Herbal
None known.

Food
None known.

DIAGNOSTIC TEST EFFECTS
May cause EKG changes and positive ANA titers and Coombs' test results. May increase SGOT (AST), SGPT (ALT), serum alkaline phosphatase, serum bilirubin, and serum LDH levels. Therapeutic serum level is 4–8 mcg/mL; toxic serum level is greater than 10 mcg/mL.

IV INCOMPATIBILITIES
Milrinone (Primacor)

IV COMPATIBILITIES
Amiodarone (Cordarone), dobutamine (Dobutrex), heparin, lidocaine, potassium chloride

SIDE EFFECTS
Frequent

PO: Abdominal pain or cramping, nausea, diarrhea, vomiting

Occasional
Dizziness, giddiness, weakness, hypersensitivity reaction (rash, urticaria, pruritus, flushing)
IV: Transient, but at times, marked hypotension
Rare
Confusion, mental depression, psychosis

SERIOUS REACTIONS

! Paradoxical, extremely rapid ventricular rate may occur during treatment of atrial fibrillation or flutter.
! Systemic lupus erythematosus-like syndrome (fever, joint pain, or pleuritic chest pain) with prolonged therapy.
! Cardiotoxic effects occur most commonly with IV administration, observed as conduction changes (50% widening of the QRS complex, frequent ventricular premature contractions, ventricular tachycardia, complete AV block).
! Prolonged PR and QT intervals and flattened T waves occur less frequently.

PEDIATRIC CONSIDERATIONS

Baseline Assessment
• Check the patient's blood pressure (B/P) and pulse for 1 full min before giving procainamide unless the patient is being monitored on a continuous EKG monitor.
• Be aware that procainamide crosses the placenta, and it is unknown whether procainamide is distributed in breast milk.
• There are no age-related precautions noted in children.
Precautions
• Use cautiously in pts with bundle-branch block, CHF, liver or renal impairment, marked AV conduction disturbances, severe digoxin toxicity, and supraventricular tachyarrhythmias.
Administration and Handling
◂ALERT▸ Know that procainamide dosage and the interval of administration are individualized based on the patient's age, clinical response, renal function, and underlying myocardial disease. Also be aware that extended-release tablets are used for maintenance therapy.
PO
Do not crush or break sustained-release tablets.
IM/IV
◂ALERT▸ May give procainamide by IM injection, IV push, or IV infusion.
• Solution normally appears clear, colorless to light yellow.
• Discard if solution darkens or appears discolored or if precipitate forms.
• When diluted with D_5W, solution is stable for up to 24 hr at room temperature or for 7 days if refrigerated.
• For IV push, dilute with 5–10 mL D_5W.
• For initial loading IV infusion, add 1 g to 50 mL D_5W to provide a concentration of 20 mg/mL.
• For IV infusion, add 1 g to 250–500 mL D_5W to provide concentration of 2–4 mg/mL. Know that the maximum concentration is 4 g/250 mL.
• For IV push, with patient in the supine position, administer at a rate not exceeding 25–50 mg/min.
• For initial loading infusion, infuse 1 mL/min for up to 25–30 min.
• For IV infusion, infuse at 1–3 mL/min.
• Check B/P every 5–10 min during infusion. If a fall in B/P

exceeds 15 mm Hg, discontinue the drug and contact the physician.
- Monitor the EKG for cardiac changes, particularly widening of the QRS complex and prolongation of PR and QT intervals. Notify the physician of any significant interval changes.
- Continuously monitor B/P and the EKG during IV administration. Continuously adjust the rate of infusion to eliminate arrhythmias.

Intervention and Evaluation

- Monitor the patient's EKG for cardiac changes, particularly widening of the QRS complex and prolongation of PR and QT intervals.
- Assess the patient's pulse for its quality and for an irregular rate.
- Monitor the patient's intake and output and serum electrolyte levels, including chloride, potassium, and sodium.
- Evaluate the patient for GI upset, headache, dizziness, or joint pain.
- Assess the patient's pattern of daily bowel activity and stool consistency.
- Assess the patient for signs of dizziness.
- Monitor the patient's B/P for signs of hypotension.
- Assess the patient's skin for a hypersensitivity reaction, especially in pts receiving high-dose therapy.
- Monitor the patient for a therapeutic serum level of 4–8 mcg/mL and a toxic serum level of greater than 10 mcg/mL.

Patient/Family Teaching

- Advise the patient/family to space drug doses evenly around the clock.
- Warn the patient/family to notify the physician if the patient experiences fever, joint pain or stiffness, or signs of upper respiratory infection.
- Caution the patient/family against abruptly discontinuing the drug. Explain to the patient that compliance with therapy is essential to control arrhythmias.
- Explain to the patient/family that the patient should not take nasal decongestants or OTC cold preparations, especially those containing stimulants, without consulting the physician for approval.
- Encourage the patient/family to restrict the patient's alcohol and salt consumption while he or she is taking procainamide.

Quinidine

kwin-ih-deen
(Apo-Quinidine [CAN], Kinidin Durules [AUS], Quinate [CAN], Quinidex)
Do not confuse with clonidine or quinine.

CATEGORY AND SCHEDULE

Pregnancy Risk Category: C

MECHANISM OF ACTION

An antiarrhythmic that decreases sodium influx during depolarization and potassium efflux during repolarization and reduces calcium transport across the myocardial cell membrane. ***Therapeutic Effect:*** Decreases myocardial excitability, conduction velocity, and contractility.

AVAILABILITY

GLUCONATE
Tablets (sustained release): 324 mg.
Injection: 80 mg/mL (50 mg/mL quinidine sulfate)
Tablets: 200 mg, 300 mg.
Tablets (sustained release): 300 mg.

INDICATIONS AND DOSAGES

▸ Maintain normal sinus rhythm after conversion of atrial fibrillation or flutter; prevention of premature atrial, AV, and ventricular contractions, paroxysmal atrial tachycardia, paroxysmal AV junctional rhythm, atrial fibrillation, atrial flutter, and paroxysmal ventricular tachycardia not associated with complete heart block

IV

Children. 2–10 mg/kg/dose q3–6h as needed. Not recommended in children.

PO

Children: 30 mg/kg/day in divided doses q4–6h. Maximum: 200 mg.

UNLABELED USES

Treatment of malaria (IV only).

CONTRAINDICATIONS

Hypersensitivity to quinidine or any related component. Complete AV block, intraventricular conduction defects (widening of QRS complex).

INTERACTIONS

Drug

Antimyasthenics: May decrease effects of these drugs on skeletal muscle.
Digoxin: May increase digoxin serum concentration.
Other antiarrhythmics, pimozide: May increase cardiac effects.
Neuromuscular blockers, oral anticoagulants: May increase effects of these drugs.
Urinary alkalizers, such as antacids: May decrease quinidine renal excretion.

Herbal

None known.

Food

Grapefruit juice: Delays absorption, decreases clearance, and inhibits metabolism of quinidine.
Acidic foods/juices: Decrease serum concentrations of quinidine, which lessens effectiveness of the drug.
Alkaline foods/juices: Increase quinidine serum concentrations leading to toxicity.

DIAGNOSTIC TEST EFFECTS

None known. Therapeutic serum level is 2–5 mcg/mL; toxic level is greater than 5 mcg/mL.

IV INCOMPATIBILITIES

Furosemide (Lasix), heparin

IV COMPATIBILITIES

Milrinone (Primacor)

SIDE EFFECTS

Frequent

Abdominal pain and cramps, nausea, diarrhea, vomiting (can be immediate and intense)

Occasional

Mild cinchonism (ringing in ears, blurred vision, hearing loss) or severe cinchonism (headache, vertigo, diaphoresis, lightheadedness, photophobia, confusion, delirium)

Rare

Hypotension (particularly with IV administration), hypersensitivity reaction (fever, anaphylaxis, photosensitivity reaction)

SERIOUS REACTIONS

! Cardiotoxic effects occur most commonly with IV administration, particularly at high concentrations, and are observed as conduction changes (50% widening of QRS complex, prolonged QT interval, flattened T waves, or disappearance of the P wave), ventricular tachycardia or flutter, frequent

premature ventricular contractions, or complete AV block.
! Quinidine-induced syncope may occur with the usual dosage.
! Severe hypotension may result from high dosages.
! Pts with atrial flutter and fibrillation may experience a paradoxical, extremely rapid ventricular rate that may be prevented by prior digitalization.
! Liver toxicity with jaundice due to drug hypersensitivity may occur.

PEDIATRIC CONSIDERATIONS

Baseline Assessment

- Check the patient's blood pressure (B/P) and pulse for 1 full min before giving quinidine unless the patient is being monitored on a continuous cardiac monitor.
- Monitor the results of the complete blood count (CBC), and BUN, serum alkaline phosphatase, bilirubin, creatinine, and SGOT (AST) and SGPT (ALT) levels for pts receiving long-term therapy.
- Use cautiously in children who have asthma, fever, or muscle weakness.

Precautions

- Use cautiously in pts with digoxin toxicity, incomplete AV block, liver or renal impairment, myasthenia gravis, myocardial depression, and sick sinus syndrome.

Administration and Handling

◂**ALERT**▸ Keep in mind that the therapeutic serum level of quinidine is 2–5 mcg/mL and the toxic level is greater than 5 mcg/mL.

PO

- Ensure that the patient does not crush or chew sustained-release tablets.
- To reduce GI upset, give quinidine with food.

IV

◂**ALERT**▸ Continuously monitor the patient's B/P and EKG waveform during IV administration and adjust the rate of the infusion as appropriate and as ordered to minimize arrhythmias and hypotension.

- Use only clear, colorless solution.
- Solution is stable for up to 24 hrs at room temperature when diluted with D_5W.
- For IV infusion, dilute 800 mg with 40 mL D_5W to provide a concentration of 16 mg/mL.
- Administer with the patient in the supine position.
- For IV infusion, give at rate of 1 mL (16 mg)/min because a rapid rate may markedly decrease arterial pressure.
- Monitor the patient's EKG for cardiac changes, particularly prolongation of the PR or QT interval and widening of the QRS complex. Notify the physician of any significant EKG changes.

Intervention and Evaluation

- Monitor the patient's complete blood count, intake and output, liver and renal function tests, and serum potassium levels.
- Assess the patient's pattern of daily bowel activity and stool consistency.
- Monitor the patient's B/P for hypotension, especially in those receiving high-dose therapy.
- Expect to discontinue the drug if the patient develops quinidine-induced syncope.
- Notify the physician immediately if the patient experiences cardiotoxic effects.

Patient/Family Teaching

- Warn the patient/family to notify the physician if the patient experiences fever, rash, ringing in the ears, unusual bleeding or bruising, or visual disturbances.

• Advise the patient/family that quinidine may cause a photosensitivity reaction. Urge the patient to avoid contact with direct sunlight or artificial light.

REFERENCES

Gunn, V. L. & Nechyba, C. (2002). The Harriet Lane handbook (16th ed.). St. Louis: Mosby.

Miller, S. & Fioravanti, J. (1997). Pediatric medications: a handbook for nurses. St. Louis: Mosby.

Taketomo, C. K., Hodding, J. H. & Kraus, D. M. (2003–2004). Pediatric dosage handbook (10th ed.). Hudson, OH: Lexi-Comp.

24 Antihyperlipidemic Agents

Cholestyramine Resin
Lovastatin
Niacin, Nicotinic Acid
Pravastatin

Uses: Antihyperlipidemics are used to lower abnormally high blood levels of cholesterol and triglycerides, which are linked with the development and progression of atherosclerosis. Effective management of cholesterol and triglycerides includes dietary modification along with pharmacologic treatment.

Action: Five subclasses of antihyperlipidemics act in different ways. *Bile acid sequestrants,* such as cholestyramine and colesevelam, bind with bile acids in the intestine, preventing their active transport and reabsorption and enhancing their excretion. By depleting hepatic bile acid, these agents increase the conversion of cholesterol to bile acids.

Hydroxymethylglutaryl coenzyme A (HMG-CoA) reductase inhibitors (statins), such as lovastatin, inhibit HMG-CoA reductase, an enzyme required for the last regulated step in cholesterol synthesis. This action reduces cholesterol synthesis in the liver.

Niacin (nicotinic acid) reduces hepatic synthesis of triglycerides and the secretion of very low-density lipoproteins by inhibiting the mobilization of free fatty acids from peripheral tissues.

COMBINATION PRODUCTS

RAVIGARD: pravastatin/aspirin (an antiplatelet) 20 mg/81 mg; 20 mg/325 mg; 40 mg/81 mg; 40 mg/325 mg; 80 mg/81 mg; 80 mg/325 mg.

Cholestyramine Resin

koh-**les**-tir-ah-meen **rez**-in
(Novo-Cholamine [CAN], Novo-Cholamine Light [CAN], Prevalite, Questran, Questran Light [AUS])
Do not confuse with Quarzan.

CATEGORY AND SCHEDULE

Pregnancy Risk Category: B

MECHANISM OF ACTION

An antihyperlipoproteinemic agent that binds with bile acids in the intestine, forming an insoluble complex. Binding results in partial removal of bile acid from the enterohepatic circulation.
Therapeutic Effect: Removes low-density lipoproteins (LDLs) and cholesterol from plasma.

PHARMACOKINETICS

Not absorbed from the GI tract. Decreases in LDLs are apparent in 5–7 days and serum cholesterol in 1 mo. Serum cholesterol returns to baseline levels about 1 mo after discontinuing drug. Excreted in feces.

AVAILABILITY

Powder: 4 g.

INDICATIONS AND DOSAGES

▸ **Primary hypercholesterolemia**

PO

Children older than 10 yrs. 2 g/day up to 8 g/day.

Children 10 yrs and younger. Initially, 2 g/day. Range: 1–4 g/day.

UNLABELED USES

Treatment of diarrhea (due to bile acids); hyperoxaluria, pruritus associated with elevated levels of bile acids.

CONTRAINDICATIONS

Complete biliary obstruction or biliary atresia, hypersensitivity to cholestyramine or tartrazine (frequently seen in aspirin hypersensitivity).

INTERACTIONS

Drug

Anticoagulants: May increase the effects of these drugs by decreasing vitamin K.

Digoxin, folic acid, penicillins, propranolol, tetracyclines, thiazides, thyroid hormones, other medications: May bind and decrease absorption of these drugs.

Oral vancomycin: Binds and decreases the effects of oral vancomycin.

Warfarin: May decrease warfarin absorption.

Herbal

None known.

Food

Fat-soluble vitamins (A, D, E, and K), iron, folic acid: May decrease absorption of these vitamins, leading to deficiency.

DIAGNOSTIC TEST EFFECTS

May increase serum alkaline phosphatase, serum magnesium, SGOT (AST), and SGPT (ALT) levels. May decrease serum calcium, potassium, and sodium levels. May prolong prothrombin time.

SIDE EFFECTS

Frequent

Constipation (may lead to fecal impaction), nausea, vomiting, stomach pain, indigestion

Occasional

Diarrhea, belching, bloating, headache, dizziness

Rare

Gallstones, peptic ulcer, malabsorption syndrome

SERIOUS REACTIONS

! GI tract obstruction, hyperchloremic acidosis, and osteoporosis secondary to calcium excretion may occur.

! High dosage may interfere with fat absorption, resulting in steatorrhea.

PEDIATRIC CONSIDERATIONS

Baseline Assessment

- Determine the patient's history of hypersensitivity to aspirin, cholestyramine, and tartrazine before beginning drug therapy.
- Check the patient's baseline electrolyte levels and serum cholesterol and triglyceride levels.
- Be aware that cholestyramine is not systemically absorbed and may interfere with maternal absorption of fat-soluble vitamins.
- There are no age-related precautions noted in children. Cholestyramine use is limited in pediatric pts younger than 10 yrs of age.

Precautions
• Use cautiously in pts with bleeding disorders, GI dysfunction (especially constipation), hemorrhoids, and osteoporosis.

Administration and Handling
PO
• Give other drugs at least 1 hr before or 4–6 hrs after cholestyramine because this drug is capable of binding drugs in the GI tract.
• Do not give cholestyramine in its dry form because it is highly irritating. Mix with 3–6 oz of fruit juice, milk, soup, or water.
• Place powder on the surface of the liquid for 1–2 min to prevent lumping, then mix thoroughly.
• When mixing the powder with carbonated beverages, use an extra large glass and stir the liquid slowly to avoid excessive foaming.
• Administer before meals.

Intervention and Evaluation
• Assess the patient's pattern of daily bowel activity and stool consistency.
• Evaluate the patient's abdominal discomfort, flatulence, and food tolerance.
• Monitor the patient's blood chemistry test results.
• Encourage the patient to drink several glasses of water between meals.

Patient/Family Teaching
• Advise the patient/family to complete a full course of therapy. Caution the patient against omitting or changing drug doses.
• Instruct the patient/family to take other drugs at least 1 hr before or 4–6 hrs after cholestyramine.
• Warn the patient/family never to take cholestyramine in its dry form.
• Teach the patient/family to mix the powder with 3–6 oz of fruit juice, milk, soup, or water. Explain to the patient/family that the powder should be placed on the surface of a liquid for 1–2 min to prevent lumping and then mixed into the liquid. Advise the patient/family to use an extra large glass and to stir the liquid slowly to avoid excessive foaming when mixing the powder with carbonated beverages.
• Instruct the patient/family to take cholestyramine before meals and to drink several glasses of water between meals.
• Encourage the patient/family to eat high-fiber foods such as fruits, whole grain cereals, and vegetables to reduce the risk of constipation.

Lovastatin

low-vah-**stah**-tin
(Altocor, Mevacor)
Do not confuse with Leustatin, Livostin, or Mivacron.

CATEGORY AND SCHEDULE
Pregnancy Risk Category: X

MECHANISM OF ACTION
An antihyperlipidemic that inhibits HMG-CoA reductase, the enzyme that catalyzes the early step in cholesterol synthesis. ***Therapeutic Effect:*** Decreases low-density lipoprotein (LDL) cholesterol, very low-density lipoprotein cholesterol, and plasma triglyceride levels; increases high-density lipoprotein cholesterol level.

PHARMACOKINETICS

Route	Onset	Peak	Duration
PO	3 days	4–6 wks	N/A

Incompletely absorbed from the GI tract (increased on empty stomach). Protein binding: greater than 95%. Hydrolyzed in liver to the active metabolite. Primarily eliminated in feces. Not removed by hemodialysis. ***Half-Life:*** 1.1–1.7 hrs.

AVAILABILITY

Tablets: 10 mg, 20 mg, 40 mg.
Tablets (extended release): 10 mg, 20 mg, 40 mg, 60 mg.

INDICATIONS AND DOSAGES

▸ Hyperlipoproteinemia
PO (EXTENDED RELEASE)
Children 10–17 yrs. 10–40 mg/day with evening meal. Start with 10 mg initially once daily and increase dose every 8–12 wks as needed. Use immediate-release formulation.

CONTRAINDICATIONS

Hypersensitivity to lovastatin or any related component. Active liver disease, pregnancy, breast-feeding, unexplained elevated liver function test results.

INTERACTIONS

Drug

Cyclosporine, erythromycin, gemfibrozil, immunosuppressants, niacin: Increases the risk of acute renal failure and rhabdomyolysis.
Erythromycin, itraconazole, ketoconazole: May increase lovastatin blood concentration, causing severe muscle inflammation, pain, and weakness.
Warfarin: Lovastatin may increase bleeding time seen with warfarin.

Herbal

St. John's wort: May decrease lovastatin serum concentrations.

Food

Grapefruit juice: Large amounts of grapefruit juice may increase the risk of side effects, such as muscle pain and weakness.

DIAGNOSTIC TEST EFFECTS

May increase serum creatine kinase and serum transaminase concentrations.

SIDE EFFECTS

Generally well tolerated. Side effects are usually mild and transient.

Frequent (9%–5%)
Headache, flatulence, diarrhea, abdominal pain or cramps, rash and pruritus

Occasional (4%–3%)
Nausea, vomiting, constipation, dyspepsia

Rare (2%–1%)
Dizziness, heartburn, myalgia, blurred vision, eye irritation

SERIOUS REACTIONS

! There is a potential for development of cataracts.

PEDIATRIC CONSIDERATIONS

Baseline Assessment

- Determine whether the female patient is pregnant before beginning lovastatin therapy.
- Assess the patient's baseline laboratory test results including serum cholesterol and triglyceride levels and liver function tests.
- Be aware that lovastatin use is contraindicated in pregnancy, because the suppression of cholesterol biosynthesis may cause fetal toxicity, and lactation.
- Be aware that it is unknown whether lovastatin is distributed in breast milk.

• Be aware that the safety and efficacy of lovastatin have not been established in children.
• Treatment of hypercholesterolemia in children is limited to children older than 10 yrs of age who, after a 6 mo–1 yr trial of diet therapy, continue to have LDL cholesterol concentrations greater than 190 mg/dL alone, or LDL cholesterol concentrations greater than 160 mg/dL and a family history of premature coronary artery disease or two or more heart disease risk factors.

Precautions

• Use cautiously in pts who also use cyclosporine, fibrates, and niacin.
• Use cautiously in pts with a history of heavy alcohol use and renal impairment

Administration and Handling

PO

Give lovastatin with meals.

Intervention and Evaluation

• Assess the patient's daily pattern of bowel activity.
• Evaluate the patient for blurred vision, dizziness, and headache.
• Assess the patient for pruritus and rash.
• Monitor the patient's serum cholesterol and triglyceride levels for a therapeutic response.
• Be alert for the onset of malaise, muscle cramping, or weakness.

Patient/Family Teaching

• Instruct the patient/family to take lovastatin with meals.
• Encourage the patient/family to follow the prescribed diet.
• Stress to the patient/family that the prescribed diet and periodic laboratory tests are essential parts of therapy.
• Urge the patient/family to avoid consuming grapefruit juice during lovastatin therapy.
• Warn the patient/family to notify the physician if the patient experiences changes in the color of his or her stool or urine, muscle pain or weakness, severe gastric upset, unusual bruising, vision changes, and yellowing of eyes or skin.

Niacin, Nicotinic Acid

(Niacor, Niaspan, Nico-400, Nicotinex)

Do not confuse with Nitro-Bid.

OTC

CATEGORY AND SCHEDULE

Pregnancy Risk Category: A (C if used at dosages above the recommended daily allowance [RDA])

MECHANISM OF ACTION

An antihyperlipidemic, water-soluble vitamin that is a component of two coenzymes needed for tissue respiration, lipid metabolism, and glycogenolysis. Inhibits synthesis of very-low-density lipoproteins. ***Therapeutic Effect:*** Reduces total and low-density lipoprotein cholesterol and triglyceride levels; Increases high-density lipoprotein cholesterol levels. Necessary for lipid metabolism, tissue respiration, and glycogenolysis.

PHARMACOKINETICS

Readily absorbed from the GI tract. Widely distributed. Excreted in breast milk. Metabolized in liver. Primarily excreted in urine. ***Half-Life:*** 45 min.

AVAILABILITY

Tablets: 50 mg, 100 mg, 250 mg, 500 mg.

Tablets (time release): 250 mg, 500 mg, 750 mg.
Capsules (time release): 125 mg, 250 mg, 400 mg, 500 mg.
Elixir: 50 mg/5 mL (contains 10% alcohol).

INDICATIONS AND DOSAGES

▸ Hyperlipidemia

PO (IMMEDIATE RELEASE)
Children. Initially, 100–250 mg/day (maximum: 10 mg/kg/day) in 3 divided doses with meals. May increase by 100 mg/day or 250 mg q2–3wks. Maximum: 2,250 mg/day.

CONTRAINDICATIONS

Hypersensitivity to niacin or any related component. Active peptic ulcer, arterial hemorrhaging, hypersensitivity to niacin or tartrazine (frequently seen in pts sensitive to aspirin), liver dysfunction, severe hypotension.

INTERACTIONS

Drug

Lovastatin, pravastatin, simvastatin: May increase the risk of acute renal failure and rhabdomyolysis.
Anticoagulants: May increase prothrombin time.

Herbal

None known.

Food

Hot drinks or alcohol: May increase flushing and pruritus.

DIAGNOSTIC TEST EFFECTS

May increase serum uric acid levels.

SIDE EFFECTS

Frequent

Flushing (especially of face and neck) occurring within 20 min of administration and lasting for 30–60 min, GI upset, pruritus

Occasional

Dizziness, hypotension, headache, blurred vision, burning or tingling of skin, flatulence, nausea, vomiting, diarrhea

Rare

Hyperglycemia, glycosuria, rash, hyperpigmentation, dry skin

SERIOUS REACTIONS

! Arrhythmias occur rarely.

PEDIATRIC CONSIDERATIONS

Baseline Assessment

- Determine whether the patient has a history of hypersensitivity to aspirin, niacin, or tartrazine before beginning drug therapy.
- Assess the patient's baseline blood glucose, serum cholesterol, and triglyceride levels and liver function test results.
- Be aware that niacin is not recommended for use during pregnancy and lactation.
- Be aware that niacin is distributed in breast milk.
- There are no age-related precautions noted in children.
- Niacin use is not recommended in children younger than 2 years of age.
- Routine use in children and adolescents is not recommended due to limited safety and efficacy information.

Precautions

- Use cautiously in pts with diabetes mellitus, gallbladder disease, gout, and a history of liver disease or jaundice.

Administration and Handling

PO
- Give niacin without regard to meals.
- Administer the drug at bedtime.

Intervention and Evaluation

• Assess the patient's degree of discomfort and flushing.
• Evaluate the patient for blurred vision, dizziness, and headache.
• Assess the patient's pattern of daily bowel activity and stool consistency.
• Monitor the patient's blood glucose levels, serum alkaline phosphatase, bilirubin, cholesterol and triglyceride, uric acid, and SGOT (AST) and SGPT (ALT) levels.
• Monitor blood glucose levels frequently, as ordered, in pts receiving insulin or oral antihyperglycemic drugs.
• Assess the patient's skin for dryness.

Patient/Family Teaching

• Advise the patient/family to take the drug at bedtime and to avoid alcohol consumption.
• Advise the patient/family that itching, flushing of the skin, sensation of warmth, and tingling may occur.
• Warn the patient/family to notify the physician if the patient experiences dark urine, dizziness, loss of appetite, nausea, vomiting, weakness, or yellowing of the skin.
• Suggest to the patient/family that the patient avoid sudden changes in posture to help prevent bouts of dizziness.

Pravastatin

pra-vah-sta-tin
(Pravachol)
Do not confuse with Prevacid or propranolol.

CATEGORY AND SCHEDULE

Pregnancy Risk Category: X

MECHANISM OF ACTION

A HMG-CoA reductase inhibitor that interferes with cholesterol biosynthesis by preventing the conversion of HMG-CoA reductase to mevalonate, a precursor to cholesterol. ***Therapeutic Effect:*** Lowers low-density lipoprotein cholesterol, very low-density lipoprotein, and plasma triglyceride levels; increases high-density lipoprotein concentration.

PHARMACOKINETICS

Poorly absorbed from the GI tract. Protein binding: 50%. Metabolized in liver (minimal active metabolites). Primarily excreted in feces via the biliary system. Not removed by hemodialysis. ***Half-Life:*** 2.7 hrs.

AVAILABILITY

Tablets: 10 mg, 20 mg, 40 mg, 80 mg.

INDICATIONS AND DOSAGES

▸ Adolescents (8 yrs of age and older) with heterozygous familial hypercholesterolemia

PO

Children 14–18 yrs. 40 mg/day.
Children 8–13 yrs. 20 mg/day.

CONTRAINDICATIONS

Hypersensitivity to pravastatin or any related component. Active liver disease or unexplained, persistent elevations of liver function test results.

INTERACTIONS

Drug

Cyclosporine, erythromycin, gemfibrozil, immunosuppressants, niacin protease inhibitors: Increases the risk of acute renal failure and rhabdomyolysis.

Herbal

None known.

Food

None known.

DIAGNOSTIC TEST EFFECTS

May increase serum creatinine kinase and transaminase concentrations.

SIDE EFFECTS

Generally well tolerated. Side effects are usually mild and transient.

Occasional (7%–4%)

Nausea, vomiting, diarrhea, constipation, abdominal pain, headache, rhinitis, rash, pruritus

Rare (3%–2%)

Heartburn, myalgia, dizziness, cough, fatigue, flu-like symptoms

SERIOUS REACTIONS

! There is a potential for malignancy and cataracts.

! Hypersensitivity occurs rarely.

PEDIATRIC CONSIDERATIONS

Baseline Assessment

- Determine whether the patient is pregnant before beginning pravastatin therapy.
- Assess the patient's baseline laboratory results including serum cholesterol and triglyceride levels and liver function test results.
- Be aware that pravastatin use is contraindicated in pregnancy because suppression of cholesterol biosynthesis may cause fetal toxicity and is also contraindicated during lactation.
- Be aware that it is unknown whether pravastatin is distributed in breast milk, but there is a risk of serious adverse reactions in breast-feeding infants.
- Be aware that the safety and efficacy of this drug have not been established in children.

Precautions

- Use cautiously in pts with a history of liver disease, severe electrolyte, endocrine, or metabolic disorders and in those who consume a substantial amount of alcohol.
- Withholding or discontinuing pravastatin may be necessary when the patient is at risk for renal failure secondary to rhabdomyolysis.

Administration and Handling

◂ ALERT ▸ Before beginning pravastatin therapy, know that the patient should be consuming a standard cholesterol-lowering diet for minimum of 3–6 mos. The patient should continue the diet throughout pravastatin therapy.

PO

- Give pravastatin without regard to meals.
- Administer in the evening.

Intervention and Evaluation

- Monitor the patient's serum cholesterol and triglyceride laboratory results for a therapeutic response.
- Monitor the patient's serum alkaline phosphatase, bilirubin, SGOT (AST), and SGPT (ALT) levels to assess liver function.
- Assess the patient's pattern of daily bowel activity and stool consistency.
- Evaluate the patient for dizziness and headache. Help the patient with ambulation if he or she experiences dizziness.
- Assess the patient for pruritus and rash.
- Assess the patient for malaise and muscle cramping or weakness. If these conditions occur and are accompanied by fever, expect that pravastatin use may be discontinued.

Patient/Family Teaching

- Advise the patient/family to follow the prescribed diet and explain that the diet is an important part of treatment.

• Stress to the patient/family that periodic laboratory tests are an essential part of therapy.
• Warn the patient/family to notify the physician if the patient experiences muscle pain or weakness, especially if accompanied by fever or malaise.
• Advise the patient/family to avoid tasks that require mental alertness or motor skills if the patient experiences dizziness.
• Urge the patient/family to use nonhormonal contraception while taking pravastatin. Explain to the patient that pravastatin is pregnancy risk category X.

REFERENCES

Gunn, V. L. & Nechyba, C. (2002). The Harriet Lane handbook (16th ed.). St. Louis: Mosby.

25 Beta-Adrenergic Blocking Agents

Atenolol
Propranolol Hydrochloride
Timolol Maleate

Uses: Beta-adrenergic blockers are used to manage hypertension, angina pectoris, arrhythmias, hypertrophic subaortic stenosis, migraine headaches, and glaucoma. They are also used to prevent myocardial infarction (MI).

Action: Beta-adrenergic blockers competitively block beta$_1$-adrenergic receptors, located primarily in the myocardium, and beta$_2$-adrenergic receptors, located primarily in bronchial and vascular smooth muscle. By occupying beta-receptor sites, these agents prevent endogenous or administered epinephrine and norepinephrine from exerting their effects. The results are basically opposite to those of sympathetic stimulation.

Effects of beta$_1$-blockade include slowed heart rate and decreased cardiac output and contractility. Effects of beta$_2$-blockade include bronchoconstriction and increased airway resistance in pts with asthma or chronic obstructive pulmonary disease. Beta-adrenergic blockers can affect cardiac rhythm and automaticity, decreasing the sinus rate and sinoatrial and atrioventricular (AV) conduction and increasing the refractory period in the AV node.

These agents decrease systolic and diastolic blood pressure. Although the exact mechanism of action of this effect is unknown, it may result from peripheral receptor blockade, decreased sympathetic outflow from the CNS, or decreased renin release from the kidneys.

All beta-adrenergic blockers mask the tachycardia that occurs with hypoglycemia. When applied to the eyes, they reduce intraocular pressure (IOP) and aqueous production.

COMBINATION PRODUCTS

COSOPT: timolol/dorzolamide (a carbonic anhydrase inhibitor) 0.5%/2%.
INDERIDE: propranolol/hydrochlorothiazide (a diuretic) 40 mg/25 mg; 80 mg/25 mg.
INDERIDE LA: propranolol/hydrochlorothiazide (a diuretic) 80 mg/50 mg; 120 mg/50 mg; 160 mg/50 mg.
TENORETIC: atenolol/chlorthalidone (a diuretic) 50 mg/25 mg; 100 mg/25 mg.
TIMOLIDE: timolol/hydrochlorothiazide (a diuretic) 10 mg/25 mg.
ZIAC: bisoprolol/hydrochlorothiazide (a diuretic) 2.5 mg/6.25 mg, 5 mg/6.25 mg, 10 mg/6.25 mg

Atenolol

ay-**ten**-oh-lol
(Apo-Atenol [CAN], AteHexal [AUS], Noten [AUS], Tenolin [CAN], Tenormin, Tensig [AUS])
Do not confuse with albuterol.

CATEGORY AND SCHEDULE

Pregnancy Risk Category: D

MECHANISM OF ACTION

A $beta_1$-adrenergic blocker that acts as an antianginal, antiarrhythmic, and antihypertensive agent by blocking $beta_1$-adrenergic receptors in cardiac tissue. ***Therapeutic Effect:*** Slows sinus node heart rate, decreasing cardiac output and blood pressure (B/P). Decreases myocardial O_2 demand.

PHARMACOKINETICS

Route	Onset	Peak	Duration
PO	1 hr	2–4 hrs	24 hrs

Incompletely absorbed from the gastrointestinal (GI) tract. Protein binding: 6%–16%. Minimal liver metabolism. Primarily excreted unchanged in urine. Moderately removed by hemodialysis.
Half-Life: Neonates: 16–35 hrs; children: 3.5–7 hrs; adults: 6–7 hrs (half-life increased in impaired renal function).

AVAILABILITY

Tablets: 25 mg, 50 mg, 100 mg.
Injection: 5 mg/10 mL.

INDICATIONS AND DOSAGES

▸ Hypertension

PO
Children. Initially, 0.8–1 mg/kg/dose once daily. The dose can range from 0.8–1.5 mg/kg/day. Maximum: 2 mg/kg/day or 100 mg/day.

UNLABELED USES

Improves survival in diabetic pts with heart disease. Treatment of hypertrophic cardiomyopathy, pheochromocytoma, and syndrome of mitral valve prolapse; prophylaxis of migraine, thyrotoxicosis, and tremors.

CONTRAINDICATIONS

Hypersensitivity to atenolol. Cardiogenic shock, overt heart failure, second- or third-degree heart block, severe bradycardia, pulmonary edema.

INTERACTIONS

Drug

Cimetidine: May increase blood atenolol concentration.
Diuretics, other hypotensives: May increase hypotensive effect of atenolol.
Insulin, oral hypoglycemics: May mask symptoms of hypoglycemia

and prolong hypoglycemic effect of insulin and oral hypoglycemics.
NSAIDs: May decrease antihypertensive effect of atenolol.
Sympathomimetics, xanthines: May mutually inhibit effects.
Herbal
None known.
Food
None known.

DIAGNOSTIC TEST EFFECTS

May increase serum ANA titer and BUN, serum creatinine, potassium, lipoprotein, triglyceride, and uric acid levels.

IV INCOMPATIBILITIES

Amphotericin complex (Abelcet, AmBisome, Amphotec)

SIDE EFFECTS

Generally well tolerated, with mild and transient side effects.
Frequent
Hypotension manifested as cold extremities, constipation or diarrhea, diaphoresis, dizziness, fatigue, headache, nausea
Occasional
Insomnia, flatulence, urinary frequency, impotence or decreased libido
Rare
Rash, arthralgia, myalgia, confusion, change in taste

SERIOUS REACTIONS

! Overdosage may produce profound bradycardia and hypotension.
! Abrupt atenolol withdrawal may result in sweating, palpitations, headache, and tremulousness.
! Atenolol administration may precipitate CHF or MI in those with cardiac disease, thyroid storm in those with thyrotoxicosis, and peripheral ischemia in those with existing peripheral vascular disease.
! Hypoglycemia may occur in pts with previously controlled diabetes.
! Thrombocytopenia, manifested as unusual bruising or bleeding, occurs rarely.

PEDIATRIC CONSIDERATIONS

Baseline Assessment
• Assess the patient's apical pulse rate and B/P immediately before giving atenolol. If the pulse is 60 beats/min or less or if the systolic B/P is less than 90 mm Hg, withhold the medication and notify the physician.
• If atenolol is being given as an antianginal agent, record the onset, type (such as dull, sharp, or squeezing), radiation, location, intensity, and duration, of anginal pain. Also, document the precipitating factors, such as emotional stress or exertion.
• Obtain the patient's baseline renal and liver function test results.
• Be aware that atenolol readily crosses the placenta and is distributed in breast milk.
• Know that atenolol use should be avoided in pregnant women during the first trimester because the drug may produce apnea, bradycardia, hypoglycemia, or hypothermia during childbirth as well as low birth-weight infants.
• Use with caution in children who have diabetes (may mask signs of hypoglycemia) or asthma.
• There are no age-related precautions noted in children.
Precautions
• Use cautiously in pts with bronchospastic disease, diabetes, hyperthyroidism, impaired renal or liver function, inadequate cardiac

function, or peripheral vascular disease.

Administration and Handling

PO

• May give without regard to meals.
• Crush tablets if necessary.

IV

• Store at room temperature.
• After reconstitution, store parenteral form for up to 48 hrs at room temperature.
• Give undiluted or dilute in 10–50 mL 0.9% NaCl or D_5W.
• Give IV push over 5 min and IV infusion over 15 min.

Intervention and Evaluation

• Monitor the patient's B/P for hypotension, pulse for bradycardia, and respirations for difficulty breathing.
• Assess the patient's pattern of daily bowel activity and stool consistency.
• Examine the patient for evidence of CHF, including distended neck veins, dyspnea, particularly on exertion or lying down, night cough, and peripheral edema.
• Monitor the patient's intake and output and weights. An increase in weight or decrease in urine output may indicate CHF.
• Assess the patient's extremities for coldness.
• Assist the patient with ambulation if dizziness occurs.

Patient/Family Teaching

• Warn the patient/family not to abruptly discontinue atenolol.
• Explain to the patient/family that compliance with therapy is essential to control angina or hypertension.
• To reduce the orthostatic effects of the drug, instruct the patient/family that the patient should rise slowly from a lying to a sitting position and permit the legs to dangle from the bed momentarily before standing.
• Warn the patient/family to avoid tasks that require alertness or motor skills until the patient's response to the drug is established.
• Advise the patient/family to report confusion, depression, dizziness, rash, or unusual bruising or bleeding to the physician.
• Teach the patient/family the correct technique to monitor the patient's B/P and pulse before taking atenolol.
• Urge the patient/family to restrict the patient's alcohol and salt intake.
• Advise the patient/family that the therapeutic antihypertensive effect of atenolol should be noted within 1–2 wks.

Propranolol Hydrochloride

pro-**pran**-oh-lol

(Apo-Propranolol [CAN], Deralin [AUS], Inderal, InnoPran XL)

Do not confuse with Adderall, Isordil, or Pravachol.

CATEGORY AND SCHEDULE

Pregnancy Risk Category: C (D if used in second or third trimester)

MECHANISM OF ACTION

An antihypertensive, antianginal, antiarrhythmic, and antimigraine agent that blocks $beta_1$- and $beta_2$-adrenergic receptors. Decreases O_2 requirements. Slows AV conduction and increases the refractory period in the AV node. ***Therapeutic Effect:*** Slows sinus heart rate, decreases cardiac output, and decreases blood pressure (B/P). Increases airway resistance.

Decreases myocardial ischemia severity. Exhibits antiarrhythmic activity.

PHARMACOKINETICS

Route	Onset	Peak	Duration
PO	1–2 hrs	N/A	6 hrs

Well absorbed from the GI tract. Protein binding: 93%. Widely distributed. Metabolized in liver. Primarily excreted in urine. Not removed by hemodialysis.
Half-Life: 3–6 hrs.

AVAILABILITY

Tablets: 10 mg, 20 mg, 40 mg, 60 mg, 80 mg.
Capsules (sustained release): 60 mg, 80 mg, 120 mg, 160 mg.
Oral Solution: 4 mg/mL, 8 mg/mL.
Solution (concentrate): 80 mg/mL.
Injection: 1 mg/mL.

INDICATIONS AND DOSAGES

▸ **Hypertension**
PO
Children. Initially, 0.5–1 mg/kg/day in divided doses q6–12h. May increase at 3- to 5-day intervals. Usual dose: 1–5 mg/kg/day. Maximum: 8 mg/kg/day.

▸ **Arrhythmias**
IV
Children. 0.01–0.1 mg/kg. Maximum (infants): 1 mg; (children): 3 mg.
Neonates. 0.01 mg/kg. May repeat q6–8h as needed. Maximum: 0.15 mg/kg/dose q6–8h.
PO
Children. Initially, 0.5–1 mg/kg/day in divided doses q6–8h. May increase q3–5 days. Usual dosage: 2–4 mg/kg/day. Maximum: 16 mg/kg/day or 60 mg/day.
Neonates. Initially, 0.25 mg/kg/dose q6–8h. May increase as needed to Maximum of 5 mg/kg/day.

▸ **Life-threatening arrhythmias**
IV
Children. 0.01–0.1 mg/kg.

▸ **Migraine headache prophylaxis**
PO
Children. 0.6–1.5 mg/kg/day in divided doses q8h. Maximum: 4 mg/kg/day.

UNLABELED USES

Treatment of adjunct anxiety, mitral valve prolapse syndrome, thyrotoxicosis.

CONTRAINDICATIONS

Hypersensitivity to propranolol or any related component. Asthma, bradycardia, cardiogenic shock, chronic obstructive pulmonary disease, heart block, Raynaud syndrome, uncompensated CHF.

INTERACTIONS

Drug

Diuretics, other hypotensives: May increase hypotensive effect.
Insulin, oral hypoglycemics: May mask symptoms of hypoglycemia and prolong the hypoglycemic effect of insulin and oral hypoglycemics.
IV phenytoin: May increase cardiac depressant effect.
NSAIDs: May decrease antihypertensive effect.
Sympathomimetics, xanthines: May mutually inhibit effects.

Herbal

None known.

Food

Natural licorice: Causes sodium and water retention and increased potassium loss.

DIAGNOSTIC TEST EFFECTS

May increase ANA titer and BUN, serum lactate dehydrogenase, serum lipoprotein, serum alkaline phosphatase, serum bilirubin, serum creatinine, serum potassium, serum uric acid, SGOT (AST), SGPT (ALT), and serum triglyceride levels.

IV INCOMPATIBILITIES
Amphotericin B complex (Abelcet, AmBisome, Amphotec)

IV COMPATIBILITIES
Alteplase (Activase), heparin, milrinone (Primacor), potassium chloride, propofol (Diprivan)

SIDE EFFECTS
Frequent
Decreased sexual ability, drowsiness, difficulty sleeping, unusual tiredness or weakness
Occasional
Bradycardia, depression, cold hands or feet, diarrhea, constipation, anxiety, nasal congestion, nausea, vomiting
Rare
Altered taste; dry eyes; itching; numbness of fingers, toes, scalp

SERIOUS REACTIONS
! May produce profound bradycardia and hypotension.
! Abrupt withdrawal may result in sweating, palpitations, headache, and tremulousness.
! May precipitate CHF and MI in pts with cardiac disease; thyroid storm in pts with thyrotoxicosis; and peripheral ischemia in pts with existing peripheral vascular disease.
! Hypoglycemia may occur in pts with previously controlled diabetes.

PEDIATRIC CONSIDERATIONS

Baseline Assessment
- Assess the patient's baseline liver and renal function test results.
- Assess the patient's apical pulse and B/P immediately before giving propranolol. If the patient's pulse rate is 60/min or less or systolic B/P is less than 90 mm Hg, withhold the medication and contact the physician.
- Document the onset, type (sharp, dull, or squeezing), radiation, location, intensity, and duration of the patient's anginal pain and its precipitating factors, such as exertion and emotional stress.
- Be aware that propranolol crosses the placenta and is distributed in breast milk and that propranolol use should be avoided during the first trimester of pregnancy. Know that propranolol use can produce apnea, bradycardia, hypoglycemia, hypothermia during delivery, and low birth-weight infants.
- Use cautiously in children who have diabetes mellitus because this drug may cause hypoglycemia.
- There are no age-related precautions noted in children.

Precautions
- Use cautiously in pts who are also receiving calcium channel blockers, especially when giving propranolol IV.
- Use cautiously in pts with diabetes and liver or renal impairment.

Administration and Handling
PO
- Crush scored tablets if necessary.
- Give at the same time each day.

IV
- Store at room temperature.
- Give undiluted for IV push.
- For IV infusion, may dilute each 1 mg in 10 mL D_5W.
- Do not exceed 1 mg/min injection rate.
- For IV infusion, give 1 mg over 10–15 min.

Intervention and Evaluation

• Assess the patient's pulse for bradycardia and an irregular rate.
• Monitor the patient's EKG for arrhythmias.
• Examine the patient's fingers for lack of color and numbness, which may indicate Raynaud syndrome.
• Evaluate the patient for signs and symptoms of CHF, including distended neck veins, dyspnea (particularly on exertion or lying down), night cough, and peripheral edema.
• Monitor the patient's intake and output. Be aware that an increase in patient weight or a decrease in patient urine output may indicate CHF.
• Assess the patient for behavioral changes, fatigue, and rash.
• Know that the therapeutic response ranges from a few days to several weeks.
• Measure the patient's B/P near the end of the dosing interval to determine whether B/P is controlled throughout the day.

Patient/Family Teaching

• Caution the patient/family against discontinuing the drug.
• Stress to the patient/family that compliance with the therapy regimen is essential to control anginal pain, arrhythmias, and hypertension.
• Instruct the patient/family that if a dose is missed, the patient should take the next scheduled dose and should not double the dose.
• Teach the patient/family to rise slowly from lying to the sitting position and wait momentarily before standing to avoid the hypotensive effect of the drug.
• Explain to the patient/family that the patient should not take any nasal decongestants or OTC cold preparations, especially those containing stimulants, without physician approval.
• Urge the patient/family to limit the patient's alcohol and salt intake.
• Advise the patient/family to avoid tasks that require mental alertness or motor skills until the patient's response to the drug is established.
• Warn the patient/family to report if the patient experiences dizziness, excessively slow pulse rate (less than 60 beats/min), or peripheral numbness.

Timolol Maleate

tim-oh-lol
(Apo-Timol [CAN], Apo-Timop [CAN], Betimol, Blocadren, Gen-Timolol [CAN], Novo-Timol [CAN], Optimol [AUS], Tenopt [AUS], Timoptic, Timoptic XE, Timoptol [AUS])
Do not confuse with atenolol or Viroptic.

CATEGORY AND SCHEDULE

Pregnancy Risk Category: C (D if used in second or third trimester)

MECHANISM OF ACTION

An antihypertensive, antimigraine, and antiglaucoma agent that blocks $beta_1$- and $beta_2$-adrenergic receptors. ***Therapeutic Effect:*** Reduces intraocular pressure by reducing aqueous humor production, reduces blood pressure (B/P), and produces negative chronotropic and inotropic activity.

PHARMACOKINETICS

Route	Onset	Peak	Duration
Eyedrops	30 min	1–2 hrs	12–24 hrs

Well absorbed from the GI tract. Protein binding: less than 10%. Minimal absorption after ophthalmic administration. Metabolized in liver. Primarily excreted in urine. Not removed by hemodialysis. ***Half-Life:*** Adults: 2-4 hrs (prolonged with renal impairment).

AVAILABILITY

Tablets: 5 mg, 10 mg, 20 mg.
Ophthalmic Solution: 0.25%, 0.5%.
Ophthalmic Gel: 0.25%, 0.5%.

INDICATIONS AND DOSAGES

OPHTHALMIC

Children. 1 drop of 0.25% solution in affected eye(s) 2 times/day. May be increased to 1 drop of 0.5% solution in affected eye(s) 2 times/day. When IOP is controlled, dosage may be reduced to 1 drop 1 time/day. If patient is switched to timolol from another antiglaucoma agent, administer concurrently for 1 day. Discontinue other agent on following day.

UNLABELED USES

Systemic: Treatment of anxiety, cardiac arrhythmias, chronic angina pectoris, hypertrophic cardiomyopathy, migraines, pheochromocytoma, thyrotoxicosis, tremors. Ophthalmic: With miotics decreases IOP in acute or chronic angle-closure glaucoma; treatment of angle-closure glaucoma during and after iridectomy, malignant glaucoma, secondary glaucoma.

CONTRAINDICATIONS

Hypersensitivity to timolol or any related component. Bronchial asthma, cardiogenic shock, chronic obstructive pulmonary disease, CHF unless secondary to tachyarrhythmias, MAOI therapy, second- or third-degree heart block, sinus bradycardia, uncontrolled cardiac failure.

INTERACTIONS

Drug

Diuretics, other hypotensives: May increase hypotensive effect.
Insulin, oral hypoglycemics: May mask symptoms of hypoglycemia and prolong hypoglycemic effects of these drugs.
NSAIDs: May decrease antihypertensive effect.
Sympathomimetics, xanthines: May mutually inhibit effects.

Herbal

None known.

Food

None known.

DIAGNOSTIC TEST EFFECTS

May increase ANA titer and BUN, serum lactate dehydrogenase, serum lipoprotein, serum alkaline phosphatase, serum bilirubin, serum creatinine, serum potassium, serum uric acid, SGOT (AST), SGPT (ALT), and serum triglyceride levels.

SIDE EFFECTS

Frequent

Decreased sexual function, drowsiness, difficulty sleeping, unusual tiredness or weakness
Ophthalmic: Eye irritation, visual disturbances

Occasional

Depression, cold hands or feet, diarrhea, constipation, anxiety, nasal congestion, nausea, vomiting

Rare

Altered taste, dry eyes, itching, numbness of fingers, toes, scalp

SERIOUS REACTIONS

! Abrupt withdrawal may result in diaphoresis, palpitations, headache, and tremulousness.

! May precipitate CHF and MI in pts with cardiac disease; thyroid storm in pts with thyrotoxicosis; and peripheral ischemia in pts with existing peripheral vascular disease.

! Hypoglycemia may occur in pts with previously controlled diabetes.

! Ophthalmic overdosage may produce bradycardia, hypotension, bronchospasm, and acute cardiac failure.

PEDIATRIC CONSIDERATIONS

Baseline Assessment

• Assess the patient's apical pulse and B/P immediately before giving timolol. If the patient's pulse is 60/min or less or systolic B/P is less than 90 mm Hg, withhold the medication and contact the physician.

• Be aware that timolol is distributed in breast milk and should not be given to breast-feeding women because of the potential for serious adverse effects on the breast-fed infant. Know that timolol use should be avoided during the first trimester of pregnancy and that the drug may produce apnea, bradycardia, hypoglycemia, hypothermia during delivery, and low birth-weight infants.

• Be aware that the safety and efficacy of timolol have not been established in children.

• The use of oral timolol is not recommended in pediatric pts.

Precautions

• Use cautiously in pts with hyperthyroidism, impaired liver or renal function, and inadequate cardiac function. Precautions also apply to oral and ophthalmic administration because of the systemic absorption of ophthalmic timolol.

Administration and Handling

OPHTHALMIC

◀ **ALERT** ▶ When using gel, invert the container and shake once before each use.

• Place a gloved finger on the patient's lower eyelid and pull it out until a pocket is formed between the eye and lower lid.

• Hold the dropper above the pocket and place the prescribed number of drops or prescribed amount of gel into the pocket. Instruct the patient to close his or her eyes gently so that medication will not be squeezed out of the sac.

• Apply gentle digital pressure to the patient's lacrimal sac at the inner canthus for 1 min after installation to lessen the risk of systemic absorption.

Intervention and Evaluation

• Assess the patient's pulse for quality and assess for bradycardia or an irregular rate.

• Monitor the patient's EKG for arrhythmias, particularly premature ventricular contractions.

• Assess the patient's pattern of daily bowel activity and stool consistency.

• Monitor the patient's B/P, heart rate, IOP (ophthalmic preparation), and liver and renal function test results.

Patient/Family Teaching

• Caution the patient/family against abruptly discontinuing timolol.

• Stress to the patient/family that compliance with the therapy regimen is essential to control angina, arrhythmias, glaucoma, and hypertension.

• Advise the patient/family to avoid tasks that require mental alertness or motor skills until the patient's response to the drug is established.

- Warn the patient/family to notify the physician if the patient experiences excessive fatigue, prolonged dizziness or headache, or shortness of breath.
- Explain to the patient/family that the patient should not use nasal decongestants and OTC cold preparations, especially those containing stimulants, without physician approval.
- Urge the patient/family to limit the patient's alcohol and salt intake.
- Teach the patient/family receiving the ophthalmic form of timolol the correct way to instill drops and obtain the patient's pulse.
- Advise the patient/family receiving the ophthalmic form of timolol that the patient may experience transient discomfort or stinging upon instillation.

REFERENCES

Gunn, V. L. & Nechyba, C. (2002). The Harriet Lane handbook (16th ed.). St. Louis: Mosby.

Miller, S. & Fioravanti, J. (1997). Pediatric medications: a handbook for nurses. St. Louis: Mosby.

Taketomo, C. K., Hodding, J. H. & Kraus, D. M. (2003–2004). Pediatric dosage handbook (10th ed.). Hudson, OH: Lexi-Comp.

26 Calcium Channel Blockers

Diltiazem Hydrochloride
Nifedipine
Verapamil Hydrochloride

Uses: Calcium channel blockers are used to treat essential hypertension, to prevent and treat angina pectoris (including vasospastic, chronic stable, and unstable forms), to prevent and control supraventricular tachyarrhythmias, and to prevent neurologic damage caused by subarachnoid hemorrhage.

Action: Calcium channel blockers inhibit the flow of extracellular calcium ions across cell membranes in cardiac and vascular tissue. They relax arterial smooth muscle, depress the rate of firing in the sinus node (the heart's normal pacemaker), slow atrioventricular conduction, and decrease the heart rate. Although they also produce negative inotropic effects, these effects are rarely seen clinically because of the reflex response. Calcium channel blockers decrease coronary vascular resistance, increase coronary blood flow, and reduce myocardial O_2 demand. The degree of action varies with the specific drug.

COMBINATION PRODUCTS

TARKA: verapamil/trandolapril (an angiotensin-converting enzyme [ACE] inhibitor) 240 mg/1 mg; 180 mg/2 mg; 240 mg/2 mg; 240 mg/4 mg.
TECZEM: diltiazem/enalapril (an ACE inhibitor) 180 mg/5 mg.

Diltiazem Hydrochloride

dill-**tie**-ah-zem
(Apo-Diltiaz [CAN], Auscard [AUS], Cardcal [AUS], Cardizem, Cardizem CD, Cartia, Cardizem LA, Coras [AUS], Dilacor XR, Diltahexal [AUS], Diltiamax [AUS], Dilzem [AUS], Novo-Diltiazem [CAN], Tiazac)
Do not confuse with Cardene or Ziac.

CATEGORY AND SCHEDULE

Pregnancy Risk Category: C

MECHANISM OF ACTION

An antianginal, antihypertensive, and antiarrhythmic agent that inhibits calcium movement across cardiac and vascular smooth muscle cell membranes. This action causes the dilation of coronary arteries, peripheral arteries, and arterioles.
Therapeutic Effect: Decreases heart rate, myocardial contractility, slows sinoatrial and atrioventricular (AV) conduction. Decreases total peripheral vascular resistance by vasodilation.

PHARMACOKINETICS

Well absorbed from the GI tract. Distributed into breast milk. Protein binding: 70%–80%. Undergoes first-pass metabolism in liver. Metabolized in liver to the active metabolite. Primarily excreted in urine. Not removed by hemodialysis. ***Half-Life:*** 3–8 hrs.

AVAILABILITY

Tablets: 30 mg, 60 mg, 90 mg, 120 mg.
Tablets (extended-release): 120 mg, 180 mg, 240 mg, 300 mg, 360 mg, 420 mg.
Capsules (sustained release): 60 mg, 90 mg, 120 mg, 180 mg, 240 mg, 300 mg, 360 mg, 420 mg.
Injection: 5 mg/mL.

INDICATIONS AND DOSAGES

▸ **Hypertension**

PO

Children. Initially 1.5–2 mg/kg/day divided in 3–4 doses. Maximum: 3.5 mg/kg/day.
Adolescents. Immediate release: 30–120 mg/dose q6–8h. Usual range 180–360 mg/day.
Extended release: 120–300 mg/day.

▸ **Antiarrhythmic**

IV

Adolescents. Initially 0.25 mg/kg bolus over 2 min, followed by continuous infusion of 5–15 mg/hr for up to 24 hrs.

CONTRAINDICATIONS

Hypersensitivity to diltiazem or any related component. Acute myocardial infarction, pulmonary congestion, severe hypotension (less than 90 mm Hg, systolic), sick sinus syndrome, and second- or third-degree AV block (except in the presence of a pacemaker).

INTERACTIONS

Drug

Beta-blockers: May have additive effect.
Carbamazepine, cyclosporine, quinidine, theophylline: May increase diltiazem blood concentration and risk of toxicity.
Digoxin: May increase serum digoxin concentration.
Procainamide, quinidine: May increase risk of QT-interval prolongation.
Cimetidine: May increase diltiazem serum concentrations.
Rifampin: May decrease diltiazem serum concentrations.

Herbal

None known.

Food

Natural licorice: May cause sodium and water retention as well as increased potassium loss.

DIAGNOSTIC TEST EFFECTS

PR interval may be increased.

IV INCOMPATIBILITIES

Acetazolamide (Diamox), acyclovir (Zovirax), aminophylline, ampicillin, ampicillin/sulbactam (Unasyn), cefoperazone (Cefobid), diazepam (Valium), furosemide (Lasix), heparin, insulin, nafcillin, phenytoin (Dilantin), rifampin (Rifadin), sodium bicarbonate

IV COMPATIBILITIES

Albumin, aztreonam (Azactam), bumetanide (Bumex), cefazolin (Ancef), cefotaxime (Claforan), ceftazidime (Fortaz), ceftriaxone (Rocephin), cefuroxime (Zinacef), cimetidine (Tagamet), ciprofloxacin (Cipro), clindamycin (Cleocin), digoxin (Lanoxin), dobutamine (Dobutrex), dopamine (Intropin), gentamicin (Garamycin), hydromorphone (Dilaudid), lidocaine, lorazepam (Ativan), metoclopramide (Reglan), metronidazole (Flagyl), midazolam (Versed), morphine, multivitamins, nitroglycerin, norepinephrine (Levophed), potassium chloride, potassium phosphate, tobramycin (Nebcin), vancomycin (Vancocin)

SIDE EFFECTS

Frequent (10%–5%)
Peripheral edema, dizziness, lightheadedness, headache, bradycardia, asthenia (loss of strength, weakness)

Occasional (5%–2%)
Nausea, constipation, flushing, altered EKG

Rare (less than 2%)
Rash, micturition disorder (polyuria, nocturia, dysuria, frequency of urination), abdominal discomfort, somnolence

SERIOUS REACTIONS

! Abrupt withdrawal may increase frequency or duration of angina.
! CHF and second- and third-degree AV block occur rarely.
! Overdosage produces nausea, drowsiness, confusion, slurred speech, and profound bradycardia.

PEDIATRIC CONSIDERATIONS

Baseline Assessment

- Concurrent sublingual nitroglycerin therapy may be used for relief of anginal pain.
- Document the onset, type (sharp, dull, or squeezing), radiation, location, intensity, and duration of anginal pain and its precipitating factors, such as exertion or emotional stress.
- Assess the patient's baseline liver and renal function and blood chemistry test results.
- Assess the patient's apical pulse and blood pressure (B/P) immediately before diltiazem is administered.
- Be aware that diltiazem is distributed in breast milk.
- There are no age-related precautions noted in children.

Precautions

- Use cautiously in pts with CHF and impaired liver or renal function.

Administration and Handling

PO

- Give diltiazem before meals and at bedtime.
- Crush tablets as needed.
- Do not crush or open sustained-release capsules.

IV

◂ALERT▸ Refer to manufacturer's information for dose concentration and infusion rates.

- Refrigerate vials.
- After dilution, solution is stable for 24 hrs.
- Add 125 mg to 100 mL D_5W or 0.9% NaCl to provide a concentration of 1 mg/mL. Add 250 mg to 250 or 500 mL diluent to provide a concentration of 0.83 or 0.45 mg/mL, respectively. The maximum concentration is 1.25 g/250 mL or 5 mg/mL.
- Infuse per dilution or rate chart provided by manufacturer.

Intervention and Evaluation

- Assist the patient with ambulation if the patient experiences dizziness.
- Assess the patient for peripheral edema behind the medial malleolus or in the sacral area in bedridden pts.
- Monitor the patient's pulse rate for bradycardia.
- For pts receiving IV diltiazem, assess B/P, the EKG, and liver and renal function test results.
- Assess the patient for signs or symptoms of asthenia or headache.

Patient/Family Teaching

- Caution the patient/family against abruptly discontinuing the medication.
- Stress to the patient/family that compliance with the treatment regimen is essential to control anginal pain.
- Instruct the patient/family to rise slowly from a lying to a sitting

position and wait momentarily before standing to avoid the hypotensive effect of diltiazem.
• Warn the patient/family to avoid tasks that require mental alertness or motor skills until the patient's response to the drug is established.
• Warn the patient/family to notify the physician if the patient experiences constipation, irregular heartbeat, nausea, pronounced dizziness, or shortness of breath.

Nifedipine

nye-**fed**-ih-peen
(Adalat CC, Adalat FT, Adalat, PA, Adalat Oros [AUS], Apo-Nifed [CAN], Nifedicol XL, Nifehexal [AUS], Novonifedin [CAN], Nyefax [AUS], Procardia)
Do not confuse with nicardipine.

CATEGORY AND SCHEDULE

Pregnancy Risk Category: C

MECHANISM OF ACTION

An antianginal and antihypertensive agent that inhibits calcium ion movement across the cell membrane, depressing contraction of cardiac and vascular smooth muscle. ***Therapeutic Effect:*** Increases heart rate and cardiac output. Decreases systemic vascular resistance and blood pressure (B/P).

PHARMACOKINETICS

Rapidly, completely absorbed from the GI tract. Protein binding: 92%–98%. Undergoes first-pass metabolism in liver. Primarily excreted in urine. Not removed by hemodialysis. ***Half-Life:*** Adults: 2–5 hrs.

AVAILABILITY

Capsules: 10 mg, 20 mg.
Tablets (extended release): 30 mg, 60 mg, 90 mg.

INDICATIONS AND DOSAGES

▸ **Hypertensive emergencies**
PO
Children. 0.25–0.5 mg/kg/dose every 4–6 hrs. Maximum: 1–2 mg/kg/day or 10 mg/dose.
▸ **Hypertrophic cardiomyopathy**
PO
Children. 0.6–0.9 mg/kg/day divided q6–8h.

UNLABELED USES

Treatment of Raynaud phenomenon.

CONTRAINDICATIONS

Hypersensitivity to nifedipine or any related component. Recent myocardial infarction (MI), advanced aortic stenosis, severe hypotension.

INTERACTIONS

Drug
Beta-blockers: May have additive effect.
Digoxin: May increase digoxin blood concentration.
Hypokalemia-producing agents: May increase the risk of arrhythmias.
Phenytoin, cyclosporine: May increase the serum concentrations of these drugs.
Delavirdine: May increase nifedipine serum concentrations.
Herbal
None known.
Food
Grapefruit and grapefruit juice: May increase nifedipine plasma concentration.

DIAGNOSTIC TEST EFFECTS

May cause positive ANA titer and direct Coombs' test results.

SIDE EFFECTS

Frequent (30%–11%)
Peripheral edema, headache, flushed skin, dizziness

Occasional (12%–6%)
Nausea, shakiness, muscle cramps and pain, drowsiness, palpitations, nasal congestion, cough, dyspnea, wheezing

Rare (5%–3%)
Hypotension, rash, pruritus, urticaria, constipation, abdominal discomfort, flatulence, sexual difficulties

SERIOUS REACTIONS

! May precipitate CHF and MI in pts with cardiac disease and peripheral ischemia.

! Overdose produces nausea, drowsiness, confusion, and slurred speech.

PEDIATRIC CONSIDERATIONS

Baseline Assessment

- Know that concurrent therapy of sublingual nitroglycerin may be used for relief of anginal pain.
- Record the onset, type (sharp, dull, or squeezing), radiation, location, intensity, and duration of anginal pain and its precipitating factors, such as exertion or emotional stress.
- Check the patient's B/P for hypotension immediately before giving nifedipine.
- Be aware that an insignificant amount of nifedipine is distributed in breast milk.
- Be cautious in using the immediate-release dosage form in children.

Precautions

- Use cautiously in pts with impaired liver or renal function.

Administration and Handling

◂ALERT▸ May give 10–20 mg sublingually as needed for an acute attack of angina.

PO

- Do not crush or break film-coated tablet or sustained-release capsule.
- Give nifedipine without regard to meals.
- Grapefruit juice may alter absorption.

SUBLINGUAL

- Capsule must be punctured, chewed, and squeezed to express liquid into the mouth.

Intervention and Evaluation

- Assist the patient with ambulation if the patient experiences dizziness or lightheadedness.
- Assess for peripheral edema behind the medial malleolus in ambulatory pts and in the sacral area in bedridden pts.
- Examine the patient's skin for flushing.
- Monitor the patient's hepatic blood chemistry test results.

Patient/Family Teaching

- Instruct the patient/family to rise slowly from a lying to a sitting position and to permit the legs to dangle from the bed momentarily before standing to reduce the hypotensive effect of nifedipine.
- Warn the patient/family to notify the physician if the patient experiences irregular heartbeat, prolonged dizziness, nausea, or shortness of breath.
- Urge the patient/family to avoid use of alcohol, grapefruit, and grapefruit juice.
- Nifedipine may rarely cause photosensitivity reactions. Caution the patient to use a broad-spectrum sunscreen and wear protective clothing when outdoors.

Verapamil Hydrochloride

ver-**ap**-ah-mill
(Anpec [AUS], Apo-Verap [CAN], Calan, Chronovera [CAN], Cordilox [AUS], Covera-HS, Isoptin, Novoveramil [CAN], Veracaps SR [AUS], Verahexal [AUS], Verelan, Verelan PM)
Do not confuse with Intropin, Virilon, Vivarin, or Voltaren.

CATEGORY AND SCHEDULE

Pregnancy Risk Category: C

MECHANISM OF ACTION

A calcium channel blocker and antianginal, antiarrhythmic, and antihypertensive agent that inhibits calcium ion entry across cardiac and vascular smooth muscle cell membranes. This action causes the dilation of coronary arteries, peripheral arteries, and arterioles. ***Therapeutic Effect:*** Decreases heart rate and myocardial contractility and slows sinoatrial and atrioventricular (AV) conduction. Decreases total peripheral vascular resistance by vasodilation.

PHARMACOKINETICS

Well absorbed from the GI tract. Protein binding: 90% (60% in neonates). Undergoes first-pass metabolism in liver. Metabolized in liver to the active metabolite. Primarily excreted in urine. Not removed by hemodialysis. ***Half-Life:*** Infants: 4–7 hrs; adults: 2–8 hrs. Increased with hepatic impairment.

AVAILABILITY

Tablets: 40 mg, 80 mg, 120 mg
Tablets (sustained release): 120 mg, 180 mg, 240 mg.
Capsules (sustained release): 100 mg (Verelan PM), 120 mg, 180 mg, 200 mg (Verelan PM), 240 mg, 300 mg (Verelan PM), 360 mg.
Injection: 2.5 mg/mL.

INDICATIONS AND DOSAGES

▸ **Supraventricular tachyarrhythmias, temporary control of rapid ventricular rate with atrial fibrillation or flutter**

IV

Children 1–15 yrs. 0.1–0.3 mg/kg/dose. Maximum: 5 mg/dose. May repeat in 30 min up to a maximum second dose of 10 mg. Not recommended for children younger than 1 yr of age.

▸ **Hypertension**

PO (PO DOSING NOT WELL ESTABLISHED IN CHILDREN)

Children. 4–8 mg/kg/day divided 3 times/day.

UNLABELED USES

Treatment of hypertrophic cardiomyopathy, vascular headaches.

CONTRAINDICATIONS

Hypersensitivity to verapamil or any related component. Atrial fibrillation or flutter and an accessory bypass tract, cardiogenic shock, heart block, sinus bradycardia, ventricular tachycardia.

INTERACTIONS

Drug

Beta-blockers: May have additive effect.
Carbamazepine, quinidine, theophylline: May increase verapamil blood concentration and risk of toxicity.
Digoxin: May increase digoxin blood concentration.
Disopyramide: May increase negative inotropic effect.

Procainamide, quinidine: May increase the risk of QT interval prolongation.

Herbal

None known.

Food

Grapefruit and grapefruit juice: May increase verapamil blood concentration.

DIAGNOSTIC TEST EFFECTS

The EKG waveform may show an increased PR interval. Therapeutic blood level is 0.08–0.3 mcg/mL.

IV INCOMPATIBILITIES

Amphotericin B complex (Abelcet, AmBisome, Amphotec), nafcillin (Nafcil), propofol (Diprivan), sodium bicarbonate

IV COMPATIBILITIES

Amiodarone (Cordarone), calcium chloride, calcium gluconate, dexamethasone (Decadron), digoxin (Lanoxin), dobutamine (Dobutrex), dopamine (Intropin), furosemide (Lasix), heparin, hydromorphone (Dilaudid), lidocaine, magnesium sulfate, metoclopramide (Reglan), milrinone (Primacor), morphine, multivitamins, nitroglycerin, norepinephrine (Levophed), potassium chloride, potassium phosphate, procainamide (Pronestyl), propranolol (Inderal)

SIDE EFFECTS

Frequent (7%)

Constipation

Occasional (4%–2%)

Dizziness, lightheadedness, headache, asthenia (loss of strength, energy), nausea, peripheral edema, hypotension

Rare (less than 1%)

Bradycardia, dermatitis or rash

SERIOUS REACTIONS

! Rapid ventricular rate in atrial flutter or fibrillation, marked hypotension, extreme bradycardia, CHF, asystole, and second- and third-degree AV block occur rarely.

PEDIATRIC CONSIDERATIONS

Baseline Assessment

- Assess and document the onset, type (such as sharp, dull, or squeezing), radiation, location, intensity, and duration of the patient's anginal pain. Also, assess and record precipitating factors, including exertion and emotional stress.
- Before giving verapamil, assess the patient's blood pressure (B/P) for signs of hypotension and pulse rate for signs of bradycardia.
- Be aware that verapamil crosses the placenta and is distributed in breast milk and that breast-feeding is not recommended for pts taking this drug.
- Do not administer verapamil to treat supraventricular tachycardia in infants.
- Avoid using the IV route in neonates and young infants because of an increased risk for hypotension, apnea, and bradycardia.

Precautions

- Use cautiously in pts with CHF, liver or renal impairment, and sick sinus syndrome.
- Use cautiously in pts also receiving beta-blocker or digoxin therapy.

Administration and Handling

PO

- Do not give with grapefruit juice.
- Give tablets that are not sustained release with or without food.
- Have the patient swallow extended-release and sustained-

released preparations whole and without chewing or crushing.
- If needed, open sustained-release capsules and sprinkle contents on applesauce. Have the patient swallow the applesauce immediately without chewing.

IV
- Store vials at room temperature.
- Give undiluted, if desired.
- Administer IV push over more than 2 min for children.
- Know that continuous EKG monitoring during IV injection is required for children.
- Monitor the patient's EKG for asystole, extreme bradycardia, heart block, PR-interval prolongation, and rapid ventricular rates. Notify the physician of significant EKG changes.
- Monitor the patient's B/P every 5–10 min or as ordered.
- Keep patient in a recumbent position for at least 1 hour after IV administration.

Intervention and Evaluation
- Assess the patient's pulse for irregular rate and rhythm and quality.

◂ALERT▸ Monitor the patient's EKG for changes, particularly PR-interval prolongation.
- Notify physician of significant PR interval prolongation or other EKG changes.
- Assist the patient with ambulation if he or she experiences dizziness.
- Assess for peripheral edema behind the medial malleolus in ambulatory pts and in the sacral area in bedridden pts.
- For pts taking the oral form of verapamil, assess stool consistency and frequency.
- Keep in mind that the therapeutic serum level for verapamil is 0.08–0.3 mcg/mL.

Patient/Family Teaching
- Caution the patient/family against abruptly discontinuing the drug.
- Stress that compliance with the treatment regimen is essential to control anginal pain.
- To avoid the orthostatic effects of verapamil, instruct the patient/family to rise slowly from a lying to a sitting position and to wait momentarily before standing.
- Advise the patient/family to avoid tasks that require mental alertness or motor skills until the patient's response to the drug is established.
- Urge the patient/family to avoid consuming grapefruit or grapefruit juice and to limit caffeine intake while taking verapamil.
- Warn the patient/family to notify the physician if the patient experiences anginal pain not reduced by the drug, constipation, dizziness, irregular heartbeats, nausea, shortness of breath, and swelling of the hands and feet.

REFERENCES

Gunn, V. L. & Nechyba, C. (2002). The Harriet Lane handbook (16th ed.). St. Louis: Mosby.
Miller, S. & Fioravanti, J. (1997). Pediatric medications: a handbook for nurses. St. Louis: Mosby.
Taketomo, C. K., Hodding, J. H. & Kraus, D. M. (2003–2004). Pediatric dosage handbook (10th ed.). Hudson, OH: Lexi-Comp.

27 Cardiac Glycosides

Digoxin
Milrinone Lactate

Uses: Cardiac glycosides are used to treat CHF, atrial fibrillation, paroxysmal atrial tachycardia, and cardiogenic shock with pulmonary edema.

Action: Cardiac glycosides act directly on the myocardium to increase the force of contraction, which leads to increased stroke volume and cardiac output. These agents also depress the firing of the sinoatrial node, decrease conduction time through the atrioventricular node, and decrease electrical impulses caused by a slow heart rate from vagal stimulation. Their ability to increase myocardial contractility may result from the improved transport of calcium, sodium, and potassium ions across cell membranes.

Digoxin

di-jox-in
(Lanoxicaps, Lanoxin)
Do not confuse with Desoxyn, doxepin, Levsinex, or Lonox.

CATEGORY AND SCHEDULE

Pregnancy Risk Category: C

MECHANISM OF ACTION

A cardiac glycoside that increases the influx of calcium from extracellular to intracellular cytoplasm. ***Therapeutic Effect:*** Potentiates the activity of the contractile cardiac muscle fibers and increases the force of myocardial contraction. Decreases conduction through the sinoatrial (SA) and atrioventricular (AV) nodes.

PHARMACOKINETICS

Readily absorbed from the GI tract. Widely distributed. Protein binding: 30%. Partially metabolized in liver. Primarily excreted in urine. Minimally removed by hemodialysis. ***Half-Life:*** Neonates: 35–45 hrs; infants/children: 18–35 hrs; adults: 36–48 hrs (half-life is dependent on age, renal and cardiac function).

AVAILABILITY

Tablets: 0.125 mg, 0.25 mg, 0.5 mg.
Capsules: 0.05 mg, 0.1 mg, 0.2 mg.
Elixir: 0.05 mg/mL (contains alcohol).
Injection: 0.25 mg/mL, 0.1 mg/mL (pediatric strength).

INDICATIONS AND DOSAGES

▸ **Rapid loading dose for the prophylactic management and treatment of CHF; control of ventricular rate in patients with atrial fibrillation; treatment and prevention of recurrent paroxysmal atrial tachycardia**

Give one-half of the total dose listed in the initial dose, then give one-quarter of the total dose in each of the next two doses at 6- to 12-hr intervals.

IV

Children older than 10 yrs. 8–12 mcg/kg.

Children 5–10 yrs. 15–30 mcg/kg.
Children 2–5 yrs. 25–35 mcg/kg.
Children 1–24 mos. 30–50 mcg/kg.
Neonates, full-term. 20–30 mcg/kg.
Neonates, premature. 15–25 mcg/kg.
PO
Children older than 10 yrs. 10–15 mcg/kg.
Children 5–10 yrs. 20–35 mcg/kg.
Children 2–5 yrs. 30–40 mcg/kg.
Children 1–24 mos. 35–60 mcg/kg.
Neonate, full-term. 25–35 mcg/kg.
Neonate, premature. 20–30 mcg/kg.

▸ **Maintenance dosage for CHF; control of ventricular rate in patients with atrial fibrillation; treatment and prevention of recurrent paroxysmal atrial tachycardia**

For children younger than 10 yrs of age, divide dose and give q12h.
PO/IV
Children. 25%–35% loading dose (20%–30% for premature neonates).

▸ **Dosage in renal impairment**

Total digitalizing dose. Decrease by 50% in end-stage renal disease.

Creatinine Clearance	Dosage
10–50 mL/min	25%–75% normal
Less than 10 mL/min	10%–25% normal

CONTRAINDICATIONS

Hypersensitivity to digoxin or any other component. Ventricular fibrillation, ventricular tachycardia unrelated to CHF, constrictive pericarditis, AV block.

INTERACTIONS

Drug

Amiodarone: May increase digoxin blood concentration and risk of toxicity and have an additive effect on the SA and AV nodes.
Amphotericin, glucocorticoids, potassium-depleting diuretics: May increase risk of toxicity resulting from hypokalemia.
Antiarrhythmics, parenteral calcium, sympathomimetics: May increase risk of arrhythmias.
Antidiarrheals, cholestyramine, colestipol, sucralfate: May decrease absorption of digoxin.
Diltiazem, fluoxetine, quinidine, verapamil, nifedipine, indomethacin, erythromycin, tetracycline, spironolactone: May increase digoxin blood concentration.
Parenteral magnesium: May cause cardiac conduction changes and heart block.

Herbal

Siberian ginseng: May increase serum digoxin levels.
St. John's wort: May decrease serum digoxin levels.

Food

None known.

DIAGNOSTIC TEST EFFECTS

None known.

IV INCOMPATIBILITIES

Amphotericin B complex (Abelcet, Amphotec, AmBisome), fluconazole (Diflucan), foscarnet (Foscavir), propofol (Diprivan)

IV COMPATIBILITIES

Cimetidine (Tagamet), diltiazem (Cardizem), furosemide (Lasix), heparin, insulin (regular), lidocaine, midazolam (Versed), milrinone (Primacor), morphine, potassium chloride, propofol (Diprivan)

SIDE EFFECTS

Sinus bradycardia, AV block, SA block, atrial or nodal ectopic beats, ventricular arrhythmias, bigeminy, trigeminy. There is a very narrow margin of safety between a therapeutic and toxic result. Signs of toxicity include vomiting, dizziness, blurred vision and halos, yellow or green vision, diplopia, flashing lights, abdominal pain, diarrhea, vertigo, disorientation, and hyperkalemia. Chronic therapy may produce mammary gland enlargement in women but is reversible when the drug is withdrawn.

SERIOUS REACTIONS

! The most common early manifestations of toxicity are GI disturbances (anorexia, nausea, and vomiting) and neurologic abnormalities (fatigue, headache, depression, weakness, drowsiness, confusion, and nightmares).

! Facial pain, personality change, and ocular disturbances (photophobia, light flashes, halos around bright objects, and yellow or green color perception) may be noted.

PEDIATRIC CONSIDERATIONS

Baseline Assessment

- Assess the patient's apical pulse for 60 sec or 30 sec if receiving maintenance therapy. If pulse is 60/min or less in adults or 70/min or less for children, withhold the drug and contact the physician.
- Expect to obtain blood samples for digoxin levels 6–8 hrs after the digoxin dose or just before the next digoxin dose.
- Be aware that digoxin crosses the placenta and is distributed in breast milk.
- Be aware that premature infants are more susceptible to toxicity.
- Be aware that neonates and children with heart, hepatic, or renal failure may have falsely elevated digoxin levels.

Precautions

- Use cautiously in patients with acute myocardial infarction, advanced cardiac disease, cor pulmonale, hypokalemia, hypothyroidism, impaired liver or renal function, incomplete AV block, and pulmonary disease.

Administration and Handling

◂ALERT▸ Avoid giving the drug by the IM route because it may cause severe local irritation and has erratic absorption. If no other route is possible, give deeply into the muscle followed by massage. Give no more than 2 mL at any one site.

◂ALERT▸ Expect to adjust the digoxin dosage in patients with renal dysfunction. Know that larger digoxin doses are often required for adequate control of ventricular rate in patients with atrial fibrillation or flutter. Administer digoxin loading dosage in several doses at 4- to 8-hr intervals.

PO

- May give without regard to meals.
- Administer digoxin 1 hr before or 2 hr after drugs that decrease the oral absorption of digoxin.
- Crush tablets if necessary.

IV

- Give undiluted or dilute with at least a 4-fold volume of Sterile Water for Injection or D_5W because less than this amount may cause a precipitate to form. Use immediately.
- Give IV infusion slowly over at least 5 min.

Intervention and Evaluation

- Monitor the patient's pulse for bradycardia and EKG for arrhythmias for 1–2 hrs after giving digoxin. Excessive slowing of the patient's pulse may be the first sign of toxicity.

• Assess the patient for signs and symptoms of digoxin toxicity, including GI disturbances and neurologic abnormalities, every 2–4 hrs during digitalization and daily during maintenance therapy.
• Monitor the patient's serum potassium and magnesium levels. Know that the therapeutic serum level of digoxin is 0.8–2 ng/mL and the toxic blood serum level is greater than 2 ng/mL.

Patient/Family Teaching

• Stress to the patient/family the importance of follow-up visits and tests.
• Teach the patient/family to take the apical pulse correctly and to notify the physician of a pulse rate of 60/min or less or a rate as indicated by the physician.
• Instruct the patient/family to recognize the signs and symptoms of toxicity and to notify physician if the patient experiences them.
• Advise the patient/family to carry or wear identification that the patient is receiving digoxin and to inform dentists or other physicians about digoxin therapy.
• Caution the patient/family not to increase or skip digoxin doses.
• Explain to the patient/family that the patient should not take OTC medications without first consulting the physician.
• Warn the patient/family to notify the physician if the patient experiences decreased appetite, diarrhea, nausea, visual changes, or vomiting.

Milrinone Lactate

mill-rih-known
(Primacor)

CATEGORY AND SCHEDULE

Pregnancy Risk Category: C

MECHANISM OF ACTION

This cardiac inotropic agent inhibits phosphodiesterase, which increases cyclic adenosine monophosphate and potentiates the delivery of calcium to myocardial contractile systems.
Therapeutic Effect: Relaxes vascular muscle, causes vasodilation. Increases cardiac output, decreases pulmonary capillary wedge pressure and vascular resistance.

PHARMACOKINETICS

Protein binding: 70%. Primarily excreted unchanged in urine.
Half-Life: Infants (after cardiac surgery): 1–5 hrs; children (after cardiac surgery): 1–4 hrs; adults: 2.4 hrs. Prolonged half-life and clearance with renal impairment.

AVAILABILITY

Injection: 1 mg/mL.
Injection (premix): 200 mcg/mL.

INDICATIONS AND DOSAGES

▸ **Short-term (less than 48 hr) management of acute heart failure.**

IV

Children (limited data). 50 mcg/kg over 15 min initially followed with a continuous infusion of 0.5–1 mcg/kg/min titrated to effect.

▸ **PALS Guidelines (2000)**

IV/INTRAOSSEOUS

Children. Loading dose of 50–75 mcg/kg over 15 min, followed by continuous infusion of 0.5–0.75 mcg/kg/min.

CONTRAINDICATIONS

Hypersensitivity to milrinone or any related component.

INTERACTIONS

Drug

Cardiac glycosides: Produces additive inotropic effects with these drugs.

Herbal

None known.

Food

None known.

DIAGNOSTIC TEST EFFECTS

None known.

IV INCOMPATIBILITIES

Furosemide (Lasix)

IV COMPATIBILITIES

Calcium gluconate, digoxin (Lanoxin), diltiazem (Cardizem), dobutamine (Dobutrex), dopamine (Intropin), heparin, lidocaine, magnesium, midazolam (Versed), nitroglycerin, potassium, propofol (Diprivan)

SIDE EFFECTS

Occasional (3%-1%)
Headache, hypotension
Rare (less than 1%)
Angina, chest pain

SERIOUS REACTIONS

! Supraventricular and ventricular arrhythmias (12%), nonsustained ventricular tachycardia (2%), and sustained ventricular tachycardia (1%) occur.

PEDIATRIC CONSIDERATIONS

Baseline Assessment

- Offer the patient emotional support, especially if the patient has become anxious as a result of experiencing difficulty breathing.
- Assess the patient's apical pulse and blood pressure (B/P) before beginning treatment and during IV therapy.
- Assess the patient's lung sounds for rales and rhonchi and check the patient's skin for edema.
- Be aware that it is unknown whether milrinone crosses the placenta or is distributed in breast milk.
- Be aware that the safety and efficacy of milrinone have not been established in children.

Precautions

- Use cautiously in patients with atrial fibrillation or flutter, a history of ventricular arrhythmias, impaired renal function, and severe obstructive aortic or pulmonic valvular disease.

Administration and Handling

IV

- Store at room temperature.
- For IV infusion, dilute 20-mg (20-mL) vial with 80 or 180 mL diluent (0.9% NaCl or D_5W) to provide a concentration of 200 or 100 mcg/mL, respectively. Maximum: 100 mg/250 mL.
- For a loading dose IV injection, administer the drug undiluted slowly over 10 min.
- Monitor the patient for arrhythmias and hypotension during IV therapy. Reduce or temporarily discontinue infusion until condition stabilizes.

Intervention and Evaluation

- Monitor the patient's B/P, cardiac output, EKG, heart rate, renal function, and serum potassium levels.
- Monitor the patient for signs and symptoms of CHF.

Patient/Family Teaching

- Warn patient/family to immediately report palpitations or chest pain.
- Explain to the patient/family that milrinone is not a cure for CHF but will help relieve symptoms.

REFERENCES

Gunn, V. L. & Nechyba, C. (2002). The Harriet Lane handbook (16th ed.). St. Louis: Mosby.

Miller, S. & Fioravanti, J. (1997). Pediatric medications: a handbook for nurses. St. Louis: Mosby.

Taketomo, C. K., Hodding, J. H. & Kraus, D. M. (2003–2004). Pediatric dosage handbook (10th ed.). Hudson, OH: Lexi-Comp.

28 Sympatholytics

Clonidine
Methyldopa
Prazosin Hydrochloride

Uses: Sympatholytics, also called adrenergic inhibitors, are used to treat mild to severe hypertension. Because these agents effectively control blood pressure (B/P), they help prevent the development and progression of serious cardiovascular complications.

Action: Sympatholytics can act centrally or peripherally. (See illustration, *Sites of Action: Sympatholytics,* page 365.) Central-acting agents, such as clonidine and methyldopa, stimulate alpha$_2$-adrenergic receptors in the cardiovascular centers of the CNS, reducing sympathetic outflow and producing antihypertensive effects. *Peripheral-acting agents,* such as doxazosin and prazosin, block alpha$_1$-adrenergic receptors in arterioles and veins, inhibiting vasoconstriction and decreasing peripheral vascular resistance, which reduces blood pressure.

COMBINATION PRODUCTS

ALDORIL: methyldopa/ hydrochlorothiazide (a diuretic) 250 mg/15 mg; 250 mg/25 mg; 500 mg/30 mg; 500 mg/50 mg.
COMBIPRES: clonidine/chlorthalidone (a diuretic) 0.1 mg/15 mg; 0.2 mg/15 mg; 0.3 mg/15 mg.
MINIZIDE: prazosin/polythiazide (a diuretic) 1 mg/0.5 mg; 2 mg/ 0.5 mg; 5 mg/0.5 mg.

Clonidine

klon-ih-deen
(Catapres, Catapres TTS, Dixarit [CAN], Duraclon)
Do not confuse with Cetapred, clomiphene, Klonopin, or quinidine.

CATEGORY AND SCHEDULE

Pregnancy Risk Category: C

MECHANISM OF ACTION

An antiadrenergic, sympatholytic agent that stimulates alpha-receptors in the brain stem, resulting in decreased sympathetic outflow that produces a decrease in vasomotor tone and heart rate. When used epidurally, clonidine prevents pain signal transmission to the brain and produces analgesia at pre– and post–alpha-adrenergic receptors in the spinal cord. ***Therapeutic Effect:*** Reduces peripheral resistance; decreases B/P, and heart rate.

PHARMACOKINETICS

Route	Onset	Peak	Duration
PO	0.5–1 hr	2–4 hrs	Up to 8 hrs

Well absorbed from the GI tract. Transdermal form best absorbed from chest, upper arm; least absorbed from thigh. Protein binding: 20%–40%. Metabolized in

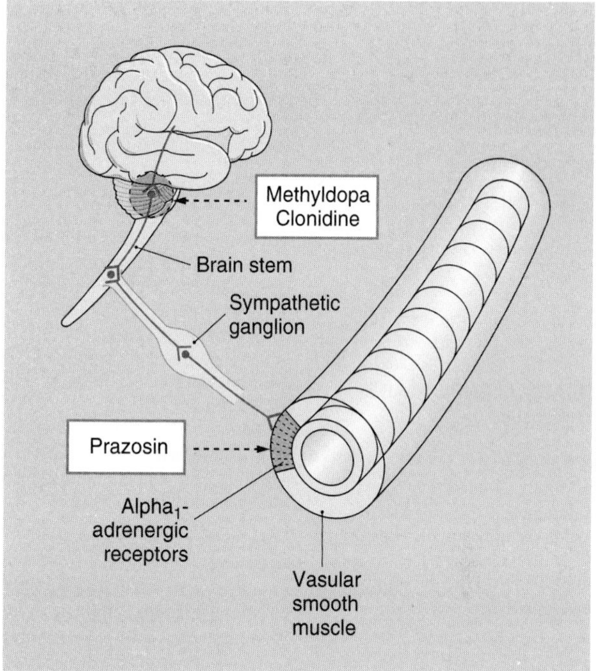

Sites of Action: Sympatholytics

Sympatholytics inhibit sympathetic nervous system (SNS) activity, which plays a major role in regulating blood pressure. Normally when the SNS is stimulated, nerve impulses travel from the cardiovascular center of the CNS to the sympathetic ganglia. From there, the impulses travel along postganglionic fibers to specific effector organs, such as the heart and blood vessels. SNS stimulation also triggers the release of norepinephrine, which acts primarily at alpha-adrenergic receptors.

Sympatholytics fall into two subclasses: central-acting alpha$_2$ agonists and peripheral-acting alpha$_1$-adrenergic antagonists. Central-acting alpha$_2$ agonists, such as methyldopa and clonidine, stimulate alpha$_2$-adrenergic receptors in the cardiovascular center of the CNS and reduce activity in the vasomotor center of the brain, interfering with sympathetic stimulation of the heart and blood vessels. This causes blood vessel dilation and decreased cardiac output, which leads to reduced blood pressure.

Peripheral-acting alpha$_1$-adrenergic antagonists, such as prazosin, inhibit the stimulation of alpha$_1$-adrenergic receptors by norepinephrine in vascular smooth muscle, interfering with SNS-induced vasoconstriction. As a result, the blood vessels dilate, reducing peripheral vascular resistance and venous return to the heart. These effects, in turn, lead to decreased blood pressure.

liver. Primarily excreted in urine. Minimal removal by hemodialysis. ***Half-Life:*** Neonates: 44–70 hrs; children: 8–12 hrs; adults: 12–16 hrs (half-life is increased with impaired renal function).

AVAILABILITY

Tablets: 0.1 mg, 0.2 mg, 0.3 mg.
Transdermal Patch: 2.5 mg (release at 0.1 mg/24 hrs), 5 mg (release at 0.2 mg/24 hrs), 7.5 mg (release at 0.3 mg/24 hrs).
Injection for Epidural Use: 100 mcg/mL, 500 mcg/mL.

INDICATIONS AND DOSAGES

▸ **Hypertension**

PO

Children. Initially 5–10 mcg/kg/day divided q8–12h. Then may increase gradually to 5–25 mcg/kg/day in divided doses q6h. Maximum: 0.9 mg/day.

▸ **Attention deficit hyperactivity disorder (ADHD)**

PO

Children. Initially, 0.05 mg/day. May increase by 0.05 mg/day q3–7days. Maximum: 0.3–0.4 mg/day.

▸ **Severe pain**

EPIDURAL

Children. Initially, 0.5 mcg/kg/hr, not to exceed adult dose of 30–40 mcg/hr.

TRANSDERMAL

Transdermal form for children can be used after oral therapy is titrated to a stable dose. Use a transdermal dose approximately equivalent to the total daily oral dose.

UNLABELED USES

ADHD, diagnosis of pheochromocytoma, opioid withdrawal, prevention of migraine headaches, treatment of dysmenorrhea or menopausal flushing.

CONTRAINDICATIONS

Hypersensitivity to clonidine or any related component. Epidural form contraindicated in those with bleeding diathesis or infection at the injection site and in those receiving anticoagulation therapy.

INTERACTIONS

Drug

Beta-blockers (used concurrently): Discontinuing these drugs may increase risk of clonidine-withdrawal hypertensive crisis.
Tricyclic antidepressants: May decrease effect of clonidine.

Herbal

None known.

Food

Natural licorice: May lead to sodium and water retention and increase potassium losses.

DIAGNOSTIC TEST EFFECTS

None known.

IV INCOMPATIBILITIES

No known drug incompatibilities

IV COMPAZTIBILITIES

Bupivacaine (Marcaine, Sensorcaine), fentanyl (Sublimaze), heparin, ketamine (Ketalar), lidocaine, lorazepam (Ativan)

SIDE EFFECTS

Frequent

Dry mouth (40%), drowsiness (33%), dizziness (16%), sedation, constipation (10%)

Occasional (5%–1%)

Depression, swelling of feet, loss of appetite, decreased sexual ability, itching eyes, dizziness, nausea, vomiting, nervousness
Transdermal: Itching, red skin, darkening of skin

Rare (less than 1%)

Nightmares, vivid dreams, cold feeling in fingers and toes

SERIOUS REACTIONS

! Overdosage produces profound hypotension, irritability, bradycardia, respiratory depression, hypothermia, miosis (pupillary constriction), arrhythmias, and apnea.

! Abrupt withdrawal may result in rebound hypertension associated with nervousness, agitation, anxiety, insomnia, hand tingling, tremor, flushing, and sweating.

PEDIATRIC CONSIDERATIONS

Baseline Assessment

- Obtain the patient's B/P immediately before giving each dose, in addition to regular monitoring. Be alert for B/P fluctuations.
- Be aware that clonidine crosses the placenta and is distributed in breast milk.
- Be aware that children are more sensitive to the effects of clonidine. Use clonidine with caution in children.
- Be aware that the medication must be tapered off over time. Stopping clonidine abruptly could lead to a hypertensive crisis.

Precautions

- Use cautiously in pts with cerebrovascular disease, chronic renal failure, Raynaud syndrome, recent myocardial infarction, severe coronary insufficiency, and thromboangiitis obliterans.

Administration and Handling

PO

- Give clonidine without regard to food.
- Tablets may be crushed.
- Give last oral dose just before bedtime.

TRANSDERMAL

- Apply transdermal system to dry, hairless area of intact skin on upper arm or chest.
- Rotate sites to prevent skin irritation.
- Do not trim patch to adjust dose.

Intervention and Evaluation

- Assess the patient's pattern of daily bowel activity and stool consistency.
- Expect to discontinue concurrent beta-blocker therapy several days before discontinuing clonidine therapy to prevent clonidine withdrawal hypertensive crisis. Also, expect to slowly reduce clonidine dosage over 2–4 days.

Patient/Family Teaching

- Recommend sips of tepid water and sugarless gum to the patient to help relieve dry mouth.
- Instruct the patient/family to rise slowly from a lying to a sitting position and permit the legs to dangle momentarily before standing to avoid the hypotensive effect of clonidine.
- Warn the patient/family that skipping doses or voluntarily discontinuing clonidine may produce severe, rebound hypertension.
- Advise the patient/family that the side effects of clonidine tend to diminish during therapy.
- Warn the patient/family to never abruptly stop taking clonidine.

Methyldopa

meth-ill-**doe**-pah

(Aldomet, Apo-Methyldopa [CAN], Hydopa [AUS], Novomedopa [CAN], Nudopa [AUS])

Do not confuse with Anzemet.

CATEGORY AND SCHEDULE

Pregnancy Risk Category: B

MECHANISM OF ACTION

An antihypertensive agent that stimulates central inhibitory alpha-adrenergic receptors and lowers arterial pressure and reduces plasma renin activity. ***Therapeutic Effect:*** Reduces standing and supine B/P.

AVAILABILITY

Tablets: 250 mg, 500 mg.
Injection: 50 mg/mg.

INDICATIONS AND DOSAGES

▸ Moderate to severe hypertension

PO

Children. Initially, 10 mg/kg/day in 2–4 divided doses. Adjust dosage at intervals of 2 days (minimum). Maximum: 65 mg/kg/day or 3 g/day, whichever is less.

IV

Children. Initially, 2–4 mg/kg/dose. May increase to 5–10 mg/kg/dose in 4–6 hrs if no response. Maximum: 65 mg/kg/day or 3 g/day, whichever is less.

CONTRAINDICATIONS

Hypersensitivity to methyldopa or any related component. Liver disease, pheochromocytoma.

INTERACTIONS

Drug

Hypotensive-producing medications: May increase the effects of methyldopa.
Lithium: May increase risk of toxicity of lithium.
MAOIs: May cause hyperexcitability.
NSAIDs, tricyclic antidepressants: May decrease the effects of methyldopa.
Sympathomimetics: May decrease the effects of sympathomimetics.

Herbal

None known.

Food

Natural licorice: May increase sodium and water retention. May lead to increased potassium losses.

DIAGNOSTIC TEST EFFECTS

May increase BUN, serum prolactin, alkaline phosphatase, bilirubin, creatinine, potassium, sodium, uric acid, SGOT (AST), and SGPT (ALT) levels. May produce false-positive Coombs' test results and prolong prothrombin time.

SIDE EFFECTS

Frequent

Peripheral edema, drowsiness, headache, dry mouth

Occasional

Mental changes (e.g., anxiety and depression), decreased sexual function or interest, diarrhea, swelling of breasts, nausea, vomiting, lightheadedness, numbness in hands or feet, rhinitis

SERIOUS REACTIONS

! Liver toxicity (abnormal liver function test results, jaundice, and hepatitis), hemolytic anemia, unexplained fever and flu-like symptoms may occur. If these conditions appear, discontinue the medication and contact the physician.

PEDIATRIC CONSIDERATIONS

Baseline Assessment

- Obtain the patient's baseline B/P, pulse, and weight.
- Infuse IV dose over 30–60 min if an infusion pump is being used.
- Check B/P every 15–30 min during IV infusion.

Precautions

- Use cautiously in pts with renal impairment.

Intervention and Evaluation
- Assess the patient's B/P and pulse closely every 30 min until stabilized.
- Monitor the patient's weight daily during initial therapy.
- Monitor the patient's liver function test results, including serum alkaline phosphatase, bilirubin, SGOT (AST), and SGPT (ALT) levels.
- Assess the patient for peripheral edema. Be aware that the first area of low extremity swelling is usually behind the medial malleolus in ambulatory pts and in the sacral area in bedridden pts.

Patient/Family Teaching
- Urge the patient/family to avoid consuming alcohol while taking methyldopa.
- Warn the patient/family to avoid tasks requiring mental alertness and motor skills until the patient's response to the drug is established.

Prazosin Hydrochloride

pray-zoe-sin
(Minipress, Prasig [AUS], Pratisol [AUS], Pressin [AUS])

CATEGORY AND SCHEDULE
Pregnancy Risk Category: C

MECHANISM OF ACTION
An antidote, antihypertensive, and vasodilator agent that selectively blocks $alpha_1$-adrenergic receptors, decreasing peripheral vascular resistance. ***Therapeutic Effect:*** Produces vasodilation of veins and arterioles; decreases total peripheral resistance; relaxes smooth muscle in bladder neck and prostate.

PHARMACOKINETICS
Well absorbed orally. Protein binding: 95%. Metabolized in the liver to active metabolites. Excreted renally. ***Half-Life:*** Adults: 2–4 hrs.

AVAILABILITY
Capsules: 1 mg, 2 mg, 5 mg.

INDICATIONS AND DOSAGES
▸ Mild to moderate hypertension
PO
Children. 5 mcg/kg/dose q6h. Gradually increase up to 25 mcg/kg/dose. Maximum: 15 mg or 400 mcg/kg/day.

UNLABELED USES
Treatment of benign prostate hypertrophy, CHF, ergot alkaloid toxicity, pheochromocytoma, Raynaud syndrome.

CONTRAINDICATIONS
Hypersensitivity to prazosin, quinazolines, or any related component.

INTERACTIONS
Drug
Estrogen, NSAIDs, sympathomimetics: May decrease the effects of prazosin.
Hypotension-producing medications: May increase antihypertensive effect.
Herbal
Licorice: Causes sodium and water retention and potassium loss.
Food
None known.

DIAGNOSTIC TEST EFFECTS
May cause false-positive for pheochromocytoma.

SIDE EFFECTS

Frequent (10%–7%)
Dizziness, drowsiness, headache, asthenia (loss of strength, energy)
Occasional (5%–4%)
Palpitations, nausea, dry mouth, nervousness
Rare (less than 1%)
Angina, urinary urgency

SERIOUS REACTIONS

! First-dose syncope, hypotension with sudden loss of consciousness, generally occurs 30–90 min after giving the initial prazosin dose of 2 mg or more, instituting a too-rapid increase in dosage or adding another hypotensive agent to therapy. First-dose syncope may be preceded by tachycardia (pulse rate of 120–160 beats/min).

PEDIATRIC CONSIDERATIONS

Baseline Assessment

• Give the first prazosin dose at bedtime. If the initial drug dose is given during the daytime, keep the patient recumbent for 3–4 hrs.
• Assess the patient's B/P and pulse immediately before each dose and every 15–30 min until stabilized. Be alert for B/P fluctuations.

Precautions

• Use cautiously in pts with chronic renal failure and impaired liver function.

Administration and Handling

PO
• Give prazosin without regard to food.
• Administer the first dose at bedtime to minimize the risk of fainting from first-dose syncope.

Intervention and Evaluation

• Monitor the patient's B/P and pulse frequently because first-dose syncope may be preceded by tachycardia.
• Assess the patient's pattern of daily bowel activity and stool consistency.
• Assist the patient with ambulation if he or she experiences dizziness.

Patient/Family Teaching

• Warn the patient/family to avoid tasks that require mental alertness or motor skills for 12–24 hrs after the first dose or any increase in dosage.
• Warn the patient/family to use caution when driving or operating machinery and when rising from a sitting or lying position.
• Advise the patient/family to notify the physician if dizziness or palpitations become bothersome.

REFERENCES

Miller, S. & Fioravanti, J. (1997). Pediatric medications: a handbook for nurses. St. Louis: Mosby.
Taketomo, C. K., Hodding, J. H. & Kraus, D. M. (2003–2004). Pediatric dosage handbook (10th ed.). Hudson, OH: Lexi-Comp.

29 Vasodilators

Hydralazine Hydrochloride
Minoxidil
Nitroglycerin
Nitroprusside Sodium

Uses: Vasodilators are used primarily to treat essential hypertension, angina pectoris, heart failure, and myocardial infarction (MI). Some of these agents are also used to manage peripheral vascular disease and to produce controlled hypotension during surgery. In addition, minoxidil is used as a hair growth stimulant.

Action: For vasodilators, the exact mechanism of action is not known. These agents directly relax smooth muscle, which reduces vascular resistance. Some of them act primarily on arterioles, others affect veins, and still others work on both types of vessels.

COMBINATION PRODUCTS

APRESAZIDE: hydralazine/hydrochlorothiazide (a diuretic) 25 mg/25 mg; 50 mg/50 mg; 100 mg/50 mg.

Hydralazine Hydrochloride

hy-**dral**-ah-zeen
(Alphapress [AUS], Apresoline, Novo-Hylazin [CAN])
Do not confuse with hydroxyzine.

CATEGORY AND SCHEDULE

Pregnancy Risk Category: C

MECHANISM OF ACTION

An antihypertensive agent with direct vasodilating effects on the arterioles. ***Therapeutic Effect:*** Decreases blood pressure (B/P) and systemic resistance.

PHARMACOKINETICS

Route	Onset	Peak	Duration
PO	20–30 min	N/A	2–4 hrs
IV	5–20 min	N/A	2–6 hrs

Well absorbed from the GI tract. Widely distributed. Protein binding: 85%–90%. Metabolized in liver to active metabolite. Primarily excreted in urine. Not removed by hemodialysis. ***Half-Life:*** Adults: 3–7 hrs (half-life increased with impaired renal function).

AVAILABILITY

Tablets: 10 mg, 25 mg, 50 mg, 100 mg.
Injection: 20 mg/mL.

INDICATIONS AND DOSAGES

▸ **Moderate to severe hypertension**

PO

Children. Initially, 0.75–1 mg/kg/day in 2–4 divided doses, not to exceed 25 mg/dose. May increase over 3–4 wks. Maximum: 7.5 mg/kg/day (5 mg/kg/day in infants).

IM/IV

Children. Initially, 0.1–0.2 mg/kg/dose (maximum: 20 mg) q4–6h as needed up to 1.7–3.5 mg/kg/day in divided doses q4–6h.

▸ **Dosage in renal impairment**

Creatinine Clearance	Dosage Interval
10–50 mL/min	q8h
Less than 10 mL/min	q8–24h

UNLABELED USES

Treatment of CHF, hypertension secondary to eclampsia and preeclampsia, primary pulmonary hypertension.

CONTRAINDICATIONS

Hypersensitivity to hydralazine or any related component. Coronary artery disease, lupus erythematosus, rheumatic heart disease, dissecting aortic aneurysm.

INTERACTIONS

Drug

Diuretics, other hypotensives: May increase hypotensive effect.
Indomethacin: May decrease hypotensive effects.

Herbal

None known.

Food

Natural licorice: May lead to sodium and water retention. May lead to increased potassium losses.

DIAGNOSTIC TEST EFFECTS

May produce positive direct Coombs' test results.

IV INCOMPATIBILITIES

Aminophylline, ampicillin (Polycillin), furosemide (Lasix)

IV COMPATIBILITIES

Dobutamine (Dobutrex), heparin, hydrocortisone (Solu-Cortef), nitroglycerin, potassium

SIDE EFFECTS

Frequent

Headache, palpitations, tachycardia (generally disappears in 7–10 days)

Occasional

GI disturbance (nausea, vomiting, diarrhea), paresthesia, fluid retention, peripheral edema, dizziness, flushed face, nasal congestion

SERIOUS REACTIONS

! High dosage may produce lupus erythematosus–like reaction, including fever, facial rash, muscle and joint aches, and splenomegaly.
! Severe orthostatic hypotension, skin flushing, severe headache, myocardial ischemia, and cardiac arrhythmias may develop.
! Profound shock may occur in cases of severe overdosage.

PEDIATRIC CONSIDERATIONS

Baseline Assessment

- Obtain the patient's B/P and pulse immediately before each hydralazine dose, in addition to regular B/P monitoring. Be alert for B/P fluctuations.
- Be aware that hydralazine crosses the placenta, and it is unknown whether hydralazine is distributed in breast milk.
- Be aware that hematomas, leukopenia, petechial bleeding, and thrombocytopenia have occurred in newborns and that these conditions resolve within 1–3 wks.
- There are no age-related precautions noted in children.
- Hydralazine has only limited use in children. It should only be used if the benefits of the medication outweigh the risks.

Precautions

- Use cautiously in pts with cerebrovascular disease and impaired renal function.

Administration and Handling

PO

- Hydralazine is best given with food or regularly spaced meals.
- Crush tablets if necessary.

IV

- Store at room temperature.
- Give undiluted if necessary.
- Give single dose over 1 min.

Intervention and Evaluation

- Monitor the patient for headache, palpitations, and tachycardia.
- Assess for peripheral edema of feet and hands. Usually the first area of lower extremity swelling is behind the medial malleolus in ambulatory pts and in the sacral area in bedridden pts.
- Assess the patient's pattern of daily bowel activity and stool consistency.

Patient/Family Teaching

- Instruct the patient/family to rise slowly from a lying to a sitting position and permit the legs to dangle from the bed momentarily before standing to reduce the hypotensive effect of hydralazine.
- Suggest to the patient/family that consuming dry toast or unsalted crackers may relieve nausea.
- With high-dose therapy, warn the patient/family to notify the physician if the patient experiences fever (lupus-like reaction) and to report joint and muscle aches.

Minoxidil

min-**ox**-ih-dill

(Apo-Gain, Loniten, Milnox, Regaine [AUS], Rogaine, Rogaine Extra Strength)

Do not confuse with Lotensin.

CATEGORY AND SCHEDULE

Pregnancy Risk Category: C

OTC (topical solution)

MECHANISM OF ACTION

An antihypertensive and hair growth stimulant that has direct action on vascular smooth muscle, producing vasodilation of arterioles. ***Therapeutic Effect:*** Decreases peripheral vascular resistance and blood pressure (B/P); increases cutaneous blood flow; stimulates hair follicle epithelium and hair follicle growth.

PHARMACOKINETICS

Route	Onset	Peak	Duration
PO	0.5 hr	2–8 hrs	2–5 days

Well absorbed from the GI tract; minimal absorption after topical application. Protein binding: None. Widely distributed. Metabolized in liver to the active metabolite. Primarily excreted in urine. Removed by hemodialysis. ***Half-Life:*** Adults: 4.2 hrs.

PHARMACOKINETICS

Tablets: 2.5 mg, 10 mg.

Topical Solution: 2% (20 mg/mL), 5% (50 mg/mL).

INDICATIONS AND DOSAGES

▸ **Severe symptomatic hypertension, hypertension associated with organ damage, hypertension that has failed to respond to maximal therapeutic dosages of a diuretic or two other antihypertensive agents**

PO

Children younger than 12 yrs. Initially, 0.1–0.2 mg/kg (5 mg maximum) daily. Gradually increase at minimum 3-day intervals of 0.1–2 mg/kg. Maintenance: 0.25–1 mg/kg/day in 1–2 doses. Maximum: 50 mg/day.

Children older than 12 yrs. Initially 5 mg once daily. Gradually increase at 3-day intervals. Maintenance: 10–40 mg/day in 1–2 doses. Maximum: 100 mg/day.

CONTRAINDICATIONS

Hypersensitivity to minoxidil or any related component and pheochromocytoma.

INTERACTIONS

Drug

Parenteral antihypertensives: May increase hypotensive effect.
NSAIDs: May decrease the effects of minoxidil.

Herbal

Natural licorice: May increase sodium and water retention. May increase potassium losses.

Food

None known.

DIAGNOSTIC TEST EFFECTS

May increase BUN, plasma renin activity, serum alkaline phosphatase, serum creatinine, and serum sodium levels. May decrease blood Hgb and Hct levels and erythrocyte count.

SIDE EFFECTS

Frequent

PO: Edema with concurrent weight gain, hypertrichosis (elongation, thickening, increased pigmentation of fine body hair) develops in 80% of pts within 3–6 wks after beginning therapy

Occasional

PO: T-wave changes but usually revert to pretreatment state with continued therapy or drug withdrawal.
Topical: Itching, skin rash, dry or flaking skin, erythema

Rare

PO: Rash, pruritus, breast tenderness in male and female, headache, photosensitivity reaction
Topical: Allergic reaction, alopecia, burning scalp, soreness at hair root, headache, visual disturbances

SERIOUS REACTIONS

! Tachycardia and angina pectoris may occur because of increased O_2 demands associated with increased heart rate and cardiac output.
! Fluid and electrolyte imbalance and CHF may be observed, especially if a diuretic is not given concurrently with minoxidil.
! Too rapid reduction in B/P may result in syncope, cerebrovascular accident, MI, and ischemia of sense organs (altered vision and hearing).
! Pericardial effusion and tamponade may be seen in those with impaired renal function not receiving dialysis.

PEDIATRIC CONSIDERATIONS

Baseline Assessment

- Assess the patient's B/P on both arms and take the patient's pulse for 1 full min immediately before giving the medication. If the patient's pulse increases 20 beats/min or more over baseline, or systolic or diastolic B/P decreases less than 20 mm Hg, withhold minoxidil and contact physician.
- Be aware that minoxidil crosses the placenta and is distributed in breast milk.
- There are no age-related precautions noted in children.

Precautions

- Use cautiously in pts with chronic CHF, coronary artery disease, recent MI (within 1 mo), and severe renal impairment.

Administration and Handling

PO
- Give without regard to food (with food if GI upset occurs).
- Crush tablets if necessary.

Intervention and Evaluation

- Monitor the patient's B/P, body weight, and serum electrolyte levels.
- Assess for peripheral edema of feet and hands. Usually the first area of low extremity swelling is behind the medial malleolus in

ambulatory pts and in the sacral area in bedridden pts.
• Assess the patient for signs and symptoms of CHF, including cool extremities, cough, dyspnea on exertion, and rales at the base of the lungs.
• Evaluate the patient for distant or muffled heart sounds by auscultation, which may indicate pericardial effusion or tamponade.

Patient/Family Teaching

• Advise the patient/family that the maximum B/P response occurs 3–7 days and reversible growth of fine body hair may begin 3–6 weeks after minoxidil treatment is initiated.
• Warn the patient/family to avoid exposure to sunlight and artificial light sources: use a broad-spectrum sunscreen and wear protective clothing.

Nitroglycerin

nigh-trow-**glih**-sir-in
(Anginine [AUS], Minitran, Nitradisc [AUS], Nitrek, Nitro-Bid, Nitro-Dur, Nitrogard, Nitroject [CAN], Nitrolingual, Nitrong-SR, NitroQuick, Nitrostat, Nitro-Tab, Rectogesic [AUS], Tansiderm Nitro [AUS], Trinipatch [CAN])
Do not confuse with Hyperstat, Nicobid, Nicoderm, Nilstat, nitroprusside, Nizoral, or nystatin.

CATEGORY AND SCHEDULE

Pregnancy Risk Category: C

MECHANISM OF ACTION

A nitrate that decreases myocardial O_2 demand. Reduces left ventricular preload and afterload. ***Therapeutic Effect:*** Dilates coronary arteries, improves collateral blood flow to ischemic areas within myocardium. IV form produces peripheral vasodilation.

PHARMACOKINETICS

Route	Onset	Peak	Duration
Sublingual	2–5 min	4–8 min	30–60 min
Transmucosal tablet	2–5 min	4–10 min	3–5 hrs
Extended-release	20–45 min	N/A	3–8 hrs
Topical	15–60 min	0.5–2 hrs	3–8 hrs
Patch	30–60 min	1–3 hrs	8–12 hrs
IV	1–2 min	N/A	3–5 min

Well absorbed after PO, sublingual, and topical administration. Undergoes extensive first-pass metabolism. Metabolized in liver and by enzymes in the bloodstream. Primarily excreted in urine. Not removed by hemodialysis. ***Half-Life:*** 1–4 min.

PHARMACOKINETICS

Tablets (sublingual): 0.3 mg, 0.4 mg, 0.6 mg.
Spray: 0.4 mg/dose.
Tablets (buccal, controlled release): 2 mg, 3 mg.
Capsules (sustained release): 2.5 mg, 6.5 mg, 9 mg.
Transdermal: 0.1 mg/hr, 0.2 mg/hr, 0.3 mg/hr, 0.4 mg/hr, 0.6 mg/hr, 0.8 mg/hr.
Topical Ointment: 2%.
Injection: 5 mg/mL.
Injection Solution (premixed): 100 mcg/mL, 200 mcg/mL, 400 mcg/mL.

INDICATIONS AND DOSAGES

▸ **Treatment of CHF associated with acute MI**

IV

Children. Initially, 0.25–0.5 mcg/kg/min; titrate by

0.5–1 mcg/kg/min every 3–5 min up to 20 mcg/kg/min.

CONTRAINDICATIONS

Allergy to adhesives (transdermal), closed-angle glaucoma, constrictive pericarditis (IV), early MI (sublingual), GI hypermotility or malabsorption (extended release), head trauma, hypersensitivity to nitrates, hypotension (IV), inadequate cerebral circulation (IV), increased intracranial pressure, pericardial tamponade (IV), postural hypotension, severe anemia, uncorrected hypovolemia (IV).

INTERACTIONS

Drug

Alcohol, antihypertensives, vasodilators: May increase risk of orthostatic hypotension.
Heparin: IV nitroglycerin may antagonize the anticoagulant effects.

Herbal

None known.

Food

None known.

DIAGNOSTIC TEST EFFECTS

May increase blood methemoglobin concentrations, urine catecholamines, and urine vanillylmandelic acid concentrations.

IV INCOMPATIBILITIES

Alteplase (Activase)

IV COMPATIBILITIES

Amiodarone (Cordarone), diltiazem (Cardizem), dobutamine (Dobutrex), dopamine (Intropin), epinephrine, famotidine (Pepcid), fentanyl (Sublimaze), furosemide (Lasix), heparin, hydromorphone (Dilaudid), insulin, labetalol (Trandate), lidocaine, lorazepam (Ativan), midazolam (Versed), milrinone (Primacor), morphine, nicardipine (Cardene), nitroprusside (Nipride), norepinephrine (Levophed), propofol (Diprivan)

SIDE EFFECTS

Frequent
Headache (may be severe) occurs mostly in early therapy, diminishes rapidly in intensity, usually disappears during continued treatment; transient flushing of face and neck; dizziness (especially if patient is standing immobile or is in a warm environment); weakness; postural hypotension
Sublingual: Burning, tingling sensation at oral point of dissolution
Ointment: Erythema, pruritus
Occasional
GI upset
Transdermal: Contact dermatitis

SERIOUS REACTIONS

! Nitroglycerin should be discontinued if blurred vision or dry mouth occurs.
! Severe postural hypotension manifested by fainting, pulselessness, cold or clammy skin, and profuse sweating may occur.
! Tolerance may occur with repeated, prolonged therapy (minor tolerance with intermittent use of sublingual tablets).
! High dose tends to produce severe headache.

PEDIATRIC CONSIDERATIONS

Baseline Assessment

• Document the onset, type (sharp, dull, or squeezing), radiation, location, intensity, and duration of anginal pain, and its precipitating factors, such as exertion and emotional stress.

• Assess the patient's apical pulse and B/P before administration and periodically after nitroglycerin dose.
• Continuously monitor the patient's EKG during IV administration.
• Be aware that it is unknown whether nitroglycerin crosses the placenta or is distributed in breast milk.
• Be aware that the safety and efficacy of nitroglycerin have not been established in children.
• IV preparations may contain alcohol and/or propylene glycol. Use with caution in neonates.

Precautions

• Use cautiously in pts with acute MI, blood volume depletion from diuretic therapy, glaucoma (contraindicated in closed-angle glaucoma), liver or renal disease, and systolic B/P less than 90 mm Hg.

Administration and Handling

IV

• Store at room temperature.
• Know that the IV form is available in ready-to-use injectable containers.
• Dilute vials in 250 or 500 mL D_5W or 0.9% NaCl to a maximum concentration of 250 mg/250 mL.
• Use microdrop or infusion pump.
• Nitroglycerin adsorbs to plastics and must be administered using special administration sets.

Intervention and Evaluation

◀ **ALERT** ▶ Remove the transdermal dosage form before cardioversion or defibrillation because the electrical current may cause arcing which can burn the patient and damage the paddles.
• Monitor the patient's B/P and heart rate.
• Examine the patient for facial or neck flushing.

Patient/Family Teaching

• Advise the patient/family to take the medication with meals if the patient experiences headache during therapy.
• Teach the patient/family to keep the drug container away from heat and moisture.
• Caution the patient/family against changing brands of nitroglycerin.
• Instruct the patient/family to rise slowly from a lying to a sitting position and dangle the legs momentarily before standing to avoid the drug's hypotensive effect.
• Urge the patient/family to avoid alcohol during nitroglycerin therapy. Explain that alcohol intensifies the drug's hypotensive effect. Warn the patient that alcohol ingested soon after taking nitroglycerin can cause an acute hypotensive episode noted by a marked drop in B/P, vertigo, and pallor.
• Caution patient to keep sublingual tablets in a tightly closed container.

Nitroprusside Sodium

nigh-troe-**pruss**-eyd
(Nipride, Nitropress)
Do not confuse with nitroglycerin.

CATEGORY AND SCHEDULE

Pregnancy Risk Category: C

MECHANISM OF ACTION

Potent vasodilator used to treat emergency hypertensive conditions; acts directly on arterial and venous smooth muscle. Decreases peripheral vascular resistance, preload, and afterload; improves cardiac output. ***Therapeutic Effect:*** Dilates coronary arteries, decreases O_2 consumption; relieves persistent chest pain.

PHARMACOKINETICS

Route	Onset	Peak	Duration
IV	1–10 min	Dependent on infusion rate	Dissipates rapidly after stopping IV

Reacts with Hgb in erythrocytes, producing cyanmethemoglobin and cyanide ions. Primarily excreted in urine. ***Half-Life:*** Less than 10 min.

AVAILABILITY

Powder for Injection: 50 mg.
Injection: 25 mg/mL.

INDICATIONS AND DOSAGES

▸ Immediate reduction of blood pressure (B/P) in hypertensive crisis, produce controlled hypotension in surgical procedures to reduce bleeding, treatment of acute CHF
IV
Children. Initially, 0.3–0.5 mcg/kg/min, then titrate to effect. Range: 0.5–10 mcg/kg/min. Maintenance: 3 mcg/kg/min. Do not exceed 10 mcg/kg/min (risk of precipitous drop in B/P).

UNLABELED USES

Control paroxysmal hypertension before and during surgery for pheochromocytoma, peripheral vasospasm caused by ergot alkaloid overdose, treatment adjunct for MI, valvular regurgitation.

CONTRAINDICATIONS

Hypersensitivity to nitroprusside or any related component. Compensatory hypertension (atrioventricular shunt or coarctation of aorta), inadequate cerebral circulation, moribund pts.

INTERACTIONS

Drug
Dobutamine: May increase cardiac output and decrease pulmonary wedge pressure.
Hypotensive-producing medications: May increase hypotensive effect.
Herbal
None known.
Food
None known.

DIAGNOSTIC TEST EFFECTS

None known.

IV INCOMPATIBILITIES

Cisatracurium (Nimbex)

IV COMPATIBILITIES

Diltiazem (Cardizem), dobutamine (Dobutrex), dopamine (Intropin), enalapril (Vasotec), heparin, insulin, labetalol (Normodyne, Trandate), lidocaine, midazolam (Versed), milrinone (Primacor), nitroglycerin, propofol (Diprivan)

SIDE EFFECTS

Occasional
Flushing of skin, increased intracranial pressure, rash, pain or redness at injection site, restlessness, headache, disorientation, nausea, vomiting, diaphoresis

SERIOUS REACTIONS

! A too rapid IV rate reduces B/P too quickly.
! Nausea, retching, diaphoresis, apprehension, headache, restlessness, muscle twitching, dizziness, palpitations, retrosternal pain, and abdominal pain may occur.

Symptoms disappear rapidly if rate of administration is slowed or temporarily discontinued.
! Overdosage produces metabolic acidosis and tolerance to the therapeutic effect.

PEDIATRIC CONSIDERATIONS

Baseline Assessment
• Continuously monitor the patient's B/P and EKG.
• Determine, with the physician, the desired B/P level. Know that the B/P is normally maintained at about 30%–40% below pretreatment levels.
• Expect to discontinue nitroprusside if the therapeutic response is not achieved within 10 min after IV infusion at 10 mcg/kg/min is initiated.
• Be aware that it is unknown whether nitroprusside crosses the placenta or is distributed in breast milk.
• Be aware that the safety and efficacy of nitroprusside have not been established in children.

Precautions
• Use cautiously in pts with hyponatremia, hypothyroidism, and severe liver or renal impairment.

Administration and Handling
IV
• Protect solution from light.
• Inspect solution, which normally appears very faint brown. Be aware that a color change from brown to blue, green, or dark red indicates drug deterioration.
• Use only freshly prepared solution. Once prepared, do not keep or use longer than 24 hrs.
• Discard unused portion.
• Reconstitute 50-mg vial with 2–3 mL D_5W or Sterile Water for Injection without preservative.
• Further dilute with 250–1,000 mL D_5W to provide concentration of 200–50 mcg/mL, respectively, up to a maximum concentration of 200 mg/250 mL.
• Wrap infusion bottle in aluminum foil immediately after mixing.
• Give by IV infusion only using the infusion rate chart provided by the manufacturer or protocol.
• Administer using an IV infusion pump or microdrip (60 gtt/mL).
• Be alert for extravasation, which produces severe pain and sloughing.

Intervention and Evaluation
• Monitor the patient's rate of infusion frequently.
• Monitor the patient's blood acid-base balance, electrolyte levels, intake and output, and laboratory results.
• Assess the patient for signs and symptoms of metabolic acidosis, including disorientation, headache, hyperventilation, nausea, vomiting, and weakness.
• Assess the patient for signs and symptoms of cyanide toxicity: psychosis, blurred vision, confusion, weakness, seizure, dilated pupils, decreased reflexes, and metabolic acidosis.
• Assess the patient for therapeutic response to medication.
• Monitor the patient's B/P for potential rebound hypertension after infusion is discontinued.

Patient/Family Teaching
• Advise the patient/family to immediately report if the patient experiences dizziness, headache, nausea, palpitations, or other unusual signs or symptoms.
• Warn the patient/family to immediately notify the physician if the patient experiences pain, redness, or swelling at the IV insertion site.

REFERENCES

Miller, S. & Fioravanti, J. (1997). Pediatric medications: a handbook for nurses. St. Louis: Mosby.

Taketomo, C. K., Hodding, J. H. & Kraus, D. M. (2003–2004). Pediatric dosage handbook (10th ed.). Hudson, OH: Lexi-Comp.

30 Vasopressors

Dobutamine Hydrochloride
Dopamine Hydrochloride
Epinephrine
Norepinephrine Bitartrate
Phenylephrine Hydrochloride

Uses: Different groups of vasopressors are used for different effects. *Alpha$_1$*-receptor stimulators, such as midodrine and phenylephrine, are used to induce vasoconstriction primarily in the skin and mucous membranes, to provide nasal decongestion, and to delay local anesthetic absorption. They are also used to increase blood pressure (B/P) in certain hypotensive states and to produce mydriasis, facilitating eye examinations and ocular surgery.

Many vasopressors, however, produce their effects by working on a combination of adrenergic receptors. In most cases, the site of action depends on the drug dose. For example, at low doses, dopamine stimulates dopaminergic receptors, dilating renal arteries. But at much higher doses, the drug stimulates alpha$_1$-receptors, causing vasoconstriction. The chart below shows how vasopressors stimulate particular receptors and produce the corresponding therapeutic effects.

Name	Receptor Specificity	Uses	Dosage Range
Dobutamine	Beta$_1$, beta$_2$, alpha$_1$	Inotropic support in cardiac compensation	2.5–10 mcg/kg/min IV
Dopamine	Beta$_1$, alpha$_1$, dopaminergic Beta$_1$: 2–10 mcg/kg/min IV Alpha$_1$: greater than 10 mcg/kg/min IV	Vasopressor, cardiac stimulant	Dopaminergic: 0.5–3 mcg/kg/min IV
Epinephrine	Beta$_1$, beta$_2$, alpha$_1$	Cardiac arrest, anaphylactic shock	Vasopressor: 1–10 mcg/min IV

(*continued*)

Name	Receptor Specificity	Uses	Dosage Range
		Cardiac arrest: 1 mg q3–5min IV during resuscitation	
Midodrine	$Alpha_1$	Vasopressor, orthostatic hypotension	10 mg PO, 3 times daily
Norepinephrine	$Beta_1$, $alpha_1$	Vasopressor	0.5–1 mcg/min up to 2–12 mcg/min IV
Phenylephrine	$Alpha_1$	Vasopressor	Initially, 10–180 mcg/min, then 40–60 mcg/min IV

Action: The sympathetic nervous system (SNS) maintains homeostasis, including the regulation of heart rate, cardiac contractility, B/P, bronchial airway tone, and carbohydrate and fatty acid metabolism. The SNS is mediated by neurotransmitters (primarily norepinephrine, epinephrine, and dopamine) that act on adrenergic receptors, which include $alpha_1$, $alpha_2$, $beta_1$, $beta_2$, and dopaminergic receptors. Vasopressors differ widely in their actions based on their specificity for these receptors:

- $Alpha_1$-receptor stimulation causes constriction of arterioles and veins.
- $Beta_1$-receptor stimulation increases the rate, force of contraction, and conduction velocity of the heart and releases renin from the kidneys.
- $Beta_2$-receptor stimulation dilates arterioles.
- Dopamine-receptor stimulation dilates renal vessels.

COMBINATION PRODUCTS

AC GEL: epinephrine/cocaine (an anesthetic).
LIDOCAINE WITH EPINEPHRINE: lidocaine (an anesthetic)/epinephrine 2%/1:50,000; 1%/1:100,000; 1%/1:200,000; 0.5%/1:2000,000.
PHENERGAN VC: phenylephrine/promethazine (an antihistamine) 5 mg/5 mg.
PHENERGAN VC WITH CODEINE: phenylephrine/promethazine (an antihistamine)/codeine (an analgesic) 6.25 mg/5 mg/10 mg.
TAC: epinephrine/tetracaine (an anesthetic)/cocaine (an anesthetic).

Dobutamine Hydrochloride

do-**byew**-ta-meen
(Dobutrex)
Do not confuse with dopamine.

CATEGORY AND SCHEDULE

Pregnancy Risk Category: B

MECHANISM OF ACTION

A direct-acting inotropic agent acting primarily on $beta_1$-adrenergic receptors.
Therapeutic Effect: Decreases preload and afterload. Enhances myocardial contractility, stroke volume, and cardiac output. Improves renal blood flow and urine output.

PHARMACOKINETICS

Route	Onset	Peak	Duration
IV	1–2 min	10 min	Length of infusion

Metabolized in tissues and liver. Primarily excreted in urine. Not removed by hemodialysis.
Half-Life: 2 min.

AVAILABILITY

Injection: 12.5 mg/mL vial.
Infusion (ready-to-use): 1 mg/mL, 2 mg/mL, 4 mg/mL.

INDICATIONS AND DOSAGES

▸ Short-term management of cardiac decompensation

IV INFUSION
Children. 2.5–15 mcg/kg/min; titrate to effect. Rarely, infusion rate up to 40 mcg/kg/min to increase cardiac output.
Neonates. 2–15 mcg/kg/min; titrate to effect.

CONTRAINDICATIONS

Hypersensitivity to dobutamine or any related component.
Hypovolemic pts, idiopathic hypertrophic subaortic stenosis, sulfite sensitivity.

INTERACTIONS

Drug

Beta-blockers: May antagonize the effects of dobutamine.
Digoxin: May increase the risk of arrhythmias, and provide additional inotropic effect.
MAOIs, oxytocics, tricyclic antidepressants: May increase the adverse effects of dobutamine, such as arrhythmias and hypertension.

Herbal

None known.

Food

None known.

DIAGNOSTIC TEST EFFECTS

Decreases serum potassium levels.

IV INCOMPATIBILITIES

Acyclovir (Zovirax), alteplase (Activase), amphotericin B complex (Abelcet, AmBisome, Amphotec), bumetanide (Bumex), cefepime (Maxipime), foscarnet (Foscavir), furosemide (Lasix), heparin, piperacillin/tazobactam (Zosyn)

IV COMPATIBILITIES

Amiodarone (Cordarone), calcium chloride, calcium gluconate, diltiazem (Cardizem), dopamine (Intropin), enalapril (Vasotec), famotidine (Pepcid), hydromorphone (Dilaudid), insulin (regular), lidocaine, lorazepam (Ativan), magnesium sulfate, midazolam (Versed), milrinone (Primacor), morphine, nitroglycerin, norepinephrine (Levophed), potassium chloride, propofol (Diprivan)

SIDE EFFECTS

Frequent (greater than 5%)
Increased heart rate and B/P

Occasional (5%–3%)
Pain at injection site

Rare (3%–1%)
Nausea, headache, anginal pain, shortness of breath, fever

SERIOUS REACTIONS

! Overdosage may produce marked increase in heart rate, 30 beats/min or higher, a marked increase in systolic B/P, 50 mm Hg or higher, anginal pain, and premature ventricular beats.

PEDIATRIC CONSIDERATIONS

Baseline Assessment

- Perform continuous cardiac monitoring of the patient to check for arrhythmias.
- Determine the patient's body weight in kilograms for dosage calculation.
- Obtain the patient's initial B/P, heart rate, and respirations.
- Correct hypovolemia before beginning dobutamine therapy.
- Be aware that it is unknown whether dobutamine crosses the placenta or is distributed in breast milk, so it is not administered to pregnant women.
- IV extravasation can occur with dobutamine. Monitor IV site often to prevent tissue damage.
- There are no age-related precautions noted in children.

Precautions

- Use cautiously in pts with atrial fibrillation and hypertension.

Administration and Handling

◂ALERT▸ Dobutamine dosage is determined by the patient's response to the drug.

◂ALERT▸ Plan to correct hypovolemia with volume expanders before dobutamine infusion. Expect to treat pts with atrial fibrillation with digoxin before infusion. Administer by IV infusion only.

IV

- Store at room temperature because freezing produces crystallization.
- Pink discoloration of solution, caused by oxidation, does not indicate loss of potency if used within the recommended time period.
- Dobutamine is a potent drug and MUST be diluted before use.
- Further diluted solution for infusion must be used within 24 hrs.
- Dilute 250-mg ampoule with 10 mL Sterile Water for Injection or D_5W for injection; the resulting solution is 25 mg/mL. Add an additional 10 mL diluent if not completely dissolved; the resulting solution is 12.5 mg/mL.
- Further dilute 250-mg vial with D_5W or 0.9% NaCl. Maximum concentration is 3.125 g/250 mL or 12.5 mg/mL.
- Use an infusion pump to control the flow rate.
- Titrate dosage to individual response, as prescribed.
- Be aware that infiltration of the IV solution causes local inflamma-

tory changes and may cause dermal necrosis.

Intervention and Evaluation

• Continuously monitor the patient for arrhythmias or changes in heart rate.
• Establish parameters with the physician for adjusting the drug rate or stopping infusion.
• Maintain accurate intake and output records. Measure the patient's urine output frequently.
• Assess the patient's serum potassium levels and dobutamine plasma levels. Keep in mind that the therapeutic range is 40–190 ng/mL.
• Continuously monitor the patient's B/P. Keep in mind that high B/P is a greater risk in pts with preexisting hypertension.
• Check the patient's cardiac output and pulmonary wedge pressure or central venous pressure frequently.
• Immediately notify the physician if the patient experiences cardiac arrhythmias, decreased urine output, or a significant increase or decrease in B/P or heart rate.

Patient/Family Teaching

• Tell the patient/family to let you know if the patient develops pain or burning at the IV site.
• Urge the patient/family to let you know if the patient experiences chest pain or palpitations during the infusion.

Dopamine Hydrochloride

dope-a-meen
(Intropin)
Do not confuse with dobutamine, Dopram, or Isoptin.
(See Color Plate)

CATEGORY AND SCHEDULE

Pregnancy Risk Category: C

MECHANISM OF ACTION

A sympathomimetic (adrenergic agonist) drug that stimulates adrenergic receptors; effects are dose dependent. Low dosages (1–5 mcg/kg/min): Stimulates dopaminergic receptors causing renal vasodilation. ***Therapeutic Effect:*** Increases renal blood flow, urine flow, sodium excretion. Low to moderate dosages (5–15 mcg/kg/min): Positive inotropic effect by direct action, release of norepinephrine.
Therapeutic Effect: Increases myocardial contractility, stroke volume, cardiac output. High dosages (greater than 15 mcg/kg/min): Stimulates alpha-receptors.
Therapeutic Effect: Increases peripheral resistance, renal vasoconstriction, and systolic and diastolic B/P.

PHARMACOKINETICS

Route	Onset	Peak	Duration
IV	1–2 min	–	Longer than 10 min

Widely distributed. Does not cross blood-brain barrier. Metabolized in liver, kidney, and plasma. Primarily excreted in urine. Not removed by hemodialysis.
Half-Life: 2 min.

AVAILABILITY

Injection: 40 mg/mL, 80 mg/mL, 160 mg/mL.
Injection (premix with dextrose): 80 mg/100 mL, 160 mg/100 mL, 320 mg/100 mL.

INDICATIONS AND DOSAGES

▸ **Prophylaxis and treatment of acute hypotension, shock that is associated with cardiac**

decompensation, myocardial infarction, open heart surgery, renal failure, trauma, treatment of low cardiac output, CHF
IV (EFFECTS ARE DOSE RELATED)
Children. 1–20 mcg/kg/min. Maximum: 50 mcg/kg/min. Low dose to maintain renal blood flow and urine output: 1–5 mcg/kg/min. Intermediate dose to increase renal blood flow, heart rate/contractility, blood pressure: 5–15 mcg/kg/min. High dose for vasoconstriction and to increase blood pressure: 15–20 mcg/kg/min.
Neonates. 1–20 mcg/kg/min.

CONTRAINDICATIONS
Hypersensitivity to dopamine or any related component. Pheochromocytoma, sulfite sensitivity, uncorrected tachyarrhythmias, ventricular fibrillation.

INTERACTIONS
Drug
Beta-blockers: May decrease the effects of dopamine.
Digoxin: May increase the risk of arrhythmias.
Ergot alkaloids: May increase vasoconstriction.
MAOIs: May increase cardiac stimulation and vasopressor effects.
Tricyclic antidepressants: May increase cardiovascular effects.
Herbal
None known.
Food
None known.

DIAGNOSTIC TEST EFFECTS
None known.

IV INCOMPATIBILITIES
Acyclovir (Zovirax), amphotericin B complex (Abelcet, AmBisome, Amphotec), cefepime (Maxipime), furosemide (Lasix), insulin

IV COMPATIBILITIES
Amiodarone (Cordarone), calcium chloride, diltiazem (Cardizem), dobutamine (Dobutrex), enalapril (Vasotec), heparin, hydromorphone (Dilaudid), labetalol (Trandate), levofloxacin (Levaquin), lidocaine, lorazepam (Ativan), methylprednisolone (Solu-Medrol), midazolam (Versed), milrinone (Primacor), morphine, nicardipine (Cardene), nitroglycerin, norepinephrine (Levophed), piperacillin tazobactam (Zosyn), potassium chloride, propofol (Diprivan)

SIDE EFFECTS
Frequent
Headache, ectopic beats, tachycardia, anginal pain, palpitations, vasoconstriction, hypotension, nausea, vomiting, dyspnea
Occasional
Piloerection or goose bumps, bradycardia, widening of QRS complex

SERIOUS REACTIONS
! High dosages may produce ventricular arrhythmias.
! Pts with occlusive vascular disease are high-risk candidates for further compromise of circulation to extremities, which may result in gangrene.
! Tissue necrosis with sloughing may occur with extravasation of IV solution.

PEDIATRIC CONSIDERATIONS
Baseline Assessment
• Determine whether the patient has been receiving MAOI therapy within last 2–3 wks because it

requires dopamine dosage reduction.
• Expect to monitor the patient with a continuous cardiac monitor to assess for arrhythmias.
• Determine the patient's weight for dosage calculation.
• Obtain the patient's initial B/P, heart rate, and respirations.
• Be aware that it is unknown whether dopamine crosses the placenta or is distributed in breast milk.
• Closely monitor pediatric pts because gangrene due to IV extravasation has been reported.
• It may take up to 1 hr to reach a steady-state concentration in pediatric pts.
• Do not administer through an umbilical arterial catheter.

Precautions
• Use cautiously in pts with ischemic heart disease and occlusive vascular disease.

Administration and Handling
◀ ALERT ▶ Expect to correct blood volume depletion before administering dopamine. Blood volume replacement may occur simultaneously with dopamine infusion.

IV
• Do not use solutions darker than slightly yellow or discolored to yellow, brown, or pink to purple because it indicates decomposition of drug.
• Know that the drug is stable for 24 hrs after dilution.
• Dilute each 5-mL (200-mg) ampule in 250–500 mL 0.9% NaCl, D_5W/0.45% NaCl, D_5W/0.45% NaCl, D_5W/lactated Ringer's or lactated Ringer's solution. Keep in mind the concentration is dependent on the dosage and the patient's fluid requirements. Remember that a 250 mL solution yields 800 mcg/mL, and a 500 mL solution yields 400 mcg/mL. The maximum concentration is 3.2 g/250 mL or 12.8 mg/mL. Know that the drug is available prediluted in 250 or 500 mL D_5W.
• Administer into large vein, such as the antecubital or subclavian vein, to prevent drug extravasation.
• Use an infusion pump to control the rate of flow.
• Titrate dosage to the desired hemodynamic values or optimum urine flow, as prescribed.

Intervention and Evaluation
• Continuously monitor the patient for cardiac arrhythmias.
• Measure the patient's urine output frequently.
• If extravasation occurs, immediately infiltrate the affected tissue with 10–15 mL 0.9% NaCl solution containing 5–10 mg phentolamine mesylate, as ordered.
• Monitor the patient's B/P, heart rate, and respirations at least every 15 min during dopamine administration.
• Assess the patient's cardiac output and pulmonary wedge pressure or central venous pressure frequently.
• Examine the patient's peripheral circulation by palpating pulses and noting the color and temperature of the extremities.
• Immediately notify the physician if the patient experiences cardiac arrhythmias, decreased peripheral circulation, marked by cold, pale, or mottled extremities, decreased urine output, and significant changes in B/P or heart rate or a failure to respond to an increase or decrease in infusion rate.
• Taper off the dopamine dosage before discontinuing the drug because abrupt cessation of dopamine therapy may result in marked hypotension.

• Be alert to excessive vasoconstriction as evidenced by decreased urine output, a disproportionate increase in diastolic B/P, and increased arrhythmias or heart rate. Slow or temporarily stop the dopamine infusion and notify the physician if excessive vasoconstriction occurs.

Patient/Family Teaching

• Tell the patient/family to let you know if the patient develops pain or burning at the IV site.
• Urge your patient/family to let you know if the patient experiences chest pain or palpitations during the infusion.

Epinephrine

eh-pih-**nef**-rin
(Adrenalin, Adrenaline Injection [AUS], EpiPen, Primatene)
Do not confuse with ephedrine.

CATEGORY AND SCHEDULE

Pregnancy Risk Category: C

MECHANISM OF ACTION

A sympathomimetic agent and adrenergic agonist that stimulates alpha-adrenergic receptors causing vasoconstriction and pressor effects, $beta_1$-adrenergic receptors, resulting in cardiac stimulation, and $beta_2$-adrenergic receptors, resulting in bronchial dilation and vasodilation. ***Therapeutic Effect:*** Relaxes smooth muscle of the bronchial tree, produces cardiac stimulation, dilates skeletal muscle vasculature.
Ophthalmic: Increases outflow of aqueous humor from the anterior eye chamber. ***Therapeutic Effect:*** Dilates pupils and constricts conjunctival blood vessels.

PHARMACOKINETICS

Route	Onset	Peak	Duration
SC	5–10 min	20 min	1–4 hrs
IM	5–10 min	20 min	1–4 hrs
Inhalation	3–5 min	20 min	1–3 hrs
Ophthalmic	1 hr	4–8 hrs	12–24 hrs

Minimal absorption after inhalation, well absorbed after parenteral administration. Metabolized in liver, other tissues, sympathetic nerve endings. Crosses placenta but not blood brain barrier. Excreted in urine. Ophthalmic: May have systemic absorption from drainage into nasal pharyngeal passages. Mydriasis occurs within several minutes and persists for several hours; vasoconstriction occurs within 5 min and lasts less than 1 hr.

AVAILABILITY

Injection in Prefilled Injector: 0.3 mg/0.3 mL, 0.15 mg/0.3 mL.
Injection: 0.1 mg/mL, 1 mg/mL.
Solution for Oral Inhalation: 2.25%, 1.125%.
Ophthalmic Solution: 0.5%, 1%, 2%.

INDICATIONS AND DOSAGES

▸ **Asystole**

IV

Children. 0.01 mg/kg (0.1 mL/kg of 1:10,000 solution). May repeat q3–5min. Subsequent doses 0.1 mg/kg (0.1 mL/kg) of a 1:1000 solution q3–5min.

▸ **Bradycardia**

IV

Children. 0.01 mg/kg (0.1 mL/kg of 1:10,000 solution) q3–5min. Maximum: 1 mg/10 mL.
Neonates: 0.01–0.03 mg/kg (0.1–0.3 mL/kg of 1:10,000 solution) q3–5 min as needed.

▸ **Asthma/bronchodilator**
SC
Children. 10 mcg/kg (0.01 mL/kg of 1:1000) Maximum: 0.5 mg or suspension (1:200) 0.005 mL/kg/dose (0.025 mg/kg/dose) to a maximum of 0.15 mL (0.75 mg for single dose) q8–12h.
▸ **Hypersensitivity reaction**
SC
Children. 0.01 mg/kg q15min for 2 doses, then q4h. Maximum single dose: 0.5 mg.
NEBULIZER
Children older than 4 yrs. 1–3 deep inhalations (0.25–0.5 mL of 2.25% racemic epinephrine diluted in 3 mL of 0.9% NaCl or L-epinephrine at an equivalent dose (half of the racemic epinephrine dose) subsequent doses no sooner than 3 hrs.
OPHTHALMIC
Children and infants: Instill 1–2 drops in eye(s) 1–2 times daily.

UNLABELED USES

Systemic: Treatment of gingival or pulpal hemorrhage, priapism. Ophthalmic: Treatment of conjunctival congestion during surgery, secondary glaucoma.

CONTRAINDICATIONS

Hypersensitivity to epinephrine or any related component. Cardiac arrhythmias, cerebrovascular insufficiency, hypertension, hyperthyroidism, ischemic heart disease, narrow-angle glaucoma, shock.

INTERACTIONS

Drug

Beta-blockers: May decrease the effects of beta-blockers.
Digoxin, sympathomimetics: May increase risk of arrhythmias.
Ergonovine, methylergonovine, oxytocin: May increase vasoconstriction.
MAOIs, tricyclic antidepressants: May increase cardiovascular effects.

Herbal

None known.

Food

None known.

DIAGNOSTIC TEST EFFECTS

May decrease serum potassium levels.

IV INCOMPATIBILITIES

Ampicillin (Omnipen, Polycillin)

IV COMPATIBILITIES

Calcium chloride, calcium gluconate, diltiazem (Cardizem), dobutamine (Dobutrex), dopamine (Intropin), fentanyl (Sublimaze), heparin, hydromorphone (Dilaudid), lorazepam (Ativan), midazolam (Versed), milrinone (Primacor), morphine, nitroglycerin, norepinephrine (Levophed), potassium chloride, propofol (Diprivan)

SIDE EFFECTS

Frequent
Systemic: Tachycardia, palpitations, nervousness
Ophthalmic: Headache, stinging, burning or other eye irritation, watering of eyes
Occasional
Systemic: Dizziness, lightheadedness, facial flushing, headache, diaphoresis, increased B/P, nausea, trembling, insomnia, vomiting, weakness
Ophthalmic: Blurred or decreased vision, eye pain
Rare
Systemic: Chest discomfort/pain, arrhythmias, bronchospasm, dry mouth or throat

SERIOUS REACTIONS

! Excessive doses may cause acute hypertension or arrhythmias.

! Prolonged or excessive use may result in metabolic acidosis due to increased serum lactic acid concentrations.

! Observe for disorientation, weakness, hyperventilation, headache, nausea, vomiting, and diarrhea.

PEDIATRIC CONSIDERATIONS

Baseline Assessment

- Obtain baseline vital signs, especially heart rate and B/P.
- Obtain a baseline EKG to monitor for arrhythmias.
- Be aware that epinephrine crosses the placenta and is distributed in breast milk.
- Use cautiously in children who have diabetes, asthma, or hypertension.
- IV extravasation may occur with epinephrine so it is important to monitor the IV site continually.
- Do not administer IM injection into the buttock.
- Maintain and assess for age-appropriate fluid intake.
- For nebulization/inhalation, use a spacer in children younger than 8 years of age.
- There are no age-related precautions noted in children.

Precautions

- Use cautiously in pts with angina pectoris, diabetes mellitus, hypoxia, myocardial infarction, psychoneurotic disorders, tachycardia, and severe liver or renal impairment.

Administration and Handling

SC

- Shake ampule thoroughly.
- Use tuberculin syringe for SC injection into the lateral deltoid region.
- Massage injection site to minimize vasoconstriction effect.

IV

- Store parenteral forms at room temperature.
- Do not use if solution appears discolored or contains a precipitate.
- For injection, dilute each 1 mg of 1:1,000 solution with 10 mL 0.9% NaCl to provide 1:10,000 solution, and inject each 1 mg or fraction thereof over longer than 1 min.
- For infusion, further dilute with 250–500 mL D_5W. Maximum concentration is 64 mg/250 mL.
- For IV infusion, give at 1–10 mcg/min, and titrate to desired response.

Intervention and Evaluation

- Monitor the patient for changes in vital signs.
- Assess the patient's lung sounds for crackles, rhonchi, and wheezing.
- Monitor the patient's arterial blood gases.
- Monitor B/P, EKG, and pulse, especially in the patient who has had cardiac arrest.

Patient/Family Teaching

- Urge the patient/family to avoid consuming an excessive amount of caffeine derivatives such as chocolate, cocoa, coffee, cola, or tea.
- Explain to the patient/family receiving the ophthalmic solution that the patient will feel a slight burning or stinging when the drug is initially administered.
- Warn the patient/family receiving the ophthalmic solution to immediately report any new symptoms such as dizziness, shortness of breath, or tachycardia because they may be a sign of systemic absorption.

Norepinephrine Bitartrate

nor-eh-pih-**nef**-rin
(Levophed)
(See Color Plate)

CATEGORY AND SCHEDULE

Pregnancy Risk Category: C

MECHANISM OF ACTION

A sympathomimetic that stimulates $beta_1$-adrenergic receptors and alpha-adrenergic receptors, increasing peripheral resistance. ***Therapeutic Effect:*** Enhances contractile myocardial force, increases cardiac output. Constricts resistance and capacitance vessels. Increases systemic B/P and coronary blood flow.

PHARMACOKINETICS

Route	Onset	Peak	Duration
IV	Rapid	1–2 min	N/A

Localized in sympathetic tissue. Metabolized in liver. Primarily excreted in urine.

AVAILABILITY

Injection: 1 mg/mL ampules.

INDICATIONS AND DOSAGES

▸ Acute hypotension unresponsive to fluid volume replacement

IV

Children. Initially, 0.05–0.1 mcg/kg/min; titrate to desired effect. Maximum: 1–2 mcg/kg/min. Range: 0.5–3 mcg/min.

CONTRAINDICATIONS

Hypersensitivity to norepinephrine or any related component. Pts with sulfite sensitivity. Hypovolemic states (unless as an emergency measure), mesenteric or peripheral vascular thrombosis, profound hypoxia.

INTERACTIONS

Drug

Beta-blockers: May have mutually inhibitory effects.
Digoxin: May increase risk of arrhythmias.
Ergonovine, oxytocin: May increase vasoconstriction.
Maprotiline, tricyclic antidepressants: May increase cardiovascular effects.
Methyldopa: May decrease the effects of methyldopa.

Herbal

None known.

Food

None known.

DIAGNOSTIC TEST EFFECTS

None known.

IV INCOMPATIBILITIES

Alkaline solutions, regular insulin.

IV COMPATIBILITIES

Amiodarone (Cordarone), calcium gluconate, diltiazem (Cardizem), dobutamine (Dobutrex), dopamine (Intropin), epinephrine, esmolol (Brevibloc), fentanyl (Sublimaze), furosemide (Lasix), haloperidol (Haldol), heparin, hydromorphone (Dilaudid), labetalol (Trandate), lorazepam (Ativan), magnesium, midazolam (Versed), milrinone (Primacor), morphine, nicardipine (Cardene), nitroglycerin, potassium chloride, propofol (Diprivan)

SIDE EFFECTS

Norepinephrine produces less pronounced and less frequent side effects than epinephrine.

Occasional (5%–3%)
Anxiety, bradycardia, awareness of slow, forceful heartbeat

Rare (2%–1%)
Nausea, anginal pain, shortness of breath, fever

SERIOUS REACTIONS

! Extravasation may produce tissue necrosis and sloughing.
! Overdosage is manifested as severe hypertension with violent headache, which may be the first clinical sign of overdosage, arrhythmias, photophobia, retrosternal or pharyngeal pain, pallor, excessive sweating, and vomiting.
! Prolonged therapy may result in plasma volume depletion.
! Hypotension may recur if plasma volume is not restored.

PEDIATRIC CONSIDERATIONS

Baseline Assessment

- Assess the patient's B/P and EKG continuously. Be alert to precipitous drops in B/P.
- Do not leave the patient alone during a norepinephrine IV infusion.
- Be alert to any patient complaint of headache.
- Be aware that norepinephrine readily crosses the placenta. Know that norepinephrine may produce fetal anoxia as a result of constriction of uterine blood vessels and uterine contraction.
- Administer medication into a large vein to prevent extravasation.
- Assess for and maintain age-appropriate fluid intake.
- There are no age-related precautions noted in children.

Precautions

- Use cautiously in pts with hypertension, hypothyroidism, and severe cardiac disease.
- Use cautiously in pts receiving concurrent MAOI therapy.

Administration and Handling

◂ALERT▸ Expect to restore blood and fluid volume before administering norepinephrine.

IV

- Do not use if solution is brown or contains precipitate.
- Store ampules at room temperature.
- Do not administer drug without dilution. Add 4 mL (4 mg) to 250 mL (16 mcg/mL). Maximum: 32 mL (32 mg) to 250 mL (128 mcg/mL).
- If available, administer infusion through a central venous catheter to avoid extravasation.
- Closely monitor the IV infusion flow rate with a microdrip or infusion pump.
- Monitor the patient's B/P every 2 min during IV infusion until the desired therapeutic response is achieved, then every 5 min during remaining IV infusion.
- Never leave the patient unattended during IV infusion.
- Plan to maintain the patient's B/P at 80–100 mm Hg in previously normotensive pts, and 30–40 mm Hg below preexisting B/P in previously hypertensive pts.
- Reduce IV infusion gradually, as prescribed. Avoid abrupt withdrawal.
- Check the peripherally inserted catheter IV site frequently for blanching, coldness, and hardness, and pallor to extremity and signs of extravasation.

Intervention and Evaluation

- Monitor the patient's IV flow rate diligently.
- Assess the patient for extravasation characterized by blanching of skin over vein and mottling and coolness of the IV site extremity. If

extravasation occurs, expect to infiltrate the affected area with 10–15 mL sterile saline containing 5–10 mg phentolamine. Know that phentolamine does not alter the pressor effects of norepinephrine.

• Assess the patient's capillary refill and the strength of his or her peripheral pulses to monitor circulation.

• Monitor the patient's intake and output hourly, or as ordered. In pts with a urine output of less than 30 mL/hr, expect to stop the infusion unless the systolic B/P falls below 70–80 mm Hg.

Patient/Family Teaching

• Instruct the patient/family to notify the nurse on duty immediately if the patient experiences burning, pain, or coolness at the IV site.

• Instruct the patient/family that vital signs need to be monitored carefully.

• Instruct the patient/family that norepinephrine needs to be protected from light.

Phenylephrine Hydrochloride

fen-ill-**eh**-frin

(AK-Dilate, Isopto Frin [AUS], Neo-Synephrine, Prefrin)

CATEGORY AND SCHEDULE

Pregnancy Risk Category: C

OTC (nasal solution, nasal spray, ophthalmic solution)

MECHANISM OF ACTION

A sympathomimetic, alpha-receptor stimulant that acts on the alpha-adrenergic receptors of vascular smooth muscle.

Therapeutic Effect: Causes vasoconstriction of arterioles of nasal mucosa or conjunctiva, activates dilator muscle of the pupil to cause contraction, and produces systemic arterial vasoconstriction.

PHARMACOKINETICS

Route	Onset	Peak	Duration
SC	10–15 min	N/A	1 hr
IM	10–15 min	N/A	0.5–2 hrs
IV	Immediate	N/A	15–20 min

Minimal absorption after intranasal or ophthalmic administration. Metabolized in liver, and GI tract. Primarily excreted in urine.

Half-Life: 2.5 hrs.

AVAILABILITY

Injection: 1% (10 mg/mL).

Nasal Solution: 0.25%, 0.5%.

Nasal Spray: 0.25%, 0.5%, 1%.

Ophthalmic Solution: 0.12%, 2.5%, 10%.

INDICATIONS AND DOSAGES

▸ **Nasal decongestant**

INTRANASAL

Children older than 12 yrs. 2–3 drops, 1–2 sprays of 0.25%–0.5% solution into each nostril q4hrs. Do not use more than 3 days.

Children 6–12 yrs. 2–3 drops or 1–2 sprays of 0.25% solution in each nostril q4hrs. Do not use more than 3 days.

Children younger than 6 yrs. 2–3 drops of 0.125% solution in each nostril. Repeat q4h as needed. Do not use for more than 3 days.

▸ **Conjunctival congestion, itching, and minor irritation, whitening of sclera**

OPHTHALMIC

Children older than 12 yrs. 1 drop of 2.5% solution, may repeat in 10–60 min as needed.

Infants younger than 1 yr. 1 drop of 2.5% solution 15–30 before procedure.

▸ **Hypotension, shock**

IM/SC

Children. 0.1 mg/kg/dose q1–2h as needed. Maximum: 5 mg.

IV BOLUS

Children. 5–20 mcg/kg/dose q10–15min as needed.

IV INFUSION

Children. 0.1–0.5 mcg/kg/min. Titrate to desired effect.

CONTRAINDICATIONS

Hypersensitivity to phenylephrine or any related component. Acute pancreatitis, heart disease, hepatitis, narrow-angle glaucoma, pheochromocytoma, severe hypertension, thrombosis, ventricular tachycardia.

INTERACTIONS

Drug

Beta-blockers: May have mutually inhibitory effects with beta-blockers.

Digoxin: May increase risk of arrhythmias with digoxin.

Ergonovine, oxytocin: May increase vasoconstriction.

MAOIs: May increase vasopressor effects.

Maprotiline, tricyclic antidepressants: May increase cardiovascular effects.

Methyldopa: May decrease effects of methyldopa.

Herbal

None known.

Food

None known.

DIAGNOSTIC TEST EFFECTS

None known.

IV INCOMPATIBILITIES

Thiopental (Pentothal)

IV COMPATIBILITIES

Amiodarone (Cordarone), dobutamine (Dobutrex), lidocaine, potassium chloride, propofol (Diprivan)

SIDE EFFECTS

Frequent

Nasal: Rebound nasal congestion due to overuse, especially when used longer than 3 days

Occasional

Mild CNS stimulation, such as restlessness, nervousness, tremors, headache, insomnia, particularly in those hypersensitive to sympathomimetics

Nasal: Stinging, burning, drying of nasal mucosa

Ophthalmic: Transient burning or stinging, brow ache, blurred vision

SERIOUS REACTIONS

! Large doses may produce tachycardia, palpitations, particularly in those with cardiac disease, lightheadedness, nausea, and vomiting.

! Prolonged nasal use may produce chronic swelling of nasal mucosa and rhinitis.

PEDIATRIC CONSIDERATIONS

Baseline Assessment

- Be sure to obtain baseline vital signs, including apical heart rate and B/P.
- Check to see if the patient has irritation of the nasal mucosa before administering the nasal preparation.
- Be aware that phenylephrine crosses the placenta and is distributed in breast milk.
- Be aware that children may exhibit increased absorption and toxicity with the nasal preparation.
- Administer phenylephrine through a large vein to prevent extravasation.

• Know that there are no age-related precautions noted with systemic use in children.

Precautions

• Use cautiously in pts with bradycardia, heart block, hyperthyroidism, and severe arteriosclerosis.
• If phenylephrine 10% ophthalmic is instilled into denuded or damaged corneal epithelium, know that corneal clouding may result.

Administration and Handling

NASAL

• Instruct the patient to blow his or her nose before giving the medication. Tilt back the patient's head and instill nasal solution drops in one nostril, as prescribed. Have the patient remain in the same position and wait 5 min before applying drops in the other nostril.
• Administer nasal spray into each nostril with the patient's head erect. Instruct the patient to sniff briskly while squeezing the container, then wait 3–5 min before blowing the nose gently.
• Rinse tip of spray bottle.

OPHTHALMIC

• Instruct patient to tilt head backward and look up.
• With a gloved finger, gently pull the patient's lower eyelid down to form a pouch and instill medication.
• Do not touch tip of applicator to eyelids or any surface.
• When lower eyelid is released, have patient keep eye open without blinking for at least 30 sec.
• Apply gentle finger pressure to the lacrimal sac, which is located at the bridge of the nose, inside the corner of the eye, for 1–2 min.
• Remove excess solution around the eye with a tissue. Wash hands immediately to remove medication on hands.

IV

• Store vials at room temperature.
• For IV push, dilute 1 mL of 10 mg/mL solution with 9 mL Sterile Water for Injection to provide a concentration of 1 mg/mL. Give over 20–30 sec.
• For IV infusion, dilute 10-mg vial with 500 mL D_5W or 0.9% NaCl to provide a concentration of 2 mcg/mL. Maximum: 500 mg/250 mL. Titrate as prescribed.

Intervention and Evaluation

• Monitor the patient's blood pressure (B/P) and heart rate.

Patient/Family Teaching

• Tell the patient/family to discontinue the drug if adverse reactions occur.
• Instruct the patient/family not to use the drug for nasal decongestion longer than 3–5 days because of the risk of rebound congestion.
• Instruct the patient/family not to use the medication if the solution is brown or precipitates.
• Warn the patient/family to discontinue the drug if the patient experiences dizziness, a feeling of irregular heartbeat, insomnia, tremor, or weakness.
• Tell the patient/family of the common side effects with all preparations of the drug.
• Warn the patient/family to discontinue ophthalmic medication and notify the physician, if the patient experiences redness or swelling of eyelids or itching.

REFERENCES

Miller, S. & Fioravanti, J. (1997). Pediatric medications: a handbook for nurses. St. Louis: Mosby.
Taketomo, C. K., Hodding, J. H. & Kraus, D. M. (2003–2004). Pediatric dosage handbook (10th ed.). Hudson: OH: Lexi-Comp.

31 Miscellaneous Cardiovascular Agents

Alprostadil (Prostaglandin E_1, PGE_1)
Digoxin Immune FAB
Sodium Polystyrene Sulfonate

Uses: Several miscellaneous agents are used primarily for their cardiovascular therapeutic effects. *Alprostadil* is used to maintain patency of the ductus arteriosus until surgery can be performed; it is also used to treat erectile dysfunction. *Digoxin immune FAB* is used as an antidote for digoxin intoxication. *Sodium polystyrene sulfonate* is used to correct hyperkalemia, which can cause serious or life-threatening arrhythmias.

Action: Each of the cardiovascular agents in this section acts in a different way. As a prostaglandin, *alprostadil* directly affects vascular and ductus arteriosus smooth muscle and relaxes trabecular smooth muscle. *Digoxin immune FAB* binds with digoxin molecules, preventing them from binding at their sites of action. Because *sodium polystyrene sulfonate* is a cation exchange resin, it releases sodium ions in exchange primarily for potassium ions and promotes potassium excretion from the body; this action prevents serious complications, such as life-threatening arrhythmias.

Alprostadil (Prostaglandin E_1, PGE_1)

ale-**pros**-tah-dill
(Caverject, Edex, Muse, Prostin VR Pediatric)

CATEGORY AND SCHEDULE

Pregnancy Risk Category: X

MECHANISM OF ACTION

A prostaglandin that directly effects vascular and ductus arteriosus smooth muscle and relaxes trabecular smooth muscle.
Therapeutic Effect: Causes vasodilation; dilates cavernosal arteries, allowing blood flow to and entrapment in the lacunar spaces of the penis.

PHARMACOKINETICS

Metabolized by oxidation in the lungs to an active metabolite. Eliminated in the urine. ***Half-Life:*** 5–10 min.

AVAILABILITY

Injection (Prostin VR Pediatric): 500 mcg/mL.
Powder for Injection: 10 mcg, 20 mcg, 40 mcg. NOTE: This is used only for impotence!
Urethral Pellet (Muse): 125 mcg, 250 mcg, 500 mcg, 1,000 mcg. NOTE: This is used only for impotence!

INDICATIONS AND DOSAGES

▸ **Maintain patency of ductus arteriosus**

IV

Neonates. Initially, 0.05–0.1 mcg/kg/min. After a therapeutic response is achieved, use the lowest dosage to maintain response. Maximum: 0.4 mcg/kg/min.

UNLABELED USES

Treatment of atherosclerosis, gangrene, pain due to severe peripheral arterial occlusive disease.

CONTRAINDICATIONS

Hypersensitivity to alprostadil or any related component. Persistent fetal circulation. Conditions predisposing to anatomic deformation of penis, hyaline membrane disease, penile implants, priapism, respiratory distress syndrome.

INTERACTIONS

Drug

Anticoagulants, including heparin, thrombolytics: May increase risk of bleeding.
Sympathomimetics: May decrease effect of alprostadil.
Vasodilators: May increase risk of hypotension.

Herbal

None known.

Food

None known.

DIAGNOSTIC TEST EFFECTS

May increase blood bilirubin levels. May decrease glucose, serum calcium, and serum potassium levels.

IV INCOMPATIBILITIES

No information available via Y-site administration.

SIDE EFFECTS

Frequent

Systemic (greater than 1%): Fever, seizures, flushing, bradycardia, hypotension, tachycardia, apnea, diarrhea, sepsis

Occasional

Systemic (less than 1%): Jitteriness, lethargy, stiffness, arrhythmias, respiratory depression, anemia, bleeding, thrombocytopenia, hematuria

SERIOUS REACTIONS

! Overdosage occurs and is manifested as apnea, flushing of the face and arms, and bradycardia.
! Cardiac arrest and sepsis occur rarely.

PEDIATRIC CONSIDERATIONS

Precautions

• Use cautiously in pts with coagulation defects, leukemia, multiple myeloma, polycythemia, severe liver disease, sickle cell disease, or thrombocythemia.
• Monitor vital signs closely when administering alprostadil.
• Therapeutic response is indicated by an increase in systemic blood pressure and pH in those with restricted systemic blood flow and acidosis.
• Some bone changes can occur. These changes are usually seen 4–6 wks after starting therapy, but have occurred as early as 9 days. These effects usually resolve over 6–12 mo after stopping therapy.

Administration and Handling

◀ **ALERT** ▶ Doses greater than 40 mcg (Edex) or 60 mcg (Caverject) are not recommended.

URETHRAL PELLET

• Refrigerate pellet unless used within 14 days.

IV

◀ **ALERT** ▶ Give by continuous IV infusion or through an umbilical artery catheter placed at the ductal opening.

• Store the parenteral form in the refrigerator.
• Dilute drug before administration. Prepare a fresh dose every 24 hrs and discard unused portions.
• Prepare a continuous IV infusion by diluting 1 mL of alprostadil, containing 500 mcg, with D_5W or 0.9% NaCl to yield a solution containing 2–20 mcg/mL. Diluting volumes can range from 25 mL to 250 mL, depending on the patient and the available infusion device.
• Infuse the lowest possible dose over the shortest possible time.
• Decrease the infusion rate immediately if a significant decrease in arterial pressure is noted via auscultation, Doppler transducer, or umbilical artery catheter.
• Discontinue the infusion immediately if signs and symptoms of overdosage, such as apnea or bradycardia, occur.

Intervention and Evaluation
• For pts with patent ductus arteriosus, monitor arterial pressure by auscultation, Doppler transducer, or umbilical artery catheter. Decrease the infusion rate immediately if a significant decrease in arterial pressure occurs. Expect to maintain continuous cardiac monitoring. Also, frequently assess the patient's heart sounds, femoral pulse (to monitor lower extremity circulation), and respiratory status.
• For pts with patent ductus arteriosus, monitor the patient for signs and symptoms of hypotension, assess blood pressure, arterial blood gas values, and temperature. If apnea or bradycardia occurs, discontinue the infusion immediately and notify the physician.

Patient/Family Teaching
• For the patient/family with patent ductus arteriosus, explain to the patient's parents the purpose of this palliative therapy.

Digoxin Immune FAB

(Digibind, DigiFab)

CATEGORY AND SCHEDULE
Pregnancy Risk Category: C

MECHANISM OF ACTION

An antidote that binds molecularly to digoxin in the extracellular space. ***Therapeutic Effect:*** Makes digoxin unavailable for binding at its site of action on cells in the body.

PHARMACOKINETICS

Route	Onset	Peak	Duration
IV	30 min	N/A	3–4 days

Widely distributed into the extracellular space. Excreted in urine. ***Half-Life:*** 15–20 hrs. Renal impairment prolongs half-life.

AVAILABILITY

Powder for Injection: 38-mg vial (Digibind), 40 mg vial (DigiFab).

INDICATIONS AND DOSAGES

▸ Treatment of potentially life-threatening digoxin overdose
Dosage varies according to amount of digoxin to be neutralized. Refer to manufacturer's dosing guidelines.
Children. Initially determine total body digoxin load (TBL):

TBL (mg) = serum digoxin level (ng/mL) × 5.6 × wt (kg) ÷ 1,000.

After determining this equation then calculate dose of digoxin immune FAB. Dose of Digibind (mg): TBL × 76. Dose of DigiFab (mg): TBL × 80. Infuse dose over 15–30 min.

CONTRAINDICATIONS

Hypersensitivity to digoxin immune FABa, ovine (sheep) proteins. Hypersensitivity to papain, chymopapain, papaya extracts, or bromelain (DigiFab only).

INTERACTIONS

Drug
None known.
Herbal
None known.
Food
None known.

DIAGNOSTIC TEST EFFECTS

May alter serum potassium levels. Serum digoxin concentration may increase precipitously and persist for up to 1 wk until the FAB–digoxin complex is eliminated from the body.

IV INCOMPATIBILITIES

None known.

SIDE EFFECTS

None known

SERIOUS REACTIONS

! As a result of digitalis toxicity, hyperkalemia may occur. Look for signs of diarrhea, paresthesia of extremities, heaviness of legs, decreased blood pressure (B/P), cold skin, grayish pallor, hypotension, mental confusion, irritability, flaccid paralysis, tented T waves, widening QRS complex, and ST depression.

! When the effect of digitalis is reversed, hypokalemia may develop rapidly. Look for muscle cramping, nausea, vomiting, hypoactive bowel sounds, abdominal distention, difficulty breathing, and postural hypotension.

! Rarely, low cardiac output and CHF may occur.

PEDIATRIC CONSIDERATIONS

Baseline Assessment

- Obtain the patient's serum digoxin level before administering the drug. If blood for the serum digoxin level was drawn less than 6 hrs before the last digoxin dose, the serum digoxin level may be unreliable.
- Know that those with impaired renal function may require longer than 1 wk before the serum digoxin assay is reliable.
- Assess the patient's mental status and muscle strength.
- Be aware that it is unknown whether digoxin immune FAB crosses the placenta or is distributed in breast milk.
- There are no age-related precautions noted in children.
- Each vial of Digibind or DigiFab will bind approximately 0.5 mg digoxin.

Precautions

- Use cautiously in pts with impaired cardiac or renal function.

Administration and Handling

IV

- Refrigerate vials.
- After reconstitution, solution is stable for 4 hrs if refrigerated.
- Use immediately after reconstitution.

- Reconstitute each 38-mg vial with 4 mL Sterile Water for Injection to provide a concentration of 9.5 mg/mL.
- Further dilute with 50 mL 0.9% NaCl.
- Infuse over 30 min. It is recommended that the solution be infused through a 0.22-μfilter.
- If cardiac arrest is imminent, may give IV push.

Intervention and Evaluation

- Closely monitor the patient's B/P, EKG, serum potassium level, and temperature during and after the drug is administered.
- Observe the patient for changes from the initial assessment. Hypokalemia may result in cardiac arrhythmias, changes in mental status, muscle cramps, muscle strength changes, or tremor. Hyponatremia may result in cold and clammy skin, confusion, and thirst.
- Assess for signs and symptoms of an arrhythmia, such as palpitations, or heart failure, such as dyspnea and edema, if the digoxin level falls below the therapeutic level.

Patient/Family Teaching

- Before discharge, review the digoxin dosages carefully with the patient/family, and make sure the patient knows how to take the drug as prescribed.
- Instruct the patient/family about any follow-up care, including serum digoxin levels.
- Make sure the patient/family knows the signs and symptoms of digoxin toxicity, including anorexia, nausea, and vomiting, as well as visual changes.

Sodium Polystyrene Sulfonate

(Kayexalate, Resonium A [AUS], SPS)

CATEGORY AND SCHEDULE

Pregnancy Risk Category: C

MECHANISM OF ACTION

An ion exchange resin that releases sodium ions in exchange primarily for potassium ions. ***Therapeutic Effect:*** Removes potassium from the blood and into the intestine so it can be expelled from the body.

AVAILABILITY

Suspension: 15 g/60 mL.
Powder for Suspension: 454 g, 480 g.

INDICATIONS AND DOSAGES

▸ Hyperkalemia

PO
Children. 1 g/kg/dose q6h.
RECTAL
Children. 1 g/kg/dose q2–6h.

CONTRAINDICATIONS

Hypersensitivity to sodium polystyrene sulfonate or any related component. Hypernatremia, intestinal obstruction, or perforation.

INTERACTIONS

Drug

Cation-donating antacids, laxatives (e.g., magnesium hydroxide): May decrease effect of sodium polystyrene sulfonate, and cause systemic alkalosis in pts with renal impairment.

Herbal

None known.

Food

None known.

DIAGNOSTIC TEST EFFECTS

May decrease serum calcium and magnesium levels.

SIDE EFFECTS

Frequent

High dosage: Anorexia, nausea, vomiting, constipation

Occasional

Diarrhea, sodium retention, marked by decreased urination, peripheral edema, and increased weight

SERIOUS REACTIONS

! Serious potassium deficiency may occur. Early signs of hypokalemia include confusion, delayed thought processes, extreme weakness, irritability, and EKG changes, including a prolonged QT interval, widening, flattening, or inversion of T waves, and prominent U waves.

! Hypocalcemia, manifested by abdominal or muscle cramps, occurs occasionally.

! Arrhythmias and severe muscle weakness may be noted.

PEDIATRIC CONSIDERATIONS

Baseline Assessment

- Keep in mind that sodium polystyrene sulfonate does not rapidly correct severe hyperkalemia; it may take hours to days. Consider other measures, such as dialysis, IV glucose and insulin, IV calcium, and IV sodium bicarbonate to correct severe hyperkalemia in a medical emergency.
- Be aware that it is unknown whether sodium polystyrene sulfonate crosses the placenta or is distributed in breast milk.
- Know that there are no age-related precautions noted in children.

Precautions

- Use cautiously in pts with edema, renal insufficiency, hypertension, and severe CHF.

Administration and Handling

PO

- Give with 20–100 mL sorbitol to aid in potassium removal, facilitate passage of resin through intestinal tract, and prevent constipation.
- Do not mix this drug with foods or liquids containing potassium.

RECTAL

- After an initial cleansing enema, insert a large rubber tube well into the sigmoid colon and tape in place.
- Introduce suspension with 100 mL sorbitol by gravity.
- Flush with 50 to 100 mL fluid and clamp.
- Retain for several hours, if possible.
- Irrigate colon with a non–sodium-containing solution to remove resin.

Intervention and Evaluation

- Monitor the patient's potassium levels frequently.
- Assess the patient's clinical condition and EKG, which is valuable in determining when treatment should be discontinued.
- In addition to checking serum potassium levels, monitor serum calcium and magnesium levels.
- Assess the patient's pattern of daily bowel activity and stool consistency. Remember that fecal impaction may occur in pts receiving high dosages of sodium polystyrene sulfonate.

Patient/Family Teaching

- Instruct the patient/family to drink the entire amount of the resin for best results.
- Explain to the patient/family that if the resin is given rectally, the patient should try to avoid

expelling the solution and try to retain the solution for several hours, if possible.

• Instruct the patient/family about which foods are rich in potassium. Plan to consult a dietician to provide dietary counseling.

REFERENCES

Miller, S. & Fioravanti, J. (1997). Pediatric medications: a handbook for nurses. St. Louis: Mosby.

Taketomo, C. K., Hodding, J. H. & Kraus, D. M. (2003–2004). Pediatric dosage handbook (10th ed.). Hudson, OH: Lexi-Comp.

32 Antianxiety Agents

Buspirone Hydrochloride
Chlordiazepoxide
Clorazepate Dipotassium
Diazepam
Doxepin Hydrochloride
Hydroxyzine
Lorazepam
Midazolam Hydrochloride

Uses: Antianxiety agents are used to treat anxiety. In addition, some benzodiazepines are used as hypnotics to induce sleep, as anticonvulsants to prevent delirium tremors during alcohol withdrawal, and as adjunctive therapy for relaxation of skeletal muscle spasms. Midazolam, a short-acting benzodiazepine, is used for preoperative sedation and relief of anxiety in short diagnostic endoscopic procedures.

Action: Although the exact mechanism of action is unknown, antianxiety agents may increase the inhibiting effect of γ-aminobutyric acid (GABA), an inhibitory neurotransmitter. Benzodiazepines, the largest and most frequently prescribed group of antianxiety agents, may inhibit nerve impulse transmission by binding to specific benzodiazepine receptors in various areas of the CNS. (See illustration, *Mechanism of Action: Benzodiazepines,* page 404.)

COMBINATION PRODUCTS

LIBRAX: chlordiazepoxide/clidinium (an anticholinergic) 5 mg/2.5 mg.
LIMBITROL: chlordiazepoxide/amitriptyline (an antidepressant) 5 mg/12.5 mg; 10 mg/25 mg.

Buspirone Hydrochloride

byew-spear-own
(BuSpar, Buspirex [CAN], Bustab [CAN])
Do not confuse with bupropion.

CATEGORY AND SCHEDULE

Pregnancy Risk Category: B

MECHANISM OF ACTION

Although the exact mechanism of action is unknown, this nonbarbiturate is thought to bind to serotonin and dopamine receptors in the CNS. The drug may also increase norepinephrine metabolism in the locus ceruleus. ***Therapeutic Effect:*** Produces antianxiety effect.

PHARMACOKINETICS

Rapidly, completely absorbed from the GI tract. Protein binding: 95%. Undergoes extensive first-pass metabolism. Metabolized in liver to the active metabolite. Primarily excreted in urine. Not removed by hemodialysis. ***Half-Life:*** 2–3 hrs. Extended with hepatic or renal impairment.

AVAILABILITY

Tablets: 5 mg, 7.5 mg, 10 mg, 15 mg, 30 mg.

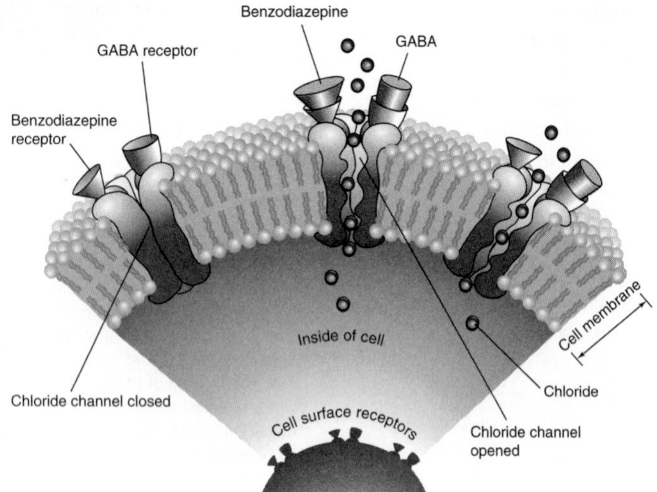

Mechanism of Action: Benzodiazepines

Benzodiazepines reduce anxiety by stimulating the action of the inhibitory neurotransmitter, γ-aminobutyric acid (GABA), in the limbic system. The limbic system plays an important role in the regulation of human behavior. Dysfunction of GABA neurotransmission in the limbic system may be linked to the development of certain anxiety disorders.

The limbic system contains a highly dense area of benzodiazepine receptors that may be linked to the antianxiety effects of benzodiazepines. These benzodiazepine receptors are located on the surface of neuronal cell membranes and are adjacent to receptors for GABA. The binding of a benzodiazepine to its receptor enhances the affinity of a GABA receptor for GABA. In the absence of a benzodiazepine, the binding of GABA to its receptor causes the chloride channel in the cell membrane to open, which increases the influx of chloride into the cell. This influx of chloride results in hyperpolarization of the neuronal cell membrane and reduces the neuron's ability to fire, which is why GABA is considered an inhibitory neurotransmitter. A benzodiazepine acts only in the presence of GABA and when it binds to a benzodiazepine receptor, the time the chloride channel remains open is prolonged. This results in greater depression of neuronal function and a reduction in anxiety.

INDICATIONS AND DOSAGES

▸ **Short-term management, up to 4 wks of anxiety disorders**

PO

Children. Initially, 5 mg/day. May increase by 5 mg/day at weekly intervals. Maximum: 60 mg/day.

UNLABELED USES

Management of panic attack, symptoms of premenstrual syndrome, including aches, pain, fatigue, irritability.

CONTRAINDICATIONS

Hypersensitivity to buspirone or any related component. MAOI therapy, severe liver or renal impairment.

INTERACTIONS

Drug

Alcohol, CNS depressants: May increase sedation.
Erythromycin, itraconazole: May increase buspirone blood concentration and risk of toxicity.
MAOIs: May increase blood pressure.

Herbal

Kava kava: May increase sedation.

Food

Grapefruit and grapefruit juice: May increase buspirone blood concentration and risk of toxicity.

DIAGNOSTIC TEST EFFECTS

None known.

SIDE EFFECTS

Frequent (12%–6%)
Dizziness, drowsiness, nausea, headache
Occasional (5%–2%)
Nervousness, fatigue, insomnia, dry mouth, lightheadedness, mood swings, blurred vision, poor concentration, diarrhea, numbness in hands and feet
Rare
Muscle pain and stiffness, nightmares, chest pain, involuntary movements

SERIOUS REACTIONS

! There is no evidence of tolerance or psychological and physical dependence or withdrawal syndrome.
! Overdosage may produce severe nausea, vomiting, dizziness, drowsiness, abdominal distention, and excessive pupil contraction.

PEDIATRIC CONSIDERATIONS

Baseline Assessment

- Offer emotional support to the anxious patient.
- Assess the patient's autonomic responses, such as cold, clammy hands; sweating, and motor responses, including agitation, trembling, and tension.
- Be aware that it is unknown whether buspirone crosses the placenta or is distributed in breast milk.
- Be aware that the safety and efficacy of buspirone have not been established in children, and it should not be used on an as-needed basis.

Precautions

- Use cautiously in pts with liver or renal impairment.

Administration and Handling

PO
- Give buspirone without regard to meals.
- Crush tablets as needed.

Intervention and Evaluation

- Plan to perform blood tests periodically to assess hepatic and renal function in pts receiving long-term therapy.
- Assist the patient with ambulation if he or she experiences drowsiness or lightheadedness.
- Evaluate the patient for a therapeutic response, including a calm facial expression and decreased restlessness and insomnia.

Patient/Family Teaching

- Explain to the patient/family that improvement may be noted in 7–10 days, but the optimum therapeutic effect generally takes 3–4 wks to appear.
- Tell the patient/family that drowsiness usually disappears during continued therapy.
- Instruct the patient/family to change position slowly from a

recumbent to a sitting position before standing to avoid dizziness.
• Warn the patient/family to avoid tasks that require mental alertness and motor skills until the patient's response to buspirone is established.
• Caution the patient/family not to take the drug with grapefruit juice. Explain that grapefruit may increase carbamazepine absorption and blood concentration.

Chlordiazepoxide

klor-dye-az-eh-**pox**-eyd
(Apo-Chlordiazepoxide [CAN], Libritabs, Librium, Lipoxide, Novopoxide [CAN])

CATEGORY AND SCHEDULE

Pregnancy Risk Category: D

MECHANISM OF ACTION

A benzodiazepine that enhances the action of GABA neurotransmission in the CNS. ***Therapeutic Effect:*** Produces anxiolytic effect.

AVAILABILITY

Capsules: 5 mg, 10 mg, 25 mg.
Injection: 100 mg (diluent provided).

INDICATIONS AND DOSAGES

▸ **Mild anxiety**

PO

Children older than 6 yrs. 5 mg 2–4 times daily. Maximum: 10 mg 2–3 times a day.

▸ **Severe anxiety**

IM/IV

Adolescent. 50–100 mg initially, followed by 25–50 mg 3–4 times a day or as needed. Maximum: 300 mg/day.

UNLABELED USES

Treatment of panic disorder, tension headache, tremors, and treatment of irritable bowel syndrome.

CONTRAINDICATIONS

Hypersensitivity to chlordiazepoxide or any related component. Acute alcohol intoxication, acute narrow-angle glaucoma. Should not be used in children younger than 6 mo of age.

INTERACTIONS

Drug

Alcohol, CNS depressants: May increase CNS depressant effect.

Herbal

Kava kava, valerian: May increase CNS depression.

Food

None known.

DIAGNOSTIC TEST EFFECTS

None known. Therapeutic serum level is 1–3 mcg/mL; toxic serum level is greater than 5 mcg/mL.

SIDE EFFECTS

Frequent

Pain with IM injection; drowsiness, ataxia, dizziness, confusion with oral dose, particularly in debilitated pts.

Occasional

Rash, peripheral edema, GI disturbances

Rare

Paradoxical CNS hyperactivity or nervousness in children (generally noted during first 2 wks of therapy, particularly noted in presence of uncontrolled pain)

SERIOUS REACTIONS

! IV route may produce pain, swelling, thrombophlebitis, and carpal tunnel syndrome.

! Abrupt or too rapid withdrawal may result in pronounced restlessness, irritability, insomnia, hand tremors, abdominal or muscle cramps, sweating, vomiting, and seizures.
! Overdosage results in somnolence, confusion, diminished reflexes, and coma.

PEDIATRIC CONSIDERATIONS

Baseline Assessment
• Assess the patient's blood pressure (B/P), pulse, and respirations immediately before giving chlordiazepoxide.
• Expect the patient to remain recumbent for up to 3 hrs after parenteral administration to reduce the hypotensive effect of the drug.
• Oral dosing is not recommended in children younger than 6 yrs of age.
• Injection is not recommended in children younger than 12 yrs of age.
• Children may be particularly sensitive to chlordiazepoxide, so use the smallest dosage possible.

Precautions
• Use cautiously in pts with impaired liver or kidney function.

Administration and Handling
◂ **ALERT** ▸ Expect to use the smallest effective chlordiazepoxide dosage in debilitated pts and pts with liver disease or low serum albumin.

Intervention and Evaluation
• Assess the patient's autonomic responses, such as cold or clammy hands, sweating, and motor responses, including agitation, trembling, and tension.
• Examine pediatric pts for a paradoxical reaction, particularly during early therapy.
• Assist the patient with ambulation if he or she experiences ataxia or drowsiness.
• Know that the therapeutic serum level for chlordiazepoxide is 1–3 mcg/mL, and the toxic serum level of chlordiazepoxide is greater than 5 mcg/mL.

Patient/Family Teaching
• Tell the patient/family that the patient may experience discomfort with IM injection.
• Explain to the patient/family that drowsiness usually disappears during continued therapy.
• Instruct the patient/family to change positions slowly from a recumbent to a sitting position before standing if the patient experiences dizziness.
• Urge the patient/family to stop smoking tobacco products. Explain to the patient that smoking reduces the drug's effectiveness.
• Warn the patient/family to avoid alcohol consumption while taking this drug.
• Caution the patient/family not to abruptly discontinue the medication after long-term therapy.

Clorazepate Dipotassium

klor-**az**-eh-payt
(Novoclopate [CAN], Tranxene)
Do not confuse with clofibrate.

CATEGORY AND SCHEDULE

Pregnancy Risk Category: D

MECHANISM OF ACTION

A benzodiazepine that depresses all levels of the CNS, including limbic and reticular formation, by binding to benzodiazepine site on the GABA receptor complex.

Modulates GABA, which is a major inhibitory neurotransmitter in the brain. ***Therapeutic Effect:*** Produces anxiolytic effect, suppresses seizure activity.

AVAILABILITY

Tablets: 3.75 mg, 7.5 mg, 15 mg. *Tablets (extended release):* 11.5 mg, 22.5 mg.

INDICATIONS AND DOSAGES

▸ Partial seizures

PO

Children older than 12 yrs. Initially, up to 7.5 mg 3 times/day. Do not increase dosage more than 7.5 mg/wk or exceed 90 mg/day.

Children 9–12 yrs. 3.75–7.5 mg/dose 2 times/day. Maximum: 60 mg/day in 2–3 divided doses.

CONTRAINDICATIONS

Hypersensitivity to clorazepate or any related component. Preexisting CNS depression, severe uncontrolled pain, acute narrow-angle glaucoma.

INTERACTIONS

Drug

Alcohol, CNS depressants: May increase CNS depressant effect.

Cimetidine: May decrease hepatic clearance.

Herbal

Kava kava, valerian: May increase CNS depression.

Food

None known.

DIAGNOSTIC TEST EFFECTS

None known. Peak therapeutic serum level is 0.12–1.5 mcg/mL; toxic serum level is greater than 5 mcg/mL.

SIDE EFFECTS

Frequent

Drowsiness

Occasional

Dizziness, GI disturbances, nervousness, blurred vision, dry mouth, headache, confusion, ataxia, rash, irritability, slurred speech

Rare

Paradoxical CNS hyperactivity or nervousness in children, excitement or restlessness in debilitated pts. Symptoms are generally noted during the first 2 wks of therapy, particularly in the presence of uncontrolled pain.

SERIOUS REACTIONS

! Abrupt or too rapid withdrawal may result in pronounced restlessness, irritability, insomnia, hand tremors, abdominal or muscle cramps, sweating, vomiting, and seizures.

! Overdosage results in somnolence, confusion, diminished reflexes, and coma.

PEDIATRIC CONSIDERATIONS

Baseline Assessment

- In the seizure patient, review the patient's history of seizure disorder, including the duration, intensity, frequency, and his or her level of consciousness.
- Observe the patient frequently for recurrence of seizure activity. Initiate seizure precautions.
- Use cautiously in children with asthma and depression.

Precautions

- Use cautiously in pts with acute alcohol intoxication and impaired liver or renal function.

Administration and Handling

◂ ALERT ▸ When replacement by another anticonvulsant is necessary, plan to decrease clorazepate gradually as therapy begins with low-replacement dosage.

Intervention and Evaluation

- Assess the patient for a paradoxical reaction, particularly during early therapy.
- Assist the patient with ambulation if he or she experiences dizziness and drowsiness.
- Evaluate the patient for a therapeutic response. In pts with seizure disorder, the therapeutic response is a decrease in intensity or frequency of seizures.
- Monitor the patient's serum level of the drug. Peak therapeutic serum level is 0.12–1.5 mcg/mL; toxic serum level is greater than 5 mcg/mL.

Patient/Family Teaching

- Caution the patient/family against abruptly withdrawing the medication after long-term use because this may precipitate seizures.
- Explain to the patient/family that strict maintenance of drug therapy is essential for seizure control.
- Tell the patient/family that drowsiness usually disappears during continued therapy.
- Warn the patient/family to avoid tasks that require mental alertness or motor skills until the patient's response to the drug is established.
- Instruct the patient/family to change positions slowly from a recumbent to a sitting position before standing, if the patient experiences dizziness.
- Urge the patient/family to stop smoking tobacco products and to avoid alcohol during clorazepate therapy. Explain to the patient that smoking reduces the drug's effectiveness.

Diazepam

dye-**az**-eh-pam
(Antenex [AUS], Apo-Diazepam [CAN], Diastat, Diazemuls [CAN], Dizac, Ducene [AUS], Valium, Valpam [AUS], Vivol [CAN])
Do not confuse with diazoxide, Ditropan, or Valcyte.

CATEGORY AND SCHEDULE

Pregnancy Risk Category: D
Controlled Substance: Schedule IV

MECHANISM OF ACTION

A benzodiazepine that depresses all levels of the CNS by binding to the benzodiazepine receptor on the GABA receptor complex, a major inhibitory neurotransmitter in the brain. ***Therapeutic Effect:*** Produces anxiolytic effect, elevates seizure threshold, produces skeletal muscle relaxation.

PHARMACOKINETICS

Route	Onset	Peak	Duration
PO	30 min	1–2 hrs	2–3 hrs
IM	15 min	30–90 min	30–90 min
IV	1–5 min	15 min	15–60 min

Well absorbed from the GI tract, including rectally. Widely distributed. Protein binding: 84%–98%. Metabolized in liver to active metabolite. Excreted in urine. Minimally removed by hemodialysis. ***Half-Life:*** Neonates: 50–95 hrs. Infants: 40–50 hrs. Children: 15–20 hrs. Adults: 20–70 hrs. Half-life is increased in elderly, liver dysfunction.

AVAILABILITY

Tablets: 2 mg, 5 mg, 10 mg.
Capsules (sustained release): 15 mg (not available in USA).
Oral Solution: 5 mg/5 mL.
Injection: 5 mg/mL.
Injectable Emulsion: 5 mg/mL (not available in USA).
Rectal Gel: 2.5 mg, 5 mg, 10 mg, 15 mg, 20 mg.

INDICATIONS AND DOSAGES

▸ **Anxiety, skeletal muscle relaxant**

PO

Children. 0.12–0.8 mg/kg/day in divided doses q6–8h.

IM/IV

Children. 0.04–0.3 mg/kg/dose q2–4h. Maximum: 0.6 mg/kg in an 8-hr period.

▸ **Preanesthesia**

IV

Children. 0.2–0.3 mg/kg 45–60 min before procedure. Maximum: 10 mg.

▸ **Status epilepticus**

IV

Children 5 yrs and older. 0.05–0.3 mg/kg/dose over 3–5 min q15–30min. Maximum: 10 mg.
Children older than 1 mo–younger than 5 yrs. 0.05–0.3 mg/kg/dose over 3–5 min q15–30min. Maximum: 5 mg.

▸ **Control of increased seizure activity in refractory epilepsy in those receiving stable medication regimens**

RECTAL GEL

Children 12 yrs and older. 0.2 mg/kg.
Children 6–11 yrs. 0.3 mg/kg.
Children 2–5 yrs. 0.5 mg/kg. Dose may be repeated in 4–12 hrs.

UNLABELED USES

Treatment of panic disorders, tension headache, tremors

CONTRAINDICATIONS

Hypersensitivity to diazepam or any related component. Comatose patient, narrow-angle glaucoma, preexisting CNS depression, respiratory depression, severe uncontrolled pain.

INTERACTIONS

Drug

Alcohol, CNS depressants: May increase CNS depressant effect.
Cimetidine, erythromycin: May decrease metabolism of diazepam, lessening effects.
Valproic acid: May increase sedative effects.

Herbal

Kava kava, valerian: May increase CNS depressant effects.

Food

Grapefruit juice: Increases amount of diazepam absorbed orally, leading to increase risk of toxicity.

DIAGNOSTIC TEST EFFECTS

May produce abnormal renal function tests and elevate serum lactate dehydrogenase, serum alkaline phosphatase, serum bilirubin, SGOT (AST), and SGPT (ALT) levels. Therapeutic serum level is 0.5–2 mcg/mL; toxic serum level is greater than 3 mcg/mL.

IV INCOMPATIBILITIES

Amphotericin B complex (AmBisome, Amphotec, Abelcet), cefepime (Maxipime), diltiazem (Cardizem), fluconazole (Diflucan), foscarnet (Foscavir), heparin, hydrocortisone (Solu-Cortef), hydromorphone (Dilaudid), meropenem (Merrem IV), potassium chloride, propofol (Diprivan), vitamins

IV COMPATIBILITIES

Dobutamine (Dobutrex), fentanyl, morphine

SIDE EFFECTS

Frequent

Pain with IM injection, drowsiness, fatigue, ataxia or muscular incoordination

Occasional

Slurred speech, orthostatic hypotension, headache, hypoactivity, constipation, nausea, blurred vision

Rare

Paradoxical CNS hyperactivity or nervousness in children, excitement or restlessness in debilitated pts, generally noted during the first 2 wks of therapy, particularly noted in the presence of uncontrolled pain

SERIOUS REACTIONS

! IV route may produce pain, swelling, thrombophlebitis, and carpal tunnel syndrome.

! Abrupt or too rapid withdrawal may result in pronounced restlessness, irritability, insomnia, hand tremors, abdominal or muscle cramps, diaphoresis, vomiting, and seizures.

! Abrupt withdrawal in pts with epilepsy may produce an increase in the frequency or severity of seizures.

! Overdosage results in somnolence, confusion, diminished reflexes, CNS depression, and coma.

PEDIATRIC CONSIDERATIONS

Baseline Assessment

- Assess the patient's blood pressure (B/P), pulse, and respirations immediately before giving diazepam.
- Know that the patient must remain recumbent for up to 3 hrs after parenteral administration to reduce the hypotensive effect of the drug.
- Assess autonomic response, including cold, clammy hands, sweating, and motor response, such as agitation, trembling, and tension for antianxiety pts.
- For pts with musculoskeletal spasm, record the duration, location, onset, and type of pain.
- Check the patient for immobility, stiffness, and swelling.
- Review the history of the seizure disorder, including duration, frequency, intensity, and length, as well as the patient's level of consciousness in pts with seizure disorder.
- Observe the patient frequently for recurrence of seizure activity, and initiate seizure precautions.
- Be aware that diazepam crosses the placenta and is distributed in breast milk. Diazepam may increase the risk of fetal abnormalities if administered during the first trimester of pregnancy.
- Chronic diazepam ingestion during pregnancy may produce withdrawal symptoms and CNS depression in neonates.
- Plan to use small initial doses with gradual increases to avoid ataxia or excessive sedation in children.
- Do not use the PO form in children less than 6 mos of age.
- Use the smallest PO dose available in children because they are more sensitive to benzodiazepines.

Precautions

- Use cautiously in pts with hypoalbuminemia or liver or renal impairment and in those who are taking other CNS depressants.

Administration and Handling

RECTAL

◂**ALERT**▸ Do not administer more than 5 times/mo or more than once every 5 days.

PO

• Give diazepam without regard to meals.
• Dilute oral concentrate with carbonated beverages, juice, or water; it may also be mixed in semisolid food, such as applesauce or pudding.
• Crush tablets as needed.
• Do not crush or break capsules.

IM

• Injection may be painful. Give IM injection deeply into the deltoid muscle.

IV

Store at room temperature. Give by IV push into tubing of a flowing IV solution as close to the vein insertion point as possible.

• Administer directly into a large vein to reduce the risk of phlebitis and thrombosis. Do not use in small veins, such as those in the wrist or dorsum of the hand.
• Administer IV at a rate not exceeding 5 mg/min. For children, give over a 3-min period; a too rapid IV infusion may result in hypotension or respiratory depression.
• Monitor respirations every 5–15 min for 2 hrs.

Intervention and Evaluation

• Monitor the patient's B/P, heart rate, and respiratory rate.
• Assess pediatric pts for a paradoxical reaction, particularly during early therapy.
• Evaluate the patient for a therapeutic response. In pts with seizure disorder, the therapeutic response is a decrease in the frequency or intensity of seizures. In antianxiety pts, the therapeutic response is a calm facial expression, decreased intensity of skeletal muscle pain, and decreased restlessness.
• Know that the therapeutic serum level for diazepam is 0.5–2 mcg/mL, and the toxic serum level for diazepam is greater than 3 mcg/mL.

Patient/Family Teaching

• Urge the patient/family to avoid consuming alcohol and to limit the patient's caffeine intake during diazepam therapy.
• Tell the patient/family that diazepam may cause drowsiness and impair the patient's ability to perform activities requiring mental alertness or motor skills.
• Explain to the patient/family that diazepam may be habit forming.
• Warn the patient/family to avoid abruptly discontinuing the drug after prolonged use.
• Tell the patient/family not to take the rectal form of the drug more than 5 times/mo or more than once every 5 days.

Doxepin Hydrochloride

dox-eh-pin

(Deptran [AUS], Novo-Doxepin [CAN], Prudoxin, Sinequan, Zonalon)

Do not confuse with doxapram, doxazosin, Doxidan, or saquinavir.

CATEGORY AND SCHEDULE

Pregnancy Risk Category: C (B for topical preparation)

MECHANISM OF ACTION

A tricyclic antidepressant, antianxiety, antineuralgic, antiulcer, and antipruritic agent that increases synaptic concentrations of norepinephrine and serotonin. ***Therapeutic Effect:*** Produces antidepressant and anxiolytic effect.

PHARMACOKINETICS

Rapidly well absorbed from the GI tract. Protein binding: 80%–85%. Metabolized in liver to the active metabolite. Primarily excreted in urine. Not removed by hemodialysis. ***Half-Life:*** Adult: 6–8 hrs.
Topical: Absorbed through skin, distributed to body tissues, metabolized to active metabolite, eliminated renally.

AVAILABILITY

Capsules: 10 mg, 25 mg, 50 mg, 75 mg, 100 mg, 150 mg.
Oral Concentrate: 10 mg/mL.
Cream: 5%.

INDICATIONS AND DOSAGES

▸ Depression, anxiety

PO
Adolescents. Initially, 25–50 mg/day as single or divided doses. May increase to 100 mg/day.
Children younger than 12 yrs. 1–3 mg/kg/day as single or divided doses.

UNLABELED USES

Treatment of neurogenic pain, panic disorder, prophylaxis for vascular headache, pruritus in idiopathic urticaria.

CONTRAINDICATIONS

Hypersensitivity to other tricyclic antidepressants, narrow-angle glaucoma, urinary retention.

INTERACTIONS

Drug

Alcohol, CNS depressants: May increase CNS and respiratory depression and have hypotensive effects.
Antithyroid agents: May increase risk of agranulocytosis.
Cimetidine: May increase doxepin blood concentration and risk of toxicity.
Clonidine, guanadrel: May decrease the effects of clonidine and guanadrel.
MAOIs: May increase the risk of hypertensive crisis, hyperthermia, and seizures.
Phenothiazines: May increase anticholinergic, sedative effects.
Sympathomimetics: May increase cardiac effects with sympathomimetics.

Herbal

None known.

Food

Fiber-rich foods: May decrease doxepin effects.
Carbonated beverages, grape juice: Oral solution is physically incompatible. Do not mix.

DIAGNOSTIC TEST EFFECTS

May alter EKG readings and blood glucose levels. Therapeutic serum level is 110–250 ng/mL; toxic serum level is greater than 300 ng/mL.

SIDE EFFECTS

Frequent
PO: Orthostatic hypotension, drowsiness, dry mouth, headache, increased appetite or weight, nausea, unusual tiredness, unpleasant taste
Occasional
PO: Blurred vision, confusion, constipation, hallucinations, difficult urination, eye pain, irregular heartbeat, fine muscle tremors, nervousness, impaired sexual function, diarrhea, increased sweating, heartburn, insomnia

Rare
Allergic reaction, alopecia, tinnitus, breast enlargement

SERIOUS REACTIONS

! High dosage may produce confusion, seizures, severe drowsiness, arrhythmias, fever, hallucinations, agitation, shortness of breath, vomiting, and unusual tiredness or weakness.

! Abrupt withdrawal from prolonged therapy may produce headache, malaise, nausea, vomiting, and vivid dreams.

PEDIATRIC CONSIDERATIONS

Baseline Assessment
- Assess the patient's blood pressure (B/P) and pulse.
- Assess EKGs in pts with a history of cardiovascular disease.
- Be aware that doxepin crosses the placenta and is distributed in breast milk.
- Be aware that the safety and efficacy of doxepin have not been established in children.

Precautions
- Use cautiously in pts with cardiac disease, diabetes mellitus, glaucoma, hiatal hernia, a history of seizures, a history of urinary obstruction or retention, hyperthyroidism, increased intraocular pressure, liver disease, prostatic hypertrophy, renal disease, and schizophrenia.

Administration and Handling
PO
- Give doxepin with food or milk if GI distress occurs.
- Dilute concentrate in 8-oz glass of grapefruit, orange, pineapple, prune, or tomato juice, milk, or water. Avoid carbonated drinks and grape juice because they are incompatible with the drug.

Intervention and Evaluation
- Monitor the patient's B/P, pulse, and weight.
- Closely supervise suicidal-risk pts during early therapy. As depression lessens, be aware that the patient's energy level generally improves, which increases the suicide potential. Assess the patient's appearance, behavior, level of interest, mood, and speech pattern.
- Monitor the patient's serum drug level. The therapeutic serum level for doxepin is 110–250 ng/mL, and the toxic serum level for doxepin is greater than 300 ng/mL.

Patient/Family Teaching
- Tell the patient/family that doxepin may cause drowsiness and dry mouth.
- Warn the patient/family to avoid tasks requiring mental alertness or motor skills until the patient's response to the drug is established.
- Urge the patient/family to avoid alcohol and limit the patient's caffeine intake while taking doxepin because these items may increase his or her appetite.
- Stress to the patient/family that the patient should avoid exposure to sunlight or artificial light sources while receiving doxepin therapy.
- Explain to the patient/family that the therapeutic effect of doxepin may be noted within 2–5 days with the maximum effect appearing within 2–3 wks.

Hydroxyzine

high-**drox**-ih-zeen
(Apo-Hydroxyzine [CAN], Atarax, Novohydroxyzin [CAN], Vistarile)
Do not confuse with hydralazine or hydroxyurea.

CATEGORY AND SCHEDULE

Pregnancy Risk Category: C

MECHANISM OF ACTION

A piperazine derivative that competes with histamine for receptor sites in the GI tract, blood vessels, and respiratory tract. Diminishes vestibular stimulation, depresses labyrinthine function. ***Therapeutic Effect:*** Produces anticholinergic, antihistaminic, and analgesic effect; relaxes skeletal muscle. Controls nausea and vomiting.

PHARMACOKINETICS

Route	Onset	Peak	Duration
PO	15–30 min	N/A	4–6 hrs

Well absorbed from the GI tract, parenteral administration. Metabolized in liver. Primarily excreted in urine. Not removed by hemodialysis. ***Half-Life:*** 20–25 hrs. Half-life is increased in elderly pts.

AVAILABILITY

Tablets: 10 mg, 25 mg, 50 mg, 100 mg.
Capsules: 25 mg, 50 mg, 100 mg.
Oral Suspension: 25 mg/5 mL.
Oral Syrup: 10 mg/5 mL.
Injection: 25 mg/mL, 50 mg/mL.

INDICATIONS AND DOSAGES

▸ Usual pediatric dosage

IM

Children. 0.5–1 mg/kg/dose q4–6h as needed.

PO

Children. 2 mg/kg/day in divided doses q6–8h.

CONTRAINDICATIONS

Hypersensitivity to hydroxyzine or any related component.

INTERACTIONS

Drug

Alcohol, CNS depressants: May increase CNS depressant effects.

MAOIs: May increase anticholinergic and CNS depressant effects.

Herbal

None known.

Food

None known.

DIAGNOSTIC TEST EFFECTS

May cause false-positive results with urine 17-hydroxycorticosteroid determinations.

SIDE EFFECTS

Side effects are generally mild and transient.

Frequent

Drowsiness, dry mouth, marked discomfort with IM injection

Occasional

Dizziness, ataxia or muscular incoordination, weakness, slurred speech, headache, agitation, increased anxiety

Rare

Paradoxical CNS hyperactivity or nervousness in children, excitement or restlessness in debilitated pts that is generally noted during the first 2 wks of therapy, particularly in the presence of uncontrolled pain

SERIOUS REACTIONS

! Hypersensitivity reaction, including wheezing, dyspnea, and chest tightness, may occur.

PEDIATRIC CONSIDERATIONS

Baseline Assessment

- Assess the patient for signs and symptoms of dehydration, including dry mucous membranes, longitudinal furrows in the tongue, and poor skin turgor, if he or she experiences excessive vomiting.
- Be aware that it is unknown whether hydroxyzine crosses the

placenta or is distributed in breast milk.
• Keep in mind that hydroxyzine use is not recommended in newborns and premature infants because of an increased risk of anticholinergic effects.
• Be aware that hydroxyzine injection and syrup may contain benzyl alcohol, large amounts of which may lead to fatal toxicity in neonates.
• Be aware that paradoxical excitement may occur in pediatric pts.
• Use cautiously in children with uncontrollable seizures.

Precautions
• Use cautiously in pts with asthma and bladder neck obstruction.

Administration and Handling
PO
• Shake oral suspension thoroughly.
• Crush scored tablets as needed, but do not crush or break capsules.
IM
◂ ALERT ▸ Do not give drug by the SC, intra-arterial, or IV route because it can cause significant tissue damage, thrombosis, and gangrene.
• Give drug undiluted IM.
• Give IM injection deeply into the gluteus maximus or the midlateral thigh in adults or the midlateral thigh in children. Use the Z-track technique of injection to prevent subcutaneous infiltration.

Intervention and Evaluation
• Plan to perform complete blood counts and blood serum chemistry tests periodically for pts receiving long-term therapy.
• Monitor the patient's lung sounds for signs of a hypersensitivity reaction, such as wheezing.
• Monitor serum electrolytes in pts with severe vomiting.
• Assess the patient for a paradoxical reaction, particularly during early therapy.
• Assist the patient with ambulation if he or she experiences drowsiness or lightheadedness.

Patient/Family Teaching
• Tell the patient/family that marked discomfort may occur with IM injection.
• Recommend taking sips of tepid water and chewing sugarless gum to help relieve dry mouth.
• Tell the patient/family that drowsiness usually diminishes with continued therapy.
• Warn the patient/family to avoid tasks that require mental alertness and motor skills until the patient's response to the drug is established.

Lorazepam

low-**raz**-ah-pam
(Apo-Lorazepam [CAN], Ativan, Novolorazepam [CAN])
Do not confuse with alprazolam.

CATEGORY AND SCHEDULE
Pregnancy Risk Category: D
Controlled Substance: Schedule IV

MECHANISM OF ACTION
A benzodiazepine that enhances the inhibitory neurotransmitter GABA neurotransmission at the CNS, affecting memory, motor, sensory, and cognitive functions. ***Therapeutic Effect:*** Produces anxiolytic, muscle relaxation, anticonvulsant, sedative, and antiemetic effect.

PHARMACOKINETICS

Route	Onset	Peak	Duration
PO	60 min	N/A	8–12 hrs
IM	30–60 min	N/A	8–12 hrs
IV	15–30 min	N/A	8–12 hrs

Well absorbed after PO and IM administration. Protein binding: 85%. Widely distributed. Metabolized in liver. Primarily excreted in urine. Not removed by hemodialysis. ***Half-Life:*** Neonates: 18–73 hrs. Children: 7–17 hrs. Adults: 10–20 hrs.

AVAILABILITY

Tablets: 0.5 mg, 1 mg, 2 mg.
Injection: 2 mg/mL, 4 mg/mL.

INDICATIONS AND DOSAGES

▸ Anxiety

PO/IV

Infants and children. 0.05 mg/kg/dose every 4–8 hrs. Maximum dose: 2 mg/dose. Range: 0.02–0.1 mg/kg.

▸ Status epilepticus

IV

Adolescents. 0.07 mg/kg over 2–5 min. Maximum: 4 mg/dose. May repeat second dose in 10–15 min.

Children. 0.1 mg/kg over 2–5 min. Maximum: 4 mg/dose. May repeat second dose of 0.05 mg/kg in 15–20 min.

Neonate. 0.05 mg/kg over 2–5 min. May repeat in 10–15 min.

UNLABELED USES

Treatment of alcohol withdrawal, adjunct to endoscopic procedures—helps to diminish patient recall, panic disorders, skeletal muscle spasms, cancer chemotherapy-induced nausea or vomiting, tension headache, tremors.

CONTRAINDICATIONS

Hypersensitivity to lorazepam or any related component. Preexisting CNS depression, narrow-angle glaucoma, severe hypotension, severe uncontrolled pain.

INTERACTIONS

Drug

Alcohol, CNS depressants: May increase CNS depressant effect.

Herbal

Kava kava, valerian: May increase CNS depression.

Food

None known.

DIAGNOSTIC TEST EFFECTS

None known. Therapeutic serum level is 50–240 ng/mL; toxic serum level is unknown.

IV INCOMPATIBILITIES

Aldesleukin (Proleukin), aztreonam (Azactam), idarubicin (Idamycin), ondansetron (Zofran), sufentanil (Sufenta)

IV COMPATIBILITIES

Bumetanide (Bumex), cefepime (Maxipime), diltiazem (Cardizem), dobutamine (Dobutrex), dopamine (Intropin), heparin, labetalol (Normodyne, Trandate), milrinone (Primacor), norepinephrine (Levophed), piperacillin/tazobactam (Zosyn), potassium, propofol (Diprivan)

SIDE EFFECTS

Frequent

Drowsiness, ataxia or incoordination, confusion. Morning drowsiness may occur initially.

Occasional

Blurred vision, slurred speech, hypotension, headache

Rare
Paradoxical CNS restlessness, excitement in debilitated pts

SERIOUS REACTIONS

! Abrupt or too rapid withdrawal may result in pronounced restlessness, irritability, insomnia, hand tremors, abdominal or muscle cramps, diaphoresis, vomiting, and seizures.
! Overdosage results in somnolence, confusion, diminished reflexes, and coma.

PEDIATRIC CONSIDERATIONS

Baseline Assessment

- Offer emotional support to the anxious patient.
- Know that the patient must remain recumbent for up to 8 hrs after parenteral administration to reduce the hypotensive effect of the drug.
- Assess the patient's autonomic responses, including cold and clammy hands and diaphoresis and motor responses, such as agitation, trembling, tension.
- Be aware that lorazepam may cross the placenta and be distributed in breast milk.
- Lorazepam may increase the risk of fetal abnormalities if administered during the first trimester of pregnancy.
- Chronic lorazepam ingestion during pregnancy may produce CNS depression in neonates, fetal toxicity, and withdrawal symptoms.
- Be aware that the safety and efficacy of this drug have not been established in children younger than 12 yrs of age.
- Injectable solutions may have benzyl alcohol, which has been linked to fatal gasping in neonates.

Precautions

- Use cautiously in neonates and pts with concomitant CNS depressant use, compromised pulmonary function, and liver or renal impairment.

Administration/Handling

PO

- Give with food.
- Crush tablets, as needed.

IM

- Give IM injection deeply into a large muscle mass, such as the gluteus maximus.

IV

- Refrigerate parenteral form, but avoid freezing.
- Do not use if precipitate forms, or solution appears discolored.
- Dilute with an equal volume of Sterile Water for Injection, 0.9% NaCl, or D_5W. To dilute a prefilled syringe, remove air from the half-filled syringe, aspirate an equal volume of diluent, pull the plunger back slightly to allow for mixing, and gently invert the syringe several times, but do not shake vigorously.
- Give by IV push into tubing of free-flowing IV infusion (0.9% NaCl or D_5W) at a rate not to exceed 2 mg/min.

Intervention and Evaluation

- Monitor the patient's blood pressure, complete blood count, and blood serum chemistry tests to assess heart rate, liver and renal function, and respiratory rate, especially during long-term therapy.
- Assess the patient for a paradoxical reaction, particularly during early therapy.
- Evaluate the patient for a therapeutic response, manifested by a calm facial expression and decreased restlessness and insomnia.

• Monitor the patient's drug serum levels. The therapeutic blood serum level for lorazepam is 50–240 ng/mL, and the toxic blood serum level of lorazepam is unknown.

Patient/Family Teaching

• Tell the patient/family that drowsiness usually disappears during continued therapy.
• Warn the patient/family to avoid tasks that require mental alertness or motor skills until the patient's response to the drug is established.
• Urge the patient/family to stop smoking tobacco products and to avoid alcohol and other CNS depressants. Explain to the patient/family that smoking reduces the effectiveness of lorazepam.
• Caution the patient/family against abruptly withdrawing the medication after long-term therapy.
• Stress to the patient/family that contraception is recommended for pts receiving long-term therapy. Teach the patient about various methods of contraception.
• Warn the patient/family to notify the physician immediately if pregnancy is suspected.

Midazolam Hydrochloride

my-**day**-zoe-lam
(Hypnovel [AUS], Versed)
Do not confuse with VePesid.

CATEGORY AND SCHEDULE

Pregnancy Risk Category: D
Controlled substance: Schedule IV

MECHANISM OF ACTION

A benzodiazepine that enhances the action of the inhibitory neurotransmitter GABA, one of the major inhibitory transmitters in the brain. ***Therapeutic Effect:*** Produces anxiolytic, hypnotic, anticonvulsant, muscle relaxant, and amnestic effect.

PHARMACOKINETICS

Route	Onset	Peak	Duration
PO	10–20 min	N/A	N/A
IM	5–15 min	15–60 min	2–6 hrs
IV	1–5 min	5–7 min	20–30 min

Well absorbed after IM, PO, or intranasal administration. Protein binding: 97%. Metabolized in liver to the active metabolite. Primarily excreted in urine. Not removed by hemodialysis. ***Half-Life:*** 1–5 hrs. Increased half-life in CHF, cirrhosis, obesity, and acute renal failure and in elderly pts.

AVAILABILITY

Injection: 1 mg/mL, 5 mg/mL.
Syrup: 2 mg/mL.

INDICATIONS AND DOSAGES

▸ **Preop sedation**

IM

Children. 0.1–0.15 mg/kg 30–60 min before surgery. Maximum: 10 mg.

IV

Children older than 12 yrs: 1–5 mg; titrate to desired effect. Do not give more than 2.5 mg over a period of 2 min.

Children 6–12 yrs. 0.025–0.05 mg/kg. Maximum: 10 mg.

Children 6 mos–5 yrs. 0.05–0.1 mg/kg. Maximum: 6 mg.

PO

Children. 0.25–0.5 mg/kg. Maximum: 20 mg.

INTRANASAL

Children: 0.2 mg/kg, may repeat in 5–15 min. Range: 0.2–0.3 mg/kg/dose.

▸ **Conscious sedation during mechanical ventilation**
IV
Children older than 32 wks. Initially, 1–2 mcg/kg/min as continuous infusion. Titrate to desired effect.
Children 32 wks and younger. Initially, 0.5 mcg/kg/min as continuous infusion. Titrate to desired effect.
▸ **Status epilepticus**
IV
Children older than 2 mos. Loading dose of 0.15 mg/kg followed by continuous infusion of 1 mcg/kg/min. Titrate. Range: 1–18 mcg/kg/min.

CONTRAINDICATIONS
Hypersensitivity to midazolam or any related component. Acute alcohol intoxication, acute narrow-angle glaucoma, coma, shock.

INTERACTIONS
Drug
Alcohol, CNS depressants: May increase CNS and respiratory depression and hypotensive effects of midazolam.
Hypotension-producing medications: May increase hypotensive effects of midazolam.
Herbal
Kava kava, valerian: May increase CNS depression.
St. John's wort: May decrease serum concentrations of oral midazolam.
Food
Grapefruit juice: Increases oral absorption.

DIAGNOSTIC TEST EFFECTS
None known.

IV INCOMPATIBILITIES
Albumin, ampicillin/sulbactam (Unasyn), amphotericin B complex (Abelcet, AmBisome, Amphotec), ampicillin (Polycillin), bumetanide (Bumex), dexamethasone (Decadron), fosphenytoin (Cerebyx), furosemide (Lasix), hydrocortisone (Solu-Cortef), methotrexate, nafcillin (Nafcil), sodium bicarbonate, sodium pentothal (thiopental), sulfamethoxazole-trimethoprim (Bactrim)

IV COMPATIBILITIES
Amiodarone (Cordarone), calcium gluconate, diltiazem (Cardizem), dobutamine (Dobutrex), dopamine (Intropin), etomidate (Amidate), fentanyl (Sublimaze), heparin, hydromorphone (Dilaudid), insulin, lorazepam (Ativan), milrinone (Primacor), morphine, nitroglycerin, norepinephrine (Levophed), potassium chloride, propofol (Diprivan)

SIDE EFFECTS
Frequent (10%–4%)
Decreased respiratory rate, tenderness at IM/IV injection site, pain during injection, desaturation, hiccups
Occasional (3%–2%)
Pain at IM injection site, hypotension, paradoxical reaction
Rare (less than 2%)
Nausea, vomiting, headache, coughing, hypotensive episodes

SERIOUS REACTIONS
! Too much or too little dosage or improper administration may result in cerebral hypoxia, agitation, involuntary movements, hyperactivity, and combativeness.
! Underventilation or apnea may produce hypoxia and cardiac arrest.
! A too-rapid IV rate, excessive doses, or a single large dose

increases the risk of respiratory depression or arrest.

PEDIATRIC CONSIDERATIONS

Baseline Assessment

- Ensure that resuscitative equipment, such as endotracheal tubes, suction, and O_2 are readily available.
- Obtain the patient's vital signs before drug administration.
- Be aware that midazolam crosses the placenta, and it is unknown whether midazolam is distributed in breast milk.
- Know that neonates are more likely to experience respiratory depression.

Precautions

- Use cautiously in pts with acute illness, CHF, liver impairment, pulmonary impairment, renal impairment, severe fluid and electrolyte imbalance, and treated open-angle glaucoma.

Administration and Handling

◂ **ALERT** ▸ Plan to individualize midazolam dosage based on the patient's age, underlying disease, medications, and desired effect.

IM

Give IM injection deeply into a large muscle mass, such as the gluteus maximus.

IV

Store vials at room temperature.

- May give undiluted or as infusion.
- Make sure resuscitative equipment, such as O_2 is readily available before IV infusion is administered.
- Administer by slow IV injection, in incremental dosages. Give each incremental dose over at least 2 min and at intervals of at least 2 min apart.
- Reduce IV infusion rate in pts older than 60 years of age who are debilitated or have chronic diseases and impaired pulmonary function.
- A too rapid IV infusion rate, excessive doses, or a single large dose increases the risk of respiratory depression or arrest.

Intervention and Evaluation

- Monitor the patient's respiratory rate and oxygen saturation continuously during parenteral administration for apnea and underventilation.
- Monitor the patient's level of sedation every 3–5 min and vital signs during the recovery period.

Patient/Family Teaching

- When giving before a procedure, let the patient/family know that the drug produces an amnesic effect.

REFERENCES

Miller, S. & Fioravanti, J. (1997). Pediatric medications: a handbook for nurses. St. Louis: Mosby.

Taketomo, C. K., Hodding, J. H. & Kraus, D. M. (2003–2004). Pediatric dosage handbook (10th ed.). Hudson, OH: Lexi-Comp.

33 Anticonvulsants

Carbamazepine
Clonazepam
Gabapentin
Lamotrigine
Oxcarbazepine
Phenobarbital
Phenytoin, Phenytoin Sodium
Primidone
Tiagabine
Topiramate
Valproic Acid, Valproate Sodium, Divalproex Sodium
Zonisamide

Uses: Anticonvulsants are used to treat seizure disorders. Seizures can be divided into two broad categories: partial seizures and generalized seizures. Partial seizures begin focally in the cerebral cortex and spread to limited areas. Simple partial seizures do not involve loss of consciousness (unless they evolve into generalized seizures) and typically last less than 1 min. Complex partial seizures involve an alteration in consciousness and usually last longer than 1 min. Generalized seizures may be convulsive or nonconvulsive and usually produce immediate loss of consciousness.

Action: Anticonvulsants can prevent or reduce excessive discharge by neurons with seizure foci or decrease the spread of excitation from seizure foci to normal neurons. Although their exact mechanism is unknown, these agents may act by suppressing sodium influx, suppressing calcium influx, or increasing the action of γ-aminobutyric acid (GABA), which inhibits neurotransmitters in the brain.

COMBINATION PRODUCTS

BELLERGAL-S: phenobarbital/ergotamine (an antimigraine)/belladonna (an anticholinergic) 40 mg/0.6 mg/0.2 mg.
DILANTIN WITH PB: phenytoin/phenobarbital (an anticonvulsant) 100 mg/15 mg; 100 mg/30 mg.

Carbamazepine

car-bah-**may**-zeh-peen
(Apo-Carbamazepine [CAN], Carbatrol, Epitol, Tegretol, Tegretol CR [CAN], Tegretol XR, Teril [AUS])
Do not confuse with Toradol or Trental.

CATEGORY AND SCHEDULE

Pregnancy Risk Category: D

MECHANISM OF ACTION

An iminostilbene derivative that decreases sodium and calcium ion influx into neuronal membranes, reducing posttetanic potentiation at synapse. ***Therapeutic Effect:*** Produces anticonvulsant effect.

PHARMACOKINETICS

Slowly, completely absorbed from the GI tract. Protein binding: 75%. Metabolized in liver to the active metabolite. Primarily excreted in urine. Not removed by hemodialysis. ***Half-Life:*** Initially 25–65 hrs, with chronic dosing 8–17 hrs; half-life is decreased with chronic use.

AVAILABILITY

Capsules (controlled release): 100 mg (Carbatrol), 200 mg (Carbatrol), 300 mg (Carbatrol).

Suspension: 100 mg/5 mL.
Tablets (chewable): 100 mg.
Tablets: 200 mg.
Tablets (controlled release): 100 mg, 200 mg, 400 mg.

INDICATIONS AND DOSAGES

▸ Seizure control

PO

Children older than 12 yrs. Initially, 200 mg 2 times/day. Increase dosage up to 200 mg/day at weekly intervals until response is attained. Maintenance: 800–1,200 mg/day. Do not exceed 1,000 mg/day in children 12–15 yrs, 1,200 mg/day in pts older than 15 yrs.

Children 6–12 yrs. Initially, 100 mg 2 times/day. Increase by 100 mg/day at weekly intervals until response is attained. Maintenance: 400–800 mg/day. Give dosages of 200 mg/day or more in 3–4 equally divided doses. Maximum: 1000 mg/day.

SUSPENSION

Children 6–12 yrs. Initially, 50 mg 4 times/day. Increase dosage slowly at weekly intervals (reduces sedation risk).

Children younger than 6 yrs. 10–20 mg/kg/day in 2–4 divided doses. Increase dosage weekly to optimal response and therapeutic levels. Maximum: 35 mg/kg/day.

UNLABELED USES

Treatment of alcohol withdrawal, bipolar disorder, diabetes insipidus, neurogenic pain, psychotic disorders.

CONTRAINDICATIONS

Hypersensitivity to carbamazepine or to any related component. Concomitant use of MAOIs, history of bone marrow depression, history of hypersensitivity to tricyclic antidepressants.

INTERACTIONS

Drug

Anticoagulants, steroids: May decrease the effects of anticoagulants and steroids.

Anticonvulsants, barbiturates, benzodiazepines, valproic acid: May increase the metabolism of anticonvulsants, barbiturates, benzodiazepines, and valproic acid.

Antipsychotics, haloperidol, tricyclic antidepressants: May increase CNS depressant effects.

Cimetidine: May increase carbamazepine blood concentration and risk of toxicity.

Clarithromycin, diltiazem, erythromycin, estrogens, propoxyphene, quinidine: May decrease the effects of clarithromycin, diltiazem, erythromycin, estrogens, propoxyphene, and quinidine.

Isoniazid: May increase metabolism of this drug, carbamazepine blood concentration, and risk of toxicity.

MAOIs: May cause convulsions and hypertensive crises.

Verapamil: May increase the toxicity of carbamazepine.

Herbal

None known.

Food

Grapefruit: May increase the absorption and blood concentration of carbamazepine.

DIAGNOSTIC TEST EFFECTS

May increase BUN, blood glucose, cholesterol, high-density lipoprotein, protein, serum alkaline phosphatase, bilirubin, SGOT (AST), SGPT (ALT), and triglyceride levels. May decrease serum calcium, triiodothyronine, and thyroxine levels and the thyroxine index. Therapeutic serum level is 4–12 mcg/mL; toxic serum level is greater than 12 mcg/mL. May produce false-positive serum tricyclic antidepressant assay.

SIDE EFFECTS

Frequent
Drowsiness, dizziness, nausea, vomiting

Occasional
Visual abnormalities, such as spots before eyes, difficulty focusing, blurred vision, dry mouth or pharynx, tongue irritation, headache, water retention, increased sweating, constipation or diarrhea

SERIOUS REACTIONS

! Toxic reactions appear as blood dyscrasias, including aplastic anemia, agranulocytosis, thrombocytopenia, leukopenia, leukocytosis, eosinophilia, cardiovascular disturbances, such as congestive heart failure, hypotension or hypertension, thrombophlebitis, arrhythmias, and dermatologic effects, such as rash, urticaria, pruritus, and photosensitivity.

! Abrupt withdrawal may precipitate status epilepticus.

PEDIATRIC CONSIDERATIONS

Baseline Assessment

- Review the history of the seizure disorder, including the duration, frequency, and intensity, of seizures, as well as the patient's level of consciousness. Initiate seizure precautions.
- Provide the patient with a quiet, dark environment and safety precautions.
- Expect to perform a complete blood count, BUN and serum iron determination, and urinalysis before beginning carbamazepine therapy and periodically during therapy.
- Be aware that carbamazepine crosses the placenta and is distributed in breast milk. Carbamazepine accumulates in fetal tissue.
- Know that behavioral changes are more likely to occur in pediatric pts taking carbamazepine.
- Be aware that higher peak serum concentrations have been seen with the suspension versus the tablet forms of carbamazepine.

Precautions

- Use cautiously in pts with impaired cardiac, liver, or renal function.

Administration and Handling

◂ALERT▸ When replacement by another anticonvulsant is necessary, plan to decrease carbamazepine gradually as therapy begins with a low replacement dose. When transferring from tablets to suspension, expect to divide the total tablet daily dose into smaller, more frequent doses of suspension. Also plan to administer extended-release tablets in 2 divided doses.

PO

- Store oral suspension and tablets at room temperature.
- Give with meals to reduce risk of GI distress.
- Shake oral suspension well. Do not administer simultaneously with other liquid medicine.
- Do not crush extended-release tablets.

Intervention and Evaluation

- Observe the seizure patient frequently for recurrence of seizure activity.
- Monitor the patient for therapeutic serum levels.

• Assess the seizure patient for clinical improvement, manifested by a decrease in the frequency and intensity of seizures.
• Assess the patient for clinical evidence of early toxic signs, such as easy bruising, fever, joint pain, mouth ulcerations, sore throat, and unusual bleeding.
• Avoid cold food or liquids, draft, hot food or liquids, jarring bed, talking, warm food or liquids, and washing the face in pts with neuralgia because it could trigger tic douloureux.
• Know that the therapeutic serum level for carbamazepine in neuralgia pts is 4–12 mcg/mL and the toxic serum level for carbamazepine in neuralgia pts is greater than 12 mcg/mL.

Patient/Family Teaching

• Caution the patient/family against abruptly withdrawing the medication after long-term use because this may precipitate seizures.
• Stress to the patient/family that strict maintenance of drug therapy is essential for seizure control.
• Tell the patient/family that drowsiness usually disappears during continued therapy.
• Warn the patient/family to avoid tasks that require mental alertness and motor skills until the patient's response to the drug is established.
• Instruct the patient/family to notify the physician if the patient experiences visual abnormalities.
• Explain to the patient/family that blood tests should be repeated frequently during the first 3 mos of therapy and at monthly intervals thereafter for 2–3 yrs.
• Teach the patient/family not to take the oral suspension of carbamazepine simultaneously with other liquid medicine.
• Caution the patient/family not to take the drug with grapefruit juice. Explain that grapefruit may increase carbamazepine absorption and blood concentration.
• Carbamazepine may cause photosensitivity reactions so it is best for the patient to use broad-spectrum sunscreens and wear protective clothing if exposure to sun is necessary.

Clonazepam

klon-**nah**-zih-pam
(Apo-Clonazepam [CAN], Clonapam [CAN], Klonopin, Paxam [AUS], Rivotril [CAN])
Do not confuse with clonidine or lorazepam.

CATEGORY AND SCHEDULE

Pregnancy Risk Category: D

MECHANISM OF ACTION

A benzodiazepine that depresses all levels of the CNS. Depresses nerve transmission in the motor cortex. ***Therapeutic Effect:*** Suppresses abnormal discharge in petite mal seizures. Produces anxiolytic effect.

PHARMACOKINETICS

Well absorbed from the GI tract. Protein binding: 85%. Metabolized in liver. Excreted in urine. Not removed by hemodialysis.
Half-Life: 18–50 hrs.

AVAILABILITY

Tablets: 0.5 mg, 1 mg, 2 mg.
Tablets (disintegrating): 0.125 mg, 0.25 mg, 0.5 mg, 1 mg, 2 mg.

INDICATIONS AND DOSAGES

▸ Anticonvulsant

PO

Infants, children younger than 10 yrs or weighing less than 30 kg. 0.01–0.03 mg/kg/day in 2–3 divided doses. Dosage may be increased in up to 0.5-mg increments at 3-day intervals until seizures are controlled. Do not exceed maintenance dosage of 0.2 mg/kg/day.

Children older than 10 yrs. Initial dose 1.5 mg in 3 divided doses. May increase by 0.5–1 mg at 3-day intervals until seizures are controlled. Maintenance: 0.05–0.2 mg/kg. Never exceed 20 mg/day.

UNLABELED USES

Adjunct treatment of seizures, tonic-clonic seizures, treatment of simple and complex partial seizures.

CONTRAINDICATIONS

Hypersensitivity to clonazepam or any related component or other benzodiazepines. Narrow-angle glaucoma, significant liver disease.

INTERACTIONS

Drug

Alcohol, CNS depressants: May increase CNS depressant effect.

Phenytoin, carbamazepine, rifampin, barbiturates: May decrease effectiveness of clonazepam.

Herbal

Kava kava: May increase CNS sedation.

Food

None known.

DIAGNOSTIC TEST EFFECTS

None known.

SIDE EFFECTS

Frequent

Mild, transient drowsiness; ataxia; behavioral disturbances, especially in children manifested as aggression, irritability, agitation

Occasional

Rash, ankle or facial edema, nocturia, dysuria, change in appetite or weight, dry mouth, sore gums, nausea, blurred vision

Rare

Paradoxical reaction, including hyperactivity or nervousness in children, particularly noted in presence of uncontrolled pain

SERIOUS REACTIONS

! Abrupt withdrawal may result in pronounced restlessness, irritability, insomnia, hand tremors, abdominal or muscle cramps, sweating, vomiting, and status epilepticus.

! Overdosage results in somnolence, confusion, diminished reflexes, and coma.

PEDIATRIC CONSIDERATIONS

Baseline Assessment

- Review the seizure patient's history of seizure disorder, including the duration, frequency, and intensity of seizures, as well as level of consciousness. Initiate seizure precautions.
- Assess the panic attack patient's autonomic responses, including cold or clammy hands, diaphoresis, and motor responses, such as agitation, trembling, tension.
- Be aware that clonazepam crosses the placenta and may be distributed in breast milk.
- Be aware that chronic clonazepam ingestion during pregnancy may produce withdrawal symptoms and CNS depression in neonates.

• Know that long-term clonazepam use may adversely affect the mental and physical development of children.
• When discontinuing the medication withdraw it from the patient gradually.

Precautions

• Use cautiously in pts with chronic respiratory disease and impaired kidney and liver function.

Administration and Handling

◂ **ALERT** ▸ When replacement by another anticonvulsant is necessary, plan to decrease clonazepam dose gradually as therapy begins with low replacement dosage.

PO

• Give clonazepam without regard to meals.
• Crush tablets, as needed.

Intervention and Evaluation

• Assess pediatric pts for paradoxical reactions, particularly during early therapy.
• Implement safety measures, and observe frequently for recurrence of seizure activity in seizure pts.
• Assist the patient with ambulation if he or she experiences ataxia or drowsiness.
• Perform complete blood counts and blood serum chemistry tests to assess liver and renal function periodically for pts receiving long-term clonazepam therapy.
• Evaluate the patient for a therapeutic response to the drug, indicated by a decrease in the frequency or intensity of seizures or, if used for panic attacks, calm facial expression and decreased restlessness.

Patient/Family Teaching

• Tell the patient/family that drowsiness usually diminishes with continued therapy.
• Warn the patient/family to avoid tasks that require mental alertness or motor skills until the patient's response to the drug is established.
• Urge the patient/family to stop smoking and to avoid alcohol. Explain to the patient that smoking reduces the effectiveness of the drug.
• Caution the patient/family against abruptly withdrawing the medication after long-term therapy.
• Stress to the patient/family that strict maintenance of drug therapy is essential for seizure control.

Gabapentin

gah-bah-**pen**-tin
(Gantin [AUS], Neurontin)
Do not confuse with Noroxin.

CATEGORY AND SCHEDULE

Pregnancy Risk Category: C

MECHANISM OF ACTION

An anticonvulsant and antineuralgic agent whose exact mechanism is unknown. May be a result of increased GABA synthesis rate, increased GABA accumulation, or binding to as yet undefined receptor sites in brain tissue. ***Therapeutic Effect:*** Produces anticonvulsant activity, reduces neuropathic pain.

PHARMACOKINETICS

Well absorbed from the GI tract (not affected by food). Protein binding: less than 5%. Widely distributed. Crosses blood-brain barrier. Primarily excreted unchanged in urine. Removed by hemodialysis. ***Half-Life:*** 5–7 hrs (half-life is increased with impaired renal function).

AVAILABILITY

Capsules: 100 mg, 300 mg, 400 mg.
Oral Solution: 250 mg/5 mL.
Tablets: 600 mg, 800 mg.

INDICATIONS AND DOSAGES

▸ **Adjunct therapy for seizure control**

PO

Children older than 12 yrs. Initially, 300 mg 3 times/day. May titrate. Range: 900–1,800 mg/day in 3 divided doses. Maximum: 3,600 mg/day.

Children 3–12 yrs. Initially, 10–15 mg/kg/day in 3 divided doses. May titrate up to 25–35 mg/kg/day (children 5–12 yrs) and 40 mg/kg/day (children 3–4 yrs). Maximum: 50 mg/kg/day.

▸ **Adjunct therapy for neuropathic pain**

PO

Children. Initially 5 mg/kg/dose at bedtime, then 5 mg/kg/dose for 2 doses on day 2, and then 5 mg/kg/dose for 3 doses on day 3. Range: 8–35 mg/kg/day in 3 divided doses.

Dosing in children older than 12 yr of age with renal failure has not been studied.

UNLABELED USES

Treatment of essential tremors, hot flashes, hyperhidrosis, migraines, psychiatric disorders.

CONTRAINDICATIONS

Hypersensitivity to gabapentin or any related component.

INTERACTIONS

Drug

Morphine, hydrocodone: May increase CNS depression.

Antacids: May decrease absorption of gabapentin—separate administration by 2 hrs.

Herbal

None known.

Food

None known.

DIAGNOSTIC TEST EFFECTS

May decrease serum WBC count. May produce false-positive urinary proteins.

SIDE EFFECTS

Frequent (19%–10%)
Fatigue, somnolence, dizziness, ataxia

Occasional (8%–3%)
Nystagmus (rapid eye movements), tremor, diplopia (double vision), rhinitis, weight gain

Rare (less than 2%)
Nervousness, dysarthria (speech difficulty), memory loss, dyspepsia, pharyngitis, myalgia

SERIOUS REACTIONS

! Abrupt withdrawal may increase seizure frequency.

! Overdosage may result in double vision, slurred speech, drowsiness, lethargy, and diarrhea.

PEDIATRIC CONSIDERATIONS

Baseline Assessment

- Review the seizure patient's history of seizure disorder, including the onset, duration, frequency, intensity, and type of seizures, as well as his or her level of consciousness. Initiate seizure precautions.
- Know that routine laboratory monitoring of serum levels of gabapentin is not necessary for safe use of the drug.
- Be aware that it is unknown whether gabapentin is distributed in breast milk.
- Be aware that the safety and efficacy of this drug have not been

established in pediatric pts younger than 3 years of age.
• Observe for changes in behavior in children taking gabapentin.

Precautions
• Use cautiously in pts with renal impairment.

Administration and Handling
◂**ALERT**▸ Keep in mind that the maximum time between drug doses should not exceed 12 hrs.
PO
• Give gabapentin without regard to meals; may give with food to avoid or reduce GI upset.
• If treatment is discontinued or anticonvulsant therapy is added, expect to make changes gradually over at least 1 wk to reduce the risk of loss of seizure control.

Intervention and Evaluation
• Provide the patient with safety measures as needed.
• Monitor the patient's behavior, especially with children, as well as body weight, renal function, and seizure duration and frequency.

Patient/Family Teaching
• Instruct the patient/family to take gabapentin only as prescribed.
• Caution the patient/family against abruptly discontinuing the drug because this may increase seizure frequency.
• Warn the patient/family to avoid tasks requiring mental alertness or motor skills because of the potential for dizziness and somnolence.
• Urge the patient/family to avoid alcohol while taking gabapentin.
• Tell the patient/family to always carry an identification card or wear an identification bracelet that displays the patient's seizure disorder and anticonvulsant therapy.

Lamotrigine

lam-**oh**-trih-geen
(Lamictal)
Do not confuse with lamivudine.

CATEGORY AND SCHEDULE
Pregnancy Risk Category: C

MECHANISM OF ACTION
An anticonvulsant whose exact mechanism is unknown. May be a result of inhibition of voltage-sensitive sodium channels, stabilizing neuronal membranes, and regulating presynaptic transmitter release of excitatory amino acids. ***Therapeutic Effect:*** Produces anticonvulsant activity.

AVAILABILITY
Tablets: 25 mg, 100 mg, 150 mg, 200 mg.
Tablets (chewable): 2 mg, 5 mg, 25 mg.

INDICATIONS AND DOSAGES
▸ **Seizure control in pts receiving enzyme-inducing antiepileptic drug (EIAEDs) but not valproate**
PO
Children older than 12 yrs. Recommended as add-on therapy: 50 mg once/day for 2 wks, followed by 100 mg/day in 2 divided doses for 2 wks. Maintenance dosage may be increased by 100 mg/day every week, up to 300–500 mg/day in 2 divided doses.
Children 2–12 yrs. 0.6 mg/kg/day in 2 divided doses for 2 wks, then 1.2 mg/kg/day in 2 divided doses for wks 3 and 4. Maintenance: 5–15 mg/kg/day. Maximum: 400 mg/day.
▸ **Seizure control in pts receiving combination therapy of valproic acid and EIAEDs**
PO
Children older than 12 yrs. 25 mg every other day for 2 wks, followed

by 25 mg once/day for 2 wks. Maintenance dosage may be increased by 25–50 mg/day q1–2wks, up to 100–400 mg/day in 2 divided doses.
Children 2–12 yrs. 0.15 mg/kg/day in 2 divided doses for 2 wks, then 0.3 mg/kg/day in 2 divided doses for wks 3 and 4. Maintenance: 1–5 mg/kg/day in 2 divided doses. Maximum: 200 mg/day.

▸ **Conversion to monotherapy**
PO
Children older than 16 yrs. Add lamotrigine 50 mg/day for 2 wks; then 100 mg/day during wks 3 and 4. Increase by 100 mg/day q1–2wks until maintenance dosage is achieved (300–500 mg/day in 2 divided doses/day). Gradually discontinue other EIAEDs over 4 wks once maintenance dose is achieved.

▸ **Renal function impairment**
Children older than 12 yrs. Same dosage as combination therapy.

▸ **Discontinuation therapy**
Children older than 12 yrs. A reduction in dosage over at least 2 wks, approximately 50% per week, is recommended.

CONTRAINDICATIONS

Hypersensitivity to lamotrigine or any related component.

INTERACTIONS

Drug

Carbamazepine, phenobarbital, phenytoin, primidone, valproic acid: Decreases lamotrigine blood concentration.
Carbamazepine, valproic acid: May increase serum levels of carbamazepine and valproic acid.
Acetaminophen: May decrease the effects of lamotrigine.

Herbal

None known.

Food

None known.

DIAGNOSTIC TEST EFFECTS

None known.

SIDE EFFECTS

Frequent
Dizziness (38%), double vision (28%), headache (29%), ataxia (muscular incoordination) (22%), nausea (19%), blurred vision (16%), somnolence, rhinitis (14%)
Occasional (10%–5%)
Rash, pharyngitis, vomiting, cough, flu syndrome, diarrhea, dysmenorrhea, fever, insomnia, dyspepsia
Rare
Constipation, tremor, anxiety, pruritus, vaginitis, sensitivity reaction

SERIOUS REACTIONS

! Abrupt withdrawal may increase seizure frequency.

PEDIATRIC CONSIDERATIONS

Baseline Assessment

- Review the patient's drug history, including use of other anticonvulsants and history of seizure disorder, along with the duration, frequency, intensity, onset, and type of seizure and level of consciousness, and other medical conditions, such as renal function impairment.
- Provide the patient with a quiet, dark environment and safety precautions.
- When titrating or starting a child on therapy, round dose down to the nearest whole tablet. Do not break tablets—use whole tablets only.

Precautions

- Use cautiously in pts with cardiac, liver, and renal function impairment.

Administration and Handling

◀ **ALERT** ▶ If the patient is currently taking valproic acid, expect to reduce lamotrigine dosage to less than half the normal dosage.

PO

- Give lamotrigine without regard to food.
- If tablets are chewed, administer a small amount of water or fruit juice to assist with swallowing because the tablets have a bitter taste.

Intervention and Evaluation

- Notify the physician promptly if the patient experiences a rash, and expect to discontinue the drug.
- Assist the patient with ambulation if he or she experiences ataxia or dizziness.
- Assess the patient for clinical improvement, manifested by a decrease in the frequency and intensity of seizures.
- Assess the patient for headache and visual abnormalities.

Patient/Family Teaching

- Instruct the patient/family to take lamotrigine only as prescribed. Caution the patient not to abruptly withdraw the medication after long-term therapy.
- Warn the patient/family to avoid alcohol and tasks that require mental alertness and motor skills until the patient's response to the drug is established.
- Tell the patient/family to carry an identification card or wear an identification bracelet to note anticonvulsant therapy.
- Stress to the patient/family that strict maintenance of drug therapy is essential for seizure control.
- Warn the patient/family to notify the physician of the first sign of fever, rash, and swelling of glands.
- Explain to the patient/family that lamotrigine may cause a photosensitivity reaction. Instruct the patient to avoid exposure to sunlight and artificial light.

Oxcarbazepine

ox-car-**bah**-zeh-peen
(Trileptal)

CATEGORY AND SCHEDULE

Pregnancy Risk Category: C

MECHANISM OF ACTION

An anticonvulsant that produces blockade of sodium channels, resulting in stabilization of hyperexcited neural membranes, inhibiting repetitive neuronal firing, and diminishing synaptic impulses. ***Therapeutic Effect:*** Prevents seizures.

PHARMACOKINETICS

Completely absorbed and extensively metabolized to active metabolite in the liver. Protein binding: 40%. Primarily excreted in urine. ***Half-Life:*** 2 hrs (metabolite: 6–10 hrs).

AVAILABILITY

Tablets: 150 mg, 300 mg, 600 mg.
Oral Suspension: 300 mg/5 mL (contains ethanol).

INDICATIONS AND DOSAGES

▸ **Adjunctive therapy**

PO

Children 4–16 yrs. 8–10 mg/kg divided in 2 doses. Maximum: 600 mg/day. Achieve maintenance dose over 2 wks based on patient's weight.

Children weighing 20–29 kg. 900 mg/day divided in 2 doses.

Children weighing 29.1–39 kg. 1,200 mg/day divided in 2 doses.

Children weighing more than 39 kg. 1,800 mg/day divided in 2 doses.

▸ Dosage in renal impairment

Creatinine clearance less than 30 mL/min. Give 50% of normal starting dose, then titrate slowly to desired dose.

UNLABELED USES

Atypical panic disorder.

CONTRAINDICATIONS

Hypersensitivity to oxcarbazepine or any related component.

INTERACTIONS

Drug

Carbamazepine, phenobarbital, phenytoin, valproic acid, verapamil: May decrease the concentration and effect of oxcarbazepine.

Felodipine, oral contraceptives: May decrease the concentration and effect of these drugs.

Phenobarbital, phenytoin: May increase the concentration and risk of toxicity of phenobarbital, phenytoin.

Herbal

None known.

Food

None known.

DIAGNOSTIC TEST EFFECTS

May increase γ-glutamyl transferase (GGT) and liver function test results. May increase or decrease blood glucose levels. May decrease serum calcium, potassium, and sodium levels.

SIDE EFFECTS

Frequent (22%–13%)

Dizziness, nausea, headache

Occasional (7%–5%)

Vomiting, diarrhea, ataxia (muscular incoordination), nervousness, dyspepsia characterized by heartburn, indigestion, epigastric pain, constipation

Rare (4%)

Tremor, rash, back pain, nosebleed, sinusitis, diplopia or double vision

SERIOUS REACTIONS

! May produce clinically significant hyponatremia.

! Potentially serious dermatologic reactions may occur, including Stevens-Johnson syndrome and Toxic Epidermal Necrolysis. Median onset of reaction was 19 days after start of drug therapy. Pts should be advised to report any skin reaction.

! Multi-organ hypersensitivity may occur with use of this medication. Median onset is 13 days after start of drug therapy. Signs may include hepatitis, nephritis, oliguria, pruritis, arthralgia and asthenia. Pts should be advised to report any skin rash, fever or other unusual symptoms.

PEDIATRIC CONSIDERATIONS

Baseline Assessment

• Review the patient's drug history, especially use of other anticonvulsants and history of seizure disorder, including duration, frequency, intensity, onset, and type of seizures, as well as his or her level of consciousness. Initiate seizure precautions.

• Provide the patient with a quiet, dark environment and safety precautions.

• Be aware that oxcarbazepine crosses the placenta and is distributed in breast milk.

• Know that there are no age-related precautions in children older than 4 years of age.

Precautions
• Use cautiously in pts with renal function impairment and sensitivity to carbamazepine.

Administration and Handling
◂ **ALERT** ▸ Plan to give all doses in a twice daily regimen.
PO
• Give oxcarbazepine without regard to food.

Intervention and Evaluation
• Assist the patient with ambulation if he or she experiences ataxia or dizziness.
• Assess the patient for headache and visual abnormalities.
• Monitor the patient's serum sodium levels. Assess the patient for signs and symptoms of hyponatremia including confusion, headache, lethargy, malaise, and nausea.
• Assess the patient for clinical improvement, manifested by a decrease in the frequency or intensity of seizures.

Patient/Family Teaching
• Caution the patient/family against abruptly discontinuing the drug because this may increase seizure activity.
• Warn the patient/family to notify the physician if the patient experiences dizziness, headache, nausea, and rash.
• Tell the patient/family that the patient may need periodic blood tests.

Phenobarbital

feen-oh-**bar**-bih-tall
(Luminal, Phenobarbitone [AUS])

CATEGORY AND SCHEDULE

Pregnancy Risk Category: D
Controlled Substance: Schedule IV

MECHANISM OF ACTION

A barbiturate that binds at the GABA receptor complex, enhancing GABA activity. ***Therapeutic Effect:*** Depresses CNS activity and the reticular activating system.

PHARMACOKINETICS

Route	Onset	Peak	Duration
PO	20–60 min	N/A	6–10 hrs
IV	5 min	30 min	4–10 hrs

Well absorbed after PO and parenteral administration. Protein binding: 35%–50%. Protein binding decreased in neonates. Rapidly, widely distributed. Metabolized in liver. Primarily excreted in urine. Moderately removed by hemodialysis. ***Half-Life:*** Neonates: 45–200 hrs. Infants: 20–133 hrs. Children: 37–73 hrs. Adults: 53–118 hrs.

AVAILABILITY

Tablets: 15 mg, 16 mg, 30 mg, 60 mg, 90 mg 100 mg.
Elixir: 20 mg/5 mL (contains alcohol).
Injection: 30 mg/mL, 60 mg/mL, 130 mg/mL.

INDICATIONS AND DOSAGES

▸ **Status epilepticus**
IV
Children, neonates. Loading dose: 15–20 mg/kg as single dose or in divided doses.

▸ **Anticonvulsant**
IV/PO
Children older than 12 yrs. 1–3 mg/kg/day in 1–2 divided doses.
Children 6–12 yrs. 4–6 mg/kg/day in 1–2 divided doses.
Children 1–5 yrs. 6–8 mg/kg/day in 1–2 divided doses.
Children younger than 1 yr. 5–6 mg/kg/day in 1–2 divided doses.

Neonates. 3–4 mg/kg/day in one dose.

▸ **Sedation**

PO/IM

Children. 2 mg/kg 3 times/day.

▸ **Hypnotic**

PO/IM/IV/SC Children.

3–5 mg/kg.

UNLABELED USES

Prophylaxis and treatment of hyperbilirubinemia.

CONTRAINDICATIONS

Hypersensitivity to phenobarbital or any related component. Porphyria, preexisting CNS depression, severe pain, and severe respiratory disease.

INTERACTIONS

Drug

Alcohol, CNS depressants: May increase the effects of phenobarbital.

Carbamazepine: May increase the metabolism of carbamazepine.

Digoxin, glucocorticoids, metronidazole, oral anticoagulants, quinidine, tricyclic antidepressants: May decrease the effects of digoxin, glucocorticoids, metronidazole, oral anticoagulants, quinidine, and tricyclic antidepressants.

Valproic acid: Decreases the metabolism and increases the concentration and risk of toxicity of phenobarbital.

Herbal

None known.

Food

None known.

DIAGNOSTIC TEST EFFECTS

May decrease serum bilirubin levels. Therapeutic serum level is 10–40 mcg/mL; toxic serum level is greater than 40 mcg/mL.

IV INCOMPATIBILITIES

Amphotericin B complex (Abelcet, AmBisome, Amphotec), hydrocortisone (Solu-Cortef), hydromorphone (Dilaudid), insulin

IV COMPATIBILITIES

Calcium gluconate, enalapril (Vasotec), fentanyl (Sublimaze), fosphenytoin (Cerebyx), morphine, propofol (Diprivan)

SIDE EFFECTS

Occasional (3%–1%)

Somnolence

Rare (less than 1%)

Confusion, paradoxical CNS hyperactivity or nervousness in children, generally noted during the first 2 wks of therapy and particularly noted in the presence of uncontrolled pain

SERIOUS REACTIONS

! Abrupt withdrawal after prolonged therapy may produce effects ranging from markedly increased dreaming, nightmares, or insomnia, tremor, sweating, and vomiting to hallucinations, delirium, seizures, and status epilepticus.

! Skin eruptions appear as a hypersensitivity reaction.

! Blood dyscrasias, liver disease, and hypocalcemia occur rarely.

! Overdosage produces cold or clammy skin, hypothermia, severe CNS depression, cyanosis, rapid pulse, and Cheyne-Stokes respirations.

! Toxicity may result in severe renal impairment.

PEDIATRIC CONSIDERATIONS

Baseline Assessment

- Assess the patient's blood pressure (B/P), pulse, and respirations

immediately before giving phenobarbital.
• Provide the patient using the drug as a hypnotic with an environment conducive to sleep, such as low lighting and quiet. As a safety precaution, raise the bed rails.
• Review the seizure patient's history of seizure disorder, including duration of seizures. Observe the patient frequently for recurrence of seizure activity. Initiate seizure precautions.
• Be aware that phenobarbital readily crosses the placenta and is distributed in breast milk.
• Keep in mind that phenobarbital lowers serum bilirubin concentrations in neonates, produces respiratory depression in neonates during labor, and may cause postpartum hemorrhage or hemorrhagic disease in newborns.
• Be aware that withdrawal symptoms may appear in neonates born to women receiving barbiturates during the last trimester of pregnancy.
• Be aware that phenobarbital use may cause paradoxical excitement in children.
• Be aware that some preparations include benzyl alcohol and administration of benzyl alcohol has been associated with fatal gasping syndrome in neonates.
• Premature infants are more sensitive to the depressant effects of phenobarbital because of immature metabolism.

Precautions

• Use cautiously in pts with liver or renal impairment.

Administration and Handling

◂ALERT▸ Expect to administer a maintenance dose 12 hrs after the loading dose.

PO
• Give phenobarbital without regard to meals.
• Crush tablets as needed.
• Elixir may be mixed with fruit juice, milk, or water.

IM
• Do not inject more than 5 mL in any one IM injection site because phenobarbital produces tissue irritation.
• Give the IM injection deeply into the gluteus maximus or the lateral aspect of the thigh.

IV
• Store vials at room temperature.
• May give undiluted, or may dilute with 0.9% NaCl, D_5W, or lactated Ringer's solution.
• Expect to adequately hydrate the patient before and immediately after infusion to decrease the risk of adverse renal effects.
• Do not inject IV solution faster than 1 mg/kg/min or give more than 30 mg/min for children and 60 mg/min for adults. Injecting too rapidly may produce marked respiratory depression and severe hypotension.
• Beware that inadvertent intra-arterial injection may result in arterial spasm with severe pain and tissue necrosis. Also know that extravasation in subcutaneous tissue may produce redness, tenderness, and tissue necrosis. If either occurs, treat the patient with 0.5% procaine solution into the affected area and apply moist heat, as ordered.

Intervention and Evaluation

• Monitor the patient's B/P, CNS status, heart rate, liver function, renal function, respiratory rate, and seizure activity.
• Monitor the patient for therapeutic serum levels (10–30 mcg/mL) of phenobarbital. The

therapeutic blood serum level of phenobarbital is 10–40 mcg/mL, and the toxic blood serum level is greater than 40 mcg/mL.

Patient/Family Teaching

- Urge the patient/family to avoid alcohol consumption and to limit caffeine intake while taking phenobarbital.
- Tell the patient/family that phenobarbital may be habit-forming.
- Caution the patient/family against abruptly discontinuing the drug.
- Warn the patient/family to avoid tasks that require mental alertness or motor skills because this drug may cause dizziness and drowsiness.

Phenytoin

phen-ih-toyn
(Dilantin, Epamin)
Do not confuse with Dilaudid or mephenytoin.

Phenytoin Sodium

(Dilantin)
(See Color Plate)

CATEGORY AND SCHEDULE

Pregnancy Risk Category: D

MECHANISM OF ACTION

An anticonvulsant and antiarrhythmic agent that stabilizes neuronal membranes in motor cortex and decreases abnormal ventricular automaticity. ***Therapeutic Effect:*** Limits spread of seizure activity. Stabilizes threshold against hyperexcitability. Decreases posttetanic potentiation and repetitive discharge. Shortens refractory period, QT interval, and action potential duration.

PHARMACOKINETICS

Slowly, variably absorbed after PO administration; slowly but completely absorbed after IM administration. Protein binding: 90%–95%; decreased protein binding in neonates. Widely distributed. Metabolized in liver. Primarily excreted in urine. Not removed by hemodialysis. ***Half-Life:*** Adults: 22 hrs.

AVAILABILITY

Capsules: 30 mg, 100 mg.
Tablets (chewable): 50 mg.
Oral Suspension: 125 mg/5 mL.
Injection: 50 mg/mL.

INDICATIONS AND DOSAGES

▸ **Status epilepticus**

IV

Children. Loading: 15–18 mg/kg. Typically start maintenance dose 12 hr after loading dose; give in 2–3 divided doses.
Children 10–16 yrs. Loading: 15–18 mg/kg. Maintenance: 6–7 mg/kg/day.
Children 7–9 yrs. Loading: 15–18 mg/kg. Maintenance: 7–8 mg/kg/day.
Children 4–6 yrs. Loading: 15–18 mg/kg. Maintenance: 7.5–9 mg/kg/day.
Children 6 mos–3 yrs. Loading: 15–18 mg/kg. Maintenance: 8–10 mg/kg/day.
Neonates. Loading: 15–20 mg/kg. Maintenance: 5–8 mg/kg/day.

▸ **Anticonvulsant**

PO

Children. Loading: 15–20 mg/kg in 3 divided doses 2–4 hrs apart. Maintenance: Same as above.

▸ **Arrhythmias**

IV

Children. Loading: 1.25 mg/kg q5min. May repeat up to total dose of 15 mg/kg.

PO/IV
Children. Maintenance: 5–10 mg/kg/day in 2–3 divided doses.

UNLABELED USES
Adjunct in treatment of tricyclic antidepressant toxicity, muscle relaxant in treatment of muscle hyperirritability, treatment of digoxin-induced arrhythmias and trigeminal neuralgia.

CONTRAINDICATIONS
Hydantoin hypersensitivity, seizures resulting from hypoglycemia.
IV: Adam-Stokes syndrome, second- and third-degree heart block, sinoatrial block, sinus bradycardia.

INTERACTIONS
Drug
Alcohol, CNS depressants: May increase CNS depression.
Amiodarone, anticoagulants, cimetidine, disulfiram, fluoxetine, isoniazid, sulfonamides: May increase phenytoin blood concentration, effects, and risk of toxicity.
Antacids: May decrease the absorption of phenytoin.
Fluconazole, ketoconazole, miconazole: May increase phenytoin blood concentration.
Glucocorticoids: May decrease the effects of glucocorticoids.
Lidocaine, propranolol: May increase cardiac depressant effects.
Valproic acid: May increase phenytoin blood concentration and decrease the metabolism of phenytoin.
Xanthine: May increase the metabolism of xanthine.
Herbal
None known.
Food
None known.

DIAGNOSTIC TEST EFFECTS
May increase blood glucose, serum γ-glutamyl transferase, and serum alkaline phosphatase levels. Therapeutic serum level is 10–20 mcg/mL; toxic serum level is greater than 20 mcg/mL.

IV INCOMPATIBILITIES
Diltiazem (Cardizem), dobutamine (Dobutrex), enalapril (Vasotec), heparin, hydromorphone (Dilaudid), insulin, lidocaine, morphine, nitroglycerin, norepinephrine (Levophed), potassium chloride, propofol (Diprivan)

SIDE EFFECTS
Frequent
Drowsiness, lethargy, confusion, slurred speech, irritability, gingival hyperplasia, hypersensitivity reaction, including fever, rash, and lymphadenopathy, constipation, dizziness, nausea
Occasional
Headache, hair growth, insomnia, muscle twitching

SERIOUS REACTIONS
! Abrupt withdrawal may precipitate status epilepticus.
! Blood dyscrasias, lymphadenopathy, and osteomalacia, caused by interference of vitamin D metabolism, may occur.
! The toxic phenytoin blood concentration of 25 mcg/mL may produce ataxia, characterized by muscular incoordination, nystagmus or rhythmic oscillation of eyes, and double vision. As the blood concentration increases, extreme lethargy to comatose states occur.

PEDIATRIC CONSIDERATIONS

Baseline Assessment

- For the patient taking anticonvulsants, review the history of seizure disorder, including the duration, frequency, intensity, and level of consciousness of seizures. Initiate seizure precautions.
- Perform a complete blood count (CBC) and blood serum chemistry tests to assess liver function before beginning phenytoin therapy and periodically during therapy. Repeat the CBC 2 wks after beginning phenytoin therapy and 2 wks after the phenytoin maintenance dose is given.
- Be aware that phenytoin crosses the placenta and is distributed in small amounts in breast milk. Know that fetal hydantoin syndrome, marked by craniofacial abnormalities, digital or nail hypoplasia, and prenatal growth deficiency, has been reported.
- Be aware that there is an increased frequency of seizures in pregnant women because of altered absorption and metabolism of phenytoin.
- Keep in mind that phenytoin use may increase the risk of hemorrhage in neonates and maternal bleeding during delivery.
- Be aware that children are more susceptible to coarsening of facial features, excess body hair, and gingival hyperplasia.

Precautions

- Use IV phenytoin extremely cautiously in pts with congestive heart failure, damaged myocardium, myocardial infarction, and respiratory depression.
- Use cautiously in pts with hyperglycemia, hypotension, impaired liver or renal function, and severe myocardial insufficiency.
- Look for signs of IV phenytoin toxicity, such as cardiovascular collapse and CNS depression.

Administration and Handling

◂**ALERT**▸ Remember that the maintenance dose is usually given 12 hrs after the loading dose.

PO

- Give phenytoin with food if GI distress occurs.
- Do not chew, open, or break capsules. Tablets may be chewed.
- Shake the oral suspension well before using.

IV

◂**ALERT**▸ Give by IV push.

- Keep in mind that a precipitate may form if the parenteral form is refrigerated, but the precipitate will dissolve at room temperature.
- Do not use if the solution is not clear or if a precipitate is present. Keep in mind that slight yellow discoloration of the parenteral form does not affect potency.
- May give undiluted or may dilute with 0.9% NaCl.
- In neonates, administer at a rate not exceeding 1–3 mg/kg/min.
- Do not give the IV injection faster than 50 mg/min for adults to avoid cardiovascular collapse and severe hypotension.
- To minimize pain from chemical irritation of the vein, flush the catheter with sterile saline solution after each bolus of phenytoin.

Intervention and Evaluation

- Observe the patient frequently for recurrence of seizure activity.
- Assess the patient for clinical improvement, manifested by a decrease in the frequency or intensity of seizures.
- Monitor the patient's blood pressure with IV use, as well as the CBC and liver or renal function test results.

• Assist the patient with ambulation if he or she experiences drowsiness or lethargy.
• Monitor the patient for therapeutic serum levels. The therapeutic serum level for phenytoin is 10–20 mcg/mL, and the toxic serum level for phenytoin is greater than 20 mcg/mL.

Patient/Family Teaching

• Warn the patient/family that the patient may experience pain with IV injection.
• Encourage the patient/family to maintain good oral hygiene care with gum massage and regular dental visits to prevent gingival hyperplasia, marked by bleeding, swelling, and tenderness of gums.
• Stress to the patient/family that a CBC should be performed every month for 1 year after the maintenance dose is established and every 3 months thereafter.
• Explain to the patient/family that the patient's urine may appear pink, red, or red-brown and that drowsiness usually diminishes with continued therapy.
• Warn the patient/family to notify the physician if the patient experiences fever, glandular swelling, skin reaction, signs of hematologic toxicity, or sore throat.
• Caution the patient/family against abruptly withdrawing the medication after long-term use because it may precipitate seizures.
• Explain to the patient/family that strict maintenance of drug therapy is essential for arrhythmia and seizure control.
• Warn the patient/family to avoid tasks that require mental alertness or motor skills until the patient's response to the drug is established.
• Urge the patient/family to avoid alcohol while taking phenytoin.

Primidone

prih-mih-doan
(Apo-Primidone [CAN], Mysoline)
Do not confuse with prednisone.

CATEGORY AND SCHEDULE

Pregnancy Risk Category: D

MECHANISM OF ACTION

A barbiturate that decreases motor activity to electrical and chemical stimulation and stabilizes the threshold against hyperexcitability. ***Therapeutic Effect:*** Produces anticonvulsant effect.

AVAILABILITY

Tablets: 50 mg, 250 mg.

INDICATIONS AND DOSAGES

▸ Anticonvulsant

Children 8 yrs and older. Initially 125–250 mg/day at bedtime. May increase by 125–250 mg/day q3–7days. Usual dose: 750–1500 mg/day in divided doses 3–4 times/day. Maximum: 2 g/day.
Children younger than 8 yrs. Initially, 50–125 mg/day at bedtime. May increase by 50–125 mg/day q3–7days. Usual dose: 10–25 mg/kg/day in divided doses.
Neonates. 12–20 mg/kg/day in divided doses.

UNLABELED USES

Treatment of essential tremor.

CONTRAINDICATIONS

Hypersensitivity to primidone or any related component and a history of bronchopneumonia or porphyria.

INTERACTIONS

Drug

Alcohol, CNS depressants: May increase the effects of primidone.
Carbamazepine: May increase the metabolism of carbamazepine.
Digoxin, glucocorticoids, metronidazole, oral anticoagulants, quinidine, tricyclic antidepressants: May decrease the effects of digoxin, glucocorticoids, metronidazole, oral anticoagulants, quinidine, and tricyclic antidepressants.
Valproic acid: Decreases the metabolism and increases the concentration and risk of toxicity of primidone.

Herbal

None known.

Food

None known.

DIAGNOSTIC TEST EFFECTS

May decrease bilirubin level. Therapeutic serum level is 4–12 mcg/mL; toxic serum level is greater than 15 mcg/mL.

SIDE EFFECTS

Frequent
Ataxia, dizziness
Occasional
Loss of appetite, drowsiness, mental changes, nausea, vomiting, paradoxical excitement
Rare
Skin rash

SERIOUS REACTIONS

! Abrupt withdrawal after prolonged therapy may produce effects ranging from markedly increased dreaming, nightmares and insomnia, tremor, sweating, and vomiting to hallucinations, delirium, seizures, and status epilepticus.
! Skin eruptions may appear as a hypersensitivity reaction.
! Blood dyscrasias, liver disease, and hypocalcemia occur rarely.
! Overdosage produces cold or clammy skin, hypothermia, and severe CNS depression followed by high fever and coma.

PEDIATRIC CONSIDERATIONS

Baseline Assessment

- Review the patient's history of seizure disorder, including duration, frequency, and intensity of seizures, as well as his or her level of consciousness. Initiate seizure precautions.
- Observe the patient frequently for recurrence of seizure activity.

Precautions

- Use cautiously in pts with liver or renal impairment.

Intervention and Evaluation

- Monitor the patient's complete blood count, neurologic status, including duration, frequency, and severity of seizures, and serum concentrations of primidone.
- Monitor the patient for therapeutic serum levels. The therapeutic serum level for primidone is 4–12 mcg/mL, and the toxic serum level for primidone is greater than 15 mcg/mL.

Patient/Family Teaching

- Caution the patient/family against abruptly withdrawing the medication after long-term use because this may precipitate seizures.
- Stress to the patient/family that strict maintenance of drug therapy is essential for seizure control.
- Tell the patient/family that drowsiness usually disappears during continued therapy.
- Instruct the patient/family to change positions slowly from a recumbent to a sitting position

before standing if the patient experiences dizziness.
• Warn the patient/family to avoid tasks that require mental alertness or motor skills until the patient's response to the drug is established.
• Urge the patient/family to avoid alcohol while taking primidone.

Tiagabine

tie-**ag**-ah-bean
(Gabitril)

CATEGORY AND SCHEDULE

Pregnancy Risk Category: C

MECHANISM OF ACTION

An anticonvulsant that blocks the reuptake of GABA in the presynaptic neurons, the major inhibitory neurotransmitter in the CNS, increasing GABA levels at postsynaptic neurons. ***Therapeutic Effect:*** Inhibits seizures.

AVAILABILITY

Tablets: 2 mg, 4 mg, 12 mg, 16 mg.

INDICATIONS AND DOSAGES

▸ **Adjunctive therapy for the treatment of partial seizures**

PO

Children 12–18 yrs. Initially, 4 mg once daily, may increase by 4 mg at week 2 and by 4–8 mg/wk thereafter. Maximum: 32 mg/day.

CONTRAINDICATIONS

Hypersensitivity to tiagabine or any related component.

INTERACTIONS

Drug

Carbamazepine, phenobarbital, phenytoin: May increase tiagabine clearance.

Valproate: May alter the effects of valproate.

Herbal

None known.

Food

None known.

DIAGNOSTIC TEST EFFECTS

None known.

SIDE EFFECTS

Frequent (34%–20%)

Dizziness, asthenia or loss of strength and energy, somnolence, nervousness, confusion, headache, infection, tremor

Occasional

Nausea, diarrhea, stomach pain, difficulty concentrating, weakness

SERIOUS REACTIONS

! Overdosage is characterized by agitation, confusion, hostility, and weakness. Full recovery occurs within 24 hrs.

PEDIATRIC CONSIDERATIONS

Baseline Assessment

• Review the patient's history of seizure disorder, including duration, frequency, and intensity of seizures, as well as his or her level of consciousness. Initiate seizure precautions.
• Observe the patient frequently for recurrence of seizure activity.
• Data on use of this medication in children younger than 12 yrs of age are limited.

Precautions

• Use cautiously in pts with liver function impairment and who concurrently use alcohol or other CNS depressants.

Intervention and Evaluation

• Plan to perform a complete blood count and blood serum chemistry tests to assess liver

and renal function periodically for pts receiving long-term therapy.
• Assist the patient with ambulation if he or she experiences dizziness.
• Assess the patient for signs of clinical improvement, manifested by a decrease in frequency or intensity of seizures.

Patient/Family Teaching

• Instruct the patient/family to change positions slowly from a recumbent to a sitting position before standing if the patient experiences dizziness.
• Warn the patient/family to avoid tasks that require mental alertness or motor skills until the patient's response to the drug is established.
• Urge the patient/family to avoid alcohol while taking tiagabine.

Topiramate

toe-**pie**-rah-mate
(Topamax)

CATEGORY AND SCHEDULE

Pregnancy Risk Category: C

MECHANISM OF ACTION

An anticonvulsant that blocks repetitive, sustained firing of neurons by enhancing the ability of GABA to induce a flux of chloride ions into the neurons; may block sodium channels. ***Therapeutic Effect:*** Decreases spread of seizure activity.

PHARMACOKINETICS

Rapidly absorbed after PO administration. Protein binding: 13%–17%. Not extensively metabolized. Primarily excreted unchanged in the urine. Removed by hemodialysis. ***Half-Life:*** Adults: 21 hrs.

AVAILABILITY

Tablets: 25 mg, 100 mg, 200 mg.
Sprinkle Capsules: 15 mg, 25 mg.

INDICATIONS AND DOSAGES

▸ **Adjunctive therapy for the treatment of partial seizures**

PO

Children 17 yrs and older. Initially, 25–50 mg for 1 wk. May increase by 25–50 mg/day at weekly intervals. Maximum: 1,600 mg/day.

Children 2–16 yrs. Initially, 1–3 mg/kg/day. Maximum: 25 mg. May increase by 1–3 mg/kg/day at weekly intervals. Maintenance: 5–9 mg/kg/day in 2 divided doses.

▸ **Tonic-clonic seizures**

PO

Children. Individual and titrated.

UNLABELED USES

Prevention of migraine headaches

CONTRAINDICATIONS

Hypersensitivity to topiramate or any related component.

INTERACTIONS

Drug

Alcohol, CNS depressants: May increase CNS depression.
Carbamazepine, phenytoin, valproic acid: May decrease topiramate blood concentration.
Carbonic anhydrase inhibitors: May increase the risk of renal calculi.
Oral contraceptives: May decrease the effectiveness of oral contraceptives.

Herbal

None known.

Food

None known.

DIAGNOSTIC TEST EFFECTS

None known.

SIDE EFFECTS

Frequent (30%–10%)
Somnolence, dizziness, ataxia, nervousness, nystagmus or involuntary eye movement, diplopia or double vision, paresthesia, nausea, tremor
Occasional (9%–3%)
Confusion, breast pain, dysmenorrhea, dyspepsia, depression, asthenia or loss of strength, pharyngitis, weight loss, anorexia, rash, back or abdominal or leg pain, difficulty with coordination, sinusitis, agitation, flu-like symptoms
Rare (3%–2%)
Mood disturbances, such as irritability and depression, dry mouth, aggressive reaction

SERIOUS REACTIONS

! Psychomotor slowing, difficulty with concentration, language problems, including word-finding difficulties, and memory disturbances occur occasionally. These reactions are generally mild to moderate but may be severe enough to require withdrawal from drug therapy.

PEDIATRIC CONSIDERATIONS

Baseline Assessment
• Review the patient's history of seizure disorder, including duration, frequency, and intensity of seizures, as well as his or her level of consciousness. Initiate seizure precautions.
• Provide the patient with a quiet, dark environment and safety precautions.
• Determine whether the patient is pregnant, sensitive to topiramate, or using other anticonvulsant medication, especially carbamazepine, carbonic anhydrase inhibitors, phenytoin, and valproic acid.
• Obtain the patient's BUN and serum creatinine levels to assess renal function.
• Instruct the female patient to use additional or alternative means of contraception if she uses oral contraceptives. Explain to the patient that topiramate decreases the effectiveness of oral contraceptives.
• Be aware that it is unknown whether topiramate is distributed in breast milk.
• Know that there are no age-related precautions noted in children older than 2 years of age.

Precautions
• Use cautiously in pts with impaired liver or renal function, a predisposition to renal calculi, and sensitivity to topiramate.

Administration and Handling
◂ **ALERT** ▸ Expect to reduce drug dosage by 50% if creatinine clearance is less than 70 mL/min in tonic-clonic seizure pts.
PO
• Do not break tablets because it produces a bitter taste.
• Give topiramate without regard to meals.
• Capsules may be swallowed whole or contents sprinkled on a teaspoonful of soft food and swallowed immediately. Do not chew.

Intervention and Evaluation
• Observe the patient frequently for recurrence of seizure activity.
• Institute seizure safety precautions.
• Assess the patient for clinical improvement, manifested by a decrease in the frequency and intensity of seizures.
• Monitor the patient's renal function test results, including BUN and serum creatinine levels.
• Assist the patient with ambulation if he or she experiences dizziness.

Patient/Family Teaching

- Warn the patient/family to avoid tasks that require mental alertness or motor skills until the patient's response to the drug is established. Keep in mind that topiramate may cause dizziness, drowsiness, or impaired thinking.
- Urge the patient/family to avoid alcohol and taking other CNS depressants while receiving topiramate therapy.
- Caution the patient/family against abruptly discontinuing the drug because this may precipitate seizures.
- Stress to the patient/family that strict maintenance of drug therapy is essential for seizure control.
- Tell the patient/family that drowsiness usually diminishes with continued therapy.
- Instruct the patient/family not to break tablets to avoid their bitter taste.
- Urge the patient/family to maintain adequate fluid intake to decrease the risk of renal stone formation.
- Warn the patient/family to notify the physician if the patient experiences blurred vision or eye pain.

Valproic Acid

val-**pro**-ick
(Depakene)

Valproate Sodium

(Depakene syrup, Epilim [AUS], Valpro [AUS])

Divalproex Sodium

(Depacon, Depakote, Epival [CAN])
(See Color Plate)

CATEGORY AND SCHEDULE

Pregnancy Risk Category: D

MECHANISM OF ACTION

An anticonvulsant, antimanic, and antimigraine agent that directly increases concentration of the inhibitory neurotransmitter GABA. ***Therapeutic Effect:*** Produces anticonvulsant effect.

PHARMACOKINETICS

Well absorbed from the GI tract. Protein binding: 80%–90%. Metabolized in liver. Primarily excreted in urine. Not removed by hemodialysis. ***Half-Life:*** 6–16 hrs. Half-life may be increased with impaired liver function and in children younger than 18 mos.

AVAILABILITY

Capsules: 250 mg (valproic acid).
Syrup: 250 mg/5 mL (valproic acid).
Tablets (delayed release): 125 mg, 250 mg, 500 mg (divalproex).
Tablets (extended release): 500 mg.
Capsules (sprinkle): 125 mg (divalproex).
Injection: 100 mg/mL.

INDICATIONS AND DOSAGES

▸ Seizures

PO

Children older than 10 yrs. Initially, 10–15 mg/kg/day in 1–3 divided doses. May increase by 5–10 mg/kg/day at weekly intervals up to 30–60 mg/kg/day (usual adult dosage: 1,000–2,500 mg/day).

IV

Children. IV dose equal to oral dose but given at a frequency of q6h.

UNLABELED USES

Treatment of myoclonic, simple partial, and tonic-clonic seizures.

CONTRAINDICATIONS

Active liver disease and hypersensitivity to valproic acid or any related component.

INTERACTIONS

Drug

Alcohol, CNS depressants: May increase CNS depressant effects.
Amitriptyline, primidone: May increase the concentration of amitriptyline and primidone.
Anticoagulants, heparin, platelet aggregation inhibitors, thrombolytics: May increase the risk of bleeding.
Carbamazepine: May decrease valproic acid blood concentration.
Liver toxic medications: May increase risk of liver toxicity.
Phenytoin: May alter phenytoin protein binding, increasing the risk of toxicity. Phenytoin may decrease the effects of valproic acid.

Herbal

None known.

Food

None known.

DIAGNOSTIC TEST EFFECTS

May increase lactate dehydrogenase, serum bilirubin, SGOT (AST), and SGPT (ALT) levels. Therapeutic serum level is 50–100 mcg/mL; toxic serum level is greater than 100 mcg/mL. May give false-positive result for urinary ketones. May alter thyroid function test results.

IV INCOMPATIBILITIES

Do not mix with any other medications.

SIDE EFFECTS

Frequent
Epilepsy: Abdominal pain, irregular menses, diarrhea, transient alopecia, indigestion, nausea, vomiting, trembling, weight change
Occasional
Epilepsy: Constipation, dizziness, drowsiness, headache, skin rash, unusual excitement, restlessness
Rare
Epilepsy: Mood changes, double vision, nystagmus, spots before eyes, unusual bleeding or bruising

SERIOUS REACTIONS

! Liver toxicity may occur, particularly in the first 6 mos of valproic acid therapy. Liver toxicity may not be preceded by abnormal liver function test results but may be noted as loss of seizure control, malaise, weakness, lethargy, anorexia, and vomiting.
! Blood dyscrasias may occur.

PEDIATRIC CONSIDERATIONS

Baseline Assessment

- Review the patient's history of seizure disorder, including duration, frequency, and intensity of seizures, as well as his or her level of consciousness. Initiate seizure precautions.
- Maintain safety measures, and provide the patient with a dark, quiet environment.
- Perform a complete blood count (CBC) with platelet count before beginning and 2 wks after valproic acid therapy and 2 wks after the valproic acid maintenance dose is given in seizure pts.
- Assess the appearance, behavior, emotional status, response to the environment, speech pattern, and thought content in manic pts.
- Be aware that valproic acid crosses the placenta and is distributed in breast milk.
- Be aware that there is an increased risk of liver toxicity in children younger than 2 years of age.

Precautions

• Use cautiously in pts with bleeding abnormalities and a history of liver disease.

Administration and Handling

◂ **ALERT** ▸ Regular release and delayed-release formulations of valproic acid are given in 2–4 divided doses and the extended-release formulation of valproic acid is given once daily.

PO

• May give with or without regard to food. Do not administer with carbonated drinks.

• May sprinkle capsule contents on applesauce and give immediately, but do not break, chew, or crush sprinkle beads.

• Delayed-release or extended-release tablets should be given whole.

IV

• Store vials at room temperature.

• Diluted solutions are stable for 24 hrs.

• Discard unused portion.

• Dilute each single dose with at least 50 mL D_5W, 0.9% NaCl, or lactated Ringer's solution.

• Infuse over 5–10 min.

• Do not exceed rate of 3 mg/kg/min (5-min infusion) or 1.5 mg/kg/min (10-min infusion). Too rapid an infusion rate increases the likelihood of side effects.

Intervention and Evaluation

• Monitor the patient's CBC and serum alkaline phosphatase, ammonia, bilirubin, SGOT (AST), and SGPT (ALT) levels.

• Observe seizure pts frequently for recurrence of seizure activity.

• Assess the seizure patient's skin for bruising and petechiae.

• Monitor the seizure patient for clinical improvement, manifested by a decrease in the frequency or intensity of seizures.

• Monitor the patient's valproic acid blood serum level. The therapeutic serum level for valproic acid is 50–100 mcg/mL, and the toxic serum level for valproic acid is greater than 100 mcg/mL.

Patient/Family Teaching

• Caution the patient/family against abruptly withdrawing the medication after long-term use because this may precipitate seizures.

• Stress to the patient/family that strict maintenance of drug therapy is essential for seizure control.

• Explain to the patient/family that drowsiness usually disappears during continued therapy.

• Warn the patient/family to avoid tasks that require mental alertness or motor skills until the patient's response to the drug is established.

• Urge the patient/family to avoid alcohol while taking valproic acid.

• Recommend to the patient/family that the patient carry an identification card or wear an identification bracelet to note anticonvulsant therapy.

• Warn the patient/family to notify the physician if the patient experiences abdominal pain, altered mental status, bleeding, easy bruising, lethargy, loss of appetite, nausea, vomiting, weakness, or yellowing of skin.

Zonisamide

zoe-**niss**-ah-mide

(Zonegran)

CATEGORY AND SCHEDULE

Pregnancy Risk Category: C

MECHANISM OF ACTION

A succinimide that may stabilize neuronal membranes and suppress neuronal hypersynchronization by action at sodium and calcium channels. ***Therapeutic Effect:*** Produces anticonvulsant effect.

PHARMACOKINETICS

Well absorbed after PO administration. Extensively bound to erythrocytes. Protein binding: 40%. Primarily excreted in urine. ***Half-Life:*** Adults: 63 hrs (plasma), 105 hrs (RBCs).

AVAILABILITY

Capsules: 25 mg, 50 mg, 100 mg.

INDICATIONS AND DOSAGES

▸ Partial seizures

PO

Children older than 16 yrs. Initially, 100 mg/day for 2 wks. May increase by 100 mg/day at intervals of 2 wks or longer. Maximum: 400 mg/day.

CONTRAINDICATIONS

Allergy to sulfonamides, zonisamide, or any related component.

INTERACTIONS

Drug

Carbamazepine, phenobarbital, phenytoin, valproic acid: May increase the metabolism and decrease the effect of zonisamide.

Herbal

None known.

Food

None known.

DIAGNOSTIC TEST EFFECTS

May increase BUN and serum creatinine levels.

SIDE EFFECTS

Frequent (17%–9%)

Somnolence, dizziness, anorexia, headache, agitation, irritability, nausea

Occasional (8%–5%)

Fatigue, ataxia, confusion, depression, memory or concentration impairment, insomnia, abdominal pain, double vision, diarrhea, speech difficulty

Rare (4%–3%)

Paresthesia, nystagmus or involuntary movement of eyeball, anxiety, rash, dyspepsia, including heartburn, indigestion, and epigastric distress, weight loss

SERIOUS REACTIONS

! Overdosage is characterized by bradycardia, hypotension, respiratory depression, and comatose state.

! Leukopenia, anemia, and thrombocytopenia occur rarely.

! Some deaths have occurred resulting from serious rashes. These rashes occurred 2–16 wks after starting therapy.

! Hyperthermia and decreased sweating have occurred in some pediatric pts.

PEDIATRIC CONSIDERATIONS

Baseline Assessment

- Review the patient's history of seizure disorder, including duration, frequency, and intensity of seizures, as well as his or her level of consciousness. Initiate seizure precautions.
- Plan to perform a complete blood count and blood serum chemistry tests to assess renal and liver function before beginning and periodically during therapy.

- Be aware that it is unknown whether zonisamide is distributed in breast milk.
- Be aware that the safety and efficacy of this drug have not been established in children younger than 16 yrs of age.

Precautions

- Use cautiously in pts with renal function impairment.

Administration and Handling

PO

- May take with or without food.
- Swallow capsules whole. Do not crush or open tablets.
- Do not give to pts allergic to sulfonamides.

Intervention and Evaluation

- Observe the patient frequently for recurrence of seizure activity.
- Assess the patient for clinical improvement, a decrease in the frequency or intensity of seizures.
- Assist the patient with ambulation if he or she experiences dizziness.

Patient/Family Teaching

- Stress to the patient/family that strict maintenance of drug therapy is essential for seizure control.
- Warn the patient/family to avoid tasks that require mental alertness or motor skills until the patient's response to the drug is established.
- Urge the patient/family to avoid alcohol while taking zonisamide.
- Warn the patient/family to notify the physician if the patient experiences abdominal or back pain, blood in urine, easy bruising, fever, rash, sore throat, or ulcers in the mouth.
- Warn the patient/family to notify the physician immediately if the patient is not sweating as usual or has an elevated temperature.
- Urge patient/family to drink adequate amounts of liquids and report any symptoms of kidney stones.

REFERENCES

Miller, S. & Fioravanti, J. (1997). Pediatric medications: a handbook for nurses. St. Louis: Mosby.

Taketomo, C. K., Hodding, J. H. & Kraus, D. M. (2003–2004). Pediatric dosage handbook (10th ed.). Hudson, OH: Lexi-Comp.

34 Antidepressants

Amitriptyline Hydrochloride
Clomipramine Hydrochloride
Desipramine Hydrochloride
Doxepin Hydrochloride
Fluoxetine Hydrochloride
Imipramine
Nortriptyline Hydrochloride
Sertraline Hydrochloride
Trazodone Hydrochloride

Uses: Antidepressants are used primarily to treat depression. In addition, imipramine is used for childhood enuresis. Clomipramine is used only for obsessive-compulsive disorder. MAOIs are rarely prescribed as initial therapy, except for patients who do not respond to, or who have contraindications for, other antidepressants.

Action: Antidepressants are classified as tricyclic antidepressants, MAOIs, or second-generation antidepressants, which include selective serotonin reuptake inhibitors and atypical antidepressants. Depression may result from decreased amounts (or effects at the receptor sites) of monoamine neurotransmitters, such as norepinephrine, serotonin, and dopamine, in the CNS.

Antidepressants block the metabolism of monoamine neurotransmitters, increasing their levels and effects at receptor sites. These agents also change the responsiveness and sensitivity of presynaptic and postsynaptic receptor sites. (See illustration, *Mechanisms of Action: Antidepressants,* page 450.)

Amitriptyline Hydrochloride

a-me-**trip**-tih-leen
(Apo-Amitriptyline [CAN], Elavil, Endep [AUS], Levate [CAN], Novo-Triptyn [CAN], Tryptanol [AUS])

Do not confuse with Mellaril or nortriptyline.

CATEGORY AND SCHEDULE
Pregnancy Risk Category: C

MECHANISM OF ACTION
This tricyclic antidepressant has strong anticholinergic activity and acts by blocking the reuptake of neurotransmitters, including norepinephrine and serotonin, at presynaptic membranes, thus increasing synaptic concentration at postsynaptic receptor sites. ***Therapeutic Effect:*** Results in antidepressant effect.

COMBINATION PRODUCTS
ETRAFON: amitriptyline/perphenazine (an antipsychotic) 10 mg/2 mg; 25 mg/2 mg; 10 mg/4 mg; 25 mg/4 mg.
LIMBITROL: amitriptyline/chlordiazepoxide (an antianxiety agent) 12.5 mg/5 mg; 25 mg/10 mg.
TRIAVIL: amitriptyline/perphenazine (an antipsychotic) 10 mg/2 mg; 25 mg/2 mg; 10 mg/4 mg; 25 mg/4 mg.

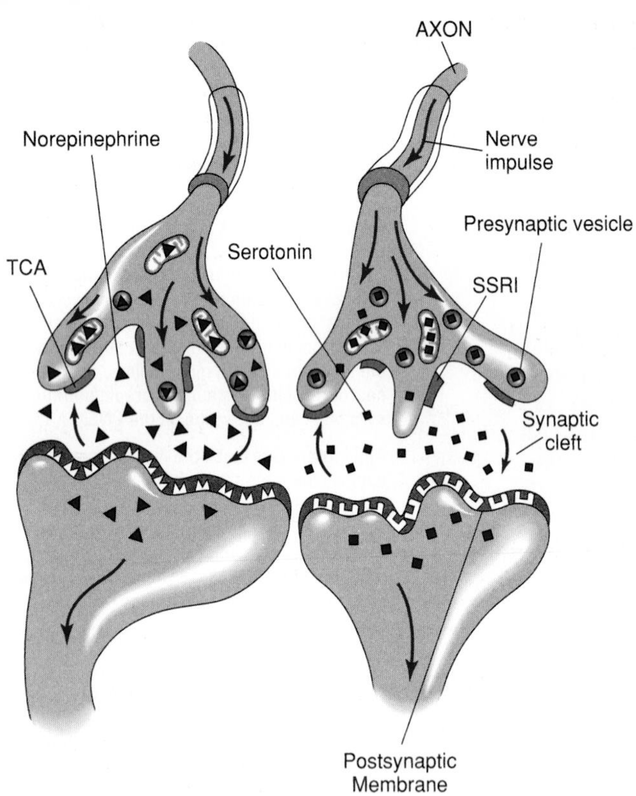

Mechanisms of Action: Antidepressants

Depression is thought to occur when levels of neurotransmitters, such as norepinephrine and serotonin, are reduced at postsynaptic receptor sites. These neurotransmitters affect a wide array of functions, including mood, obsessions, appetite, and anxiety.

Antidepressants work by increasing the availability of these neurotransmitters at postsynaptic membranes and by enhancing and prolonging their effects. As a result, these agents improve mood, reduce anxiety, and minimize obsessions.

Antidepressants typically are classified as tricyclic antidepressants (TCAs), monoamine oxidase inhibitors (not shown), selective serotonin reuptake inhibitors (SSRIs), and atypical antidepressants (not shown). TCAs, such as amitriptyline and desipramine, primarily block norepinephrine reuptake at presynaptic membranes, thereby increasing the norepinephrine concentration at synapses and making more available at postsynaptic receptors (A).

SSRIs, such as fluoxetine and paroxetine, selectively inhibit serotonin uptake at presynaptic membranes. This action leads to increased serotonin availability at postsynaptic receptors (B).

PHARMACOKINETICS

Rapid, well absorbed from GI tract. Protein binding: 90%. Metabolized in liver, undergoes first-pass metabolism. Primarily excreted in urine. Not dialyzable. ***Half-Life:*** Adults: 10–26 hrs.

AVAILABILITY

Tablets: 10 mg, 25 mg, 50 mg, 75 mg, 100 mg, 150 mg.
Injection: 10 mg/mL.

INDICATIONS AND DOSAGES

▸ Depression

PO

Children 6–12 yrs. 1 mg/kg/day in 3 divided doses.
Adolescents. 25–50 mg/day. Increase gradually to 100 mg/day. Maximum: 200 mg/day.

UNLABELED USES

Relieves neuropathic pain, such as that experienced by patients with diabetic neuropathy and postherpetic neuralgia, as well as that experienced by those being treated for bulimia nervosa. Also used for migraine prophylaxis.

CONTRAINDICATIONS

Hypersensitivity to amitriptyline or any related component. Narrow-angle glaucoma, acute recovery period after myocardial infarction, within 14 days of MAOI ingestion.

INTERACTIONS

Drug

Antithyroid agents: May increase the risk of agranulocytosis.
Cimetidine, valproic acid: May increase amitriptyline blood concentration and the risk for amitriptyline toxicity.
Clonidine, guanadrel: May decrease effects of clonidine and guanadrel.
CNS depressants, including alcohol, anticonvulsants, barbiturates, phenothiazines, and sedative-hypnotics: May increase the hypotensive effects, respiratory depression, and sedation caused by amitriptyline.
MAOIs: May increase the risk of hypertensive crisis, as evidenced by seizures, and a hyperpyresis with these drugs.
Phenothiazines: May increase sedative and anticholinergic effects of amitriptyline.
Sympathomimetics: May increase cardiac effects with sympathomimetics.

Herbal

St. John's wort: May increase serious side effects.

Food

None known.

DIAGNOSTIC TEST EFFECTS

May alter EKG readings (flattens T wave) or increase or decrease blood glucose levels. Peak therapeutic serum level is 120–250 ng/mL; toxic serum level is greater than 500 ng/mL.

SIDE EFFECTS

Frequent

Dizziness, drowsiness, dry mouth, orthostatic hypotension, headache, increased appetite or weight, nausea, unusual tiredness, unpleasant taste

Occasional

Blurred vision, confusion, constipation, hallucinations, delayed micturition, eye pain, arrhythmias, fine muscle tremors, parkinsonian syndrome, nervousness, diarrhea, increased sweating, heartburn, insomnia

Rare
Hypersensitivity, alopecia, tinnitus, breast enlargement

SERIOUS REACTIONS

! High amitriptyline dosage may produce confusion, seizures, severe drowsiness, irregular heartbeat, fever, hallucinations, agitation, shortness of breath, vomiting, and unusual tiredness or weakness.
! Abrupt withdrawal from prolonged therapy may produce headache, malaise, nausea, vomiting, and vivid dreams.
! Blood dyscrasias and cholestatic jaundice occur rarely.

PEDIATRIC CONSIDERATIONS

Baseline Assessment

- Assess the patient's psychological status by observing and documenting his or her appearance, behavior, interest in the environment, level of contentment, and sleep patterns.
- Expect to periodically obtain a complete blood count as well as blood serum chemistry profile for patients receiving long-term therapy.
- Be aware that amitriptyline crosses the placenta and is minimally distributed in breast milk.
- Be aware that children are more sensitive to an increased drug dosage and have a higher risk for amitriptyline toxicity.
- Be aware that amitriptyline may increase body weight. Obese or heavy children and adolescents may be better managed with another agent.

Precautions

- Use cautiously in patients with cardiovascular disease, diabetes mellitus, glaucoma, hiatal hernia, a history of seizures, a history of urinary retention or obstruction, hyperthyroidism, increased intraocular pressure, liver disease, prostatic hypertrophy, renal disease, and schizophrenia.

Administration and Handling

PO
- Give with food or milk if GI distress occurs.

IM
- Give by IM injection only if PO administration is not feasible.
- If crystals form in the ampule, immerse it in hot water for 1 min.
- Give deep IM injection slowly.

Intervention and Evaluation

- Closely supervise patients at risk for committing suicide during early therapy. As the patient's depression lessens, his or her energy level will improve, thereby increasing the likelihood of suicide attempts.
- Assess the patient's appearance, behavior, level of interest, mood, and speech pattern to determine the therapeutic effect of the drug.
- Expect to monitor the patient's blood pressure and pulse to watch for the occurrence of arrhythmias and hypotension.

Patient/Family Teaching

- Caution the patient/family not to abruptly discontinue the drug.
- Advise the patient/family to change positions slowly to avoid the hypotensive effect of the drug.
- Explain to the patient/family that the patient will develop a tolerance to the postural hypotensive, sedative, and anticholinergic effects of amitriptyline during early therapy.
- Tell the patient/family that the maximum therapeutic effect may be noted in 2–4 wks.
- Advise the patient/family that the patient may develop sensitivity to sunlight.

• Urge the patient/family to report any visual disturbances.
• Warn the patient/family to avoid tasks that require alertness or motor skills until the patient's response to the drug is established.
• Suggest to the patient/family that sips of tepid water and chewing sugarless gum may relieve dry mouth.

Clomipramine Hydrochloride

klow-**mih**-prah-meen
(Anafranil, Apo-Clomipramine [CAN], Clopram [AUS], Novo-Clopamine [CAN], Placil [AUS])
Do not confuse with alfentanil, chlorpromazine, clomiphene, enalapril, or nafarelin.

CATEGORY AND SCHEDULE

Pregnancy Risk Category: C

MECHANISM OF ACTION

A tricyclic antidepressant that blocks the reuptake of neurotransmitters, such as norepinephrine and serotonin, at CNS presynaptic membranes, increasing their availability at postsynaptic receptor sites. ***Therapeutic Effect:*** Reduces obsessive-compulsive behavior.

AVAILABILITY

Capsules: 25 mg, 50 mg, 75 mg.

INDICATIONS AND DOSAGES

▸ Obsessive-compulsive disorder

PO

Children 10 yrs and older. Initially, 25 mg/day. Gradually increase dose over the first 2 wks of therapy. May give in divided doses. May gradually increase up to maximum of 200 mg/day.

UNLABELED USES

Treatment of bulimia, cataplexy associated with narcolepsy, mental depression, neurogenic pain, panic disorder.

CONTRAINDICATIONS

Hypersensitivity to clomipramine or any related component. Acute recovery period after myocardial infarction, within 14 days of MAOI ingestion

INTERACTIONS

Drug

Alcohol, CNS depressants: May increase CNS and respiratory depression and the hypotensive effects of clomipramine.
Antithyroid agents: May increase the risk of agranulocytosis.
Cimetidine: May increase clomipramine blood concentration and risk of toxicity.
Clonidine, guanadrel: May decrease the effects of clonidine and guanadrel
MAOIs: May increase the risk of convulsions, hyperpyresis, and hypertensive crisis.
Phenothiazines: May increase the anticholinergic and sedative effects of clomipramine.
Sympathomimetics: May increase cardiac effects.

Herbal

None known.

Food

None known.

DIAGNOSTIC TEST EFFECTS

May alter blood glucose levels and EKG readings.

SIDE EFFECTS

Frequent

Drowsiness, fatigue, dry mouth, blurred vision, constipation, sexual dysfunction (42%), ejaculatory failure (20%), impotence, weight gain (18%), delayed micturition, postural hypotension, excessive sweating, disturbed concentration, increased appetite, urinary retention

Occasional

GI disturbances, such as nausea, GI distress, and metallic taste, asthenia, aggressiveness, muscle weakness

Rare

Paradoxical reactions (agitation, restlessness, nightmares, insomnia, extrapyramidal symptoms, particularly fine hand tremor), laryngitis, seizures

SERIOUS REACTIONS

! High dosage may produce cardiovascular effects, including severe postural hypotension, dizziness, tachycardia, palpitations, and arrhythmias, and seizures. High dosage may also result in altered temperature regulation, such as hyperpyrexia or hypothermia.

! Abrupt withdrawal from prolonged therapy may produce headache, malaise, nausea, vomiting, and vivid dreams.

! Anemia has been noted.

PEDIATRIC CONSIDERATIONS

Baseline Assessment

- Observe for neuroleptic malignant syndrome (fever, increased breathing and heartbeat, sweating, loss of urinary control, and muscle stiffness).

Precautions

- Use cautiously in patients with cardiac disease, diabetes mellitus, glaucoma, hiatal hernia, a history of seizures, a history of urinary obstruction or retention, hyperthyroidism, increased intraocular pressure, liver disease, prostatic hypertrophy, renal disease, and schizophrenia.

Intervention and Evaluation

- Closely supervise suicidal-risk patients during early therapy. As depression lessens, the patient's energy level improves, which increases the suicide potential.
- Assess the patient's appearance, behavior, level of interest, mood, and speech pattern.
- Monitor complete blood count results to assess for signs of anemia and agranulocytosis.
- Monitor EKG tracings for arrhythmias.

Patient/Family Teaching

- Advise the patient/family that clomipramine may cause blurred vision, constipation, and dry mouth.
- Warn the patient/family to change positions slowly, especially in the beginning of therapy, to avoid or lessen postural hypotension.
- Advise the patient/family that the patient will develop a tolerance to the drug's anticholinergic effect, postural hypotension, and sedative effects during early therapy.
- Explain to the patient/family that the maximum therapeutic effect of clomipramine may be noted in 2–4 wks.
- Caution the patient/family against abruptly discontinuing the medication.
- Warn the patient/family to avoid tasks that require mental alertness or motor skills until the patient's response to the drug is established.
- Urge the patient/family to avoid alcohol while taking clomipramine.

Desipramine Hydrochloride

deh-**sip**-rah-meen
(Apo-Desipramine [CAN], Norpramin, Novo-Desipramine [CAN], Pertofrane [AUS])
Do not confuse with disopyramide or imipramine.

CATEGORY AND SCHEDULE

Pregnancy Risk Category: C

MECHANISM OF ACTION

A tricyclic antidepressant that increases the synaptic concentration of norepinephrine and/or serotonin by inhibiting their reuptake by presynaptic membranes. Strong anticholinergic activity. ***Therapeutic Effect:*** Produces antidepressant effect.

PHARMACOKINETICS

Rapidly well absorbed from the GI tract. Protein binding: 90%. Metabolized in liver. Primarily excreted in urine. Minimally removed by hemodialysis. ***Half-Life:*** Adults: 12–27 hrs.

AVAILABILITY

Tablets: 10 mg, 25 mg, 50 mg, 75 mg, 100 mg, 150 mg.

INDICATIONS AND DOSAGES

▸ Depression

PO

Children older than 12 yrs. Initially, 25–50 mg/day. May gradually increase to 100 mg/day. Maximum: 150 mg/day.
Children 6–12 yrs. 1–3 mg/kg/day. Maximum: 5 mg/kg/day.

UNLABELED USES

Treatment of attention deficit hyperactivity disorder, bulimia nervosa, cataplexy associated with narcolepsy, cocaine withdrawal, neurogenic pain, panic disorder.

CONTRAINDICATIONS

Hypersensitivity to desipramine or any related component. Narrow-angle glaucoma, use of MAOIs within 14 days.

INTERACTIONS

Drug

Alcohol, CNS depressants: May increase CNS and respiratory depression and the hypotensive effects of desipramine.
Antithyroid agents: May increase risk of agranulocytosis.
Cimetidine: May increase desipramine blood concentration and risk of toxicity.
Clonidine, guanadrel: May decrease the effects of clonidine and guanadrel.
MAOIs: May increase the risk of hyperpyrexia, hypertensive crisis, and seizures.
Phenothiazines: May increase the anticholinergic and sedative effects of desipramine.
Phenytoin: May decrease desipramine blood concentration.
Sympathomimetics: May increase the cardiac effects.

Herbal

St. John's wort: May have additive effects.

Food

None known.

DIAGNOSTIC TEST EFFECTS

May alter blood glucose levels and EKG readings. Therapeutic serum level is 115–300 ng/mL; toxic serum level is greater than 1,000 ng/mL.

SIDE EFFECTS

Frequent

Drowsiness, fatigue, dry mouth, blurred vision, constipation, delayed micturition, postural hypotension, diaphoresis, disturbed concentration, increased appetite, urinary retention.

Occasional
GI disturbances, such as nausea, GI distress, metallic taste sensation

Rare
Paradoxical reaction, marked by agitation, restlessness, nightmares, insomnia, extrapyramidal symptoms, particularly fine hand tremor

SERIOUS REACTION

! High dosage may produce confusion, seizures, severe drowsiness, arrhythmias, fever, hallucinations, agitation, shortness of breath, vomiting, and unusual tiredness or weakness.

! Abrupt withdrawal from prolonged therapy may produce severe headache, malaise, nausea, vomiting, and vivid dreams.

PEDIATRIC CONSIDERATIONS

Baseline Assessment

- Plan to perform a complete blood count and blood serum chemistry tests to assess liver and renal function periodically for patients receiving long-term therapy.
- Be aware that desipramine crosses the placenta and is minimally distributed in breast milk.
- Be aware that desipramine use is not recommended in children younger than 6 yrs of age.
- Be aware that desipramine may be a cardiac toxicity risk in children younger than 12 yrs of age.

Precautions

- Use cautiously in patients with cardiac conduction disturbances, cardiovascular disease, hyperthyroidism, seizure disorders, and urinary retention and in patients who are taking thyroid replacement therapy.

Administration and Handling

PO

- Give with food or milk if GI distress occurs.

Intervention and Evaluation

- Supervise the suicidal-risk patient closely during early therapy because as the patient's depression lessens and his or her energy level improves, the risk for suicide increases.
- Assess the patient's appearance, behavior, level of interest, mood, and speech pattern.
- Monitor the patient for therapeutic desipramine serum levels. Know that the therapeutic serum level for desipramine is 115–300 ng/mL and the toxic serum level for desipramine is greater than 400 ng/mL.
- Expect to perform and monitor EKGs if the patient has a history of arrhythmias.

Patient/Family Teaching

- Instruct the patient/family to change positions slowly to avoid the drug's hypotensive effect.
- Explain to the patient/family that tolerance to the drug's anticholinergic and sedative effects as well as postural hypotension usually develops during early therapy.
- Advise the patient/family that the drug's maximum therapeutic effect may be noted in 2–4 wks.
- Caution the patient/family against abruptly discontinuing the medication.

Doxepin Hydrochloride

dox-eh-pin
(Deptran [AUS], Novo-Doxepin [CAN], Prudoxin, Sinequan, Zonalon)

Do not confuse with doxapram, doxazosin, Doxidan, or saquinavir.

CATEGORY AND SCHEDULE
Pregnancy Risk Category: C (B topical)

MECHANISM OF ACTION
A tricyclic antidepressant, antianxiety, antineuralgic, antipruritic, and antiulcer agent that increases synaptic concentrations of norepinephrine and serotonin. ***Therapeutic Effect:*** Produces antidepressant and anxiolytic effect.

PHARMACOKINETICS
Rapidly well absorbed from the GI tract. Protein binding: 80%–85%. Metabolized in liver to active metabolite. Primarily excreted in urine. Not removed by hemodialysis. ***Half-Life:*** Adults: 6–8 hrs.
Topical: Absorbed through skin, distributed to body tissues, metabolized to active metabolite, eliminated renally.

AVAILABILITY
Capsules: 10 mg, 25 mg, 50 mg, 75 mg, 100 mg, 150 mg.
Oral Concentrate: 10 mg/mL.
Cream: 5%.

INDICATIONS AND DOSAGES
▸ Depression or anxiety
PO
Children younger than 12 yrs.
1–3 mg/kg/day in single or divided doses.
Adolescents. Begin with 25–50 mg/day in single or divided doses. May increase gradually to 100 mg/day.

UNLABELED USES
Treatment of neurogenic pain, panic disorder, prophylaxis vascular headache, pruritus in idiopathic cold urticaria.

CONTRAINDICATIONS
Hypersensitivity to doxepin or any related component or to other tricyclic depressants. Narrow-angle glaucoma, urine retention.

INTERACTIONS
Drug
Alcohol, CNS depressants: May increase CNS and respiratory depression and the hypotensive effects of doxepin.
Antithyroid agents: May increase the risk of agranulocytosis.
Cimetidine: May increase doxepin blood concentration and risk of toxicity.
Clonidine, guanadrel: May decrease the effects of clonidine and guanadrel.
MAOIs: May increase the risk of convulsions, hyperpyrexia, and hypertensive crisis.
Phenothiazines: May increase the anticholinergic and sedative effects of doxepin.
Sympathomimetics: May increase cardiac effects.
Herbal
St. John's wort: May have additive effects.
Food
None known.

DIAGNOSTIC TEST EFFECTS
May alter blood glucose levels and EKG readings. Therapeutic serum level is 110–250 ng/mL; toxic serum level is greater than 500 ng/mL.

SIDE EFFECTS

Frequent

PO: Orthostatic hypotension, drowsiness, dry mouth, headache, increased appetite or weight, nausea, unusual tiredness, unpleasant taste

Topical: Edema at application site, increased itching or eczema, burning, stinging of skin, altered taste, dizziness, drowsiness, dry skin, dry mouth, fatigue, headache, thirst

Occasional

PO: Blurred vision, confusion, constipation, hallucinations, difficult urination, eye pain, irregular heartbeat, fine muscle tremors, nervousness, impaired sexual function, diarrhea, increased sweating, heartburn, insomnia

Topical: Anxiety, skin irritation or cracking, nausea

Rare

Allergic reaction, alopecia, tinnitus, breast enlargement

Topical: Fever

SERIOUS REACTIONS

! High dosage may produce confusion, seizures, severe drowsiness, fast or slow irregular heartbeat, fever, hallucinations, agitation, shortness of breath, vomiting, and unusual tiredness or weakness.

! Abrupt withdrawal from prolonged therapy may produce headache, malaise, nausea, vomiting, and vivid dreams.

PEDIATRIC CONSIDERATIONS

Baseline Assessment

• Assess the patient's blood pressure (B/P), and pulse.

• In patients with a history of cardiovascular disease, monitor the EKG.

• Be aware that doxepin crosses the placenta and is distributed in breast milk.

• Be aware that the safety and efficacy of this drug have not been established in children.

Precautions

• Use cautiously in patients with cardiac disease, diabetes mellitus, glaucoma, hiatal hernia, a history of seizures, a history of urinary obstruction or retention, hyperthyroidism, increased intraocular pressure, liver disease, prostatic hypertrophy, renal disease, and schizophrenia.

Administration and Handling

PO

• Give with food or milk, if GI distress occurs.

• Dilute concentrate in an 8-oz glass of fruit juice, such as grapefruit, orange, pineapple, or prune, or milk or water. Avoid diluting in carbonated drinks because they are incompatible with doxepin.

Intervention and Evaluation

• Monitor the patient's B/P, pulse, and weight.

• Closely supervise suicidal-risk patients during early therapy. As depression lessens, be aware that the patient's energy level generally improves, which increases the suicide potential.

• Assess the patient's appearance, behavior, level of interest, mood, and speech pattern.

• Monitor the patient for therapeutic serum levels. Know that the therapeutic serum level for doxepin is 110–250 ng/mL and the toxic serum level for doxepin is greater than 500 ng/mL.

Patient/Family Teaching

• Advise the patient/family that doxepin may cause drowsiness or decrease the patient's ability to perform tasks requiring mental

alertness or physical coordination. Warn the patient to avoid tasks that require mental alertness and motor skills until his or her response to the drug is established.
• Warn the patient/family to change positions slowly, especially early in therapy, to avoid postural hypotension.
• Advise the patient/family that doxepin may cause dry mouth and increased appetite.
• Urge the patient/family to avoid alcohol and limit caffeine intake while taking doxepin.
• Caution the patient/family to avoid exposure to sunlight or artificial light sources.
• Explain to the patient/family that the therapeutic effect of doxepin may be noted within 2–5 days with the maximum effect noted within 2–3 wks.

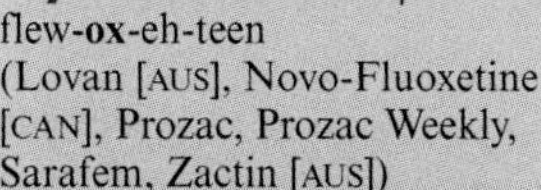

Fluoxetine Hydrochloride

flew-**ox**-eh-teen
(Lovan [AUS], Novo-Fluoxetine [CAN], Prozac, Prozac Weekly, Sarafem, Zactin [AUS])
Do not confuse with fluvastatin, Prilosec, Proscar, ProSom, or Serophene.
(See Color Plate)

CATEGORY AND SCHEDULE

Pregnancy Risk Category: C

MECHANISM OF ACTION

A psychotherapeutic agent that selectively inhibits serotonin uptake in the CNS, enhancing serotonergic function. ***Therapeutic Effect:*** Resulting enhancement of synaptic activity produces antidepressant, antiobsessional, and antibulimic effect.

PHARMACOKINETICS

Well absorbed from the GI tract. Crosses blood-brain barrier. Protein binding: 94%. Metabolized in liver to the active metabolite. Primarily excreted in urine. Not removed by hemodialysis. ***Half-Life:*** Adults: 2–3 days. Metabolite: 7–9 days.

AVAILABILITY

Capsules: 10 mg, 20 mg, 40 mg, 90 mg (Prozac Weekly).
Liquid: 20 mg/5 mL.
Tablets: 10 mg, 20 mg.

INDICATIONS AND DOSAGES

▸ **Depression, obsessive-compulsive disorder**

PO

Children 7–17 yrs. Initially, 5–10 mg/day. Titrate upward as needed (20 mg/day usual dosage). Maximum: 40 mg/day.

UNLABELED USES

Treatment of hot flashes.

CONTRAINDICATIONS

Hypersensitivity to fluoxetine or any related component. Avoid giving within 14 days of MAOI ingestion.

INTERACTIONS

Drug

Alcohol, CNS depressants: Antagonize CNS depressant effect.
Highly protein-bound medications, including oral anticoagulants: May displace highly protein-bound drugs from protein-binding sites.
MAOIs: May produce serotonin syndrome.
Phenytoin: May increase blood concentration and risk of toxicity of phenytoin.

Herbal

St. John's wort: May have additive effect.

Food
None known.

DIAGNOSTIC TEST EFFECTS
None known.

SIDE EFFECTS
Frequent (more than 10%)
Headache, asthenia (loss of strength), inability to sleep, anxiety, nervousness, drowsiness, nausea, diarrhea, decreased appetite
Occasional (9%–2%)
Dizziness, tremor, fatigue, vomiting, constipation, dry mouth, abdominal pain, nasal congestion, diaphoresis
Rare (less than 2%)
Flushed skin, lightheadedness, decreased ability to concentrate

SERIOUS REACTIONS
! Overdosage may produce seizures, nausea, vomiting, excessive agitation, and restlessness.

PEDIATRIC CONSIDERATIONS
Baseline Assessment
- Expect to perform baseline and periodic complete blood counts and liver and renal function tests for patients receiving long-term therapy.
- Be aware that it is unknown whether fluoxetine crosses the placenta or is distributed in breast milk.
- Be aware that children may be more sensitive to the drug's behavioral side effects, such as insomnia and restlessness.
- Be aware that use of fluoxetine in children and adolescents has been linked to suicide.

Precautions
- Use cautiously in patients with cardiac dysfunction, diabetes, and seizure disorder.
- Use cautiously in patients at high risk for suicide.

Administration and Handling
◀ALERT▶ Expect to use lower or less frequent doses in patients with liver or renal impairment, those who have concurrent disease, and those who are taking multiple medications.
PO
- Give fluoxetine with food or milk if GI distress occurs.

Intervention and Evaluation
- Closely supervise suicidal-risk patients during early therapy. As depression lessens, the patient's energy level improves, which increases the suicide potential.
- Assess the patient's appearance, behavior, level of interest, mood, and speech pattern.
- Assess the patient's pattern of daily bowel activity and stool consistency.
- Assess the patient's skin for the appearance of rash.
- Monitor the patient's blood glucose, serum alkaline phosphatase, bilirubin, sodium, SGOT (AST), and SGPT (ALT) levels.

Patient/Family Teaching
- Explain to the patient/family that the maximum therapeutic response of the drug may require 4 wks or more of therapy.
- Caution the patient/family against abruptly discontinuing the medication.
- Warn the patient/family to avoid tasks that require mental alertness or motor skills until the patient's response to the drug is established.
- Urge the patient/family to avoid alcohol while taking fluoxetine.
- Instruct the patient/family to take the last dose of the drug before 4 PM to avoid insomnia.

Imipramine

ih-**mih**-prah-meen
(Apo-Imipramine [CAN], Melipramine [AUS], Tofranil, Tofranil-PM)
Do not confuse with desipramine.

CATEGORY AND SCHEDULE

Pregnancy Risk Category: D

MECHANISM OF ACTION

A tricyclic antibulimic, anticataplectic, antidepressant, antinarcoleptic, antineuralgic, antineuritic, and antipanic agent that blocks the reuptake of neurotransmitters, such as norepinephrine and serotonin, at presynaptic membranes, increasing their concentration at postsynaptic receptor sites. ***Therapeutic Effect:*** Results in antidepressant effect. Anticholinergic effect controls nocturnal enuresis.

AVAILABILITY

Tablets: 10 mg, 25 mg, 50 mg.
Capsules: 75 mg, 100 mg, 125 mg, 150 mg.

INDICATIONS AND DOSAGES

▸ Depression

PO

Children younger than 12 yrs. 1.5 mg/kg/day. May increase 1 mg/kg q3–4days. Maximum: 5 mg/kg/day.
Children older than 12 yrs. 25–50 mg/day. May increase gradually. Maximum: 200 mg/day in single or divided doses.

▸ Childhood enuresis

PO

Children older than 6 yrs. Initially, 10–25 mg at bedtime. May increase by 25 mg/day. Maximum 6–12 yrs: 50 mg. Maximum older than 12 yrs: 75 mg.

▸ Adjunct in the treatment of cancer pain

PO

Children older than 6 yrs. Initially, 0.2–0.4 mg/kg at bedtime. Maximum: 1–3 mg/kg/dose at bedtime.

UNLABELED USES

Treatment of attention-deficit hyperactivity disorder, cataplexy associated with narcolepsy, neurogenic pain, panic disorder.

CONTRAINDICATIONS

Hypersensitivity to imipramine or any related component. Acute recovery period after myocardial infarction, within 14 days of MAOI ingestion. Narrow-angle glaucoma.

INTERACTIONS

Drug

Alcohol, CNS depressants: May increase CNS and respiratory depression and the hypotensive effects of imipramine.
Antithyroid agents: May increase the risk of agranulocytosis.
Cimetidine: May increase imipramine blood concentration and risk of toxicity.
Clonidine, guanadrel: May decrease the effects of clonidine and guanadrel.
MAOIs: May increase the risk of hyperpyrexia, hypertensive crisis, and seizures.
Phenothiazines: May increase anticholinergic and sedative effects of imipramine.
Phenytoin: May decrease imipramine blood concentration.
Sympathomimetics: May increase the cardiac effects.

Herbal

Ginkgo biloba: May decrease seizure threshold.

St. John's wort: May have additive effect.

Food

None known.

DIAGNOSTIC TEST EFFECTS

May alter blood glucose levels and EKG readings. Therapeutic serum level is 225–300 ng/mL; toxic serum level is greater than 500 ng/mL.

SIDE EFFECTS

Frequent

Drowsiness, fatigue, dry mouth, blurred vision, constipation, delayed micturition, postural hypotension, diaphoresis, disturbed concentration, increased appetite, urinary retention, photosensitivity

Occasional

GI disturbances, such as nausea, and a metallic taste sensation

Rare

Paradoxical reaction, marked by agitation, restlessness, nightmares, insomnia, extrapyramidal symptoms, particularly fine hand tremors

SERIOUS REACTIONS

! High dosage may produce cardiovascular effects, such as severe postural hypotension, dizziness, tachycardia, palpitations, arrhythmias and seizures. High dosage may also result in altered temperature regulation, including hyperpyrexia or hypothermia.

! Abrupt withdrawal from prolonged therapy may produce headache, malaise, nausea, vomiting, and vivid dreams.

PEDIATRIC CONSIDERATIONS

Baseline Assessment

• Expect to perform a complete blood count and blood serum chemistry tests to assess blood glucose level, liver, and renal function periodically for patients receiving long-term therapy.

• Plan to perform a baseline EKG, if the patient is at risk for arrhythmias.

• Be aware that Tofranil-PM capsules should not be administered to children because of the risk of overdosage.

• Never abruptly discontinue long-term therapy in children.

Precautions

• Use cautiously in patients with cardiac disease, diabetes mellitus, glaucoma, hiatal hernia, a history of seizures, a history or urinary obstruction or retention, hyperthyroidism, increased intraocular pressure, liver disease, prostatic hypertrophy, renal disease, and schizophrenia.

Administration and Handling

PO

• Give with food or milk if GI distress occurs.

• Do not crush or break film-coated tablets.

Intervention and Evaluation

• Closely supervise suicidal-risk patients during early therapy. As depression lessens, be aware that the patient's energy level generally improves, which increases the suicide potential.

• Assess the patient's appearance, behavior, level of interest, mood, and speech pattern.

• Assess the patient's pattern of daily bowel activity and stool consistency.

• Monitor the patient's blood pressure for hypotension and the pulse for irregularities that may represent an arrhythmia.

• Palpate the patient's bladder for evidence of urinary retention.

• Monitor the patient's therapeutic serum levels of imipramine. Know that the therapeutic serum level for imipramine is 225–300 ng/mL, and the toxic serum level of imipramine is greater than 500 ng/mL.

Patient/Family Teaching

• Instruct the patient/family to change positions slowly to avoid the hypotensive effect of the drug.
• Explain to the patient/family that a tolerance to anticholinergic effects, postural hypotension, and sedative effects usually develops during early therapy.
• Tell the patient/family that the therapeutic effect of the drug may be noted within 2–5 days with the maximum effect noted within 2–3 wks.
• Suggest to the patient/family that taking sips of tepid water and chewing sugarless gum may relieve dry mouth.
• Caution the patient/family against abruptly discontinuing the medication.
• Warn the patient/family to avoid tasks that require mental alertness or motor skills until the patient's response to the drug is established.

Nortriptyline Hydrochloride

nor-**trip**-teh-leen
(Allegron [AUS], Aventyl, Norventyl, Pamelor)
Do not confuse with Ambenyl, amitriptyline, or Bentyl.

CATEGORY AND SCHEDULE

Pregnancy Risk Category: D

MECHANISM OF ACTION

A tricyclic compound that blocks reuptake of neurotransmitters (norepinephrine and serotonin) at neuronal presynaptic membranes, increasing availability at postsynaptic receptor sites.
Therapeutic Effect: Resulting enhancements of synaptic activity produces antidepressant effect.

AVAILABILITY

Capsules: 10 mg, 25 mg, 50 mg, 75 mg.
Oral Solution: 10 mg/5 mL.

INDICATIONS AND DOSAGES

▸ Depression

PO

Children older than 12 yrs. 30–50 mg/day in 3–4 divided doses. Maximum: 150 mg/day.
Children 6–12 yrs. 10–20 mg/day in 3–4 divided doses.

▸ Enuresis

PO

Children older than 11 yrs. 25–35 mg/day.
Children 8–11 yrs. 10–20 mg/day.
Children 6–7 yrs. 10 mg/day.

UNLABELED USES

Treatment of neurogenic pain, panic disorder, prophylaxis of migraine headache.

CONTRAINDICATIONS

Hypersensitivity to nortriptyline or any related component. Acute recovery period after myocardial infarction, within 14 days of MAOI ingestion, angle closure glaucoma.

INTERACTIONS

Drug

Alcohol, CNS depressants: May increase CNS and respiratory depression and hypotensive effects.
Antithyroid agents: May increase the risk of agranulocytosis.

Cimetidine: May increase the blood concentration and risk of toxicity with nortriptyline.
Clonidine, guanadrel: May decrease the effects of clonidine and guanadrel
MAOIs: May increase the risk of convulsions, hyperpyrexia, and hypertensive crisis.
Phenothiazines: May increase the anticholinergic and sedative effects of nortriptyline.
Sympathomimetics: May increase cardiac effects.

Herbal
St. John's wort: May increase serious side effects.

Food
None known.

DIAGNOSTIC TEST EFFECTS

May alter blood glucose levels and EKG readings. Therapeutic serum level 50–150 ng/mL.

SIDE EFFECTS

Frequent
Drowsiness, fatigue, dry mouth, blurred vision, constipation, delayed micturition, postural hypotension, excessive sweating, disturbed concentration, increased appetite, urine retention

Occasional
GI disturbances, including nausea, GI distress, metallic taste sensation, photosensitivity

Rare
Paradoxical reaction (agitation, restlessness, nightmares, insomnia), extrapyramidal symptoms, particularly fine hand tremors

SERIOUS REACTIONS

! High dosage may produce cardiovascular effects, such as severe postural hypotension, dizziness, tachycardia, palpitations, arrhythmias, and seizures. High dosage may also result in altered temperature regulation, such as hyperpyrexia or hypothermia.

! Abrupt withdrawal from prolonged therapy may produce headache, malaise, nausea, vomiting, and vivid dreams.

PEDIATRIC CONSIDERATIONS

Baseline Assessment
- Plan to perform a complete blood count and blood serum chemistry tests to assess glucose levels and liver and renal function periodically for patients receiving long-term therapy.
- Assess the patient's EKG for arrhythmias.

Precautions
- Use cautiously in patients with cardiac disease, diabetes mellitus, glaucoma, hiatal hernia, a history of seizures, a history of urinary obstruction and retention, hyperthyroidism, increased intraocular pressure, liver disease, prostatic hypertrophy, renal disease, and schizophrenia.

Administration and Handling
PO
- Give nortriptyline with food or milk if GI distress occurs.

Intervention and Evaluation
- Closely supervise suicidal-risk patients during early therapy. As depression lessens, the patient's energy level improves, which increases the suicide potential.
- Assess the patient's appearance, behavior, level of interest, mood, and speech pattern.
- Assess the patient's pattern of daily bowel activity and stool consistency. Help the patient to avoid constipation by stressing the consumption of high-fiber foods and fluids.

• Monitor the patient's blood pressure for hypotension and pulse for irregularities that could indicate an arrhythmia.
• Palpate the patient's bladder for signs of urine retention, and monitor his or her urine output.
• Monitor the patient's therapeutic serum levels of nortriptyline. Know that the therapeutic serum level is 50–150 ng/mL.

Patient/Family Teaching

• Instruct the patient/family to change positions slowly to avoid the hypotensive effect of nortriptyline.
• Advise the patient/family that a tolerance to anticholinergic effects, postural hypotension, and sedative effects usually develops during early therapy.
• Tell the patient/family that the therapeutic effect of nortriptyline may be noted in 2 wks or longer.
• Caution the patient/family that photosensitivity to sunlight may occur. Encourage the patient to use sunscreen and wear protective clothing.
• Suggest to the patient/family that taking sips of tepid water and chewing sugarless gum may relieve dry mouth.
• Warn the patient/family to notify the physician if the patient experiences visual disturbances.
• Caution the patient/family against abruptly discontinuing the medication.
• Warn the patient/family to avoid tasks that require mental alertness or motor skills until the patient's response to the drug is established.

Sertraline Hydrochloride

sir-trah-leen
(Zoloft)

Do not confuse with Serentil.

CATEGORY AND SCHEDULE

Pregnancy Risk Category: C

MECHANISM OF ACTION

An antidepressant, antipanic, and obsessive-compulsive adjunct agent that blocks the reuptake of the neurotransmitter serotonin at CNS neuronal presynaptic membranes, increasing its availability at postsynaptic receptor sites. ***Therapeutic Effect:*** Produces antidepressant effect, reduces obsessive-compulsive behavior, decreases anxiety.

PHARMACOKINETICS

Incompletely, slowly absorbed from the GI tract; food increases absorption. Protein binding: 98%. Widely distributed. Undergoes extensive first-pass metabolism in liver to the active compound. Excreted in urine, eliminated in feces. Not removed by hemodialysis. ***Half-Life:*** 26 hrs.

AVAILABILITY

Tablets: 25 mg, 50 mg, 100 mg.
Oral Concentrate: 20 mg/mL.

INDICATIONS AND DOSAGES

▸ Antidepressant, obsessive-compulsive disorder

PO

Children 13–17 yrs. Initially, 50 mg/day with morning or evening meal. May increase by 50 mg/day at 7-day intervals. Maximum: 200 mg/day.
Children 6–12 yrs. Initially, 25 mg/day. May increase by 25–50 mg/day at 7-day intervals. Maximum: 200 mg/day.

CONTRAINDICATIONS

Hypersensitivity to sertraline or any related component. During or within 14 days of MAOI antidepressant therapy.

INTERACTIONS

Drug

Highly protein-bound medications (e.g., digoxin, warfarin): May increase the blood concentration and risk of toxicity with highly protein-bound medications.
MAOIs: May cause agitation, confusion, hyperpyretic convulsions, and serotonin syndrome, marked by diaphoresis, diarrhea, fever, mental changes, restlessness, shivering.

Herbal

St. John's wort: May increase the risk of adverse effects.

Food

None known.

DIAGNOSTIC TEST EFFECTS

May increase SGOT (AST), SGPT (ALT), serum total cholesterol, and triglyceride levels. May decrease serum uric acid levels.

SIDE EFFECTS

Frequent (26%–12%)
Headache, nausea, diarrhea, insomnia, drowsiness, dizziness, fatigue, rash, dry mouth
Occasional (6%–4%)
Anxiety, nervousness, agitation, tremor, dyspepsia, excessive sweating, vomiting, constipation, abnormal ejaculation, change in vision, change in taste
Rare (less than 3%)
Flatulence, urinary frequency, paresthesia, hot flashes, chills

SERIOUS REACTIONS

None known.

PEDIATRIC CONSIDERATIONS

Baseline Assessment

- Plan to perform complete blood counts and liver and renal function tests periodically for patients receiving long-term therapy.
- Be aware that it is unknown whether sertraline crosses the placenta or is distributed in breast milk.
- There are no age-related precautions in children older than 6 yrs of age.
- The safety and effectiveness of sertraline has not been established in children.
- Be aware that withdrawal symptoms can occur if the medication is stopped abruptly.
- Be aware that the use of sertraline in children and adolescents has been linked to suicide.

Precautions

- Use cautiously in patients with cardiac disease, liver impairment, and seizure disorders.
- Use cautiously in patients who have had a recent myocardial infarction and in suicidal-risk patients.

Administration and Handling

PO

- Give sertraline with food or milk if GI distress occurs.

Intervention and Evaluation

- Closely supervise suicidal-risk patients during early therapy. As depression lessens, the patient's energy level improves, which increases the suicide potential.
- Assess the patient's appearance, behavior, level of interest, mood, and speech pattern.
- Monitor the patient's pattern of daily bowel activity and stool consistency.
- Assist the patient with ambulation if he or she experiences dizziness.

Patient/Family Teaching

- Suggest to the patient/family that taking sips of tepid water and

chewing sugarless gum may relieve dry mouth.
• Warn the patient/family to notify the physician if the patient becomes pregnant or experiences fatigue, headache, sexual dysfunction, or tremor.
• Tell the patient/family to avoid tasks that require mental alertness or motor skills until the patient's response to the drug is established.
• Explain to the patient/family to take the drug with food if the patient experiences nausea.
• Urge the patient/family to avoid alcohol while taking sertraline.
• Explain to the patient/family not to take OTC medications without consulting the physician.

Trazodone Hydrochloride

tra-zoh-doan
(Desyrel)
Do not confuse with Delsym or Zestril.

CATEGORY AND SCHEDULE
Pregnancy Risk Category: C

MECHANISM OF ACTION
An antidepressant that blocks the reuptake of serotonin by CNS presynaptic neuronal membranes, increasing its availability at postsynaptic neuronal receptor sites. ***Therapeutic Effect:*** Produces antidepressant effect.

PHARMACOKINETICS
Well absorbed from the GI tract. Protein binding: 85%–95%. Metabolized in liver. Primarily excreted in urine. Unknown whether removed by hemodialysis. ***Half-Life:*** Adults: 5–9 hrs.

AVAILABILITY
Tablets: 50 mg, 100 mg, 150 mg, 300 mg.

INDICATIONS AND DOSAGES
▸ Antidepressant
PO
Children 6–18 yrs. Initially, 1.5–2 mg/kg/day in divided doses. May increase gradually to 6 mg/kg/day in 3 divided doses.
Adolescents. Initially, 25–50 mg/day. May increase to 100–150 mg/day in 2–3 divided doses.

UNLABELED USES
Treatment of neurogenic pain.

CONTRAINDICATIONS
Hypersensitivity to trazodone or any related component.

INTERACTIONS
Drug
Alcohol, CNS depressant-producing medications: May increase CNS depression.
Antihypertensives: May increase effects of antihypertensives.
Digoxin, phenytoin: May increase blood concentration of digoxin and phenytoin.
Fluoxetine: May increase trazodone serum concentrations.
Herbal
St. John's wort: May increase the adverse effects of trazodone.
Food
None known.

DIAGNOSTIC TEST EFFECTS
May decrease serum leukocyte and neutrophil counts.

SIDE EFFECTS
Frequent (9%–3%)
Drowsiness, dry mouth, lightheadedness or dizziness, headache, blurred vision, nausea or vomiting

Occasional (3%–1%)
Nervousness, fatigue, constipation, generalized aches and pains, mild hypotension

SERIOUS REACTIONS

! Priapism, marked by painful, prolonged penile erection, decreased or increased libido, retrograde ejaculation, and impotence have been noted rarely.

! Trazodone appears to be less cardiotoxic than other antidepressants, although arrhythmias may occur in patients with preexisting cardiac disease.

PEDIATRIC CONSIDERATIONS

Baseline Assessment

- Plan to perform complete blood counts and liver and renal function tests periodically for patients receiving long-term therapy.
- Be aware that trazodone crosses the placenta and is minimally distributed in breast milk.
- Be aware that the safety and efficacy of trazodone have not been established in children younger than 6 yrs of age.

Precautions

- Use cautiously in patients with arrhythmias and cardiac disease.

Administration and Handling

PO

- Give trazodone shortly after a meal or snack to reduce the risk of dizziness or lightheadedness.
- Crush tablets, as needed.

Intervention and Evaluation

- Closely supervise suicidal-risk patients during early therapy. As depression lessens, be aware that the patient's energy level generally improves, which increases the suicide potential.
- Assess the patient's appearance, behavior, level of interest, mood, and speech pattern.
- Monitor the patient's serum neutrophil and WBC counts. Stop administering the drug, as ordered, if these levels fall below normal.
- Assist the patient with ambulation if he or she experiences dizziness or lightheadedness.
- Assess EKG for arrhythmias.

Patient/Family Teaching

- Teach the patient/family that the patient may take trazodone after a meal or snack to try to avoid feeling dizzy or lightheaded.
- Teach the patient/family that the patient may take trazodone at bedtime if he or she experiences drowsiness while taking the drug.
- Warn the patient/family to immediately notify the physician if the patient experiences painful, prolonged penile erections.
- Instruct the patient/family to change positions slowly to avoid the hypotensive effect of the drug.
- Tell the patient/family that a tolerance to the anticholinergic and sedative effects of the drug usually develops during early therapy.
- Explain to the patient/family that the patient may develop photosensitivity to sunlight during trazodone therapy.
- Suggest to the patient/family that taking sips of tepid water and chewing sugarless gum may relieve dry mouth.
- Warn the patient/family to notify the physician if the patient experiences visual disturbances.
- Caution the patient/family against abruptly discontinuing the medication.

• Warn the patient/family to avoid tasks that require mental alertness or motor skills until the patient's response to the drug is established.
• Urge the patient/family to avoid alcohol while taking trazodone.

REFERENCES

Miller, S. & Fioravanti, J. (1997). Pediatric medications: a handbook for nurses. St. Louis: Mosby.
Taketomo, C. K., Hodding, J. H. & Kraus, D. M. (2003–2004). Pediatric dosage handbook (10th ed.). Hudson, OH: Lexi-Comp.

35 Antiemetics

Chlorpromazine
Dimenhydrinate
Dolasetron
Granisetron
Meclizine
Metoclopramide
Ondansetron Hydrochloride
Prochlorperazine
Trimethobenzamide Hydrochloride

Uses: Antiemetics are used to suppress vomiting (emesis). Resulting from chemotherapy, motion sickness, and other causes, emesis is a complex reflex caused by activation of the vomiting center in the medulla oblongata.

Action: Each subclass of antiemetics has a different mechanism of action. *Serotonin antagonists,* such as ondansetron, block serotonin receptors peripherally on vagal nerve terminals and centrally in the chemoreceptor trigger zone (CTZ). *Dopamine antagonists,* such as chlorpromazine, block dopamine receptors in the CTZ. *Anticholinergics,* such as scopolamine, block muscarinic receptors in the pathway from the inner ear to the vomiting center. *Antihistamines,* such as dimenhydrinate, block histamine (H_1) and muscarinic receptors in the pathway from the inner ear to the vomiting center. In addition, *palonosetron* antagonizes 5-hydroxytryptamine$_3$ (HT_3) receptors in the CTZ and peripherally.

Chlorpromazine

klor-**pro**-mah-zeen
(Chlorpromanyl [CAN], Largactil [CAN], Thorazine)
Do not confuse with chlorpropamide, thiamide, or thioridazine.

CATEGORY AND SCHEDULE

Pregnancy Risk Category: C

MECHANISM OF ACTION

A phenothiazine that blocks dopamine neurotransmission at postsynaptic dopamine receptor sites. Possesses strong anticholinergic, sedative, antiemetic effects; moderate extrapyramidal effects; slight antihistamine action.
Therapeutic Effect: Reduces psychosis; relieves nausea and vomiting; controls intractable hiccups and porphyria.

AVAILABILITY

Injection: 25 mg/mL.
Solution (concentrate): 100 mg/mL, 30 mg/mL.
Suppository: 25 mg, 100 mg.
Syrup: 10 mg/5 mL.
Tablets: 10 mg, 25 mg, 50 mg, 100 mg, 200 mg.

INDICATIONS AND DOSAGES

▸ **Psychosis**

IM/IV
Children older than 6 mos.
0.5–1 mg/kg q6–8h. Maximum (in children younger than 5 yrs): 40 mg/day. Maximum (in children 5–12 yrs): 75 mg/day.

PO
Children older than 6 mos.
0.5–1 mg/kg q4–6h.

▸ **Severe nausea or vomiting**
IM/IV
Children. 0.5–1 mg/kg q6–8h. Maximum (in children younger than 5 yrs): 40 mg/day. Maximum (in children 5–12 yrs): 75 mg/day.
PO
Children. 0.5–1 mg/kg q4–6h.
RECTAL
Children. 1 mg/kg q6–8h.

UNLABELED USES

Treatment of choreiform movement of Huntington's disease.

CONTRAINDICATIONS

Hypersensitivity to chlorpromazine or any related component. Bone marrow depression, comatose states, severe cardiovascular disease, severe CNS depression, subcortical brain damage.

INTERACTIONS

Drug

Alcohol, CNS depressants: May increase respiratory depression and the hypotensive effects of chlorpromazine.
Antithyroid agents: May increase the risk of agranulocytosis.
Extrapyramidal symptom–producing medications: Increased risk of extrapyramidal symptoms.
Hypotensives: May increase hypotension.
Levodopa: May decrease the effects of levodopa.
Lithium: May decrease the absorption of chlorpromazine and produce adverse neurologic effects.
MAOIs, tricyclic antidepressants: May increase the anticholinergic and sedative effects of chlorpromazine.

Herbal

None known.

Food

None known.

DIAGNOSTIC TEST EFFECTS

May produce false-positive pregnancy test and phenylketonuria. EKG changes may occur, including Q- and T-wave disturbances. Therapeutic serum level is 50–300 mcg/mL; toxic serum level is greater than 750 mcg/mL.

SIDE EFFECTS

Frequent
Drowsiness, blurred vision, hypotension, abnormal color vision, difficulty in night vision, dizziness, decreased sweating, constipation, dry mouth, nasal congestion
Occasional
Difficulty urinating, increased skin sensitivity to sun, skin rash, decreased sexual function, swelling or pain in breasts, weight gain, nausea, vomiting, stomach pain, tremors

SERIOUS REACTIONS

! Extrapyramidal symptoms appear to be dose related, particularly with high dosages, and are divided into 3 categories: akathisia, including inability to sit still, tapping of feet, and the urge to move around; parkinsonian symptoms, such as masklike face, tremors, shuffling gait, and hypersalivation; and acute dystonias, including torticollis or neck muscle spasm, opisthotonos or rigidity of back muscles, and oculogyric crisis or rolling back of eyes.
! Dystonic reaction may also produce profuse sweating and pallor.
! Tardive dyskinesia, including protrusion of tongue, puffing of cheeks, and chewing or puckering of the mouth, occurs rarely and may be irreversible.
! Abrupt withdrawal after long-term therapy may precipitate

nausea, vomiting, gastritis, dizziness, and tremors.
! Blood dyscrasias, particularly agranulocytosis or mild leukopenia, may occur. Blood dyscrasias may lower seizure threshold.

PEDIATRIC CONSIDERATIONS

Baseline Assessment

- Avoid skin contact with solution to prevent contact dermatitis.
- Assess the patient for signs and symptoms of dehydration including dry mucous membranes, longitudinal furrows in the tongue, and poor skin turgor.
- Assess the patient's appearance, behavior, emotional status, response to environment, speech pattern, and thought content.
- Extrapyramidal reactions are more common in pediatric patients who suffer from acute illnesses.

Precautions

- Use cautiously in patients with alcohol withdrawal, glaucoma, history of seizures, hypocalcemia (increases susceptibility to dystonias), impaired cardiac, liver, renal, or respiratory function, prostatic hypertrophy, and urinary retention.

Intervention and Evaluation

- Monitor the patient's blood pressure for hypotension.
- Assess the patient for extrapyramidal symptoms.
- Monitor the patient for signs of tardive dyskinesia, such as tongue protrusion.
- Regularly check the patient's complete blood count, as ordered, for blood dyscrasias.
- Monitor serum calcium levels to determine whether hypocalcemia is present.
- Supervise the suicidal-risk patient closely during early therapy because as the patient's depression lessens and his or her energy level improves, the risk for suicide increases.
- Assess the patient for therapeutic response, including increased ability to concentrate, improvement in self-care, an interest in surroundings, and a relaxed facial expression.
- Monitor the patient's therapeutic serum level. Know that the therapeutic serum level for chlorpromazine is 50–300 mcg/mL and the toxic serum level is greater than 750 mcg/mL.

Patient/Family Teaching

- Explain to the patient/family that a full therapeutic response may take up to 6 wks to appear.
- Advise the patient/family that the patient's urine may darken.
- Caution the patient/family against abruptly withdrawing from long-term drug therapy.
- Warn the patient/family to notify the physician if the patient experiences visual disturbances.
- Advise the patient/family that drowsiness generally subsides during continued therapy.
- Warn the patient/family to avoid tasks that require mental alertness or motor skills until the patient's response to the drug is established.
- Urge the patient/family to avoid alcohol while taking chlorpromazine.
- Instruct the patient/family to avoid exposure to sunlight.

Dimenhydrinate 

die-men-**high**-drin-ate
(Dramamine)

CATEGORY AND SCHEDULE

Pregnancy Risk Category: B
OTC

MECHANISM OF ACTION

An antihistamine and anticholinergic that competes for H_1 receptor sites on effector cells of the GI tract, blood vessels, and respiratory tract. The anticholinergic action diminishes vestibular stimulation and depresses labyrinthine function. ***Therapeutic Effect:*** Prevents symptoms of motion sickness.

AVAILABILITY

Chewable Tablets: 50 mg.
Tablets: 50 mg.

INDICATIONS AND DOSAGES

▸ Motion sickness

PO

Children older than 12 yrs. 50–100 mg q4–6h. Maximum: 400 mg/day.
Children 6–12 yrs. 25–50 mg q6–8h. Maximum: 150 mg/day.
Children 2–5 yrs. 12.5–25 mg q6–8h. Maximum: 75 mg/day.

CONTRAINDICATIONS

Hypersensitivity to dimenhydrinate or any related component.

INTERACTIONS

Drug

Aminoglycosides: Masks signs and symptoms of ototoxicity associated with aminoglycosides.
CNS depressants: Increases sedation with CNS depressants.
Other anticholinergics: Increases anticholinergic effect with other anticholinergics.

Herbal

None known.

Food

None known.

DIAGNOSTIC TEST EFFECTS

None known.

SIDE EFFECTS

Occasional

Hypotension, palpitations, tachycardia, headache, drowsiness, dizziness, paradoxical stimulation, especially in children, anorexia, constipation, dysuria, blurred vision, ringing in the ears, wheezing, chest tightness

Rare

Photosensitivity, rash, urticaria

SERIOUS REACTIONS

None significant.

PEDIATRIC CONSIDERATIONS

Baseline Assessment

- Assess the patient's other medical conditions, such as asthma, glaucoma, prostatic hypertrophy, and seizures.
- Establish the patient's medication history, especially concurrent use of other anticholinergics and CNS depressants.

Precautions

- Use cautiously in patients with asthma, bladder neck obstruction, a history of seizures, narrow-angle glaucoma, and prostatic hypertrophy.

Administration and Handling

PO

- Give with water.

Intervention and Evaluation

- Monitor the patient's blood pressure and for a paradoxical reaction, especially in children, and signs and symptoms of motion sickness.

Patient/Family Teaching

- Warn the patient/family to avoid tasks requiring mental alertness or motor skills until the patient's response to the drug is established.
- Tell the patient/family that dimenhydrinate may cause drowsiness and dry mouth.

• Urge the patient/family to avoid alcohol during dimenhydrinate therapy.
• Caution the patient/family to avoid prolonged sun exposure because this may cause a photosensitivity reaction.

Dolasetron

dole-**ah**-seh-tron
(Anzemet)
Do not confuse with Aldomet.

CATEGORY AND SCHEDULE

Pregnancy Risk Category: B

MECHANISM OF ACTION

An antiemetic that exhibits selective 5-HT_3 receptor antagonism. Action may occur centrally in the CTZ or peripherally on the vagal nerve terminals. ***Therapeutic Effect:*** Prevents nausea and vomiting.

PHARMACOKINETICS

Oral form readily absorbed from the GI tract. Protein binding: 69%–77%. Metabolized in liver. Primarily excreted in urine. Unknown whether removed by hemodialysis. ***Half-Life:*** 5–10 hrs.

AVAILABILITY

Tablets: 50 mg, 100 mg.
Injection: 20 mg/mL.

INDICATIONS AND DOSAGES

▸ **Prevention of chemotherapy-induced nausea and vomiting**

IV
Children 1–16 yrs. 1.8 mg/kg as a single dose 30 min before chemotherapy. Maximum: 100 mg.

PO
Children 2–16 yrs. 1.8 mg/kg within 1 hr of chemotherapy. Maximum: 100 mg.

▸ **Treatment and prevention of postoperative nausea or vomiting**

IV
Children 2–16 yrs. 0.35 mg/kg. Maximum: 12.5 mg. Give approximately 15 min before cessation of anesthesia or as soon as nausea presents.

PO
Children 2–16 yrs. 1.2 mg/kg. Maximum: 100 mg within 2 hrs of surgery.

UNLABELED USES

Radiation therapy–induced nausea and vomiting.

CONTRAINDICATIONS

Hypersensitivity to dolasetron or any related component.

INTERACTIONS

Drug

Cimetidine: Increased activity of dolasetron.
Rifampin: May decrease effectiveness of dolasetron.
Atenolol: May increase cardiac complications.

Herbal

None known.

Food

None known.

DIAGNOSTIC TEST EFFECTS

May alter liver function tests.

IV INCOMPATIBILITIES

No information available via Y-site administration.

SIDE EFFECTS

Frequent (10%–5%)
Headache, diarrhea, fatigue

Occasional (5%–1%)
Fever, dizziness, tachycardia, dyspepsia

SERIOUS REACTIONS

! Overdose may produce a combination of CNS stimulation and depressant effects.
! May prolong the QTc interval when used in patients with hypokalemia and hypomagnesemia and patients receiving antiarrhythmic medications or diuretics.

PEDIATRIC CONSIDERATIONS

Baseline Assessment

- Assess the patient for signs and symptoms of dehydration, including dry mucous membranes, longitudinal furrows in the tongue, and poor skin turgor, if he or she experiences excessive vomiting.
- Be aware that it is unknown whether dolasetron is distributed in breast milk.
- Be aware that the safety and efficacy of this drug have not been established in children younger than 2 yrs.

Precautions

- Use cautiously in patients with congenital QT syndrome, hypokalemia, hypomagnesemia, and prolongation of cardiac conduction intervals.
- Use cautiously in patients taking diuretics with the potential for inducing electrolyte disturbances and antiarrhythmics that may lead to QT prolongation and those receiving cumulative high-dose anthracycline therapy.

Administration and Handling

PO

- Do not cut, break, or chew film-coated tablets.
- For children 2–16 yrs of age, mix injection form in apple or apple-grape juice, if needed, for oral dosing at 1.8 mg/kg up to a maximum of 100 mg.

IV

- Store vials at room temperature.
- After dilution, store solution for up to 24 hrs at room temperature or up to 48 hrs if refrigerated.
- May dilute in 0.9% NaCl, D_5W, D_5W with 0.45% NaCl, D_5W with lactated Ringer's solution, lactated Ringer's solution, or 10% mannitol injection to 50 mL.
- Can be given as IV push as rapidly as 100 mg/30 sec.
- Give intermittent IV infusion or piggyback over 15 min.

Intervention and Evaluation

- Monitor the patient for therapeutic relief from nausea or vomiting.
- Monitor the EKG for high-risk patients.
- Maintain a quiet, supportive atmosphere.
- Offer the patient emotional support.

Patient/Family Teaching

- Tell postoperative patient/family to report nausea as soon as it occurs. Know that prompt administration of the drug increases its effectiveness.
- Warn the patient/family not to cut, break, or chew film-coated tablets.
- Teach the patient/family other methods of reducing nausea, such as lying quietly and avoiding strong odors.

Granisetron

gran-**is**-eh-tron
(Kytril)

CATEGORY AND SCHEDULE

Pregnancy Risk Category: B

MECHANISM OF ACTION

An antiemetic that selectively blocks serotonin stimulation at receptor sites on abdominal vagal afferent nerve and CTZ. ***Therapeutic Effect:*** Prevents nausea, vomiting.

PHARMACOKINETICS

Route	Onset	Peak	Duration
IV	1–3 min	N/A	24 hrs

Rapidly, widely distributed to tissues. Protein binding: 65%. Metabolized in liver to the active metabolite. Excreted in urine, eliminated in feces. ***Half-Life:*** Adults: 3–4 hrs. Adult cancer patients: 10–12 hrs.

AVAILABILITY

Tablets: 1 mg.
Injection: 1 mg/mL.
Oral Solution: 1 mg/5 mL.

INDICATIONS AND DOSAGES

▸ Prophylaxis of chemotherapy-induced nausea and vomiting

IV

Children 2 yrs and older.
10 mcg/kg/dose (or 1 mg/dose) given within 30 min of chemotherapy.

▸ Postoperative nausea or vomiting

PO

Children 4 yrs and older. 20–40 mcg/kg as a single postoperative dose. Maximum: 1 mg.

UNLABELED USES

Prophylaxis of nausea or vomiting associated with cancer radiotherapy and radiation therapy.

CONTRAINDICATIONS

Hypersensitivity to granisetron or any related component.

INTERACTIONS

Drug

Liver enzyme inducers: May decrease the effects of granisetron.

Herbal

None known.

Food

None known.

DIAGNOSTIC TEST EFFECTS

May increase SGOT (AST) and SGPT (ALT) levels.

IV INCOMPATIBILITIES

Amphotericin B (Fungizone)

IV COMPATIBILITIES

Allopurinol (Aloprim), bumetanide (Bumex), calcium gluconate, carboplatin (Paraplatin), cisplatin (Platinol), cyclophosphamide (Cytoxan), cytarabine (ARA-C), dacarbazine (DTIC), dexamethasone (Decadron), diphenhydramine (Benadryl), docetaxel (Taxotere), doxorubicin (Adriamycin), etoposide (VePesid), gemcitabine (Gemzar), magnesium, mitoxantrone (Novantrone), paclitaxel (Taxol), potassium

SIDE EFFECTS

Frequent (21%–14%)

Headache, constipation, asthenia (loss of strength)

Occasional (8%–6%)

Diarrhea, abdominal pain

Rare (less than 2%)

Altered taste, hypersensitivity reaction

SERIOUS REACTIONS

None known.

PEDIATRIC CONSIDERATIONS

Baseline Assessment

- Ensure that granisetron is given to the patient within 30 min of the start of chemotherapy.

• Be aware that it is unknown whether granisetron is distributed in breast milk.
• Be aware that the safety and efficacy of granisetron have not been established in children younger than 2 yrs of age.

Precautions

• Use cautiously in patients younger than 2 yrs of age.

Administration and Handling

◂ **ALERT** ▸ Administer only on days of chemotherapy, as prescribed.

IV

• Solution normally appears clear and colorless. Inspect for particulates and discoloration.
• Store at room temperature.
• After dilution, solution is stable for at least 24 hrs at room temperature.
• Give undiluted or dilute with 20–50 mL 0.9% NaCl or D_5W. Do not mix with other medications.
• Give undiluted as IV push over 30 sec.
• For IV piggyback, infuse over 5–20 min depending on volume of diluent used.

Intervention and Evaluation

• Monitor the patient for therapeutic effect.
• Assess the patient for headache.
• Assess the patient's daily pattern of bowel activity and stool consistency.

Patient/Family Teaching

• Tell the patient/family that granisetron is effective shortly after administration and that the drug prevents nausea and vomiting.
• Explain to the patient/family that a transitory taste disorder may occur.
• Help the patient/family use other methods of reducing nausea and vomiting, such as lying quietly and avoiding strong odors.

Meclizine

mek-lih-zeen
(Antivert, Bonamine [CAN], Bonine)

CATEGORY AND SCHEDULE

Pregnancy Risk Category: B
OTC

MECHANISM OF ACTION

An anticholinergic that reduces labyrinth excitability and diminishes vestibular stimulation of labyrinth, affecting the CTZ. Possesses anticholinergic activity. ***Therapeutic Effect:*** Reduces nausea, vomiting, vertigo.

PHARMACOKINETICS

Route	Onset	Peak	Duration
PO	30–60 min	N/A	12–24 hrs

Well absorbed from the GI tract. Widely distributed. Metabolized in liver. Primarily excreted in urine. ***Half-Life:*** 6 hrs.

AVAILABILITY

Tablets: 12.5 mg, 25 mg, 50 mg.
Tablets (chewable): 25 mg.

INDICATIONS AND DOSAGES

▸ **Motion sickness**

PO

Children 12 yrs and older. 2.5–25 mg 1 hr before travel. May repeat q12–24h. May require a dose of 50 mg.

▸ **Vertigo**

PO

Children 12 yrs and older. 25–100 mg/day in divided doses, as needed.

CONTRAINDICATIONS

Hypersensitivity to meclizine or any related component.

INTERACTIONS

Drug

Alcohol, CNS depression–producing medications: May increase CNS depressant effect.

Herbal

None known.

Food

None known.

DIAGNOSTIC TEST EFFECTS

May suppress wheal and flare reactions to antigen skin testing, unless meclizine discontinued 4 days before testing.

SIDE EFFECTS

Frequent

Drowsiness

Occasional

Blurred vision, dry mouth, nose, or throat

SERIOUS REACTIONS

! Children may experience dominant paradoxical reaction, including restlessness, insomnia, euphoria, nervousness, and tremors.

! Overdosage in children may result in hallucinations, convulsions, and death.

! Hypersensitivity reaction, marked by eczema, pruritus, rash, cardiac disturbances, and photosensitivity, may occur.

! Overdosage may vary from CNS depression, such as sedation, apnea, cardiovascular collapse, or death, to severe paradoxical reaction, including hallucinations, tremor, or seizures.

PEDIATRIC CONSIDERATIONS

• Be aware that it is unknown whether meclizine crosses the placenta or is distributed in breast milk. Keep in mind that meclizine use may produce irritability in breast-feeding infants.

• Be aware that children may be more sensitive to the drug's anticholinergic effects, such as dry mouth.

• Be aware that young children are more prone to excitability with this medication.

Precautions

• Use cautiously in patients with narrow-angle glaucoma and obstructive diseases of the GI or GU tract.

Administration and Handling

PO

• Give meclizine without regard to meals.

• Crush scored tablets as needed.

• Do not crush, open, or break capsule form.

Intervention and Evaluation

• Monitor the patient's blood pressure.

• Monitor pediatric patients closely for a paradoxical reaction.

• Monitor the serum electrolytes in patients experiencing severe vomiting.

• Assess the patient's mucous membranes and skin turgor to evaluate his or her hydration status.

Patient/Family Teaching

• Explain to the patient/family that a tolerance to the drug's sedative effect may occur.

• Warn the patient/family to avoid tasks that require mental alertness or motor skills until the patient's response to the drug is established.

• Explain to the patient/family that the patient should expect dizziness, drowsiness, and dry mouth as responses to the drug.

• Warn the patient/family to avoid alcohol during meclizine therapy.

• Suggest to the patient/family that taking sips of tepid water and chewing sugarless gum may help relieve dry mouth.

• Tell the patient/family that coffee or tea may help reduce drowsiness.

Metoclopramide

meh-tah-**klo**-prah-myd
(Apo-Metoclop [CAN], Pramin [AUS], Reglan)
Do not confuse with Renagel.

CATEGORY AND SCHEDULE

Pregnancy Risk Category: B

MECHANISM OF ACTION

A dopamine receptor antagonist that stimulates motility of the upper GI tract. Decreases reflux into esophagus. Raises threshold activity of CTZ. ***Therapeutic Effect:*** Accelerates intestinal transit and gastric emptying. Produces antiemetic activity.

PHARMACOKINETICS

Route	Onset	Peak	Duration
PO	30–60 min	N/A	N/A
IM	10–15 min	N/A	N/A
IV	1–3 min	N/A	N/A

Well absorbed from GI tract. Metabolized in liver. Protein binding: 30%. Primarily excreted in urine. Not removed by hemodialysis. ***Half-Life:*** 2.5–6 hrs.

AVAILABILITY

Tablets: 5 mg, 10 mg.
Syrup: 5 mg/5 mL.
Injection: 5 mg/mL.

INDICATIONS AND DOSAGES

▸ Symptomatic gastroesophageal reflux

PO

Children. 0.4–0.8 mg/kg/day in 4 divided doses.

▸ Prevention of cancer chemotherapy-induced nausea and vomiting

IV

Children. 1–2 mg/kg/dose 30 min before chemotherapy; repeat q2h for 2 doses, then q3h as needed.

▸ To facilitate small bowel intubation (single dose)

IV

Children 6–14 yrs. 2.5–5 mg.
Children younger than 6 yrs. 0.1 mg/kg.
Children older than 14 yrs. 10 mg over 1–2 minutes.

▸ Postoperative nausea and vomiting

IV

Children older than 14 yrs. 10 mg; repeat q6–8h as needed.
Children 14 yrs and younger. 0.1–0.2 mg/kg/dose; repeat q6–8h as needed.

▸ Dosage in renal impairment

Creatinine Clearance	% of normal dose
40–50 mL/min	75%
10–40 mL/min	50%
Less than 10 mL/min	25%–50%

UNLABELED USES

Prophylaxis of aspiration pneumonia, treatment of drug-related postoperative nausea and vomiting, persistent hiccups, slow gastric emptying, vascular headaches.

CONTRAINDICATIONS

Hypersensitivity to metoclopramide or any related component. Concurrent use of medications likely to produce extrapyramidal reactions, GI hemorrhage, GI obstruction or perforation, history of seizure disorders, pheochromocytoma.

INTERACTIONS

Drug

Alcohol: May increase CNS depressant effect.
CNS depressants: May increase sedative effect.
MAOIs: May increase hypertension episodes.

Herbal

None known.

Food

None known.

DIAGNOSTIC TEST EFFECTS

May increase aldosterone and prolactin concentrations

IV INCOMPATIBILITIES

Allopurinol (Aloprim), cefepime (Maxipime), doxorubicin liposome (Doxil), furosemide (Lasix), propofol (Diprivan)

IV COMPATIBILITIES

Dexamethasone, diltiazem (Cardizem), diphenhydramine (Benadryl), fentanyl (Sublimaze), heparin, hydromorphone (Dilaudid), morphine, potassium chloride

SIDE EFFECTS

Frequent (10%)
Drowsiness, restlessness, fatigue, lassitude
Occasional (3%)
Dizziness, anxiety, headache, insomnia, breast tenderness, altered menstruation, constipation, rash, dry mouth, galactorrhea, gynecomastia
Rare (less than 3%)
Hypotension or hypertension, tachycardia

SERIOUS REACTIONS

! Extrapyramidal reactions occur most frequently in children and young adults (18–30 yrs) receiving large doses (2 mg/kg) during cancer chemotherapy and is usually limited to akathisia or motor restlessness, involuntary limb movement, and facial grimacing.

PEDIATRIC CONSIDERATIONS

Baseline Assessment

- Assess the patient taking metoclopramide as an antiemetic for signs of dehydration, such as dry mucous membranes, longitudinal furrows in tongue, and poor skin turgor.
- Be aware that metoclopramide crosses the placenta and is distributed in breast milk.
- Be aware that children are more susceptible to having dystonia reactions.
- There is an increased incidence of extrapyramidal reactions and CNS effects when metoclopramide is administered to children.

Precautions

- Use cautiously in patients with cirrhosis, congestive heart failure, and impaired renal function.

Administration and Handling

◂ ALERT ▸ May give PO, IM, IV push, or IV infusion.

◂ ALERT ▸ Know that doses of 2 mg/kg or more or an increase in length of therapy may result in a greater incidence of side effects.

PO

- Give 30 min before meals and at bedtime.
- Crush tablets as needed.

IV

- Store vials at room temperature.
- After dilution, IV piggyback infusion is stable for 48 hrs.
- Dilute doses greater than 10 mg in 50 mL D_5W, 0.9% NaCl, or lactated Ringer's solution.
- Infuse over at least 15 min.
- May give slow IV push at rate of 10 mg over 1–2 min.

• A too-rapid IV injection may produce intense feelings of anxiety or restlessness, followed by drowsiness.

Intervention and Evaluation

• Monitor the patient for anxiety, extrapyramidal symptoms, and restlessness during IV administration.
• Assess the patient's pattern of daily bowel activity and stool consistency.
• Assess the patient for periorbital edema.
• Assess the patient's skin for rash and urticaria.
• Evaluate the patient for therapeutic response from gastroparesis, such as relief from nausea, persistent fullness after meals, and vomiting.
• Monitor the patient's blood pressure, heart rate, and BUN and serum creatinine levels to assess renal function.

Patient/Family Teaching

• Warn the patient/family to avoid tasks that require mental alertness or motor skills until the patient's response to the drug is established.
• Tell the patient/family to notify the physician if the patient experiences involuntary eye, facial, or limb movement or signs of an extrapyramidal reaction.
• Urge the patient/family to avoid alcohol during metoclopramide therapy.

Ondansetron Hydrochloride

on-**dan**-sah-tron
(Zofran)
Do not confuse with Zantac and Zosyn.

CATEGORY AND SCHEDULE

Pregnancy Risk Category: B

MECHANISM OF ACTION

An antiemetic and antinausea agent that blocks serotonin, both peripherally on vagal nerve terminals and centrally in the CTZ. ***Therapeutic Effect:*** Prevents nausea and vomiting.

PHARMACOKINETICS

Readily absorbed from the GI tract. Protein binding: 70%–76%. Metabolized in liver. Primarily excreted in urine. Unknown whether removed by hemodialysis. ***Half-Life:*** 2–5 hrs.

AVAILABILITY

Tablets: 4 mg, 8 mg, 24 mg.
Oral Disintegrating Tablets: 4 mg, 8 mg.
Oral Solution: 4 mg/5 mL.
Injection: 2 mg/mL.
Injection (premix): 32 mg/50 mL.

INDICATIONS AND DOSAGES

▸ Prevention of chemotherapy-induced nausea and vomiting

IV

Children 4–18 yrs. 0.15 mg/kg/dose given 30 min before chemotherapy, then 4 and 8 hrs after chemotherapy.

PO

Children older than 11 yrs. 24 mg as a single dose 30 min before starting chemotherapy or 8 mg q8h (first dose 30 min before chemotherapy) then q12h for 1–2 days.

Children 4–11 yrs. 4 mg 30 min before chemotherapy and 4 and 8 hrs after chemotherapy, then 4 mg q8h for 1–2 days.

▸ Prevention of postoperative nausea, vomiting

IM/IV

Children weighing less than 40 kg. 0.1 mg/kg.

Children weighing 10 kg and more. 4 mg.

UNLABELED USES
Treatment of postoperative nausea, vomiting.

CONTRAINDICATIONS
Hypersensitivity to ondansetron or any related component.

INTERACTIONS
Drug
None known.
Herbal
None known.
Food
None known.

DIAGNOSTIC TEST EFFECTS
May transiently increase serum bilirubin, SGOT (AST), and SGPT (ALT) levels.

IV INCOMPATIBILITIES
Acyclovir (Zovirax), allopurinol (Aloprim), aminophylline, amphotericin B (Fungizone), amphotericin B complex (Abelcet, AmBisome, Amphotec), ampicillin (Polycillin), ampicillin/sulbactam (Unasyn), cefepime (Maxipime), cefoperazone (Cefobid), fluorouracil, lorazepam (Ativan), meropenem (Merrem IV), methylprednisolone (Solu-Medrol)

IV COMPATIBILITIES
Carboplatin (Paraplatin), cisplatin (Platinol), cyclophosphamide (Cytoxan), cytarabine (Cytosar), dacarbazine (DTIC-Dome), daunorubicin (Cerubidine), dexamethasone (Decadron), diphenhydramine (Benadryl), docetaxel (Taxotere), dopamine (Intropin), etoposide (VePesid), gemcitabine (Gemzar), heparin, hydromorphone (Dilaudid), ifosfamide (Ifex), magnesium, mannitol, mesna (Mesnex), methotrexate, metoclopramide (Reglan), mitomycin (Mutamycin), mitoxantrone (Novantrone), morphine, paclitaxel (Taxol), potassium chloride, teniposide (Vumon), topotecan (Hycamtin), vinblastine (Velban), vincristine (Oncovin), vinorelbine (Navelbine)

SIDE EFFECTS
Frequent (13%–5%)
Anxiety, dizziness, drowsiness, headache, fatigue, constipation, diarrhea, hypoxia, urinary retention
Occasional (4%–2%)
Abdominal pain, xerostomia or diminished saliva secretion, fever, feeling of cold, redness and pain at injection site, paresthesia, weakness
Rare (less than 1%)
Hypersensitivity reaction, including rash and itching, blurred vision

SERIOUS REACTIONS
! Overdose may produce a combination of CNS stimulation and depressant effects.

PEDIATRIC CONSIDERATIONS
Baseline Assessment
- Assess the patient for signs and symptoms of dehydration, including dry mucous membranes, longitudinal furrows in the tongue, and poor skin turgor, if he or she experiences excessive vomiting.
- Monitor serum bilirubin, SGOT (AST), and SGPT (ALT) levels.
- Be aware that it is unknown whether ondansetron crosses the placenta or is distributed in breast milk.
- Be aware that the safety and efficacy of ondansetron have not been established in children.

Administration and Handling

◀ **ALERT** ▶ Give all oral doses 30 min before chemotherapy and repeat at 8-hr intervals, as prescribed.

PO

Give ondansetron without regard to food.

IM

Inject into a large muscle mass, such as the gluteus maximus.

IV

- Store at room temperature.
- Solution is stable for 48 hrs after dilution.
- May give undiluted as IV push.
- For IV infusion, dilute with 50 mL D_5W or 0.9% NaCl before administration.
- Give IV push over 2–5 min.
- Give IV infusion over 15 min.

Intervention and Evaluation

- Offer the patient emotional support.
- Assess and record the patient's bowel sounds for peristalsis, and his or her daily pattern of bowel activity and stool consistency.
- Evaluate the patient's mental status.

Patient/Family Teaching

- Explain to the patient/family that relief from nausea and vomiting generally occurs shortly after drug administration.
- Urge the patient/family to avoid alcohol and barbiturates while taking ondansetron.
- Warn the patient/family to notify the physician if the patient experiences persistent vomiting.
- Advise the patient/family that ondansetron may cause dizziness or drowsiness.
- Teach the patient/family other methods of reducing nausea and vomiting, including lying quietly and avoiding strong odors.

Prochlorperazine

pro-klor-**pear**-ah-zeen
(Compazine, Stemetil [CAN], Stemzine [AUS])

Do not confuse with chlorpromazine or Copaxone.

CATEGORY AND SCHEDULE

Pregnancy Risk Category: C

MECHANISM OF ACTION

A phenothiazine that acts centrally to inhibit or block dopamine receptors in the CTZ and peripherally to block the vagus nerve in the GI tract. ***Therapeutic Effect:*** Relieves nausea and vomiting.

PHARMACOKINETICS

Route (Antiemetic)	Onset	Peak	Duration
Tablets, syrup	30–40 min	N/A	3–4 hrs
Extended-release	30–40 min	N/A	10–12 hrs
Rectal	60 min	N/A	3–4 hrs

Variably absorbed after PO administration. Widely distributed. Metabolized in liver and GI mucosa. Primarily excreted in urine. Unknown whether removed by hemodialysis. ***Half-Life:*** Adults: 23 hrs.

AVAILABILITY

Tablets: 5 mg, 10 mg.
Capsules (sustained release): 10 mg, 15 mg.
Suppository: 2.5 mg, 5 mg, 25 mg.
Syrup: 5 mg/5 mL.
Injection: 5 mg/mL.

INDICATIONS AND DOSAGES

▸ **Antiemetic**

PO

Children weighing more than 10 kg. 0.4 mg/kg/day in 3–4 divided doses.

▸ **Rectal**
Children weighing more than 10 kg. 0.4 mg/kg/day in 3–4 divided doses.
IM
Children weighing more than 10 kg. 0.1–0.15 mg/kg/dose.
▸ **Psychosis**
PO
Children 2–12 yrs. 2.5 mg 2–3 times/day. Maximum 2–5 yrs: 20 mg. Maximum 6–12 yrs: 25 mg.

CONTRAINDICATIONS

Hypersensitivity to prochlorperazine or any related component. Bone marrow suppression, CNS depression, coma, narrow-angle glaucoma, severe hypotension or hypertension, severe liver or cardiac impairment.

INTERACTIONS

Drug

Alcohol, CNS depressants: May increase CNS and respiratory depression and hypotensive effects of prochlorperazine.
Antihypertensives: May increase hypotension.
Antithyroid agents: May increase the risk of agranulocytosis.
Extrapyramidal symptom-producing medications: May increase extrapyramidal symptoms.
Levodopa: May decrease the effects of levodopa.
Lithium: May decrease the absorption of prochlorperazine and produce adverse neurologic effects.
MAOIs, tricyclic antidepressants: May increase the anticholinergic and sedative effects of prochlorperazine.

Herbal

None known.

Food

None known.

DIAGNOSTIC TEST EFFECTS

None known.

SIDE EFFECTS

Frequent

Drowsiness, hypotension, dizziness, fainting occur frequently after first dose, occasionally after subsequent dosing, and rarely with oral dosage.

Occasional

Dry mouth, blurred vision, lethargy, constipation/diarrhea, muscular aches, nasal congestion, peripheral edema, urinary retention

SERIOUS REACTIONS

! Extrapyramidal symptoms appear to be dose-related, particularly with high dosage, and are divided into 3 categories: akathisia, marked by the inability to sit still, tapping of feet, and the urge to move around; parkinsonian symptoms, including masklike face, tremors, shuffling gait, and hypersalivation; and acute dystonias, such as torticollis or neck muscle spasm, opisthotonos or rigidity of back muscles, and oculogyric crisis or rolling back of eyes. Dystonic reaction may also produce profuse sweating or pallor.
! Tardive dyskinesia, manifested by protrusion of the tongue, puffing of cheeks, and chewing or puckering of the mouth occurs rarely and may be irreversible.
! Abrupt withdrawal after long-term therapy may precipitate nausea, vomiting, gastritis, dizziness, and tremors.
! Blood dyscrasias, particularly agranulocytosis and mild leukopenia, and sore mouth, gums, or throat may occur.
! Prochlorperazine use may lower seizure threshold.

PEDIATRIC CONSIDERATIONS

Baseline Assessment

- Avoid skin contact with prochlorperazine solution because it may cause contact dermatitis.
- Assess the patient with nausea and vomiting for signs and symptoms of dehydration including dry mucous membranes, longitudinal furrows in the tongue, and poor skin turgor.
- Assess the psychotic patient's appearance, behavior, emotional status, response to the environment, speech pattern, and thought content.
- Be aware that prochlorperazine crosses the placenta and is distributed in breast milk.
- Be aware that the safety and efficacy of this drug have not been established in children younger than 2 yrs of age or weighing less than 9 kg.
- Never administer this medication to a child SC; tissue damage may occur.

Precautions

- Use cautiously in patients with Parkinson's disease and seizures and in patients younger than 2 yrs of age.

Administration and Handling

PO

- Give prochlorperazine without regard to meals.

PARENTERAL

- Note that the patient must remain recumbent for 30–60 min after drug administration, with his or her head in a low position with legs raised to minimize the hypotensive effect of the drug.

RECTAL

- Moisten suppository with cold water before inserting well into rectum.

IM

- Administer IM injections into a large muscle mass.
- Be aware that the IM solution contains sulfites which may cause an allergic reaction.

Intervention and Evaluation

- Monitor the patient's blood/pressure for hypotension.
- Assess the patient for extrapyramidal symptoms.
- Monitor the patient's complete blood count for blood dyscrasias.
- Evaluate the patient's fine tongue movement because it may be an early sign of tardive dyskinesia.
- Closely supervise suicidal-risk patients during early therapy. As depression lessens, be aware that the patient's energy level generally improves, which increases the suicide potential.
- Assess the patient for therapeutic response, improvement in self-care, increased ability to concentrate, interest in surroundings, and a relaxed facial expression.

Patient/Family Teaching

- Urge the patient/family to avoid alcohol and limit caffeine intake while taking prochlorperazine.
- Advise the patient/family that prochlorperazine may impair the patient's ability to perform tasks requiring mental alertness or physical coordination, such as driving.

Trimethobenzamide Hydrochloride

try-meth-oh-**benz**-ah-mide

(Tigan)

CATEGORY AND SCHEDULE

Pregnancy Risk Category: C

MECHANISM OF ACTION

An anticholinergic that acts at the CTZ in the medulla oblongata in the CNS. ***Therapeutic Effect:*** Relieves nausea and vomiting.

PHARMACOKINETICS

Route	Onset	Peak	Duration
PO	10–40 min	N/A	3–4 hrs
IM	15–30 min	N/A	2–3 hrs

Partially absorbed from the GI tract. Distributed primarily to liver. Metabolic fate unknown. Excreted in urine. ***Half-Life:*** Adults: 7–9 hrs.

AVAILABILITY

Capsules: 300 mg.
Suppositories: 100 mg, 200 mg.
Injection: 100 mg/mL.

INDICATIONS AND DOSAGES

▸ Control of nausea, vomiting

PO

Children weighing 13–41 kg. 100–200 mg 3–4 times/day.

RECTAL

Children weighing 13–41 kg. 100–200 mg 3–4 times/day.

Children weighing less than 13 kg. 100 mg 3–4 times/day. Do not use in premature or newborn infants.

CONTRAINDICATIONS

Hypersensitivity to benzocaine or similar local anesthetics; parenteral form in children, suppositories in premature infants or neonates.

INTERACTIONS

Drug

CNS depression–producing medications: May increase CNS depression.

Herbal

None known.

Food

None known.

DIAGNOSTIC TEST EFFECTS

None known.

SIDE EFFECTS

Frequent

Drowsiness

Occasional

Blurred vision, diarrhea, dizziness, headache, muscle cramps

Rare

Skin rash, seizures, depression, opisthotonus, Parkinson's syndrome, Reye's syndrome, marked by vomiting, seizures

SERIOUS REACTIONS

! Hypersensitivity reaction manifested as extrapyramidal symptoms, including muscle rigidity, and allergic skin reactions occurs rarely.

! Children may experience dominant paradoxical reaction, marked by restlessness, insomnia, euphoria, nervousness, or tremors.

! Overdosage may vary from CNS depression, manifested by sedation, apnea, cardiovascular collapse, and death to severe paradoxical reaction, characterized by hallucinations, tremor, and seizures.

PEDIATRIC CONSIDERATIONS

Baseline Assessment

- Assess the patient for signs and symptoms of dehydration, including dry mucous membranes, longitudinal furrows in the tongue, and poor skin turgor, if the patient experiences excessive vomiting.
- Be aware that it is unknown whether trimethobenzamide crosses the placenta or is distributed in breast milk.

• There are no age-related precautions noted in children.
• Avoid the parenteral form in children and suppositories in neonates.

Precautions

• Use cautiously in patients with dehydration, electrolyte imbalance, or high fever.

Administration and Handling

◀ **ALERT** ▶ Do not use the IV route because it produces severe hypotension.

PO

• Give trimethobenzamide without regard to meals.
• Do not crush, open, or break capsule form.

IM

• Give IM injection deeply into a large muscle mass, preferably the upper outer gluteus maximus.

RECTAL

• If suppository is too soft, chill for 30 min in the refrigerator or run cold water over the foil wrapper.
• Moisten suppository with cold water before inserting well into rectum.

Intervention and Evaluation

• Monitor the patient's blood pressure.
• Assess pediatric patients closely for signs of a paradoxical reaction.
• Monitor serum electrolytes in patients with severe vomiting.
• Measure the patient's intake and output; assess any emesis.
• Assess the patient's mucous membranes and skin turgor to evaluate hydration status.
• Observe the patient for extrapyramidal symptoms, such as hypersensitivity.

Patient/Family Teaching

• Tell the patient/family that trimethobenzamide use causes drowsiness. Warn the patient to avoid tasks requiring mental alertness or physical coordination.
• Warn the patient/family to notify the physician if the patient experiences headache or visual disturbances.
• Instruct the patient/family that dry mouth is an expected response to the medication. Suggest to the patient that taking sips of tepid water or chewing sugarless gum may relieve dry mouth.
• Teach the patient/family other methods of reducing nausea and vomiting, including lying quietly and avoiding strong odors.
• Tell the patient/family that relief from nausea or vomiting generally occurs within 30 min of drug administration.

REFERENCES

Miller, S. & Fioravanti, J. (1997). Pediatric medications: a handbook for nurses. St. Louis: Mosby.

Taketomo, C. K., Hodding, J. H. & Kraus, D. M. (2003–2004). Pediatric dosage handbook (10th ed.). Hudson, OH: Lexi-Comp.

36 Antimigraine Agents

Dihydroergotamine
Ergotamine
Tartrate

Uses: Antimigraine agents are used to treat migraine headaches with aura (also called classic migraine) or without aura (also called common migraine) in patients age 18 or older. The goal of treatment includes the relief of headache and accompanying symptoms and a return to baseline functioning. Antimigraine agents are commonly used with nondrug measures, such as lifestyle modification and avoidance of headache triggers.

Action: Two groups of antimigraine agents work by different mechanisms. *Triptans,* selectively stimulate serotonin (5-HT) receptors that inhibit neuropeptide release and vasodilation. Both actions are believed to reduce the pain associated with vascular headaches. *Ergot alkaloids,* such as ergotamine and dihydroergotamine, interact with neurotransmitter receptors, including serotonergic, dopaminergic, and alpha-adrenergic receptors. More specifically, they may stimulate specific subtypes of serotonin receptors. However, their exact mechanism of action is unknown.

Dihydroergotamine Ergotamine Tartrate

er-**got**-a-meen
(Ergodryl Mono [AUS], Ergomar Medihaler Ergotamine [CAN] Cafergot, Ergomar, Wigraine)
dihydroergotamine
(D.H.E., Dihydergot [AUS], Ergomar [CAN], Migranal)

CATEGORY AND SCHEDULE

Pregnancy Risk Category: X

MECHANISM OF ACTION

An ergotamine derivative, alpha-adrenergic blocker that directly stimulates vascular smooth muscle. May also have antagonist effects on serotonin. ***Therapeutic Effect:*** Peripheral and cerebral vasoconstriction.

PHARMACOKINETICS

Slow, incomplete absorption from the GI tract; rapid, extensive absorption rectally (ergotamine). Caffeine increases ergotamine absorption. Well absorbed nasally (dihydroergotamine). Protein binding: greater than 90% (dihydroergotamine). Undergoes extensive first-pass metabolism in liver. Metabolized to active metabolite. Eliminated in feces via biliary system. ***Half-Life:*** 21 hrs.

AVAILABILITY

Tablets: 1 mg, with 100 mg caffeine
Tablets (sublingual): 2 mg.

Injection: 1 mg/mL.
Nasal Spray: 0.5 mg/spray.
Suppository: 2 mg, with 100 mg caffeine.

INDICATIONS AND DOSAGES

▸ PO/sublingual (ergotamine)
Children. 1 mg at onset of headache, then 1 mg q30min. Maximum: 3 mg/episode.
IM/SC (DIHYDROERGOTAMINE)
Children: 1 mg at onset of headache, then 1 mg q1h. Maximum: 3 mg/day or 6 mg/wk.
INTRANASAL (DIHYDROERGOTAMINE)
Children: 1 spray into each nostril. Repeat in 15 min if needed. Maximum: 4 sprays/day or 8 sprays/wk.

CONTRAINDICATIONS

Hypersensitivity to ergotamine, dihydroergotamine, caffeine, or any related component. Pregnancy, coronary artery disease, hypertension, impaired liver or renal function, malnutrition, peripheral vascular diseases, such as thromboangiitis obliterans, syphilitic arteritis, severe arteriosclerosis, thrombophlebitis, Raynaud's disease, sepsis, severe pruritus.

INTERACTIONS

Drug

Beta-blockers, erythromycin: May increase the risk of vasospasm.
Ergot alkaloids, systemic vasoconstrictors: May increase pressor effect.
Nitroglycerin: May decrease the effect of nitroglycerin.
Protease inhibitors: May lead to severe peripheral ischemia.

Herbal

None known.

Food

None known.

DIAGNOSTIC TEST EFFECTS

None known.

SIDE EFFECTS

Occasional (5%–2%)
Cough, dizziness
Rare (less than 2%)
Muscle pain, fatigue, diarrhea, upper respiratory infection, dyspepsia
Nasal Spray: Pharyngitis, rhinitis, sneezing, nasal edema
Injection: Pleural pulmonary fibrosis, retroperitoneal fibrosis

SERIOUS REACTIONS

! Prolonged administration or excessive dosage may produce ergotamine poisoning manifested as nausea, vomiting, weakness of the legs, pain in limb muscles, numbness and tingling of fingers or toes, precordial pain, tachycardia or bradycardia, and hypertension or hypotension.
! Localized edema and itching due to vasoconstriction of peripheral arteries and arterioles may occur.
! Feet or hands will become cold, pale, and numb.
! Muscle pain will occur when walking and later even at rest.
! Gangrene may occur.
! Occasionally confusion, depression, drowsiness, and seizures appear.

PEDIATRIC CONSIDERATIONS

Baseline Assessment

- Determine the patient's history of peripheral vascular disease and liver or renal impairment.
- Carefully perform an assessment of the patient's peripheral circulation, including the temperature,

color, and strength of pulses in the extremities.
• Determine whether the patient is pregnant.
• Determine the duration, location, onset, and precipitating symptoms of the patient's migraine.
• Be aware that ergotamine use is contraindicated in pregnancy as it produces uterine stimulant action resulting in possible fetal death or retarded fetal growth and increases vasoconstriction of the placental vascular bed.
• Be aware that ergotamine is distributed in breast milk and may prohibit lactation.
• Be aware that ergotamine use may produce diarrhea or vomiting in the neonate.
• Keep in mind that ergotamine may be used safely in children older than 6 yrs, but only use when the patient is unresponsive to other medication.
• Keep in mind that dihydroergotamine should be used in children older than 12 yrs of age and only when the patient is unresponsive to other medications.

Administration and Handling

SUBLINGUAL
• Place under tongue and allow the tablet to dissolve, then swallow. Do not administer with water.

INTRANASAL
• Before administration, the nasal spray applicator should be primed (pumped 4 times). Spray once into each nostril; avoid deep inhalation through the nose while spraying or immediately after use. Do not tilt the head back.

IM/SC
• Administer undiluted.

Intervention and Evaluation

• Monitor the patient closely for evidence of ergotamine overdosage as result of prolonged administration or excessive dosage.

Patient/Family Teaching

• Instruct the patient/family to begin taking ergotamine at the first sign of a migraine headache.
• Tell the patient/family to notify the physician if the ergotamine dosage does not relieve vascular headaches, or if the patient experiences irregular heartbeat, nausea, numbness or tingling of the fingers and toes, pain or weakness of the extremities, and vomiting.
• Warn the patient/family to avoid pregnancy and to report any suspected pregnancy immediately to the physician. Explain to the patient that this drug is contraindicated in pregnancy. Teach the patient about other methods of contraception.

37 Antiparkinson Agents

Amantadine Hydrochloride

Uses: Antiparkinson agents are used to treat Parkinson's disease. They're prescribed to reduce parkinsonian signs and symptoms, to correct the disease-induced dopamine deficit, or both. In addition, some drugs in this class have other indications. For example, amantadine is used to treat viral respiratory infections and control extrapyramidal reactions.

Amantadine Hydrochloride

ah-**man**-tih-deen
(Endantadine [CAN], PMS-Amantadine [CAN], Symmetrel)

CATEGORY AND SCHEDULE

Pregnancy Risk Category: C

MECHANISM OF ACTION

A dopaminergic agonist that blocks the uncoating of influenza A virus, preventing penetration into the host, and inhibiting M2 protein in the assembly of progeny virions. Amantadine blocks the reuptake of dopamine into presynaptic neurons and causes direct stimulation of postsynaptic receptors. ***Therapeutic Effect:*** Antiviral and antiparkinson activity.

PHARMACOKINETICS

Rapidly, completely absorbed from the GI tract. Protein binding: 67%. Widely distributed. Primarily excreted in urine. Minimally removed by hemodialysis. ***Half-Life:*** 11-15 hrs (half-life decreased in impaired renal function).

AVAILABILITY

Capsule: 100 mg.
Syrup: 50 mg/5 mL.
Tablets: 100 mg.

INDICATIONS AND DOSAGES

▸ **Prophylaxis, symptomatic treatment of respiratory illness due to influenza A virus**

PO

Children 9-12 yrs. 100 mg 2 times/day. Maximum: 200 mg/day.
Children 1-8 yrs. 5 mg/kg/day 2 times/day. Maximum: 200 mg/day.

▸ **Dosage in renal impairment**

Dose and frequency are modified based on creatinine clearance.

Creatinine Interval Clearance	
30-50 mL/min	Give once daily.
15-29 mL/min	Give every other day.
Less than 15 mL/min	Give dose once weekly.

UNLABELED USES

Treatment of attention-deficit hyperactivity disorder and of fatigue associated with multiple sclerosis.

CONTRAINDICATIONS

Hypersensitivity to amantadine or any related component.

INTERACTIONS

Drug

Anticholinergics, antihistamines, phenothiazine, tricyclic antidepressants: May increase anticholinergic effects of amantadine.

Hydrochlorothiazide, triamterene: May increase amantadine blood concentration and risk for toxicity.
CNS stimulants: Additive stimulant effect.

Herbal
None known.

Food
None known.

DIAGNOSTIC TEST EFFECTS
None known.

SIDE EFFECTS
Frequent (10%–5%)
Nausea, dizziness, poor concentration, insomnia, nervousness
Occasional (5%–1%)
Orthostatic hypotension, anorexia, headache, livedo reticularis evidenced by reddish blue, netlike blotching of skin, blurred vision, urinary retention, dry mouth or nose
Rare
Vomiting, depression, irritation or swelling of eyes, rash

SERIOUS REACTIONS
! Congestive heart failure (CHF), leukopenia, and neutropenia occur rarely.
! Hyperexcitability, convulsions, and ventricular arrhythmias may occur.

PEDIATRIC CONSIDERATIONS

Baseline Assessment
- When treating infections caused by the influenza A virus, expect to obtain specimens for viral diagnostic tests before giving the first dose. Therapy may begin before test results are known.
- Be aware that it is unknown whether amantadine crosses the placenta or is distributed in breast milk.
- There are no age-related precautions noted in children younger than 1 yr of age.

Precautions
- Use cautiously in patients with cerebrovascular disease, CHF, a history of seizures, liver disease, orthostatic hypotension, peripheral edema, recurrent eczematoid dermatitis, and renal dysfunction and those receiving CNS stimulants.

Administration and Handling
PO
◂ **ALERT** ▸ Give as a single dose or in 2 divided doses.
- May give without regard to food.
- Administer nighttime dose several hours before bedtime to prevent insomnia.

Intervention and Evaluation
- Expect to monitor the patient's intake and output and renal function tests, if ordered.
- Check for peripheral edema. Assess the patient's skin for blotching or rash.
- Evaluate the patient's food tolerance and episodes of nausea or vomiting.
- Assess the patient for dizziness.

Patient/Family Teaching
- Advise the patient/family to continue therapy for the full length of treatment and to evenly space drug doses around the clock.
- Explain to the patient/family that the patient should not take any medications, including OTC drugs, without first consulting the physician.
- Warn the patient/family to avoid alcoholic beverages.
- Caution the patient/family not to drive, use machinery, or engage in other activities that require mental

acuity if the patient is experiencing dizziness or blurred vision.

- Teach the patient/family to get up slowly from a sitting or lying position.
- Stress to the patient/family that the patient should notify the physician of new symptoms, especially any blurred vision, dizziness, nausea or vomiting, and skin blotching or rash.
- Tell the patient/family to take the nighttime dose several hours before bedtime to prevent insomnia.

REFERENCES

Miller, S. & Fioravanti, J. (1997). Pediatric medications: a handbook for nurses. St. Louis: Mosby.

Taketomo, C. K., Hodding, J. H. & Kraus, D. M. (2003–2004). Pediatric dosage handbook (10th ed.). Hudson, OH: Lexi-Comp.

38 Antipsychotics

Haloperidol
Thioridazine
Thiothixene
Trifluoperazine Hydrochloride

Uses: Antipsychotics are used primarily to manage psychotic illness, especially in patients with increased psychomotor activity. They are also used to treat the manic phase of bipolar disorder, behavioral problems in children, nausea and vomiting, intractable hiccups, anxiety, and agitation. In addition, these agents are used to potentiate the effects of narcotics and, as adjuncts, to treat tetanus.

Action: Antipsychotic agents produce effects at all levels of the CNS. Although their exact mechanism of action is unknown, they may antagonize the action of dopamine as a neurotransmitter in the basal ganglia and limbic system. Antipsychotics may block postsynaptic dopamine receptors, inhibit dopamine release, or increase dopamine turnover.

This class of drugs can be divided into phenothiazines and nonphenothiazines. Besides their use in treating the symptoms of psychiatric illness, some have antiemetic, antinausea, antihistamine, anticholinergic, or sedative effects.

Haloperidol

hal-oh-**pear**-ih-dawl
(Apo-Haloperidol [CAN], Haldol, Novoperidol [CAN], Peridol [CAN], Serenace [AUS])
Do not confuse with Halcion, Halog, or Stadol.

CATEGORY AND SCHEDULE

Pregnancy Risk Category: C

MECHANISM OF ACTION

An antipsychotic, antiemetic, and antidyskinetic agent that competitively blocks postsynaptic dopamine receptors, interrupts nerve impulse movement, and increases turnover of brain dopamine. ***Therapeutic Effect:*** Produces tranquilizing, strong extrapyramidal and antiemetic effects and weak anticholinergic and sedative effects.

PHARMACOKINETICS

Readily absorbed from the GI tract. Crosses the placenta and appears in breast milk. Protein binding: 92%. Extensively metabolized in liver. Primarily excreted in urine. Not removed by hemodialysis. ***Half-Life:*** Adults: PO 12–37 hrs; IM 17–25 hrs, IV 10–19 hrs.

AVAILABILITY

Tablets: 0.5 mg, 1 mg, 2 mg, 5 mg, 10 mg, 20 mg.
Oral Concentrate: 2 mg/mL.
Injection: 5 mg/mL.
Injection (decanoate): 50 mg/mL, 100 mg/mL.

INDICATIONS AND DOSAGES

▸ **Treatment of psychoses, Tourette's disorder, severe behavioral problems in children, emergency sedation of severely agitated or delirious patients**

PO

Children 3–12 yrs weighing 15–40 kg. Initially, 0.25–0.5 mg/day in 2–3 divided doses. May increase by 0.25–0.5 mg q5–7 days. Maximum: 0.15 mg/kg/day.

IM/IV (LACTATE)

Children 6–12 yrs. 1–3 mg/dose q4–8h. Maximum: 0.15 mg/kg/day.

UNLABELED USES

Treatment of Huntington's chorea, infantile autism, nausea or vomiting associated with cancer chemotherapy.

CONTRAINDICATIONS

Hypersensitivity to haloperidol or any related component. Bone marrow suppression, CNS depression, narrow-angle glaucoma, parkinsonism, severe cardiac or liver disease.

INTERACTIONS

Drug

Alcohol, CNS depressants: May increase CNS depression.
Epinephrine: May block alpha-adrenergic effects.
Extrapyramidal symptom (EPS)–producing medications: May increase EPSs.
Lithium: May increase neurologic toxicity.
Fluoxetine: May increase toxic effects.
Carbamazepine, phenobarbital, rifampin: May decrease effectiveness of haloperidol.

Herbal

None known.

Food

Coffee, tea: May lead to precipitation if mixed with oral concentrate.

DIAGNOSTIC TEST EFFECTS

None known. Therapeutic serum level is 0.2–1 mcg/mL; toxic serum level is greater than 1 mcg/mL.

IV INCOMPATIBILITIES

Allopurinol (Aloprim), amphotericin B complex (Abelcet, AmBisome, Amphotec), cefepime (Maxipime), fluconazole (Diflucan), foscarnet (Foscavir), heparin, nitroprusside (Nipride), piperacillin-tazobactam (Zosyn)

IV COMPATIBILITIES

Dobutamine (Dobutrex), dopamine (Intropin), fentanyl (Sublimaze), hydromorphone (Dilaudid), lidocaine, lorazepam (Ativan), midazolam (Versed), morphine, nitroglycerin, norepinephrine (Levophed), propofol (Diprivan)

SIDE EFFECTS

Frequent

Blurred vision, constipation, orthostatic hypotension, dry mouth, swelling or soreness of female breasts, peripheral edema

Occasional

Allergic reaction, difficulty urinating, decreased thirst, dizziness, decreased sexual function, drowsiness, nausea, vomiting, photosensitivity, lethargy

SERIOUS REACTIONS

! Extrapyramidal symptoms appear to be dose-related and may be noted in first few days of therapy.
! Marked drowsiness and lethargy, excessive salivation, and fixed stare may be mild to severe in intensity.

! Less frequently seen are severe akathisia or motor restlessness and acute dystonias, such as torticollis or neck muscle spasm, opisthotonos or rigidity of back muscles, and oculogyric crisis or rolling back of eyes.

! Tardive dyskinesia or protrusion of tongue, puffing of cheeks, chewing or puckering of the mouth may occur during long-term administration or after drug discontinuance and may be irreversible. The risk is greater in female geriatric patients. Abrupt withdrawal after long-term therapy may provoke signs of transient dyskinesia.

PEDIATRIC CONSIDERATIONS

Baseline Assessment

• Assess the patient's appearance, behavior, emotional status, response to environment, speech pattern, and thought content.

• Be aware that haloperidol crosses the placenta and is distributed in breast milk.

• Be aware that children are more susceptible to dystonias and haloperidol use is not recommended in children younger than 3 yrs or those who weigh less than 15 kg.

• Be aware that a possible consequence of using haloperidol is neuroleptic malignant syndrome (e.g., fever, fast heartbeat, increased respiratory rate, seizures, and loss of urinary control).

Precautions

• Use cautiously in patients with cardiovascular disease, a history of seizures, and liver or renal dysfunction.

Administration and Handling

PO

• Give haloperidol without regard to meals.

• May give with food or milk if GI upset occurs.

• Oral concentrate may be mixed with 2 oz of water or acidic beverage. Do not mix with coffee or tea.

• Crush scored tablets as needed.

IM

• Patient must remain recumbent for 30–60 min in head-low position with the legs raised to minimize the hypotensive effect.

• Prepare haloperidol decanoate IM injection using 21-gauge needle.

• Do not exceed maximum volume of 3 mL per IM injection site.

• Give IM injection deeply and slowly into the upper, outer quadrant of the gluteus maximus.

IV

◂ ALERT ▸ Only haloperidol lactate is given IV.

• Discard if precipitate forms or discoloration occurs.

• Store at room temperature.

• Protect from light; do not freeze.

• May give undiluted for IV push.

• Flush with at least 2 mL 0.9% NaCl before and after administration.

• May add to 30–50 mL of most solutions, but D_5W is preferred.

• Give IV push at rate of 5 mg/min.

• Infuse IV piggyback over 30 min.

• For IV infusion, up to 25 mg/hr has been used, titrated to patient response.

Intervention and Evaluation

• Closely supervise suicidal-risk patients during early therapy. As depression lessens, the patient's energy level improves, which increases the suicide potential.

• Monitor the patient for fine tongue movement, a masklike facial expression, rigidity, and tremor.

• Assess the patient for a therapeutic response, including improvement in self-care, increased ability to concentrate, interest in surroundings, and relaxed facial expression.

• Know that the therapeutic serum level for haloperidol is 0.2–1 mcg/mL, and the toxic serum level of haloperidol is greater than 1 mcg/mL.

Patient/Family Teaching

• Tell the patient/family that the drug's full therapeutic effect may take up to 6 wks to appear.
• Caution the patient/family against abruptly withdrawing from long-term drug therapy.
• Suggest sips of tepid water and sugarless gum to patients to help relieve dry mouth.
• Tell the patient/family that drowsiness generally subsides during continued therapy.
• Warn the patient/family to avoid tasks that require mental alertness or motor skills until the patient's response to the drug is established.
• Urge the patient/family to avoid alcohol during haloperidol therapy.
• Warn the patient/family to notify the physician if the patient experiences muscle stiffness.
• Caution the patient/family to avoid exposure to sunlight and any conditions that may cause dehydration or be overheating because of an increased risk of heat stroke.

Thioridazine

thigh-oh-**rid**-ah-zeen
(Aldazine [AUS], Apo-Thioridazine [CAN]
Do not confuse with Mebaral, thiothixene, or Thorazine.

CATEGORY AND SCHEDULE

Pregnancy Risk Category: C

MECHANISM OF ACTION

A phenothiazine that blocks dopamine at postsynaptic receptor sites. Possesses strong anticholinergic, sedative effects. ***Therapeutic Effect:*** Suppresses behavioral response in psychosis, reducing locomotor activity and aggressiveness and suppressing conditioned responses.

AVAILABILITY

Tablets: 10 mg, 15 mg, 25 mg, 50 mg, 100 mg, 150 mg, 200 mg.
Oral Solution (concentrate): 30 mg/mL, 100 mg/mL.

INDICATIONS AND DOSAGES

▸ Psychosis

PO

Children older than 12 yrs. Initially, 25–100 mg 3 times/day. Gradually increase. Maximum: 800 mg/day.
Children 2–12 yrs. Initially, 0.5 mg/kg/day in 2–3 divided doses. Maximum: 3 mg/kg/day.

UNLABELED USES

Behavioral problems in children, dementia, depressive neurosis.

CONTRAINDICATIONS

Hypersensitivity to thioridazine or any related component. Drugs that prolong QT interval, cardiac arrhythmias, severe CNS depression, narrow-angle glaucoma, blood dyscrasias, liver or cardiac impairment.

INTERACTIONS

Drug

Alcohol, CNS depressants: May increase respiratory depression and the hypotensive effects of thioridazine.
Antithyroid agents: May increase the risk of agranulocytosis.

Extrapyramidal symptom (EPS)–producing medications: May increase EPSs.
Hypotensives: May increase hypotension.
Levodopa: May decrease the effects of levodopa.
Lithium: May decrease the absorption of thioridazine and produce adverse neurologic effects.
MAOIs, tricyclic antidepressants: May increase the anticholinergic and sedative effects of thioridazine.
Drugs that prolong the QTc interval, fluoxetine, fluvoxamine, paroxetine: Increase the risk for serious adverse effects including sudden death.

Herbal

None known.

Food

None known.

DIAGNOSTIC TEST EFFECTS

May cause EKG changes. Therapeutic serum level is 0.2–2.6 mcg/mL; toxic blood serum level is not established.

SIDE EFFECTS

Generally well tolerated with only mild and transient effects

Occasional

Drowsiness during early therapy, dry mouth, blurred vision, lethargy, constipation or diarrhea, nasal congestion, peripheral edema, urinary retention

Rare

Ocular changes, skin pigmentation in those taking high dosages for prolonged periods, photosensitivity

SERIOUS REACTIONS

! Prolongation of the QT interval may produce torsades de pointes, a form of ventricular tachycardia, and sudden death.

PEDIATRIC CONSIDERATIONS

Baseline Assessment

- Avoid skin contact with solution because it can cause contact dermatitis.
- Assess the patient's appearance, behavior, emotional status, response to environment, speech pattern, and thought content.
- Plan to obtain a baseline EKG and to measure the QT interval. Calculate the QTc interval.
- Do not use in children less than 2 yrs of age.
- Be aware that a possible consequence of thioridazine is neuroleptic malignant syndrome.

Precautions

- Use cautiously in patients with seizures.

Intervention and Evaluation

- Assess the patient for EPSs.
- Monitor the patient's blood pressure, complete blood count, EKG, eye examinations, liver function test results, including serum alkaline phosphatase, bilirubin, potassium, SGOT (AST), and SGPT (ALT) levels.
- Monitor the patient for fine tongue movement, which may be an early sign of tardive dyskinesia.
- Closely supervise suicidal-risk patients during early therapy. As depression lessens, the patient's energy level improves, which increases the suicide potential.
- Assess the patient for a therapeutic response, an improvement in self-care, an increased ability to concentrate, an interest in his or her surroundings, and a relaxed facial expression.
- Know the therapeutic serum level for thioridazine is 0.2–2.6 mcg/mL, and the toxic serum level for thioridazine is not established.

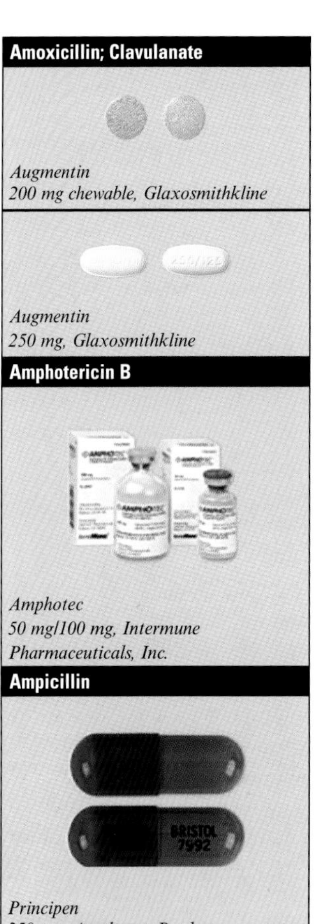

Amoxicillin; Clavulanate

Augmentin
200 mg chewable, Glaxosmithkline

Augmentin
250 mg, Glaxosmithkline

Amphotericin B

Amphotec
50 mg/100 mg, Intermune Pharmaceuticals, Inc.

Ampicillin

Principen
250 mg, Apothecon Products

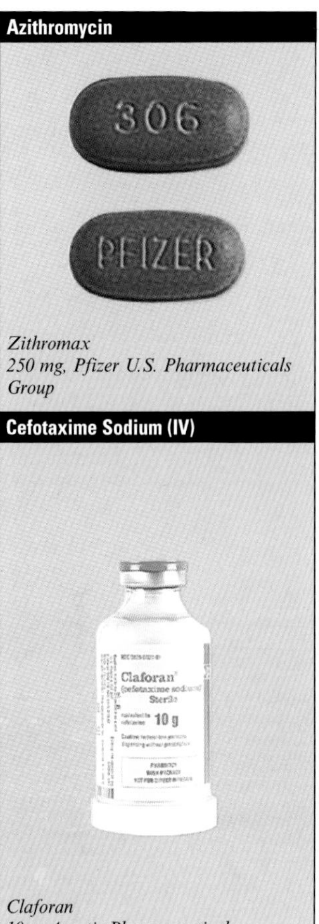

Azithromycin

Zithromax
250 mg, Pfizer U.S. Pharmaceuticals Group

Cefotaxime Sodium (IV)

Claforan
10 g, Aventis Pharmaceuticals

Cefuroxime Axetil (IV and PO)

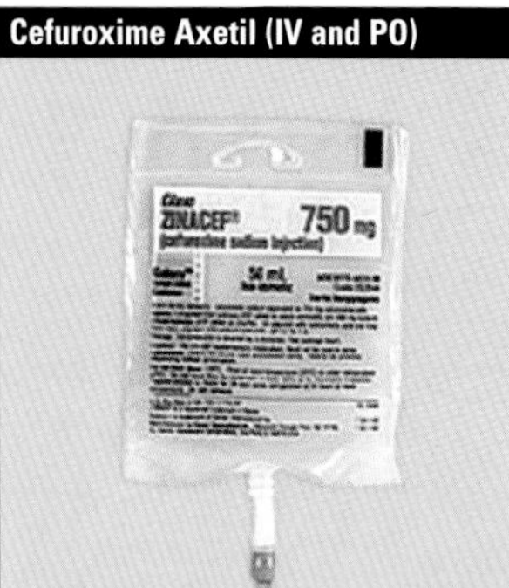

Zinacef
750 mg/50 ml, Glaxo Wellcome Inc.

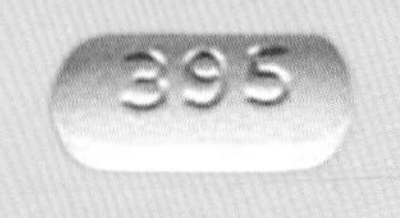

Ceftin
125 mg, Lifecycle Pharmaceuticals

Cimetidine (ch. 49) – Trade Name:

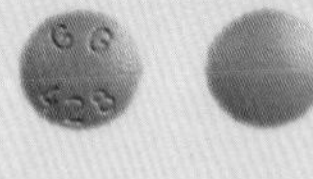

Cimetidine
300 mg, Geneva Pharmaceuticals, Inc.

Ciprofloxacin Hydrochloride (PO Form)

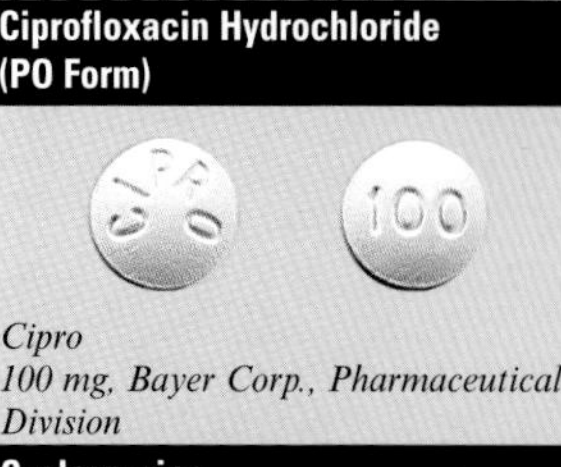

Cipro
100 mg, Bayer Corp., Pharmaceutical Division

Cyclosporine

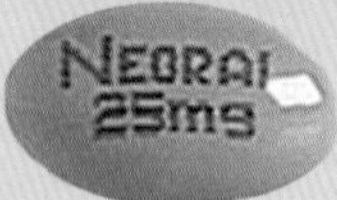

Neoral
25 mg, Novartis Pharmaceuticals Corporation

Dopamine Hydrochloride

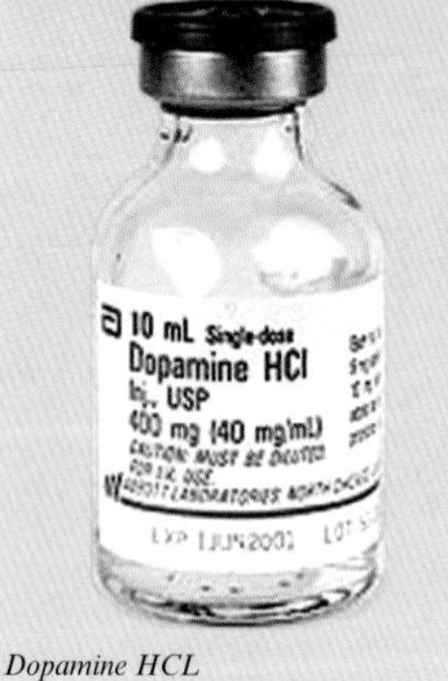

Dopamine HCL
400 mg, Abbott Laboratories

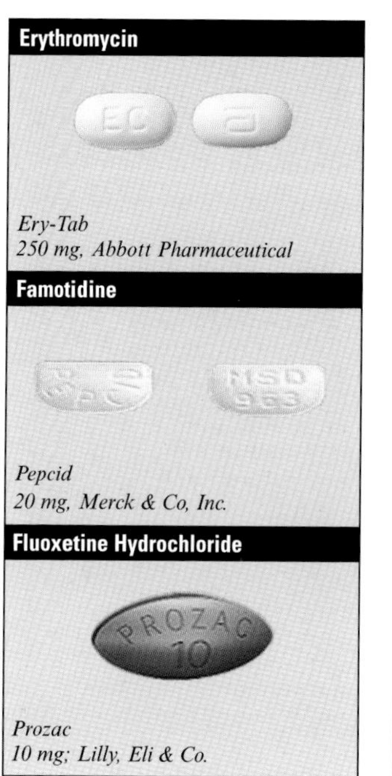

Erythromycin

Ery-Tab
250 mg, Abbott Pharmaceutical

Famotidine

Pepcid
20 mg, Merck & Co, Inc.

Fluoxetine Hydrochloride

Prozac
10 mg; Lilly, Eli & Co.

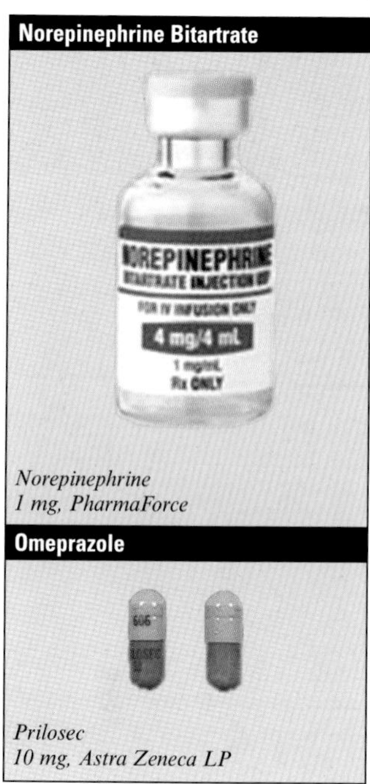

Norepinephrine Bitartrate

Norepinephrine
1 mg, PharmaForce

Omeprazole

Prilosec
10 mg, Astra Zeneca LP

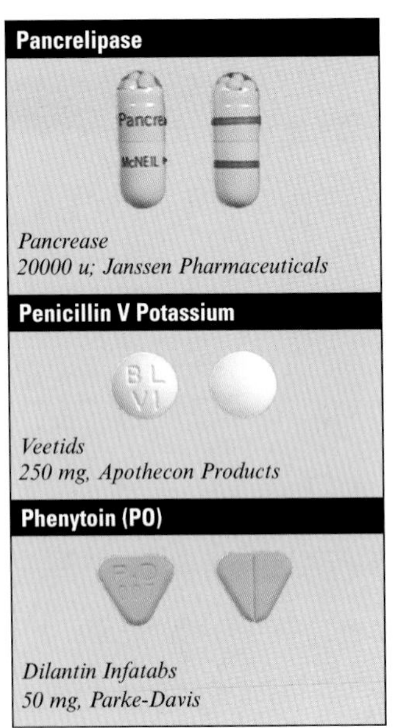

Pancrelipase

Pancrease
20000 u; Janssen Pharmaceuticals

Penicillin V Potassium

Veetids
250 mg, Apothecon Products

Phenytoin (PO)

Dilantin Infatabs
50 mg, Parke-Davis

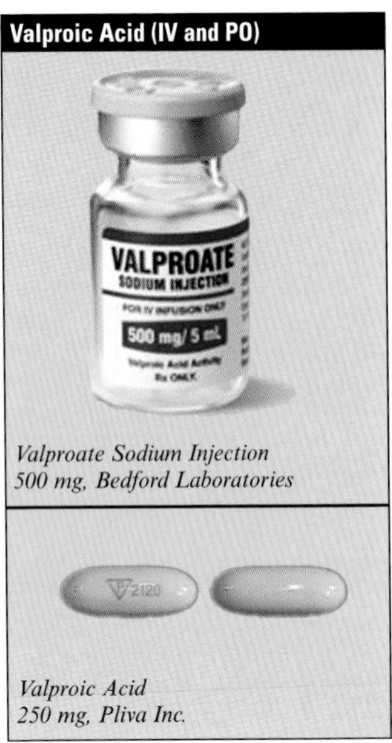

Valproic Acid (IV and PO)

Valproate Sodium Injection
500 mg, Bedford Laboratories

Valproic Acid
250 mg, Pliva Inc.

Patient/Family Teaching

• Tell the patient/family that the drug's full therapeutic effect may take up to 6 wks to appear.
• Explain to the patient/family that the patient's urine may darken.
• Caution the patient/family against abruptly withdrawing from long-term drug therapy.
• Warn the patient/family to notify the physician if the patient experiences visual disturbances.
• Suggest to the patient that sips of tepid water and sugarless gum may help relieve dry mouth.
• Explain to the patient/family that drowsiness generally subsides during continued therapy.
• Warn the patient/family to avoid tasks that require mental alertness or motor skills until the patient's response to the drug is established.
• Urge the patient/family to avoid alcohol and exposure to artificial light and sunlight during thioridazine therapy.

Thiothixene

thigh-oh-**thicks**-een
(Navane)
Do not confuse with thioridazine.

CATEGORY AND SCHEDULE

Pregnancy Risk Category: C

MECHANISM OF ACTION

An antipsychotic that blocks postsynaptic dopamine receptor sites in brain. Has alpha-adrenergic blocking effects; depresses release of hypothalamic and hypophyseal hormones. ***Therapeutic Effect:*** Suppresses behavioral response in psychosis.

PHARMACOKINETICS

Well absorbed from the GI tract after IM administration. Widely distributed. Metabolized in liver. Primarily excreted in urine. Unknown whether removed by hemodialysis. ***Half-Life:*** Adults 34 hrs.

AVAILABILITY

Capsules: 1 mg, 2 mg, 5 mg, 10 mg, 20 mg.
Oral Concentrate: 5 mg/mL.

INDICATIONS AND DOSAGES

▸ Psychosis

PO

Children older than 12 yrs. Initially, 2 mg 3 times/day. Maximum: 60 mg/day.

CONTRAINDICATIONS

Blood dyscrasias, CNS depression, circulatory collapse, comatose states, history of seizures.

INTERACTIONS

Drug

Alcohol, CNS depressants: May increase CNS and respiratory depression, and increase hypotension.
Extrapyramidal symptom–producing medications: May increase risk of EPSs.
Levodopa: May inhibit the effects of levodopa.
Quinidine: May increase cardiac effects with quinidine.

Herbal

Kava kava, St. John's wort, valerian: May increase CNS depression.

Food

None known.

DIAGNOSTIC TEST EFFECTS

May decrease serum uric acid.

SIDE EFFECTS

Expected

Hypotension, dizziness, and fainting occur frequently after the first injection, occasionally after subsequent injections, and rarely with oral dosage.

Frequent

Transient drowsiness, dry mouth, constipation, blurred vision, nasal congestion

Occasional

Diarrhea, peripheral edema, urinary retention, nausea

Rare

Ocular changes, skin pigmentation alterations with those taking high dosage for prolonged periods, photosensitivity

SERIOUS REACTIONS

! Akathisia or motor restlessness and anxiety is the most frequently noted EPS.

! Occurring less frequently is akinesia or rigidity, tremor, salivation, a masklike facial expression, and reduced voluntary movements.

! Infrequently noted are dystonias including torticollis or neck muscle spasm, opisthotonos or rigidity of the back muscles, and oculogyric crisis or rolling back of the eyes.

! Tardive dyskinesia, characterized by protrusion of the tongue, puffing of the cheeks, and chewing or puckering of the mouth, occurs rarely but may be irreversible. The risk of tardive dyskinesia is greater in female geriatric patients.

! Grand mal seizures may occur in epileptic patients, with a higher risk noted with IM administration.

! Neuroleptic malignant syndrome occurs rarely.

PEDIATRIC CONSIDERATIONS

Baseline Assessment

- Assess the patient's appearance, behavior, emotional status, response to the environment, speech pattern, and thought content.
- Be aware that thiothixene crosses the placenta and is distributed in breast milk.
- Be aware that children may develop EPSs or neuromuscular symptoms, especially dystonias.

Precautions

- Use cautiously in patients during alcohol withdrawal and exposure to extreme heat and in those with severe cardiovascular disorders.

Administration and Handling

PO

- Give thiothixene without regard to meals.
- Avoid skin contact with the oral solution because it can cause contact dermatitis.

Intervention and Evaluation

- Closely supervise suicidal-risk patients during early therapy. As depression lessens, the patient's energy level improves, which increases the suicide potential.
- Monitor the patient's blood pressure (B/P) for hypotension.
- Evaluate the patient for peripheral edema.
- Assess the patient's pattern of daily bowel activity and stool consistency.
- Monitor the patient for EPS, tardive dyskinesia, and potentially fatal, rare neuroleptic malignant syndrome, such as altered mental status, fever, irregular pulse or B/P, and muscle rigidity.
- Assess the patient for a therapeutic response, an improvement in self-care, an increased ability to concentrate, an interest in his or

her surroundings, and a relaxed facial expression.

Patient/Family Teaching

- Tell the patient/family that the drug's full therapeutic effect may take up to 6 wks to appear.
- Warn the patient/family to notify the physician if the patient experiences visual disturbances.
- Suggest to the patient that sips of tepid water and sugarless gum may to help relieve dry mouth.
- Explain to the patient/family that drowsiness generally subsides during continued therapy.
- Warn the patient/family to avoid tasks that require mental alertness or motor skills until the patient's response to the drug is established.
- Urge the patient/family to avoid alcohol, exposure to artificial light or direct sunlight, and other CNS depressants during thiothixene therapy.

Trifluoperazine Hydrochloride

try-floo-oh-**pear**-ah-zeen
(Apo-Trifluoperazine [CAN], Stelazine)

Do not confuse with selegiline or triflupromazine.

CATEGORY AND SCHEDULE

Pregnancy Risk Category: C

MECHANISM OF ACTION

A phenothiazine derivative that blocks dopamine at postsynaptic receptor sites. Possesses strong extrapyramidal, antiemetic action; weak anticholinergic, and sedative effects. ***Therapeutic Effect:*** Suppresses behavioral response in psychosis, reducing locomotor activity or aggressiveness; suppresses conditioned responses.

AVAILABILITY

Oral Concentrate: 10 mg/mL.
Tablets: 1 mg, 2 mg, 5 mg, 10 mg.

INDICATIONS AND DOSAGES

▸ Psychotic disorders

PO

Children older than 12 yrs. Initially, 2–5 mg 1–2 times/day. Range: 15–20 mg/day. Maximum: 40 mg/day.

Children 6–12 yrs. Initially, 1 mg 1–2 times/day. Maintenance: Up to 15 mg/day.

CONTRAINDICATIONS

Hypersensitivity to trifluoperazine or any related component. Bone marrow suppression, circulatory collapse, narrow-angle glaucoma, severe cardiac or liver disease, severe hypertension or hypotension.

INTERACTIONS

Drug

Alcohol, CNS depressants: May increase CNS and respiratory depression and the hypotensive effects of trifluoperazine.

Antithyroid agents: May increase the risk of agranulocytosis.

Extrapyramidal symptom (EPS)–producing medications: May increase EPSs.

Hypotensives: May increase hypotension.

Levodopa: May decrease the effects of levodopa.

Lithium: May decrease the absorption of trifluoperazine and produce adverse neurologic effects.

MAOIs, tricyclic antidepressants: May increase anticholinergic and sedative effects of trifluoperazine.

Herbal

None known.

Food

None known.

DIAGNOSTIC TEST EFFECTS

May cause EKG changes.

SIDE EFFECTS

Frequent

Hypotension, dizziness, and fainting occur frequently after the first injection, occasionally after subsequent injections, and rarely with oral dosage.

Occasional

Drowsiness during early therapy, dry mouth, blurred vision, lethargy, constipation or diarrhea, nasal congestion, peripheral edema, urinary retention

Rare

Ocular changes, skin pigmentation in those taking high dosages for prolonged periods

SERIOUS REACTIONS

! EPSs appear to be dose-related, particularly high dosage, and are divided into three categories: akathisia or the inability to sit still, tapping of feet, the urge to move around; parkinsonian symptoms, such as a masklike face, tremors, shuffling gait, and hypersalivation; and acute dystonias such as torticollis or neck muscle spasm, opisthotonos or rigidity of the back muscles, and oculogyric crisis or rolling back of the eyes.

! Dystonic reaction may also produce profuse diaphoresis and pallor.

! Tardive dyskinesia, marked by protrusion of the tongue, puffing of the cheeks, and chewing or puckering of the mouth, occurs rarely but may be irreversible.

! Abrupt withdrawal after long-term therapy may precipitate nausea, vomiting, gastritis, dizziness, and tremors.

! Blood dyscrasias, particularly agranulocytosis, and mild leukopenia may occur.

! May lower seizure threshold.

PEDIATRIC CONSIDERATIONS

Baseline Assessment

- Avoid skin contact with oral concentrate because it may cause contact dermatitis.
- Assess the patient's appearance, behavior, emotional status, response to the environment, speech pattern, and thought content.
- Do not administer this medication to children younger than 6 yrs of age.
- The IM route should not be used with children.
- A possible consequence of trifluoperazine is neuroleptic malignant syndrome.

Precautions

- Use cautiously in patients with Parkinson's disease and seizure disorders.

Administration and Handling

PO

- Oral concentrate must be diluted in 2–4 oz of carbonated beverage, juice, pudding, or water.
- Do not take antacids within 1 hr of trifluoperazine.

Intervention and Evaluation

- Monitor the patient's blood pressure for hypotension.
- Assess the patient for EPS.
- Monitor the patient's WBC count for blood dyscrasias manifested as anemia, neutropenia, pancytopenia, or thrombocytopenia.
- Monitor the patient for abnormal movement in the trunk, neck, or extremities, fine tongue movement that may be early sign of tardive dyskinesia, gait changes, or tremors.

• Supervise the suicidal-risk patient closely during early therapy. As the patient's depression lessens, his or her energy level improves, increasing suicide potential.
• Monitor the patient's target behaviors.
• Assess the patient for a therapeutic response, an improvement in self-care, an increased ability to concentrate, an interest in his or her surroundings, and a relaxed facial expression.

Patient/Family Teaching

• Teach the patient/family to dilute the oral concentrate in 2–4 oz of carbonated beverage, juice, pudding, or water.
• Instruct the patient/family not to take antacids within 1 hr of trifluoperazine.
• Urge the patient/family to avoid alcohol and excessive exposure to artificial light and sunlight during trifluoperazine therapy.
• Tell the patient/family that trifluoperazine may cause drowsiness. Warn the patient to avoid tasks requiring mental alertness or motor skills until the patient's response to the drug is established.
• Instruct the patient/family to rise slowly from a lying or sitting position to prevent hypotension.

REFERENCES

Miller, S. & Fioravanti, J. (1997). Pediatric medications: a handbook for nurses. St. Louis: Mosby.
Taketomo, C. K., Hodding, J. H. & Kraus, D. M. (2003–2004). Pediatric dosage handbook (10th ed.). Hudson, OH: Lexi-Comp.

39 CNS Stimulants

Atomoxetine
Dexmethylphenidate Hydrochloride
Dextroamphetamine Sulfate
Methylphenidate Hydrochloride
Pemoline

Uses: Most CNS stimulants are used to treat attention deficit hyperactivity disorder (ADHD), primarily in children age 6 and older. In addition, dextroamphetamine is used for short-term treatment of obesity.

Action: In this classification, specific subgroups and individual agents act by different mechanisms. *Amphetamines*, such as dextroamphetamine, promote the release and action of norepinephrine and dopamine by blocking reuptake from synapses; they also inhibit the action of monoamine oxidase. *Methylphenidate* blocks the reuptake mechanisms of dopaminergic neurons. *Pemoline* blocks the reuptake of dopamine at neurons in the cerebral cortex and subcortical structures.

Atomoxetine

ah-toe-**mocks**-eh-teen
(Strattera)

CATEGORY AND SCHEDULE

Pregnancy Risk Category: C

MECHANISM OF ACTION

A norepinephrine reuptake inhibitor that enhances noradrenergic function by selective inhibition of the presynaptic norepinephrine transporter. ***Therapeutic Effect:*** Improves symptoms of ADHD.

PHARMACOKINETICS

Rapidly absorbed after oral administration. Protein binding: 98%, primarily albumin. Eliminated primarily in urine with a lesser amount excreted in feces. Not removed by hemodialysis. ***Half-Life:*** 4–5 hrs found in the major population, 22 hrs in 7% of Caucasians, and in 2% of African-Americans. Half-life is increased in moderate to severe liver insufficiency.

AVAILABILITY

Capsules: 10 mg, 18 mg, 25 mg, 40 mg, 60 mg.

INDICATIONS AND DOSAGES

▸ **ADHD**

PO

Children weighing 70 kg and more. 40 mg once daily. May increase after a minimum of 3 days to 80 mg as a single daily dose or in divided doses. Maximum: 100 mg.

Children weighing less than 70 kg. Initially, 0.5 mg/kg/day. May increase to 1.2 mg/kg/day after minimum of 3 days. Maximum: 1.4 mg/kg/day.

CONTRAINDICATIONS

Hypersensitivity to atomoxetine or any related component. Concurrent use of MAOIs or within 2 wks of discontinuing an MAOI, narrow-angle glaucoma.

INTERACTIONS

Drug

Fluoxetine, paroxetine, quinidine: May increase atomoxetine blood concentration.
MAOIs: May increase toxic effects.
Midazolam: May increase midazolam concentrations.
Albuterol: May increase cardiovascular effects.

Herbal

None known.

Food

None known.

DIAGNOSTIC TEST EFFECTS

None known.

SIDE EFFECTS

Frequent
Headache, dyspepsia (epigastric distress, heartburn), nausea, vomiting, fatigue, reduced appetite, dizziness, changes in mood
Occasional
Increase in heart rate and blood pressure, weight loss, slowing of growth
Rare
Insomnia, sexual dysfunction in adults (desire, performance, satisfaction)

SERIOUS REACTIONS

! Urinary retention or urinary hesitance may occur.
! In an overdose, gastric emptying and repeated activated charcoal may prevent systemic absorption.

PEDIATRIC CONSIDERATIONS

Baseline Assessment

• Assess the patient's blood pressure and pulse before beginning atomoxetine therapy, after dose increases, and periodically while receiving therapy.
! Be aware that it is unknown whether atomoxetine is excreted in breast milk.
! Be aware that the safety and efficacy of atomoxetine have not been established in children younger than 6 yrs.
! Monitor pediatric patients' height and weight carefully during therapy, as growth may be affected.

Precautions

◂ALERT▸ Avoid concurrent use of medications that can increase heart rate or blood pressure.
• Use cautiously in patients with cardiovascular disease, hypertension, moderate or severe liver impairment, a risk of urinary retention, and tachycardia.

Administration and Handling

◂ALERT▸ Reduce atomoxetine dosage to 50% in those with moderate liver impairment and to 25% in those with severe liver impairment.
PO
• Give atomoxetine without regard to meals.

Intervention and Evaluation

• Monitor the patient's urinary output. A patient complaint of an inability to urinate (urinary retention) or hesitancy may be a related adverse reaction.
• Assist the patient with ambulation if he or she experiences dizziness.
• Be alert to mood changes in the patient.
• Monitor the fluid and electrolyte status in patients experiencing significant vomiting.

Patient/Family Teaching

• Advise the patient/family to avoid tasks that require mental alertness and motor skills until the patient's response to the drug is established.

• Instruct the patient/family to take the last dose of the day early in the evening to avoid insomnia.
• Warn the patient/family to notify the physician if the patient experiences fever, nervousness, palpitations, skin rash, or vomiting.

Dexmethylphenidate Hydrochloride

dex-meh-thyl-**fen**-ih-date
(Focalin)

CATEGORY AND SCHEDULE

Pregnancy Risk Category: C
Controlled Substance: Schedule II

MECHANISM OF ACTION

A piperidine derivative B that blocks the reuptake mechanisms of norepinephrine and dopamine into presynaptic neurons. Increases the release of these neurotransmitters into the synaptic cleft. ***Therapeutic Effect:*** Decreases motor restlessness and enhances attention span. Increases motor activity and mental alertness. Diminishes sense of fatigue and enhances spirit.

PHARMACOKINETICS

Route	Onset	Peak	Duration
PO	N/A	N/A	4–5 hrs

Readily absorbed from the GI tract. Plasma concentrations increase rapidly. Metabolized in liver. Excreted unchanged in urine. ***Half-Life:*** 2.2 hrs.

AVAILABILITY

Tablets: 2.5 mg, 5 mg, 10 mg.

INDICATIONS AND DOSAGES

▸ ADHD

PO

Patients new to dexmethylphenidate or methylphenidate. 2.5 mg twice daily (5 mg/day). May adjust dosage in 2.5- to 5-mg increments. Maximum: 20 mg/day.

Patients currently taking methylphenidate. 1.25 mg twice daily (2.5 mg/day). Maximum: 20 mg/day.

CONTRAINDICATIONS

Hypersensitivity to dexmethylphenidate or any related component. Diagnosis or family history of Tourette's syndrome or glaucoma, a history of marked agitation, anxiety, or tension, within 14 days after discontinuation of an MAOI, patients with motor tics.

INTERACTIONS

Drug

Amitriptyline, phenobarbital, phenytoin, primidone: Downward dosage adjustments of amitriptyline, phenobarbital, phenytoin, and primidone may be necessary.
CNS stimulants: May have an additive effect.
MAOIs: May increase the effects of dexmethylphenidate.
Warfarin: May inhibit the metabolism of warfarin.

Herbal

None known.

Food

None known.

DIAGNOSTIC TEST EFFECTS

None known.

SIDE EFFECTS

Frequent

Abdominal discomfort

Occasional
Anorexia, fever, nausea
Rare
Blurred vision, difficulty with accommodation, motor, vocal tics, insomnia, tachycardia

SERIOUS REACTIONS

! Withdrawal after chronic therapy may unmask symptoms of the underlying disorder.
! Dexmethylphenidate may lower the seizure threshold in those with history of seizures.
! Overdosage produces excessive sympathomimetic effects, including vomiting, tremors, hyperreflexia, seizures, confusion, hallucinations, and diaphoresis.
! Prolonged administration to children may produce temporary suppression of normal weight gain.

PEDIATRIC CONSIDERATIONS

Baseline Assessment
- Obtain baseline height and weight, and plan to weigh the patient regularly to monitor for growth retardation.
- Be aware that it is unknown if dexmethylphenidate is excreted in breast milk.
- Be aware that children are more susceptible to development of abdominal pain, anorexia, insomnia, and weight loss.
- Be aware that chronic dexmethylphenidate use may inhibit growth in children.
- Know that in psychotic children, dexmethylphenidate use may exacerbate symptoms of behavior disturbance and thought disorder.

Precautions
- Use cautiously in patients with cardiovascular disease, psychosis, and seizure disorders.
- Avoid dexmethylphenidate use in those with a history of substance abuse.

Administration and Handling
PO
- Do not give drug in the afternoon or evening because it can cause insomnia.
- Crush tablets, as needed.
- May give dexmethylphenidate with or without food.

Intervention and Evaluation
- Plan to perform a complete blood count to assess WBC, differential, and platelet count routinely during therapy.
- Discontinue or reduce dexmethylphenidate dose if paradoxical return of attention deficit occurs.

Patient/Family Teaching
- Warn the patient/family to avoid tasks that require mental alertness or motor skills until the patient's response to the drug is established.
- Tell the patient/family to notify the physician of any increase in seizures, fever, nervousness, palpitations, and vomiting occurs.
- Instruct the patient/family to take the last dose of the day several hours before retiring to prevent insomnia.

Dextroamphetamine sulfate

dex-tro-am-**fet**-ah-meen
(Dexedrine)
Do not confuse with dextran, dextromethorphan, or Excedrin.

CATEGORY AND SCHEDULE

Pregnancy Risk Category: C
Controlled Substance: Schedule II

MECHANISM OF ACTION
An amphetamine that enhances release and action of catecholamines (dopamine and norepinephrine) by blocking reuptake and inhibiting monoamine oxidase. ***Therapeutic Effect:*** Increases motor activity and mental alertness; decreases drowsiness, and fatigue.

AVAILABILITY
Tablets: 5 mg, 10 mg.
Capsules (sustained release): 5 mg, 10 mg, 15 mg.

INDICATIONS AND DOSAGES
▸ Narcolepsy
PO
Children older than 12 yrs. Initially, 10 mg/day. Increase by 10 mg at weekly intervals until a therapeutic response achieved. Maximum: 60 mg/day.
Children 6–12 yrs. Initially, 5 mg/day. Increase by 5 mg/day at weekly intervals until therapeutic response is achieved. Maximum: 60 mg/day.
▸ Attention deficit disorder (ADD)
PO
Children 6 yrs and older. Initially, 5 mg 1–2 times/day. Increase by 5 mg/day at weekly intervals until therapeutic response is achieved. Maximum: 40 mg/day.
Children 3–5 yrs. Initially, 2.5 mg/day. Increase by 2.5 mg/day at weekly intervals until therapeutic response is achieved. Maximum: 40 mg/day.
▸ Appetite suppressant
PO
Children 12 yrs and older. 5–30 mg daily in divided doses of 5–10 mg each dose, given 30–60 min before meals. Extended-release: 1 capsule in morning.

CONTRAINDICATIONS
Hypersensitivity to dextroamphetamine or any related component. Advanced arteriosclerosis, agitated states, glaucoma, a history of drug abuse, a history of hypersensitivity to sympathomimetic amines, hyperthyroidism, moderate to severe hypertension, symptomatic cardiovascular disease, within 14 days after discontinuation of an MAOI.

INTERACTIONS
Drug
Beta-blockers: May increase risk of bradycardia, heart block, and hypertension.
CNS stimulants: May increase the effects of dextroamphetamine.
Digoxin: May increase the risk of arrhythmias with this drug.
MAOIs: May prolong and intensify the effects of dextroamphetamine.
Meperidine: May increase the risk of hypotension, respiratory depression, seizures, and vascular collapse.
Tricyclic antidepressants: May increase cardiovascular effects.
Herbal
St. John's wort: May increase serious side effects.
Food
Acidic juices, acidic food, vitamin C: Decrease absorption of dextroamphetamine.

DIAGNOSTIC TEST EFFECTS
May increase plasma corticosteroid concentrations.

SIDE EFFECTS
Frequent
Irregular pulse, increased motor activity, talkativeness, nervousness, mild euphoria, insomnia

Occasional
Headache, chills, dry mouth, GI distress, worsening depression in patients who are clinically depressed, tachycardia, palpitations, chest pain

SERIOUS REACTIONS

! Overdose may produce skin pallor or flushing, arrhythmias, and psychosis.
! Abrupt withdrawal after prolonged administration of high dosage may produce lethargy (may last for weeks).
! Prolonged administration to children with ADD may produce a temporary suppression of normal weight and height patterns.

PEDIATRIC CONSIDERATIONS

Baseline Assessment
• This medication is not recommended for those children who are 3 yrs of age or younger.
• Use of this medication in psychotic children may worsen symptoms of behavior and thought disorders.
• This medication may potentially inhibit growth in children.
• Be aware that the tablet and capsule forms contain tartrazine.
• Be aware that dextroamphetamine has a potential for abuse.
Intervention and Evaluation
• Monitor the patient for CNS overstimulation, an increase in blood pressure, and weight loss.
Patient/Family Teaching
• Advise the patient/family that normal dosage levels may produce tolerance to the drug's anorexic mood-elevating effects within a few weeks.
• Warn the patient/family to avoid performing tasks that require mental alertness or motor skills until the patient's response to the drug is established.
• Suggest to the patient/family that sips of tepid water and sugarless gum may relieve dry mouth.
• Instruct the patient/family to take dextroamphetamine early in the day.
• Caution the patient/family that this drug may mask signs and symptoms of extreme fatigue.
• Warn the patient/family to notify the physician if the patient experiences decreased appetite, dizziness, dry mouth, or pronounced nervousness.

Methylphenidate Hydrochloride

meh-thyl-**fen**-ih-date
(Attenta [AUS], Concerta, Metadate, Ritalin, Ritalin LA, Ritalin SR)
Do not confuse with Rifadin.

CATEGORY AND SCHEDULE

Pregnancy Risk Category: C
Controlled Substance: Schedule II

MECHANISM OF ACTION

A piperidine derivative B that blocks reuptake mechanisms of dopaminergic neurons. ***Therapeutic Effect:*** Decreases motor restlessness; enhances the ability to pay attention. Increases motor activity and mental alertness; diminishes sense of fatigue; enhances spirit; produces mild euphoria.

PHARMACOKINETICS

Onset	Peak	Duration
Immediate release	2 hrs	3–5 hrs
Sustained release	4–7 hrs	3–8 hrs
Extended-release	N/A	8–12 hrs

Slowly, incompletely absorbed from the GI tract. Protein binding: 15%. Metabolized in liver. Excreted in urine, eliminated in feces via biliary system. Unknown if removed by hemodialysis. ***Half-Life:*** 2–4 hrs.

AVAILABILITY

Capsules (extended release): 10 mg (Metadate CD), 20 mg (Metadate CD), 20 mg (Ritalin LA), 30 mg (Metadate CD), 30 mg (Ritalin LA), 40 mg (Ritalin LA).
Tablets: 5 mg (Ritalin), 10 mg (Ritalin), 20 mg (Ritalin).
Tablets (chewable): 2.5 mg (Methylin), 5 mg (Methylin), 10 mg (Methylin).
Tablets (extended release): 10 mg (Metadate ER, Methylin ER), 18 mg (Concerta), 20 mg (Metadate ER, Methylin ER), 27 mg (Concerta), 36 mg (Concerta), 54 mg (Concerta).
Tablets (sustained release): 20 mg (Ritalin SR).

INDICATIONS AND DOSAGES

▸ ADHD

PO

Children older than 6 yrs. Initially, 2.5–5 mg before breakfast and lunch. May increase by 5–10 mg/day at weekly intervals. Maximum: 60 mg/day.

CONCERTA

Initially, 18 mg once daily. May increase by 18 mg/day at weekly intervals. Maximum: 54 mg/day.

METADATE CD

Initially, 20 mg/day. May increase by 20 mg/day at 7-day intervals. Maximum: 60 mg/day.

RITALIN LA

Initially, 20 mg/day. May increase by 10 mg/day at 7-day intervals. Maximum: 60 mg/day.

▸ Narcolepsy

PO

Children older than 12 yrs. 10 mg 2–3 times/day. Range: 10–60 mg/day.

UNLABELED USES

Treatment of secondary mental depression.

CONTRAINDICATIONS

Hypersensitivity to methylphenidate or any related component. Glaucoma, motor tics; Tourette's syndrome; patients with marked agitation or tension anxiety, within 14 days after discontinuation of an MAOI.

INTERACTIONS

Drug

CNS stimulants: May have an additive effect.
MAOIs: May increase the effects of methylphenidate.
Clonidine: May increase EKG effects.
Tricyclic antidepressants, selective serotonin reuptake inhibitors, phenylbutazone, warfarin, phenytoin, phenobarbital, primidone: May increase serum concentrations and toxic effects of these drugs.

Herbal

St. John's wort: May increase serious side effects.

Food

None known.

DIAGNOSTIC TEST EFFECTS

None known.

SIDE EFFECTS

Frequent

Nervousness, insomnia, anorexia

Occasional

Dizziness, drowsiness, headache, nausea, stomach pain, fever, rash, joint pain

Rare

Blurred vision, Tourette's syndrome, marked by uncontrolled vocal outbursts, repetitive body movements, and tics

SERIOUS REACTIONS

! Prolonged administration to children with attention deficit disorder may produce a temporary suppression of normal weight gain pattern.

! Overdose may produce tachycardia, palpitations, cardiac irregularities, chest pain, psychotic episode, seizures, and coma.

! Hypersensitivity reactions and blood dyscrasias occur rarely.

PEDIATRIC CONSIDERATIONS

Baseline Assessment

• Obtain baseline height and weight, and plan to weigh the patient regularly to monitor for growth retardation.

• Be aware that it is unknown if methylphenidate crosses the placenta or is distributed in breast milk.

• Be aware that children may be more susceptible to development of abdominal pain, anorexia, decreased weight, and insomnia. Chronic methylphenidate use may inhibit growth in children.

• Do not abruptly discontinue this medication.

Precautions

• Use cautiously in patients with acute stress reaction, emotional instability, a history of drug dependence, hypertension, and seizures.

Administration and Handling

◂ALERT▸ Be aware that the sustained-release forms (Metadate SR and Ritalin SR) may be given once the daily dose is titrated; the regular tablets and the titrated 8-hr dosage correspond to sustained-release size.

PO

• Do not give drug in the afternoon or evening because the drug can cause insomnia.

• Do not crush or break sustained-release capsules.

• Crush tablets as needed.

• Give dose 30–45 min before meals.

• Open Metadate CD and sprinkle on applesauce, if desired.

Intervention and Evaluation

• Perform a complete blood count to assess WBC count, differential, and platelet count routinely during therapy.

• Discontinue or reduce methylphenidate dosage if a paradoxical return of attention deficit occurs.

Patient/Family Teaching

• Warn the patient/family to avoid tasks that require mental alertness or motor skills until the patient's response to the drug is established.

• Suggest to the patient/family that taking sips of tepid water and chewing sugarless gum may relieve dry mouth.

• Warn the patient/family to notify the physician if the patient experiences any increase in seizures, fever, nervousness, palpitations, skin rash, or vomiting.

• Instruct the patient/family to take the last dose of methylphenidate in the early morning to avoid insomnia.

• Urge the patient/family to avoid consuming caffeine during methylphenidate therapy.
• Caution the patient/family against abruptly discontinuing the drug after prolonged use.

Pemoline

pem-oh-leen
(Cylert)

CATEGORY AND SCHEDULE

Pregnancy Risk Category: B
Controlled Substance: Schedule IV

MECHANISM OF ACTION

A CNS stimulant that blocks reuptake of dopaminergic neurons at cerebral cortex and subcortical structures.
Therapeutic Effect: Reduces motor restlessness, increases mental alertness, provides mood elevation, and reduces sense of fatigue.

AVAILABILITY

Tablets: 18.75 mg, 37.5 mg, 75 mg.
Tablets (chewable): 37.5 mg.

INDICATIONS AND DOSAGES

▸ **Attention deficit disorder**

PO

Children 6 yrs and older. Initially, 37.5 mg/day given as a single dose in morning. May increase by 18.75 mg at weekly intervals until a therapeutic response is achieved. Range: 56.25–75 mg/day. Maximum: 112.5 mg/day.

CONTRAINDICATIONS

Hypersensitivity to pemoline or any related component. A family history of Tourette's disorder, impaired liver function, patients with motor tics.

INTERACTIONS

Drug

CNS-stimulation medications: May increase CNS stimulation.

Herbal

None known.

Food

None known.

DIAGNOSTIC TEST EFFECTS

May increase lactate dehydrogenase, SGOT (AST), and SGPT (ALT) levels.

SIDE EFFECTS

Frequent

Anorexia, insomnia

Occasional

Nausea, abdominal discomfort, diarrhea, headache, dizziness, drowsiness

SERIOUS REACTIONS

! Dyskinetic movements of tongue, lips, face, and extremities, visual disturbances, and rash have occurred.
! Large doses may produce extreme nervousness and tachycardia.
! Hepatic effects, such as hepatitis and jaundice, appear to be reversible when drug is discontinued.
! Prolonged administration to children with attention deficit disorder may produce a temporary suppression of weight and height patterns.

PEDIATRIC CONSIDERATIONS

Baseline Assessment

• Perform blood serum hepatic enzyme tests before beginning pemoline therapy and periodically during therapy.

• Obtain baseline height and weight, and plan to weigh the patient regularly to monitor for growth retardation.
• Be aware that this medication is not intended for those younger than 6 yrs of age.
• This medication seems to be more effective as children age and mature. Be aware that dosages will need to be continually monitored and adjusted to maintain effectiveness.

Precautions

• Use cautiously in patients with a history of drug abuse, hypertension, psychosis, renal impairment, and seizures.

Patient/Family Teaching

• Urge the patient/family to avoid alcohol and caffeine during pemoline therapy.
• Tell the patient/family that pemoline may cause dizziness and impair the patient's ability to perform tasks requiring mental alertness or motor skills.
• Explain to the patient/family that pemoline may be habit-forming. Caution the patient against abruptly discontinuing the medication.
• Warn the patient/family to notify the physician if the patient experiences dark urine, gastrointestinal complaints, loss of appetite, or yellow skin.

REFERENCES

Miller, S. & Fioravanti, J. (1997). Pediatric medications: a handbook for nurses. St. Louis: Mosby.
Taketomo, C. K., Hodding, J. H. & Kraus, D. M. (2003–2004). Pediatric dosage handbook (10th ed.). Hudson, OH: Lexi-Comp.

40 Narcotic Analgesics

Codeine Phosphate, Codeine Sulfate
Fentanyl
Hydromorphone Hydrochloride
Meperidine Hydrochloride
Methadone Hydrochloride
Morphine Sulfate
Oxycodone

Uses: Narcotic analgesics are used to relieve moderate to severe pain related to surgery, myocardial infarction, burns, cancer, and other conditions. These agents may be used as an adjunct to anesthesia, either as preoperative medication or as an intraoperative supplement to anesthesia. They are also used for obstetric analgesia. Codeine may be prescribed for its antitussive effects. Opium tinctures can be used to control severe diarrhea. Although methadone can relieve severe pain, it is used primarily as part of heroin detoxification.

Action: All narcotic analgesics bind to opioid receptors and have actions similar to those of morphine, which is why they are also referred to as *opioid* analgesics. (See illustration, *Mechanism of Action: Narcotic Analgesics,* page 516.) These agents produce major effects on the CNS (causing analgesia, drowsiness, mood changes, mental clouding, analgesia without loss of consciousness, nausea, and vomiting) and the GI tract (reducing hydrochloric acid secretion; biliary, pancreatic, and intestinal secretions; and propulsive peristalsis). They also depress respirations and cause cardiovascular effects such as peripheral vasodilation, decreased peripheral resistance, and inhibited baroreceptors reflexes.

COMBINATION PRODUCTS

CAPITAL WITH CODEINE: acetaminophen (a non-narcotic analgesic)/codeine 120 mg/12 mg per 5 mL.

PERCOCET: oxycodone/acetaminophen (a non-narcotic analgesic) 2.5 mg/325 mg; 5 mg/325 mg; 5 mg/500 mg; 7.5 mg/325 mg; 7.5 mg/500 mg; 10 mg/325 mg; 10 mg/650 mg.

PERCODAN: oxycodone/aspirin (a non-narcotic analgesic) 2.25 mg/325 mg; 4.5 mg/325 mg.

PHENERGAN WITH CODEINE: codeine/promethazine (an antihistamine) 10 mg/6.25 mg

PHENERGAN VC WITH CODEINE: codeine/promethazine (an antihistamine)/phenylephrine (a vasopressor) 10 mg/6.25 mg/5 mg.

ROBITUSSIN AC: codeine/guaifenesin (an antitussive) 10 mg/100 mg.

ROXICET: oxycodone/acetaminophen (a non-narcotic analgesic) 5 mg/500 mg.

TYLENOL WITH CODEINE: acetaminophen (a non-narcotic analgesic)/codeine 120 mg/12 mg per 5 mL; 300 mg/15 mg; 300 mg/30 mg; 300 mg/60 mg.

TYLOX: oxycodone/acetaminophen (a non-narcotic analgesic) 5 mg/500 mg.

Codeine Phosphate

koe-deen
(Actacode [AUS], Codeine, Codeine Linctus [AUS])

Codeine Sulfate

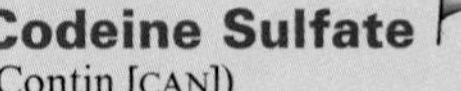

(Contin [CAN])
Do not confuse with Lodine.

CATEGORY AND SCHEDULE

Pregnancy Risk Category: C (D if used for prolonged periods or at high dosages at term)
Controlled substance: Schedule II (analgesic), Schedule III (fixed-combination form)

MECHANISM OF ACTION

An opioid agonist that binds at opiate receptor sites in the CNS. Has direct action in the medulla. ***Therapeutic Effect:*** Inhibits ascending pain pathways, altering perception of and response to pain; suppresses cough reflex.

AVAILABILITY

Tablets: 15 mg, 30 mg, 60 mg.
Solution: 15 mg/5 mL.
Injection: 30 mg, 60 mg.

INDICATIONS AND DOSAGES

▸ Analgesia

PO/SC/IM
Children. 0.5–1 mg/kg q4–6h. Maximum: 60 mg/dose.

▸ Antitussive

PO
Children 12 yrs and older. 10–20 mg q4–6h. Maximum: 120 mg/day.
Children 6–11 yrs. 5–10 mg q4–6h. Maximum 60 mg/day.
Children 2–5 yrs. 2.5–5 mg q4–6h. Maximum 30 mg/day.

▸ Dosage in renal impairment

Creatinine Clearance	Dosage
10–50 mL/min	75% dose
Less than 10 mL/min	50% dose

UNLABELED USES

Treatment of diarrhea.

CONTRAINDICATIONS

Hypersensitivity to codeine or any related component.

INTERACTIONS

Drug

Alcohol, CNS depressants: May increase CNS or respiratory depression, and hypotension.
MAOIs May produce severe, fatal reaction unless dosage reduced by one quarter.

Herbal

None known.

Food

None known.

DIAGNOSTIC TEST EFFECTS

May increase serum amylase and lipase levels.

SIDE EFFECTS

Frequent

Constipation, drowsiness, nausea, vomiting

Occasional

Paradoxical excitement, confusion, pounding heartbeat, facial flushing, decreased urination, blurred vision, dizziness, dry mouth, headache, hypotension, decreased appetite, redness, burning, pain at injection site

Rare

Hallucinations, depression, stomach pain, insomnia

SERIOUS REACTIONS

! Too frequent use may result in paralytic ileus.

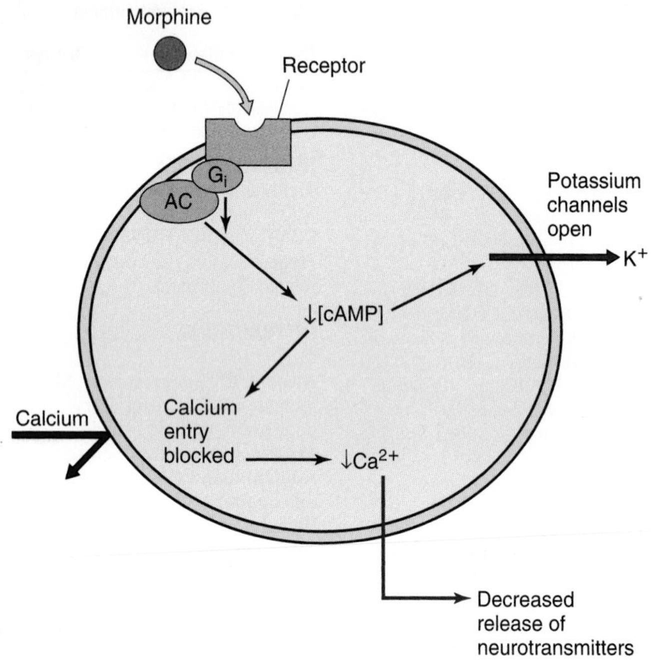

Mechanism of Action: Narcotic Analgesics

Narcotic analgesics bind to three types of opioid receptors: mu, kappa, and delta. They produce analgesia primarily by activating mu receptors. However, they also engage with and activate kappa and delta receptors, producing other effects, such as sedation and vasomotor stimulation.

When morphine or another narcotic analgesic binds to opioid receptors, activation occurs. The receptors send signals to the enzyme adenyl cyclase (AC) to slow activity by way of G-proteins (G_i). Decreased AC activity causes less cyclic adenosine monophosphate (cAMP) to be produced. A secondary messenger substance, cAMP, is important for regulating cell membrane channels. A reduced cAMP level allows fewer potassium ions to leave the cell and blocks calcium ions from entering the cell. This ion imbalance—especially the reduced intracellular calcium level—ultimately decreases the release of neurotransmitters from the cell, thereby blocking or reducing pain impulse transmission.

! Overdosage results in cold or clammy skin, confusion, convulsions, decreased blood pressure, restlessness, pinpoint pupils, bradycardia, respiratory depression, decreased level of consciousness, and severe weakness.
! Tolerance to analgesic effect and physical dependence may occur with repeated use.

PEDIATRIC CONSIDERATIONS

Baseline Assessment

• Assess the duration, location, onset, and type of pain.

• Keep in mind that the effect of medication is reduced if a full pain response recurs before the next dose.

• Assess the frequency, severity, and type of cough and sputum production.

• Be aware that parenteral doses are not recommended for children who weigh less than 50 kg.

• Be aware that codeine is not used as an antitussive in children younger than 2 yrs of age.

• Be aware that codeine is not used as an oral suspension in children younger than 6 yrs of age.

• Be aware that some preparations of codeine are prepared with sulfite. Do not give this preparation to those with a sulfite allergy.

Precautions

• Use extremely cautiously in patients with acute alcoholism, anoxia, CNS depression, hypercapnia, respiratory depression, respiratory dysfunction, seizures, shock and untreated myxedema.

• Use cautiously in patients with acute abdominal conditions, Addison's disease, chronic obstructive pulmonary disease, hypothyroidism, impaired liver function, increased intracranial pressure, prostatic hypertrophy, and urethral stricture.

Administration and Handling

◂ **ALERT** ▸ Be aware that ambulatory patients and those not in severe pain may experience dizziness, hypotension, nausea, and vomiting more frequently than patients in the supine position or with severe pain.

◂ **ALERT** ▸ Expect to reduce the initial dosage in those with hypothyroidism, Addison's disease, or renal insufficiency and in debilitated patients and those receiving concurrent CNS depressants.

Intervention and Evaluation

• Assess the patient's pattern of daily bowel activity and stool consistency.

• Increase the patient's fluid intake and environmental humidity to help improve viscosity of lung secretions.

• Encourage deep breathing and coughing exercises.

• Assess the patient for clinical improvement. Record the onset of relief of cough or pain.

Patient/Family Teaching

• Instruct the patient/family to change positions slowly to avoid orthostatic hypotension.

• Warn the patient/family to avoid tasks that require mental alertness or motor skills until the patient's response to the drug is established.

• Explain to the patient/family that drug dependence or tolerance may occur with prolonged use of high dosages.

• Urge the patient/family to avoid alcohol during codeine therapy.

• Tell the patient/family to report the onset of pain because the effect of drug is reduced if a full pain response recurs before next dose.

Fentanyl

fen-**tah**-nil

(Actiq, Duragesic, Sublimaze)

Do not confuse with alfentanil.

CATEGORY AND SCHEDULE

Pregnancy Risk Category: C (D if used for prolonged periods or at high dosages at term)

Controlled Substance: Schedule II

MECHANISM OF ACTION

An opioid, narcotic agonist that binds at opiate receptor sites within the CNS, reducing stimuli from sensory nerve endings. ***Therapeutic Effect:*** Increases pain threshold, alters pain reception, inhibits ascending pain pathways.

PHARMACOKINETICS

Route	Onset	Peak	Duration
IM	7–15 min	20–30 min	1–2 hrs
IV	1–2 min	3–5 min	0.5–1 hr
Trans-dermal	6–8 hrs	24 hrs	72 hrs
Trans-mucosal	5–15 min	20–30 min	1–2 hrs

Well absorbed after topical or IM administration. Transmucosal absorbed through mucosal tissue of mouth and GI tract. Protein binding: 80%–85%. Metabolized in liver. Primarily eliminated via the biliary system. ***Half-Life:*** IV: 2–4 hrs. Transdermal: 17 hrs. Transmucosal: 6.6 hrs.

AVAILABILITY

Injection: 50 mcg/mL.
Transdermal Patch: 25 mcg/hr, 50 mcg/hr, 75 mcg/hr, 100 mcg/hr.
Lozenges: 200 mcg, 400 mcg, 600 mcg, 800 mcg, 1,200 mcg, 1,600 mcg.

INDICATIONS AND DOSAGES

▸ Sedation (minor procedures or analgesia)

IM/IV

Children older than 12 yrs. 0.5–1 mcg/kg/dose; may repeat after 30–60 min.
Children 1–12 yrs. 1–2 mcg/kg/dose; may repeat after 30–60 min.
Children younger than 1 yr. 1–4 mcg/kg/dose; may repeat every 2–4 hrs.

▸ Preoperative sedation, adjunct regional anesthesia, postoperative pain

IM/IV

Children older than 12 yrs. 50–100 mcg/dose.

▸ Adjunct to general anesthesia

IV

Children older than 12 yrs. 2–50 mcg/kg slow IV infusion.

TRANSDERMAL

Children older than 12 yrs. Initially, 25 mcg/hr system. May increase after 3 days.

TRANSMUCOSAL

Children. 200–400 mcg for breakthrough cancer pain.

▸ Continuous analgesia

IV

Children 1–12 yrs. Bolus of 1–2 mcg/kg, then 1 mcg/kg/hr. Range: 1–5 mcg/kg/hr. Titrate to effect.
Children younger than 1 yr. Bolus of 1–2 mcg/kg, then 0.5–1 mcg/kg/hr. Titrate to effect.

▸ Dosage in renal impairment

Creatinine Clearance	Dosage
10–50 mL/min	75% of dose
Less than 10 mL/min	50% of dose

CONTRAINDICATIONS

Hypersensitivity to fentanyl or any related component. Increased intracranial pressure, severe liver or renal impairment, severe respiratory depression.
Transdermal: Patients with hypersensitivity to adhesives.

INTERACTIONS

Drug

Benzodiazepines: May increase the risk of hypotension and respiratory depression.

Buprenorphine: May decrease the effects of fentanyl.
Central nervous system (CNS) depressants: May increase respiratory depression and hypotension.

Herbal

None known.

Food

None known.

DIAGNOSTIC TEST EFFECTS

May increase serum amylase levels and plasma lipase concentrations.

IV INCOMPATIBILITIES

Phenytoin (Dilantin)

IV COMPATIBILITIES

Atropine, bupivacaine (Marcaine, Sensorcaine), clonidine (Duraclon), diltiazem (Cardizem), diphenhydramine (Benadryl), dobutamine (Dobutrex), dopamine (Intropin), droperidol (Inapsine), heparin, hydromorphone (Dilaudid), ketorolac (Toradol), lorazepam (Ativan), metoclopramide (Reglan), midazolam (Versed), milrinone (Primacor), morphine, nitroglycerin, norepinephrine (Levophed), ondansetron (Zofran), potassium chloride, propofol (Diprivan)

SIDE EFFECTS

Frequent

Transdermal (10%–3%): Headache, itching skin, nausea, vomiting, sweating, difficulty breathing, confusion, dizziness, drowsiness, diarrhea, constipation, decreased appetite
IV: Postoperative drowsiness, nausea, vomiting

Occasional

Transdermal (3%–1%): Chest pain, irregular heartbeat, redness, itching, swelling of skin, fainting, agitation, tingling or burning of skin
IV: Postoperative confusion, blurred vision, chills, orthostatic hypotension, constipation, difficulty urinating

SERIOUS REACTIONS

! Overdosage or too rapid IV administration results in severe respiratory depression, skeletal and thoracic muscle rigidity causing apnea, laryngospasm, bronchospasm, cold and clammy skin, cyanosis, and coma.
! Tolerance to the drug's analgesic effect may occur with repeated use.

PEDIATRIC CONSIDERATIONS

Baseline Assessment

- Make sure resuscitative equipment and an opiate antagonist (naloxone 0.5 mcg/kg) is readily available before administering the drug.
- Establish the patient's baseline blood pressure (B/P) and respiration rate.
- Assess the duration, intensity, location, and type of pain the patient is experiencing.
- Be aware that fentanyl readily crosses the placenta and that it is unknown whether fentanyl is distributed in breast milk. Know that fentanyl may prolong labor if administered in the latent phase of the first stage of labor or before the cervix has dilated 4–5 cm.
- Be aware that respiratory depression may occur in the neonate if the mother received opiates during labor.
- Be aware that the safety and efficacy of the fentanyl patch have not been established in children younger than 12 yrs of age.
- Be aware that the transdermal form of fentanyl is not

recommended in children younger than 12 yrs or children younger than 18 yrs and weighing less than 50 kg.
• Be aware that neonates are more susceptible to the respiratory depressant effects of fentanyl.
• Be aware that rapid IV infusion may lead to muscle rigidity affecting respiration.

Precautions
• Use cautiously in patients with bradycardia, head injuries, impaired consciousness, and liver, renal, or respiratory disease.
• Use cautiously in patients who use MAOIs within 14 days of fentanyl administration.

Administration and Handling
◀ **ALERT** ▶ Keep in mind that fentanyl may be combined with a local anesthetic, such as bupivacaine.

IV
• Store the parenteral form at room temperature.
• For initial anesthesia induction dosage, give a small amount, via a tuberculin syringe, as prescribed.
• Give by slow IV push, over 1–2 min.
• Too rapid IV infusion increases the risk that the patient will experience severe adverse reactions, such as anaphylaxis, marked by bronchospasm, cardiac arrest, laryngospasm, peripheral circulatory collapse, and skeletal and thoracic muscle rigidity resulting in apnea.
• An opiate antagonist, such as naloxone, should be readily available during fentanyl administration.

TRANSDERMAL
• Apply to a nonhairy area of intact skin of the upper torso of the patient.
• Use a flat, nonirritated site.
• Firmly press the patch onto the patient's skin evenly for 10–20 sec, ensuring that the adhesion is in full contact with skin and that the edges are completely sealed.
• Use only water to cleanse the patient's patch site before application because soap and oils may irritate the skin.
• Rotate sites of application.
• Carefully fold used patches so that they adhere to themselves; discard in secure receptacle.

TRANSMUCOSAL
• Patient should suck lozenge vigorously. Do not bite lozenge.

Intervention and Evaluation
• Assist the patient with ambulation.
• Encourage the patient to cough, turn, and deep breathe every 2 hrs.
• Monitor the patient's B/P, heart rate, oxygen saturation, and respiratory rate.
• Assess the patient for relief of pain.

Patient/Family Teaching
• Urge the patient/family to avoid alcohol and not to take any other medications during fentanyl therapy without first notifying the physician.
• Warn the patient/family to avoid tasks requiring mental alertness or motor skills until the patient's response to the drug is established.
• Teach the patient/family the proper application of the transdermal fentanyl patch.
• Tell the patient/family to use fentanyl as directed to avoid overdosage. Explain to the patient that there is a potential for physical dependence on the drug with prolonged use.
• Instruct the patient/family to discontinue fentanyl slowly after long-term use.

Hydromorphone Hydrochloride

high-dro-**more**-phone
(Dilaudid, Dilaudid HP, Hydromorph Contin [CAN])

CATEGORY AND SCHEDULE

Pregnancy Risk Category C (D if used for prolonged periods or at high dosages at term)
Controlled Substance: Schedule II

MECHANISM OF ACTION

An opioid agonist that binds at opiate receptor sites in the CNS. ***Therapeutic Effect:*** Reduces intensity of pain stimuli coming from sensory nerve endings, altering pain perception and emotional response to pain; suppresses cough reflex.

PHARMACOKINETICS

Route	Onset	Peak	Duration
PO	30 min	90–120 min	4 hrs
SC	15 min	30–90 min	4 hrs
IM	15 min	30–60 min	4–5 hrs
IV	10–15 min	15–30 min	2–3 hrs
Rectal	15–30 min	N/A	N/A

Well absorbed from the GI tract, after IM administration. Widely distributed. Metabolized in liver. Excreted in urine. ***Half-Life:*** Adults 1–3 hrs.

AVAILABILITY

Tablets: 2 mg, 4 mg, 8 mg.
Liquid: 5 mg/5 mL.
Injection: 1 mg/mL, 2 mg/mL, 4 mg/mL, 10 mg/mL.
Suppository: 3 mg.

INDICATIONS AND DOSAGES

▸ Analgesic

IV

Children weighing more than 50 kg (opioid-naïve). 0.2–0.6 mg q2–4h as needed.
Children weighing less than 50 kg (opioid-naïve). 0.015 mg/kg/dose q3–6h as needed.

PO

Children weighing 50 kg and more. 1–2 mg q3–4h as needed. Range: 2–8 mg/dose.
Children older than 6 mos, weighing less than 50 kg. 0.03–0.08 mg/kg/dose q3–4h as needed

▸ Antitussive

PO

Children older than 12 yrs. 1 mg q3–4h as needed.
Children 6–12 yrs. 0.5 mg q3–4h as needed.

CONTRAINDICATIONS

Hypersensitivity to hydromorphone or any related component.

INTERACTIONS

Drug

Alcohol, CNS depressants: May increase CNS or respiratory depression, hypotension.
MAOIs: May produce severe, fatal reaction; plan to reduce dose to one quarter usual dose.

Herbal

None known.

Food

None known.

DIAGNOSTIC TEST EFFECTS

May increase serum amylase levels and plasma lipase concentrations.

IV INCOMPATIBILITIES

Amphotericin B complex (Abelcet, AmBisome, Amphotec), cefazolin (Ancef, Kefzol), diazepam

(Valium), phenobarbital, phenytoin (Dilantin)

IV COMPATIBILITIES

Diltiazem (Cardizem), diphenhydramine (Benadryl), dobutamine (Dobutrex), dopamine (Intropin), fentanyl (Sublimaze), furosemide (Lasix), heparin, lorazepam (Ativan), magnesium sulfate, metoclopramide (Reglan), midazolam (Versed), milrinone (Primacor), morphine, propofol (Diprivan)

SIDE EFFECTS

Frequent
Drowsiness, dizziness, hypotension, decreased appetite
Occasional
Confusion, diaphoresis, facial flushing, urinary retention, constipation, dry mouth, nausea, vomiting, headache, pain at injection site
Rare
Allergic reaction, depression

SERIOUS REACTIONS

! Overdosage results in respiratory depression, skeletal muscle flaccidity, cold or clammy skin, cyanosis, extreme somnolence progressing to seizures, stupor, and coma.
! Tolerance to analgesic effect and physical dependence may occur with repeated use.
! Prolonged duration of action and cumulative effect may occur in patients with impaired liver or renal function.

PEDIATRIC CONSIDERATIONS

Baseline Assessment
- Obtain the patient's vital signs before administering hydromorphone.
- Withhold the medication, and notify the physician if the respirations are 12/min or fewer in an adult patient or 20/min or fewer in children.
- Assess the duration, location, onset, and type of pain.
- Know that the effect of hydromorphone is reduced if the patient experiences full pain before the next dose.
- Assess the frequency, severity, and type of cough the patient experiences.
- Be aware that hydromorphone readily crosses the placenta, and it is unknown whether hydromorphone is distributed in breast milk.
- Be aware that hydromorphone use may prolong labor if administered in the latent phase of the first stage of labor or before cervical dilation of 4–5 cm has occurred.
- Be aware that respiratory depression may occur in the neonate if the mother receives opiates during labor. Regular use of opiates during pregnancy may produce withdrawal symptoms in the neonate, including diarrhea, excessive crying, fever, hyperactive reflexes, irritability, seizures, sneezing, tremors, vomiting, and yawning.
- Be aware that pediatric patients younger than 2 yrs of age may be more susceptible to respiratory depression.
- Be aware that rapid IV infusion is associated with respiratory depression, circulatory collapse, and hypotension. Have naloxone on hand for IV administration.

Precautions
- Use extremely cautiously in patients with acute alcoholism, anoxia, CNS depression, hypercapnia, respiratory depression or dysfunction, seizures, shock, and untreated myxedema.
- Use cautiously in patients with acute abdominal conditions,

Addison's disease, chronic obstructive pulmonary disease, hypothyroidism, impaired liver function, increased intracranial pressure, prostatic hypertrophy, and urethral stricture.

Administration and Handling

◂ALERT▸ Keep in mind that the side effects of hydromorphone depend on the dosage amount and route of administration but occur infrequently with oral antitussives.

• Know that patients who are ambulatory or not in severe pain may experience dizziness, hypotension, nausea, and vomiting more frequently than those in the supine position or having severe pain.

PO

• Give hydromorphone without regard to meals.

• Crush tablets, as needed.

SC/IM

• Use short 30-gauge needle for SC injection.

• Administer slowly, rotating injection sites.

• Know that patients with circulatory impairment experience a higher risk of overdosage because of delayed absorption of repeated SC or IM injections.

IV

◂ALERT▸ Be aware that a high concentration injection (10 mg/mL) should be used only in patients currently receiving high doses of another opiate agonist for severe, chronic pain caused by cancer or tolerance to opiate agonists.

• Store at room temperature; protect from light.

• Slight yellow discoloration of parenteral form does not indicate loss of potency.

• May give undiluted as IV push.

• May further dilute with 5 mL Sterile Water for Injection or 0.9% NaCl.

• Administer IV push very slowly over 2–5 min.

• Be aware that rapid IV administration increases the risk of a severe anaphylactic reaction, marked by apnea, cardiac arrest, and circulatory collapse.

RECTAL

• Refrigerate suppositories.

• Moisten suppository with cold water before inserting well up into rectum.

Intervention and Evaluation

• Monitor and assess the patient's vital signs.

• Assess the patient for cough and pain relief.

• Auscultate the patient's lungs for adventitious breath sounds.

• Increase the patient's fluid intake and environmental humidity to decrease the viscosity of patient lung secretions.

• Assess the patient's pattern of daily bowel activity and stool consistency, especially with long-term use.

• Initiate deep breathing and coughing exercises, particularly in patients with impaired pulmonary function.

• Assess the patient for clinical improvement and record the onset of relief of cough or pain.

Patient/Family Teaching

• Urge the patient/family to avoid alcohol during hydromorphone therapy.

• Warn the patient/family to avoid tasks that require mental alertness and motor skills until the patient's response to the drug is established.

• Explain to the patient/family that drug dependence and tolerance may occur with prolonged use at high dosages.

• Instruct the patient/family to change positions slowly to avoid orthostatic hypotension.

• Tell the patient/family to alert you to pain at its onset because the effect of hydromorphone is reduced if the patient experiences full pain before the next dose.

Meperidine Hydrochloride

meh-**pear**-ih-deen
(Demerol, Pethidine Injection [AUS])

CATEGORY AND SCHEDULE

Pregnancy Risk Category: B (D if used for prolonged periods or at high dosages at term)
Controlled Substance: Schedule II

MECHANISM OF ACTION

A narcotic agonist that binds with opioid receptors within the CNS. ***Therapeutic Effect:*** Alters processes, affecting pain perception and emotional response to pain.

PHARMACOKINETICS

Route	Onset	Peak	Duration
PO	15 min	60 min	2–4 hrs
SC	10–15 min	30–50 min	2–4 hrs
IM	10–15 min	30–50 min	2–4 hrs
IV	less than 5 min	5–7 min	2–3 hrs

Variably absorbed from the GI tract, well absorbed after IM administration. Protein binding: 60%–80%. Widely distributed. Metabolized in liver to the active metabolite. Primarily excreted in urine. Not removed by hemodialysis. ***Half-Life:*** Premature infants 3–60 hrs. Neonates 5–31 hrs. Infants 2 hrs. Children 3 hrs. Adults 2.4–4 hrs. Metabolite: Adults 8–16 hrs.

AVAILABILITY

Tablets: 50 mg, 100 mg.
Syrup: 50 mg/5 mL.
Injection: 25 mg/mL, 50 mg/mL, 75 mg/mL, 100 mg/mL.

INDICATIONS AND DOSAGES

▸ **Pain**

IM/SC/IV

Children. 0.5–2 mg/kg/dose q3–4h. Do not exceed single pediatric dose of 100 mg.

▸ **Dosage in renal impairment**

Creatinine Clearance	% Normal Dose
10–50 mL/min	75
Less than 10 mL/min	50

CONTRAINDICATIONS

Hypersensitivity to meperidine or any related component. Delivery of premature infant, diarrhea due to poisoning, those receiving MAOIs in past 14 days.

INTERACTIONS

Drug

Alcohol, CNS depressants: May increase CNS or respiratory depression and hypotension.
MAOIs: May produce severe, fatal reaction; plan to reduce dose to one quarter the usual dose.

Herbal

Valerian: May increase CNS depression.

Food

None known.

DIAGNOSTIC TEST EFFECTS

May increase serum amylase and lipase levels.

IV INCOMPATIBILITIES

Allopurinol (Aloprim), amphotericin B complex (Abelcet, AmBisome, Amphotec), cefepime (Maxipime), cefoperazone (Cefobid), doxorubicin liposome (Doxil), furosemide (Lasix), idarubicin (Idamycin), nafcillin (Nafcil)

IV COMPATIBILITIES

Bumetanide (Bumex), diltiazem (Cardizem), dobutamine (Dobutrex), dopamine (Intropin), heparin, insulin, lidocaine, magnesium, oxytocin (Pitocin), potassium

SIDE EFFECTS

Frequent
Sedation, decreased blood pressure (B/P), diaphoresis, flushed face, dizziness, nausea, vomiting, constipation

Occasional
Confusion, irregular heartbeat, tremors, decreased urination, abdominal pain, dry mouth, headache, irritation at injection site, euphoria, dysphoria

Rare
Allergic reaction, marked by rash and itching, insomnia

SERIOUS REACTIONS

! Overdosage results in respiratory depression, skeletal muscle flaccidity, cold or clammy skin, cyanosis, and extreme somnolence progressing to convulsions, stupor, and coma. The overdosage antidote is 0.4 mg naloxone (Narcan).

! Accumulation of the active metabolite (normeperidine) can occur in patients with hepatic or renal impairment or with continuous infusions. This may precipitate twitches, tremors, or seizures.

! Tolerance to the drug's analgesic effect and physical dependence may occur with repeated use.

PEDIATRIC CONSIDERATIONS

Baseline Assessment

- Place patient in a recumbent position before giving parenteral meperidine.
- Assess the duration, location, onset, and type of pain the patient is experiencing.
- Obtain the patient's vital signs before giving meperidine.
- Withhold the medication and notify the physician if the respirations are 12/min or fewer in an adult patient or 20/min or fewer in children.
- Know that the effects of meperidine are reduced if the patient experiences full pain before the next dose of the drug.
- Be aware that meperidine crosses the placenta and is distributed in breast milk.
- Be aware that respiratory depression may occur in the neonate if the mother received opiates during labor. Regular use of opiates during pregnancy may produce withdrawal symptoms in the neonate, such as diarrhea, excessive crying, fever, hyperactive reflexes, irritability, seizures, sneezing, tremors, vomiting, and yawning.
- Be aware that children may experience paradoxical excitement.
- Know that children younger than 2 yrs of age are more susceptible to the respiratory depressant effects of meperidine.
- Be aware that rapid IV infusion of meperidine can cause respiratory depression, circulatory collapse, and hypotension. Have naloxone on hand.

Precautions

- Use cautiously in patients with acute abdominal conditions, cor pulmonale, a history of seizures, increased intracranial pressure, liver or renal impairment,

respiratory abnormalities, and supraventricular tachycardia.
• Use cautiously in debilitated patients.

Administration and Handling

◀ **ALERT** ▶ Be aware that the side effects of meperidine are dependent on the dosage amount and route of administration.
• Be aware that the IV boluses may cause euphoria in some patients.
• Know that patients who are ambulatory and not in severe pain may experience dizziness, nausea, and vomiting more frequently than those in the supine position or having severe pain.

◀ **ALERT** ▶ Keep in mind that the IM route is preferred over the SC route because the SC injection can produce induration, local irritation, and pain.

PO
• Give meperidine without regard to meals.
• Dilute syrup in a glass of water to prevent an anesthetic effect on the mucous membranes.

SC/IM
• Inject slowly.
• Know that patients with circulatory impairment experience a higher risk of overdosage because of delayed absorption of repeated injection.

IV

◀ **ALERT** ▶ Give by slow IV push or infusion.
• Store at room temperature.
• May give undiluted or may dilute in D_5W, lactated Ringer's solution, a dextrose-saline combination, such as 2.5%, 5%, or 10% dextrose with 0.45% or 0.9% NaCl, Ringer's solution, or molar sodium lactate diluent for IV injection or infusion.
• Administer IV push very slowly, over 2–3 min.
• Be aware that rapid IV administration increases risk of severe anaphylactic reaction, marked by apnea, cardiac arrest, and circulatory collapse.

Intervention and Evaluation

• Monitor the patient's vital signs 15–30 min after SC/IM dose and 5–10 min after IV dose. Monitor for decreased B/P, as well as a change in quality and rate of pulse.
• Monitor the patient's pain level and sedation.
• Assess the patient's pattern of daily bowel activity and stool consistency.
• Evaluate the patient for adequate voiding.
• Initiate deep breathing and coughing exercises, particularly in patients with impaired pulmonary function.

Patient/Family Teaching

• Instruct the patient/family to take meperidine before the pain fully returns, within prescribed intervals.
• Explain to the patient/family that discomfort may occur with injection.
• Instruct the patient/family to change positions slowly to avoid orthostatic hypotension.
• Urge the patient/family to increase the patient's fluid intake and consumption of fiber or bulking agents to prevent constipation.
• Tell the patient/family that dependence on and tolerance to the drug may occur with prolonged use of high doses.
• Urge the patient/family to avoid alcohol and other CNS depressants while taking meperidine.
• Warn the patient/family to avoid tasks that require mental alertness or motor skills until the patient's response to the drug is established.

Methadone Hydrochloride

meth-ah-doan
(Dolophine, Metadol [CAN], Methadose, Physeptone [AUS])

CATEGORY AND SCHEDULE

Pregnancy Risk Category: B (D if used for prolonged periods or at high dosages at term)
Controlled Substance: Schedule II

MECHANISM OF ACTION

A narcotic agonist that binds with opioid receptors within the CNS. ***Therapeutic Effect:*** Alters processes affecting analgesia and emotional response to acute withdrawal syndrome.

PHARMACOKINETICS

Route	Onset	Peak	Duration
PO	30–60 min	0.5–1 hr	6–8 hrs
SC	10–15 min	1–2 hrs	4–6 hrs
IM	10–15 min	1–2 hrs	4–6 hrs

Well absorbed after IM injection. Protein binding: 80%–85%. Metabolized in liver. Primarily excreted in urine. Not removed by hemodialysis. ***Half-Life:*** Adults 15–25 hrs.

AVAILABILITY

Tablets: 5 mg, 10 mg.
Tablets (dispersible): 40 mg.
Oral Solution: 5 mg/5 mL, 10 mg/5 mL.
Oral Concentrate: 10 mg/mL.
Injection: 10 mg/mL.

INDICATIONS AND DOSAGES

▸ Analgesia

PO

Children. 0.05–0.2 mg/kg/dose q6–8hr as needed. Maximum: 10 mg/dose.

SC/IM

Children. Initially, 0.1 mg/kg/dose q4h for 2–3 doses, then q6–12h. Maximum: 10 mg/dose.

CONTRAINDICATIONS

Hypersensitivity to opioids, delivery of premature infant, during labor, diarrhea due to poisoning.

INTERACTIONS

Drug

Alcohol, CNS depressants: May increase CNS or respiratory depression and hypotension.
MAOIs May produce a severe, fatal reaction; plan to reduce to one quarter usual dose.

Herbal

Valerian: May increase CNS depression.

Food

None known.

DIAGNOSTIC TEST EFFECTS

May increase serum amylase and lipase levels.

SIDE EFFECTS

Frequent

Sedation, decreased blood pressure, diaphoresis, flushed face, constipation, dizziness, nausea, vomiting

Occasional

Confusion, decreased urination, pounding heartbeat, stomach cramps, visual changes, dry mouth, headache, decreased appetite, nervousness, inability to sleep

Rare

Allergic reaction, such as rash or itching

SERIOUS REACTIONS

! Overdosage results in respiratory depression, skeletal muscle flaccidity, cold or clammy skin, cyanosis, extreme somnolence progressing to convulsions, stupor, and coma. The antidote for overdosage is 0.4 mg naloxone.

! Tolerance to the drug's analgesic effect and physical dependence may occur with repeated use.

PEDIATRIC CONSIDERATIONS

Baseline Assessment

- Place the patient in the recumbent position before giving parenteral methadone.
- Obtain the patient's vital signs before giving the medication.
- Withhold the medication, and notify the physician if respirations are 12/minor fewer in an adult patient or 20/min or fewer in children.
- Be aware that methadone crosses the placenta and is distributed in breast milk.
- Be aware that respiratory depression may occur in the neonate if the mother received opiates during labor. Know that regular use of opiates during pregnancy may produce withdrawal symptoms in the neonate, such as diarrhea, excessive crying, fever, hyperactive reflexes, irritability, seizures, sneezing, tremors, vomiting, and yawning.
- Be aware that children may experience paradoxical excitement.
- Be aware that children younger than 2 yrs of age are more susceptible to the respiratory depressant effects of methadone.
- Be aware that to prevent withdrawal symptoms in a child the medication must be tapered gradually.

Precautions

- Use extremely cautiously in patients with acute abdominal conditions, cor pulmonale, a history of seizures, impaired liver or renal function, increased intracranial pressure, respiratory abnormalities, and supraventricular tachycardia.
- Use cautiously in debilitated patients.

Administration and Handling

PO

- Give methadone without regard to meals.
- Dilute syrup in a glass of water to prevent an anesthetic effect on mucous membranes.

SC/IM

◂ALERT▸ Be aware that the IM route is preferred over the SC route because the SC route can produce induration, local irritation, and pain.

- Do not use if the solution appears cloudy or contains a precipitate.
- Inject slowly.
- Know that patients with circulatory impairment have a higher risk of overdosage because of delayed absorption of repeated SC or IM injections.

Intervention and Evaluation

- Monitor the patient's vital signs 15–30 min after a SC/IM dose and 5–10 min after an IV dose.
- Know that oral methadone is one-half as potent as parenteral methadone.
- Assess the patient for adequate voiding.
- Assess the patient for clinical improvement, and record the onset of relief of pain.
- Provide support to the patient in a detoxification program. Monitor

the patient for withdrawal symptoms.

Patient/Family Teaching

• Urge the patient/family to avoid alcohol.

• Caution the patient/family against abruptly discontinuing the drug after prolonged use.

• Explain to the patient/family that methadone may cause drowsiness and dry mouth.

• Warn the patient/family that methadone may impair the patient's ability to perform activities requiring mental alertness and motor skills.

Morphine Sulfate

(Anamorph [AUS], Astramorph, Avinza, Duramorph, Infumorph, Kadian, Kapanol [AUS], M-Eslon, Morphine Mixtures [AUS], MS Contin, MSIR, MS Mono [AUS], Oramorph SR, RMS, Roxanol, Statex [CAN])

Do not confuse with hydromorphone or Roxicet.

CATEGORY AND SCHEDULE

Pregnancy Risk Category: C (D if used for prolonged periods or at high dosages at term)
Controlled Substance: Schedule II

MECHANISM OF ACTION

A narcotic agonist that binds with opioid receptors within the CNS. ***Therapeutic Effect:*** Alters processes affecting pain perception and emotional response to pain; produces generalized CNS depression.

PHARMACOKINETICS

Route	Onset	Peak	Duration
Tablets	N/A	1 hr	3–5 hrs
Oral solution	N/A	1 hr	3–5 hrs
Epidural	N/A	1 hr	12–20 hrs
Extended-release tablets	N/A	3–4 hrs	8–12 hrs
Rectal	N/A	0.5–1 hr	3–7 hrs
SC	N/A	1.1–5 hrs	3–5 hrs
IM	5–30 min	0.5–1 hr	3–5 hrs
IV	Rapid	0.3 hr	3–5 hrs

Variably absorbed from the GI tract. Readily absorbed after SC or IM administration. Protein binding: 20%–35%. Widely distributed. Metabolized in liver. Primarily excreted in urine. Removed by hemodialysis. ***Half-Life:*** Adults 2–3 hrs.

AVAILABILITY

Capsules (sustained release): 20 mg (Kadian), 30 mg (Kadian), 50 mg (Kadian), 60 mg (Kadian), 100 mg (Kadian).

Capsules (extended release): 30 mg (Avinza), 60 mg (Avinza), 90 mg (Avinza), 120 mg (Avinza).

Solution for Injection: 0.5 mg/mL, 1 mg/mL, 2 mg/mL, 4 mg/mL, 5 mg/mL, 8 mg/mL, 10 mg/mL, 15 mg/mL, 25 mg/mL, 50 mg/mL.

Solution for Injection (preservative free): 0.5 mg/mL, 1 mg/mL, 10 mg/mL, 25 mg/mL, 50 mg/mL.

Epidural and Intrathecal via Infusion Device: 10 mg/mL (Infumorph), 25 mg/mL (Infumorph).

Epidural, Intrathecal, IV Infusion: 0.5 mg/mL (Astramorph, Duramorph), 1 mg/mL (Astramorph, Duramorph), 4 mg/mL (Astramorph, Duramorph).

IV Infusion (via patient-controlled analgesia): 1 mg/mL, 5 mg/mL.
Oral Solution: 10 mg/5 mL (Roxanol), 20 mg/5 mL (Roxanol), 20 mg/mL (Roxanol), 100 mg/5 mg (Roxanol).
Suppository: 5 mg, 10 mg, 20 mg, 30 mg (RMS).
Tablets: 15 mg/30 mg (MSIR).
Tablets (extended release): 15 mg (MS Contin, Oramorph SR), 30 mg (MS Contin, Oramorph SR), 60 mg (MS Contin, Oramorph SR), 100 mg (MS Contin, Oramorph SR), 200 mg (MS Contin, Oramorph SR).

INDICATIONS AND DOSAGES

▸ Pain

PO
Children (sustained-release). 0.3–0.6 mg/kg/dose q12h as needed.
Children (prompt release). 0.2–0.5 mg/kg/dose q4–6h as needed.
IV/IM/SC
Children. 0.1–0.2 mg/kg/dose q2–4h as needed. Maximum: 15 mg/dose.
IV CONTINUOUS INFUSION
Children. 0.02–2.6 mg/kg/hr.

CONTRAINDICATIONS

Hypersensitivity to morphine or any related component. Severe respiratory depression, acute or severe asthma, severe liver or renal impairment, GI obstruction.

INTERACTIONS

Drug

Alcohol, CNS depressants: May increase CNS or respiratory depression and hypotension.
MAOIs: May produce severe, fatal reaction; plan to reduce dose to one quarter of usual dose.

Herbal

None known.

Food

None known.

DIAGNOSTIC TEST EFFECTS

May increase serum amylase and lipase levels.

IV INCOMPATIBILITIES

Amphotericin B complex (Abelcet, AmBisome, Amphotec), cefepime (Maxipime), doxorubicin liposome (Doxil), thiopental

IV COMPATIBILITIES

Amiodarone (Cordarone), bumetanide (Bumex), bupivacaine (Marcaine, Sensorcaine), diltiazem (Cardizem), dobutamine (Dobutrex), dopamine (Intropin), heparin, lidocaine, lorazepam (Ativan), magnesium, midazolam (Versed), milrinone (Primacor), nitroglycerin, potassium, propofol (Diprivan)

SIDE EFFECTS

Frequent

Sedation, decreased blood pressure (B/P), diaphoresis, flushed face, constipation, dizziness, drowsiness, nausea, vomiting

Occasional

Allergic reaction, such as rash and itching, difficulty breathing, confusion, pounding heartbeat, tremors, decreased urination, stomach cramps, vision changes, dry mouth, headache, decreased appetite, pain/burning at injection site

Rare

Paralytic ileus

SERIOUS REACTIONS

! Overdosage results in respiratory depression, skeletal muscle flaccidity, cold or clammy skin, cyanosis, and extreme somnolence progressing to convulsions, stupor, and coma.

! Tolerance to analgesic effects and physical dependence may occur with repeated use.

! Prolonged duration of action and cumulative effect may occur in those with impaired liver and renal function.

PEDIATRIC CONSIDERATIONS

Baseline Assessment

- Place the patient in a recumbent position before giving parenteral morphine.
- Assess the duration, location, onset, and type of pain the patient is experiencing.
- Obtain the patient's vital signs before giving morphine.
- Withhold the medication and notify the physician if respirations are 12/min or fewer in the adult patient or 20/min or fewer in children.
- Be aware that the effect of the medication is reduced if the patient experiences full pain before the next dose.
- Be aware that morphine crosses the placenta and is distributed in breast milk.
- Be aware that morphine may prolong labor if administered in the latent phase of the first stage of labor or before cervical dilation of 4–5 cm has occurred. Respiratory depression may occur in the neonate if the mother received opiates during labor.
- Be aware that regular use of opiates during pregnancy may produce withdrawal symptoms in the neonate, such as diarrhea, excessive crying, fever, hyperactive reflexes, irritability, seizures, sneezing, tremors, vomiting, and yawning.
- Be aware that children may experience paradoxical excitement.
- Be aware that children younger than 2 yrs of age are more susceptible to the respiratory depressant effects of morphine.
- Be aware that rapid IV infusion can lead to respiratory depression, cardiovascular collapse, and hypotension. Have naloxone on hand.

Precautions

- Use extremely cautiously in patients with chronic obstructive pulmonary disease, cor pulmonale, head injury, hypoxia, hypercapnia, increased intracranial pressure, preexisting respiratory depression, and severe hypotension.
- Use cautiously in patients with Addison's disease, alcoholism, biliary tract disease, CNS depression, hypothyroidism, pancreatitis, prostatic hypertrophy, seizure disorders, toxic psychosis, and urethral stricture.
- Use cautiously in debilitated patients.

Administration and Handling

◂ **ALERT** ▸ Expect to reduce the drug dosage in debilitated patients and those receiving concurrent CNS depressants. Titrate to desired effect, as prescribed.

◂ **ALERT** ▸ Be aware that the side effects of morphine are dependent on the dosage amount and route of administration.

- Know that patients who are ambulatory and not in severe pain may experience dizziness, nausea, and vomiting more frequently than those in the supine position or having severe pain.

PO

- Mix the liquid form with fruit juice to improve taste.
- Do not crush, open, or break extended-release capsules.

• May mix Kadian with applesauce immediately before administration.
SC/IM
• Give injection slowly, rotating injection sites.
• Know that patients with circulatory impairment experience a higher risk of overdosage because of delayed absorption of repeated injections.
IV
• Store at room temperature.
• May give undiluted as IV push.
• For IV push, may dilute 2.5–15 mg morphine in 4–5 mL Sterile Water for Injection.
• For continuous IV infusion, dilute to concentration of 0.1–1 mg/mL in D_5W and give through a controlled infusion device.
• Always administer very slowly. Be aware that rapid IV administration increases the risk of a severe anaphylactic reaction, marked by apnea, cardiac arrest, and circulatory collapse.
RECTAL
• If suppository is too soft, chill for 30 min in the refrigerator or run cold water over the foil wrapper.
• Moisten suppository with cold water before inserting well into rectum.

Intervention and Evaluation
• Monitor the patient's vital signs 5–10 min after IV administration and 15–30 min after SC or IM injection.
• Be alert for decreased patient respirations or B/P.
• Evaluate the patient for difficulty voiding.
• Assess the patient's pattern of daily bowel activity and stool consistency.
• Initiate deep breathing and coughing exercises, particularly in patients with impaired pulmonary function.
• Assess the patient for clinical improvement, and record the onset of pain relief.
• Consult with the physician if the patient's pain relief is not adequate.

Patient/Family Teaching
• Tell the patient/family that discomfort may occur with injection.
• Instruct the patient/family to change positions slowly to avoid orthostatic hypotension.
• Warn the patient/family to avoid tasks that require mental alertness or motor skills until the patient's response to the drug is established.
• Urge the patient/family to avoid alcohol and CNS depressants during morphine therapy.
• Explain to the patient/family that dependence and tolerance may occur with prolonged use of high morphine doses.

Oxycodone

ox-ih-**koe**-doan
(Endone [AUS], Intensol, OxyContin, OxyFast, OxyIR, Percolone, Roxicodone, Supeudol [CAN])
Do not confuse with oxybutynin.

CATEGORY AND SCHEDULE

Pregnancy Risk Category: B (D if used for prolonged periods or at high dosages at term)
Controlled Substance: Schedule II

MECHANISM OF ACTION

An opioid analgesic that binds with opioid receptors within the CNS. ***Therapeutic Effect:*** Alters processes affecting pain perception and emotional response to pain.

PHARMACOKINETICS

Route	Onset	Peak	Duration
Immediate-release tablets	N/A	N/A	4–5 hrs
Controlled-release tablets	N/A	N/A	12 hrs

Moderately absorbed from the GI tract. Protein binding: 38%–45%. Widely distributed. Metabolized in liver. Excreted in urine. Unknown whether removed by hemodialysis. ***Half-Life:*** Adults: 2–3 hrs (controlled-release: 3.2 hrs).

AVAILABILITY

Capsules (immediate release): 5 mg (OxyIR).
Oral Concentrate: 20 mg/mL (OxyFast, Roxicodone, Intensol).
Oral Solution: 5 mg/mL (Roxicodone).
Tablets (immediate release): 5 mg (Percolone, Roxicodone), 15 mg (Percolone, Roxicodone), 30 mg (Percolone, Roxicodone).
Tablets (controlled release): 10 mg (OxyContin), 20 mg (OxyContin), 40 mg (OxyContin), 80 mg (OxyContin), 160 mg (OxyContin).

INDICATIONS AND DOSAGES

▸ **Analgesia**

PO

Children. 0.05–0.15 mg/kg/dose q4–6h as needed.

CONTRAINDICATIONS

Hypersensitivity to oxycodone or any related component. Pts with hypercarbia, paralytic ileus, severe or acute asthma.

INTERACTIONS

Drug

Alcohol, CNS depressants: May increase CNS or respiratory depression and hypotension.
MAOIs: May produce severe, fatal reaction; expect to reduce dose to one quarter usual dose.

Herbal

None known.

Food

None known.

DIAGNOSTIC TEST EFFECTS

May increase serum amylase and lipase levels.

SIDE EFFECTS

Frequent

Drowsiness, dizziness, hypotension, anorexia

Occasional

Confusion, diaphoresis, facial flushing, urinary retention, constipation, dry mouth, nausea, vomiting, headache

Rare

Allergic reaction, depression, paradoxical CNS hyperactivity or nervousness in children, excitement and restlessness in debilitated patients

SERIOUS REACTIONS

! Overdose results in respiratory depression, skeletal muscle flaccidity, cold or clammy skin, cyanosis, and extreme somnolence progressing to convulsions, stupor, and coma.

! Liver toxicity may occur with overdosage of acetaminophen component.

! Tolerance to analgesic effect and physical dependence may occur with repeated use.

PEDIATRIC CONSIDERATIONS

Baseline Assessment

- Assess the duration, location, onset, and type of pain the patient is experiencing.
- Know that the effect of oxycodone is reduced if the patient experiences full pain before the next dose.
- Obtain the patient's vital signs before giving the medication.
- Withhold the medication and notify the physician if are 12/min or fewer in the adult patient or 20/min or fewer in children.
- Be aware that oxycodone readily crosses the placenta and is distributed in breast milk.
- Be aware that respiratory depression may occur in the neonate if the mother received opiates during labor.
- Be aware that regular use of opiates during pregnancy may produce withdrawal symptoms in the neonate, including irritability, diarrhea, excessive crying, fever, hyperactive reflexes, irritability, seizures, sneezing, tremors, vomiting, and yawning.
- Be aware that children may experience paradoxical excitement.
- Be aware that children younger than 2 yrs of age are more susceptible to the respiratory depressant effects of oxycodone.

Precautions

- Use extremely cautiously in patients with acute alcoholism, anoxia, CNS depression, hypercapnia, respiratory depression or dysfunction, seizures, shock, and untreated myxedema.
- Use cautiously in patients with acute abdominal conditions, Addison's disease, chronic obstructive pulmonary disease, hypothyroidism, impaired liver function, increased intracranial pressure, prostatic hypertrophy, and urethral stricture.

Administration and Handling

◂ **ALERT** ▸ Be aware that the effects of oxycodone are dependent on the dosage amount.

- Know that ambulatory patients and patients not in severe pain may experience dizziness, hypotension, nausea, and vomiting more frequently than those in the supine position or having severe pain.

PO

- Give oxycodone without regard to meals.
- Crush immediate-release tablets as needed.
- Have the patient swallow controlled-release tablets whole; do not crush, break, or chew.

Intervention and Evaluation

- Palpate the patient's bladder for urine retention.
- Monitor the patient's pattern of daily bowel activity and stool consistency.
- Initiate deep breathing and coughing exercises, particularly in patients with impaired pulmonary function.
- Monitor the patient's blood pressure, mental status, respiratory rate, and pain relief.

Patient/Family Teaching

- Tell the patient/family that oxycodone may cause drowsiness and dry mouth.
- Warn the patient/family to avoid performing tasks that require mental alertness or motor skills.
- Urge the patient/family to avoid alcohol while taking oxycodone.
- Caution the patient/family that oxycodone use may be habit forming.

• Instruct the patient/family not to break, chew, or crush controlled-release tablets.
• Instruct the patient/family to take oxycodone before the pain fully returns, within prescribed intervals.

REFERENCES

Miller, S. & Fioravanti, J. (1997). Pediatric medications: a handbook for nurses. St. Louis: Mosby.
Taketomo, C. K., Hodding, J. H. & Kraus, D. M. (2003–2004). Pediatric dosage handbook (10th ed.). Hudson, OH: Lexi-Comp.

41 Narcotic Antagonists

Naloxone Hydrochloride

Uses: Narcotic antagonists are primarily used to reverse the respiratory depression caused by narcotic overdosage. Naloxone is the drug of choice for reversal of respiratory depression. In patients with severe respiratory depression, treatment requires additional measures, including oxygen administration and mechanical ventilation.

Action: By displacing narcotics (opioid agonists) at receptor sites in the CNS, narcotic antagonists prevent and reverse their effects on mu receptors. For example, they increase respiration and reverse sedative effects.

COMBINATION PRODUCTS

SUBOXONE: naloxone/buprenorphine (a non-narcotic analgesic) 0.5 mg/2 mg; 2 mg/8 mg.

Naloxone Hydrochloride

nay-**lox**-own

(Narcan)

Do not confuse with Norcuron.

CATEGORY AND SCHEDULE

Pregnancy Risk Category: B

MECHANISM OF ACTION

A narcotic antagonist that displaces opiates at opiate-occupied receptor sites in the CNS. ***Therapeutic Effect:*** Blocks narcotic effects. Reverses opiate-induced sleep or sedation. Increases respiratory rate, returns depressed blood pressure (B/P) to normal rate.

PHARMACOKINETICS

Route	Onset	Peak	Duration
SC	2–5 min	N/A	20–60 min
IM	2–5 min	N/A	20–60 min
IV	1–2 min	N/A	20–60 min

Well absorbed after SC or IM administration. Crosses the placenta. Metabolized in liver. Primarily excreted in urine. ***Half-Life:*** 60–100 min.

AVAILABILITY

Injection: 0.02 mg/mL, 0.4 mg/mL, 1 mg/mL.

INDICATIONS AND DOSAGES

▸ **Opioid toxicity**

SC/IM/IV

Children 5 yrs and older or weighing 20 kg or more. 2 mg/dose; if no response may repeat q2–3min. May need to repeat q20–60 min.

Children younger than 5 yrs or weighing less than 20 kg. 0.1 mg/kg, repeat q2–3min. May need to repeat q20–60min.

▸ **Postanesthesia narcotic reversal**

IV

Children. 0.01 mg/kg, may repeat q2–3min.

▸ **Neonatal opioid-induced depression**

IV/IM/SC

Neonates. 0.01 mg/kg. May repeat q2–3min as needed. May need to repeat q1–2h.

CONTRAINDICATIONS

Hypersensitivity to naloxone or any related component. Respiratory depression due to nonopiate drugs.

INTERACTIONS

Drug

Butorphanol, nalbuphine, opioid agonist analgesics, pentazocine: Reverses the analgesic and side effects and may precipitate withdrawal symptoms of butorphanol, nalbuphine, opioid agonist analgesics, and pentazocine.

Herbal

None known.

Food

None known.

DIAGNOSTIC TEST EFFECTS

None known.

IV INCOMPATIBILITIES

Amphotericin B complex (Abelcet, AmBisome, Amphotec)

IV COMPATIBILITIES

Heparin, ondansetron (Zofran), propofol (Diprivan)

SIDE EFFECTS

None known, little or no pharmacologic effect in absence of narcotics

SERIOUS REACTIONS

! Too rapid reversal of narcotic depression may result in signs of opioid withdrawal including nausea, vomiting, tremulousness, sweating, increased B/P, and tachycardia.

! Excessive dosage in postoperative patients may produce significant reversal of analgesia, excitement, and tremulousness.

! Hypotension or hypertension, ventricular tachycardia and fibrillation, and pulmonary edema may occur in patients with cardiovascular disease.

PEDIATRIC CONSIDERATIONS

Baseline Assessment

• Maintain the patient's airway.
• Obtain the body weight of pediatric patients to calculate expected drug dosage.
• Be aware that it is unknown whether naloxone crosses the placenta or is distributed in breast milk.
• Be aware that naloxone may be given through an endotracheal tube if no other access is available.
• There are no age-related precautions noted in children.

Precautions

• Use cautiously in patients with chronic cardiac or pulmonary disease and coronary artery disease.
• Use cautiously in postoperative patients—to avoid potential cardiovascular complications—and in patients suspected of being opioid dependent.
• In patients receiving long-term treatment with opioids, watch for signs of withdrawal including: nausea, vomiting, abdominal cramps, lacrimation, rhinorrhea, piloerection, anxiety, restlessness, increased temperature, and diaphoresis.

Administration and Handling

◂ **ALERT** ▸ The American Academy of Pediatrics recommends an initial dose of 0.1 mg/kg for infants and children 5 yrs of age and younger and weighing less than 20 kg. For children older than 5 yrs or weighing more than 20 kg, the recommended initial dose is 2 mg.

IM

• Give IM injection in upper, outer quadrant of buttock.

IV

- Store parenteral form at room temperature.
- Use mixture within 24 hrs; discard unused solution.
- Protect from light; is stable in D_5W or 0.9% NaCl at 4 mcg/mL for 24 hrs.
- May dilute 1 mg/mL with 50 mL Sterile Water for Injection to provide a concentration of 0.02 mg/mL.
- For continuous IV infusion, dilute each 2 mg naloxone with 500 mL D_5W or 0.9% NaCl, producing solution containing 0.004 mg/mL.
- May administer undiluted.
- Give each 0.4 mg as IV push over 15 sec.
- Use the 0.4 mg/mL and 1 mg/mL concentration for injection for adults and the 0.02 mg/mL concentration for neonates.

Intervention and Evaluation

- Monitor the patient's vital signs, especially the depth, rate, and rhythm of respirations, during and frequently after administration.
- Carefully observe the patient after a satisfactory response because the duration of opiate use may exceed the duration of naloxone use, resulting in recurrence of respiratory depression.
- Assess patient for increased pain after administration of naloxone caused by reversal of the analgesic effects

Patient/Family Teaching

- Instruct the patient/family to let you know if the patient experiences pain or feelings of increased sedation.
- Review the potential source of opiate overdose—whether it was caused by taking too much of a drug or if the drug overdose was intentional.

REFERENCES

Miller, S. & Fioravanti, J. (1997). Pediatric medications: a handbook for nurses. St. Louis: Mosby.

Taketomo, C. K., Hodding, J. H. & Kraus, D. M. (2003–2004). Pediatric dosage handbook (10th ed.). Hudson, OH: Lexi-Comp.

42 Non-Narcotic Analgesics

Acetaminophen
Aspirin (Acetylsalicylic Acid, ASA)
Buprenorphine Hydrochloride
Nalbuphine Hydrochloride

Uses: Non-narcotic analgesics are used to relieve mild to moderate pain. Acetaminophen and salicylates, such as aspirin, also have anti-inflammatory and antipyretic effects. By virtue of its action on platelet function, aspirin is also used to prevent and treat diseases associated with hypercoagulability and to reduce the risk of stroke and myocardial infarction.

Action: Different non-narcotic analgesics act in distinct ways. *Agonist-antagonists,* such as nalbuphine, primarily act as antagonists at mu receptors and as agonists at kappa receptors. Although these agents have less abuse potential and cause less respiratory depression than narcotic analgesics, they generally produce weaker analgesic effects. (See illustration, *Mechanism of Action: Agonist-Antagonists,* page 540.) *Acetaminophen* may act by inhibiting prostaglandin synthesis in the CNS. *Salicylates,* such as aspirin, inhibit cyclooxygenase, thereby inhibiting prostaglandin synthesis in the CNS and periphery.

COMBINATION PRODUCTS

AGGRENOX: aspirin/dipyridamole (an antiplatelet agent) 25 mg/200 mg.
ANEXSIA: acetaminophen/hydrocodone (a narcotic analgesic) 500 mg/6 mg; 650 mg/7.5 mg; 660 mg/10 mg.
CAPITAL WITH CODEINE: acetaminophen/codeine (a narcotic analgesic) 120 mg/12 mg per 5 mL.
DARVOCET A 500: acetaminophen/propoxyphene (a narcotic analgesic) 500 mg/100 mg.
DARVOCET-N: acetaminophen/propoxyphene (a narcotic analgesic) 325 mg/50 mg; 650 mg/100 mg.
FIORICET: acetaminophen/caffeine (a CNS stimulant)/butabarbital (a sedative-hypnotic) 325 mg/40 mg/50 mg.
FIORINAL: aspirin/butabarbital (a sedative-hypnotic)/caffeine (a CNS stimulant) 325 mg/50 mg/40 mg.
LORTAB: acetaminophen/hydrocodone (a narcotic analgesic) 500 mg/2.5 mg; 500 mg/5 mg; 500 mg/7.5 mg.
LORTAB/ASA: aspirin/hydrocodone (a narcotic analgesic) 325 mg/5 mg.
LORTAB ELIXIR: acetaminophen/hydrocodone (a narcotic analgesic) 167 mg/2.5 mg per 5 mL.
NORCO: acetaminophen/hydrocodone (a narcotic analgesic) 325 mg/10 mg.
PERCOCET: acetaminophen/oxycodone (a narcotic analgesic) 325 mg/5 mg.
PERCODAN: aspirin/oxycodone (a narcotic analgesic) 325 mg/2.25 mg; 325 mg/4.5 mg.

PRAVIGARD: aspirin/pravastatin (an antihyperlipidemic) 81 mg/20 mg; 325 mg/20 mg; 81 mg/40 mg; 325 mg/40 mg; 81 mg/80 mg; 325 mg/80 mg.
ROXICET: acetaminophen/oxycodone (a narcotic analgesic) 325 mg/5 mg.
SUBOXONE: buprenorphine/naloxone (a narcotic antagonist) 2 mg/0.5 mg; 8 mg/2 mg.
TYLENOL WITH CODEINE: acetaminophen/codeine (a narcotic analgesic) 120 mg/12 mg per 5 mL; 300 mg/15 mg; 300 mg/30 mg; 300 mg/60 mg.
TYLOX: acetaminophen/oxycodone (a narcotic analgesic) 500 mg/5 mg.
ULTRACET: acetaminophen/tramadol (a non-narcotic analgesic) 325 mg/37.5 mg.
VICODIN: acetaminophen/hydrocodone (a narcotic analgesic) 500 mg/5 mg.
VICODIN ES: acetaminophen/hydrocodone (a narcotic analgesic) 750 mg/7.5 mg.
VICODIN HP: acetaminophen/hydrocodone (a narcotic analgesic) 660 mg/10 mg.

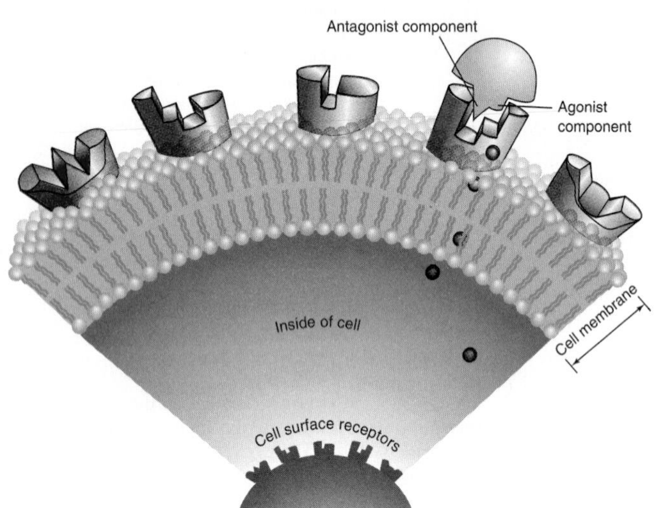

Mechanism of Action: Agonist-Antagonists

Cell membranes have different types of opioid receptors, such as mu, kappa, and delta receptors. Opioid agonist-antagonists, such as butorphanol and nalbuphine, work by stimulating one type of receptor, while simultaneously blocking another type. As agonists, they work primarily by activating kappa receptors to produce analgesia and other effects such as CNS and respiratory depression, decreased GI motility, and euphoria. As antagonists, they compete with opioids at mu receptors, helping to reverse or block some of the other effects of agonists.

ZYDONE: acetaminophen/ hydrocodone (a narcotic analgesic) 400 mg/5 mg; 400 mg/7.5 mg; 400 mg/10 mg.

Acetaminophen

ah-see-tah-**min**-oh-fen
(Abenol [CAN], Apo-Acetaminophen [CAN], Atasol [CAN], Dymadon [AUS], Feverall, Panadol [AUS], Panamax [AUS], Paralgin [AUS], Setamol [AUS], Tempra, Tylenol)
Do not confuse with Fiorinal, Hycodan, Indocin, Percodan, or Tuinal.

CATEGORY AND SCHEDULE

Pregnancy Risk Category: B
OTC

MECHANISM OF ACTION

A central analgesic whose exact mechanism is unknown, but appears to inhibit prostaglandin synthesis in the nervous CNS and, to a lesser extent, block pain impulses through peripheral action. Acetaminophen acts centrally on the hypothalamic heat-regulating center, producing peripheral vasodilation (heat loss, skin erythema, and sweating). ***Therapeutic Effect:*** Results in antipyresis. Produces analgesic effects.

PHARMACOKINETICS

Route	Onset	Peak	Duration
PO	15–30 min	1–1.5 hrs	4–6 hrs

Rapidly, completely absorbed from GI tract; rectal absorption variable. Protein binding: 20%–50%. Widely distributed to most body tissues. Metabolized in liver; excreted in urine. Removed by hemodialysis. ***Half-Life:*** 1–4 hrs (half-life is increased in those with liver disease, neonates; decreased in children).

AVAILABILITY

Capsules: 80 mg, 160 mg, 325 mg, 500 mg.
Drops: 100 mg/mL.
Elixir: 100 mg/mL, 130 mg/ 5 mL, 160 mg/ 5 mL, 500 mg/ 5 mL.
Liquid: 32 mg/mL, 100 mg/mL, 160 mg/ 5 mL.
Suppository: 80 mg, 120 mg, 325 mg, 650 mg.
Suspension: 100 mg/mL, 160 mg/ 5 mL.
Syrup: 160 mg/ 5 mL.
Tablets: 80 mg, 160 mg, 325 mg, 500 mg, 650 mg.
Tablets (chewable): 80 mg, 160 mg.
Tablets (controlled release): 650 mg.

INDICATIONS AND DOSAGES

▸ **Analgesia and antipyresis**

PO

Children. 10–15 mg/kg/dose q4–6h as needed. Maximum: 5 doses/ 24 hrs.
Neonates. 10–15 mg/kg/dose q6–8h as needed. Maximum: 90 mg/kg/day.

RECTAL

Children. 10–20 mg/kg/dose q4–6h as needed.
Neonates. 10–15 mg/kg/dose q6–8h as needed.

▸ **Dosage in renal impairment**

Creatinine Clearance	Frequency
10–50 mL/min	q6h
Less than 10 mL/min	q8h

CONTRAINDICATIONS

Active alcoholism, liver disease, or viral hepatitis, all of which increase the risk of hepatotoxicity.

INTERACTIONS

Drug

Alcohol (chronic use), hepatotoxic medications (e.g., phenytoin), liver enzyme inducers (e.g., cimetidine): May increase risk of hepatotoxicity with prolonged high dose or single toxic dose.
Warfarin: May increase the risk of bleeding with regular use.

Herbal

None known.

Food

None known.

DIAGNOSTIC TEST EFFECTS

May increase prothrombin time (may indicate hepatotoxicity) and serum bilirubin, SGOT (AST), and SGPT (ALT) levels. Therapeutic serum level is 10–30 mcg/mL; toxic serum level is greater than 200 mcg/mL.

SIDE EFFECTS

Rare
Hypersensitivity reaction

SERIOUS REACTIONS

! Acetaminophen toxicity is the primary serious reaction.
! Early signs and symptoms of acetaminophen toxicity include anorexia, nausea, diaphoresis, and generalized weakness within the first 12–24 hrs.
! Later signs of acetaminophen toxicity include vomiting, right upper quadrant tenderness, and elevated liver function test results within 48–72 hrs after ingestion.
! The antidote to acetaminophen toxicity is acetylcysteine.

PEDIATRIC CONSIDERATIONS

Baseline Assessment

- Assess onset, type, location, and duration of pain before acetaminophen is given for analgesia. The effect of the medication is reduced if a full pain response recurs before the next dose.
- Expect to obtain the patient's vital signs before giving any of the fixed combinations of acetaminophen. If respirations are 12/min or fewer (20/min or fewer in children), withhold the medication and contact the physician.
- Acetaminophen crosses the placenta and is distributed in breast milk.
- Acetaminophen is routinely used in all stages of pregnancy and appears safe for short-term use.
- Be sure to check for sulfite allergies before administering acetaminophen to a child.
- There are no age-related precautions noted in children.

◂ALERT▸ Children may receive repeat doses 4–5 times/day to a maximum of 5 doses in 24 hrs.

Precautions

- Use cautiously in patients with glucose-6-phosphate dehydrogenase deficiency, phenylketonuria, sensitivity to acetaminophen, or severe impaired renal function.

Administration and Handling

PO

- Give without regard to meals.
- Tablets may be crushed.

RECTAL

- Moisten suppository with cold water before inserting well up into the rectum.

Intervention and Evaluation

- Assess for clinical improvement and relief of pain or fever.
- Monitor serum levels. A therapeutic serum level is 10–30

mcg/mL; a toxic serum level is greater than 200 mcg/mL.

Patient/Family Teaching

• Caution the patient/family to consult with the physician before using acetaminophen in children younger than 2 yrs of age and before oral use for more than 5 days in children or more than 10 days in adults, or if fever lasts for more than 3 days. Monitor the patient for severe or recurrent pain or high, continuous fever, which may indicate a serious illness.

Aspirin (Acetylsalicylic Acid, ASA)

ass-purr-in

(Ascriptin, Aspro [AUS], Bayer, Bex [AUS], Bufferin, Disprin [AUS], Ecotrin, Entrophen [CAN], Halfprin, Novasen [CAN], Solprin [AUS], Spren [AUS])

CATEGORY AND SCHEDULE

Pregnancy Risk Category: C (D if full dose used in third trimester of pregnancy)

OTC

MECHANISM OF ACTION

A nonsteroidal salicylate that inhibits prostaglandin synthesis, acts on the hypothalamus heat-regulating center, and blocks prostaglandin synthetase action. ***Therapeutic Effect:*** Reduces inflammatory response and intensity of pain stimulus reaching sensory nerve endings. Decreases elevated body temperature. Inhibits platelet aggregation.

AVAILABILITY

Route	Onset	Peak	Duration
PO	1 hr	2–4 hrs	24 hrs

Rapidly, completely absorbed from GI tract; enteric-coated absorption delayed; rectal absorption delayed and incomplete. Protein binding: High. Widely distributed. Rapidly hydrolyzed to salicylate. ***Half-Life:*** Aspirin: 15–20 min; salicylate half-life is 2–3 hrs at low dose and greater than 20 hrs at high dose.

AVAILABILITY

Tablets: 81 mg, 325 mg, 500 mg, 650 mg.
Tablets (chewable): 81 mg.
Tablets (enteric coated): 81 mg, 162 mg, 325 mg, 500 mg, 650 mg, 975 mg.
Tablets (controlled release): 650 mg, 800 mg, 975 mg.
Suppository: 60 mg, 120 mg, 200 mg, 300 mg, 600 mg.

INDICATIONS AND DOSAGES

▸ **Analgesic, antipyretic**

PO/RECTAL

Children. 10–15 mg/kg/dose q4–6h. Maximum: 4 g/day.

▸ **Anti-inflammatory**

PO

Children. 60–90 mg/kg/day in divided doses, then 80–100 mg/kg/day.

▸ **Kawasaki disease**

PO

Children. 80–100 mg/kg/day in divided doses q6h.

UNLABELED USES

Prophylaxis against thromboembolism, treatment of Kawasaki disease.

CONTRAINDICATIONS

Allergy to tartrazine dye, bleeding disorders, chickenpox or flu in children and teenagers, GI bleeding or ulceration, history of hypersensitivity to aspirin or NSAIDs, impaired liver function.

INTERACTIONS

Drug

Alcohol, NSAIDs: May increase the risk of adverse GI effects, including ulceration.
Antacids, urinary alkalinizers: Increase the excretion of aspirin.
Anticoagulants, heparin, thrombolytics: Increase the risk of bleeding.
Insulin, oral hypoglycemics: Large doses of aspirin may increase the effect of insulin or oral hypoglycemics.
Methotrexate, zidovudine: May increase the risk of toxicity of these drugs.
Ototoxic medications, vancomycin: May increase the risk of ototoxicity of aspirin.
Platelet aggregation inhibitors, valproic acid: May increase the risk of bleeding.
Probenecid, sulfinpyrazone: May decrease the effect of these drugs.

Herbal

None known.

Food

None known.

DIAGNOSTIC TEST EFFECTS

May alter serum alkaline phosphatase, SGOT (AST), SGPT (ALT), and serum uric acid levels. May prolong bleeding time and prothrombin time. May decrease blood levels of cholesterol, serum potassium, triiodothyronine and thyroxine levels.

SIDE EFFECTS

Occasional

GI distress, including abdominal distention, cramping, heartburn, and mild nausea; allergic reaction, including bronchospasm, pruritus, and urticaria

SERIOUS REACTIONS

! High doses of aspirin may produce GI bleeding and gastric mucosal lesions.
! High doses of aspirin may produce low-grade toxicity characterized by ringing in the ears, generalized pruritus (may be severe), headache, dizziness, flushing, tachycardia, hyperventilation, sweating, and thirst.
! Toxic aspirin levels may be reached quickly in dehydrated, febrile children. Marked toxicity is manifested as hyperthermia, restlessness, abnormal breathing patterns, convulsions, respiratory failure, and coma.

PEDIATRIC CONSIDERATIONS

Baseline Assessment

- Do not give aspirin to children or teenagers who have chickenpox or flu as this increases the risk of development of Reye syndrome.
- Do not use aspirin that smells of vinegar because this odor indicates chemical breakdown in the medication.
- Assess the duration, location, and type of inflammation or pain.
- Inspect the appearance of affected joints for deformities, immobility, and skin condition.
- The therapeutic serum aspirin level for antiarthritic effect is 20–30 mg/dl. Aspirin toxicity occurs if levels are greater than 30 mg/dl.

• Be aware that aspirin readily crosses the placenta and is distributed in breast milk.
• Be aware that aspirin may decrease fetal birth weight, increase the incidence of hemorrhage, neonatal mortality, and stillbirths, and prolong gestation and labor.
• Be aware that aspirin use should be avoided during the last trimester of pregnancy because the drug may adversely affect the fetal cardiovascular system, causing premature closure of the ductus arteriosus.
• Use caution in giving aspirin to children with acute febrile illness because this increases the risk of development of Reye syndrome.

Precautions
• Use cautiously in patients with chronic renal insufficiency or vitamin K deficiency.
• Use cautiously in those patients diagnosed with the "aspirin triad" of asthma, nasal polyps, and rhinitis.

Administration and Handling
PO
• Do not crush or break enteric-coated or sustained-release forms.
• May give with water, milk, or meals if GI distress occurs.
RECTAL
• Refrigerate suppositories.
• If the suppository is too soft, chill it for 30 min in the refrigerator or run cold water over the foil wrapper.
• Moisten the suppository with cold water before inserting well into the rectum.

Intervention and Evaluation
• Monitor the patient's urine pH levels for signs of sudden acidification, indicated by a pH of 6.5–5.5. Sudden acidification may cause the serum salicylate level to greatly increase, leading to toxicity.
• Assess the patient's skin for evidence of bruising.
• If aspirin is given as an antipyretic, assess the patient's temperature directly before and 1 hr after giving the medication.
• Evaluate the patient for a therapeutic response to the drug manifested as improved grip strength, increased joint mobility, reduced joint tenderness, and relief of pain, stiffness, or swelling.

Patient/Family Teaching
• Instruct the patient/family not to crush or chew sustained-release or enteric-coated aspirin.
• Caution the patient/family to report ringing in the ears or persistent GI pain to the physician.
• Advise the patient/family that the therapeutic anti-inflammatory effect of aspirin should be noticed within 1–3 wks.

Buprenorphine Hydrochloride

byew-**pren**-or-phen
(Buprenex, Subutex, Temgesic [CAN])

CATEGORY AND SCHEDULE

Pregnancy Risk Category: C
Controlled Substance: Schedule V (opioid agonist), Schedule III (tablet)

MECHANISM OF ACTION

An opioid agonist that binds with opioid receptors within the CNS. ***Therapeutic Effect:*** Alters pain perception, emotional response to pain.

AVAILABILITY

Injection: 0.3 mg/mL.
Tablets (sublingual): 2 mg, 8 mg.

INDICATIONS AND DOSAGES

▸ **Analgesic**

IM/IV

Children older than 12 yrs. 0.3 mg q6–8h as needed. May repeat once in 30–60 min. Range: 0.15–0.6 mg q4–8h as needed.

Children 2–12 yrs. 2–6 mcg/kg q4–6h as needed.

▸ **Opioid dependence**

SUBLINGUAL

Children older than 16 yrs. Initially, 12–16 mg/day. Begin at least 4 hrs after the last use of heroin or short-acting opioid. Maintenance: 16 mg/day. Range: 4–24 mg/day. Patients should be switched to a buprenorphine and naloxone combination.

CONTRAINDICATIONS

None significant.

INTERACTIONS

Drug

CNS depressants, MAOIs: May increase CNS or respiratory depression and hypotension.

Other opioid analgesics: May decrease the effects of other opioid analgesics.

Herbal

Kava kava, St. John's wort, valerian: May increase CNS depression.

Food

None significant.

DIAGNOSTIC TEST EFFECTS

May increase serum amylase and lipase.

SIDE EFFECTS

Frequent

Injection (greater than 10%): Sedation

Tablet: Headache, pain, insomnia, anxiety, depression, nausea, abdominal pain, constipation, back pain, weakness, rhinitis, withdrawal syndrome, infection, sweating

Occasional

Injection: Hypotension, respiratory depression, dizziness, headache, vomiting, nausea, vertigo

SERIOUS REACTIONS

! Overdosage results in cold, clammy skin, weakness, confusion, severe respiratory depression, cyanosis, pinpoint pupils, and extreme somnolence progressing to convulsions, stupor, and coma.

PEDIATRIC CONSIDERATIONS

Baseline Assessment

- Assess the duration, location, onset, and type of pain.
- Know that the effect of buprenorphine is reduced if full pain recurs before next dose.

Precautions

- Use cautiously in patients with impaired liver function and in patients with possible neurologic injury.

Administration and Handling

IV

- Administer slowly over at least 2 min.

PO

Place tablet under the patient's tongue until dissolved. If 2 or more tablets are needed, may place all under the tongue at the same time.

Intervention and Evaluation

- Monitor the patient for changes in blood pressure, rate and quality of pulse, and respiration.
- Have the patient initiate deep breathing and coughing exercises, particularly in patients with impaired pulmonary function.
- Assess the patient for clinical improvement, and record the onset of pain relief.

Patient/Family Teaching

- Instruct the patient/family to change positions slowly to avoid dizziness.
- Warn the patient/family to avoid tasks requiring mental alertness or motor skills until the patient's response to the drug is established.

Nalbuphine Hydrochloride

nail-**byew**-phin
(Nubain)
Do not confuse with Navane.

CATEGORY AND SCHEDULE

Pregnancy Risk Category: B (D if used for prolonged periods or at high dosages at term)

MECHANISM OF ACTION

A narcotic agonist and antagonist that binds with opioid receptors within the CNS. May displace opioid agonists and competitively inhibit their action; may precipitate withdrawal symptoms.
Therapeutic Effect: Alters pain perception and emotional response to pain.

PHARMACOKINETICS

Route	Onset	Peak	Duration
SC	less than 15 min	N/A	3–6 hrs
IM	less than 15 min	60 min	3–6 hrs
IV	2–3 min	30 min	3–6 hrs

Well absorbed after SC or IM administration. Protein binding: 50%. Metabolized in liver. Primarily eliminated in feces via biliary secretion. ***Half-Life:*** 2–5 hrs.

AVAILABILITY

Injection: 10 mg/mL, 20 mg/mL.

INDICATIONS AND DOSAGES

▸ **Analgesia**

SC/IM/IV

Children. 0.1–0.15 mg/kg q3–6h as needed. Maximum: 20 mg/dose (safety of this medication has not been established in children).

CONTRAINDICATIONS

Hypersensitivity to nalbuphine or any related component.
Respirations less than 12/min.

INTERACTIONS

Drug

Alcohol, CNS depressants: May increase CNS or respiratory depression and hypotension.
Buprenorphine: Effects may be decreased with this drug.
MAOIs: May produce severe reaction; plan to reduce dose to one quarter usual dose.

Herbal

None known.

Food

None known.

DIAGNOSTIC TEST EFFECTS

May increase serum amylase and lipase levels.

IV INCOMPATIBILITIES

Amphotericin B complex (Abelcet, AmBisome, Amphotec), cefepime (Maxipime), docetaxel (Doxil), methotrexate, nafcillin (Nafcil), piperacillin/tazobactam (Zosyn), sargramostim (Leukine, Prokine), sodium bicarbonate

IV COMPATIBILITIES

Diphenhydramine (Benadryl), droperidol (Inapsine), glycopyrrolate (Robinul), hydroxyzine (Vistaril), ketorolac (Toradol), lidocaine, midazolam (Versed), propofol (Diprivan)

SIDE EFFECTS

Frequent (35%)
Sedation

Occasional (9%–3%)
Sweaty or clammy feeling, nausea, vomiting, dizziness, vertigo, dry mouth, headache

Rare (1% or less)
Restlessness, crying, euphoria, hostility, confusion, numbness, tingling, flushing, paradoxical reaction

SERIOUS REACTIONS

! Abrupt withdrawal after prolonged use may produce symptoms of narcotic withdrawal, marked by abdominal cramping, rhinorrhea, lacrimation, anxiety, increased temperature, and piloerection or goose bumps.
! Overdose results in severe respiratory depression, skeletal muscle flaccidity, cyanosis, extreme somnolence progressing to convulsions, stupor, and coma.
! Tolerance to analgesic effect and physical dependence may occur with chronic use.

PEDIATRIC CONSIDERATIONS

Baseline Assessment

- Obtain the patient's vital signs before giving nalbuphine.
- Withhold the medication and notify the physician if respirations are 12/min or fewer in the adult patient or 20/min or fewer in children.
- Assess the duration, location, onset, and type of pain the patient is experiencing.
- Know that the effect of the medication is reduced if the patient experiences full pain before the next dose.
- Know that nalbuphine has a low abuse potential.
- Be aware that nalbuphine readily crosses the placenta and is distributed in breast milk. Breast-feeding is not recommended in this patient population.
- Be aware that children may experience paradoxical excitement.
- Be aware that children younger than 2 yrs of age are more susceptible to respiratory depression.
- Be aware that the safety of nalbuphine has not been firmly established in children.

Precautions

- Use cautiously in patients with head trauma, increased intracranial pressure, liver or renal impairment, recent biliary tract surgery, recent myocardial infarction, and respiratory depression.
- Use cautiously in pregnant patients and patients suspected of being opioid dependent.

Administration and Handling

◀ **ALERT** ▶ Keep in mind that nalbuphine dosage is based on the patient's concurrent use of other medications, physical condition, and severity of pain.

IM
Rotate IM injection sites.

IV

- Store at room temperature.
- May give undiluted.
- For IV push, administer each 10 mg over 3–5 min.

Intervention and Evaluation

- Monitor the patient for change in blood pressure, pulse rate or quality, and respirations.
- Assess the patient's pattern of daily bowel activity and stool consistency.
- Initiate deep breathing and coughing exercises, particularly in patients with impaired pulmonary function.

• Assess the patient for clinical improvement and record the onset of relief of pain.
• Consult the physician if the patient's pain relief is not adequate.

Patient/Family Teaching

• Urge the patient/family to avoid alcohol during nalbuphine therapy.
• Warn the patient/family that nalbuphine use may cause drowsiness and impair the patient's ability to perform activities requiring mental alertness or motor skills.
• Tell the patient/family that nalbuphine may cause dry mouth.
• Caution the patient/family that nalbuphine use may be habit forming.
• Tell the patient/family to alert you to the onset of pain because the effect of the medication is reduced if the patient experiences full pain before the next dose.

REFERENCES

Miller, S. & Fioravanti, J. (1997). Pediatric medications: a handbook for nurses. St. Louis: Mosby.
Taketomo, C. K., Hodding, J. H. & Kraus, D. M. (2003–2004). Pediatric dosage handbook (10th ed.). Hudson, OH: Lexi-Comp.

43 Nonsteroidal Anti-Inflammatory Drugs (NSAIDs)

Diclofenac
Flurbiprofen
Ibuprofen
Indomethacin
Ketorolac Tromethamine
Naproxen, Naproxen Sodium
Piroxicam

Uses: NSAIDs relieve the pain and inflammation of musculoskeletal disorders, such as rheumatoid arthritis, osteoarthritis, and ankylosing spondylitis. They are also used to provide analgesia for mild to moderate pain and to reduce fever. However, many of these agents are not suited for long-term therapy because of toxicity.

Action: The exact mechanism of action of the NSAIDs in relieving inflammation, pain, and fever is unknown. They may work by inhibiting cyclooxygenase, the enzyme responsible for prostaglandin synthesis. Also, these agents may inhibit other mediators of inflammation, such as leukotrienes. In addition, they may have a direct action on the heat-regulating center of the hypothalamus, which may contribute to their antipyretic effects.

COMBINATION PRODUCTS

ARTHROTEC: diclofenac/misoprostol (an antisecretory gastric protectant) 50 mg/200 mcg; 75 mg/200 mcg.
CHILDREN'S ADVIL COLD: ibuprofen/pseudoephedrine (a nasal decongestant) 100 mg/15 mg/5 mL.
VICOPROFEN: ibuprofen/hydrocodone (a narcotic analgesic) 200 mg/7.5 mg.

Diclofenac

dye-**klo**-feh-nak
(Cataflam, Diclohexal [AUS], Diclotek [CAN], Fenac [AUS], Novo-Difenac [CAN], Solaraze, Voltaren, Voltaren Emulgel [AUS], Voltaren Rapid [AUS], Voltaren XR)
Do not confuse with Diflucan, Duphalac, or Verelan.

CATEGORY AND SCHEDULE

Pregnancy Risk Category: B (D if used in third trimester or near delivery [oral]; C ophthalmic solution; B topical preparation)

MECHANISM OF ACTION

A NSAID that inhibits prostaglandin synthesis and the intensity of pain stimulus reaching sensory nerve endings. Constricts iris sphincter. ***Therapeutic Effect:*** Produces analgesic and anti-inflammatory effect. Prevents miosis during cataract surgery.

PHARMACOKINETICS

Route	Onset	Peak	Duration
PO	30 min	2–3 hrs	Up to 8 hrs

Completely absorbed from the GI tract; penetrates cornea after ophthalmic administration (may be systemically absorbed). Widely distributed. Protein binding: greater than 99%. Metabolized in liver. Primarily excreted in urine. Minimally removed by hemodialysis. ***Half-Life:*** Adults: 1.2–2 hrs.

AVAILABILITY

Gel: 3%.
Tablets: 50 mg (Cataflam).
Tablets (delayed release): 25 mg, 50 mg, 75 mg.
Tablets (extended release): 100 mg.
Ophthalmic Solution: 0.1%.

INDICATIONS AND DOSAGES

▸ **Usual pediatric dosage**

Children. 2–3 mg/kg/day in divided doses 2–4 times/day.

▸ **Actinic keratoses**

TOPICAL

Adolescents. Apply 2 times/day to lesion for 60–90 days.

UNLABELED USES

Ophthalmic: Reduces occurrence and severity of cystoid macular edema after cataract surgery.
PO: Treatment of vascular headaches.

CONTRAINDICATIONS

Hypersensitivity to aspirin, diclofenac, and NSAIDs. Porphyria. Active GI bleeding or ulcers.

INTERACTIONS

Drug

Acetylcholine, carbachol: Ophthalmic diclofenac may decrease the effects of acetylcholine and carbachol.
Antihypertensives, diuretics: May decrease the effects of antihypertensives and diuretics.
Aspirin, salicylates: May increase the risk of GI bleeding and side effects.
Bone marrow depressants: May increase the risk of hematologic reactions.
Epinephrine, other antiglaucoma medications: May decrease the antiglaucoma effect of these drugs.
Heparin, oral anticoagulants, thrombolytics: May increase the effects of heparin, oral anticoagulants, and thrombolytics.
Lithium: May increase the blood concentration and risk of toxicity of lithium.
Methotrexate: May increase the risk of toxicity of methotrexate.
Probenecid: May increase diclofenac blood concentration.

Herbal

Ginkgo biloba: May increase the risk of bleeding.

Food

None known.

DIAGNOSTIC TEST EFFECTS

May increase BUN, lactate dehydrogenase (LDH), serum potassium, urine protein, serum alkaline phosphatase, creatinine, and transaminase levels. May decrease serum uric acid levels.

SIDE EFFECTS

Frequent (9%–4%)
PO: Headache, abdominal cramping, constipation, diarrhea, nausea, dyspepsia
Occasional (3%–1%)
PO: Flatulence, dizziness, epigastric pain
Rare (less than 1%)
PO: Rash, peripheral edema or fluid retention, visual disturbances, vomiting, drowsiness

SERIOUS REACTIONS

! Overdosage may result in acute renal failure.
! In pts treated chronically, peptic ulcer disease, GI bleeding, gastritis, a severe hepatic reaction, marked by jaundice, nephrotoxicity, characterized by hematuria, dysuria, or proteinuria, and a severe hypersensitivity reaction, manifested by

bronchospasm or facial edema, occur rarely.

PEDIATRIC CONSIDERATIONS

Baseline Assessment

• Assess the duration, location, onset, and type of inflammation or pain the patient is experiencing.
• Inspect the appearance of the patient's affected joints for deformity, immobility, and skin condition.
• Plan to obtain baseline BUN, LDH, serum potassium, urine protein, serum alkaline phosphatase, creatinine, and transaminase as well as serum uric acid levels.
• Be aware that diclofenac crosses the placenta, and it is unknown whether the drug is distributed in breast milk.
• Be aware that diclofenac use should be avoided during the last trimester of pregnancy because the drug may adversely affect the fetal cardiovascular system, causing premature closure of the ductus arteriosus.
• Be aware that the safety and efficacy of diclofenac have not been established in children.

Precautions

• Use cautiously in pts with congestive heart failure, a history of GI disease, hypertension, and impaired liver or renal function.
• Avoid applying diclofenac topical gel to children, eyes, exfoliative dermatitis, infants, infections, neonates, and open skin wounds.

Administration and Handling

PO

• Do not crush or break enteric-coated form.
• May give with food, milk, or antacids if the patient experiences GI distress.

Intervention and Evaluation

• Monitor the patient for dyspepsia and headache.
• Assess the patient's pattern of daily bowel activity and stool consistency.
• Evaluate the patient for therapeutic response, improved grip strength, increased joint mobility, reduced joint tenderness, and relief of pain, stiffness, and swelling.

Patient/Family Teaching

• Instruct the patient/family to swallow the diclofenac tablet whole and not to crush or chew tablets.
• Warn the patient/family to avoid alcohol and aspirin during diclofenac therapy because these substances increase the risk of GI bleeding.
• Instruct the patient/family to take diclofenac with food or milk if the patient experiences GI upset.
• Warn the patient/family to notify the physician if the patient experiences black stools, changes in vision, itching, persistent headache, skin rash, or weight gain.
• Instruct the patient/family not to use hydrogel soft contact lenses during ophthalmic diclofenac therapy.
• Warn the patient/family to notify the physician if the patient experiences a rash during diclofenac topical therapy.
• Instruct the female patient to notify the physician if she suspects pregnancy or plans to become pregnant.

Flurbiprofen

fleur-bih-pro-fen
(Ansaid, Froben [CAN], Ocufen, Strepfen [AUS])

CATEGORY AND SCHEDULE

Pregnancy Risk Category: B (D if used in third trimester or near delivery; C ophthalmic solution)

MECHANISM OF ACTION

A phenylalkanoic acid that produces analgesic and anti-inflammatory effects by inhibiting prostaglandin synthesis. Relaxes iris sphincter. ***Therapeutic Effect:*** Reduces inflammatory response and the intensity of pain stimulus reaching sensory nerve endings. Prevents or reduces miosis.

PHARMACOKINETICS

Well absorbed from the GI tract, penetrates the cornea after ophthalmic administration, which may be systemically absorbed. Widely distributed. Protein binding: 99%. Metabolized in liver. Primarily excreted in urine. ***Half-Life:*** 3–4 hrs.

AVAILABILITY

Tablets: 50 mg, 100 mg.
Ophthalmic Solution: 0.03%.

INDICATIONS AND DOSAGES

OPHTHALMIC
Children. 1 drop q30min starting 2 hrs before surgery for total of 4 doses.

CONTRAINDICATIONS

History of hypersensitivity to aspirin or NSAIDs, active peptic ulcer, chronic inflammation of GI tract, GI bleeding disorders, GI ulceration.

INTERACTIONS

Drug

Acetylcholine, carbachol: Ophthalmic flurbiprofen may decrease the effects of acetylcholine and carbachol.
Antihypertensives, diuretics: May decrease the effects of antihypertensives and diuretics.
Aspirin, salicylates: May increase the risk of GI bleeding and side effects.
Bone marrow depressants: May increase the risk of hematologic reactions.
Epinephrine, other antiglaucoma medications: May decrease antiglaucoma effect.
Heparin, oral anticoagulants, thrombolytics: May increase the effects of heparin, oral anticoagulants, and thrombolytics.
Lithium: May increase the blood concentration and risk of toxicity of lithium.
Methotrexate: May increase the risk of toxicity of methotrexate.
Probenecid: May increase flurbiprofen blood concentration.

Herbal

Feverfew: May have decreased effect.
Ginkgo biloba: May increase the risk of bleeding.

Food

None known.

DIAGNOSTIC TEST EFFECTS

May increase bleeding time and serum lactate dehydrogenase, serum alkaline phosphatase, and serum transaminase levels.

SIDE EFFECTS

Occasional
Ophthalmic: Burning, stinging on instillation, keratitis, elevated intraocular pressure

Rare (less than 3%)
Blurred vision, flushed skin, dizziness, drowsiness, nervousness, insomnia, unusual weakness, constipation, decreased appetite, vomiting, confusion

SERIOUS REACTIONS

! Overdosage may result in acute renal failure.
! In pts treated chronically, peptic ulcer, GI bleeding, gastritis, severe hepatic reaction, marked by jaundice, nephrotoxicity, hematuria, dysuria, proteinuria, severe hypersensitivity reaction, characterized by bronchospasm and facial edema, and cardiac arrhythmias occur rarely.

PEDIATRIC CONSIDERATIONS

Baseline Assessment
- Assess the duration, location, onset, and type of inflammation or pain the patient is experiencing.
- Inspect the appearance of the patient's affected joints for deformity, immobility, and skin condition.
- Be aware that flurbiprofen crosses the placenta, and it is unknown whether the drug is distributed in breast milk.
- Be aware that flurbiprofen use should be avoided during the last trimester of pregnancy as the drug may adversely affect the fetal cardiovascular system causing premature closure of ductus arteriosus.
- Be aware that the safety and efficacy of flurbiprofen have not been established in children.

Precautions
- Use cautiously in pts with a history of GI tract disease, impaired liver or renal function, or a predisposition to fluid retention, soft contact lens wearers, and surgical pts with bleeding tendencies.

Administration and Handling
OPHTHALMIC
- Place a gloved finger on the patient's lower eyelid, and pull it out until a pocket is formed between the eye and lower lid.
- Hold the dropper above the pocket, and place the prescribed number of drops into the pocket.
- Close the patient's eye gently and apply digital pressure to the lacrimal sac for 1–2 min to minimize drainage into the nose and throat, reducing the risk of systemic effects.
- Remove excess solution with tissue.

Intervention and Evaluation
- Monitor the patient for dizziness, dyspepsia, and headache.
- Assess the patient's pattern of daily bowel activity and stool consistency.
- For pts taking oral flurbiprofen, monitor the patient's complete blood count, BUN, serum alkaline phosphatase, bilirubin, creatinine, SGOT (AST), and SGPT (ALT) levels. Check stools for occult blood.
- Perform periodic eye examinations in pts on ophthalmic flurbiprofen therapy.
- Evaluate the patient for therapeutic response, improved grip strength, increased joint mobility, and relief of pain, stiffness, and swelling.

Patient/Family Teaching
- Warn the patient/family to avoid alcohol and aspirin during flurbiprofen therapy. These substances increase the risk of GI bleeding.
- Warn the patient/family to notify the physician if the patient experiences edema, GI distress, headache, rash, or visual disturbances.

• Tell the patient taking ophthalmic flurbiprofen that his or her eye may momentarily sting during drug instillation.
• Instruct the patient to notify the physician if she suspects pregnancy or plans to become pregnant.

Ibuprofen

eye-byew-**pro**fen
(Act-3 [AUS], Advil, Apo-Ibuprofen, Brufen [AUS], Codral Period Pain [AUS], Motrin, Novoprofen [CAN], Nuprin, Nurofen [AUS], Rafen [AUS])

CATEGORY AND SCHEDULE

Pregnancy Risk Category: B (D if used in third trimester or near delivery)
OTC (Tablets: 200 mg; Oral Suspension: 100 mg/5 mL)

MECHANISM OF ACTION

An NSAID that inhibits prostaglandin synthesis. Produces vasodilation in hypothalamus. ***Therapeutic Effect:*** Produces analgesic and anti-inflammatory effect, decreases elevated body temperature.

PHARMACOKINETICS

Route	Onset	Peak	Duration
PO (analgesic)	0. 5 hr	N/A	4–6 hrs
PO (anti-rheumatic)	2 days	1–2 wks	N/A

Rapidly absorbed from the GI tract. Protein binding: greater than 90%. Metabolized in liver. Primarily excreted in urine. Not removed by hemodialysis. ***Half-Life:*** Children: 1–2 hrs. Adults: 2–4 hrs.

AVAILABILITY

Capsules: 200 mg.
Tablets: 100 mg, 200 mg (OTC), 300 mg, 400 mg, 600 mg, 800 mg.
Tablets (chewable): 50 mg, 100 mg.
Oral Suspension: 100 mg/5 mL (OTC).
Oral Drops: 40 mg/mL.

INDICATIONS AND DOSAGES

▸ **Fever, minor aches, pain**
PO
Children. 5–10 mg/kg/dose q6–8h. Maximum: 40 mg/kg/day. OTC: 7.5 mg/kg/dose q6–8h. Maximum: 40 mg/kg/day.
▸ **Menstrual pain**
PO
Adolescents. 200–400 mg divided q4–6h. Maximum: 1.2 g/day.
▸ **Juvenile arthritis**
PO
Children. 30–70 mg/kg/24 hrs in 3–4 divided doses. Maximum in children weighing less than 20 kg: 400 mg/day. Maximum in children weighing 20–30 kg: 600 mg/day. Maximum in children weighing greater than 30–40 kg: 800 mg/day.

UNLABELED USES

Treatment of psoriatic arthritis, vascular headaches.

CONTRAINDICATIONS

History of hypersensitivity to aspirin or NSAIDs, active peptic ulcer, chronic inflammation of GI tract, GI bleeding disorders, GI ulceration.

INTERACTIONS

Drug

Antihypertensives, diuretics: May decrease the effects of antihypertensives and diuretics.

Aspirin, salicylates: May increase the risk of GI bleeding and side effects.
Bone marrow depressants: May increase the risk of hematologic reactions.
Heparin, oral anticoagulants, thrombolytics: May increase the effects of heparin, oral anticoagulants, and thrombolytics.
Lithium: May increase the blood concentration and risk of toxicity of lithium.
Methotrexate: May increase the risk of toxicity of methotrexate.
Probenecid: May increase ibuprofen blood concentration.

Herbal

Feverfew: May decrease the effects of feverfew.
Ginkgo biloba: May increase the risk of bleeding.

Food

None known.

DIAGNOSTIC TEST EFFECTS

May prolong bleeding time. May alter blood glucose levels. May increase BUN, liver function test results, and serum creatinine and potassium levels. May decrease blood Hgb and Hct.

SIDE EFFECTS

Occasional (9%–3%)

Nausea with or without vomiting, dyspepsia, including heartburn, indigestion, and epigastric pain, dizziness, rash

Rare (less than 3%)

Diarrhea or constipation, flatulence, abdominal cramping or pain, itching

SERIOUS REACTIONS

! Acute overdosage may result in metabolic acidosis.
! Peptic ulcer disease, GI bleeding, gastritis, and severe hepatic reaction (cholestasis, jaundice) occur rarely.
! Nephrotoxicity, including dysuria, hematuria, proteinuria, and nephrotic syndrome and severe hypersensitivity reaction, particularly in those with systemic lupus erythematosus; other collagen diseases occur rarely.

PEDIATRIC CONSIDERATIONS

Baseline Assessment

- Assess the duration, location, onset, and type of inflammation or pain the patient is experiencing.
- Inspect the appearance of the patient's affected joints for deformity, immobility, and skin condition.
- Be aware that it is unknown whether ibuprofen crosses the placenta or is distributed in breast milk.
- Be aware that ibuprofen use should be avoided during the third trimester of pregnancy, as this drug may adversely affect the fetal cardiovascular system causing premature closure of ductus arteriosus.
- Be aware that the safety and efficacy of this drug have not been established in children younger than 6 mos of age.
- Children with asthma are at higher risk for developing hypersensitivity reactions.

Precautions

- Use cautiously in pts with congestive heart failure, concurrent anticoagulant use, dehydration, GI disease, such as GI bleeding or ulcers, hypertension, and impaired liver or renal function.

Administration and Handling

PO

- Do not crush or break enteric-coated form.
- Give ibuprofen with antacids, food, or milk if the patient experiences GI distress.

Intervention and Evaluation

- Monitor the patient for dyspepsia and nausea.
- Monitor the patient's complete blood count, platelet count, and serum alkaline phosphatase, bilirubin, creatinine, SGOT (AST), and SGPT (ALT) levels.
- Assess the patient's pattern of daily bowel activity and stool consistency.
- Examine the patient's skin for rash.
- Evaluate the patient for therapeutic response, improved grip strength, increased joint mobility, reduced joint tenderness, and relief of pain, stiffness, and swelling.
- Monitor the patient's body temperature for fever.

Patient/Family Teaching

- Warn the patient/family to avoid alcohol and aspirin during ibuprofen therapy. These substances increase the risk of GI bleeding.
- Instruct the patient/family to take ibuprofen with antacids, food, or milk if the patient experiences GI upset.
- Teach the patient/family not to chew or crush enteric-coated ibuprofen tablets.
- Tell the patient/family that ibuprofen use may cause dizziness.

Indomethacin

in-doe-**meth**-ah-sin
(Apo-Indomethacin [CAN], Arthrexin [AUS], Indocid [CAN], Indocin, Indocin-SR, Novomethacin [CAN])

CATEGORY AND SCHEDULE

Pregnancy Risk Category: B (D if used after 34 wks' gestation, close to delivery, or longer than 48 hrs)

MECHANISM OF ACTION

A nonsteroidal anti-inflammatory that produces analgesic and anti-inflammatory effects by inhibiting prostaglandin synthesis.
Therapeutic Effect: Reduces inflammatory response and intensity of pain stimulus reaching sensory nerve endings. Patent ductus in neonates: Inhibits prostaglandin synthesis, increases sensitivity of premature ductus to dilating effects of prostaglandins.
Therapeutic Effect: Causes closure of patent ductus arteriosus.

PHARMACOKINETICS

Incomplete absorption in neonates after oral administration. Oral absorption in adults is rapid. Protein binding: 99%. Metabolized in the liver. Eliminated 60% in urine and 33% in feces. ***Half life:*** Neonates: 11–20 hrs, Adults: 2–11 hrs.

AVAILABILITY

Capsules: 25 mg, 50 mg.
Capsules (sustained release): 75 mg.
Oral Suspension: 25 mg/5 mL.
Suppository: 50 mg.
Powder for Injection: 1 mg.

INDICATIONS AND DOSAGES

▸ **Moderate to severe rheumatoid arthritis, osteoarthritis, ankylosing spondylitis**

PO

Children. 1–2 mg/kg/day in 2 or 4 divided doses. Maximum: 150–200 mg/day.

RECTAL

Children. Initially, 1.5–2.5 mg/kg/day, up to 4 mg/kg/day. Do not exceed 150–200 mg/day.

▸ **Patent ductus arteriosus**

IV

Neonates. Initially, 0.2 mg/kg.

Neonates older than 7 days. 0.25 mg/kg for 2nd and 3rd doses at 12- to 24-hr intervals.
Neonates 2–7 days. 0.2 mg/kg for 2nd and 3rd doses at 12- to 24-hr intervals.
Neonates younger than 48 hrs. 0.1 mg/kg for 2nd and 3rd doses at 12- to 24-hr intervals.

UNLABELED USES

Treatment of fever resulting from malignancy, pericarditis, psoriatic arthritis, rheumatic complications associated with Paget's disease of bone, vascular headache.

CONTRAINDICATIONS

Hypersensitivity to aspirin, indomethacin, or other NSAIDs, active GI bleeding and ulcers, impaired renal function, thrombocytopenia. Premature neonates with necrotizing enterocolitis, impaired renal function, intraventricular hemorrhage, active bleeding or thrombocytopenia.

INTERACTIONS

Drug

Aminoglycosides: May increase the blood concentration of these drugs in neonates.
Antihypertensives, diuretics: May decrease the effects of antihypertensives and diuretics.
Aspirin, salicylates: May increase the risk of GI bleeding and side effects.
Bone marrow depressants: May increase the risk of hematologic reactions.
Heparin, oral anticoagulants, thrombolytics: May increase the effects of heparin, oral anticoagulants, and thrombolytics.
Lithium: May increase the blood concentration and risk of toxicity of lithium.
Methotrexate: May increase the toxicity of methotrexate.
Probenecid: May increase indomethacin blood concentration.
Triamterene: Do not give concurrently with this drug as this may potentiate acute renal failure.

Herbal

Feverfew: The effect of this herb may be decreased.
Ginkgo biloba: May increase the risk of bleeding.

Food

None known.

DIAGNOSTIC TEST EFFECTS

May prolong bleeding time. May alter blood glucose levels. May increase liver function test results and BUN, serum creatinine, and potassium levels. May decrease sodium levels and platelet count.

IV INCOMPATIBILITIES

Amino acid injection, calcium gluconate, cimetidine (Tagamet), dobutamine (Dobutrex), dopamine (Intropin), gentamicin (Garamycin), tobramycin (Nebcin)

IV COMPATIBILITIES

Insulin, potassium

SIDE EFFECTS

Frequent (11%–3%)
Headache, nausea, vomiting, dyspepsia, as well as heartburn, indigestion, and epigastric pain, dizziness
Occasional (less than 3%)
Depression, tinnitus, diaphoresis, drowsiness, constipation, diarrhea
Patent ductus arteriosus: bleeding disturbances
Rare
Increased blood pressure, confusion, hives, itching, rash, blurred vision

SERIOUS REACTIONS

! Paralytic ileus and ulceration of esophagus, stomach, duodenum, or small intestine may occur.
! In those with impaired renal function, hyperkalemia along with worsening of impairment may occur.
! May aggravate depression or psychiatric disturbances, epilepsy, and parkinsonism.
! Nephrotoxicity, including dysuria, hematuria, proteinuria, and nephrotic syndrome, occurs rarely.
! In patent ductus arteriosus, acidosis, apnea, bradycardia, and alkalosis occur rarely.

PEDIATRIC CONSIDERATIONS

Baseline Assessment

- Know that indomethacin use may mask signs of infection.
- Assess the duration, location, onset, and type of fever, inflammation, or pain the patient is experiencing.
- Inspect the appearance of the patient's affected joints for deformity, immobility, and skin condition.
- Expect to obtain baseline laboratory values, especially a complete blood count and blood chemistry tests, including prothrombin time, a PTT, and liver and renal function studies.
- In neonates with patent ductus arteriosus, assess baseline heart sounds. For murmurs, note the location, intensity, quality, and timing.
- In neonates with patent ductus arteriosus, never administer IV indomethacin rapidly. This can lead to a reduction in mesenteric artery and cerebral blood flow, which may lead to the development of necrotizing enterocolitis.
- Never administer indomethacin with antacids.
- Children who have asthma may be at increased risk for having an allergic response to indomethacin.

Precautions

- Use cautiously in pts with cardiac dysfunction, concurrent anticoagulant therapy, epilepsy, hypertension, and liver or renal impairment.

Administration and Handling

PO

- Give indomethacin after meals or with antacids or food.
- Do not crush sustained-release capsules.

RECTAL

- If suppository is too soft, chill for 30 min in refrigerator or run cold water over the foil wrapper.
- Moisten suppository with cold water before inserting into rectum.

IV

◂ ALERT ▸ IV injection is the preferred route for neonatal pts with patent ductus arteriosus. May give dose PO by nasogastric tube or rectally.

◂ ALERT ▸ May give up to 3 doses at 12- to 24-hr intervals.

- IV solutions made without preservatives should be used immediately.
- Use IV solution immediately after reconstitution. IV solution normally appears clear; discard if cloudy or if precipitate forms.
- Discard unused portion.
- To 1-mg vial, add 1 to 2 mL preservative-free Sterile Water for Injection or 0.9% NaCl to provide concentration of 1 mg or 0. 5 mg/mL, respectively.
- Do not further dilute.
- Administer over 5–10 sec.
- Restrict the patient's fluid intake, as ordered.

Intervention and Evaluation

- Monitor the patient for dyspepsia and nausea.
- Assist the patient with ambulation if he or she experiences dizziness.
- Evaluate the patient for therapeutic response, improved grip strength, increased joint mobility, reduced joint tenderness, and relief of pain, stiffness, and swelling.
- Monitor the patient's BUN, serum alkaline phosphatase, bilirubin, creatinine, potassium, SGOT (AST), and SGPT (ALT) levels.
- Monitor the blood pressure, EKG, heart rate and, platelet count, serum sodium and blood glucose levels, and urine output in neonatal pts. Assess heart sounds for the presence of a murmur or changes in intensity.

Patient/Family Teaching

- Warn the patient/family to avoid alcohol and aspirin during indomethacin therapy. These substances increase the risk of GI bleeding.
- Instruct the patient/family to swallow capsules whole and not to chew, open, or crush capsules.
- Teach the patient/family to take indomethacin with food or milk if the patient experiences GI upset.
- Warn the patient/family to avoid tasks that require mental alertness or motor skills until the patient's response to the drug is established.

Ketorolac Tromethamine

key-**tore**-oh-lack

(Acular, Acular PF, Toradol)

Do not confuse with Acthar.

CATEGORY AND SCHEDULE

Pregnancy Risk Category: C (D if used in third trimester)

MECHANISM OF ACTION

An NSAID that inhibits prostaglandin synthesis and reduces prostaglandin levels in aqueous humor. ***Therapeutic Effect:*** Reduces intensity of pain stimulus reaching sensory nerve endings, reduces intraocular inflammation.

PHARMACOKINETICS

Route	Onset	Peak	Duration
PO	30–60 min	1.5–4 hrs	4–6 hrs
IV/IM	30 min	1–2 hrs	4–6 hrs

Readily absorbed from the GI tract and after IM administration. Protein binding: greater than 99%. Partially metabolized, primarily in liver. Primarily excreted in urine. Not removed by hemodialysis. ***Half-Life:*** 3.8–6.3 hrs, half-life is increased with impaired renal function.

AVAILABILITY

Tablets: 10 mg.
Injection: 15 mg/mL, 30 mg/mL.
Ophthalmic Solution: 0.4%, 0.5%.

INDICATIONS AND DOSAGES

▸ **Analgesic for short-term relief of mild to moderate pain (multiple dosing)**

IV/IM

Children 2–16 yrs. 0. 5 mg/kg q6h. Limited information exists on this dosage. Do not use for more than 5 days.

▸ **Analgesic (single dose)**

IM

Children 2–16 yrs. 0.5–1 mg/kg. Limited information exists on this dosage.

IV

Children. 0.5–1 mg/kg. Limited information exists on this dosage.

UNLABELED USES
Ophthalmic: Prophylaxis or treatment of ocular inflammation.

CONTRAINDICATIONS
History of hypersensitivity to aspirin or NSAIDs, active peptic ulcer disease, chronic inflammation of the GI tract, GI bleeding disorders, GI ulceration. Advanced renal impairment, preoperative use, pts at risk for bleeding or thrombocytopenia.

INTERACTIONS
Drug
Antihypertensives, diuretics: May decrease the effects of antihypertensives.
Aspirin, salicylates: May increase the risk of GI bleeding and side effects.
Bone marrow depressants: May increase the risk of hematologic reactions.
Heparin, oral anticoagulants, thrombolytics: May increase the effects of heparin, oral anticoagulants, and thrombolytics.
Lithium:
May increase the blood concentration and risk of toxicity of lithium.
Methotrexate: May increase the risk of toxicity of methotrexate.
Probenecid: May increase ketorolac blood concentration.
Herbal
Feverfew: The effects of this herb may be decreased.
Ginkgo biloba: May increase the risk of bleeding.
Food
None known.

DIAGNOSTIC TEST EFFECTS
May prolong bleeding time. May increase liver function test results.

IV INCOMPATIBILITIES
Promethazine (Phenergan)

IV COMPATIBILITIES
Fentanyl (Sublimaze), hydromorphone (Dilaudid), morphine, nalbuphine (Nubain)

SIDE EFFECTS
Frequent (17%–12%)
Headache, nausea, abdominal cramping/pain, dyspepsia (heartburn, indigestion, epigastric pain)
Occasional (9%–3%)
Diarrhea
Ophthalmic: Transient stinging and burning
Rare (3%–1%)
Constipation, vomiting, flatulence, stomatitis
Ophthalmic: Ocular irritation, allergic reactions, superficial ocular infection, keratitis

SERIOUS REACTIONS
! GI bleeding, perforation, and peptic ulcer occur infrequently.
! Nephrotoxicity, including glomerular nephritis, interstitial nephritis, and nephrotic syndrome may occur in pts with preexisting impaired renal function.
! Acute hypersensitivity reaction, such as fever, chills, and joint pain, occurs rarely.

PEDIATRIC CONSIDERATIONS
Baseline Assessment
- Assess the duration, location, onset, and type of pain the patient is experiencing.
- Be aware that it is unknown if ketorolac is excreted in breast milk.
- Be aware that ketorolac use should be avoided during the third trimester of pregnancy because the

drug may adversely affect the fetal cardiovascular system causing premature closure of a ductus arteriosus.

• Be aware that the safety and efficacy of ketorolac have not been established in children, but doses of 0.5 mg/kg have been used.

• Be aware that use for longer than 5 days total is not advised in children because of increased adverse effects.

Precautions

• Use cautiously in pts with a history of GI tract disease, impaired liver or renal function, and a predisposition to fluid retention.

Administration and Handling

◀ **ALERT** ▶ Be aware that the combined duration of IM, IV, and PO administration should not exceed 5 days. May give as single dose, routine, or as-needed schedule, as prescribed.

PO

• Give ketorolac with antacids, food, or milk if the patient experiences GI distress.

IM

• Give injection deeply and slowly into a large muscle mass.

IV

• Give undiluted as IV push over at least 15 sec.

OPHTHALMIC

• Place a gloved finger on the patient's lower eyelid and pull it out until a pocket is formed between the eye and lower lid.

• Hold the dropper above the pocket and place the prescribed number of drops in the pocket.

• Close the patient's eye gently and apply digital pressure to the lacrimal sac for 1–2 min to minimize drainage into the nose and throat, reducing the risk of systemic effects.

• Remove excess solution with tissue.

Intervention and Evaluation

• Monitor the patient's liver and renal function, BUN, serum alkaline phosphatase, bilirubin, creatinine, SGOT (AST), SGPT (ALT) levels, and assess complete blood count and urine output.

• Evaluate the patient for therapeutic response, improved grip strength, increased joint mobility, reduced joint tenderness, and relief of pain, stiffness, and swelling.

• Be alert to signs of bleeding, which may also occur with the ophthalmic route because of systemic absorption.

Patient/Family Teaching

• Warn the patient/family to avoid alcohol and aspirin during ketorolac therapy with oral or ophthalmic ketorolac, which increase the tendency to bleed.

• Instruct the patient/family to take ketorolac with food or milk if the patient experiences GI upset.

• Warn the patient/family to avoid tasks that require mental alertness or motor skills until the patient's response to the drug is established.

• Advise the patient/family receiving ophthalmic ketorolac that transient burning and stinging may occur upon instillation.

• Instruct the patient/family receiving ophthalmic ketorolac not to administer the drug while wearing soft contact lenses.

• Tell the patient to inform the physician if she suspects pregnancy or plans to become pregnant.

Naproxen

nah-**prox**-en
(Crysanal [AUS], EC-Naprosyn, Inza [AUS], Naprelan, Naprosyn, Naxen [CAN])
naproxen sodium
(Aleve, Anaprox, Apo-Napro [CAN], Naprogesic [AUS], Novonaprox [CAN])

CATEGORY AND SCHEDULE

Pregnancy Risk Category: B (D if used in third trimester or near delivery)
OTC (gelcaps, 200 mg tablets)

MECHANISM OF ACTION

An NSAID that produces analgesic and anti-inflammatory effects by inhibiting prostaglandin synthesis. ***Therapeutic Effect:*** Reduces inflammatory response and intensity of pain stimulus reaching sensory nerve endings.

PHARMACOKINETICS

Route	Onset	Peak	Duration
PO (analgesic)	Less than 1 hr	N/A	7 hrs or less
PO (anti-rheumatic)	14 days or less	2–4 wks	N/A

Completely absorbed from the GI tract. Protein binding: 99%. Metabolized in liver. Primarily excreted in urine. Not removed by hemodialysis. ***Half-Life:*** Children: 8–10 hrs. Adults: 13 hrs.

AVAILABILITY

Gelcaps: 220 mg (OTC).
Tablets: 200 mg (OTC), 250 mg, 375 mg, 500 mg.
Tablets (delayed release): 375 mg, 500 mg.
Oral Suspension: 125 mg/5 mL.

INDICATIONS AND DOSAGES

▸ Juvenile rheumatoid arthritis (naproxen only)
PO
Children. 10–15 mg/kg/day in 2 divided doses. Maximum: 1,000 mg/day.

▸ Analgesic
PO
Children older than 2 yrs. 5–7 mg/kg/dose given q8–12hrs.

UNLABELED USES

Treatment of vascular headaches.

CONTRAINDICATIONS

Hypersensitivity to aspirin, naproxen, or other NSAIDs. Active GI bleeding, ulcer disease.

INTERACTIONS

Drug

Antihypertensives, diuretics: May decrease the effects of antihypertensives and diuretics.
Aspirin, salicylates: May increase the risk of GI bleeding and side effects.
Bone marrow depressants: May increase risk of hematologic reactions.
Heparin, oral anticoagulants, thrombolytics: May increase the effects of heparin, oral anticoagulants, and thrombolytics.
Lithium: May increase the blood concentration and risk of toxicity of lithium.
Methotrexate: May increase the risk of toxicity of methotrexate.
Probenecid: May increase naproxen blood concentration.

Herbal

Feverfew: May decrease the effects of feverfew.
Ginkgo biloba: May increase the risk of bleeding.

Food

None known.

DIAGNOSTIC TEST EFFECTS

May prolong bleeding time and alter blood glucose levels. May increase liver function test results. May decrease serum sodium and uric acid levels.

SIDE EFFECTS

Frequent (9%–4%)
Nausea, constipation, abdominal cramps/pain, heartburn, dizziness, headache, drowsiness
Occasional (3%–1%)
Stomatitis, diarrhea, indigestion
Rare (less than 1%)
Vomiting, confusion

SERIOUS REACTIONS

! Peptic ulcer disease, GI bleeding, gastritis, and severe hepatic reaction, such as cholestasis and jaundice, occur rarely.
! Nephrotoxicity, including dysuria, hematuria, proteinuria, and nephrotic syndrome, and severe hypersensitivity reaction, marked by fever, chills, and bronchospasm, occur rarely.

PEDIATRIC CONSIDERATIONS

Baseline Assessment

- Assess the duration, location, onset, and type of inflammation or pain that the patient is experiencing.
- Inspect the appearance of the patient's affected joints for deformity, immobility, and skin condition.
- Be aware that naproxen crosses the placenta and is distributed in breast milk.
- Be aware that naproxen use should be avoided during the third trimester of pregnancy as this drug may adversely affect the fetal cardiovascular system causing premature closing of a ductus arteriosus.
- Be aware that the safety and efficacy of naproxen have not been established in children younger than 2 yrs of age.
- Be aware that children older than 2 yrs of age are at an increased risk of developing skin rash during naproxen therapy.
- Be aware that children with asthma are at increased risk of developing hypersensitivity reactions.

Precautions

- Use cautiously in pts with cardiac disease, GI disease, and impaired liver or renal function.
- Use cautiously in pts concurrently on anticoagulant therapy.

Administration and Handling

◂ALERT▸ Be aware that each 275- or 550-mg tablet of naproxen sodium equals 250 or 500 mg naproxen, respectively.

PO

- Have patient swallow enteric-coated form whole; scored tablets may be broken or crushed.
- May give naproxen with food, milk, or antacids if the patient experiences GI distress.

Intervention and Evaluation

- Assist the patient with ambulation if he or she experiences dizziness.
- Monitor the patient's complete blood count, and particularly platelet count, BUN, Hgb, Hct, serum alkaline phosphatase, bilirubin, creatinine, SGOT (AST), and SGPT (ALT) levels to assess liver and renal function.
- Assess the patient's pattern of daily bowel activity and stool consistency.
- Evaluate the patient for therapeutic response, improved grip strength, increased joint mobility, reduced joint tenderness, and relief of pain, stiffness, and swelling.

Patient/Family Teaching

- Instruct the patient/family to take naproxen with food or milk if the patient experiences GI upset.
- Caution the patient/family to avoid alcohol and aspirin during naproxen therapy. These substances increase the risk of GI bleeding.
- Warn the patient/family to notify the physician if the patient experiences black stools, persistent headache, rash, visual disturbances, and weight gain.
- Warn the patient/family to avoid tasks that require mental alertness or motor skills until the patient's response to the drug is established.
- Tell the patient/family to inform the physician if the patient suspects pregnancy or plans to become pregnant.

Piroxicam

purr-**ox**-i-kam

(Apo-Piroxicam [CAN], Candyl-D [AUS], Feldene, Fexicam [CAN], Mobilis [AUS], Novopirocam [CAN], Pirohexal-D [AUS], Rosig [AUS], Rosig-D [AUS])

CATEGORY AND SCHEDULE

Pregnancy Risk Category: B (D if used in third trimester)

MECHANISM OF ACTION

An NSAID that produces analgesic and anti-inflammatory effects by inhibiting prostaglandin synthesis. ***Therapeutic Effect:*** Reduces inflammatory response and intensity of pain stimulus reaching sensory nerve endings.

PHARMACOKINETICS

Well absorbed. Protein binding: 99%. Metabolized in the liver. Excreted as metabolites and unchanged in the urine.

AVAILABILITY

Capsules: 10 mg, 20 mg.

INDICATIONS AND DOSAGES

▸ **Acute or chronic rheumatoid arthritis, osteoarthritis**

PO

Children. 0.2–0.3 mg/kg/day once daily. Maximum: 15 mg/day.

UNLABELED USES

Treatment of acute gouty arthritis, ankylosing spondylitis, dysmenorrhea.

CONTRAINDICATIONS

History of hypersensitivity to aspirin or NSAIDs, active peptic ulcer disease, chronic inflammation of the GI tract, GI bleeding disorders, GI ulceration.

INTERACTIONS

Drug

Antihypertensives, diuretics: May decrease the effects of antihypertensives and diuretics.

Aspirin, salicylates: May increase the risk of GI bleeding and side effects.

Bone marrow depressants: May increase the risk of hematologic reactions.

Heparin, oral anticoagulants, thrombolytics: May increase the effects of heparin, oral anticoagulants, and thrombolytics.

Lithium: May increase the blood concentration and risk of toxicity of lithium.

Methotrexate: May increase the risk of toxicity of methotrexate.

Probenecid: May increase piroxicam blood concentration.

Herbal

Feverfew: May decrease the effects of feverfew.

Ginkgo biloba: May increase the risk of bleeding.
St. John's wort: May increase the risk of phototoxicity.

Food

None known.

DIAGNOSTIC TEST EFFECTS

May increase serum transaminase activity. May decrease serum uric acid levels.

SIDE EFFECTS

Frequent (9%–4%)

Dyspepsia, nausea, dizziness

Occasional (3%–1%)

Diarrhea, constipation, abdominal cramping/pain, flatulence, stomatitis

Rare (less than 1%)

Increased blood pressure, hives, painful or difficult urination, ecchymosis, blurred vision, insomnia

SERIOUS REACTIONS

! Peptic ulcer disease, GI bleeding, gastritis, and severe hepatic reaction, such as cholestasis and jaundice, occur rarely.

! Nephrotoxicity, including dysuria, hematuria, proteinuria, and nephrotic syndrome, and a severe hypersensitivity reaction, marked by fever, chills, and bronchospasm, occur rarely.

! Hematologic toxicity, characterized by anemia, leukopenia, eosinophilia, and thrombocytopenia, may occur rarely with long-term treatment.

PEDIATRIC CONSIDERATIONS

Baseline Assessment

- Assess the duration, location, onset, and type of inflammation or pain that the patient is experiencing.
- Inspect the appearance of the patient's affected joints for deformity, immobility, and skin condition.
- Expect to obtain a baseline complete blood count (CBC) and serum chemistry tests, especially BUN, serum alkaline phosphatase, bilirubin, creatinine, SGOT (AST), and SGPT (ALT) levels to assess liver and renal function.

Precautions

- Use cautiously in pts with GI disease, hypertension, and impaired cardiac or liver function.
- Use cautiously in pts concurrently receiving anticoagulant therapy.

Administration and Handling

PO

- Do not crush or break capsule form.
- May give piroxicam with antacids, food, or milk if the patient experiences GI distress.

Intervention and Evaluation

- Monitor the patient for GI distress and nausea.
- Monitor the patient's CBC and liver and renal function test results.
- Assess the patient's pattern of daily bowel activity and stool consistency.
- Evaluate the patient for therapeutic response, improved grip strength, increased joint mobility, reduced joint tenderness, and relief of pain, stiffness, and swelling.

Patient/Family Teaching

- Warn the patient/family to avoid tasks that require mental alertness or motor skills until the patient's response to the drug is established.
- Instruct the patient/family to take piroxicam with antacids, food, or milk if the patient experiences GI upset.
- Caution the patient/family to avoid alcohol and aspirin during

piroxicam therapy. These substances increase the risk of GI bleeding.

- Tell the patient to inform the physician if she suspects pregnancy or plans to become pregnant.
- Caution patient/family that exposure to sunlight may cause severe sunburn: the patient should wear broad sunscreen products and protective clothing.

REFERENCES

Miller, S. & Fioravanti, J. (1997). Pediatric medications: a handbook for nurses. St. Louis: Mosby.

Taketomo, C. K., Hodding, J. H. & Kraus, D. M. (2003–2004). Pediatric dosage handbook (10th ed.). Hudson, OH: Lexi-Comp.

44 Sedative-Hypnotics

Chloral hydrate
Flurazepam Hydrochloride
Temazepam
Triazolam

Uses: Sedative-hypnotics are used to treat insomnia, which includes difficulty falling asleep initially, frequent awakening, and awakening too early. Benzodiazepines, such as flurazepam and triazolam, are the most widely used agents. As sedative-hypnotics, they have largely replaced barbiturates because they offer greater safety and a lower risk of drug dependence.

Action: Sedatives decrease motor activity, moderate excitement, and have calming effects. Hypnotics produce drowsiness and enhance the onset and maintenance of sleep, resembling natural sleep. *Benzodiazepines* potentiate γ-aminobutyric acid (GABA), which inhibits impulse transmission in the reticular formation in the brain. They increase the total sleep time by decreasing sleep latency (time before the onset of sleep), the number of awakenings, and the time spent in the awake stage of sleep (light sleep).

Chloral Hydrate

klor-al **high**-drate
(Aquachloral Supprettes, PMS-Chloral Hydrate [CAN], Somnote)

CATEGORY AND SCHEDULE

Pregnancy Risk Category: C
Schedule IV

MECHANISM OF ACTION

A nonbarbiturate chloral derivative that produces CNS depression. ***Therapeutic Effect:*** Induces quiet, deep sleep, with only a slight decrease in respiration and blood pressure (B/P).

AVAILABILITY

Capsules: 500 mg.
Syrup: 500 mg/5 mL.
Suppository: 500 mg, 648 mg.

INDICATIONS AND DOSAGES

▸ Premedication for dental or medical procedures

PO/RECTAL

Children. 50–75 mg/kg/dose 30–60 before procedure; up to 1 g total for infants and 2 g total for children.

Neonates. 25 mg/kg/dose before procedure. Use caution when administering repeated doses because of increased chances of toxicity.

▸ Premedication for electroencephalogram

PO/RECTAL

Children. 25-50 mg/kg/dose 30–60 min before procedure.

▸ Hypnotic

PO

Children. 50 mg/kg. Maximum dose: 1 g.

IV CONTRAINDICATIONS

Marked hepatic impairment, presence of gastritis, renal impairment,

severe cardiac disease.
Hypersensitivity to chloral hydrate or any related component.
Presence of esophagitis or gastric or duodenal ulcers.

INTERACTIONS

Drug

Alcohol, CNS depressants: May increase the effects of chloral hydrate.
IV furosemide: This drug, given within 24 hrs after chloral hydrate, may alter B/P and cause diaphoresis.
Warfarin: May increase the effect of warfarin.
Cyclophosphamide, ifosfamide: May increase toxicity of these products.

Herbal

None known.

Food

None known.

DIAGNOSTIC TEST EFFECTS

None known.

SIDE EFFECTS

Occasional
Gastric irritation, including nausea, vomiting, flatulence, and diarrhea, rash, sleepwalking
Rare
Headache, paradoxical CNS hyperactivity or nervousness in children, particularly noted when given in presence of pain

SERIOUS REACTIONS

! Overdosage may produce somnolence, confusion, slurred speech, severe incoordination, respiratory depression, and coma.
! Tolerance and psychological dependence may occur by second week of therapy.

PEDIATRIC CONSIDERATIONS

Baseline Assessment

- Assess the patient's B/P, pulse, and respirations immediately before beginning chloral hydrate administration.
- Raise the patient's bed rails and provide call bell.
- Provide the patient with an environment conducive to sleep. For example, offer a back rub, quiet environment, and low lighting.
- Expect to obtain baseline chemistry laboratory values to assess renal and liver function.
- Monitor pediatric patients for respiratory depression.
- Be aware that the half-life of chloral hydrate decreased with increasing postconceptional age.

Precautions

- Use cautiously in patients with clinical depression and a history of drug abuse.

Intervention and Evaluation

- Monitor the patient's mental status and vital signs.
- Dilute the drug dose in water to decrease gastric irritation.
- Assess the patient's sleep pattern, including time it takes to fall asleep and nocturnal awakenings.
- Assess pediatric patients for paradoxical reaction, such as excitability.
- Evaluate the patient for a therapeutic response to insomnia, a decrease in the number of nocturnal awakenings, and an increase in length of sleep.
- Be aware that chloral hydrate does not have analgesic properties.
- Use with caution in neonates because drug and metabolites may accumulate and lead to increased toxicity. Prolonged use in neonates has been associated with hyperbilirubinemia.

Patient/Family Teaching

- Instruct the patient/family to take the chloral hydrate capsule with a full glass of fruit juice or water.
- Teach the patient/family to swallow capsules whole and not to chew them.
- Tell the patient/family not to drive if the patient is taking chloral hydrate before a procedure.
- Caution the patient/family against abruptly withdrawing the medication after long-term use.
- Tell the patient/family that dependence and tolerance may occur with prolonged use.

Flurazepam Hydrochloride

flur-**ah**-zah-pam
(Apo-Flurazepam [CAN], Dalmane)
Do not confuse with Dialume.

CATEGORY AND SCHEDULE

Pregnancy Risk Category: X
Controlled Substance: Schedule IV

MECHANISM OF ACTION

A benzodiazepine that enhances the action of inhibitory neurotransmitter c GABA. ***Therapeutic Effect:*** Produces a hypnotic effect due to CNS depression.

PHARMACOKINETICS

Route	Onset	Peak	Duration
PO	15–20 min	3–6 hrs	7–8 hrs

Well absorbed from the GI tract. Protein binding: 97%. Crosses blood-brain barrier. Widely distributed. Metabolized in liver to the active metabolite. Primarily excreted in urine. Not removed by hemodialysis. ***Half-Life:*** 2.3 hrs (adults); metabolite: 40–114 hrs.

AVAILABILITY

Capsules: 15 mg, 30 mg.

INDICATIONS AND DOSAGES

▸ Insomnia

PO

Children older than 15 yrs. 15 mg at bedtime.

CONTRAINDICATIONS

Hypersensitivity to flurazepam or any related component. Pregnancy, preexisting respiratory depression, acute alcohol intoxication, and acute narrow-angle glaucoma

INTERACTIONS

Drug

Alcohol, CNS depressants: May increase CNS depressant effect.
Ritonavir: Increases metabolism of ritonavir.

Herbal

Kava kava, valerian: May increase CNS depression.

Food

None known.

DIAGNOSTIC TEST EFFECTS

None known.

SIDE EFFECTS

Frequent

Drowsiness, dizziness, ataxia, sedation
Morning drowsiness may occur initially.

Occasional

GI disturbances, nervousness, blurred vision, dry mouth, headache, confusion, skin rash, irritability, slurred speech

Rare
Paradoxical CNS excitement or restlessness, particularly noted in debilitated patients

SERIOUS REACTIONS

! Abrupt or too rapid withdrawal after long-term use may result in pronounced restlessness and irritability, insomnia, hand tremors, abdominal or muscle cramps, sweating, vomiting, and seizures.
! Overdosage results in somnolence, confusion, diminished reflexes, and coma.

PEDIATRIC CONSIDERATIONS

Baseline Assessment
- Assess the patient's blood pressure, pulse, and respirations immediately before beginning flurazepam administration.
- Raise the patient's bed rails and place the call bell within reach.
- Provide the patient with an environment conducive to sleep. For example, offer a back rub, quiet environment, and low lighting.
- Be aware that flurazepam crosses the placenta and may be distributed in breast milk.
- Be aware that chronic flurazepam ingestion during pregnancy may produce withdrawal symptoms and CNS depression in neonates.
- Be aware that the safety and efficacy of flurazepam have not been established in children younger than 15 yrs of age.

Precautions
- Use cautiously in patients with impaired liver or renal function.

Administration and Handling
PO
- Give flurazepam without regard to meals.
- If desired, empty capsules and mix with food.

Intervention and Evaluation
- Assess patients for a paradoxical reaction, such as excitability, particularly during early therapy.
- Evaluate the patient for a therapeutic response to insomnia, a decrease in the number of nocturnal awakenings, and an increase in length of sleep.

Patient/Family Teaching
- Tell the patient/family that smoking reduces the effectiveness of the drug.
- Caution the patient/family against abruptly withdrawing the medication after long-term use.
- Explain to the patient/family that the patient may have disturbed sleep for 1–2 nights after discontinuing the drug.
- Instruct the patient/family to notify the physician if the patient becomes pregnant or plans to become pregnant. Explain to the patient/family that flurazepam is pregnancy risk category X and the drug cannot be taken because of its risk factor.
- Urge the patient/family to avoid alcohol and other CNS depressants during flurazepam therapy.
- Advise the patient/family that flurazepam use may be habit forming.

Temazepam

tem-**az**-eh-pam
(Apo-Temazepam [CAN], Novo-Temazepam [CAN], PMS-Temazepam [CAN], Restoril)
Do not confuse with Vistaril or Zestril.

CATEGORY AND SCHEDULE

Pregnancy Risk Category: X
Controlled Substance: Schedule IV

MECHANISM OF ACTION

A benzodiazepine that enhances the action of the inhibitory neurotransmitter dGABA. ***Therapeutic Effect:*** Produces a hypnotic effect due to CNS depression.

PHARMACOKINETICS

Well absorbed from the GI tract. Protein binding: 96%. Widely distributed. Crosses blood-brain barrier. Metabolized in liver. Primarily excreted in urine. Not removed by hemodialysis. ***Half-Life:*** 4-18 hrs (adults).

AVAILABILITY

Capsules: 7.5 mg, 15 mg, 30 mg.

INDICATIONS AND DOSAGES

▸ **Insomnia**

PO

Children older than 18 yrs. 15–30 mg at bedtime.

CONTRAINDICATIONS

Hypersensitivity to temazepam or any related component. CNS depression, narrow-angle glaucoma, severe uncontrolled pain, and sleep apnea.

INTERACTIONS

Drug

Alcohol, CNS depressants: May increase CNS depressant effect.

Herbal

Kava kava, valerian: May increase CNS effects.

Food

None known.

DIAGNOSTIC TEST EFFECTS

None known.

SIDE EFFECTS

Frequent

Drowsiness, sedation, rebound insomnia that may occur for 1–2 nights after the drug is discontinued, dizziness, confusion, euphoria

Occasional

Weakness, anorexia, diarrhea

Rare

Paradoxical CNS excitement, restlessness, particularly noted in debilitated patients

SERIOUS REACTIONS

! Abrupt or too rapid withdrawal may result in pronounced restlessness, irritability, insomnia, hand tremors, abdominal or muscle cramps, diaphoresis, vomiting, and seizures.

! Overdosage results in somnolence, confusion, diminished reflexes, respiratory depression, and coma.

PEDIATRIC CONSIDERATIONS

Baseline Assessment

- Determine whether the patient is pregnant before beginning temazepam therapy.
- Assess the patient's blood pressure, pulse, and respirations before temazepam administration.
- Provide the patient with an environment conducive to sleep. For example, offer a back rub, low lighting, and a quiet environment.
- Assess the patient's baseline sleep pattern, including time to fall asleep and nocturnal awakenings.
- Be aware that temazepam crosses the placenta and may be distributed in breast milk.
- Be aware that chronic temazepam ingestion during pregnancy may produce withdrawal symptoms and CNS depression in neonates.
- Be aware that temazepam use is not recommended in

children younger than 18 yrs of age.

Precautions

• Use cautiously in patients with a potential for drug dependence and mental impairment.

Administration and Handling

PO

• Give temazepam without regard to meals.

• Capsules may be emptied and mixed with food.

Intervention and Evaluation

• Assess debilitated patients for a paradoxical reaction, particularly during early drug therapy.

• Monitor the patient's cardiovascular, mental, and respiratory statuses.

• Evaluate the patient for a therapeutic response, a decrease in the number of nocturnal awakenings, and an increase in the length of sleep.

Patient/Family Teaching

• Urge the patient/family to avoid alcohol and other CNS depressants.

• Advise the patient/family that temazepam may cause daytime drowsiness.

• Warn the patient/family to avoid activities requiring mental alertness or motor skills until the patient's response to the drug is established.

• Instruct the patient/family to take temazepam about 30 min before bedtime.

• Caution the patient/family to notify the physician if the patient becomes pregnant or plans to become pregnant during temazepam therapy.

Triazolam

try-**aye**-zoe-lam
(Apo-Triazo [CAN], Halcion)
Do not confuse with Haldol or Healon.

CATEGORY AND SCHEDULE

Pregnancy Risk Category: X
Controlled Substance: Schedule IV

MECHANISM OF ACTION

A benzodiazepine that enhances the action of the inhibitory neurotransmitter GABA. ***Therapeutic Effect:*** Produces a hypnotic effect due to CNS depression.

AVAILABILITY

Tablets: 0.125 mg, 0.25 mg.

INDICATIONS AND DOSAGES

▸ Hypnotic

PO

Children older than 18 yrs.
0.125–0.25 mg at bedtime.

CONTRAINDICATIONS

Hypersensitivity to triazolam or any related component. CNS depression, narrow-angle glaucoma, pregnancy or lactation, severe uncontrolled pain, and sleep apnea.

INTERACTIONS

Drug

Alcohol, CNS depressants: May increase CNS depressant effect.
Cimetidine, erythromycin: May decrease metabolism of triazolam.
Protease inhibitors: May increase triazolam serum concentrations.
Ketoconazole, itraconazole: May increase intensity and duration of triazolam effects.

Herbal

Kava kava, valerian: May increase CNS depression.

Food

Grapefruit or grapefruit juice: May alter the absorption of triazolam.

DIAGNOSTIC TEST EFFECTS

None known.

SIDE EFFECTS

Frequent

Drowsiness, sedation, dry mouth, headache, dizziness, nervousness, lightheadedness, incoordination, nausea

Occasional

Euphoria, tachycardia, abdominal cramps, visual disturbances

Rare

Paradoxical CNS excitement, restlessness, particularly noted in debilitated patients

SERIOUS REACTIONS

! Abrupt or too rapid withdrawal may result in pronounced restlessness, irritability, insomnia, hand tremors, abdominal or muscle cramps, diaphoresis, vomiting, and seizures.

! Overdosage results in somnolence, confusion, diminished reflexes, respiratory depression, and coma.

PEDIATRIC CONSIDERATIONS

Baseline Assessment

• Determine whether the patient is pregnant before beginning triazolam therapy.
• Assess the patient's vital signs immediately before triazolam administration.
• Raise the patient's bed rails and provide a call bell.
• Provide the patient with an environment conducive to sleep. For example, offer a back rub, quiet environment, and low lighting.
• No dosing in those younger than 18 yrs.

Precautions

• Use cautiously in patients with a potential for drug abuse.

Administration and Handling

PO

• Give triazolam without regard to meals.
• Crush tablets as needed.
• Keep in mind that grapefruit juice may alter absorption.

Intervention and Evaluation

• Assess the patient's sleep pattern.
• Assess debilitated patients for a paradoxical reaction, particularly during early drug therapy.
• Monitor the patient's cardiovascular, mental, and respiratory status and liver function with prolonged triazolam use.
• Evaluate the patient for a therapeutic response, a decrease in the number of nocturnal awakenings, and an increase in the length of sleep.

Patient/Family Teaching

• Urge the patient/family to avoid alcohol and other CNS depressants.
• Inform the patient/family that triazolam may cause drowsiness.
• Warn the patient/family to avoid activities requiring mental alertness or motor skills until the patient's response to the drug is established.
• Caution the patient/family to notify the physician if the patient becomes pregnant, or plans to become pregnant during triazolam therapy.
• Tell the patient/family that triazolam may cause dry mouth and

physical or psychological dependence.
• Explain to the patient/family that smoking reduces the effectiveness of the drug.
• Inform the patient/family that rebound insomnia may occur when this drug is discontinued after short-term therapy. Explain further to the patient that the patient may experience disturbed sleep patterns for 1–2 nights after discontinuing triazolam.
• Urge the patient/family to avoid consuming grapefruit or grapefruit juice during triazolam therapy. Explain to the patient/family that these foods decrease the absorption of triazolam.

REFERENCES

Miller, S. & Fioravanti, J. (1997). Pediatric medications: a handbook for nurses. St. Louis: Mosby.
Taketomo, C. K., Hodding, J. H. & Kraus, D. M. (2003–2004). Pediatric dosage handbook (10th ed.). Hudson, OH: Lexi-Comp.

45 Skeletal Muscle Relaxants

Baclofen
Dantrolene Sodium

Uses: Skeletal muscle relaxants are used as adjuncts to rest and physical therapy. *Baclofen and dantrolene* are used to treat spasticity characterized by heightened muscle tone, spasm, and loss of dexterity caused by multiple sclerosis, cerebral palsy, spinal cord lesions, or stroke.

Action: *Central-acting skeletal muscle relaxants* work by a mechanism that is not fully understood. They may act at various levels of the CNS to depress polysynaptic reflexes, and their sedative effect may be responsible for their ability to relax muscles. *Baclofen* may mimic the actions of γ-aminobutyric acid on spinal neurons; it does not directly affect skeletal muscles. *Dantrolene* acts directly on skeletal muscles, relieving spasticity.

Baclofen

back-low-fin
(Apo-Baclofen [CAN], Baclo [AUS], Clofen [AUS], Kemstro, Liotec [CAN])
Do not confuse with Bactroban, Beclovent, or lisinopril.

CATEGORY AND SCHEDULE

Pregnancy Risk Category: C

MECHANISM OF ACTION

A skeletal muscle relaxant that inhibits transmission of reflexes at the spinal cord level. ***Therapeutic Effect:*** Relieves muscle spasticity.

PHARMACOKINETICS

Well absorbed from the GI tract. Protein binding: 30%. Partially metabolized in liver. Primarily excreted in urine. ***Half-Life:*** 2.5–4 hrs. Intrathecal: 1.5 hrs.

AVAILABILITY

Tablets: 10 mg, 20 mg.
Ampules: 500 mcg/mL.
Oral Disintegrating Tablet: 10 mg, 20 mg.

INDICATIONS AND DOSAGES

▸ **Musculoskeletal spasm**

PO

Children 2–7 yrs. Initially 10–15 mg/day in divided dose q8h. May increase at 3-day intervals by 5–15 mg/day. Maximum: 40 mg/day.

Children 8 yrs and older. Titrate as above. Maximum: 60 mg/day.

▸ **Intrathecal Average Daily Dose**

Children older than 12 yrs. Usual dose 300–800 mcg/day.

Children 12 yrs or younger. Usual dose 100–300 mcg/day.

UNLABELED USES

Treatment of trigeminal neuralgia. Cerebral palsy, Parkinson's disease, skeletal muscle spasm due to rheumatic disorders, stroke.

CONTRAINDICATIONS

Hypersensitivity to baclofen or any related component.

INTERACTIONS

Drug

CNS depressants, including alcohol: Potentiate effects when used with other CNS depressants, including alcohol.

Lithium: May decrease the effect of lithium.

Herbal

None known.

Food

None known.

DIAGNOSTIC TEST EFFECTS

May increase serum alkaline phosphatase, blood glucose, SGOT (AST), and SGPT (ALT) levels.

SIDE EFFECTS

Frequent (greater than 10%)

Transient drowsiness, weakness, dizziness, lightheadedness, nausea, vomiting

Occasional (10%–2%)

Headache, paresthesia of hands and feet, constipation, anorexia, hypotension, confusion, nasal congestion

Rare (less than 1%)

Paradoxical CNS excitement and restlessness, slurred speech, tremor, dry mouth, diarrhea, nocturia, impotence

SERIOUS REACTIONS

! Abrupt baclofen withdrawal may produce hallucinations and seizures.

! Baclofen overdosage results in blurred vision, convulsions, myosis, mydriasis, severe muscle weakness, strabismus, respiratory depression, and vomiting.

PEDIATRIC CONSIDERATIONS

Baseline Assessment

- Record the duration, location, onset, and type of muscular spasm.
- Evaluate the patient for signs and symptoms of immobility, stiffness, or swelling.
- Be aware that it is unknown whether baclofen crosses the placenta or is distributed in breast milk.
- Be aware that the safety and efficacy of baclofen have not been established in children younger than 12 yrs of age.

Precautions

- Use cautiously in patients with a history of stroke, diabetes mellitus, epilepsy, impaired renal function, and preexisting psychiatric disorders.
- Be aware that abrupt discontinuation of continuous use of intrathecal baclofen may lead to high fever, altered mental status, exaggerated rebound spasticity, and muscle rigidity. In rare cases, rhabdomyolysis, multiple organ failure, and death have occurred.

Administration and Handling

PO

- Give without regard to meals.
- Tablets may be crushed.

Intervention and Evaluation

- Assess the patient for a paradoxical reaction.
- Assist the patient with ambulation at all times.
- Expect to obtain blood counts and liver and renal function tests periodically for those receiving long-term therapy.
- Evaluate the patient for a therapeutic response, such as decreased intensity of skeletal muscle pain.
- Assess the patient for signs and symptoms of developing infection.

Patient/Family Teaching

- Explain to the patient/family that the side effect of drowsiness usually diminishes with continued therapy.

• Warn the patient/family to avoid tasks that require mental alertness or motor skills until the patient's response to baclofen is established.
• Caution the patient/family against abruptly discontinuing baclofen after long-term therapy.
• Urge the patient/family to avoid alcohol and CNS depressants.

Dantrolene Sodium

dan-trow-lean
(Dantrium)
Do not confuse with Daraprim.

CATEGORY AND SCHEDULE
Pregnancy Risk Category: C

MECHANISM OF ACTION

A skeletal muscle relaxant that reduces muscle contraction by interfering with release of calcium ions. Reduces calcium ion concentration. ***Therapeutic Effect:*** Dissociates excitation-contraction coupling. Interferes with the catabolic process associated with malignant hyperthermic crisis.

PHARMACOKINETICS

Poorly absorbed from the GI tract. Protein binding: High. Metabolized in liver. Primarily excreted in feces via bile. ***Half-Life:*** IV: 4–8 hrs. PO: 8.7 hrs (adults) and 7.3 (children).

AVAILABILITY

Capsules: 25 mg, 50 mg, 100 mg.
Powder for Injection: 20-mg vial.

INDICATIONS AND DOSAGES

▸ Spasticity
PO
Children. Initially, 0.5 mg/kg 2 times/day. Increase to 0.5 mg/kg 3–4 times/day, then increase by 0.5 mg/kg/day up to 3 mg/kg 2–4 times/day. Maximum: 400 mg/day.

▸ Prevention of malignant hyperthermia crisis
PO
Children. 4–8 mg/kg/day in 3–4 divided doses 1–2 days before surgery; give last dose 3–4 hrs before surgery.
IV INFUSION
Children. Infuse 2.5 mg/kg over 1 hr approximately 1.25 hrs before surgery.

▸ Management of malignant hyperthermia crisis
IV
Children. Initially a minimum of 1 mg/kg rapid IV; may repeat up to total cumulative dose of 10 mg/kg. May follow with 4–8 mg/kg/day PO in 4 divided doses up to 3 days after crisis.

UNLABELED USES

Relief of exercise-induced pain in patients with muscular dystrophy, treatment of flexor spasms and neuroleptic malignant syndrome.

CONTRAINDICATIONS

Hypersensitivity to dantrolene or any related component. Active liver disease.

INTERACTIONS

Drug
CNS depressants: May increase CNS depression with short-term use.
Liver toxic medications: May increase the risk of liver toxicity with chronic use.
Verapamil: May increase incidence of hyperkalemia and myocardial depression.
Estrogen: Increased incidence of hepatotoxicity.

Herbal
None known.
Food
None known.

DIAGNOSTIC TEST EFFECTS

May alter liver function tests.

IV INCOMPATIBILITIES

None known.

SIDE EFFECTS

Frequent
Drowsiness, dizziness, weakness, general malaise, diarrhea, which may be severe
Occasional
Confusion, headache, insomnia, constipation, urinary frequency
Rare
Paradoxical CNS excitement or restlessness, paresthesia, tinnitus, slurred speech, tremor, blurred vision, dry mouth, diarrhea, nocturia, impotence

SERIOUS REACTIONS

! There is a risk of liver toxicity, most notably in females, those older than 35 yrs of age, and those taking other medications concurrently.
! Overt hepatitis noted most frequently between the 3rd and 12th mo of therapy.
! Overdosage results in vomiting, muscular hypotonia, muscle twitching, respiratory depression, and seizures.

PEDIATRIC CONSIDERATIONS

Baseline Assessment

- Plan to obtain the patient's baseline liver function tests, including serum alkaline phosphatase, SGOT (AST), SGPT (ALT), and total bilirubin levels.
- Record the duration, location, onset, and type of muscular spasm the patient is experiencing.
- Examine the patient for immobility, stiffness, and swelling.
- Be aware that dantrolene readily crosses the placenta and should not be used in breast-feeding mothers.
- There are no age-related precautions noted in children older than 5 yrs of age.
- This medication is not recommended for long-term use in children younger than 5 yrs of age.
- Be aware that dantrolene should not be reconstituted with bacteriostatic water.

Precautions

- Use cautiously in patients with a history of previous liver disease and impaired cardiac or pulmonary function.

Administration and Handling

◂ **ALERT** ▸ Begin with low-dose therapy, as prescribed, then increase gradually at 4- to 7-day intervals to reduce incidence of side effects.

PO
Give dantrolene without regard to meals.

IV

- Store at room temperature.
- Use within 6 hrs after reconstitution.
- Solution normally appears clear, colorless.
- Discard if cloudy or precipitate is present.
- Reconstitute 20-mg vial with 60 mL Sterile Water for Injection to provide a concentration of 0.33 mg/mL.
- For IV infusion, administer over 1 hr.
- Diligently monitor for extravasation because of the high pH of the IV preparation. May produce severe complications.

Intervention and Evaluation

- Assist the patient with ambulation.

• Perform periodic blood counts and liver and renal function tests, as ordered, in patients receiving long-term therapy.
• Evaluate the patient for a therapeutic response or decreased intensity of skeletal muscle pain or spasm.

Patient/Family Teaching

• Explain to the patient/family that drowsiness usually diminishes with continued therapy.
• Caution the patient/family to avoid tasks that require mental alertness or motor skills until the patient's response to the drug is established.
• Urge the patient/family to avoid alcohol or other depressants while taking dantrolene.
• Warn the patient/family to notify the physician if the patient experiences bloody or tarry stools, continued weakness, diarrhea, fatigue, itching, nausea, or skin rash.

REFERENCES

Miller, S. & Fioravanti, J. (1997). Pediatric medications: a handbook for nurses. St. Louis: Mosby.
Taketomo, C. K., Hodding, J. H. & Kraus, D. M. (2003–2004). Pediatric dosage handbook (10th ed.). Hudson, OH: Lexi-Comp.

46 Miscellaneous CNS Agents

Flumazenil
Fluvoxamine Maleate

Uses: Miscellaneous CNS agents have a wide variety of uses. *Flumazenil* is used as an antidote for benzodiazepine overdosage. *Fluvoxamine* is used to treat obsessive-compulsive disorder.

Action: Most of these miscellaneous agents act on receptors in the CNS. *Flumazenil* antagonizes the effect of benzodiazepines on γ-aminobutyric acid (GABA) receptors in the CNS. *Fluvoxamine* selectively inhibits serotonin reuptake by neurons in the CNS.

Flumazenil

flew-**maz**-ah-nil
(Anexate [CAN], Romazicon)

CATEGORY AND SCHEDULE

Pregnancy Risk Category: C

MECHANISM OF ACTION

An antidote that antagonizes the effect of benzodiazepines on the GABA receptor complex in the CNS. ***Therapeutic Effect:*** Reverses sedative effect of benzodiazepines.

PHARMACOKINETICS

Route	Onset	Peak	Duration
IV	1–2 min	6–10 min	less than 1 hr

Duration and degree of benzodiazepine reversal are related to dosage and plasma concentration. Protein binding: 50%. Metabolized by liver; excreted by liver. Less than 1% excreted in urine.

AVAILABILITY

Injection: 0.1 mg/mL.

INDICATIONS AND DOSAGES

Reversal of conscious sedation, in general anesthesia

IV

Children and neonates. Initially, 0.01 mg/kg. Maximum: 0.2 mg. May repeat after 45 sec and then every minute. Maximum cumulative dose: 0.05 mg/kg or 1 mg.

Benzodiazepine overdose

IV

Children and neonates. Initially, 0.01 mg/kg. Maximum: 0.2 mg. May repeat in 45 sec, then at 60-sec intervals. Maximum cumulative dose: 1 mg.

CONTRAINDICATIONS

Hypersensitivity to flumazenil or any related component. Anticholinergic signs, arrhythmias, cardiovascular collapse, a history of hypersensitivity to benzodiazepines, those showing signs of a serious cyclic antidepressant overdose manifested by motor abnormalities, those who have been given a benzodiazepine for control of a potentially life-threatening condition, such as control of intracranial pressure and status epilepticus.

INTERACTIONS

Drug

Toxic effects, such as seizures and arrhythmias, of drugs taken in overdose, especially tricyclic antidepressants, may emerge with reversal of the sedative effect of benzodiazepines.

Herbal

None known.

Food

None known.

DIAGNOSTIC TEST EFFECTS

None known.

IV INCOMPATIBILITIES

No information available via Y-site administration.

IV COMPATIBILITIES

Aminophylline, cimetidine (Tagamet), dobutamine (Dobutrex), dopamine (Intropin), famotidine (Pepcid), heparin, lidocaine, procainamide (Pronestyl), ranitidine (Zantac)

SIDE EFFECTS

Frequent (11%–4%)

Agitation, anxiety, dry mouth, dyspnea, insomnia, palpitations, tremors, headache, blurred vision, dizziness, ataxia, nausea, vomiting, pain at injection site, diaphoresis

Occasional (3%–1%)

Fatigue, flushing, auditory disturbances, thrombophlebitis, skin rash

Rare (less than 1%)

Hives, itching, hallucinations

SERIOUS REACTIONS

! Toxic effects, such as seizures and arrhythmias, of other drugs taken in overdose, especially tricyclic antidepressants, may emerge with reversal of sedative effect of benzodiazepines.

! May provoke panic attack in those with history of panic disorder.

PEDIATRIC CONSIDERATIONS

Baseline Assessment

- Obtain arterial blood gas measurements before and at 30-min intervals during IV flumazenil administration.
- Prepare to intervene in reestablishing the patient's airway and assisting ventilation because the drug may not fully reverse ventilatory insufficiency induced by benzodiazepines.
- Know that the effects of flumazenil may wear off before the effects of benzodiazepines wear off.
- Be aware that it is unknown whether flumazenil crosses the placenta or is distributed in breast milk. Flumazenil use is not recommended during labor and delivery.
- There are no age-related precautions noted in children.

Precautions

- Use cautiously in pts with alcoholism, drug dependence, head injury, and impaired liver function.

Administration and Handling

- Compatible with D_5W, lactated Ringer's solution, and 0.9% NaCl.

◂ **ALERT** ▸ If resedation occurs, repeat dose at 20-min intervals. Maximum: 1 mg, given as 0.2 mg/min, at any one time, 3 mg in any 1 hr.

IV

- Store parenteral form at room temperature.
- Discard after 24 hrs once the medication is drawn into a syringe or is mixed with any solutions or if a particulate or discoloration is noted.

• Rinse spilled medication from skin with cool water.
• Give over 15 sec, as prescribed, for reversal of conscious sedation or general anesthesia.
• Give over 30 sec, as prescribed, for benzodiazepine overdose.
• Administer through a freely running IV infusion into a large vein because local injection produces pain and inflammation at the injection site.

Intervention and Evaluation

• Properly manage the patient's airway and assisted breathing, maintain circulatory access and support, perform internal decontamination by lavage and charcoal, and provide adequate clinical evaluation.
• Monitor the patient for reversal of the benzodiazepine effect.
• Assess the patient for possible hypoventilation, resedation, and respiratory depression.
• Assess the patient closely for return of unconsciousness or narcosis for at least 1 hr after patient is fully alert.

Patient/Family Teaching

• Warn the patient/family to avoid tasks requiring mental alertness or motor skills until at least 24 hrs after discharge.
• Instruct the patient/family to avoid taking nonprescription drugs until at least 18–24 hrs after discharge.

Fluvoxamine Maleate

flew-**vox**-ah-meen
(Faverin [AUS], Luvox)

CATEGORY AND SCHEDULE

Pregnancy Risk Category: C

MECHANISM OF ACTION

An antidepressant, antiobsessional agent that selectively inhibits serotonin neuronal uptake in the CNS. ***Therapeutic Effect:*** Produces antidepressant and antiobsessive effects.

AVAILABILITY

Tablets: 25 mg, 50 mg, 100 mg.

INDICATIONS AND DOSAGES

◂Obsessive compulsive disorder

PO

Children 8–17 yrs. 25 mg at bedtime; increase by 25 mg q4–7days. Doses greater than 50 mg/day in 2 divided doses. Maximum: 200 mg/day.

UNLABELED USES

Treatment of depression, bulimia nervosa, panic disorder, social phobia.

CONTRAINDICATIONS

Hypersensitivity to fluvoxamine or any related component. Within 14 days of MAOI ingestion.

INTERACTIONS

Drug

Benzodiazepines, carbamazepine, clozapine, theophylline: May increase the blood concentration and risk of toxicity of benzodiazepines, carbamazepine, clozapine, and theophylline.
Lithium, tryptophan: May enhance serotonergic effects.
MAOIs: May produce serious reactions, including hyperthermia, rigidity, and myoclonus.
Tricyclic antidepressants: May increase fluvoxamine blood concentration.
Warfarin: May increase the effects of warfarin.

Herbal

St. John's wort: May have an additive effect.

Food

None known.

DIAGNOSTIC TEST EFFECTS

None known.

SIDE EFFECTS

Frequent

Nausea (40%), headache, somnolence, insomnia (21%–22%)

Occasional (14%–8%)

Nervousness, dizziness, diarrhea or loose stools, dry mouth, asthenia or loss of strength, weakness, dyspepsia, constipation, abnormal ejaculation

Rare (6%–3%)

Anorexia, anxiety, tremor, vomiting, flatulence, urinary frequency, sexual dysfunction, taste change

SERIOUS REACTIONS

! Overdosage may produce seizures, nausea, vomiting, excessive agitation, and extreme restlessness.

PEDIATRIC CONSIDERATIONS

Baseline Assessment

- Plan to perform baseline blood serum chemistry tests to assess liver function.
- Be aware that there may be a possible increase in potentiating suicide in adolescents/children.

Precautions

- Use cautiously in pts with impaired liver or renal function.

Administration and Handling

◂ **ALERT** ▸ Expect to use lower or less frequent dosing in pts with impaired liver function.

Intervention and Evaluation

- Closely supervise suicidal-risk pts during early therapy. As depression lessens, the patient's energy level improves, which increases the suicide potential.
- Assess the patient's appearance, behavior, level of interest, mood, and speech pattern.
- Assist the patient with ambulation if he or she experiences dizziness and somnolence.
- Assess the patient's pattern of daily bowel activity and stool consistency.

Patient/Family Teaching

- Tell the patient/family that the maximum therapeutic response may require 4 wks or more to appear.
- Suggest to the patient/family that taking sips of tepid water and chewing sugarless gum may relieve dry mouth.
- Caution the patient/family not to abruptly discontinue the medication.
- Warn the patient/family to avoid tasks that require mental alertness or motor skills until the patient's response to the drug is established.

REFERENCES

Miller, S. & Fioravanti, J. (1997). Pediatric medications: a handbook for nurses. St. Louis: Mosby.

Taketomo, C. K., Hodding, J. H. & Kraus, D. M. (2003–2004). Pediatric dosage handbook (10th ed.). Hudson, OH: Lexi-Comp.

47 Anticholinergics and Antispasmodics

Atropine Sulfate
Dicyclomine Hydrochloride
Glycopyrrolate
Hyoscyamine
Scopolamine

Uses: Anticholinergic and antispasmodic agents are used to treat a wide variety of GI conditions that involve bowel irritability and increased tone (spasticity) or motility of the GI tract.

Action: Also known as parasympatholytics, antimuscarinics, and muscarinic blockers, anticholinergics and antispasmodics competitively block the actions of acetylcholine at muscarinic receptors. Through this action, they reduce GI tone and motility and suppress gastric acid secretion.

COMBINATION PRODUCTS

LOMOTIL: atropine sulfate/diphenoxylate hydrochloride (an antidiarrheal) 0.025 mg/2.5 mg.

Atropine Sulfate

See antiarrhythmic agents

Dicyclomine Hydrochloride

dye-**sigh**-clo-meen
(Bentyl, Bentylol [CAN], Formulex [CAN], Lomine [CAN], Merbentyl [AUS])
Do not confuse with Aventyl, Benadryl, doxycycline, or dyclonine.

CATEGORY AND SCHEDULE

Pregnancy Risk Category: B

MECHANISM OF ACTION

A GI antispasmodic and anticholinergic agent that directly acts as a relaxant on smooth muscle. ***Therapeutic Effect:*** Reduces tone and motility of the GI tract.

PHARMACOKINETICS

Route	Onset	Peak	Duration
PO	1–2 hrs	N/A	4 hrs

Readily absorbed from the GI tract. Widely distributed. Metabolized in liver. Mostly eliminated in the urine. ***Half-Life:*** 9–10 hrs.

AVAILABILITY

Capsules: 10 mg.
Tablets: 20 mg.
Syrup: 10 mg/5 mL.
Injection: 10 mg/mL.

INDICATIONS AND DOSAGES

▸ **Functional disturbances of GI motility**

PO

Children older than 2 yrs. 10 mg 3–4 times/day.
Children 6 mos–2 yrs. 5 mg 3–4 times/day.

CONTRAINDICATIONS

Hypersensitivity to dicyclomine or any related component. Bladder neck obstruction resulting from prostatic hypertrophy, cardiospasm, intestinal atony, myasthenia gravis in those not treated with neostigmine, narrow-angle glaucoma, obstructive disease of the GI tract, paralytic ileus, severe ulcerative colitis, tachycardia secondary to cardiac insufficiency or thyrotoxicosis, toxic megacolon, unstable cardiovascular status in acute hemorrhage.

INTERACTIONS

Drug

Antacids, antidiarrheals: May decrease the absorption of dicyclomine.
Anticholinergics: May increase the effects of dicyclomine.
Antiglaucoma drugs: May decrease effectiveness of antiglaucoma drugs.
Ketoconazole: May decrease the absorption of ketoconazole.
Potassium chloride: May increase the severity of GI lesions with the wax matrix formulation of potassium chloride.

Herbal

None known.

Food

None known.

DIAGNOSTIC TEST EFFECTS

None known.

SIDE EFFECTS

Frequent

Dry mouth, sometimes severe, constipation, decreased sweating ability

Occasional

Blurred vision, intolerance to light, urinary hesitancy, drowsiness with high dosage, agitation, excitement

Rare

Confusion, hypersensitivity reaction, increased intraocular pressure, nausea, vomiting, unusual tiredness

SERIOUS REACTIONS

! Overdosage may produce temporary paralysis of ciliary muscle, pupillary dilation, tachycardia, palpitation, hot, dry, or flushed skin, absence of bowel sounds, hyperthermia, increased respiratory rate, EKG abnormalities, nausea, vomiting, a rash over the face or upper trunk, CNS stimulation, and psychosis, marked by agitation, restlessness, rambling speech, visual hallucination, paranoid behavior, and delusions, followed by depression.

PEDIATRIC CONSIDERATIONS

Baseline Assessment

- Instruct the patient to void before giving the medication to reduce the risk of urinary retention.
- Be aware that it is unknown whether dicyclomine crosses the placenta or is distributed in breast milk.
- Be aware that infants and young children are more susceptible to the toxic effects of the drug.
- Dicyclomine is not recommended in infants younger than 6 mos of age.
- The IM route is not recommended in children.
- Be aware that children with spastic paralysis, brain damage, or Down syndrome are at a greater risk for experiencing side effects.

Precautions

- Use extreme caution in pts with autonomic neuropathy, diarrhea, known or suspected GI infections, and mild to moderate ulcerative colitis.
- Use cautiously in pts with chronic obstructive pulmonary disease, CHF, coronary artery disease, esophageal reflux or

hiatal hernia associated with reflux esophagitis, gastric ulcer, hyperthyroidism, hypertension, liver or renal disease, and tachyarrhythmias.
• Use cautiously in infants.

Administration and Handling

• Store capsules, tablets, syrup, and parenteral form at room temperature.

PO

Dilute oral solution with an equal volume of water just before administration.
• May give dicyclomine without regard to meals although food may slightly decrease absorption.

Intervention and Evaluation

• Assess the patient's pattern of daily bowel activity and stool consistency.
• Evaluate the patient for urinary retention.
• Monitor changes in the patient's blood pressure and body temperature.
• Be alert for fever because it increases the risk of hyperthermia.
• Assess the patient's bowel sounds for peristalsis and mucous membranes and skin turgor to evaluate hydration status.
• Encourage adequate fluid intake.

Patient/Family Teaching

• Tell the patient/family not to become overheated during exercise in hot weather because this may cause heat stroke.
• Urge the patient/family to avoid hot baths and saunas.
• Warn the patient/family to avoid tasks that require mental alertness or motor skills until the patient's response to the drug is established.
• Instruct the patient/family not to take antacids or antidiarrheals within 1 hr of taking this medication as these drugs decrease the effectiveness of dicyclomine.
• Instruct the patient/family to avoid alcohol or alcohol-containing products.
• Caution patient/family that this medication may cause dry mouth. Frequent sips of water may help.

Glycopyrrolate

gly-ko-**pie**-roll-ate
(Robinul, Robinul Forte, Robinul Injection [AUS])

CATEGORY AND SCHEDULE

Pregnancy Risk Category: B

MECHANISM OF ACTION

A quaternary anticholinergic that inhibits action of acetylcholine at postganglionic parasympathetic sites in smooth muscle, secretory glands, and the CNS. ***Therapeutic Effect:*** Reduces salivation and excessive secretions of respiratory tract; reduces gastric secretions and acidity.

AVAILABILITY

Injection: 0.2 mg/mL.
Tablet: 1 mg, 2 mg.

INDICATIONS AND DOSAGES

▸ **Preoperative**

IM

Children 2 yrs and older. 4.4 mcg/kg 30–60 min before a procedure.
Children younger than 2 yrs. 4.4–8.8 mcg/kg 30–60 minutes before a procedure.

▸ **Reversal of muscarinic effects of cholinergic agents**

IV

Children. 0.2 mg for each 1 mg neostigmine or 5 mg pyridostigmine administered.

▸ **Control of secretions**
PO
Children. 40–100 mcg/kg/dose 3–4 times in 24 hrs.
IM/IV
Children. 4–10 mcg/kg/dose 3–4 times in 24 hrs.

CONTRAINDICATIONS
Hypersensitivity to glycopyrrolate or any related component. Acute hemorrhage, myasthenia gravis, narrow-angle glaucoma, obstructive uropathy, paralytic ileus, tachycardia, ulcerative colitis.

INTERACTIONS
Drug
Antacids, antidiarrheals: May decrease the absorption of glycopyrrolate.
Anticholinergics, phenothiazines, meperidine, amantadine, quinidine: May increase the effects of glycopyrrolate.
Ketoconazole: May decrease the absorption of ketoconazole.
Potassium chloride: May increase the severity of GI lesions with potassium chloride.
Herbal
None known.
Food
None known.

DIAGNOSTIC TEST EFFECTS
May decrease serum uric acid levels.

IV INCOMPATIBILITIES
None known.

IV COMPATIBILITIES
Diphenhydramine (Benadryl), droperidol (Inapsine), hydromorphone (Dilaudid), hydroxyzine (Vistaril), lidocaine, midazolam (Versed), morphine, promethazine (Phenergan)

SIDE EFFECTS
Frequent
Dry mouth, decreased sweating, constipation
Occasional
Blurred vision, bloated feeling, urinary hesitancy, drowsiness with high dosage, headache, intolerance to light, loss of taste, nervousness, flushing, insomnia, impotence, mental confusion or excitement, particularly in children
Parenteral form: temporary lightheadedness, local irritation
Rare
Dizziness, faintness

SERIOUS REACTIONS
! Overdosage may produce temporary paralysis of ciliary muscle, pupillary dilation, tachycardia, palpitation, hot, dry, or flushed skin, absence of bowel sounds, hyperthermia, increased respiratory rate, EKG abnormalities, nausea, vomiting, a rash over the face or upper trunk, CNS stimulation, and psychosis, marked by agitation, restlessness, rambling speech, visual hallucination, paranoid behavior, and delusions, followed by depression.

PEDIATRIC CONSIDERATIONS
Baseline Assessment
- Instruct the patient to void before giving the medication to reduce the risk of urinary retention.
- Perform a careful health history that screens for the presence of myasthenia gravis, narrow-angle glaucoma, obstructive uropathy, tachyarrhythmias, and ulcerative colitis.
- Be aware that infants or children with spastic paralysis, brain injury, and Down syndrome are at

increased risk to the side effects of this medication.

Precautions

• Use cautiously in pts with CHF, diarrhea, fever, GI infections, hyperthyroidism, liver or renal disease, and reflux esophagitis.

Intervention and Evaluation

• Assess the patient's pattern of daily bowel activity and stool consistency.
• Palpate the patient's bladder for signs of urine retention, and monitor his or her urine output.
• Monitor the patient's blood pressure, body temperature, and heart rate.
• Assess the patient's bowel sounds for peristalsis and mucous membranes and skin turgor to evaluate hydration status.
• Encourage adequate fluid intake.
• Be alert for fever because of an increased risk of hyperthermia.

Patient/Family Teaching

• Inform the patient/family that glycopyrrolate use may cause dry mouth.
• Instruct the patient/family to take glycopyrrolate 30 min before meals. Explain that food decreases the absorption of glycopyrrolate.
• Instruct the patient/family not to become overheated during exercise in hot weather as this may result in heat stroke.
• Urge the patient/family to avoid hot baths and saunas.
• Warn the patient/family to avoid tasks that require mental alertness or motor skills until the patient's response to the drug is established.
• Instruct the patient/family not to take antacids or antidiarrheals within 1 hr of taking this medication as these drugs decrease effectiveness of glycopyrrolate.

Hyoscyamine

high-oh-**sigh**-ah-meen
(Anaspaz, Buscopan [CAN], Cystospaz, Levsin, Levsinex, NuLev)
Do not confuse with Anaprox.

CATEGORY AND SCHEDULE

Pregnancy Risk Category: C

MECHANISM OF ACTION

A GI antispasmodic and anticholinergic agent that inhibits the action of acetylcholine at postganglionic (muscarinic) receptor sites. ***Therapeutic Effect:*** Decreases secretions (bronchial, salivary, sweat glands, gastric juices) and reduces motility of the GI and urinary tracts.

AVAILABILITY

Tablets: 0.125 mg, 0.15 mg.
Tablets (sublingual): 0.125 mg.
Tablets (extended release): 0.375 mg.
Tablets (oral disintegrating): 0.125 mg.
Capsules (time release): 0.375 mg.
Drops and Oral Solution: 0.125 mg/ml
Elixir: 0.125 mg/5 ml.
Injection: 0.5 mg/ml.

INDICATIONS AND DOSAGES

▸ **GI tract disorders**

IM/SC
Children older than 12 yrs. 0.25–0.5 mg q4h for 1–4 doses.
PO/SUBLINGUAL
Children older than 12 yrs. 0.125–0.25 mg q4h. Maximum: 1.5 or 0.375–0.75 mg q12h, time-release capsule.
Children 2–12 yrs. 0.0625–0.125 mg q4h as needed. Maximum: 0.75 mg/day.

Children younger than 2 yrs. Drops: dose q4h, using drop formulation.

CONTRAINDICATIONS

Hypersensitivity to hyoscyamine or any related component. GI or GU obstruction, myasthenia gravis, narrow-angle glaucoma, paralytic ileus, severe ulcerative colitis.

INTERACTIONS

Drug

Antacids, antidiarrheals: May decrease the absorption of hyoscyamine.
Anticholinergics: May increase the effects of hyoscyamine.
Ketoconazole: May decrease the absorption of this drug.
Potassium chloride: May increase the severity of GI lesions with this drug.

Herbal

None known.

Food

None known.

DIAGNOSTIC TEST EFFECTS

None known.

SIDE EFFECTS

Frequent
Dry mouth (sometimes severe), decreased sweating, constipation
Occasional
Blurred vision, bloated feeling, urinary hesitancy, drowsiness with high dosage, headache, intolerance to light, loss of taste, nervousness, flushing, insomnia, impotence, mental confusion or excitement, particularly in children
Parenteral form: temporary lightheadedness, local irritation
Rare
Dizziness, faintness

SERIOUS REACTIONS

! Overdosage may produce temporary paralysis of ciliary muscle, pupillary dilation, tachycardia, palpitations, hot, dry, or flushed skin, absence of bowel sounds, hyperthermia, increased respiratory rate, EKG abnormalities, nausea, vomiting, a rash over the face or upper trunk, CNS stimulation, and psychosis, marked by agitation, restlessness, rambling speech, visual hallucinations, paranoid behavior, and delusions, followed by depression.

PEDIATRIC CONSIDERATIONS

Baseline Assessment

- Instruct the patient to void before giving the medication to reduce the risk of urine retention.
- Use caution in children with spastic paralysis.
- Monitor the patient's pulse, anticholinergic effects, urine output, and GI symptoms.

Precautions

- Use cautiously in pts with cardiac arrhythmias, chronic lung disease, CHF, hyperthyroidism, and neuropathy.

Administration and Handling

PO

- Give hyoscyamine without regard to meals.
- Crush or chew tablets.
- Extended-release capsule should be swallowed whole.

PARENTERAL

- May give undiluted.

Intervention and Evaluation

- Assess the patient's pattern of daily bowel activity and stool consistency.
- Palpate the patient's bladder for signs of urine retention, and monitor his or her urine output.

- Monitor changes in the patient's blood pressure and body temperature.
- Be alert for fever because of an increased risk of hyperthermia.
- Assess the patient's bowel sounds for peristalsis and mucous membranes and skin turgor to evaluate hydration status.
- Encourage adequate fluid intake.

Patient/Family Teaching

- Advise the patient/family that hyoscyamine may cause dry mouth. Urge the patient to maintain good oral hygiene habits as the lack of saliva may increase risk of cavities.
- Warn the patient/family to notify the physician if the patient experiences constipation, difficulty urinating, eye pain, or rash.
- Urge the patient/family to avoid hot baths and saunas.
- Caution the patient/family to avoid tasks that require mental alertness or motor skills until the patient's response to the drug is established.

Scopolamine

See antiemetics

REFERENCES

Miller, S. & Fioravanti, J. (1997). Pediatric medications: a handbook for nurses. St. Louis: Mosby.

Taketomo, C. K., Hodding, J. H. & Kraus, D. M. (2003–2004). Pediatric dosage handbook (10th ed.). Hudson, OH: Lexi-Comp.

48 Antidiarrheals

Bismuth Subsalicylate
Diphenoxylate Hydrochloride with Atropine Sulfate
Loperamide Hydrochloride
Nitazoxanide

Uses: Antidiarrheals are used to treat acute diarrhea and chronic diarrhea of inflammatory bowel disease. The goal of antidiarrheal therapy is to determine and treat the underlying cause of diarrhea, replenish fluids and electrolytes, relieve GI cramping, and reduce the passage of unformed stools. Some antidiarrheals are also used to reduce fluid from ileostomies.

Action: Systemic and local antidiarrheals act in different ways. *Systemic agents,* such as diphenoxylate, act at receptors in enteric smooth muscles, disrupting peristaltic movements, decreasing GI motility, and decreasing the transit time of intestinal contents. *Local agents,* such as bismuth subsalicylate, adsorb toxic substances and fluids to large surface areas of particles in the preparation. Some of these agents coat and protect irritated intestinal walls. They may also have local anti-inflammatory action. Nitazoxanide interferes with an enzyme-dependent reaction that is essential for anaerobic metabolism in *Cryptosporidium parvum* and *Giardia lamblia,* two organisms responsible for diarrhea.

COMBINATION PRODUCTS

HELIDAC: bismuth/metronidazole (an anti-infective)/tetracycline (an anti-infective) 262 mg/250 mg/500 mg.
IMODIUM ADVANCED: loperamide/simethicone (an antiflatulent) 2 mg/125 mg.
LOMOTIL: diphenoxylate/atropine (an anticholinergic and antispasmodic) 2.5 mg/0.025 mg.

Bismuth Subsalicylate

bis-muth sub-sal-**ih**-sah-late
(Bismed [CAN], Pepto-Bismol, Kaopectate)

CATEGORY AND SCHEDULE

Pregnancy Risk Category: C
OTC

MECHANISM OF ACTION

An antinauseant and antiulcer agent that absorbs water and toxins in the large intestine and forms a protective coat in the intestinal mucosa. Also possesses antisecretory and antimicrobial effects. ***Therapeutic Effect:*** Prevents diarrhea. Helps treat *Helicobacter pylori*–associated peptic ulcer disease.

AVAILABILITY

Tablets: 262 mg.
Tablets (chewable): 262 mg, 300 mg.
Suspension: 87 mg/5 mL, 130 mg/5 mL, 262 mg/5 mL, 525 mg/5 mL.

INDICATIONS AND DOSAGES

▸ **Diarrhea, gastric distress**

PO

Children 9–12 yrs. 1 tablet or 15 mL (262 mg/15 mL concentration) q30–60min up to 8 doses/24 hrs.
Children 6–8 yrs. Two-thirds of a tablet or 10 mL (262 mg/15 mL concentration) q30–60min up to 8 doses/24 hrs.
Children 3–5 yrs. One-third of a tablet or 5 mL (262 mg/15 mL concentration) q30–60min up to 8 doses/24 hrs.

▸ **Chronic infantile diarrhea: Bismuth subsalicylate**

PO

Infants 48–70 mos. 10 mL (262 mg/15 mL concentration) q4h.
Infants 24–48 mos. 5 mL (262 mg/15 mL concentration) q4h.
Infants 2–24 mos. 2.5 mL (262 mg/15 mL concentration) q4h.

UNLABELED USES

Prevents traveler's diarrhea.

CONTRAINDICATIONS

Hypersensitivity to bismuth, salicylates, or any related component. Pts with chicken pox or influenza. Bleeding ulcers, gout, hemophilia, hemorrhagic states, renal function impairment.

INTERACTIONS

Drug

Anticoagulants, heparin, thrombolytics: May increase the risk of bleeding.
Insulin, oral hypoglycemics: Large doses may increase the effects of insulin and oral hypoglycemics.
Other salicylates: May increase the risk of toxicity.
Tetracyclines: May decrease the absorption of tetracyclines.

Herbal

Willow bark: May increase the risk of toxicity.

Food

None known.

DIAGNOSTIC TEST EFFECTS

May alter serum alkaline phosphatase, SGOT (AST), SGPT (ALT), and uric acid levels. May decrease serum potassium levels. May prolong prothrombin time.

SIDE EFFECTS

Frequent
Grayish black stools
Rare
Constipation

SERIOUS REACTIONS

! Debilitated pts and infants may develop impaction.

PEDIATRIC CONSIDERATIONS

Baseline Assessment

- Before administration, assess the patient's abdomen for signs of tenderness, rigidity, and the presence of bowel sounds.
- Determine when the patient last had a bowel movement, and find out the amount and consistency.
- Be cautious in children who have viral illness, especially chicken pox or influenza.
- Be aware of the salicylate amount when using this medication in children.

Precautions

- Use cautiously in diabetic pts.

Intervention and Evaluation

- Encourage the patient to maintain adequate fluid intake.
- Assess the patient's bowel sounds for peristaltic activity.
- Assess the patient's pattern of daily bowel activity and stool consistency.

Patient/Family Teaching

• Explain to the patient/family that the patient's stool may appear black or gray.
• Instruct the patient/family to chew tablets thoroughly before swallowing.
• Warn the patient/family to avoid this drug if the patient is taking aspirin or other salicylates because of an increased risk for toxicity.
• Instruct the patient/family to ask the physician about taking bismuth if the patient is taking anticoagulants, because this drug combination can dangerously prolong the bleeding time.

Diphenoxylate Hydrochloride with Atropine Sulfate

dye-pen-**ox**-e-late
(Lofenoxal [AUS], Lomotil, Lonox)
Do not confuse with Lamictal, Lanoxin, Loprox, or Lovenox.

CATEGORY AND SCHEDULE

Pregnancy Risk Category: C

MECHANISM OF ACTION

A meperidine derivative that acts locally and centrally to reduce intestinal motility.

PHARMACOKINETICS

Well absorbed from the GI tract. Metabolized in liver to the active metabolite. Primarily eliminated in feces. ***Half-Life:*** 2.5 hrs; metabolite: 12–24 hrs.

AVAILABILITY

Tablets: 2.5 mg diphenoxylate and 0.025 mg atropine sulfate.
Liquid: 2.5 mg diphenoxylate and 0.025 mg atropine sulfate per 5 mL.

INDICATIONS AND DOSAGES

▸ Antidiarrheal

PO
Children 9–12 yrs. 2 mg 5 times/day.
Children 6–8 yrs. 2 mg 4 times/day.
Children 2–5 yrs. 2 mg 3 times/day.

CONTRAINDICATIONS

Hypersensitivity to diphenoxylate, atropine, or any related component. Children younger than 2 yrs of age, dehydration, jaundice, narrow-angle glaucoma, severe liver disease.

INTERACTIONS

Drug

Alcohol, CNS depressants: May increase the effects of diphenoxylate hydrochloride with atropine sulfate.
Anticholinergics: May increase the effects of atropine.
MAOIs: May precipitate hypertensive crisis.

Herbal

St. John's wort: May increase the effects of diphenoxylate/atropine.

Food

None known.

DIAGNOSTIC TEST EFFECTS

May increase serum amylase levels.

SIDE EFFECTS

Frequent

Drowsiness, lightheadedness, dizziness, nausea

Occasional

Headache, dry mouth

Rare

Flushing, tachycardia, urinary retention, constipation,

paradoxical reaction, marked by restlessness and agitation, blurred vision

SERIOUS REACTIONS

! Dehydration may predispose to toxicity.
! Paralytic ileus, toxic megacolon, marked by constipation, decreased appetite, and stomach pain with nausea or vomiting occur rarely.
! A severe anticholinergic reaction, manifested by severe lethargy, hypotonic reflexes, and hyperthermia, may result in severe respiratory depression and coma.

PEDIATRIC CONSIDERATIONS

Baseline Assessment

• Check the patient's baseline hydration status. Assess the mucous membranes, skin turgor, and urinary output.
• Perform a baseline abdominal assessment, checking for abdominal tenderness, distension, and guarding, as well as the presence and activity of bowel sounds.
• Be aware that it is unknown whether the drug crosses the placenta or is distributed in breast milk.
• Be aware that this drug is not recommended for use in children because of increased susceptibility to toxicity that can cause respiratory depression.
• Do not use this medication in children younger than 2 yrs of age.
• Only the liquid component is recommended for use in children younger than 13 yrs of age.
• Use extreme caution in children who have acute colitis or infectious diarrhea.
• Do not exceed recommended doses in children; reduce dose as soon as symptoms are controlled.
• If no improvement is seen within 48 hrs of initiation of treatment, this drug is not likely to be effective.

Precautions

• Use cautiously in pts with acute ulcerative colitis, cirrhosis, liver or renal disease, and renal impairment.

Administration and Handling

PO

• Give without regard to meals. If GI irritation occurs, give with food or meals.
• Administer the liquid form to children 2 to 12 yrs of age using a graduated dropper for accurate measurement.

Intervention and Evaluation

• Encourage the patient to maintain adequate fluid intake.
• Assess the patient's bowel sounds for peristalsis.
• Assess the patient's pattern of daily bowel activity and stool consistency, and record time of evacuation.
• Evaluate the patient for abdominal disturbances.
• Discontinue the medication if the patient experiences abdominal distention.

Patient/Family Teaching

• Warn the patient/family to avoid tasks that require mental alertness or motor skills until the patient's response to the drug is established.
• Urge the patient/family to avoid alcohol and barbiturates during drug therapy.
• Tell the patient/family to notify the physician if the patient experiences abdominal distention, fever, palpitations, or persistent diarrhea.

Loperamide Hydrochloride

low-**pear**-ah-myd
(Apo-Loperamide [CAN], Gastro-Stop [AUS], Imodium A-D, Loperacap [CAN], Novo-Loperamide [CAN])
Do not confuse with Ionamin.

CATEGORY AND SCHEDULE

Pregnancy Risk Category: B
OTC tablets, liquid

MECHANISM OF ACTION

An antidiarrheal that directly affects the intestinal wall muscles. ***Therapeutic Effect:*** Slows intestinal motility, prolongs transit time of intestinal contents by reducing fecal volume, diminishing loss of fluid and electrolytes, and increasing viscosity and bulk of stool.

PHARMACOKINETICS

Poorly absorbed from the GI tract. Protein binding: 97%. Metabolized in liver. Eliminated in feces and excreted in urine. Not removed by hemodialysis. ***Half-Life:*** 9.1–14.4 hrs.

AVAILABILITY

Tablets: 2 mg (OTC).
Tablets (chewable): 2 mg (OTC).
Capsules: 2 mg.
Liquid: 1 mg/5 mL (OTC).

INDICATIONS AND DOSAGES

▸ Acute diarrhea

PO

Children 9–12 yrs weighing more than 30 kg. Initially, 2 mg 3 times/day for 24 hrs.
Children 6–8 yrs weighing 20–30 kg. Initially, 2 mg 2 times/day for 24 hrs.
Children 2–5 yrs weighing 13–20 kg. Initially, 1 mg 3 times/day for 24 hrs. Maintenance: 1 mg/10 kg only after loose stool.

▸ Chronic diarrhea

PO

Children. 0.08–0.24 mg/kg/day in 2–3 divided doses. Maximum: 2 mg/dose.

▸ Traveler's diarrhea

PO

Children 9–11 yrs. Initially, 2 mg, then 1 mg after each loose bowel movement. Maximum: 6 mg/day for 2 days.
Children 6–8 yrs. Initially, 1 mg, then 1 mg after each loose bowel movement. Maximum: 4 mg/day for 2 days.

CONTRAINDICATIONS

Hypersensitivity to loperamide or any related component. Acute ulcerative colitis (may produce toxic megacolon), diarrhea associated with pseudomembranous enterocolitis resulting from broad-spectrum antibiotics or with organisms that invade intestinal mucosa, such as *Escherichia coli*, shigella, and salmonella, pts who must avoid constipation, bloody diarrhea.

INTERACTIONS

Drug

Opioid (narcotic) analgesics: May increase the risk of constipation.

Herbal

None known.

Food

None known.

DIAGNOSTIC TEST EFFECTS

None known.

SIDE EFFECTS

Rare

Dry mouth, drowsiness, abdominal discomfort, allergic reaction, such as rash and itching

SERIOUS REACTIONS

! Toxicity results in constipation, GI irritation, including nausea and vomiting, and CNS depression. Activated charcoal is the treatment for toxicity.

PEDIATRIC CONSIDERATIONS

Baseline Assessment

- Do not administer to the patient in the presence of bloody diarrhea or temperature greater than 101°F.
- Ask the patient if he or she has a history of ulcerative colitis.
- Expect to obtain stool specimens for culture and sensitivity and ova and parasites if infectious diarrhea is suspected.
- Be aware that it is unknown whether loperamide crosses the placenta or is distributed in breast milk.
- Be aware that loperamide use is not recommended in children younger than 6 yrs of age; infants younger than 3 mos of age are more susceptible to CNS effects.
- Be aware that children with diarrhea should maintain adequate hydration.

Precautions

- Use cautiously in pts with fluid and electrolyte depletion and liver impairment.

Intervention and Evaluation

- Encourage the patient to maintain adequate fluid intake.
- Assess the patient's bowel sounds for peristalsis.
- Assess the patient's pattern of daily bowel activity and stool consistency.
- Withhold the drug and notify the physician promptly if the patient experiences abdominal distention, pain, or fever.

Patient/Family Teaching

- Caution the patient/family not to exceed the prescribed dose.
- Tell the patient/family that loperamide may cause dry mouth.
- Urge the patient/family to avoid alcohol during loperamide therapy.
- Instruct the patient/family to avoid tasks that require mental alertness or motor skills until the patient's response to the drug is established.
- Warn the patient/family to notify the physician if the patient experiences abdominal distention and pain, diarrhea that does not stop within 3 days, or fever.

Nitazoxanide

nye-tay-**zocks**-ah-nide
(Alinia)

CATEGORY AND SCHEDULE

Pregnancy Risk Category: B

MECHANISM OF ACTION

An antiparasitic that interferes with the body's reaction to pyruvate ferredoxin oxidoreductase, an enzyme essential for anaerobic energy metabolism. ***Therapeutic Effect:*** Produces antiprotozoal activity, reducing or terminating diarrheal episodes.

PHARMACOKINETICS

Rapidly hydrolyzed to an active metabolite. Protein binding: 99%. Excreted in the urine, bile, and feces. ***Half-Life:*** 2–4 hrs.

AVAILABILITY

Powder for Oral Suspension: 100 mg/5 mL (contains sucrose).

INDICATIONS AND DOSAGES

▸ **Diarrhea**

PO

Children 5–11 yrs. 200 mg (10 mL) q12h for 3 days.
Children 1–4 yrs. 100 mg (5 mL) q12h for 3 days.

CONTRAINDICATIONS

A history of sensitivity to nitazoxanide, aspirin, and salicylates

INTERACTIONS

Drug
None known.
Herbal
None known.
Food
None known.

DIAGNOSTIC TEST EFFECTS

May increase serum creatinine and SGPT (ALT) levels.

SIDE EFFECTS

Occasional (8%)
Abdominal pain
Rare (2%–1%)
Diarrhea, vomiting, headache

SERIOUS REACTIONS

! None known.

PEDIATRIC CONSIDERATIONS

Baseline Assessment

- Establish the patient's baseline blood glucose and electrolyte levels, blood pressure, and weight.
- Assess the patient for dehydration.
- Be aware that it is unknown whether nitazoxanide is distributed in breast milk.
- Be aware that the safety and efficacy of nitazoxanide have not been established in children older than 11 yrs of age or younger than 1 yr of age.

Precautions

- Use cautiously in pts with biliary or liver disease, GI disorders, and renal impairment.

Administration and Handling

PO

- Store unreconstituted powder at room temperature.
- Reconstitute oral suspension with 48 mL water to provide a concentration of 100 mg/5 mL.
- Shake vigorously to suspend powder.
- Reconstituted solution is stable for 7 days at room temperature.
- Give with food.

Intervention and Evaluation

- Evaluate the diabetic patient's blood glucose levels.
- Assess the patient's electrolyte levels for abnormalities that may have been caused by diarrhea.
- Weigh the patient each day.
- Encourage the patient to maintain adequate fluid intake.
- Assess the patient's bowel sounds for peristalsis.
- Assess the patient's pattern of daily bowel activity and stool consistency.

Patient/Family Teaching

- Tell older children with diabetes mellitus and their parents that the oral suspension of nitazoxanide contains 1.48 g of sucrose per 5 mL.
- Explain to the patient/family that nitazoxanide therapy should significantly improve the patient's symptoms.
- Instruct the patient/family to make sure the drug is taken with food.

REFERENCES

Miller, S. & Fioravanti, J. (1997). Pediatric medications: a handbook for nurses. St. Louis: Mosby.

Taketomo, C. K., Hodding, J. H. & Kraus, D. M. (2003–2004). Pediatric dosage handbook (10th ed.). Hudson, OH: Lexi-Comp.

49 Histamine (H_2) Antagonists

Cimetidine
Famotidine
Ranitidine,
Ranitidine Bismuth Citrate

Uses: Histamine (H_2) antagonists are used for short-term treatment of duodenal ulcer and active benign gastric ulcer and for maintenance therapy of duodenal ulcer. They are also used to treat pathologic hypersecretory conditions, such as Zollinger-Ellison syndrome and gastroesophageal reflux disease (GERD). In addition, these agents are used to prevent upper GI tract bleeding in critically ill pts.

Action: H_2 antagonists inhibit gastric acid secretion by interfering with histamine at H_2–receptors in parietal cells. (See illustration, *Sites of Action: Drugs Used to Treat GERD,* page 601.) They also inhibit acid secretion, which is regulated by the hormone gastrin, whether the secretion is basal (fasting), nocturnal, or stimulated by food or fundic distention. H_2 antagonists decrease the volume and H_2 concentration of gastric juices.

COMBINATION PRODUCTS

PEPCID COMPLETE: famotidine/ calcium chloride (an antacid)/ magnesium hydroxide (an antacid) 10 mg/800 mg/165 mg.

Cimetidine

sih-**met**-ih-deen
(Apo-Cimetidine [CAN], Cimehexal [AUS], Magicul [AUS], Novo-Cimetine [CAN], Peptol [CAN], Sigmetadine [AUS], Tagamet, Tagamet HB)
Do not confuse with simethicone.
(See Color Plate)

CATEGORY AND SCHEDULE

Pregnancy Risk Category: B
OTC Tablets: 100 mg

MECHANISM OF ACTION

An antiulcer and gastric acid secretion inhibitor that inhibits histamine action at H_2–receptor sites of parietal cells. ***Therapeutic Effect:*** Inhibits gastric acid secretion during fasting, at night, or when stimulated by food, caffeine, or insulin.

PHARMACOKINETICS

Well absorbed from the GI tract. Protein binding: 15%–20%. Widely distributed. Metabolized in liver. Primarily excreted in urine. Not removed by hemodialysis. ***Half-Life:*** Neonates 3–4 hrs; children: 1.5 hrs; adults 2 hrs. Half-life is increased with impaired renal function.

AVAILABILITY

Tablets: 200 mg (OTC), 300 mg, 400 mg, 800 mg.
Oral Liquid: 300 mg/ 5 mL.
Injection: 150 mg/mL.

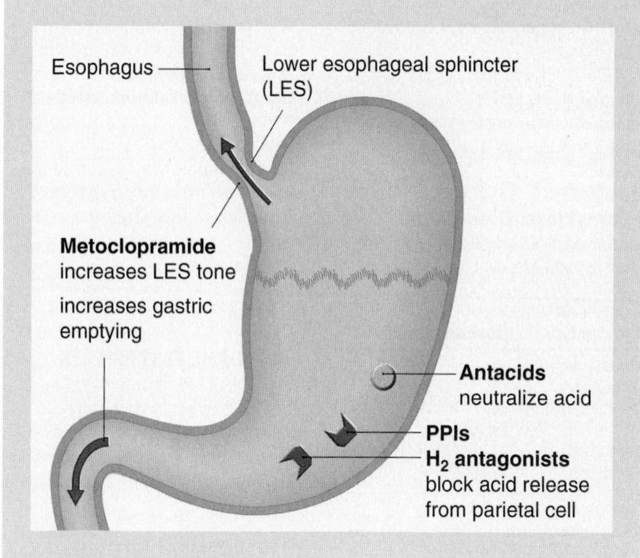

Sites of Action: Drugs Used to Treat GERD

Gastroesophageal reflux disease (GERD) occurs when acidic stomach contents regurgitate into the esophagus, causing heartburn. The disorder may result from weakness or incompetence of the lower esophageal sphincter (LES). Because the malfunctioning LES makes the reflux leave the esophagus and reenter the stomach slowly, the esophageal mucosa is exposed to the acid for a long time. The enzymatic action of parietal cells in the stomach makes the reflux highly acidic thus, GERD causes irritation and possible erosion of the esophageal mucosa.

Treatment of GERD can include drugs from several classes: histamine (H_2) antagonists, proton pump inhibitors (PPIs), the miscellaneous GI agent metoclopramide, and antacids. H_2 antagonists, such as cimetidine, act in the parietal cells of the stomach. Normally, H_2-receptor stimulation results in gastric acid secretion. By blocking these receptors, H_2 antagonists decrease the amount and acidity of gastric secretion, including secretion that occurs with fasting, food consumption at night, and stomach distension.

PPIs, such as esomeprazole, also suppress gastric acid secretion. However, they do it by inhibiting the hydrogen-potassium adenosine triphosphatase (H^+/K^+–ATPase) enzyme system, which is located on the surface of parietal cells and controls their gastric acid secretion. PPIs block acid secretion that results from fasting or stomach distension caused by food ingestion.

Metoclopramide increases the tone and motility of the upper GI tract. It works by stimulating the release of acetylcholine from GI nerve endings, which improves LES tone and leads to decreased reflux. The drug also stimulates gastric emptying, which reduces gastric contents.

Antacids, such as aluminum hydroxide, act primarily in the stomach by chemically combining with the hydrogen ions (H^+) in gastric acid and raising the pH of gastric contents. They do not prevent reflux. However, they make the reflux less acidic, so it causes less damage to the esophageal mucosa.

INDICATIONS AND DOSAGES

▸ Gastric hypersecretory conditions

IM/IV/PO

Children. 20–40 mg/kg/day in divided doses q6h.

Infants. 10–20 mg/kg/day in divided doses q6–12h.

Neonates. 5–10 mg/kg/day in divided doses q8–12h.

▸ Dosage in renal impairment

Based on 5–10 mg/kg/dose in children or 300 mg dose in adults.

Creatinine Clearance	Dosage Interval
Greater than 40 mL/min	q6h
20–40 mL/min	q8h or decrease dose by 25%
Less than 20 mL/min	q12h or decrease dose by 50%

Give after hemodialysis and q12h between dialysis period.

UNLABELED USES

Prophylaxis of aspiration pneumonia, treatment of acute urticaria, chronic warts, upper GI tract bleeding.

CONTRAINDICATIONS

Hypersensitivity to cimetidine or any related component.

INTERACTIONS

Drug

Antacids: May decrease the absorption of cimetidine, so do not give within 30 min–1 hr.

Calcium channel blockers, cyclosporine, lidocaine, metoprolol, metronidazole, oral anticoagulants, oral hypoglycemics, phenytoin, propranolol, theophylline, tricyclic antidepressants: May decrease the metabolism and increase the blood concentrations of calcium channel blockers, cyclosporine, lidocaine, metoprolol, metronidazole, oral anticoagulants, oral hypoglycemics, phenytoin, propranolol, theophylline, and tricyclic antidepressants.

Ketoconazole: May decrease the absorption of ketoconazole, so give at least 2 hrs after.

Herbal

None known.

Food

None known.

DIAGNOSTIC TEST EFFECTS

Interferes with skin tests using allergen extracts. May increase prolactin, serum creatinine, and transaminase levels. May decrease parathyroid hormone concentration.

IV INCOMPATIBILITIES

Allopurinol (Aloprim), amphotericin B complex (AmBisome, Amphotec, Abelcet), cefepime (Maxipime)

IV COMPATIBILITIES

Aminophylline, diltiazem (Cardizem), furosemide (Lasix), heparin, hydromorphone (Dilaudid), insulin (regular), lidocaine, lorazepam (Ativan), midazolam (Versed), morphine, potassium chloride, propofol (Diprivan)

SIDE EFFECTS

Occasional (4%–2%)

Headache

Severely ill and impaired renal function: Confusion, agitation, psychosis, depression, anxiety, disorientation, hallucinations (effects reverse 3–4 days after discontinuance).

Rare (less than 2%)
Diarrhea, dizziness, drowsiness, headache, nausea, vomiting, gynecomastia, rash, impotence

SERIOUS REACTIONS

! Rapid IV infusion may produce cardiac arrhythmias and hypotension.

PEDIATRIC CONSIDERATIONS

Baseline Assessment

• Do not administer antacids concurrently. Separate administration of drugs by 1 hr.
• Be aware that cimetidine crosses the placenta and is distributed in breast milk.
• Be aware that, in infants, cimetidine use may suppress gastric acidity, inhibit drug metabolism, and produce CNS stimulation.
• Be aware that, in children, long-term use may induce cerebral toxicity and affect the hormonal system.

Precautions

• Use cautiously in pts with impaired liver and renal function.

Administration and Handling

PO
• Give cimetidine without regard to meals, but keep in mind that it is best given after meals and at bedtime.
• Do not administer within 1 hr of antacids.
IM
• Administer undiluted.
• Inject deep into a large muscle mass, such as the gluteus maximus muscle.
IV
• Store at room temperature.
• Reconstituted IV preparation is stable for 48 hrs at room temperature.
• Dilute each 300 mg (2 mL) with 18 mL 0.9% NaCl, 0.45% NaCl, 0.2% NaCl, D_5W, $D_{10}W$, Ringer's solution, or lactated Ringer's solution to a total volume of 20 mL.
• For IV push, administer over not less than 2 min to prevent arrhythmias and hypotension.
• For intermittent IV (piggyback) administration, infuse over 15–20 min.
• For IV infusion, dilute with 100–1,000 mL 0.9% NaCl, D_5W, or other compatible solution, and infuse over 24 hrs.

Intervention and Evaluation

• Monitor the patient's blood pressure for hypotension during IV infusion.
• Assess the patient for GI bleeding manifested as blood in the stool and hematemesis.
• Check mental status of severely ill pts and pts with impaired renal function.

Patient/Family Teaching

• Warn the patient/family that IM administration may produce transient discomfort at the injection site.
• Instruct the patient/family not to take antacids within 1 hr of PO cimetidine administration.
• Warn the patient/family to avoid tasks that require mental alertness or motor skills until the patient's response to the drug is established.
• Urge the patient/family to avoid smoking.
• Caution the patient/family to notify the physician if the patient experiences any blood in emesis or stool or dark, tarry stool.

Famotidine

fah-mow-**tih**-deen
(Mylanta AR, Novo-Famotidine [CAN], Pepcid, Pepcid AC, Pepcidine [AUS], Pepcid RPD, Ulcidine [CAN])
(See Color Plate)

CATEGORY AND SCHEDULE

Pregnancy Risk Category: B
OTC (Tablets, 10 mg)

MECHANISM OF ACTION

An antiulcer and gastric acid secretion inhibitor that inhibits histamine action at H_2-receptors of parietal cells. ***Therapeutic Effect:*** Inhibits gastric acid secretion when fasting, at night, or when stimulated by food, caffeine, or insulin.

PHARMACOKINETICS

Route	Onset	Peak	Duration
PO	1 hr	1–4 hrs	10–12 hrs
IV	1 hr	0.5–3 hrs	10–12 hrs

Rapidly, incompletely absorbed from the GI tract. Protein binding: 15%–20%. Partially metabolized in liver. Primarily excreted in urine. Not removed by hemodialysis. ***Half-Life:*** 3.3–2.5 hrs (children).

AVAILABILITY

Tablets: 10 mg (OTC), 20 mg, 40 mg.
Tablet (chewable): 10 mg.
Tablets (oral disintegrating): 20 mg, 40 mg.
Gelcaps: 10 mg (OTC).
Powder for Oral Suspension: 40 mg/5 mL.
Injection: 10 mg/mL, 20 mg/50 mL NaCl infusion.

INDICATIONS AND DOSAGES

▸ **Acute therapy—duodenal ulcer**

PO

Children 1–16 yrs. 0.5 mg/kg/day at bedtime or divided twice daily. Maximum: 40 mg.

▸ **GERD**

PO

Children 1–16 yrs. 1 mg/kg/day in 2 divided doses. Maximum: 80 mg/day.
Infants 3–12 mos. 0.5 mg/kg/dose twice daily.
Neonates and infants younger than 3 mos. 0.5 mg/kg/dose once daily.

▸ **Usual parenteral dosage**

IV

Children. 0.25 mg/kg q12h. Maximum: 40 mg/day.

▸ **Dosage in renal impairment**

Creatinine Clearance	Dosing Frequency
10–50 mL/min	q24h
Less than 10 mL/min	q36–48h

UNLABELED USES

Autism, prophylaxis for aspiration pneumonitis.

CONTRAINDICATIONS

Hypersensitivity to famotidine or any related component.

INTERACTIONS

Drug

Antacids: May decrease the absorption of famotidine; do not give within 30 min–1 hr.
Ketoconazole, triamterene, delavirdine, itraconazole, cefpodoxime, indomethacin: May decrease the absorption of these drugs, give at least 2 hrs after.

Herbal

None known.

Food

None known.

DIAGNOSTIC TEST EFFECTS

Interferes with skin tests using allergen extracts. May increase liver enzyme levels.

IV INCOMPATIBILITIES

Amphotericin B complex (Abelcet, Amphotec, AmBisome), cefepime (Maxipime), furosemide (Lasix), piperacillin/tazobactam (Zosyn)

IV COMPATIBILITIES

Calcium gluconate, dobutamine (Dobutrex), dopamine (Intropin), heparin, hydromorphone (Dilaudid), insulin (regular), lidocaine, lorazepam (Ativan), magnesium sulfate, midazolam (Versed), morphine, nitroglycerin, norepinephrine (Levophed), potassium chloride, potassium phosphate, propofol (Diprivan)

SIDE EFFECTS

Occasional (5%)
Headache
Rare (2% or less)
Constipation, diarrhea, dizziness

SERIOUS REACTIONS

None known.

PEDIATRIC CONSIDERATIONS

Baseline Assessment

• Do not administer antacids concurrently. Separate administration of drugs by 30 min–1 hr.
• Be aware that it is unknown whether famotidine crosses the placenta or is distributed in breast milk.
• There are no age-related precautions noted in children.

Precautions

• Use cautiously in pts with impaired liver or renal function.

Administration and Handling

PO
• Store tablets and suspension at room temperature.
• After reconstitution, oral suspension is stable for 30 days at room temperature.
• Give famotidine without regard to meals but keep in mind that it is best given before meals or at bedtime.
• Shake suspension well before use.
• Pepcid RPD dissolves under the tongue; does not require water for dosing.

IV
• Refrigerate unreconstituted vials.
• IV solution normally appears clear, colorless.
• After dilution, IV solution is stable for 48 hrs at room temperature.
• For IV push, dilute 20 mg with 5–10 mL 0.9% NaCl, D_5W, $D_{10}W$, lactated Ringer's solution, or 5% sodium bicarbonate.
• For intermittent IV piggyback infusion, dilute with 50–100 mL D_5W or 0.9% NaCl.
• IV push should be given over at least 2 min.
• Infuse IV piggyback over 15–30 min.

Intervention and Evaluation

• Monitor the patient's pattern of daily bowel activity and stool consistency.
• Assess the patient for constipation, diarrhea, and headache.

Patient/Family Teaching

• Tell the patient/family that the patient may take famotidine without regard to meals or antacids, but that it is best taken before meals.
• Warn the patient/family to notify the physician if the patient experiences headache.

• Urge the patient/family to avoid consuming excessive amounts of aspirin and coffee.
• Instruct the patient/family to contact the physician if the patient experiences persistent acid indigestion, heartburn, or sour stomach despite the medication.

Ranitidine

rah-**nih**-tih-deen
(Apo-Ranitidine [CAN], Novo-Ranidine [CAN], Zantac, Zantac-75, Zantac EFFERdose)
Do not confuse with Xanax, Ziac, or Zyrtec.

Ranitidine Bismuth Citrate

(Tritec)

CATEGORY AND SCHEDULE

Pregnancy Risk Category: B
OTC (Tablets, 75 mg)

MECHANISM OF ACTION

An antiulcer agent that inhibits histamine action at H_2-receptors of gastric parietal cells. ***Therapeutic Effect:*** Inhibits gastric acid secretion when fasting, at night, or when stimulated by food, caffeine, or insulin. Reduces volume and hydrogen ion concentration of gastric juice.

PHARMACOKINETICS

Rapidly absorbed from the GI tract. Protein binding: 15%. Widely distributed. Metabolized in liver. Primarily excreted in urine. Not removed by hemodialysis. ***Half-Life:*** 1.8–2 hrs (children 3.5–16 yrs).

AVAILABILITY

Tablets: 75 mg (OTC), 150 mg, 300 mg, 400 mg (bismuth citrate).
Tablets (effervescent): 150 mg.
Capsules: 150 mg, 300 mg.
Syrup: 15 mg/mL.
Granules (effervescent): 150 mg.
Injection (vial): 25 mg/mL.
Injection (infusion premix): 0.5 mg/mL, 50 mL infusion.

INDICATIONS AND DOSAGES

▸ **Duodenal, gastric ulcers, GERD**
PO
Children. 2–4 mg/kg/day in divided doses 2 times/day. Maximum: 300 mg/day.
▸ **Erosive esophagitis**
PO
Children. 4–10 mg/kg/day in 2 divided doses. Maximum: 600 mg/day.
▸ **Usual parenteral dosage**
IV
Children. 2–4 mg/kg/day in divided doses q6–8h. Maximum: 200 mg/day.
▸ **Usual neonatal dosage**
IV
Neonates. Initially, 1.5 mg/kg/dose as a loading dose, then 1.5–2 mg/kg/day in divided doses q12h.
PO
Neonates. 2 mg/kg/day in divided doses q12h.
▸ **Dosage in renal impairment**
Creatinine clearance less than 50 mL/min. Reduce dose by 50%.
Creatinine clearance less than 10 mL/min. Reduce dose by 75%.

UNLABELED USES

Prophylaxis of aspiration pneumonia.

CONTRAINDICATIONS

Hypersensitivity to ranitidine or any related component. History of acute porphyria.

INTERACTIONS

Drug

Antacids: May decrease the absorption of ranitidine; do not give within 1 hr.
Ketoconazole, itraconazole: May decrease the absorption of these drugs; therefore give at least 2 hrs after.

Herbal

None known.

Food

None known.

DIAGNOSTIC TEST EFFECTS

Interferes with skin tests using allergen extracts. May increase liver function enzyme, γ-glutamyl transpeptidase, and serum creatinine levels.

IV INCOMPATIBILITIES

Amphotericin B complex (Abelcet, AmBisome, Amphotec)

IV COMPATIBILITIES

Diltiazem (Cardizem), dobutamine (Dobutrex), dopamine (Intropin), heparin, hydromorphone (Dilaudid), insulin, lidocaine, lorazepam (Ativan), morphine, norepinephrine (Levophed), potassium chloride, propofol (Diprivan)

SIDE EFFECTS

Occasional (2%)
Diarrhea
Rare (1%)
Constipation, headache (may be severe)

SERIOUS REACTIONS

! Reversible hepatitis and blood dyscrasias occur rarely.

PEDIATRIC CONSIDERATIONS

Baseline Assessment

- Expect to obtain baseline blood chemistry tests including BUN, serum alkaline phosphatase, bilirubin, creatinine, SGOT (AST), and SGPT (ALT) levels to assess liver and renal function.
- Be aware that it is unknown whether ranitidine crosses the placenta or is distributed in breast milk.
- Never administer ranitidine to children by IV push. This may result in arrhythmias, cardiac arrest, or hypotension.
- There are no age-related precautions noted in children.

Precautions

- Use cautiously in pts with impaired liver and renal function.

Administration and Handling

PO

- Give ranitidine without regard to meals, but it is best given after meals or at bedtime.
- Do not administer within 1 hr of magnesium- or aluminum-containing antacids because they decrease ranitidine absorption by 33%.

IM

- May be given undiluted.
- Give deep IM injection into a large muscle mass, such as the gluteus maximus.

IV

- IV solutions normally appear clear, colorless to yellow; slight darkening does not affect potency.
- IV infusion (piggyback) is stable for 48 hrs at room temperature. Discard if discolored or precipitate forms.
- For IV push, dilute each 50 mg with 20 mL 0.9% NaCl or D_5W.
- For intermittent IV infusion (piggyback), dilute each 50 mg with 50 mL 0.9% NaCl or D_5W.
- For IV infusion, dilute with 250–1,000 mL 0.9% NaCl or D_5W.
- Administer IV push over a minimum of 5 min to prevent arrhythmias and hypotension.

• Infuse IV piggyback over 15–20 min.
• Give IV infusion over 24 hrs.

Intervention and Evaluation

• Monitor the patient's serum alkaline phosphatase, bilirubin, SGOT (AST), and SGPT (ALT) levels.

Patient/Family Teaching

• Tell the patient/family that smoking decreases the effectiveness of ranitidine.
• Instruct the patient/family not to take ranitidine within 1 hr of magnesium- or aluminum-containing antacids.
• Warn the patient/family that transient burning or itching may occur with IV administration.
• Instruct the patient/family to notify the physician if the patient experiences headache during ranitidine therapy.
• Urge the patient/family to avoid alcohol and aspirin during ranitidine therapy.

REFERENCES

Miller, S. & Fioravanti, J. (1997). Pediatric medications: a handbook for nurses. St. Louis: Mosby.
Taketomo, C. K., Hodding, J. H. & Kraus, D. M. (2003–2004). Pediatric dosage handbook (10th ed.). Hudson, OH: Lexi-Comp.

50 Laxatives

Bisacodyl
Cascara Sagrada
Docusate, Docusate Sodium
Lactulose
Magnesium, Magnesium Chloride, Magnesium Citrate, Magnesium Hydroxide, Magnesium Oxide, Magnesium Protein Complex, Magnesium Sulfate
Methylcellulose
Polycarbophil
Polyethylene Glycol-Electrolyte Solution (PEG-ES)
Psyllium
Senna

Uses: Laxatives are used for short-term treatment of constipation and for colon evacuation before rectal or bowel examinations. They are also used to prevent straining, such as after anorectal surgery or myocardial infarction; to prevent fecal impaction; and to reduce painful elimination, such as in pts with a recent episiotomy, hemorrhoids, or anorectal lesions. In addition, these agents are helpful in modifying ileostomy effluent and in removing ingested poisons.

Action: Laxatives ease or stimulate defecation by three basic mechanisms: they attract and retain fluid in the colonic contents through their hydrophilic or osmotic properties; they act directly or indirectly on the mucosa to decrease water and sodium absorption; or they increase intestinal motility and decrease water and sodium absorption. (See illustration, *Mechanisms of Action: Laxatives,* page 611.)

- *Bulk-forming laxatives,* such as psyllium and polycarbophil, act primarily in the small and large intestines. They retain water in the stool and may bind with water and ions in the colonic lumen to soften feces and increase stool bulk. They may also increase colonic bacteria growth, which increases fecal mass. Typically, they produce a soft stool in 1–3 days.
- *Osmotic laxatives,* including lactulose, act in the colon like saline laxatives. Their osmotic action may be enhanced in the distal ileum and colon by bacterial metabolism to lactate and other organic acids. This decreases the pH and increases the osmotic pressure, which in turn increases the stool water content and softens the stool. They produce a soft stool in 1–3 days.
- *Stimulant laxatives,* such as bisacodyl and senna, act in the colon. They enhance water and electrolyte accumulation in the colonic lumen, which enhances intestinal motility, and may also act directly on the intestinal mucosa. Most of them produce a semifluid stool in 6–12 hrs. However, bisacodyl suppositories act in 15–60 min.

- *Surfactant laxatives,* such as docusate, act in the small and large intestines. By their surfactant action, they hydrate and soften stool, helping fat and water penetrate it. They produce a soft stool in 1–3 days.

COMBINATION PRODUCTS

FERRO-SEQUELS: docusate/ferrous fumarate (a hematinic) 100 mg/150 mg.
GELUSIL: magnesium hydroxide/aluminum hydroxide (an antacid)/simethicone (an antiflatulent) 200 mg/200 mg/25 mg.
GENTLAX-S: senna/docusate (a laxative) 8.6 mg/50 mg.
HALEY'S M-O: magnesium/mineral oil (a lubricant laxative) 300 mg/1.25 mL.
PEPCID COMPLETE: magnesium hydroxide/famotidine (a histamine [H_2] antagonist)/calcium chloride (an antacid) 165 mg/10 mg/800 mg.
SENOKOT-S: senna/docusate (a laxative) 8.6 mg/50 mg.

Bisacodyl

bise-ah-**co**-dahl
(Apo-Bisacodyl [CAN], Bisalax [AUS], Dulcolax)

CATEGORY AND SCHEDULE

Pregnancy Risk Category: C
OTC

MECHANISM OF ACTION

A GI stimulant that has a direct effect on colonic smooth musculature by stimulating the intramural nerve plexi. ***Therapeutic Effect:*** Promotes fluid and ion accumulation in colon to increase peristalsis and promote a laxative effect.

PHARMACOKINETICS

Route	Onset	Peak	Duration
PO	6–12 hrs	N/A	N/A
Rectal	15–60 min	N/A	N/A

Minimal absorption after PO or rectal administration. Metabolized in the liver. Absorbed drug excreted in urine; remainder eliminated in feces. Conjugated drug excreted in breast milk, bile and urine.

AVAILABILITY

Tablets (enteric coated): 5 mg.
Suppository: 10 mg.
Enema: 10 mg/30 mL.

INDICATIONS AND DOSAGES

▸ Laxative

PO

Children 12 yrs and older. 5–15 mg/day as a single dose. Maximum: 30 mg.
Children 3–12 yrs. 5–10 mg or 0.3 mg/kg at bedtime or after breakfast.

RECTAL

Children 12 yrs and older. 10 mg to induce bowel movement.
Children 2–11 yrs. 5–10 mg as a single dose.
Children younger than 2 yrs. 5 mg.

CONTRAINDICATIONS

Hypersensitivity to bisacodyl or any related component. Abdominal pain, appendicitis, intestinal obstruction, nausea, undiagnosed rectal bleeding, vomiting. Should not be used in pregnancy or lactation.

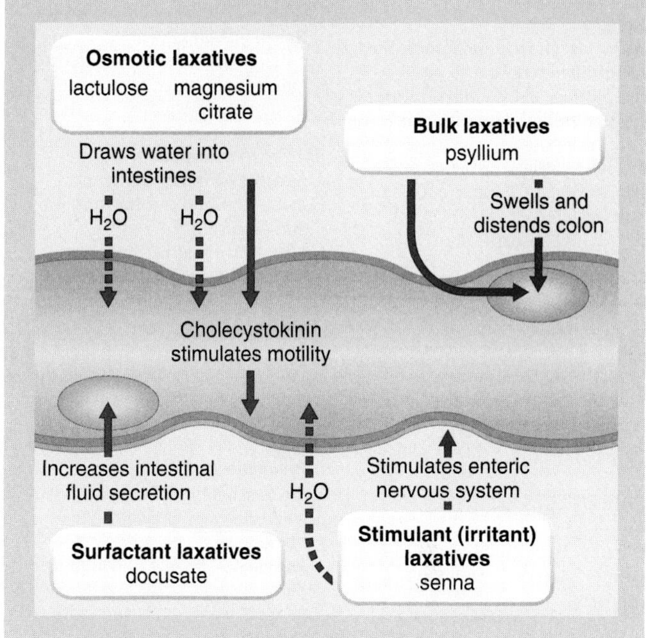

Mechanisms of Action: Laxatives

Laxatives ease or stimulate defecation. Typically, they are classified by their mechanism of action as bulk-forming, osmotic, stimulant, or surfactant laxatives.

Bulk-forming laxatives, such as psyllium, act in the small and large bowel. Because ingredients in these laxatives are undigestible, they remain within the stool and increase the fecal mass by drawing in water. These agents also enhance bacterial growth in the colon, further adding to the fecal mass.

Osmotic laxatives, such as lactulose, draw water into the intestinal lumen, causing the fecal mass to soften and swell. This osmotic action may be enhanced by the metabolism of colonic bacteria to lactate and other organic acids. These acids decrease colonic pH and increase colonic motility.

Stimulant (or irritant) laxatives, such as senna, act on the intestinal wall to increase water and electrolytes in the intestinal lumen. In addition, they directly irritate the colon, increasing motility.

Surfactant laxatives (or fecal softeners), such as docusate, reduce the surface tension of the stool, allowing water to enter it. These laxatives may also help to increase water and electrolyte excretion into the intestinal lumen, softening and increasing the fecal mass.

INTERACTIONS

Drug

Antacids, cimetidine, famotidine, ranitidine: May cause rapid dissolution of bisacodyl, producing abdominal cramping, and vomiting.
PO medications: May decrease transit time of concurrently administered PO medications, decreasing absorption of bisacodyl.

Herbal

None known.

Food

Milk: May cause rapid dissolution of bisacodyl.

DIAGNOSTIC TEST EFFECTS

None known.

SIDE EFFECTS

Frequent

Some degree of abdominal discomfort, nausea, mild cramps, faintness

Occasional

Rectal administration may produce burning of rectal mucosa, mild proctitis

SERIOUS REACTIONS

! Long-term use may result in laxative dependence, chronic constipation, and loss of normal bowel function.
! Chronic use or overdosage may result in electrolyte or metabolic disturbances, such as hypokalemia, hypocalcemia, metabolic acidosis or alkalosis, as well as persistent diarrhea, malabsorption, and weight loss. Electrolyte and metabolic disturbances may produce vomiting and muscle weakness.

PEDIATRIC CONSIDERATIONS

Baseline Assessment

- Before administration, assess the patient's abdomen for signs of tenderness or rigidity and the presence of bowel sounds.
- Try to determine when the patient last had a bowel movement, and find out the amount and consistency.
- Be aware that it is unknown whether bisacodyl crosses the placenta or is distributed in breast milk.
- Avoid bisacodyl use in children younger than 6 yrs of age as this patient population is usually unable to describe symptoms or more severe side effects.

Precautions

- Know that excessive use may lead to fluid and electrolyte imbalance.

Administration and Handling

PO

- Give bisacodyl on an empty stomach for faster action.
- Offer 6–8 glasses of water daily to aid in stool softening.
- Administer tablets whole; do not chew or crush.
- Avoid giving within 1 hr of antacids, milk, or other oral medications.

RECTAL

- If suppository is too soft, chill for 30 min in the refrigerator or run cold water over the foil wrapper.
- Moisten suppository with cold water before inserting well into rectum.

Intervention and Evaluation

- Encourage the patient to maintain adequate fluid intake.
- Assess the patient's bowel sounds for peristalsis.

• Assess the patient's pattern of daily bowel activity and stool consistency and record time of evacuation.
• Assess the patient for abdominal disturbances.
• Monitor serum electrolyte levels in pts exposed to excessive, frequent, or prolonged use of bisacodyl.

Patient/Family Teaching

• Tell the patient/family to institute measures to promote defecation such as increasing the patient's fluid intake, exercising, and eating a high-fiber diet.
• Instruct the patient/family not to take antacids, milk, or other medications within 1 hr of taking bisacodyl as these substances may decrease the effectiveness of bisacodyl.
• Warn the patient/family to notify the physician if the patient experiences unrelieved constipation, dizziness, muscle cramps or pain, rectal bleeding, or weakness.

Cascara Sagrada

cass-**care**-ah sah-**graud**-ah
(Cascara Sagrada)

CATEGORY AND SCHEDULE

Pregnancy Risk Category: C

MECHANISM OF ACTION

A GI stimulant that increases peristalsis by a direct effect on the colonic smooth musculature and by stimulating intramural nerve plexi. ***Therapeutic Effect:*** Promotes fluid and ion accumulation in the colon to promote a laxative effect.

AVAILABILITY

Tablets: 325 mg.
Liquid: (18% alcohol).

INDICATIONS AND DOSAGES

▸ Laxative

PO LIQUID

Children older than 12 yrs. 5 mL/day at bedtime.
Children 2–11 yrs. 2.5 mL/day, 1–3 mL as a single dose.
Infants. 1.25 mL/day, 0.5–2 mL as a single dose.

CONTRAINDICATIONS

Abdominal pain, appendicitis, intestinal obstruction, nausea, vomiting, fecal impaction, GI bleeding, congestive heart failure.

INTERACTIONS

Drug

PO medications: May decrease transit time of concurrently administered oral medication, decreasing the absorption of cascara sagrada.

Herbal

None known.

Food

None known.

DIAGNOSTIC TEST EFFECTS

May increase blood glucose levels. May decrease serum calcium and potassium levels.

SIDE EFFECTS

Frequent

Pink-red, red-violet, red-brown, or yellow-brown discoloration of urine

Occasional

Some degree of abdominal discomfort, nausea, mild cramps, faintness

SERIOUS REACTIONS

! Long-term use may result in laxative dependence, chronic constipation, and loss of normal bowel function.

! Chronic use or overdosage may result in electrolyte disturbances, such as hypokalemia, hypocalcemia, metabolic acidosis or alkalosis, persistent diarrhea, malabsorption, and weight loss. Electrolyte disturbance may produce vomiting and muscle weakness.

PEDIATRIC CONSIDERATIONS

Baseline Assessment

- Before administration, assess the patient's abdomen for signs of tenderness or rigidity and the presence of bowel sounds.
- Try to determine when the patient last had a bowel movement, and find out the amount and consistency.

Intervention and Evaluation

- Encourage the patient to maintain adequate fluid intake.
- Assess the patient's bowel sounds for peristalsis.
- Assess the patient's pattern of daily bowel activity and stool consistency, and record time of evacuation.
- Assess the patient for abdominal disturbances.
- Monitor serum electrolyte levels in pts exposed to excessive, frequent, or prolonged use of cascara sagrada.

Patient/Family Teaching

- Explain to the patient/family that the patient's urine may temporarily turn pink-red, red-violet, red-brown, or yellow-brown.
- Tell the patient/family to institute measures to promote defecation such as increasing the patient's fluid intake, exercising, and eating a high-fiber diet.
- Instruct the patient/family not to take other oral medications within 1 hr of taking cascara sagrada as these substances may decrease the effectiveness of cascara sagrada because of increased peristalsis.
- Warn the patient/family not to use cascara sagrada if the patient experiences abdominal pain, nausea, or vomiting longer than 1 week.
- Tell the patient/family that the liquid form contains alcohol.

Docusate

dock-cue-sate
(Coloxyl [AUS], Pro-Cal-Sof, Surfak)
docusate sodium
(Colace, Diocto, Selax [CAN], SoFlax [CAN], Surfak)

CATEGORY AND SCHEDULE

Pregnancy Risk Category: C
OTC

MECHANISM OF ACTION

A bulk-producing laxative that decreases surface film tension by mixing liquid and bowel docusate contents. ***Therapeutic Effect:*** Increases infiltration of liquid to form a softer stool.

PHARMACOKINETICS

Minimal absorption from the GI tract. Acts in small and large intestines. Results occur 1–2 days after first dose, may take 3–5 days.

AVAILABILITY

Capsules: 50 mg (sodium), 100 mg (sodium), 240 mg (calcium), 250 mg (sodium).
Tablets: 100 mg (sodium).
Syrup: 50 mg/15 mL (sodium), 60 mg/15 mL (sodium).
Liquid: 150 mg/15 mL (sodium).

INDICATIONS AND DOSAGES

▸ Stool softener

PO

Children older than 12 yrs. 50–500 mg/day in 1–4 divided doses.
Children 6–12 yrs. 40–150 mg/day in 1–4 divided doses.
Children 3–5 yrs. 20–60 mg/day in 1–4 divided doses.
Children younger than 3 yrs. 10–40 mg in 1–4 divided doses.

CONTRAINDICATIONS

Hypersensitivity to docusate or any related component. Acute abdominal pain, concomitant use of mineral oil, intestinal obstruction, nausea, vomiting.

INTERACTIONS

Drug

Danthron, mineral oil: May increase the absorption of danthron or mineral oil.
Aspirin: May increase the GI toxicity of aspirin.

Herbal

None known.

Food

None known.

DIAGNOSTIC TEST EFFECTS

None known.

SIDE EFFECTS

Occasional

Mild GI cramping, throat irritation with liquid preparation

Rare

Rash

SERIOUS REACTIONS

! None known.

PEDIATRIC CONSIDERATIONS

Baseline Assessment

• Before administration, assess the patient's abdomen for signs of tenderness or rigidity and the presence of bowel sounds.
• Try to determine when the patient last had a bowel movement, and find out the amount and consistency.
• Be aware that it is unknown whether docusate is distributed in breast milk.
• Be aware that docusate use is not recommended in children younger than 6 yrs of age.

Administration and Handling

• Drink 6–8 glasses of water daily to aid in stool softening.
• Give each dose with a full glass of water or fruit juice.
• Administer docusate liquid with infant formula, fruit juice, or milk to mask the bitter taste.

Intervention and Evaluation

• Encourage the patient to maintain adequate fluid intake.
• Assess the patient's bowel sounds for peristalsis.
• Assess the patient's pattern of daily bowel activity and stool consistency, and record time of evacuation.
• Assess the patient for abdominal disturbances.

Patient/Family Teaching

• Advise the patient/family to institute measures to promote defecation such as increasing the patient's fluid intake, exercising, and eating a high-fiber diet.
• Warn the patient/family to notify the physician if the patient experiences unrelieved constipation, dizziness, muscle cramps or pain, rectal bleeding, and weakness.

Lactulose

lack-tyoo-lows
(Acilac [CAN], Actilax [AUS], Constulose, Duphalac [CAN], Enulose, Generlac, Genlac [AUS], Kristalose, Laxilose [CAN])
Do not confuse with lactose.

CATEGORY AND SCHEDULE
Pregnancy Risk Category: B

MECHANISM OF ACTION
A lactose derivative that retains ammonia in colon and decreases the serum ammonia concentration, producing an osmotic effect. ***Therapeutic Effect:*** Promotes increased peristalsis and bowel evacuation, expelling ammonia from the colon.

PHARMACOKINETICS

Route	Onset	Peak	Duration
PO	24–48 hrs	N/A	N/A
Rectal	30–60 min	N/A	N/A

Poorly absorbed from the GI tract. Acts in colon. Primarily excreted in feces.

AVAILABILITY
Syrup: 10 g/15 mL.
Packets: 10 g, 20 g.

INDICATIONS AND DOSAGES
▸ Constipation
PO
Children. 7.5 mL/day after breakfast.
▸ Portal-systemic encephalopathy
PO
Children. 40–90 mL/day in divided doses 3–4 times daily to produce 2–3 soft stools/day.
Infants. 2.5–10 mL/day in divided doses 3–4 times daily to produce 2–3 soft stools/day.

CONTRAINDICATIONS
Hypersensitivity to lactulose or any related component. Abdominal pain, appendicitis, nausea, vomiting, pts consuming a galactose-free diet.

INTERACTIONS
Drug
PO medication: May decrease transit time of concurrently administered oral medication, decreasing absorption.
Oral antibiotics: May decrease effectiveness of lactulose.
Herbal
None known.
Food
None known.

DIAGNOSTIC TEST EFFECTS
May decrease serum potassium levels.

SIDE EFFECTS
Occasional
Cramping, flatulence, increased thirst, abdominal discomfort
Rare
Nausea, vomiting

SERIOUS REACTIONS
! Diarrhea indicates overdosage.
! Long-term use may result in laxative dependence, chronic constipation, and loss of normal bowel function.

PEDIATRIC CONSIDERATIONS
Baseline Assessment
• Before administration, assess the patient's abdomen for signs of tenderness or rigidity and the presence of bowel sounds.

• Try to determine when the patient last had a bowel movement, and find out the amount and consistency.
• Plan to obtain baseline serum ammonia levels.
• Assess the patient's baseline mental status, and look for signs of high ammonia levels, such as asterixis.
• Be aware that it is unknown whether lactulose crosses the placenta or is distributed in breast milk.
• Be aware that lactulose use should be avoided in children younger than 6 yrs of age because this patient population is usually unable to describe symptoms.

Precautions

• Use cautiously in pts with diabetes mellitus.

Administration and Handling

PO

• Store solution at room temperature.
• Solution normally appears pale yellow to yellow in color and viscous in consistency. Cloudy, darkened solution does not indicate potency loss.
• Drink juice, milk, or water with each dose to aid in stool softening and increase palatability.

RECTAL

• Lubricate anus with petroleum jelly before enema insertion.
• Insert carefully, to prevent damage to the rectal wall, with nozzle toward navel.
• Squeeze container until entire dose is expelled.
• Retain liquid until definite lower abdominal cramping is felt.

Intervention and Evaluation

• Encourage the patient to maintain adequate fluid intake.
• Assess the patient's bowel sounds for peristalsis.
• Assess the patient's pattern of daily bowel activity and stool consistency, and record time of evacuation.
• Assess the patient for abdominal disturbances.
• Monitor serum electrolyte levels in pts exposed to excessive, frequent, or prolonged use of lactulose.
• Obtain periodic serum ammonia levels, looking for a reduction.
• Assess the patient's mental status, and monitor for signs of reduced ammonia levels, such as lessening of asterixis.

Patient/Family Teaching

• Instruct the patient/family to retain the liquid until cramping is felt.
• Tell the patient/family that evacuation occurs in 24–48 hrs of the initial drug dose.
• Instruct the patient/family to institute measures to promote defecation such as increasing the patient's fluid intake, exercising, and eating a high-fiber diet.

Magnesium

mag-**nee**-zee-um

Magnesium Chloride

(Citro-Mag [CAN], Phillips' Magnesia Tablets [CAN], Slow-Mag)

Magnesium Citrate

(Citrate of Magnesia, Citroma)

Magnesium Hydroxide

(MOM)

Magnesium Oxide
(Mag-Ox 400, Maox 420)

Magnesium Protein Complex
(Mg-PLUS)

Magnesium Sulfate
(Epsom salt, magnesium sulfate injection)

Do not confuse with manganese sulfate.

CATEGORY AND SCHEDULE
Pregnancy Risk Category: B

MECHANISM OF ACTION
An antacid, anticonvulsant, electrolyte, and laxative.
Antacid: Acts in stomach to neutralize gastric acid. ***Therapeutic Effect:*** Increases pH.
Laxative: Osmotic effect primarily in small intestine. Draws water into intestinal lumen. ***Therapeutic Effect:*** Produces distention; promotes peristalsis and bowel evacuation.
Systemic dietary supplement or replacement: Found primarily in intracellular fluids. Essential for enzyme activity, nerve conduction, and muscle contraction.
Anticonvulsant: Blocks neuromuscular transmission, amount of acetylcholine released at motor end plate. ***Therapeutic Effect:*** Produces seizure control.

PHARMACOKINETICS
Antacid, laxative: Minimal absorption through intestine. Absorbed dose primarily excreted in urine.
Systemic: Widely distributed. Primarily excreted in urine.

AVAILABILITY
MAGNESIUM CHLORIDE
Tablets (delayed release): 64 mg (Slow-Mag).
MAGNESIUM CITRATE
Solution: 300 mL (290 mg/5 mL).
MAGNESIUM HYDROXIDE
Liquid: 400 mg/5 mL, 800 mg/5 mL.
Chewable Tablets: 311 mg.
MAGNESIUM OXIDE
Tablets: 400 mg (Mag-Ox).
MAGNESIUM SULFATE
Premix Solution: 10 mg/mL, 20 mg/mL, 40 mg/mL, 80 mg/mL.
Injection Solution: 125 mg/mL, 500 mg/mL.

INDICATIONS AND DOSAGES
▸ **Hypomagnesemia (magnesium sulfate)**
IM/IV
Neonates. 25–50 mg/kg/dose q8–12h for 2–3 doses.
Children. 25–50 mg/kg/dose q4–6h for 3–4 doses. Maximum single dose: 2 g.
PO
Children. 10–20 mg/kg (elemental magnesium)/dose 4 times/day.
▸ **Hypertension, seizures (magnesium sulfate)**
IM/IV
Children. 20–100 mg/kg/dose q4–6h as needed.
▸ **Torsades de pointes (magnesium sulfate)**
IV
Children and neonates. 25–50 mg/kg/dose. Maximum: 2 g.
▸ **Laxative (magnesium hydroxide 400 mg/5 mL strength).**
PO
Children older than 12 yrs. 150–300 mL.
Children 6–12 yrs. 100–150 mL.
Children younger than 6 yrs. 2–4 mL/kg in single or divided doses.

▸ **Laxative (magnesium hydroxide)**
PO
Children 12 yrs and older. 30–60 mL/day.
Children 6–11 yrs. 15–30 mL/day.
Children 2–5 yrs. 5–15 mL/day.
Children younger than 2 yrs. 0.5 mL/kg/dose.

▸ **Antacid (magnesium hydroxide)**
PO
Children. 2.5–5 mL/dose (liquid) or 311 mg (tablet) up to 4 times/day.

CONTRAINDICATIONS

General: Hypersensitivity to magnesium salts or any related component. Severe renal impairment.
Antacids: Appendicitis or symptoms of appendicitis, ileostomy, intestinal obstruction, severe renal impairment.
Laxative: Appendicitis, colostomy, CHF, hypersensitivity, ileostomy, intestinal obstruction, undiagnosed rectal bleeding.
Systemic: Heart block, myocardial damage, renal failure.

INTERACTIONS

Drug

Antacids
Ketoconazole, tetracyclines: May decrease the absorption of ketoconazole and tetracyclines.
Methenamine: May decrease the effects of methenamine.
Antacids, laxatives
Digoxin, oral anticoagulants, phenothiazines: May decrease the effects of digoxin, oral anticoagulants, and phenothiazines.
Tetracyclines: May form nonabsorbable complex with tetracyclines.
Systemic
(dietary supplement, replacement)
Calcium: May neutralize the effects of magnesium.
CNS depression-producing medications: May increase CNS depression.
Digoxin: May cause changes in cardiac conduction or heart block with digoxin.

Herbal

None known.

Food

None known.

DIAGNOSTIC TEST EFFECTS

Antacid: May increase gastric pH.
Laxative: May decrease serum potassium level.
Systemic (dietary supplement, replacement): None known.

IV INCOMPATIBILITIES

Amphotericin B complex (Abelcet, AmBisome, Amphotec), cefepime (Maxipime)

IV COMPATIBILITIES

Amikacin (Amikin), cefazolin (Ancef), cefepime (Maxipime), ciprofloxacin (Cipro), dobutamine (Dobutrex), enalapril (Vasotec), gentamicin, heparin, hydromorphone (Dilaudid), insulin, milrinone (Primacor), morphine, piperacillin/tazobactam (Zosyn), potassium chloride, propofol (Diprivan), tobramycin (Nebcin), vancomycin (Vancocin)

SIDE EFFECTS

Frequent
Antacid: Chalky taste, diarrhea, laxative effect
Occasional
Antacid: Nausea, vomiting, stomach cramps
Antacid, laxative: Prolonged use or large dose with renal impairment may cause increased magnesium levels, marked by dizziness, irregular heartbeat, mental changes, tiredness, and weakness

Laxative: Cramping, diarrhea, increased thirst, gas
Systemic (dietary supplement, replacement): Reduced respiratory rate, decreased reflexes, flushing, hypotension, decreased heart rate

SERIOUS REACTIONS

! Magnesium as an antacid or laxative has no known serious reactions.
! Systemic use of magnesium may produce a prolonged PR interval and widening of QRS intervals.
! Magnesium may cause loss of deep tendon reflexes, heart block, respiratory paralysis, and cardiac arrest. The antidote is 10–20 mL 10% calcium gluconate (5–10 mEq of calcium).

PEDIATRIC CONSIDERATIONS

Baseline Assessment

- Determine whether the patient is sensitive to magnesium.
- Assess for the presence of GI pain. Note its pattern, duration, quality, intensity, location, and areas of radiation, as well as factors that relieve or worsen the pain.
- Assess the amount, color, and consistency of the stool of the patient taking magnesium as a laxative.
- Assess the pattern of daily bowel activity and evaluate bowel sounds for peristalsis in the patient taking magnesium as a laxative.
- Assess the patient for history of recent abdominal surgery, nausea, vomiting, and weight loss.
- Assess the BUN and serum creatinine and magnesium levels of the patient taking magnesium for systemic use.
- Be aware that it is unknown whether the antacid forms of magnesium are distributed in breast milk.
- Be aware that parenteral magnesium readily crosses the placenta and is distributed in breast milk for 24 hrs after magnesium therapy is discontinued.
- Be aware that continuous IV infusion increases the risk of magnesium toxicity in the neonate.
- Be aware that IV administration of magnesium should not be used for 2 hrs preceding delivery.

Precautions

- Use cautiously in children younger than 6 yrs of age. The safety of magnesium use in this patient population is unknown.
- When magnesium is given as an antacid, use cautiously in pts with chronic diarrhea, colostomy, diverticulitis, ulcerative colitis, and undiagnosed GI or rectal bleeding.
- When magnesium is given as a laxative, use cautiously in pts with diabetes mellitus or pts consuming a low-salt diet because some magnesium supplements contain sugar or sodium.
- When magnesium is given for systemic use, use cautiously in pts with severe renal impairment.

Administration and Handling

PO (ANTACID)

◂ **ALERT** ▸ Keep in mind that antacids may be given up to 4 times/day.

- Shake suspension well before use.
- Make sure that chewable tablets are chewed thoroughly before swallowing and are followed by a full glass of water.

PO (LAXATIVE)

- Drink a full glass of liquid (8 oz) with each dose to prevent dehydration.
- Follow dose with citrus carbonated beverage or fruit juice to improve flavor.

• Refrigerate citrate of magnesia to retain potency and palatability.
IM
For infants and children, do not exceed 200 mg/mL (20%) as prescribed.
IV
• Store at room temperature.
• Must dilute to avoid exceeding 20 mg/mL concentration.
• For IV infusion, do not exceed magnesium sulfate concentration of 200 mg/mL (20%).
• Do not exceed IV infusion rate of 150 mg/min.

Intervention and Evaluation
• Assess the patient taking a magnesium antacid for relief of gastric distress.
• Monitor renal function of the patient taking a magnesium antacid, especially if dosing is long-term or frequent.
• Monitor the patient taking a magnesium laxative for constipation or diarrhea.
• Ensure that the patient taking a magnesium laxative maintains adequate fluid intake.
• Monitor the EKG and BUN and serum creatinine and magnesium levels in pts taking systemic magnesium.
• Test the knee-jerk and patellar reflexes before giving repeat parenteral doses of systemic magnesium because these reflexes are used as indicators of CNS depression. Know that a suppressed reflex may be a sign of impending respiratory arrest. Make sure that patellar reflexes are present, with a respiratory rate greater than 16/min, before giving each parenteral dose.
• Provide seizure precautions to the patient taking systemic magnesium.

Patient/Family Teaching
• Instruct the patient/family to take magnesium antacids at least 2 hrs apart from other medications.
• Tell the patient/family not to take magnesium antacids for longer than 2 wks, unless directed by the physician.
• Instruct the peptic ulcer disease patient to take magnesium antacids 1 and 3 hr after meals and at bedtime for 4–6 wks. Teach the patient/family to chew tablets thoroughly followed with a glass of water or to shake suspensions well.
• Warn the patient/family that repeat dosing or large doses of magnesium antacids may have a laxative effect.
• Instruct the patient/family taking magnesium laxatives to drink a full glass (8 oz) of liquid to aid stool softening.
• Tell the patient/family taking magnesium laxatives that these drugs are for short-term use only.
• Warn the patient/family taking magnesium laxatives not to use the drug if the patient experiences abdominal pain, nausea, or vomiting.
• Warn the patient/family taking systemic magnesium to notify the physician if the patient experiences any signs of hypermagnesemia, including confusion, cramping, dizziness, irregular heartbeat, lightheadedness, or unusual tiredness or weakness.

Methylcellulose

meth-ill-**cell**-you-los
(Citrucel, Cologel)
Do not confuse with Citracal.

CATEGORY AND SCHEDULE
Pregnancy Risk Category: C
OTC

MECHANISM OF ACTION

A bulk-forming laxative that dissolves and expands in water.
Therapeutic Effect: Provides increased bulk, moisture content in stool, increasing peristalsis, and bowel motility.

PHARMACOKINETICS

Route	Onset	Peak	Duration
PO	12–24 hrs	N/A	N/A

The full effect may not be evident for 2–3 days. Acts in small and large intestines.

AVAILABILITY

Powder: 2 g/scoop.
Tablets: 500 mg.

INDICATIONS AND DOSAGES

▸ **Laxative**

PO

Children 6–12 yrs. ½ scoop (8 g) in 8 oz of cold water once daily.
Children older than 12 yrs. 1 scoop (1 heaping tbsp) in 8 oz of cold water 1–3 times daily.

CONTRAINDICATIONS

Abdominal pain, dysphagia, nausea, partial bowel obstruction, symptoms of appendicitis, vomiting.

INTERACTIONS

Drug

Digoxin, oral anticoagulants, salicylates: May decrease the effects of digoxin, oral anticoagulants, and salicylates by decreasing absorption.
Potassium-sparing diuretics, potassium supplements: May interfere with the effects of potassium-sparing diuretics and potassium supplements.

Herbal

None known.

Food

None known.

DIAGNOSTIC TEST EFFECTS

May increase blood glucose levels. May decrease serum potassium levels.

SIDE EFFECTS

Rare

Some degree of abdominal discomfort, nausea, mild cramps, griping, faintness

SERIOUS REACTIONS

! Esophageal or bowel obstruction may occur if administered with insufficient liquid (less than 250 mL or 1 full glass).

PEDIATRIC CONSIDERATIONS

Baseline Assessment

- Before administration, assess the patient's abdomen for signs of tenderness or rigidity and the presence of bowel sounds.
- Try to determine when the patient last had a bowel movement, and find out the amount and consistency.
- This drug may be used safely in pregnancy.
- Be aware that the safety and efficacy of methylcellulose have not been established in children younger than 6 yrs of age. Methylcellulose use is not recommended in this age group.

Administration and Handling

PO

- Instruct the patient to drink 6–8 glasses of water daily to aid in stool softening.
- Methylcellulose is not to be swallowed in dry form; mix with at least 1 full glass (8 oz) of liquid.

Intervention and Evaluation

- Encourage the patient to maintain adequate fluid intake.
- Assess the patient's bowel sounds for peristalsis.
- Assess the patient's pattern of daily bowel activity and stool consistency, and record time of evacuation.
- Monitor serum electrolyte levels in pts exposed to excessive, frequent, or prolonged use of methylcellulose.

Patient/Family Teaching

- Tell the patient/family to institute measures to promote defecation such as increasing the patient's fluid intake, exercising, and eating a high-fiber diet.
- Instruct the patient/family to take each dose with a full glass of water.
- Warn the patient/family that inadequate fluid intake may cause choking or swelling in the throat.

Polycarbophil

polly-**car**-bow-fill
(FiberCon, Replens [CAN])

CATEGORY AND SCHEDULE

Pregnancy Risk Category: C
OTC

MECHANISM OF ACTION

A bulk-forming laxative and antidiarrheal.
Laxative: Retains water in intestine, opposes dehydrating forces of the bowel. ***Therapeutic Effect:*** Promotes well-formed stools.
Antidiarrheal: Absorbs fecal-free water, restores normal moisture level, provides bulk. ***Therapeutic Effect:*** Forms gel, produces formed stool.

PHARMACOKINETICS

Route	Onset	Peak	Duration
PO	12–72 hrs	N/A	N/A

Acts in small and large intestines.

AVAILABILITY

Tablets: 500 mg, 625 mg.
Tablets (chewable): 625 mg.

INDICATIONS AND DOSAGES

▸ Laxative, antidiarrheal

PO

Children older than 12 yrs. 1 g 1–4 times/day or as needed. Maximum: 4 g/24 hrs.
Children 6–12 yrs. 500 mg 1–4 times/day, or as needed. Maximum: 2 g/24 hrs.
Children younger than 6 yrs. Consult product labeling—product directions vary.

CONTRAINDICATIONS

Abdominal pain, dysphagia, nausea, partial bowel obstruction, symptoms of appendicitis, vomiting.

INTERACTIONS

Drug

Digoxin, oral anticoagulants, salicylates, tetracyclines: May decrease the effects of digoxin, salicylates, and tetracyclines.
Potassium-sparing diuretics, potassium supplements: May interfere with the effects of potassium-sparing diuretics and potassium supplements.

Herbal

None known.

Food

None known.

DIAGNOSTIC TEST EFFECTS

May increase blood glucose levels. May decrease serum potassium levels.

SIDE EFFECTS

Rare

Some degree of abdominal discomfort, nausea, mild cramps, griping, faintness

SERIOUS REACTIONS

! Esophageal or bowel obstruction may occur if administered with less than 250 mL or 1 full glass of liquid.

PEDIATRIC CONSIDERATIONS

Baseline Assessment

- Before administration, assess the patient's abdomen for signs of tenderness or rigidity and the presence of bowel sounds.
- Try to determine when the patient last had a bowel movement, and find out the amount and consistency.
- This drug may be used safely in pregnancy.
- Be aware that polycarbophil use is not recommended in children younger than 6 yrs of age.

Administration and Handling

◂ALERT▸ For severe diarrhea, give every ½ hr up to the maximum daily dosage; for laxative, give with 8 oz of liquid, as prescribed.

Intervention and Evaluation

- Encourage the patient to maintain adequate fluid intake.
- Assess the patient's bowel sounds for peristalsis.
- Assess the patient's pattern of daily bowel activity and stool consistency, and record time of evacuation.
- Monitor serum electrolyte levels in pts exposed to excessive, frequent, or prolonged use of polycarbophil.

Patient/Family Teaching

- Tell the patient/family to institute measures to promote defecation such as increasing the patient's fluid intake, exercising, and eating a high-fiber diet.
- Instruct the patient/family to drink 6–8 glasses of water daily when using polycarbophil as a laxative to aid in stool softening.

Polyethylene Glycol-Electrolyte Solution (PEG-ES)

poly-**eth**-ah-leen

(CoLyte, GoLYTELY, Klean-Prep [CAN], MiraLax, NuLytely, Peglyte [CAN], Pro-Lax [CAN])

CATEGORY AND SCHEDULE

Pregnancy Risk Category: C

MECHANISM OF ACTION

A laxative that has an osmotic effect. ***Therapeutic Effect:*** Induces diarrhea and cleanses the bowel without depleting electrolytes.

PHARMACOKINETICS

Indication	Onset	Peak	Duration
Bowel cleansing	1–2 hrs	N/A	N/A
Constipation	2–4 days	N/A	N/A

AVAILABILITY

Powder for Oral Solution. (Colyte, GoLYTELY, NuLytely)

CoLytely: 4000 mL

GoLytely: 4000 mL

NuLytely: 4000 mL

MiraLax: 14 oz, 27 oz

INDICATIONS AND DOSAGES

▸ **Bowel evacuant**

PO/NASOGASTRIC

Children. 25–40 mL/kg/hr until rectal effluent clear.

CONTRAINDICATIONS

Hypersensitivity to polyethylene glycol or any component. Bowel perforation, gastric retention, GI obstruction, toxic colitis, toxic ileus, megacolon.

INTERACTIONS

Drug

PO medications: May decrease the absorption of oral medications if given within 1 hr because they may be flushed from GI tract.

Herbal

None known.

Food

None known.

DIAGNOSTIC TEST EFFECTS

None known.

SIDE EFFECTS

Frequent (50%)

Some degree of abdominal fullness, nausea, bloating

Occasional (10%–1%)

Abdominal cramping, vomiting, anal irritation

Rare (less than 1%)

Urticaria, rhinorrhea, dermatitis

SERIOUS REACTIONS

None known.

PEDIATRIC CONSIDERATIONS

Baseline Assessment

• Do not give oral medication within 1 hr of the initiation of polyethylene therapy or the oral medication may not be adequately be absorbed before GI cleansing.

• Be aware that it is unknown whether polyethylene crosses the placenta or is distributed in breast milk.

• There are no age-related precautions noted in children.

• Be aware that pts with impaired gag reflex who are prone to regurgitation or aspiration should be observed very closely during administration. Use with caution in these pts.

Precautions

• Use cautiously in pts with ulcerative colitis.

Administration and Handling

PO

• Refrigerate reconstituted solutions; use within 48 hrs.

• May use tap water to prepare solution. Shake vigorously several minutes to ensure complete dissolution of powder.

• Give nothing by mouth 3 hrs or more before ingestion of solution. Give clear liquids only after administration.

• May give via nasogastric tube.

• Rapid drinking preferred. Chilled solution is more palatable.

Intervention and Evaluation

• Assess the patient's bowel sounds for peristalsis.

• Assess the patient's pattern of daily bowel activity and stool consistency, and record time of evacuation.

• Assess the patient for abdominal disturbances.

• Monitor the patient's blood glucose, BUN, and serum electrolyte levels and urine osmolality.

Patient/Family Teaching

• Tell the patient/family to chill the solution to make it more palatable, and encourage fast ingestion.

• Instruct the patient/family to fast for 3 hrs before taking the drug and to only ingest clear liquids afterward, as prescribed.

• Warn the patient/family to notify the physician if the patient experiences severe abdominal pain or bloating.

Psyllium

sill-ee-um

(Fiberall, Hydrocil, Konsyl, Metamucil, Perdiem, Prodiem Plain [CAN])

CATEGORY AND SCHEDULE

Pregnancy Risk Category: B

OTC

MECHANISM OF ACTION

A bulk-forming laxative in powder or wafer form that dissolves and swells in water and provides increased bulk and moisture content in the stool. ***Therapeutic Effect:*** Increased bulk promotes peristalsis and bowel motility.

PHARMACOKINETICS

Route	Onset	Peak	Duration
PO	12–24 hrs	2–3 days	N/A

Acts in small and large intestines.

AVAILABILITY

Powder: 3.4 g/dose, 3.5 g/dose, 6 g/dose (Konsyl).

Granules: 2.5 g/tsp (Serutan), 4.03 g/tsp (Perdiem).

Wafer: 3.4 g/dose (Metamucil).

Capsules: 0.52 g/capsule (Metamucil).

INDICATIONS AND DOSAGES

▸ **Laxative**

PO

Children older than 11 yrs. 1–2 rounded tsp, packet, or wafer in 4 oz of water 1–4 times/day.

Children 6–11 yrs. ½–1 tsp in 4 oz of water 1–3 times/day.

CONTRAINDICATIONS

Hypersensitivity to psyllium or any related component. Fecal impaction and GI obstruction.

INTERACTIONS

Drug

Digoxin, oral anticoagulants, salicylates: May decrease the effects of digoxin, oral anticoagulants, and salicylates by decreasing absorption.

Potassium-sparing diuretics, potassium supplements: May interfere with the effects of potassium-sparing diuretics and potassium supplements.

Herbal

None known.

Food

None known.

DIAGNOSTIC TEST EFFECTS

May increase blood glucose levels. May decrease serum potassium levels.

SIDE EFFECTS

Rare

Some degree of abdominal discomfort, nausea, mild cramps, griping, faintness

SERIOUS REACTIONS

! Esophageal or bowel obstruction may occur if administered with insufficient liquid (less than 250 mL or 1 full glass of liquid).

PEDIATRIC CONSIDERATIONS

Baseline Assessment

• Before administration, assess the patient's abdomen for signs of tenderness or rigidity and the presence of bowel sounds.
• Try to determine when the patient last had a bowel movement, and find out the amount and consistency.
• This drug may be used safely in pregnancy.
• Be aware that the safety and efficacy of psyllium have not been established in children younger than 6 yrs of age.

Precautions

• Use cautiously in pts with esophageal strictures, intestinal adhesions, stenosis, and ulcers.

Administration and Handling

PO
• Drink 6–8 glasses of water daily to aid in stool softening.
• Do not swallow in dry form; mix with at least 1 full glass (8 oz) of liquid.

Intervention and Evaluation

• Encourage the patient to maintain adequate fluid intake.
• Assess the patient's bowel sounds for peristalsis.
• Assess the patient's pattern of daily bowel activity and stool consistency, and record time of evacuation.
• Assess the patient for abdominal disturbances.
• Monitor serum electrolyte levels in pts exposed to excessive, frequent, or prolonged use of psyllium.

Patient/Family Teaching

• Tell the patient/family to institute measures to promote defecation such as increasing the patient's fluid intake, exercising, and eating a high-fiber diet.
• Instruct the patient/family to take each dose with a full glass of water.
• Warn the patient/family that inadequate fluid intake may cause choking or swelling in the throat.

Senna

sen-ah
(Senokot, Senolax)

CATEGORY AND SCHEDULE

Pregnancy Risk Category: C
OTC

MECHANISM OF ACTION

A GI stimulant that has a direct effect on intestinal smooth musculature by stimulating the intramural nerve plexi. ***Therapeutic Effect:*** Increases peristalsis and promotes laxative effect.

PHARMACOKINETICS

Route	Onset	Peak	Duration
PO	6–12 hrs	N/A	N/A
Rectal	0.5–2 hrs	N/A	N/A

Minimal absorption after PO administration. Hydrolyzed to active form by enzymes of colonic flora. Absorbed drug metabolized in liver; eliminated in feces via the biliary system.

AVAILABILITY

Granules: 15 mg/tsp.
Liquid: 25 mg/15 mL, 33.3 mg/mL.
Syrup: 8.8 mg/5 mL.
Tablets: 8.6 mg, 15 mg, 25 mg.
Tablets (chewable): 10 mg, 15 mg.

INDICATIONS AND DOSAGES

▸ Constipation

PO (TABLETS)

Children older than 12 yrs. 2 tablets at bedtime up to 4 tablets 2 times/day.
Children 6–12 yrs. 1 tablet at bedtime up to 2 tablets 2 times/day.
Children 2–5 yrs. ½ tablet at bedtime up to 1 tablet 2 times/day.

PO (SYRUP)

Children older than 12 yrs. 10–15 mL at bedtime up to 15 mL 2 times/day.
Children 6–12 yrs. 5–7.5 mL at bedtime up to 7.5 mL 2 times/day.
Children 2–5 yrs. 2.5–3.75 mL at bedtime up to 3.75 mL 2 times/day.

PO (GRANULES)

Children older than 12 yrs. 1 tsp at bedtime up to 2 tsp 2 times/day.
Children 6–12 yrs. ½ teaspoon at bedtime up to 1 tsp 2 times/day.
Children 2–5 yrs. ¼ tsp at bedtime up to ½ tsp 2 times/day.

CONTRAINDICATIONS

Hypersensitivity to senna or any related component. Abdominal pain, appendicitis, intestinal obstruction, nausea, vomiting.

INTERACTIONS

Drug

PO medications: May decrease transit time of concurrently administered oral medication, decreasing absorption of senna.
Docusate: May increase the absorption of senna.

Herbal

None known.

Food

None known.

DIAGNOSTIC TEST EFFECTS

May increase blood glucose levels. May decrease serum potassium levels.

SIDE EFFECTS

Frequent

Pink-red, red-violet, red-brown, or yellow-brown discoloration of urine

Occasional

Some degree of abdominal discomfort, nausea, mild cramps, griping, faintness

SERIOUS REACTIONS

! Long-term use may result in laxative dependence, chronic constipation, and loss of normal bowel function.

! Chronic use or overdosage may result in electrolyte disturbances, such as hypokalemia, hypocalcemia, and metabolic acidosis or alkalosis, persistent diarrhea, malabsorption, and weight loss. Electrolyte disturbance may produce vomiting, muscle weakness.

PEDIATRIC CONSIDERATIONS

Baseline Assessment

- Before administration, assess the patient's abdomen for signs of tenderness or rigidity and the presence of bowel sounds.
- Try to determine when the patient last had a bowel movement, and find out the amount and consistency.
- Be aware that it is unknown whether senna is distributed in breast milk.
- Be aware that the safety and efficacy of senna have not been established in children younger than 6 yrs of age.

Precautions

- Use cautiously for extended periods longer than 1 wk.

Administration and Handling

PO

- Give senna on an empty stomach for faster results.

• Offer the patient at least 6–8 glasses of water daily to aid in stool softening.
• Avoid giving within 1 hr of other oral medication because it decreases drug absorption.

Intervention and Evaluation

• Encourage the patient to maintain adequate fluid intake.
• Assess the patient's bowel sounds for peristalsis.
• Assess the patient's pattern of daily bowel activity and stool consistency, and record time of evacuation.
• Assess the patient for GI disturbances.
• Monitor serum electrolyte levels in pts exposed to excessive, frequent, or prolonged use of senna.

Patient/Family Teaching

• Explain to the patient/family that the patient's urine may turn pink-red, red-violet, red-brown, or yellow-brown.
• Instruct the patient/family to institute measures to promote defecation such as increasing the patient's fluid intake, exercising, and eating a high-fiber diet.
• Instruct the patient/family not to take other oral medications within 1 hr of taking senna as these substances may decrease the effectiveness of senna.
• Tell the patient/family that the laxative effect of senna generally occurs in 6–12 hrs but may take 24 hrs to appear, and the senna suppository produces evacuation in 30 min–2 hrs.

REFERENCES

Miller, S. & Fioravanti, J. (1997). Pediatric medications: a handbook for nurses. St. Louis: Mosby.
Taketomo, C. K., Hodding, J. H. & Kraus, D. M. (2003–2004). Pediatric dosage handbook (10th ed.). Hudson, OH: Lexi-Comp.

51 Proton Pump Inhibitors

Lansoprazole
Omeprazole

Uses: Proton pump inhibitors (PPIs) are used to treat various gastric disorders, including gastric and duodenal ulcers, gastroesophageal reflux disease (GERD), and pathologic hypersecretory conditions.

Action: PPIs suppress gastric acid secretion by specifically inhibiting the hydrogen-potassium-adenosine triphosphatase (H^+/K^+–ATPase) enzyme system found at the secretory surface of gastric parietal cells. This enzyme system is considered the acid pump of the gastric mucosa. (See illustration, *Sites of Action: Drugs Used to Treat GERD,* page 000.) PPIs do not have anticholinergic or histamine-receptor antagonistic properties.

Lansoprazole

lan-sew-**prah**-zoll
(Prevacid, Zoton [AUS])
Do not confuse with Pepcid, Pravachol, or Prevpac.

CATEGORY AND SCHEDULE

Pregnancy Risk Category: B

MECHANISM OF ACTION

A PPI that selectively inhibits parietal cell membrane enzyme system H^+, K^+, –ATPase or the proton pump. ***Therapeutic Effect:*** Suppresses gastric acid secretion.

PHARMACOKINETICS

Dosage	Onset	Peak	Duration
15 mg	2–3 hrs	N/A	24 hrs
30 mg	1–2 hrs	N/A	longer than 24 hrs

Once leaving the stomach, rapid and complete absorption (food may decrease absorption). Protein binding: 97%. Distributed primarily to the gastric parietal cells, converted to two active metabolites. Extensively metabolized in liver. Eliminated from the body in bile and urine. Not removed by hemodialysis. ***Half-Life:*** Children: 1.2–1.5 hrs; adult: 1.5 hrs. Half-life is increased in those with liver impairment.

AVAILABILITY

Capsules (extended release): 15 mg, 30 mg.
Tablets (oral disintegrating): 15 mg, 30 mg.
Granules for Oral Suspension: 15 mg/pack; 30 mg/pack.
Injection: 30 mg/vial.

INDICATIONS AND DOSAGES

Duodenal ulcer

PO

Children 12 yrs and older. 15 mg/day, before eating, preferably in the morning, for up to 4 wks.

Erosive esophagitis

PO

Children 12 yrs and older. 30 mg/day, before eating, for up to 8 wks. If healing does not occur within 8 wks (5%–10%), may give for additional 8 wks. Maintenance: 15 mg/day.

Gastric ulcer

PO

Children 12 yrs and older: 30 mg/day for up to 8 wks.

Healed duodenal ulcer, GERD

PO

Children 12 yrs and older: 15 mg/day for up to 8 wks.

Usual pediatric dosage

Children 3 mos–14 yrs weighing less than 10 kg. 7.5 mg/day.
Children 3 mos–14 yrs weighing 10–20 kg. 15 mg/day.
Children 3 mos–14 yrs weighing more than 20 kg. 30 mg/day.

Helicobacter pylori

PO

Children 12 yrs and older: 30 mg 2 times/day for 10 days (with amoxicillin and clarithromycin).

CONTRAINDICATIONS

Hypersensitivity to lansoprazole or any related component.

INTERACTIONS

Drug

Ampicillin, digoxin, iron salts, ketoconazole: May interfere with the absorption of ampicillin, digoxin, iron salts, and ketoconazole.

Sucralfate: May delay the absorption of lansoprazole; give lansoprazole 30 min before sucralfate.

Herbal

None known.

Food

None known.

DIAGNOSTIC TEST EFFECTS

May increase lactate dehydrogenase, serum alkaline phosphatase, bilirubin, cholesterol, creatinine, SGOT (AST), SGPT (ALT), triglyceride, and uric acid levels. May produce abnormal albumin/globulin ratio, electrolyte balance, and platelet, RBC, and WBC counts. May increase blood Hgb and Hct.

SIDE EFFECTS

Occasional (3%–2%)

Diarrhea, abdominal pain, rash, pruritus, altered appetite

Rare (1%)

Nausea, headache

SERIOUS REACTIONS

! Bilirubinemia, eosinophilia, and hyperlipemia occur rarely.

PEDIATRIC CONSIDERATIONS

Baseline Assessment

- Obtain the patient's baseline laboratory values, including complete blood count and blood chemistry.
- Assess the patient's medication history, especially for the use of sucralfate.
- Be aware that it is unknown whether lansoprazole is distributed in breast milk.
- Be aware that the safety and efficacy of lansoprazole have not been established in children.

Precautions

- Use cautiously in pts with impaired liver function.

Administration and Handling

PO

- Give lansoprazole while the patient is fasting or before meals because food diminishes absorption.
- Instruct the patient not to chew or crush delayed-release capsules.
- If the patient has difficulty swallowing capsules, open capsules and sprinkle granules on 1 tbsp of applesauce. Instruct the patient to swallow immediately.

Intervention and Evaluation

- Monitor the patient's ongoing laboratory results.

• Assess the patient for therapeutic response, such as relief of GI symptoms.
• Assess the patient for abdominal pain, diarrhea, and nausea.

Patient/Family Teaching

• Instruct the patient/family not to chew or crush delayed-release capsules.
• Teach pts/families that if the patient has difficulty swallowing the lansoprozole capsule to open it, sprinkle the granules on 1 tbsp of applesauce, and swallow immediately.
• Instruct patient/family to take lansoprazole 30 min before sucralfate.

Omeprazole

oh-**mep**-rah-zole
(Losec [CAN], Maxor [AUS], Prilosec, Prilosec DR)
Do not confuse with prilocaine, Prinivil, or Prozac.
(See Color Plate)

CATEGORY AND SCHEDULE

Pregnancy Risk Category: C

MECHANISM OF ACTION

A benzimidazole that is converted to active metabolites that irreversibly bind to and inhibit H^+/K^+-ATPase, an enzyme on the surface of gastric parietal cells. Inhibits hydrogen ion transport into gastric lumen. ***Therapeutic Effect:*** Increases gastric pH, reduces gastric acid production.

PHARMACOKINETICS

Route	Onset	Peak	Duration
PO	1 hr	2 hrs	72 hrs

Rapidly absorbed from the GI tract. Protein binding: 99%. Primarily distributed into gastric parietal cells. Metabolized extensively in liver. Primarily excreted in urine. Unknown whether removed by hemodialysis. ***Half-Life:*** 0.5–1 hr (increased in pts with decreased liver function).

AVAILABILITY

Capsules (delayed release): 10 mg, 20 mg, 40 mg.

INDICATIONS AND DOSAGES

Children. Dosage has not been established, but a starting dose of 0.6–0.7 mg/kg/day in the morning has been suggested. Another dose 12 hrs later may be administered if necessary. An effective range is 0.7–3.5 mg/kg/day.
Children older than 2 yrs weighing less than 20 kg. 10 mg once daily.
Children weighing more than 20 kg. 20 mg once daily (per manufacturer's recommendations)

UNLABELED USES

Prevention and treatment of NSAID-induced ulcers, treatment of active benign gastric ulcers, *H. pylori*–associated duodenal ulcer with amoxicillin and clarithromycin.

CONTRAINDICATIONS

Hypersensitivity to omeprazole or any related component.

INTERACTIONS

Drug

Diazepam, oral anticoagulants, phenytoin: May increase the blood concentration of diazepam, oral anticoagulants, and phenytoin.
Digoxin, didanosine: May increase absorption of these drugs.

Methotrexate: May decrease the elimination of methotrexate, leading to increased toxicity.
Ketoconazole, itraconazole, iron salts, ampicillin: May decrease effectiveness of these drugs.

Herbal
None known.

Food
None known.

DIAGNOSTIC TEST EFFECTS

May increase serum alkaline phosphatase, SGOT (AST), and SGPT (ALT) levels.

SIDE EFFECTS

Frequent (7%)
Headache
Occasional (3%–2%)
Diarrhea, abdominal pain, nausea
Rare (less than 2%)
Dizziness, asthenia or loss of strength, vomiting, constipation, upper respiratory infection, back pain, rash, cough

SERIOUS REACTIONS

None known.

PEDIATRIC CONSIDERATIONS

Baseline Assessment

- Expect to obtain baseline serum chemistry laboratory values, particularly serum alkaline phosphatase, SGOT (AST), and SGPT (ALT) levels, to assess liver function.
- Be aware that it is unknown whether omeprazole crosses the placenta or is distributed in breast milk.
- Be aware that the safety and efficacy of omeprazole have not been established in children.

Administration and Handling

PO

- Give omeprazole before meals.
- Do not crush or open capsules; capsules should be swallowed whole.

Intervention and Evaluation

- Evaluate the patient for therapeutic response, relief of GI symptoms.
- Assess the patient for diarrhea, discomfort, and nausea.

Patient/Family Teaching

- Warn the patient/family to notify the physician if the patient experiences headache during omeprazole therapy.
- Instruct the patient/family to swallow omeprazole capsules whole and not to open or crush them.
- Teach the patient/family to take omeprazole capsules before eating.

REFERENCES

Miller, S. & Fioravanti, J. (1997). Pediatric medications: a handbook for nurses. St. Louis: Mosby.
Taketomo, C. K., Hodding, J. H. & Kraus, D. M. (2003–2004). Pediatric dosage handbook (10th ed.). Hudson, OH: Lexi-Comp.

52 Miscellaneous Gastrointestinal Agents

Mesalamine (5-Aminosalicylic Acid, 5-ASA)
Pancreatin, Pancrelipase
Simethicone

Uses: Because miscellaneous GI agents come from different classes, their uses vary greatly. As GI anti-inflammatory agents, drugs such as *mesalamine* are prescribed to manage ulcerative colitis; other indications include proctosigmoiditis and proctitis (mesalamine) and inflammatory bowel disease and rheumatoid arthritis. *Pancreatin and pancrelipase* are used to replace or supplement pancreatic enzymes in chronic pancreatitis and other disorders; they can also treat steatorrhea caused by certain conditions. The antiflatulent *simethicone* is used to treat flatulence, gastric bloating, postoperative gas pain, and other conditions that may cause gas retention.

Action: Miscellaneous GI agents act in different ways. Among the other GI anti-inflammatory drugs, *mesalamine* acts locally to inhibit the production of arachidonic acid metabolites and *olsalazine* is converted to mesalamine by colonic bacteria. *Pancreatin and pancrelipase* act by replacing endogenous pancreatic enzymes. The antiflatulent *simethicone* changes the surface tension of gas bubbles, allowing easier gas elimination.

COMBINATION PRODUCTS

EXTRA STRENGTH MAALOX: simethicone/magnesium hydroxide (an antacid)/aluminum hydroxide (an antacid) 20 mg/200 mg/200 mg; 40 mg/400 mg/400 mg.
GELUSIL: simethicone/aluminum hydroxide (an antacid)/magnesium hydroxide (an antacid) 25 mg/200 mg/200 mg.
IMODIUM ADVANCED: simethicone/loperamide (an antidiarrheal) 125 mg/2 mg.
MAALOX PLUS: simethicone/aluminum hydroxide (an antacid)/magnesium hydroxide (an antacid) 25 mg/200 mg/200 mg.
MYLANTA: simethicone/magnesium hydroxide (an antacid)/aluminum hydroxide (an antacid) 20 mg/200 mg/200 mg; 40 mg/400 mg/400 mg.
SILAIN-GEL: 25 mg simethicone/285 mg magnesium hydroxide (an antacid)/282 mg aluminum hydroxide (an antacid).

Mesalamine (5-Aminosalicylic Acid, 5-ASA)

mess-**al**-ah-meen
(Asacol, Fiv-ASA, Mesasal [CAN], Pentasa, Rowasa, Salofalk [CAN])
Do not confuse with Os-Cal.

CATEGORY AND SCHEDULE

Pregnancy Risk Category: B

MECHANISM OF ACTION
A salicylic acid derivative that produces a local inhibitory effect on arachidonic acid metabolite production, which is increased in pts with chronic inflammatory bowel disease. ***Therapeutic Effect:*** Blocks prostaglandin production, diminishes inflammation in colon.

PHARMACOKINETICS
Poorly absorbed from colon. Moderately absorbed from the GI tract. Metabolized in liver to the active metabolite. Unabsorbed portion eliminated in feces; absorbed portion excreted in urine. Unknown whether removed by hemodialysis. ***Half-Life:*** 0.5–1.5 hrs; metabolite: 5–10 hrs.

AVAILABILITY
Tablets (delayed release): 400 mg.
Capsules (controlled release): 250 mg.
Suppository: 500 mg.
Rectal Suspension: 4 g/60 mL.

INDICATIONS AND DOSAGES
▸ Ulcerative colitis, proctosigmoiditis, proctitis
PO (ASACOL)
Children. 50 mg/kg/day q6–12h.
PO (PENTASA)
Children. 50 mg/kg/day q8–12h.

CONTRAINDICATIONS
Hypersensitivity to mesalamine, any related component, or salicylates.

INTERACTIONS
Drug
Digoxin: Decreases the amount of digoxin that is absorbed.
Herbal
None known.
Food
None known.

DIAGNOSTIC TEST EFFECTS
May increase BUN, serum alkaline phosphatase, creatinine, SGOT (AST), and SGPT (ALT) levels.

SIDE EFFECTS
Generally well tolerated, with only mild and transient effects.
Frequent (greater than 6%)
PO: Abdominal cramps or pain, diarrhea, dizziness, headache, nausea, vomiting, rhinitis, unusual tiredness
Rectal: Abdominal or stomach cramps, flatulence, headache, nausea
Occasional (6%–2%)
PO: Hair loss, decreased appetite, back or joint pain, flatulence, acne
Rectal: Hair loss
Rare (less than 2%)
Rectal: Anal irritation

SERIOUS REACTIONS
! Sulfite sensitivity in susceptible pts noted as cramping, headache, diarrhea, fever, rash, hives, itching, and wheezing. Discontinue drug immediately.
! Hepatitis, pancreatitis, and pericarditis occur rarely with oral dosage.

PEDIATRIC CONSIDERATIONS
Baseline Assessment
- Expect to obtain baseline BUN, serum alkaline phosphatase, creatinine, SGOT (AST), and SGPT (ALT) levels.
- Ask the patient if he or she has an allergy to sulfa-based products before administering the drug.
- Be aware that it is unknown whether mesalamine crosses the placenta or is distributed in breast milk.

• Be aware that the safety and efficacy of mesalamine have not been established in children.

Precautions

• Use cautiously in pts with preexisting renal disease and sulfasalazine sensitivity.

Administration and Handling

◂ **ALERT** ▸ Store rectal suspension, suppository, and oral forms at room temperature.

PO

Have patient swallow tablets whole; do not break the outer coating of the tablet.

• Give mesalamine without regard to food.

Intervention and Evaluation

• Encourage the patient to maintain adequate fluid intake.

• Assess the patient's bowel sounds for peristalsis.

• Assess the patient's pattern of daily bowel activity and stool consistency, and record time of evacuation.

• Evaluate the patient for abdominal disturbances.

• Assess the patient's skin for rash and urticaria.

• Discontinue the medication if cramping, diarrhea, fever, or rash occurs.

Patient/Family Teaching

• Warn the patient/family to avoid tasks that require mental alertness or motor skills until the patient's response to the drug is established.

• Tell the patient/family that mesalamine use may discolor the patient's urine yellow-brown.

• Explain to the patient/family that mesalamine suppositories stain fabrics.

Pancreatin

pan-kree-**ah**-tin

(Ku-Zyme, Pancreatin)

Pancrelipase

pan-kree-**lie**-pace

(Cotazym, Cotazym-S Forte [AUS], Creon, Pancrease [CAN], Pancrease MT, Ultrase, Viokase)

(See Color Plate)

CATEGORY AND SCHEDULE

Pregnancy Risk Category: C

MECHANISM OF ACTION

A digestive enzyme that replaces endogenous pancreatic enzymes. ***Therapeutic Effect:*** Assists in digestion of protein, starch, and fats.

AVAILABILITY

Pancreatic enzymes

Product	Dosage Form	Lip-ase USP Units	Pro-tease USP units	Amy-lase USP units
Creon 5	Capsule, delayed release, enteric coated microspheres	5000	18750	16600
Creon 10	Capsule, delayed release, enteric coated microspheres	10000	37500	33200
Creon 20	Capsule, delayed release, enteric coated microspheres	20000	75000	66400
Lipram 4500	Capsule, delayed release, enteric coated microspheres	4500	25000	20000
Lipram PN 16	Capsule, delayed release, enteric coated microspheres	16000	48000	48000
Libram PN 10	Capsule, delayed release, enteric coated microspheres	10000	30000	30000
Lipram CR 10	Capsule, delayed release, enteric coated microspheres	10000	37500	33200
Lipram CR 20	Capsule, delayed release, enteric coated microspheres	20000	75000	66400
Lipram UL 12	Capsule, delayed release, enteric coated microspheres	12000	39000	39000
Lipram UL 18	Capsule, delayed release, enteric coated microspheres	18000	58500	58500
Lipram UL 20	Capsule, delayed release, enteric coated microspheres	20000	65000	65000
Pancrease	Capsule, enteric coated microspheres	4500	25000	20000
Buffered, enteric coated microspheres		16000	52000	52000
Ultrase	Capsule, enteric coated microspheres	4500	25000	20000
Pancrease MT 4	Capsule, enteric coated microtablets	4000	12000	12000
Pancrease MT 10	Capsule, enteric coated microtablets	10000	30000	30000
Pancrease MT 16	Capsule, enteric coated microtablets	16000	48000	48000
Pancrease MT 20	Capsule, enteric coated microtablets	20000	44000	56000
Pancrecarb MS-4	Buffered, enteric coated microspheres	4000	25000	25000
Pancrecarb MS-8	Buffered, enteric coated microspheres	8000	45000	40000
Pancrecarb MS-16 Ultrase MT 12	Capsule, enteric coated minitablets	12000	39000	39000
Ultrase MT 18	Capsule, enteric coated minitablets	18000	58500	58500
Ultrase MT 20	Capsule, enteric coated minitablets	20000	65000	65000
Viokase	Powder	16800 (per 0.7 g)	70000 (per 0.7 g)	70000 (per 0.7 g)
Viokase 8	Tablet	8000	30000	30000
Viokase 16	Tablet	16000	60000	60000

INDICATIONS AND DOSAGES

▸ Pancreatic enzyme replacement or supplement when enzymes are absent or deficient, such as with chronic pancreatitis, cystic fibrosis, or ductal obstruction from cancer of the pancreas or common bile duct, reduces malabsorption, treatment of steatorrhea associated with bowel resection or postgastrectomy syndrome

PO

Children 7–12 yrs. 4,000–12,000 USP U lipase with meals and snacks.
Children 1–6 yrs. 4,000–8,000 USP U lipase with meals, 4,000 USP U lipase with snacks.
Infants 6 mo–1 yr. 2,000 USP U lipase with meals and snacks.

CONTRAINDICATIONS

Hypersensitivity to pancreatin, pancrelipase, or any related component. Acute pancreatitis, exacerbation of chronic pancreatitis, hypersensitivity to pork or bovine protein.

INTERACTIONS

Drug

Antacids: May decrease the effects of pancreatin and pancrelipase.
Iron supplements: May decrease the absorption of iron supplements.
H_2 antagonists (cimetidine, ranitidine): May increase effectiveness of pancreatic enzyme preparations.

Herbal

None known.

Food

Avoid use with alkaline foods (milk, custard, or ice cream).

DIAGNOSTIC TEST EFFECTS

May increase serum uric acid levels.

SIDE EFFECTS

Rare

Allergic reaction, mouth irritation, shortness of breath, wheezing

SERIOUS REACTIONS

! Excessive dosage may produce nausea, cramping, and diarrhea.
! Hyperuricosuria and hyperuricemia have been reported with extremely high dosages.

PEDIATRIC CONSIDERATIONS

Baseline Assessment

- Know that spilling Viokase powder on the hands may irritate the skin.
- Know that inhaling powder may irritate mucous membranes and produce bronchospasm.
- Be aware that it is unknown whether pancreatin and pancrelipase cross the placenta or are distributed in breast milk.
- Be aware that the dose of pancreatin or pancrelipase must be individualized to the patient.
- Know that these products are not bioequivalent.

Precautions

- Use pancreatin and pancrelipase cautiously because inhalation of the drug's powder form may precipitate an asthma attack.

Administration and Handling

PO

- Give pancreatin or pancrelipase before or with meals or snacks.
- Crush tablets as needed. Do not crush the enteric-coated form.
- After administration to infants, use a swab or gauze-covered finger to sweep away granules that may be left between the cheek and the gums. Leaving granules there may lead to mouth ulceration/irritation.

Intervention and Evaluation

• Evaluate the patient for therapeutic relief from GI symptoms.
• Advise the patient not to change brands of the drug without first consulting the physician.

Patient/Family Teaching

• Instruct the patient/family not to chew capsules or tablets to minimize irritation to mouth, lips, and tongue. May open capsule and spread over applesauce, mashed fruit, or rice cereal.
• Warn the patient/family not to spill Viokase powder on the hands because it may irritate skin.
• Instruct the patient/family to avoid inhaling powder because it may irritate mucous membranes and produce bronchospasm.

Simethicone

sye-**meth**-ih-cone
(Alka-Seltzer Gas Relief, Gas-X, Genasym, Maalox AntiGas, Mylanta Gas, Ovol [CAN], Phazyme)

CATEGORY AND SCHEDULE

Pregnancy Risk Category: C
OTC

MECHANISM OF ACTION

An antiflatulent that changes surface tension of gas bubbles, allowing easier elimination of gas. ***Therapeutic Effect:*** Disperses, prevents formation of gas pockets in the GI tract.

PHARMACOKINETICS

Does not appear to be absorbed from GI tract. Excreted unchanged in feces.

AVAILABILITY

Softgel: 125 mg, 180 mg.
Oral Suspension Drops: 40 mg/0.6 mL.
Tablets (chewable): 80 mg, 125 mg.

INDICATIONS AND DOSAGES

▸ Antiflatulent

PO

Children older than 12 yrs. 40–125 mg after meals and at bedtime. Maximum: 500 mg/day.
Children 2–12 yrs. 40 mg 4 times/day.
Children younger than 2 yrs. 20 mg 4 times/day.

UNLABELED USES

Adjunct to bowel radiography and gastroscopy.

CONTRAINDICATIONS

Hypersensitivity to simethicone or any related component.

INTERACTIONS

Drug

None known.

Herbal

None known.

Food

None known.

DIAGNOSTIC TEST EFFECTS

None known.

SIDE EFFECTS

None known.

SERIOUS REACTIONS

None known.

PEDIATRIC CONSIDERATIONS

Baseline Assessment

• Before administration, assess the patient's abdomen for signs of tenderness or rigidity and the presence of bowel sounds.

• Determine when the patient last had a bowel movement, and find out the amount and consistency.
• Be aware that it is unknown whether simethicone crosses the placenta or is distributed in breast milk.
• This drug may be used safely in children.

Administration and Handling

PO
• Give simethicone after meals and at bedtime as needed. Chew tablets thoroughly before swallowing.
• Shake suspension well before using.

Intervention and Evaluation

• Evaluate the patient for a therapeutic response manifested as relief of abdominal bloating and flatulence.

Patient/Family Teaching

• Urge the patient/family to avoid carbonated beverages during simethicone therapy.
• Instruct the patient/family to chew tablets thoroughly before swallowing.

REFERENCES

Miller, S. & Fioravanti, J. (1997). Pediatric medications: a handbook for nurses. St. Louis: Mosby.

Taketomo, C. K., Hodding, J. H. & Kraus, D. M. (2003–2004). Pediatric dosage handbook (10th ed.). Hudson, OH: Lexi-Comp.

53 Anticoagulants

Enoxaparin Sodium
Heparin Sodium
Warfarin Sodium

Uses: Subclasses of anticoagulants have somewhat different indications. *Heparin* is used to treat pulmonary embolism, evolving stroke, and massive deep vein thrombosis (DVT). It is also used as an adjunct to thrombolytics to treat acute myocardial infarction (MI) and in low doses to prevent postoperative venous thrombosis. *Low-molecular-weight (LMW) heparins* are used to prevent DVT after hip or knee replacement surgery and to treat DVT, ischemic stroke, pulmonary embolism, and non–Q-wave MI. *Thrombin inhibitors* are prescribed for preventing and treating thrombosis in heparin-induced thrombocytopenia (HIT) and for preventing HIT during percutaneous coronary procedures. *Warfarin* is used to prevent venous thrombosis and associated pulmonary embolism.

Action: Each anticoagulant subclass acts by a different mechanism. *Heparin* combines with antithrombin III, accelerating the anticoagulant cascade that prevents thrombosis formation. (See illustration, *Sites and Mechanisms of Action: Hematologic Agents,* page 642.) It inhibits the action of thrombin and factor Xa. By preventing the conversion of fibrinogen to fibrin, heparin prevents the formation of fibrin clots. *LMW heparins,* such as enoxaparin, are composed of shorter molecules than those in standard heparin.

Enoxaparin Sodium

en-**ox**-ah-pear-in
(Klexane [CAN], Lovenox)
Do not confuse with Lotronex.

CATEGORY AND SCHEDULE

Pregnancy Risk Category: B

MECHANISM OF ACTION

A low-molecular-weight heparin that potentiates the action of antithrombin III and inactivates coagulation factor Xa. ***Therapeutic Effect:*** Produces anticoagulation. Does not significantly influence bleeding time, prothrombin time, or activated partial thromboplastin time (aPTT).

PHARMACOKINETICS

Route	Onset	Peak	Duration
SC	N/A	3–5 hrs	12 hrs

Well absorbed after SC administration. Eliminated

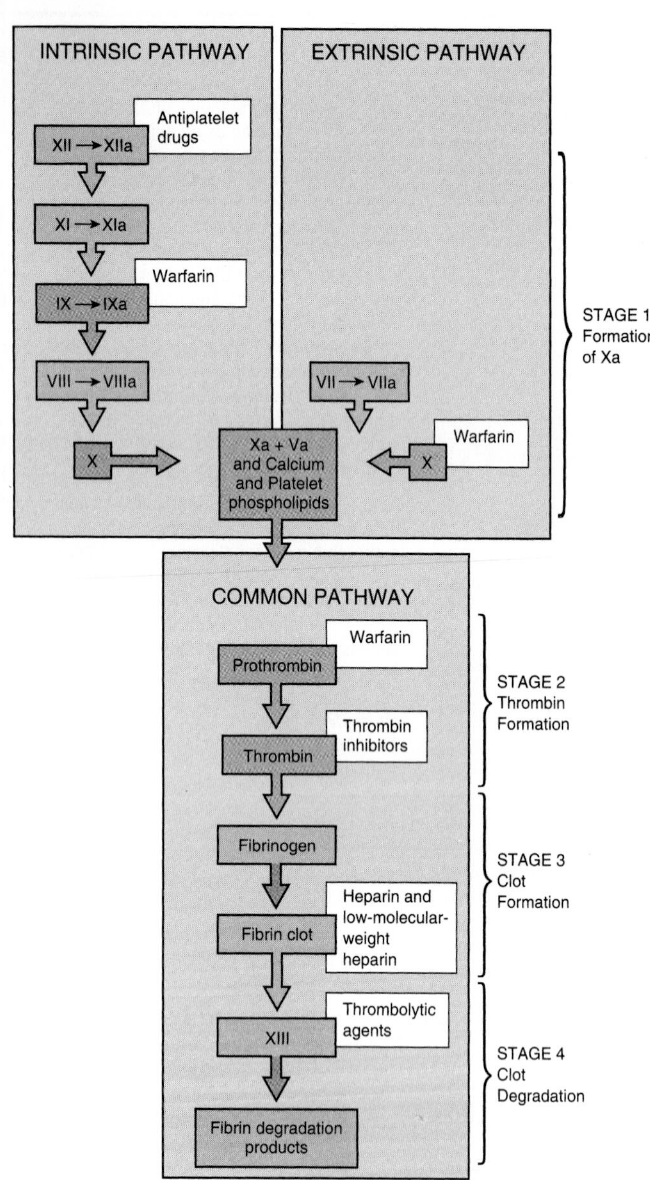
INTRINSIC PATHWAY
EXTRINSIC PATHWAY
Antiplatelet drugs
XII → XIIa
XI → XIa
Warfarin
IX → IXa
VIII → VIIIa
X
VII → VIIa
Warfarin
X
Xa + Va and Calcium and Platelet phospholipids
STAGE 1 Formation of Xa
COMMON PATHWAY
Warfarin
Prothrombin
Thrombin inhibitors
Thrombin
STAGE 2 Thrombin Formation
Fibrinogen
Heparin and low-molecular-weight heparin
Fibrin clot
STAGE 3 Clot Formation
Thrombolytic agents
XIII
Fibrin degradation products
STAGE 4 Clot Degradation

Sites and Mechanisms of Action: Hematologic Agents

Hemostasis causes the formation of a fibrin-platelet meshwork (clot) to stop bleeding. It results from activation of the coagulation cascade, which consists of intrinsic, extrinsic, and common pathways. Drugs that affect hemostasis include anticoagulants and antiplatelets (which prevent clot formation) and thrombolytics (which dissolve already formed clots).

Different anticoagulants act at various points in the cascade. For example, heparin enhances antithrombin III in the plasma to inactivate factor Xa. As a result, prothrombin cannot be converted to thrombin, which prevents fibrinogen from forming fibrin, a major clot component. Low-molecular-weight heparins also inactivate factor Xa and thrombin by enhancing antithrombin III, ultimately preventing fibrinogen from forming fibrin. Thrombin inhibitors, reversibly inhibit thrombin by binding to its receptor sites. This action prevents the conversion of fibrinogen to a fibrin clot. Warfarin depletes vitamin K–dependent factors X, IX, VII, and prothrombin. Consequently new clots cannot form, and preexisting clots cannot extend.

Antiplatelet drugs inhibit platelet aggregation—and clotting—in different ways. Platelet aggregation and adhesion starts at the beginning of the clotting cascade that ultimately results in inactivated factor X. Aspirin inhibits cyclooxygenase and blocks the production of thromboxane A_2, a substance that causes vasoconstriction and platelet aggregation. Adenosine diphosphate (ADP) receptor antagonists block ADP receptors on platelets, inhibiting their aggregation. Glycoprotein (GP) IIb/IIIa receptor inhibitors prevent fibrinogen from binding to GP IIb/IIIa receptors on platelets, rapidly inhibiting platelet aggregation.

Thrombolytic agents, such as streptokinase, break down clots that have already formed. They trigger the conversion of plasminogen to plasmin, an enzyme that dissolves fibrin clots into fibrin degradation products.

---

primarily in urine. Not removed by hemodialysis. ***Half-Life:*** 4.5 hrs in adults.

AVAILABILITY

Injection: 30 mg/0.3 mL, 40 mg/0.4 mL, 60 mg/0.6 mL, 80 mg/0.8 mL, 100 mg/1 mL, 120 mg/0.8 mL, 150 mg/1 mL, prefilled syringes.

INDICATIONS AND DOSAGES

▸ Usual dosage for children

SC

Infants older than 2 mos and children younger than 18 yrs. 0.5 mg/kg q12h (prophylaxis); 1 mg/kg q12h (treatment).

Infants younger than 2 mos. 0.75 mg/kg q12h (prophylaxis); 1.5 mg/kg q12h (treatment).

▸ Dosage in renal impairment

Clearance decreased when creatinine clearance is less than 30 mL/min. Monitor antifactor Xa activity; adjust dosage.

UNLABELED USES

Prevents DVT after general surgical procedures.

CONTRAINDICATIONS

Hypersensitivity to enoxaparin or any related component. Active major bleeding, concurrent heparin therapy, hypersensitivity to heparin or pork products, thrombocytopenia associated with positive in vitro test for antiplatelet antibody.

INTERACTIONS

Drug

Anticoagulants, platelet inhibitors: May increase bleeding.

Herbal

None known.

Food
None known.

DIAGNOSTIC TEST EFFECTS
Reversible increases in lactate dehydrogenase, serum alkaline phosphatase, SGOT (AST), and SGPT (ALT) levels.

SIDE EFFECTS
Occasional (4%–1%)
Injection site hematoma, nausea, peripheral edema

SERIOUS REACTIONS
! Accidental overdosage may lead to bleeding complications ranging from local ecchymoses to major hemorrhage. Antidote: Protamine sulfate (1% solution) should be equal to the dose of enoxaparin injected. One mg protamine sulfate neutralizes 1 mg enoxaparin. A second dose of 0.5 mg/mg protamine sulfate may be given if aPTT tested 2–4 hrs after the first injection remains prolonged.

PEDIATRIC CONSIDERATIONS
Baseline Assessment
- Assess the patient's complete blood count (CBC).
- Examine the patient's list of allergies, especially to heparin or pork products.
- Be aware that enoxaparin should be used with caution in pregnant women, particularly during the last trimester of pregnancy and immediately postpartum. Enoxaparin use increases the risk of maternal hemorrhage.
- Be aware that it is unknown whether enoxaparin is excreted in breast milk.
- Be aware that the safety and efficacy of enoxaparin have not been established in children.

Precautions
- Use cautiously in pts with conditions with increased risk of hemorrhage, a history of recent GI ulceration and hemorrhage, a history of heparin-induced thrombocytopenia, impaired renal function, and uncontrolled arterial hypertension.

Administration and Handling
◀ **ALERT** ▶ Do not mix with other injections or infusions. Do not give IM.
◀ **ALERT** ▶ Give initial dose as soon as possible after surgery but not more than 24 hrs after surgery.
SC
- The parenteral form normally appears clear and colorless to pale yellow.
- Store at room temperature.
- Instruct the patient to lie down before administering by deep SC injection.
- Inject between left and right anterolateral and left and right posterolateral abdominal wall.
- Introduce the entire length of the needle (½ inch) into a skin fold held between the thumb and forefinger, holding the skin fold during injection.

Intervention and Evaluation
- Periodically monitor the patient's CBC and stool for occult blood; there is no need for daily monitoring in pts with normal presurgical coagulation parameters.
- Assess the patient for any sign of bleeding, including bleeding at injection or surgical sites, bleeding from gums, blood in stool, bruising, hematuria, and petechiae.

Patient/Family Teaching
- Tell the patient/family that the usual length of therapy is 7–10 days.
- Instruct the patient/family to let you know if the patient experi-

ences bleeding from the surgical site, chest pain, or dyspnea.

- Tell the patient/family to use an electric razor and soft toothbrush to prevent bleeding during enoxaparin therapy.
- Explain to the patient/family that the patient should not take any medications, including OTC drugs, especially aspirin, without consulting the physician.
- Warn the patient/family to notify you if the patient experiences black or red stool, coffee-ground vomitus, dark or red urine, or red-speckled mucus from cough.
- Tell female pts that their menstrual flow may be heavier than usual.

Heparin Sodium

hep-ah-rin

(Hepalean [CAN], Heparin injection B.P. [AUS], Heparin Leo, Uniparin [AUS])

Do not confuse with Hespan.

CATEGORY AND SCHEDULE

Pregnancy Risk Category: C

MECHANISM OF ACTION

A blood modifier that interferes with blood coagulation by blocking conversion of prothrombin to thrombin and fibrinogen to fibrin. ***Therapeutic Effect:*** Prevents further extension of existing thrombi or new clot formation. No effect on existing clots.

PHARMACOKINETICS

Erratically absorbed after SC and IM administration. Protein binding: Very high. Does not cross the placenta or appear in breast milk. Metabolized in liver and removed from circulation via uptake by reticuloendothelial system. Primarily excreted in urine. Not removed by hemodialysis. ***Half-Life:*** 1–6 hrs, affected by renal/hepatic function, malignancy, infections, and obesity.

AVAILABILITY

Injection: 10 units/mL, 100 units/mL, 1,000 units/mL, 2,500 units/mL, 5,000 units/mL, 7,500 units/mL, 10,000 units/mL, 20,000 units/mL, 40,000 units/mL, 25,000 units/500 mL infusion.

INDICATIONS AND DOSAGES

▸ **Line flushing**

IV

Children. 100 units q6–8h.

Infants weighing less than 10 kg. 10 units q6–8h.

▸ **Prophylaxis of venous thrombosis, pulmonary embolism, peripheral arterial embolism, atrial fibrillation with embolism**

INTERMITTENT IV

Children older than 1 yr. Initially, 50–100 units/kg, then 50–100 units q4h.

IV INFUSION

Children older than 1 yr. Loading dose: 75 units/kg over 10 min, then 20 units/kg/hr with adjustments according to activated partial thromboplastin time (aPTT).

Children younger than 1 yr. Loading dose: 75 units/kg over 10 min, then 28 units/kg/hr with adjustments according to APPT.

CONTRAINDICATIONS

Hypersensitivity to heparin or any related component. Intracranial hemorrhage, severe hypotension, severe thrombocytopenia, subacute bacterial endocarditis, uncontrolled bleeding.

INTERACTIONS

Drug

Anticoagulants, platelet aggregation inhibitors, thrombolytics: May increase the risk of bleeding.
Antithyroid medications, cefoperazone, cefotetan, valproic acid: May cause hypoprothrombinemia.
Probenecid: May increase the effects of heparin.

Herbal

Feverfew, ginkgo biloba: May have additive effect.

Food

None known.

DIAGNOSTIC TEST EFFECTS

May increase free fatty acid, SGOT (AST), and SGPT (ALT) levels. May decrease serum cholesterol and triglyceride levels.

IV INCOMPATIBILITIES

Amiodarone (Cordarone), amphotericin B complex (Abelcet, AmBisome, Amphotec), ciprofloxacin (Cipro), dacarbazine (DTIC), diazepam (Valium), dobutamine (Dobutrex), doxorubicin (Adriamycin), droperidol (Inapsine), filgrastim (Neupogen), gentamicin (Garamycin), haloperidol (Haldol), idarubicin (Idamycin), labetalol (Trandate), nicardipine (Cardene), phenytoin (Dilantin), quinidine, tobramycin (Nebcin), vancomycin (Vancocin)

IV COMPATIBILITIES

Aminophylline, ampicillin/sulbactam (Unasyn), aztreonam (Azactam), calcium gluconate, cefazolin (Ancef), ceftazidime (Fortaz), ceftriaxone (Rocephin), digoxin (Lanoxin), diltiazem (Cardizem), dopamine (Intropin), enalapril (Vasotec), famotidine (Pepcid), fentanyl (Sublimaze), furosemide (Lasix), hydromorphone (Dilaudid), insulin, lidocaine, lorazepam (Ativan), magnesium sulfate, methylprednisolone (Solu-Medrol), midazolam (Versed), milrinone (Primacor), morphine, nitroglycerin, norepinephrine (Levophed), oxytocin (Pitocin), piperacillin/tazobactam (Zosyn), procainamide (Pronestyl), propofol (Diprivan)

SIDE EFFECTS

Occasional

Itching, burning, particularly on soles of feet, caused by vasospastic reaction

Rare

Pain, cyanosis of extremity 6–10 days after initial therapy, lasts 4–6 hrs; hypersensitivity reaction, including chills, fever, pruritus, urticaria, asthma, rhinitis, lacrimation, and headache

SERIOUS REACTIONS

! Bleeding complications ranging from local ecchymoses to major hemorrhage occur more frequently with high-dose therapy, intermittent IV infusion, and in women older than 60 yrs of age.
! Antidote: Protamine sulfate 1–1.5 mg for every 100 units heparin SC if overdosage occurred before 30 min, 0.5–0.75 mg for every 100 units heparin SC if overdosage occurred within 30–60 min, 0.25–0.375 mg for every 100 units heparin SC if 2 hrs have elapsed since overdosage, or 25–50 mg if heparin given by IV infusion.

PEDIATRIC CONSIDERATIONS

Baseline Assessment

• Cross-check heparin dose with another nurse before administering to the patient. Determine the patient's aPTT before administering heparin, and 24 hrs after heparin therapy, then 24–48 hrs for the first week of heparin therapy or until the maintenance dose is established.

• Monitor the patient's aPTT 1–2 times/wk for 3–4 wks. In long-term therapy, monitor the patient's aPTT 1–2 times/mo.

• Be aware that heparin should be used with caution in pregnant women, particularly during the last trimester of pregnancy and immediately postpartum because heparin increases the risk of maternal hemorrhage.

• Be aware that heparin does not cross the placenta and is not distributed in breast milk.

• There are no age-related precautions noted in children.

• Be aware that the benzyl alcohol preservative may cause gasping syndrome in infants.

Precautions

• Use cautiously in pts receiving IM injections, peptic ulcer disease, or severe liver or renal disease, in those who have had recent invasive or surgical procedures, and in women during menstruation.

Administration and Handling

◂ **ALERT** ▸ Do not give by IM injection because it may cause pain, hematoma, ulceration, and erythema.

SC

◂ **ALERT** ▸ Keep in mind that the SC route is used for low-dose therapy.

• After withdrawing heparin from the vial, change the needle before injection to prevent leakage along the needle track.

• Inject the heparin dose above the iliac crest or in the abdominal fat layer. Do not inject within 2 in of the umbilicus or any scar tissue.

• Withdraw the needle rapidly and apply prolonged pressure at the injection site without massaging. Rotate injection sites.

IV

◂ **ALERT** ▸ Be aware that continuous IV therapy is preferred because intermittent IV therapy produces a higher incidence of bleeding abnormalities.

• Store at room temperature.

• Dilute IV infusion in isotonic sterile saline, D_5W, or lactated Ringer's solution.

• Invert the IV bag at least 6 times to ensure mixing and to prevent pooling of the medication.

• Use a constant-rate IV infusion pump.

Intervention and Evaluation

• Monitor the patient's aPTT diligently. The therapeutic heparin dosage causes an aPTT of 1.5–2.5 times normal.

• Assess the patient's Hct, platelet count, SGOT (AST) and SGPT (ALT) levels, and stool and urine cultures for occult blood, regardless of route of administration.

• Determine the patient's discharge during menses and monitor for an increase.

• Assess the patient's gums for erythema and gingival bleeding, skin for bruises or petechiae, and urine for hematuria.

• Examine the patient for excessive bleeding from minor cuts and scratches.

• Evaluate the patient for abdominal or back pain, a decrease in blood pressure, an increase in pulse rate, and severe headache, which may be evidence of hemorrhage.

• Check the patient's peripheral pulses for loss of peripheral circulation.

• Avoid giving IM injections of other medications to the patient because of the potential for hematomas.

• When converting to Coumadin therapy, monitor the patient's prothrombin time (PT) results, as ordered. Keep in mind that the PT will be 10%–20% higher while heparin is given concurrently.

Patient/Family Teaching

• Tell the patient/family to use an electric razor and soft toothbrush to prevent bleeding during heparin therapy.
• Explain to the patient/family that the patient should not take any medications, including OTC drugs, without consulting the physician.
• Warn the patient/family to notify the physician if the patient experiences black or red stool, coffee-ground vomitus, dark or red urine, or red-speckled mucus from cough.
• Suggest to the patient/family that the patient should carry or wear identification noting he or she is receiving anticoagulant therapy.
• Stress to the patient/family that the patient should inform his or her dentist and other physicians of heparin therapy.

Warfarin Sodium

war-fair-in
(Coumadin, Marevan [AUS], Warfilone [CAN])
Do not confuse with Kemadrin.

CATEGORY AND SCHEDULE

Pregnancy Risk Category: X

MECHANISM OF ACTION

A coumarin derivative that interferes with hepatic synthesis of vitamin K–dependent clotting factors, resulting in depletion of coagulation factors II, VII, IX, and X. ***Therapeutic Effect:*** Prevents further extension of formed existing clot; prevents new clot formation or secondary thromboembolic complications.

PHARMACOKINETICS

Route	Onset	Peak	Duration
PO	1.5–3 days	5–7 days	N/A

Well absorbed from the GI tract. Metabolized in liver. Primarily excreted in urine. Not removed by hemodialysis. ***Half-Life:*** 1.5–2.5 days (varies by individual).

AVAILABILITY

Tablets: 1 mg, 2 mg, 2.5 mg, 3 mg, 4 mg, 5 mg, 6 mg, 7.5 mg, 10 mg.
Injection: 5-mg vials.

INDICATIONS AND DOSAGES

▸ Anticoagulant

PO

Children. Initially, 0.1–0.2 mg/kg (maximum 10 mg). Maintenance: 0.05–0.34 mg/kg/day. Dose is adjusted according to the desired international normalizing ratio (INR) for the patient.

UNLABELED USES

Prophylaxis against recurrent cerebral embolisms and myocardial reinfarction, treatment adjunct in transient ischemic attacks.

CONTRAINDICATIONS

Hypersensitivity to warfarin or any related component. Neurosurgical procedures, open wounds, pregnancy, severe hypertension, severe liver or renal damage, uncontrolled bleeding, ulcers.

INTERACTIONS

Drug

Acetaminophen, allopurinol, amiodarone, anabolic steroids, andro-

gens, aspirin, cefamandole, cefoperazone, chloral hydrate, chloramphenicol, cimetidine, clofibrate, danazol, dextrothyroxine, diflunisal, disulfiram, erythromycin, fenoprofen, gemfibrozil, indomethacin, methimazole, metronidazole, oral hypoglycemics, phenytoin, plicamycin, propylthiouracil, quinidine, salicylates, sulfinpyrazone, sulfonamides, sulindac: Warfarin increases the effects of aforementioned drugs.
Barbiturates, carbamazepine, cholestyramine, colestipol, estramustine, estrogens, griseofulvin, primidone, rifampin, vitamin K: Warfarin decreases the effects of aforementioned drugs.

Herbal

Feverfew, garlic, ginkgo biloba, ginseng: May increase the risk of bleeding.
St. John's wort, Coenzyme Q10: May decrease the effectiveness of warfarin.

Food

Vitamin K–containing foods: May decrease the anticoagulant effect of warfarin.

DIAGNOSTIC TEST EFFECTS

None known.

SIDE EFFECTS

Occasional

GI distress, such as nausea, anorexia, abdominal cramps, and diarrhea

Rare

Hypersensitivity reaction, including dermatitis and urticaria, especially in those sensitive to aspirin

SERIOUS REACTIONS

! Bleeding complications ranging from local ecchymoses to major hemorrhage may occur. Drug should be discontinued immediately and vitamin K or phytonadione administered. Mild hemorrhage: 2.5–10 mg PO/IM/IV. Severe hemorrhage: 10–15 mg IV and repeated q4h, as necessary.
! Hepatotoxicity, blood dyscrasias, necrosis, vasculitis, and local thrombosis occur rarely.

PEDIATRIC CONSIDERATIONS

Baseline Assessment

- Cross-check warfarin dose with another nurse before administering the drug to the patient.
- Determine the patient's INR before administration and daily after therapy initiation. When stabilized, follow with INR determination every 4–6 wks.
- Be aware that warfarin use is contraindicated in pregnancy because it will cause fetal and neonatal hemorrhage and intrauterine death.
- Be aware that warfarin crosses the placenta and is distributed in breast milk.
- Be aware that children are more susceptible to the effects of warfarin.

Precautions

- Use cautiously in pts at risk for hemorrhage and pts with active tuberculosis, diabetes, gangrene, heparin-induced thrombocytopenia, and necrosis.

Administration and Handling

◂ **ALERT** ▸ Remember that the dosage is highly individualized, based on prothrombin time and INR.

PO

- Crush scored tablets as needed.
- Give warfarin without regard to food. If GI upset occurs, give with food.

Intervention and Evaluation

- Monitor the patient's INR reports diligently.
- Assess the patient's Hct, platelet count, SGOT (AST) and SGPT (ALT) levels, and stool and urine cultures for occult blood, regardless of route of administration.
- Evaluate the patient for abdominal or back pain, a decrease in blood pressure, an increase in pulse rate, and severe headache because these may be a sign of hemorrhage.
- Determine the patient's discharge during menses and monitor for an increase.
- Assess the patient's area of thromboembolus for color and temperature.
- Check the patient's peripheral pulses.
- Assess the patient's gums for erythema and gingival bleeding, skin for bruises and petechiae, and urine for hematuria.
- Examine the patient for excessive bleeding from minor cuts or scratches.

Patient/Family Teaching

- Instruct the patient/family to take warfarin exactly as prescribed.
- Caution the patient/family against taking or discontinuing any other medication except on the advice of the physician.
- Urge the patient/family to avoid alcohol, drastic dietary changes, and salicylates.
- Teach the patient/family not to change from one brand of the drug to another.
- Instruct the patient/family to consult the physician before having dental work or surgery.
- Explain to the patient/family that the patient's urine may become red-orange.
- Tell the patient/family to use an electric razor and soft toothbrush to prevent bleeding during warfarin therapy.
- Explain to the patient/family that the patient should not take any medications, including OTC drugs, without consulting the physician.
- Warn the patient/family to notify the physician if the patient experiences black stool, bleeding, brown, dark, or red urine, coffee-ground vomitus, or red-speckled mucus from cough.

REFERENCES

Taketomo, C. K., Hodding, J. H. & Kraus, D. M. (2003–2004). Pediatric dosage handbook (10th ed.). Hudson, OH: Lexi-Comp.

Factor VIII (Antihemophilic Factor, AHF)
Factor IX Complex

Uses: Antihemophilic agents are used to prevent or treat bleeding episodes in pts with hemophilia A, in which factor VIII activity is deficient, or hemophilia B (also called Christmas disease), in which factor IX complex activity is deficient.

Action: Antihemophilic agents promote hemostasis by activating the intrinsic or extrinsic pathway of the coagulation cascade. Factor VIII prevents bleeding by replacing this clotting factor, which is needed to transform prothrombin into thrombin. Factor IX complex raises the plasma level of factor IX, restoring hemostasis in pts with factor IX deficiency.

Antihemophilic Factor (Factor VIII, AHF)

(Alphanate, Hyate, Bioclate, Humate-P, Kogenate, Monoclate-P)

CATEGORY AND SCHEDULE

Pregnancy Risk Category: C

MECHANISM OF ACTION

An antihemophilic agent that assists in conversion of prothrombin to thrombin, essential for blood coagulation, Replaces missing clotting factor. ***Therapeutic Effect:*** Produces hemostasis, corrects or prevents bleeding episodes.

AVAILABILITY

Injection: Actual number of antihemolytic factor units listed on each vial.

INDICATIONS AND DOSAGES

▸ **Prevention and treatment of bleeding in pts with hemophilia A factor XIII deficiency, hypofibrinogenemia, von Willebrand disease**

Dosage is highly individualized, based on patient weight, severity of bleeding, coagulation studies.

UNLABELED USES

Treatment of disseminated intravascular coagulation.

CONTRAINDICATIONS

Hypersensitivity to any component. Hypersensitivity to mouse protein (Hemofil M, Monarc M, Monoclate-P).

INTERACTIONS

Drug

None known.

Herbal

None known.

Food

None known.

DIAGNOSTIC TEST EFFECTS

None known.

IV INCOMPATIBILITIES

Do not mix with other IV solutions or medications.

SIDE EFFECTS

Occasional

Allergic reaction, including fever, chills, urticaria, wheezing, slight hypotension, nausea, and a feeling of chest tightness, stinging at injection site, dizziness, dry mouth, headache, unpleasant taste

SERIOUS REACTIONS

! There is a risk of transmitting viral hepatitis.

! Possibility of intravascular hemolysis occurring if large or frequent doses used with blood group A, B, or AB.

PEDIATRIC CONSIDERATIONS

Baseline Assessment

- Avoid overinflation of cuff when monitoring the patient's blood pressure (B/P). Take blood pressure manually, avoiding automatic blood pressure cuffs.
- Remove adhesive tape from any pressure dressing on the patient very carefully and slowly.

Precautions

- Use cautiously in pts with liver disease and in pts with blood type A, B, or AB. If large doses are given to pts with these blood types, expect to monitor the blood hematocrit and direct Coombs' test results to check for hemolytic anemia. If hemolytic anemia occurs, expect to give transfusions with type O blood.

Administration and Handling

IV

- Refer to individual vials for specific storage requirements.
- Warm concentrate and diluent to room temperature.
- Gently agitate or rotate to dissolve. Do not shake vigorously. Complete dissolution may take 5–10 min.
- Filter before administration.
- Administer IV at rate of approximately 2 mL/min. Can give up to 10 mL/min.

Intervention and Evaluation

- Monitor the patient's IV site for oozing.
- Assess the patient for allergic reactions.
- Assess the patient's urine for hematuria.
- Monitor the patient's vital signs.
- Assess the patient for complaints of abdominal or back pain or severe headache, a decrease in B/P, and an increase in pulse rate.
- Determine whether the patient has an increase in the amount of discharge during menses.
- Assess the patient's skin for bruises and petechiae.
- Examine the patient for excessive bleeding from minor cuts or scratches.
- Assess the patient's gums for erythema and gingival bleeding.
- Evaluate the patient for therapeutic reduction of swelling and restricted joint movement and relief of pain.

Patient/Family Teaching

- Tell the patient/family to use an electric razor and soft toothbrush to prevent bleeding.
- Warn the patient/family to notify the physician if the patient experiences any sign of black or red stool, coffee-ground emesis, dark or red urine, or red-speckled mucus from cough.

Factor IX Complex

Benefix, Proplex T, Konyne

CATEGORY AND SCHEDULE

Pregnancy Risk Category: C

MECHANISM OF ACTION

A blood modifier that raises plasma levels of factor IX and restores hemostasis in pts with factor IX deficiency. ***Therapeutic Effect:*** Increases blood clotting factors II, VII, IX, and X.

AVAILABILITY

Injection: Number of units indicated on each vial.

INDICATIONS AND DOSAGES

▸ Reversal of anticoagulant effect of coumarin anticoagulants, treatment of bleeding caused by hemophilia B, treatment of bleeding in pts with hemophilia A who have factor VIII inhibitors

Amount of factor IX required is individualized. Dosage depends on degree of deficiency, level of each factor desired, weight of patient, and severity of bleeding.

CONTRAINDICATIONS

Sensitivity to mouse protein.

INTERACTIONS

Drug

Aminocaproic acid: May increase the risk of thrombosis.

Herbal

None known.

Food

None known.

DIAGNOSTIC TEST EFFECTS

None known.

IV INCOMPATIBILITIES

Do not mix with any other medications.

SIDE EFFECTS

Rare

Mild hypersensitivity reaction, marked by, fever, chills, a change in blood pressure (B/P) and pulse rate, rash, and urticaria

SERIOUS REACTIONS

! High risk of venous thrombosis during postoperative period.

! Acute hypersensitivity reaction or anaphylactic reaction may occur.

! Risk of transmitting viral hepatitis and other viral diseases.

PEDIATRIC CONSIDERATIONS

Baseline Assessment

• Assess the results of the patient's coagulation studies and the extent of existing bleeding, joint pain, overt bleeding or bruising, and swelling.

Precautions

• Use cautiously in pts with liver impairment, recent surgery, and sensitivity to factor IX.

Administration and Handling

IV

• Store in refrigerator.

• Know that reconstituted solution is stable for 12 hrs at room temperature.

• Begin administration within 3 hrs of reconstitution.

• Do not refrigerate reconstituted solution.

• Before reconstitution, warm diluent to room temperature.

• Gently agitate the vial until the powder is completely dissolved to prevent the removal of active components during administration through filter.

• Administer by slow IV push or IV infusion.

• Filter before administration.

• Infuse slowly, not to exceed 3 mL/min. Too rapid an IV infusion may produce a change in B/P and pulse rate, headache, flushing, and tingling sensation.

Intervention and Evaluation

• Monitor the patient's intake and output and vital signs.
• Assess the patient for a hypersensitivity reaction.
• Monitor the results of the patient's coagulation studies closely.
• Avoid IM or SC injections.
• Monitor the patient's IV site for oozing every 5–15 min for 1–2 hrs after administration.
• Report any evidence of hematuria or change in the patient's vital signs immediately.

Patient/Family Teaching

• Tell the patient/family to use an electric razor and soft toothbrush to prevent bleeding.
• Warn the patient/family to notify the physician if the patient experiences any sign of black or red stool, coffee-ground emesis, dark or red urine, and red-speckled mucus from cough.
• Caution the patient/family against using OTC medications without physician approval.
• Instruct the patient/family to carry identification that indicates the patient's condition or disease.

55 Antiplatelet Agents

Aspirin
Dipyridamole

Uses: Most antiplatelet agents are used to prevent myocardial infarction (MI) or stroke, repeat MI, and stroke in pts with transient ischemic attacks. The glycoprotein IIb/IIIa receptor inhibitors are used to prevent ischemic events in pts with acute coronary syndrome and those undergoing percutaneous coronary intervention.

Action: Antiplatelet drugs inhibit platelet aggregation by different mechanisms. *Aspirin* irreversibly inhibits cyclooxygenase, thereby blocking the synthesis of thromboxane A_2.

COMBINATION PRODUCTS

AGGRENOX: dipyridamole/aspirin (an antiplatelet agent) 200 mg/25 mg.

ASPIRIN: see Central Nervous System Agents, Chapter 42.

Dipyridamole

die-pie-**rid**-ah-mole
(Apo-Dipyridamole [CAN], Novodipiradol [CAN], Persantin [AUS], Persantin 100 [AUS], Persantin SR [AUS], Persantine)
Do not confuse with Aggrastat, disopyramide, or Periactin.

CATEGORY AND SCHEDULE

Pregnancy Risk Category: B

MECHANISM OF ACTION

A blood modifier and platelet aggregation inhibitor that inhibits the activity of adenosine deaminase and phosphodiesterase, enzymes causing accumulation of adenosine and cyclic adenosine monophosphate. ***Therapeutic Effect:*** Inhibits platelet aggregation, may cause coronary vasodilation.

PHARMACOKINETICS

Slowly, variably absorbed from the GI tract. Widely distributed. Protein binding: 91%–99%. Metabolized in liver. Primarily eliminated via biliary excretion. ***Half-Life:*** 10–15 hrs.

AVAILABILITY

Tablets: 25 mg, 50 mg, 75 mg.
Injection: 5 mg/mL.

INDICATIONS AND DOSAGES

▸ **Prevention of thromboembolic disorders**
PO
Children. 3–6 mg/kg/day in 3 divided doses.

▸ **Investigational use to treat proteinuria**
PO
Children. 4–10 mg/kg/day.

UNLABELED USES

Prophylaxis of myocardial reinfarction, treatment of transient ischemic attacks.

CONTRAINDICATIONS

Hypersensitivity to dipyridamole or any related component.

INTERACTIONS

Drug

Anticoagulants, aspirin, heparin, salicylates, thrombolytics: May increase the risk of bleeding with anticoagulants, aspirin, heparin, salicylates, and thrombolytics.

Herbal

None known.

Food

None known.

DIAGNOSTIC TEST EFFECTS

None known.

IV INCOMPATIBILITIES

No information available via Y-site administration.

SIDE EFFECTS

Frequent (14%)
Dizziness

Occasional (6%–2%)
Abdominal distress, headache, rash

Rare (less than 2%)
Diarrhea, vomiting, flushing, pruritus

SERIOUS REACTIONS

! Overdosage produces peripheral vasodilation, resulting in hypotension.

PEDIATRIC CONSIDERATIONS

Baseline Assessment

- Assess the patient for chest pain.
- Obtain the patient's baseline blood pressure (B/P) and pulse.
- When used as an antiplatelet, check the patient's hematologic laboratory levels.
- Be aware that dipyridamole is distributed in breast milk.
- Be aware that the safety and efficacy of dipyridamole have not been established in children.

Precautions

- Use cautiously in pts with hypotension.

Administration and Handling

PO

- Give when patient has an empty stomach with a full glass of water.

IV

- Dilute to at least 1:2 ratio with 0.9% NaCl or D_5W for a total volume of 20–50 mL because undiluted solution may cause irritation.
- Infuse over 4 min.
- Inject thallium within 5 min after dipyridamole infusion, as prescribed.

Intervention and Evaluation

- Assist the patient with ambulation if he or she experiences dizziness.
- Monitor the patient's heart sounds by auscultation.
- Assess the patient's B/P for hypotension.
- Examine the patient's skin for erythema and rash.

Patient/Family Teaching

- Urge the patient/family to avoid alcohol during dipyridamole therapy.
- Suggest dry toast and unsalted crackers to the patient to relieve nausea.
- Tell the patient/family that the therapeutic response may not be achieved before 2–3 months of continuous therapy.
- Warn the patient/family to use caution when getting up suddenly from a lying or sitting position.

REFERENCES

Taketomo, C. K., Hodding, J. H. & Kraus, D. M. (2003–2004). Pediatric dosage handbook (10th ed.). Hudson, OH: Lexi-Comp.

56 Hematinics

Ferrous Fumarate, Ferrous Gluconate, Ferrous Sulfate
Iron Dextran

Uses: Hematinics (iron supplements) are used to prevent and treat iron deficiency, which may result from improper diet, pregnancy, impaired absorption, or prolonged blood loss.

Action: Hematinics provide supplementary iron to ensure adequate supplies for the formation of hemoglobin, which is needed for erythropoiesis and oxygen transport.

COMBINATION PRODUCTS

FERRO-SEQUELS: ferrous fumarate/docusate (a stool softener) 150 mg/100 mg.

Ferrous Fumarate

fair-us **fume**-ah-rate
(Feostat, Femiron, Palafer [CAN])

Ferrous Gluconate

fair-us **glue**-kuh-nate
(Apo-Ferrous Gluconate [CAN], Fergon, Ferralet, Simron)

Ferrous Sulfate

fair-us **sul**-fate
(Apo-Ferrous Sulfate [CAN], Feosol, Fer-In-Sol, Ferro-Gradumet [AUS], Slow-Fe)

CATEGORY AND SCHEDULE

Pregnancy Risk Category: A
OTC

MECHANISM OF ACTION

An enzymatic mineral that acts as an essential component in the formation of Hgb, myoglobin, and enzymes. ***Therapeutic Effect:*** Necessary for effective erythropoiesis and for transport and utilization of O_2.

PHARMACOKINETICS

Absorbed in duodenum and upper jejunum; 10% absorbed in those with normal iron stores, increased to 20%–30% in those with inadequate iron stores. Primarily bound to serum transferrin. Excreted in urine, sweat, and sloughing of intestinal mucosa and by menses. ***Half-Life:*** 6 hrs.

AVAILABILITY

Ferrous fumarate (33% elemental iron)
Tablets: 200 mg, 324 mg, 325 mg, 350 mg.
Tablets (chewable): 100 mg.
Tablets (controlled release): 150 mg.
Suspension: 100 mg/ 5 mL.
Ferrous gluconate (12% elemental iron)
Tablets: 240 mg, 246 mg, 300 mg, 325 mg.
Ferrous sulfate (20% elemental iron)
Tablets: 300 mg, 324 mg, 325 mg.
Elixir: 220 mg/5 mL.
Oral Drops: 75 mg/0.6 mL.
Ferrous sulfate exsiccated (30% of elemental iron)
Tablets: 200 mg.
Tablets (slow release): 160 mg.

INDICATIONS AND DOSAGES

▸ **Iron deficiency**
PO
Children. 3–6 mg/kg/day elemental iron in 1–3 divided doses.

▸ **Prophylaxis, iron deficiency**
PO
Children. 1–2 mg/kg/day elemental iron. Maximum: 15 mg elemental iron/day.

CONTRAINDICATIONS

Hypersensitivity to iron salts or any related component. Hemochromatosis, hemosiderosis, hemolytic anemias, peptic ulcer, regional enteritis, ulcerative colitis.

INTERACTIONS

Drug

Antacids, calcium supplements, pancreatin, pancrelipase: May decrease the absorption of ferrous fumarate, ferrous gluconate, and ferrous sulfate.
Etidronate, quinolones, tetracyclines: May decrease the absorption of etidronate, quinolones, and tetracyclines.

Herbal

None known.

Food

Eggs, cereals, dietary fiber, tea, coffee, milk: Inhibit ferrous fumarate absorption.

DIAGNOSTIC TEST EFFECTS

May increase serum bilirubin. May decrease serum calcium levels. May obscure occult blood in stools.

SIDE EFFECTS

Occasional
Mild, transient nausea
Rare
Heartburn, anorexia, constipation or diarrhea

SERIOUS REACTIONS

! Large doses may aggravate existing GI tract disease, such as peptic ulcer disease, regional enteritis, and ulcerative colitis.
! Severe iron poisoning occurs mostly in children and is manifested as vomiting, severe abdominal pain, diarrhea, dehydration, followed by hyperventilation, pallor or cyanosis, and cardiovascular collapse.

PEDIATRIC CONSIDERATIONS

Baseline Assessment

• Use dropper or straw and allow the drug solution to drop on the back of the patient's tongue to prevent mucous membrane and teeth staining with liquid preparation.
• Know that eggs and milk inhibit drug absorption.
• Be aware that ferrous fumarate, ferrous sulfate, and ferrous gluconate cross the placenta and are distributed in breast milk.
• Keep medication out of reach of children. Overdosage can be fatal.
• There are no age-related precautions noted in children.

Precautions

• Use cautiously in pts with bronchial asthma and iron hypersensitivity.

Administration and Handling

◂**ALERT**▸ Keep in mind that dosage is expressed in terms of elemental iron. Elemental iron content for ferrous fumarate is 33% (99 mg iron/300 mg tablet); ferrous gluconate is 11.6% (35 mg iron/300 mg tablet); ferrous sulfate is 20% (60 mg iron/300 mg tablet).
PO
• Store all forms, including tablets, capsules, suspension, and drops at room temperature.
• Give between meals with water unless GI discomfort occurs; if so, give with meals.
• To avoid transient staining of mucous membranes and teeth, place liquid on back of tongue with dropper or straw.

• Avoid simultaneous administration of antacids or tetracycline.
• Do not crush sustained-release preparations.

Intervention and Evaluation

• Monitor the patient's blood Hgb, ferritin, reticulocyte count, serum iron level, and total iron-binding capacity.
• Assess the patient's daily pattern of bowel activity and stool consistency.
• Evaluate the patient for clinical improvement, and record relief of iron deficiency symptoms, fatigue, headache, irritability, pallor, and paresthesia of extremities.

Patient/Family Teaching

• Tell the patient/family that the patient's stools will darken in color.
• Teach the patient/family to take the drug after meals or with food if the patient experiences GI discomfort.
• Instruct the patient/family not to take the drug within 2 hrs of antacids because antacids prevent the absorption of this drug.
• Teach the patient/family not to take the drug with milk or eggs.

Iron Dextran

iron **dex**-tran
(Dexiron [CAN], INFeD, Infufer [CAN])

CATEGORY AND SCHEDULE

Pregnancy Risk Category: C

MECHANISM OF ACTION

A trace element and essential component of formation of Hgb. Necessary for effective erythropoiesis and O_2 transport capacity of blood. Serves as cofactor of several essential enzymes. ***Therapeutic Effect:*** Replenishes Hgb and depleted iron stores.

PHARMACOKINETICS

Readily absorbed after IM administration. Major portion of absorption occurs within 72 hrs; remainder within 3–4 wks. Iron is bound to protein to form hemosiderin, ferritin, or transferrin. No physiologic system of elimination. Small amounts lost daily in shedding of skin, hair, and nails and in feces, urine, and perspiration. Not dialyzable. ***Half-Life:*** 5–20 hrs.

AVAILABILITY

Injection: 50 mg/mL.

INDICATIONS AND DOSAGES

▸ Iron deficiency anemia (no blood loss)

IM/IV

Children. Weight (kg) × 4.5 (desired Hgb – patient's Hgb g%) = mg Fe. Maximum: 5 mg/kg or 100 mg for infants and children. Maximum daily IM dose: infants weighing less than 5 kg 25 mg; children weighing 5–10 kg 50 mg; children weighing more than 10 kg 100 mg.

CONTRAINDICATIONS

Hypersensitivity to iron dextran or any related component. All anemias except iron deficiency anemia, including pernicious, aplastic, normocytic, and refractory.

INTERACTIONS

Drug

None known.

Herbal

None known.

Food

None known.

DIAGNOSTIC TEST EFFECTS

None known.

IV INCOMPATIBILITIES

No information available via Y-site administration.

SIDE EFFECTS

Frequent

Allergic reaction, such as rash and itching, backache, muscle pain, chills, dizziness, headache, fever, nausea, vomiting, flushed skin, pain or redness at injection site, brown discoloration of skin, metallic taste

SERIOUS REACTIONS

! Anaphylaxis has occurred during the first few minutes after injection, causing death on rare occasions.

! Leukocytosis and lymphadenopathy occur rarely.

PEDIATRIC CONSIDERATIONS

Baseline Assessment

- Do not give concurrently with oral iron form because excessive iron may produce excessive iron storage, called hemosiderosis.
- Be alert to pts with rheumatoid arthritis or iron deficiency anemia as acute exacerbation of joint pain and swelling may occur.
- Know that inguinal lymphadenopathy may occur with IM injection.
- Assess the patient for adequate muscle mass before injecting medication.
- Be aware that iron dextran may cross the placenta in some form and trace amounts of the drug are distributed in breast milk.
- Use cautiously in children who have juvenile rheumatoid arthritis.
- Do not use with premature infants or infants younger than 4 mos of age.
- There are no age-related precautions noted in children.

Precautions

- Use extremely cautiously in pts with serious liver impairment.
- Use cautiously in pts with bronchial asthma, a history of allergies, and rheumatoid arthritis.

Administration and Handling

◂ALERT▸ Know that a test dose is generally given before the full dosage; stay with patient for several minutes after injection because of the potential for an anaphylactic reaction.

◂ALERT▸ Plan to discontinue the oral iron form before administering iron dextran. Know that the dosage is expressed in terms of milligrams of elemental iron, degree of anemia, patient weight, and the presence of any bleeding. Expect to use periodic hematologic determinations as guide to therapy.

IM

- Draw up medication with one needle; use a new needle for injection to minimize skin staining.
- Administer IM injection deep in the upper outer quadrant of buttock only.
- Use the Z-tract technique by displacing subcutaneous tissue lateral to injection site before inserting the needle to minimize skin staining.

IV

Store at room temperature.

- May give undiluted or dilute in 0.9% NaCl for infusion.
- Do not exceed IV administration rate of 50 mg/min (1 mL/min). A too rapid IV infusion rate may produce flushing, chest pain, shock, hypotension, and tachycardia.

- Keep patient recumbent for 30–45 minutes after IV administration to avoid postural hypotension.

Intervention and Evaluation

- Monitor the patient's IM site for abscess formation, atrophy, brownish skin color, necrosis, and swelling.
- Evaluate the patient for inflammation, pain, and soreness at or near the IM injection site.
- Examine the patient's IV site for phlebitis.
- Monitor the patient's serum ferritin levels.

Patient/Family Teaching

- Tell the patient/family that the patient may experience pain and brown staining of the skin at the injection site.
- Caution the patient/family that oral iron should not be taken when the patient is receiving iron injections.
- Instruct the patient/family that the patient's stools may become black with iron therapy. Explain that this side effect is harmless unless accompanied by abdominal cramping or pain, red streaking, and sticky consistency of stool.
- Warn the patient/family to notify the physician if the patient experiences abdominal cramping or pain, back pain, fever, headache, or red streaking or a sticky consistency of stool.
- Suggest gum, hard candy, and maintaining good oral hygiene to prevent or reduce the metallic taste.

REFERENCES

Miller, S. & Fioravanti, J. (1997). Pediatric medications: a handbook for nurses. St. Louis: Mosby.

57 Hematopoietic Agents

Epoetin Alfa
Filgrastim

Uses: Hematopoietic agents are used to accelerate neutrophil repopulation after cancer chemotherapy, to accelerate bone marrow recovery after autologous bone marrow transplant, and to stimulate erythrocyte production in pts with chronic renal failure.

Action: Hematopoietic agents act by stimulating the proliferation and differentiation of hematopoietic growth factors (naturally occurring hormones) and by enhancing the function of mature forms of neutrophils, monocytes, macrophages, and erythrocytes.

Epoetin Alfa

eh-po-ee-tin
(Epogen, Eprex [CAN], Procrit)
Do not confuse with Neupogen.

CATEGORY AND SCHEDULE

Pregnancy Risk Category: C

MECHANISM OF ACTION

A glycoprotein that stimulates division and differentiation of erythroid progenitor cells in bone marrow. ***Therapeutic Effect:*** Induces erythropoiesis, releases reticulocytes from marrow.

PHARMACOKINETICS

Well absorbed after SC administration. After administration, an increase in reticulocyte count is seen within 10 days; increases in blood Hgb and Hct and RBC count are seen within 2–6 wks. ***Half-Life:*** Neonates 11–17 hrs. Adults 4–13 hrs.

AVAILABILITY

Injection: 2,000 units/mL, 3,000 units/mL, 4,000 units/mL, 10,000 units/mL, 20,000 units/mL, 40,000 units/mL.

INDICATIONS AND DOSAGES

▸ **Chemotherapy pts**

IV/SC

Children. 150 units/kg/dose 3 times/wk. Maximum: 1,200 units/kg/wk.

▸ **Anemia of prematurity**

SC

Neonates. 25–100 units/kg/dose 3 times/wk or 100 units/kg/dose 5 times/wk or 200 units/kg/dose every other day for 10 doses.

UNLABELED USES

Prevents anemia in pts donating blood before elective surgery or autologous transfusion, treatment of anemia associated with neoplastic diseases.

CONTRAINDICATIONS

History of sensitivity to mammalian cell–derived products or human albumin, uncontrolled hypertension, neutropenia in newborns.

INTERACTIONS

Drug

Heparin: May need to increase heparin. An increase in RBC volume may enhance blood clotting.

Herbal
None known.
Food
None known.

DIAGNOSTIC TEST EFFECTS

May decrease bleeding time, iron concentration, and serum ferritin. May increase BUN, serum phosphorus, potassium, serum creatinine, serum uric acid, and sodium levels.

IV INCOMPATIBILITIES

Do not mix with any other medications.

SIDE EFFECTS

Cancer pts on chemotherapy
Frequent (20%–17%)
Fever, diarrhea, nausea, vomiting, edema
Occasional (13%–11%)
Asthenia (loss of strength, energy), shortness of breath, paresthesia
Rare (5%–3%)
Dizziness, trunk pain

SERIOUS REACTIONS

! Hypertensive encephalopathy, thrombosis, cerebrovascular accident, myocardial infarction, and seizures have occurred rarely.
! Hyperkalemia occurs occasionally in pts with chronic renal failure, usually in those who do not conform to medication compliance, dietary guidelines, and frequency of dialysis.

PEDIATRIC CONSIDERATIONS

Baseline Assessment
• Assess the patient's blood pressure (B/P) before giving the drug. Know that 80% of pts with chronic renal failure have a history of hypertension. Expect that B/P often rises during early therapy in pts with history of hypertension.
• Assess the patient's serum iron, keeping in mind that the transferrin saturation should be greater than 20%, and serum ferritin should be greater than 100 ng/mL, before and during therapy.
• Consider that all pts will eventually need supplemental iron therapy.
• Establish the patient's baseline complete blood count (CBC), and especially note the patient's blood Hct.
• Monitor the patient aggressively for increased B/P. Know that 25% of pts taking medication require antihypertensive therapy and dietary restrictions.
• Be aware that it is unknown whether epoetin alfa crosses the placenta or is distributed in breast milk.
• Be aware that the safety and efficacy of epoetin alfa have not been established in children younger than 12 years of age.
• Be aware that epoetin alfa therapy can lead to polycythemia if Hct is not monitored and dosage is adjusted as needed.
Precautions
• Use cautiously in pts with a history of seizures and known porphyria, an impairment of erythrocyte formation in bone marrow.
Administration and Handling
◂ **ALERT** ▸ Avoid excessive agitation of vial; do not shake because it can cause foaming.
◂ **ALERT** ▸ Be aware that pts receiving azidothymidine with serum erythropoietin levels greater than 500 milliunits are likely not to respond to therapy.

SC
Use 1 dose per vial; do not reenter vial. Discard unused portion.
May be mixed in a syringe with bacteriostatic 0.9% NaCl with benzyl alcohol 0.9% (Bacteriostatic Saline) at a 1:1 ratio. Know that benzyl alcohol acts as a local anesthetic and may reduce injection site discomfort.

IV

- Refrigerate vials. Vigorous shaking may denature medication, rendering it inactive.
- No reconstitution necessary.
- May be given as an IV bolus.

Intervention and Evaluation

- Monitor the patient's blood Hct level diligently. Reduce the drug dosage if the patient's Hct level increases more than 4 points in 2 weeks.
- Assess the patient's CBC routinely.
- Monitor the patient's body temperature, especially in cancer pts receiving chemotherapy and zidovudine-treated HIV pts, and BUN, phosphorus, potassium, serum creatinine, and serum uric acid levels, especially in pts with chronic renal failure.

Patient/Family Teaching

- Stress to the patient/family that frequent blood tests will be needed to determine the correct drug dosage.
- Warn the patient/family to notify the physician if the patient experiences severe headache.
- Caution the patient/family to avoid any potentially hazardous activity during the first 90 days of therapy as there is an increased risk of seizure development in renal pts during the first 90 days of epoetin alfa therapy.

Filgrastim

fill-grass-tim
(Neupogen)
Do not confuse with ezpogen and Nutramigen.

CATEGORY AND SCHEDULE

Pregnancy Risk Category: C

MECHANISM OF ACTION

A biologic modifier that stimulates production, maturation, and activation of neutrophils. ***Therapeutic Effect:*** Activates neutrophils to increase their migration and cytotoxicity.

PHARMACOKINETICS

Readily absorbed after SC administration. Not removed by hemodialysis. ***Half-Life:*** 3.5 hrs.

AVAILABILITY

Vials for Injection: 300 mcg, 480 mcg
Prefilled syringes: 300 mcg/0.5 mL, 480 mcg/0.8mL

INDICATIONS AND DOSAGES

▸ Usual pediatric dose

IV/SC
Children. 5–10 mcg/kg/day once daily up to 14 days until absolute neutrophil count (ANC) is 10,000/mm^3
Neonates. 5–10 mcg/kg/day once daily for 3–5 days (investigational therapy).

UNLABELED USES

Treatment of AIDS-related neutropenia; chronic, severe neutropenia; drug-induced neutropenia; myelodysplastic syndrome.

CONTRAINDICATIONS
Hypersensitivity to *Escherichia coli*–derived proteins. Use 24 hrs before or after cytotoxic chemotherapy, use with other drugs that may result in lowered platelet count.

INTERACTIONS
Drug
None known.
Herbal
None known.
Food
None known.

DIAGNOSTIC TEST EFFECTS
May increase lactate dehydrogenase concentrations, leukocyte (leukocyte alkaline phosphatate) scores, and serum alkaline phosphatase and uric acid levels.

IV INCOMPATIBILITIES
Amphotericin (Fungizone), cefepime (Maxipime), cefotaxime (Claforan), cefoxitin (Mefoxin), ceftizoxime (Cefizox), ceftriaxone (Rocephin), cefuroxime (Zinacef), clindamycin (Cleocin), dactinomycin (Cosmegen), etoposide (VePesid), fluorouracil, furosemide (Lasix), heparin, mannitol, methylprednisolone (Solu-Medrol), mitomycin (Mutamycin), prochlorperazine (Compazine)

IV COMPATIBILITIES
Bumetanide (Bumex), calcium gluconate, hydromorphone (Dilaudid), lorazepam (Ativan), morphine, potassium chloride

SIDE EFFECTS
Frequent
Nausea or vomiting (57%), mild to severe bone pain (22%) occurs more frequently in those receiving a high dose via IV form, less frequently in low-dose, SC form; alopecia (18%), diarrhea (14%), fever (12%), fatigue (11%)
Occasional (9%–5%)
Anorexia, dyspnea, headache, cough, skin rash
Rare (less than 5%)
Psoriasis, hematuria/proteinuria, osteoporosis

SERIOUS REACTIONS
! Chronic administration occasionally produces chronic neutropenia and splenomegaly.
! Thrombocytopenia, myocardial infarction, and arrhythmias occur rarely.
! Adult respiratory distress syndrome may occur in septic pts.

PEDIATRIC CONSIDERATIONS
Baseline Assessment
- Obtain a complete blood count (CBC) before filgrastim therapy and twice weekly thereafter.
- Be aware that it is unknown if filgrastim crosses the placenta or is distributed in breast milk.
- There are no age-related precautions noted in children.

Precautions
- Use cautiously in pts with gout, malignancy with myeloid characteristics due to the potential of granulocyte colony-stimulating factor to act as a growth factor, preexisting cardiac conditions, and psoriasis.

Administration and Handling
◀ **ALERT** ▶ May be given by SC injection or short IV infusion (15–30 min) or by continuous IV infusion.
◀ **ALERT** ▶ Begin at least 24 hrs after the last dose of chemotherapy; discontinue at least 24 hrs before the next dose of chemotherapy.
◀ **ALERT** ▶ Begin at least 24 hrs after

the last dose of chemotherapy and at least 24 hrs after bone marrow infusion.

SC

Store in refrigerator, but remove before use and allow to warm to room temperature.

- Aspirate syringe before injecting the drug to avoid intra-arterial administration.

IV

- Refrigerate vials.
- Know that the drug is stable for up to 24 hrs at room temperature, provided vial contents are clear and contain no particulate matter. Be aware that the drug remains stable if accidentally exposed to freezing temperature.
- Use single-dose vial, do not reenter vial. Do not shake.
- Dilute with 10–50 mL D_5W to concentration of 15 mcg/mL and higher. For concentration from 5–15 mcg/mL, add 2 mL of 5% albumin to each 50 mL D_5W to provide a final concentration of 2 mg/mL. Do not dilute to a final concentration of less than 5 mcg/mL.
- For intermittent infusion (piggyback), infuse over 15–30 min.
- For continuous infusion, give single dose over 4–24 hrs.
- In all situations, flush the IV line with D_5W before and after administration.

Intervention and Evaluation

- In septic pts, be alert to adult respiratory distress syndrome.
- Closely monitor pts with preexisting cardiac conditions.
- Monitor the patient's blood pressure (B/P) because a transient decrease in B/P may occur. Also assess his or her temperature, CBC, hepatic enzyme studies, and blood Hct and serum uric acid levels.

Patient/Family Teaching

- Warn the patient/family to notify the physician if the patient experiences chest pain, chills, fever, palpitations, or severe bone pain.
- Instruct the patient/family to avoid situations that might place them at risk for contracting an infectious disease, such as influenza.

REFERENCES

Miller, S. & Fioravanti, J. (1997). Pediatric medications: a handbook for nurses. St. Louis: Mosby.

Taketomo, C. K., Hodding, J. H. & Kraus, D. M. (2003–2004). Pediatric dosage handbook (10th ed.). Hudson, OH: Lexi-Comp.

58 Plasma Expanders

Albumin, Human
Dextran, Low Molecular Weight (Dextran 40);
Dextran, High Molecular Weight (Dextran 75)
Hetastarch

Uses: Plasma expanders are used to treat hypovolemia, to expand plasma volume and maintain cardiac output in shock or impending shock, and to treat hypoproteinemia-induced edema or decreased intravascular volume.

Action: Plasma expanders stay in the vascular space and restore plasma volume by maintaining the colloidal osmotic pressure.

Albumin, Human

al-byew-min
(Albumex [AUS], Albuminar, Albutein, Buminate, Plasbumin)

CATEGORY AND SCHEDULE

Pregnancy Risk Category: C

MECHANISM OF ACTION

A plasma protein fraction that acts as a blood volume expander. ***Therapeutic Effect:*** Provides a temporary increase in blood volume, reduces hemoconcentration and blood viscosity.

PHARMACOKINETICS

Route	Onset	Peak	Duration
IV	15 min	N/A	N/A

Distributed throughout extracellular fluid. Onset of action: 15 min provided the patient is well hydrated. ***Half-Life:*** 15–20 days.

AVAILABILITY

Injection: 5%, 20%, 25%.

INDICATIONS AND DOSAGES

Hypovolemia
IV
Children. 0.5–1 g/kg/dose (10–20 mL/kg/dose of 5% albumin) over 30–120 min. Maximum: 6 g/kg/day.
Neonates. 0.5 g/kg/dose (10 mL/kg/dose of 5% albumin); dosage range: 0.25–0.5 g/kg/dose (5–10 mL/kg/dose of 5% albumin).

▸ Hypoproteinemia
IV
Children. 0.5–1 g/kg/dose (10–20 mL/kg/dose of 5% albumin) over 30–120 minutes; repeat in 1–2 days.

▸ Burns
IV
Children. Initially, begin with administration of large volumes of crystalloid infusion to maintain plasma volume. After 24 hrs, an initial dose of 25 g with dosage adjusted to maintain plasma albumin concentration of 2–2.5 g/100 mL.

▸ Hyperbilirubinemia, erythroblastosis fetalis
IV
Infants. 1 g/kg 1–2 hrs before transfusion.

CONTRAINDICATIONS

Heart failure, a history of allergic reaction to albumin, hypervolemia, normal serum albumin, pulmonary edema, severe anemia.

INTERACTIONS

Drug
None known.

Herbal
None known.
Food
None known.

DIAGNOSTIC TEST EFFECTS

May increase serum alkaline phosphatase concentrations.

IV INCOMPATIBILITIES

Midazolam (Versed), vancomycin (Vancocin), verapamil (Isoptin)

IV COMPATIBILITIES

Diltiazem (Cardizem), lorazepam (Ativan)

SIDE EFFECTS

Occasional
Hypotension
Rare
High-dose, repeated therapy may result in altered vital signs, chills, fever, increased salivation, nausea, vomiting, urticaria, tachycardia

SERIOUS REACTIONS

! Fluid overload evidenced by signs and symptoms including headache, weakness, blurred vision, behavioral changes, incoordination, and isolated muscle twitching may occur.
! Congestive heart failure as evidenced by rapid breathing, rales, wheezing, coughing, increased blood pressure (B/P), and distended neck veins may occur.

PEDIATRIC CONSIDERATIONS

Baseline Assessment
- Expect to obtain B/P, pulse, and respirations immediately before administration.
- Ensure adequate hydration before albumin is administered.
- Be aware that it is unknown whether albumin crosses the placenta or is distributed in breast milk.
- There are no age-related precautions noted in children.

Precautions
- Use cautiously in pts with liver or renal impairment, hypertension, normal serum albumin concentration, poor heart function, or pulmonary disease.
- Use with caution in pts requiring sodium restriction.

Administration and Handling
IV
◂ALERT▸ Be aware that the dosage is based on the patient's condition and the duration of administration is based on the patient's response.
- Store at room temperature. Albumin normally appears as a clear, brownish, odorless, and moderate viscous fluid.
- Do not use if solution has been frozen, appears turbid, contains sediment or is not used within 4 hrs of opening the vial.
- Make a 5% solution from a 25% solution by adding 1 volume of 25% solution to 4 volumes of 0.9% NaCl or D_5W (NaCl preferred). Do not use sterile water for injection because life-threatening acute renal failure and hemolysis can occur.
- Give by IV infusion. The rate is variable and depends on the therapeutic use, the patient's blood volume, and the concentration of solute.
- Give 5% solution at 5–10 mL/min; 25% is usually given at 2–3 mL/min.
- Administer 5% solution undiluted; 25% solution may be administered undiluted or diluted with 0.9% NaCl or D_5W. Dilution with NaCl is preferred.

• May give without regard to patient blood group or Rh factor.

Intervention and Evaluation

• Monitor B/P for hypertension or hypotension.
• Assess the patient frequently for signs and symptoms of fluid overload and pulmonary edema.
• Check the patient's skin for flushing and urticaria.
• Monitor the patient's intake and output and, in particular, watch for decreased urine output.
• Assess for a therapeutic response as evidenced by increased B/P and decreased edema.

Patient/Family Teaching

• Advise the patient/family to immediately report difficulty breathing or skin itching or rash.

Dextran, Low Molecular Weight (Dextran 40)

dex-tran
(Gentran, Rheomacrodex [CAN])

Dextran, High Molecular Weight (Dextran 75)

(Macrodex)

CATEGORY AND SCHEDULE

Pregnancy Risk Category: C

MECHANISM OF ACTION

A branched polysaccharide that produces plasma volume expansion due to a high colloidal osmotic effect. Draws interstitial fluid into the intravascular space. May also increase blood flow in microcirculation. ***Therapeutic Effect:*** Increases central venous pressure, cardiac output, stroke volume, blood pressure (B/P), urine output, capillary perfusion, and pulse pressure. Decreases heart rate, peripheral resistance, and blood viscosity. Corrects hypovolemia.

AVAILABILITY

Injection: 10% dextran 40 in NaCl or D_5W, 6% dextran 70 in NaCl.

INDICATIONS AND DOSAGES

▸ Volume expansion, shock

IV

Children. Total dose not to exceed 20 mL/kg on day 1, 10 mL/kg/day thereafter. Do not use continuously for more than 5 days.

CONTRAINDICATIONS

Hypersensitivity to dextrans or any related component. Hypervolemia, renal failure. severe bleeding disorders, severe CHF, severe thrombocytopenia.

INTERACTIONS

Drug

None known.

Herbal

None known.

Food

None known.

DIAGNOSTIC TEST EFFECTS

Prolongs bleeding time, depresses platelet count. Decreases factors VIII, V, and IX.

IV INCOMPATIBILITIES

Do not add any medications to dextran solution.

SIDE EFFECTS

Occasional

Mild hypersensitivity reaction, including urticaria, nasal congestion, wheezing

SERIOUS REACTIONS

! Severe or fatal anaphylaxis, manifested by marked hypotension or cardiac or respiratory arrest, may occur early during IV infusion, generally in those not previously exposed to IV dextran.

PEDIATRIC CONSIDERATIONS

Baseline Assessment

• Expect to obtain baseline laboratory values, such bleeding time, platelet count, and clotting factors.
• Be aware that dehydration can lead to renal failure. Monitor and assess for adequate fluid intake.

Precautions

• Use cautiously in pts with chronic liver disease and extreme dehydration.

Administration and Handling

◂**ALERT**▸ Therapy should not continue longer than 5 days.

IV

• Store at room temperature.
• Use only clear solutions.
• Discard partially used containers.
• Give by IV infusion only.
• Monitor the patient closely during the first minutes of infusion for an anaphylactic reaction.
• Monitor the patient's vital signs every 5 min.
• Monitor the patient's urine flow rates during administration. Discontinue dextran 40 and give an osmotic diuretic, as prescribed, if oliguria or anuria occurs to minimize vascular overloading.
• Monitor the patient's central venous pressure (CVP) when given by rapid infusion. Immediately discontinue the drug and notify the physician if there is a precipitous rise in CVP caused by overexpansion of blood volume.
• Monitor the patient's B/P diligently during infusion. Stop the infusion immediately if marked hypotension occurs, a sign of imminent anaphylactic reaction.
• Discontinue drug until blood volume adjusts via diuresis if evidence of blood volume overexpansion occurs.

Intervention and Evaluation

• Monitor the patient's urine output closely. An increase in output generally occurs in oliguric pts after dextran administration. Discontinue dextran until the patient experiences diuresis if there is no increase in urine output observed after 500 mL dextran is infused.
• Monitor the patient for signs of fluid overload, such as peripheral or pulmonary edema, and symptoms of impending CHF.
• Assess the patient's lung sounds for crackles.
• Monitor the patient's CVP to detect overexpansion of blood volume.
• Monitor the patient's vital signs and observe the patient closely for signs of an allergic reaction.
• Assess the patient for overt bleeding, especially at the surgical site, as well as for bruising and petechiae development, particularly after surgery or in pts receiving anticoagulant therapy.

Patient/Family Teaching:

• Instruct the patient/family to let you know if the patient experiences bleeding from the surgical site, chest pain, or dyspnea.
• Tell the patient/family to use an electric razor and soft toothbrush to prevent bleeding during dextran therapy.
• Explain to the patient/family that the patient should not take any medications, including OTC drugs, especially aspirin, without consulting the physician.

• Warn the patient/family to notify you if the patient experiences black or red stool, coffee-ground emesis, dark or red urine, or red-speckled mucus from cough.
• Tell the female patient/family that the patient's menstrual flow may be heavier than usual.

Hetastarch

het-ah-starch
(Hespan, Hextend)

CATEGORY AND SCHEDULE

Pregnancy Risk Category: C

MECHANISM OF ACTION

A plasma volume expander that exerts osmotic pull on tissue fluids. ***Therapeutic Effect:*** Reduces hemoconcentration and blood viscosity, increases circulating blood volume.

PHARMACOKINETICS

Smaller molecules (less than 50,000 molecular weight) rapidly excreted by kidneys; larger molecules (greater than 50,000 molecular weight) slowly degraded to smaller sized molecules, then excreted. ***Half-Life:*** 17 days.

AVAILABILITY

Injection: 6 g/100 mL 0.9% NaCl, 500 mL infusion container.

INDICATIONS AND DOSAGES

▸ Usual pediatric dosage

Children. 10 mL/kg/dose; the total daily dose should not surpass 20 mL/kg.

CONTRAINDICATIONS

Hypersensitivity to hetastarch or any related component. Anuria, oliguria, severe bleeding disorders, severe CHF, severe renal failure, lactic acidosis, or leukapheresis.

INTERACTIONS

Drug

None significant.

Herbal

None known.

Food

None known.

DIAGNOSTIC TEST EFFECTS

May prolong bleeding and clotting times, partial thromboplastin time, and prothrombin time (PT). May decrease blood hematocrit concentration.

IV INCOMPATIBILITIES

Amikacin (Amikin), ampicillin (Polycillin), cefazolin (Ancef, Kefzol), cefotaxime (Claforan), cefoxitin (Mefoxin), gentamicin (Garamycin), ranitidine (Zantac), tobramycin (Nebcin)

SIDE EFFECTS

Rare

Allergic reaction resulting in vomiting, mild temperature elevation, chills, itching, submaxillary and parotid gland enlargement, peripheral edema of lower extremities, mild flu-like symptoms, headache, muscle aches

SERIOUS REACTIONS

! Fluid overload, marked by headache, weakness, blurred vision, behavioral changes, incoordination, and isolated muscle twitching, and pulmonary edema, manifested by rapid breathing, crackles, wheezing, coughing, increased blood pressure, and distended neck veins may occur.
! An anaphylactic reaction may be observed as periorbital edema, urticaria, and wheezing.

PEDIATRIC CONSIDERATIONS

Baseline Assessment

• Expect to obtain baseline laboratory tests, including coagulation studies and complete blood count.
• Assess the patient's vital signs, including blood pressure and central venous pressure (CVP).
• Be aware that children with a history of liver disease or thrombocytopenia may experience anaphylactic reactions when taking hetastarch.

Precautions

• Use cautiously in pts with CHF, liver disease, pulmonary edema, sodium-restricted diets, and thrombocytopenia.
• Use cautiously in the very young.

Administration and Handling

IV

• Store solutions at room temperature.
• Solution normally appears clear, pale yellow to amber. Do not use if discolored a deep turbid brown or if precipitate forms.
• Administer only by IV infusion.
• Do not add drugs or mix with other IV fluids.
• In acute hemorrhagic shock, administer at rate approaching 1.2 g/kg (20 mL/kg) per hr, as prescribed. Expect to use slower rates for burns or septic shock.
• Monitor the patient's CVP when given by rapid infusion. If there is a precipitous rise in CVP, immediately discontinue the drug, as prescribed, to prevent overexpansion of blood volume.

Intervention and Evaluation

• Monitor the patient for signs of fluid overload, such as peripheral and pulmonary edema and impending CHF symptoms.
• Assess the patient's lung sounds for crackles and wheezing.
• During leukapheresis, monitor the patient's aPTT, complete blood count, particularly Hct and Hgb, fluid intake and output, leukocyte and platelet counts, and PT.
• Monitor the patient's CVP to detect overexpansion of blood volume.
• Monitor the patient's urine output closely. An increase in output generally occurs in oliguric pts after administration.
• Assess the patient for itching, periorbital edema, wheezing, and urticaria, signs of an allergic reaction.
• Monitor the patient for anuria, any change in output ratio, and oliguria.
• Monitor the patient for bleeding from surgical or trauma sites.

Patient/Family Teaching

• Tell the patient/family to use an electric razor and soft toothbrush to prevent bleeding.
• Warn the patient/family to notify the physician if the patient experiences any sign of black or red stool, coffee-ground vomitus, dark or red urine, or red-speckled mucus from cough.

REFERENCES

Miller, S. & Fioravanti, J. (1997). Pediatric medications: a handbook for nurses. St. Louis: Mosby.
Taketomo, C. K., Hodding, J. H. & Kraus, D. M. (2003–2004). Pediatric dosage handbook (10th ed.). Hudson, OH: Lexi-Comp.

59 Miscellaneous Hematologic Agents

Aminocaproic Acid

Uses: Miscellaneous hematologic agents serve different purposes. *Aminocaproic acid* is used to treat excessive bleeding from hyperfibrinolysis or urinary fibrinolysis.

Action: Each miscellaneous agent acts in a different way on the hematologic system. *Aminocaproic acid* inhibits the activation of plasminogen activator substances and blocks antiplasmin activity by inhibiting fibrinolysis.

Aminocaproic Acid

ah-meen-oh-kah-**pro**-ick
(Amicar)
Do not confuse with amikacin or Amikin.

CATEGORY AND SCHEDULE

Pregnancy Risk Category: C

MECHANISM OF ACTION

A systemic hemostatic that acts as an antifibrinolytic and antihemorrhagic by inhibiting the activation of plasminogen activator substances. ***Therapeutic Effect:*** prevents fibrin clots from forming.

AVAILABILITY

Tablets: 500 mg.
Syrup: 250 mg/mL.
Injection: 250 mg/mL.

INDICATIONS AND DOSAGES

▸ Acute bleeding

PO/IV INFUSION
Children. 3 g/m^2 over the first hour, then 1 g/m^2/hr. Maximum daily dose: 18 g/m^2/24 hrs.
PO/IV BOLUS
Children. 100–200 mg/kg loading dose. Maintenance: 100 mg/kg/dose q6h. Maximum daily dose: 30 g.

▸ Dosage in renal impairment

Decrease dose to 25% of normal.

UNLABELED USES

Prevents reoccurrence of subarachnoid hemorrhage, prevents hemorrhage in hemophiliacs after dental surgery.

CONTRAINDICATIONS

Hypersensitivity to aminocaproic acid or any related component. Evidence of active intravascular clotting process, disseminated intravascular coagulation without concurrent heparin therapy, hematuria of upper urinary tract origin (unless benefits outweigh risk). Parenteral: newborns.

INTERACTIONS

Drug

Oral contraceptives, estrogens, factor IX: Increased risk of thrombosis.

Herbal

None known.

Food

None known.

DIAGNOSTIC TEST EFFECTS

May elevate serum potassium level.

IV INCOMPATIBILITIES

Sodium lactate. Do not mix with other medications.

SIDE EFFECTS

Occasional

Nausea, diarrhea, cramps, decreased urination, decreased blood pressure (B/P), dizziness, headache, muscle fatigue and weakness, myopathy, bloodshot eyes

SERIOUS REACTIONS

! Too rapid IV administration produces tinnitus, skin rash, arrhythmias, unusual tiredness, and weakness.

! Rarely, a grand mal seizure occurs, generally preceded by weakness, dizziness, and headache.

PEDIATRIC CONSIDERATIONS

Precautions

- Use cautiously in pts with hyperfibrinolysis or impaired cardiac, liver, or renal disease.
- Injection contains benzyl alcohol. Large amounts of benzyl alcohol may cause a potentially fatal toxicity in neonates.

Administration and Handling

◀ **ALERT** ▶ Expect to administer a reduced aminocaproic acid dose if the patient has cardiac, renal, or liver impairment.

IV

Dilute each 1 g in up to 50 mL 0.9% NaCl, D_5W, Ringer's solution, or Sterile Water for Injection. Do not use Sterile Water for Injection in pts with subarachnoid hemorrhage.

Do not give by direct injection. Give only by IV infusion.

Infuse 5 g or less over the first hour in 250 mL of solution. Give each succeeding 1 g over 1 hr in 50–100 mL solution.

Monitor the patient for hypotension during infusion.

Be aware that rapid infusion may produce arrhythmias, including bradycardia.

Intervention and Evaluation

- Assess the patient for severe and continuous muscular pain or weakness, which may indicate myopathy.
- Monitor creatine kinase and SGOT (AST) serum levels frequently to determine whether myopathy is present. Myopathy is characterized by an increase in serum creatine kinase and SGOT (AST) levels.
- Monitor the patient's B/P, heart rate and rhythm, and pulse rate. Any abdominal or back pain, decrease in B/P, increase in pulse rate, and severe headache may be evidence of hemorrhage. Assess the quality of the patient's peripheral pulses.
- Check for bruising of the skin, excessive bleeding from minor cuts or scratches, and petechiae.
- Monitor the patient for an increase in menstrual flow.
- Evaluate the patient's gums for erythema and gingival bleeding.
- Examine the patient's urine output for hematuria.

Patient/Family Teaching

- Instruct the patient/family to report any signs of red or dark urine, black or red stool, coffee-ground vomit, or red-speckled mucus produced from a cough.

60 Adrenocortical Steroids

Betamethasone
Cortisone Acetate
Dexamethasone
Fludrocortisone
Hydrocortisone, Hydrocortisone Acetate, Hydrocortisone Sodium Phosphate, Hydrocortisone Valerate, Sodium Succinate
Methylprednisolone, Methylprednisolone Acetate, Methylprednisolone Sodium Succinate
Prednisolone
Prednisone
Triamcinolone, Triamcinolone Acetonide, Triamcinolone Diacetate, Triamcinolone Hexacetonide

Uses: Adrenocortical steroids are used as replacement therapy in adrenal insufficiency, including Addison disease. Because these agents have anti-inflammatory and immunosuppressant properties, they are also used to treat the symptoms of multiorgan diseases and conditions, such as rheumatoid arthritis, osteoarthritis, severe psoriasis, ulcerative colitis, lupus erythematosus, anaphylactic shock, and status asthmaticus and to prevent the rejection of transplanted organs.

Action: Adrenocortical steroids suppress the migration of polymorphonuclear leukocytes and reverse increased capillary permeability by their anti-inflammatory effects. They suppress the immune system by decreasing lymphatic system activity.

COMBINATION PRODUCTS

BLEPHAMIDE: prednisolone/sulfacetamide (an anti-infective) 0.2%/10%.

CIPRO HC OTIC: hydrocortisone/ciprofloxacin (an anti-infective) 1%/0.2%.

CIPRODEX OTIC: dexamethasone/ciprofloxacin (an anti-infective) 0.1%/0.3%.

CORTISPORIN: hydrocortisone/neomycin (an anti-infective)/polymyxin (an anti-infective) 5 mg/10,000 units/5 mg; 10 mg/10,000 units/5 mg.

DEXACIDIN: dexamethasone/neomycin (an anti-infective)/polymyxin (an anti-infective): 0.1%/3.5 mg/10,000 units per g or mL.

LOTRISONE: betamethasone/clotrimazole (an antifungal) 0.05%/1%.

MAXITROL: dexamethasone/neomycin (an anti-infective)/

polymyxin (an anti-infective) 0.1%/3.5 mg/10,000 units per g or mL.
MYCO-II: triamcinolone/nystatin (an antifungal) 0.1%/100,000 units/g.
MYCOLOG II: triamcinolone/nystatin (an antifungal) 0.1%/100,000 units/g.
MYCO-TRIACET: triamcinolone/nystatin (an antifungal) 0.1%/100,000 units/g.
TOBRADEX: dexamethasone/tobramycin (an aminoglycoside) 1%/3%.
VASOCIDIN: prednisolone/sulfacetamide (an anti-infective) 0.25%/10%.

Betamethasone

bay-tah-**meth**-a-sone
(Betaderm [CAN], Beta-Val, Betnesol [CAN], Celestone, Diprolene, Diprosone, Luxig Foam)

CATEGORY AND SCHEDULE

Pregnancy Risk Category: C (D if used in first trimester)

MECHANISM OF ACTION

An adrenocorticosteroid that controls the rate of protein synthesis, depresses migration of polymorphonuclear leukocytes and fibroblasts, reduces capillary permeability, and prevents or controls inflammation. ***Therapeutic Effect:*** Decreases tissue response to the inflammatory process.

AVAILABILITY

Aerosol: 0.1%.
Cream: 0.1%, 0.05%.
Foam: 0.12%.
Gel: 0.05%
Injection: 4 mg/mL (Celestone), 3 mg/mL (Celestone Soluspan)
Lotion: 0.1%, 0.05%
Ointment: 0.05%, 0.1%.
Syrup: 0.6 mg/5 mL.
Tablet: 0.6 mg.

INDICATIONS AND DOSAGES

▸ **Anti-inflammatory, immunosuppressant, corticosteroid replacement therapy**

PO/IM
Adolescents. 0.6–7.2 mg/day in divided doses.
Children. 0.0175–0.25 mg/kg/day in 3–4 divided doses.
TOPICAL
Adolescents and children. Apply a thin amount to affected area 1–3 times daily.

CONTRAINDICATIONS

Hypersensitivity to betamethasone, systemic fungal infections.

INTERACTIONS

Drug

Amphotericin: May increase hypokalemia.
Digoxin: May increase the toxicity of digoxin secondary to hypokalemia.
Diuretics, insulin, oral hypoglycemics, potassium supplements: May decrease the effects of diuretics, insulin, oral hypoglycemics, and potassium supplements.
Hepatic enzyme inducers: May decrease the effect of betamethasone.
Live virus vaccines: May decrease the patient's antibody response to vaccine, increase vaccine side effects, and potentiate virus replication.

Herbal

None known.

Food

None known.

DIAGNOSTIC TEST EFFECTS

May decrease serum calcium, potassium, and thyroxine levels. May increase blood glucose, serum lipid, amylase, and sodium levels.

SIDE EFFECTS

Frequent

Systemic: Increased appetite, abdominal distention, nervousness, insomnia, false sense of well-being
Foam: Burning, stinging, pruritus

Occasional

Systemic: Dizziness, facial flushing, diaphoresis, decreased or blurred vision, mood swings
Topical: Allergic contact dermatitis, purpura or blood-containing blisters, thinning of skin with easy bruising, telangiectasis or raised dark red spots on skin

SERIOUS REACTIONS

! When taken in excessive quantities, systemic hypercorticism and adrenal suppression may occur.

PEDIATRIC CONSIDERATIONS

Baseline Assessment

- Determine if the patient has a hypersensitivity to any corticosteroids and sulfite.
- Obtain the patient's baseline blood pressure (B/P), blood glucose and serum electrolyte levels, height, and weight.
- Evaluate the results of initial tests, such as a tuberculosis skin test, radiographs, and EKG.
- Determine whether the patient has diabetes mellitus, and anticipate an increase in his or her antidiabetic drug regimen due to raised blood glucose levels.
- Find out whether the patient takes digoxin, and if so plan to draw blood for measurement of serum digoxin levels.
- Be aware that use in children may result in increased systemic absorption.
- Be aware that topical use in children should be limited to the least amount that is effective.

Precautions

- Use cautiously in pts at increased risk of peptic ulcer disease and pts with cirrhosis, hypothyroidism, cirrhosis, and nonspecific ulcerative colitis.

Administration and Handling

PO

- Give betamethasone with milk or food because it decreases GI upset.
- Give single doses before 9 A.M.; multiple doses should be given at evenly spaced intervals.

TOPICAL

- Gently cleanse area before application.
- Use occlusive dressings only as ordered.
- Apply sparingly and rub into area thoroughly.
- When using aerosol, spray area 3 sec from 15 cm distance; avoid inhalation.

Intervention and Evaluation

- Monitor the patient's blood glucose, B/P, and electrolyte levels. If the patient takes digoxin, closely follow his or her digoxin levels.
- Apply topical preparation sparingly. Do not use topical betamethasone on broken skin or in areas of infection and do not apply to the face, inguinal areas, or wet skin.

Patient/Family Teaching

- Instruct the patient/family to take betamethasone with food or milk.
- Teach the patient/family to take a single daily dose in the morning.

• Caution the patient/family against abruptly discontinuing the drug.
• Instruct the patient/family to apply topical preparations in a thin layer.
• Explain that steroids often cause mood swings, ranging from euphoria to depression.

Cortisone Acetate

kore-tih-zone
(Cortate [AUS], Cortone [CAN])
Do not confuse with Cort-Dome.

CATEGORY AND SCHEDULE

Pregnancy Risk Category: C (D if used in the first trimester)

MECHANISM OF ACTION

An adrenocortical steroid that inhibits the accumulation of inflammatory cells at inflammation sites, phagocytosis, lysosomal enzyme release, and synthesis and release of mediators of inflammation. ***Therapeutic Effect:*** Prevents or suppresses cell-mediated immune reactions. Decreases or prevents tissue response to inflammatory process.

AVAILABILITY

Tablets: 25 mg.

INDICATIONS AND DOSAGES

Dosage is dependent on the condition being treated and patient response.

▸ **Anti-inflammatory, immunosuppressive**
PO
Children. 2.5–10 mg/kg/day in divided doses q6–8h.

▸ **Physiologic replacement**
PO
Children. 0.5–0.75 mg/kg/day in divided doses q8h.

CONTRAINDICATIONS

Hypersensitivity to any corticosteroid, use with live virus vaccine, peptic ulcers (except in life-threatening situations), systemic fungal or viral infections, serious infections.

INTERACTIONS

Drug
Amphotericin: May increase hypokalemia.
Digoxin: May increase the toxicity of digoxin caused by hypokalemia.
Diuretics, insulin, oral hypoglycemics, potassium supplements: May decrease the effects of diuretics, insulin, oral hypoglycemics, and potassium supplements.
Hepatic enzyme inducers: May decrease the effects of cortisone.
Live virus vaccines: May decrease the patient's antibody response to vaccine, increase vaccine side effects, and potentiate virus replication.
Herbal
None known.
Food
None known.

DIAGNOSTIC TEST EFFECTS

May decrease serum calcium, potassium, and thyroxine levels. May increase blood glucose, serum lipid, amylase, and sodium levels.

SIDE EFFECTS

Frequent
Insomnia, heartburn, nervousness, abdominal distention, increased sweating, acne, mood swings, increased appetite, facial flushing, delayed wound healing, increased

susceptibility to infection, diarrhea or constipation

Occasional

Headache, edema, change in skin color, frequent urination

Rare

Tachycardia, allergic reaction, such as rash and hives, psychological changes, hallucinations, depression

SERIOUS REACTIONS

! The serious reactions of long-term therapy are hypocalcemia, hypokalemia, muscle wasting in arms and legs, osteoporosis, spontaneous fractures, amenorrhea, cataracts, glaucoma, peptic ulcer, and CHF.

! Abrupt withdrawal after long-term therapy may cause anorexia, nausea, fever, headache, joint pain, rebound inflammation, fatigue, weakness, lethargy, dizziness, and orthostatic hypertension.

PEDIATRIC CONSIDERATIONS

Baseline Assessment

- Determine whether the patient is hypersensitive to any of the corticosteroids.
- Obtain the patient's baseline blood pressure, blood glucose and serum electrolyte levels, height, and weight.
- Determine whether the patient has diabetes mellitus, and anticipate an increase in his or her antidiabetic drug regimen because of raised blood glucose levels.
- Find out whether the patient takes digoxin, and if so plan to draw blood for measurement of serum digoxin levels.
- Be aware that chronic use of this medication in children may interrupt growth patterns and maturation.

Precautions

- Use cautiously in pts with cirrhosis, CHF, history of tuberculosis (because it may reactivate the disease), hypertension, hypothyroidism, nonspecific ulcerative colitis, psychosis, seizure disorders, and thromboembolic disorders.
- Discontinue prolonged therapy slowly.

Intervention and Evaluation

- Be alert to signs of infection caused by reduced immune response, including fever, sore throat, or vague symptoms.
- For those receiving long-term therapy, monitor for signs and symptoms of hypocalcemia, such as muscle twitching, cramps, positive Chvostek or Trousseau sign, or hypokalemia, including weakness and muscle cramps, numbness or tingling, especially in the lower extremities, nausea and vomiting, irritability, and EKG changes.
- Assess the patient's ability to sleep and emotional status.

Patient/Family Teaching

- Instruct the patient/family not to change the dose or schedule of cortisone.
- Caution the patient/family against discontinuing the drug. Taper off cortisone under medical supervision.
- Warn the patient/family to notify the physician if the patient experiences fever, muscle aches, sore throat, and sudden weight gain or swelling.
- Tell the patient/family to inform the patient's dentist and other physicians of cortisone therapy now or within the past 12 mos.
- Explain that steroids often cause mood swings, ranging from euphoria to depression.

Dexamethasone

dex-a-**meth**-a-sone
(Decadron, Dexasone [CAN], Dexmethsone [AUS], Diodex [CAN], Hexadrol [CAN], Maxidex)
Do not confuse with desoximetasone, dextromethorphan, or Maxzide.

CATEGORY AND SCHEDULE
Pregnancy Risk Category: C (D if used in the first trimester)

MECHANISM OF ACTION
A long-acting glucocorticoid that inhibits accumulation of inflammatory cells at inflammation sites, phagocytosis, lysosomal enzyme release, and synthesis and release of mediators of inflammation. ***Therapeutic Effect:*** Prevents and suppresses cell and tissue immune reactions and the inflammatory process.

PHARMACOKINETICS
Rapidly, completely absorbed from the GI tract after PO administration. Widely distributed. Protein binding: High. Metabolized in liver. Primarily excreted in urine and bile. Minimally removed by hemodialysis. ***Half-Life:*** 3–4.5 hrs.

AVAILABILITY
Tablets: 0.25 mg, 0.5 mg, 0.75 mg, 1 mg, 1.5 mg, 2 mg, 4 mg, 6 mg.
Elixir: 0.5 mg/5 mL, 1 mg/mL.
Oral Solution: 0.5 mg/5 mL, 0.5 mg/0.5 mL.
Injection: 4 mg/mL.
Injection (suspension, long acting): 8 mg/mL, 16 mg/mL.
Inhalant, Intranasal, Ophthalmic: Solution, suspension, ointment.
Topical: Aerosol, cream.

INDICATIONS AND DOSAGES
▸ Anti-inflammatory
PO/IM/IV
Children. 0.08–0.3 mg/kg/day in divided doses q6–12h.

▸ Cerebral edema
PO/IM/IV
Children. Loading dose of 1–2 mg/kg, then 1–1.5 mg/kg/day in divided doses q4–6h. Maximum: 16 mg/day.

▸ Chemotherapy antiemetic
IV
Children. 10 mg/m^2/dose (maximum: 20 mg), then 5 mg/m^2/dose q6h.

▸ Physiologic replacement
PO/IM/IV
Children. 0.03–0.15 mg/kg/day in divided doses q6–12h.

▸ Airway edema or extubation
PO/IM/IV
Children. 0.5–2 mg/kg/day in divided doses q6h.
IV
Neonates. 0.25 mg/kg/dose 4 hrs before a scheduled extubation, then follow every 8 hrs for 3 doses. Maximum: 1 mg/kg/day.

▸ Meningitis
IV
Adolescents and children. 0.15 mg/kg/dose q6h for 4 days.

▸ Usual ophthalmic dosage, ocular inflammatory conditions
OINTMENT
Children. Thin coating 3–4 times/day.
SUSPENSION
Children. Initially, 2 drops q1h while awake and q2h at night for 1 day, then reduce to 3–4 times/day.

CONTRAINDICATIONS
Hypersensitivity to dexamethasone or any related component. Active untreated infections, fungal, tuberculosis, or viral diseases of the eye.

INTERACTIONS

Drug

Amphotericin: May increase hypokalemia.
Digoxin: May increase the toxicity of this drug caused by hypokalemia.
Diuretics, insulin, oral hypoglycemics, potassium supplements: May decrease the effects of diuretics, insulin, oral hypoglycemics, and potassium supplements.
Hepatic enzyme inducers: May decrease the effects of dexamethasone.
Live virus vaccines: May decrease the patient's antibody response to vaccine, increase vaccine side effects, and potentiate virus replication.

Herbal

None known.

Food

None known.

DIAGNOSTIC TEST EFFECTS

May decrease serum calcium, potassium, and thyroxine levels. May increase blood glucose, serum lipid, amylase, and sodium levels.

IV INCOMPATIBILITIES

Ciprofloxacin (Cipro), daunorubicin (Cerubidine), idarubicin (Idamycin), midazolam (Versed)

IV COMPATIBILITIES

Aminophylline, cimetidine (Tagamet), cisplatin (Platinol), cyclophosphamide (Cytoxan), cytarabine (Cytosar), docetaxel (Taxotere), doxorubicin (Adriamycin), etoposide (VePesid), granisetron (Kytril), heparin, hydromorphone (Dilaudid), lorazepam (Ativan), morphine, ondansetron (Zofran), paclitaxel (Taxol), potassium chloride, propofol (Diprivan)

SIDE EFFECTS

Frequent

Inhalation: Cough, dry mouth, hoarseness, throat irritation
Intranasal: Burning, mucosal dryness
Ophthalmic: Blurred vision
Systemic: Insomnia, facial swelling or cushingoid appearance, moderate abdominal distention, indigestion, increased appetite, nervousness, facial flushing, diaphoresis

Occasional

Inhalation: Localized fungal infection, such as thrush
Intranasal: Crusting inside nose, nosebleed, sore throat, ulceration of nasal mucosa.
Ophthalmic: Decreased vision, watering of eyes, eye pain, burning, stinging, redness of eyes, nausea, vomiting
Systemic: Dizziness, decreased or blurred vision
Topical: Allergic contact dermatitis, purpura or blood-containing blisters, thinning of skin with easy bruising, telangiectasis or raised dark red spots on skin

Rare

Inhalation: Increased bronchospasm, esophageal candidiasis
Intranasal: Nasal and pharyngeal candidiasis, eye pain
Systemic: General allergic reaction, such as rash and hives, pain, redness, swelling at injection site, psychological changes, false sense of well-being, hallucinations, depression

SERIOUS REACTIONS

! The serious reactions of long-term therapy are muscle wasting, especially in the arms and legs, osteoporosis, spontaneous fractures, amenorrhea, cataracts, glaucoma, peptic ulcer disease, and CHF.

! Abrupt withdrawal after long-term therapy may cause severe joint pain, severe headache, anorexia, nausea, fever, rebound inflammation, fatigue, weakness, lethargy, dizziness, and orthostatic hypotension.

! The serious reactions with the ophthalmic form of dexamethasone are glaucoma, ocular hypertension, and cataracts.

PEDIATRIC CONSIDERATIONS

Baseline Assessment

- Determine whether the patient is hypersensitive to any corticosteroids.
- Obtain the patient's baseline blood pressure, blood glucose and serum electrolyte levels, height, and weight.
- Evaluate the results of initial tests, such as a tuberculosis skin test, radiographs, and EKG.
- Determine whether the patient has diabetes mellitus, and anticipate an increase in his or her antidiabetic drug regimen because of raised blood glucose levels.
- Find out whether the patient takes digoxin, and if so plan to draw blood for measurement of serum digoxin levels.
- Be aware that dexamethasone crosses the placenta and is distributed in breast milk.
- Be aware that prolonged treatment with high-dose therapy may decrease cortisol secretion and short-term growth rate in children.
- Be aware that children taking this medication should not receive immunizations until they have reached full immune system recovery.

Precautions

- Use cautiously in pts with cirrhosis, CHF, diabetes mellitus, hypertension, hyperthyroidism, ocular herpes simplex, osteoporosis, peptic ulcer disease, respiratory tuberculosis, seizure disorders, ulcerative colitis, and untreated systemic infections and in pts at high risk of thromboembolus.
- Use cautiously in pts receiving long-term therapy as prolonged ophthalmic dexamethasone use may result in cataracts or glaucoma.

Administration and Handling

PO

- Give dexamethasone with milk or food.

IM

- Give IM injection deeply, preferably in the gluteus maximus.

IV

◂ALERT▸ Dexamethasone sodium phosphate may be given by IV push or IV infusion.

- For IV push, give over 1–4 min.
- For IV infusion, mix with 0.9% NaCl or D_5W and infuse over 15–30 min.
- For neonate, solution must be preservative free.
- IV solution must be used within 24 hrs.

OPHTHALMIC

- Place a gloved finger on the patient's lower eyelid and pull it out until a pocket is formed between the patient's eye and lower lid.
- Hold the dropper above the pocket and place the correct number of drops—¼–½ inch ointment—into the pocket. Close the patient's eye gently.
- For the ophthalmic solution apply digital pressure to the lacrimal sac for 1–2 min to minimize the drainage to the nose and

throat, thereby reducing the risk of systemic effects.
• For the ophthalmic ointment, close the patient's eye for 1–2 min. Instruct the patient to roll his or her eyeball to increase the contact area of drug to eye.
• Remove excess solution or ointment around the patient's eye with a tissue.
• Use ointment at night to reduce the frequency of solution administration.
• Taper the drug dosage off slowly when discontinuing the drug.
TOPICAL
• Gently cleanse the area before application.
• Use occlusive dressings only as ordered.
• Apply sparingly and rub into the area thoroughly.

Intervention and Evaluation

• Monitor the patient's intake and output and record his or her daily body weight.
• Evaluate the patient for edema.
• Evaluate the patient's food tolerance. Assess the patient's pattern of daily bowel activity.
• Report any hyperacidity the patient experiences promptly.
• Check the patient's vital signs at least 2 times/day.
• Be alert to signs and symptoms of infection such as fever, sore throat, or vague symptoms.
• Monitor the patient's electrolyte levels.
• Assess the patient's ability to sleep and emotional status.
• Monitor the patient for hypercalcemia, including cramps and muscle twitching, or hypokalemia, including irritability, numbness or tingling, especially in the lower extremities, muscle cramps and weakness, and nausea and vomiting.

Patient/Family Teaching

• Caution the patient/family against abruptly discontinuing the drug and changing the drug dose or schedule. Explain to the patient/family that the drug dose must be tapered gradually under medical supervision.
• Warn the patient/family to notify the physician if the patient experiences fever, muscle aches, sore throat, and sudden weight gain or swelling.
• Explain to the patient/family that any severe stress, including serious infection, surgery, or trauma, may require an increase in dexamethasone dosage.
• Tell the patient/family to inform the patient's dentist and other physicians of dexamethasone therapy now or within past 12 mos.
• Instruct the patient/family using topical dexamethasone to apply the drug after a bath or shower for best absorption.
• Explain that steroids often cause mood swings, ranging from euphoria to depression.

Fludrocortisone

floo-droe-**kor**-tih-sone
(Florinef)
Do not confuse with Fioricet or Flurinol.

CATEGORY AND SCHEDULE

Pregnancy Risk Category: C

MECHANISM OF ACTION

A mineralocorticoid that acts at distal tubules. ***Therapeutic Effect:*** Increases potassium and hydrogen ion excretion, sodium reabsorption, and water retention.

PHARMACOKINETICS

Well absorbed from the GI tract. Protein binding: 42%. Widely distributed. Metabolized in liver and kidney. Primarily excreted in urine. ***Half-Life:*** 3.5 hrs.

AVAILABILITY

Tablets: 0.1 mg.

INDICATIONS AND DOSAGES

▸ Usual pediatric dosage

Children. 0.05–0.1 mg/day.

UNLABELED USES

Treatment of acidosis in renal tubular disorders, idiopathic orthostatic hypotension.

CONTRAINDICATIONS

Hypersensitivity to fludrocortisone or any related component. CHF, systemic fungal infection.

INTERACTIONS

Drug

Digoxin: May increase the risk of toxicity of digoxin caused by hypokalemia.

Hypokalemia-causing medications: May increase the effects of fludrocortisone.

Liver enzyme inducers (e.g., phenytoin): May increase the metabolism of fludrocortisone.

Sodium-containing medications: May increase blood pressure (B/P), incidence of edema, and serum sodium levels.

Herbal

None known.

Food

None known.

DIAGNOSTIC TEST EFFECTS

May increase serum sodium levels. May decrease blood Hct and serum potassium levels.

SIDE EFFECTS

Frequent

Increased appetite, exaggerated sense of well-being, abdominal distention, weight gain, insomnia, mood swings.

High-dose, prolonged therapy, too rapid withdrawal: Increased susceptibility to infection, with masked signs and symptoms, delayed wound healing, hypokalemia, hypocalcemia, GI distress, diarrhea or constipation, hypertension.

Occasional

Frontal or occipital headache, dizziness, menstrual difficulty or amenorrhea, gastric ulcer development.

Rare

Hypersensitivity reaction.

SERIOUS REACTIONS

! The serious reactions of long-term therapy are muscle wasting, especially in the arms and legs, osteoporosis, spontaneous fractures, amenorrhea, cataracts, glaucoma, peptic ulcer disease, and CHF.

! Abruptly withdrawing the drug after long-term therapy may cause anorexia, nausea, fever, headache, joint pain, rebound inflammation, fatigue, weakness, lethargy, dizziness, and orthostatic hypotension.

PEDIATRIC CONSIDERATIONS

Baseline Assessment

- Obtain the patient's baseline B/P, chest radiograph, EKG, blood glucose and serum electrolyte levels, and weight.
- Be aware that it is unknown whether fludrocortisone crosses the placenta or is distributed in breast milk.

- Be aware that fludrocortisone use in children may cause growth suppression and inhibition of endogenous steroid production.

Precautions
- Use cautiously in pts with edema, hypertension, and impaired renal function.

Administration and Handling
PO
- Give fludrocortisone with food or milk.

Intervention and Evaluation
- Monitor the patient's B/P, and blood glucose, serum renin, and electrolyte levels.
- Taper the drug dosage slowly if fludrocortisone is to be discontinued.

Patient/Family Teaching
- Warn the patient/family not to alter the drug dose or schedule. Also caution the patient not to abruptly discontinue the drug. Explain to the patient that fludrocortisone dosages must be tapered gradually.
- Tell the patient/family to notify the physician if the patient experiences continuing headaches, fever, muscle aches, sore throat, or sudden weight gain or swelling.
- Instruct the patient/family to maintain careful personal hygiene and to avoid exposure to disease or trauma.
- Explain that severe stress such as serious infection, surgery, or trauma may require the fludrocortisone dosage to be increased.
- Explain that steroids often cause mood swings, ranging from euphoria to depression.

Hydrocortisone

high-droe-**core**-tah-sewn
(Colifoam [AUS], Cortef cream [AUS], Cortic cream [AUS], Derm-Aid cream [AUS], Dermaid [AUS], Dermaid soft cream [AUS], Egocort cream [AUS], Hycor [AUS], Hycor eye ointment [AUS], Siquent Hycor [AUS], Squibb HC [AUS], WestCort)

CATEGORY AND SCHEDULE

Pregnancy Risk Category: C (D if used in first trimester)
OTC (Hydrocortisone 0.5% and 1% Cream, Gel, and Ointment)

MECHANISM OF ACTION

An adrenal corticosteroid that inhibits accumulation of inflammatory cells at inflammation sites, phagocytosis, lysosomal enzyme release, and synthesis or release of mediators of inflammation. ***Therapeutic Effect:*** Prevents or suppresses cell-mediated immune reactions. Decreases or prevents tissue response to the inflammatory process.

PHARMACOKINETICS

Route	Onset	Peak	Duration
IV	N/A	4–6 hrs	8–12 hrs

Well absorbed after all routes of administration. Widely distributed. Metabolized in liver. ***Half-Life:*** Plasma: 1.5–2 hrs; biologic: 8–12 hrs.

AVAILABILITY

Hydrocortisone
Gel: 1%, 2%.
Lotion: 0.25%, 0.5%, 1%, 2%, 2.5%.

Cream: 0.5%, 1%, 2.5%.
Ointment: 0.5%, 1%, 2.5%.
Topical Solution: 1%.
Oral Suspension: 10 mg/ 5 mL.
Hydrocortisone Sodium Phosphate
Injection: 50 mg/mL.
Hydrocortisone Sodium Succinate
Injection: 100 mg, 250 mg, 500 mg, 1,000 mg.
Hydrocortisone Acetate
Injection: 25 mg/mL, 50 mg/mL.
Suppository: 10 mg, 25 mg, 30 mg.
Cream: 0.5%, 1%.
Ointment: 0.5%, 1%.
Hydrocortisone Valerate
Cream: 0.2%.

INDICATIONS AND DOSAGES

▸ Acute adrenal insufficiency
IV/IM
Children. 1–2 mg/kg/dose bolus, then 150–250 mg/day in divided doses q6–8h.
Infants. 1–2 mg/kg/dose bolus, then 25–150 mg/day in divided doses q6–8h.

▸ Anti-inflammatory and immunosuppression
PO
Children. 2.5–10 mg/kg/day in divided doses q6–8h.
IM/IV
Children. 1–5 mg/kg/day in divided doses q12–24h.

▸ Physiologic replacement
IM
Children. 0.25–0.35 mg/kg/day as a single daily dose.
PO
Children. 0.5–0.75 mg/kg/day in divided doses q8h.

▸ Status asthmaticus
IV
Children. Loading dose 4–8 mg/kg/dose once. Maintenance: 0.5–2 mg/kg/dose q6h.

▸ Shock (use sodium succinate)
IV
Children 12 yrs and older. 100–500 mg q6h.
Children younger than 12 yrs. 50 mg/kg. May repeat in 4 hrs, then q24h as needed.

▸ Inflammation
RECTAL
Adolescents and children. 1 application daily for 2–3 wks.

▸ Adjunctive treatment of ulcerative colitis
Adolescents and children. 1 enema nightly for 21 days or until remission.
TOPICAL
Adolescents and children. Apply sparingly 2–4 times/day.

CONTRAINDICATIONS

Hypersensitivity to hydrocortisone or any related component. Fungal, tubercular, or viral skin lesions, serious infections.

INTERACTIONS

Drug

Amphotericin: May increase hypokalemia.
Digoxin: May increase the risk of toxicity of this drug caused by hypokalemia.
Diuretics, insulin, oral hypoglycemics, potassium supplements: May decrease the effects of diuretics, insulin, oral hypoglycemics, and potassium supplements.
Liver enzyme inducers: May decrease the effects of hydrocortisone.
Live virus vaccines: May decrease the patient's antibody response to vaccine, increase vaccine side effects, and potentiate virus replication.

Herbal

None known.

Food
None known.

DIAGNOSTIC TEST EFFECTS
May decrease serum calcium, potassium, and thyroxine levels. May increase blood glucose levels, serum lipids, amylase, and sodium levels.

IV INCOMPATIBILITIES
Ciprofloxacin (Cipro), diazepam (Valium), idarubicin (Idamycin), midazolam (Versed), phenytoin (Dilantin)

IV COMPATIBILITIES
Aminophylline, amphotericin, calcium gluconate, cefepime (Maxipime), digoxin (Lanoxin), diltiazem (Cardizem), diphenhydramine (Benadryl), dopamine (Intropin), insulin, lidocaine, lorazepam (Ativan), magnesium sulfate, morphine, norepinephrine (Levophed), procainamide (Pronestyl), potassium chloride, propofol (Diprivan)

SIDE EFFECTS
Frequent
Insomnia, heartburn, nervousness, abdominal distention, diaphoresis, acne, mood swings, increased appetite, facial flushing, delayed wound healing, increased susceptibility to infection, diarrhea or constipation
Occasional
Headache, edema, change in skin color, frequent urination
Topical: Itching, redness, irritation
Rare
Tachycardia, allergic reaction rash and hives, psychic changes, hallucinations, depression
Topical: Allergic contact dermatitis, purpura
Systemic: Absorption more likely with occlusive dressings or extensive application in young children

SERIOUS REACTIONS
! The serious reactions of long-term therapy are hypocalcemia, hypokalemia, muscle wasting, especially in arms and legs, osteoporosis, spontaneous fractures, amenorrhea, cataracts, glaucoma, peptic ulcer disease, and CHF.
! Abruptly withdrawing the drug after long-term therapy may cause anorexia, nausea, fever, headache, sudden severe joint pain, rebound inflammation, fatigue, weakness, lethargy, dizziness, and orthostatic hypotension.

PEDIATRIC CONSIDERATIONS

Baseline Assessment
• Determine whether the patient has a hypersensitivity to any corticosteroids.
• Obtain the patient's baseline blood pressure, blood glucose and serum electrolyte levels, height, and weight.
• Evaluate the results of initial tests, such as a tuberculosis skin test, radiographs, and EKG.
• Determine whether the patient has diabetes mellitus, and anticipate an increase in his or her antidiabetic drug regimen because of raised blood glucose levels.
• Find out whether the patient takes digoxin, and if so plan to draw blood for measurement of serum digoxin levels.
• Be aware that hydrocortisone crosses the placenta and is distributed in breast milk.
• Be aware that chronic hydrocortisone use during the first trimester

of pregnancy may produce cleft palate in the neonate.
• Be aware that breast-feeding is contraindicated in this patient population.
• Be aware that prolonged treatment or high dosages may decrease the cortisol secretion and short-term growth rate in children.

Precautions
• Use cautiously in pts with cirrhosis, CHF, diabetes mellitus, hypertension, hyperthyroidism, osteoporosis, peptic ulcer, seizure disorders, thromboembolic tendencies, thrombophlebitis, and ulcerative colitis.

Administration and Handling

IV
• Store at room temperature.
• After reconstitution, use hydrocortisone sodium succinate solution within 72 hrs. Use immediately if further diluted with D_5W, 0.9% NaCl, or other compatible diluent.
• Once reconstituted, hydrocortisone sodium succinate solution is stable for 72 hrs at room temperature.
• May further dilute hydrocortisone sodium succinate solution with D_5W or 0.9% NaCl. For IV push, dilute to 50 mg/mL; for intermittent infusion, dilute to 1 mg/mL.
• Administer hydrocortisone sodium succinate solution IV push over 3–5 min. Give intermittent infusion over 20–30 min.

TOPICAL
• Gently cleanse area before application.
• Use occlusive dressings only as ordered.
• Apply sparingly, and rub into area thoroughly.

RECTAL
• Shake homogeneous suspension well.
• Instruct the patient to lie on his or her left side with the left leg extended and the right leg flexed.
• Gently insert the applicator tip into the rectum, pointed slightly toward the umbilicus, and slowly instill the medication.

Intervention and Evaluation
• Examine the patient for edema.
• Be alert to signs and symptoms of infection such as fever and sore throat that indicate a reduced immune response.
• Assess the patient's daily pattern of bowel activity.
• Monitor the patient's electrolyte levels.
• Observe the patient for evidence of hypocalcemia, such as cramps or muscle twitching, or hypokalemia, such as EKG changes, irritability, nausea and vomiting, numbness or tingling of the lower extremities, and weakness.
• Evaluate the patient's ability to sleep and emotional status.

Patient/Family Teaching
• Warn the patient/family to notify the physician if the patient experiences fever, muscle aches, sore throat, or sudden weight gain or swelling.
• Instruct the patient/family to consult with the physician before the patient takes aspirin or any other medication during hydrocortisone therapy.
• Urge the patient/family to avoid alcohol and limit the patient's caffeine intake during hydrocortisone therapy.
• Tell the patient/family to notify the patient's dentist and other physicians of his or her use of cortisone therapy now or within past 12 mos.

• Caution the patient/family against overuse of joints injected for symptomatic relief.
• Instruct the patient/family to apply topical hydrocortisone valerate after a bath or shower for best absorption. Teach the patient/family not to cover the affected area with any coverings, plastic pants, or tight diapers unless the physician instructs otherwise.
• Warn the patient/family to avoid getting the medication in contact with the patient's eyes.
• Explain that steroids often cause mood swings, ranging from euphoria to depression.

Methylprednisolone

meth-ill-pred-**niss**-oh-lone
(Medrol)

Methylprednisolone Acetate

(Depo-Medrol, Depo-Nisolone [AUS])

Methylprednisolone Sodium Succinate

(A-methaPred, Solu-Medrol)
Do not confuse with Mebaral or medroxyprogesterone.

CATEGORY AND SCHEDULE

Pregnancy Risk Category: C

MECHANISM OF ACTION

An adrenal corticosteroid that suppresses migration of polymorphonuclear leukocytes and reverses increased capillary permeability. ***Therapeutic Effect:*** Decreases inflammation.

PHARMACOKINETICS

Route	Onset	Peak	Duration
PO	N/A	1–2 hrs	30–36 hrs
IM	N/A	4–8 days	1–4 wks

Well absorbed from the GI tract after IM administration. Widely distributed. Metabolized in liver. Excreted in urine. Removed by hemodialysis. ***Half-Life:*** Longer than 3.5 hrs.

AVAILABILITY

Tablets: 2 mg, 4 mg, 8 mg, 16 mg, 24 mg, 32 mg.
Succinate
Powder for Injection: 40 mg, 125 mg, 500 mg, 1 g, 2 g.
Acetate
Injection: 20 mg/mL, 40 mg/mL, 80 mg/mL.

INDICATIONS AND DOSAGES

▸ **Anti-inflammatory or immunosuppressive**
PO/IM/IV (NOTE ONLY SODIUM SUCCINATE SALT MAY BE GIVEN IV)
Children. 0.5–1.7 mg/kg/day in divided doses q6–12h.
▸ **Status asthmaticus**
IV
Children. Loading dose of 2 mg/kg/dose followed by 0.5–1 mg/kg/dose q6h.
▸ **Lupus nephritis**
IV
Children. 30 mg/kg given over 30 min every other day for 6 doses.
▸ **Acute spinal cord injury**
IV
Children. 30 mg/kg given over 15 min. May be followed in 45 min with a continuous IV infusion of 5.4 mg/kg/hr for 23 hrs.

CONTRAINDICATIONS

Hypersensitivity to methylprednisolone or any related component. Administration of live virus vaccines, systemic fungal infection.

INTERACTIONS

Drug

Amphotericin: May increase hypokalemia.
Digoxin: May increase the risk of toxicity of this drug caused by hypokalemia
Diuretics, insulin, oral hypoglycemics, potassium supplements: May decrease the effects of diuretics, insulin, oral hypoglycemics, and potassium supplements.
Liver enzyme inducers: May decrease the effects of methylprednisolone.
Live virus vaccines: May decrease the patient's antibody response to vaccine, increase vaccine side effects, and potentiate virus replication.

Herbal

None known.

Food

None known.

DIAGNOSTIC TEST EFFECTS

May decrease serum calcium, potassium, and thyroxine levels. May increase blood glucose, serum lipid, amylase, and sodium levels.

IV INCOMPATIBILITIES

Ciprofloxacin (Cipro), diltiazem (Cardizem), docetaxel (Taxotere), etoposide (VePesid), filgrastim (Neupogen), gemcitabine (Gemzar), paclitaxel (Taxol), potassium chloride, propofol (Diprivan), vinorelbine (Navelbine)

IV COMPATIBILITIES

Dopamine (Intropin), heparin, midazolam (Versed), theophylline

SIDE EFFECTS

Frequent
Insomnia, heartburn, nervousness, abdominal distention, diaphoresis, acne, mood swings, increased appetite, facial flushing, GI distress, delayed wound healing, increased susceptibility to infection, diarrhea or constipation
Occasional
Headache, edema, tachycardia, change in skin color, frequent urination, depression
Rare
Psychosis, increased blood coagulability, hallucinations

SERIOUS REACTIONS

! The serious reactions of long-term therapy are hypocalcemia, hypokalemia, muscle wasting, especially in arms and legs, osteoporosis, spontaneous fractures, amenorrhea, cataracts, glaucoma, peptic ulcer disease, and CHF.
! Abruptly withdrawing the drug after long-term therapy may cause anorexia, nausea, fever, headache, sudden severe joint pain, rebound inflammation, fatigue, weakness, lethargy, dizziness, and orthostatic hypotension.

PEDIATRIC CONSIDERATIONS

Baseline Assessment

- Determine whether the patient has a hypersensitivity to any corticosteroids.
- Obtain the patient's baseline blood pressure (B/P), blood glucose and serum electrolyte levels, height, and weight.
- Evaluate the results of initial tests, such as a tuberculosis skin test, radiographs, and EKG.
- Determine whether the patient has diabetes mellitus, and antici-

pate an increase in his or her antidiabetic drug regimen because of raised blood glucose levels.

• Find out whether your patient takes digoxin, and if so plan to draw blood for measurement of serum digoxin levels.

• Be aware that methylprednisolone crosses the placenta and is distributed in breast milk.

• Be aware that chronic methylprednisolone use in the first trimester of pregnancy may cause cleft palate in the neonate.

• Be aware that breast-feeding is contraindicated in this patient population.

• Be aware that prolonged treatment or high dosages may decrease cortisol secretion and short-term growth rate in children.

• Be cautious to not confuse Solu-Cortef (hydrocortisone sodium succinate) with Solu-Medrol.

Precautions

• Use cautiously in pts with cirrhosis, CHF, diabetes mellitus, hypertension, hypothyroidism, thromboembolic disorders, and ulcerative colitis.

Administration and Handling

◂ ALERT ▸ Individualize the drug dose based on the disease, patient, and response.

PO

• Give methylprednisolone with food or milk.

• Give single doses before 9 A.M.; give multiple doses at evenly spaced intervals.

IM

• Methylprednisolone acetate should not be further diluted.

• Methylprednisolone sodium succinate should be reconstituted with bacteriostatic water for injection.

• Give deep IM injection in gluteus maximus.

IV

• Store vials at room temperature.

• Follow directions with a Mix-o-vial.

• For infusion, add to D_5W or 0.9% NaCl.

• Give IV push over 2–3 min.

• Give IV piggyback over 10–20 min.

• Do not give methylprednisolone acetate via IV infusion.

Intervention and Evaluation

• Monitor the patient's intake and output, and record the patient's daily weight.

• Assess the patient for edema.

• Evaluate the patient's pattern of daily bowel activity.

• Check the patient's vital signs at least 2 times/day.

• Be alert to signs and symptoms of infection such as fever, sore throat, or vague symptoms.

• Monitor the patient's electrolytes.

• Observe the patient for evidence of hypocalcemia, such as cramps, muscle twitching, or hypokalemia, such as EKG changes, irritability, nausea and vomiting, numbness or tingling of lower extremities, or weakness.

• Assess the patient's ability to sleep and emotional status.

• Check the patient's laboratory results for blood coagulability and clinical evidence of thromboembolism.

Patient/Family Teaching

• Instruct the patient/family to take oral methylprednisolone with food or milk.

• Caution the patient/family against abruptly discontinuing the drug or changing the drug dose or schedule. Explain to the patient/family that methylprednisolone doses must be tapered gradually under medical supervision.

• Warn the patient/family to notify the physician if the patient experiences fever, muscle aches, sore throat, or sudden weight gain or swelling.
• Tell the patient/family to maintain good personal hygiene and to avoid exposure to disease or trauma. Explain to the patient/family that severe stress, such as serious infection, surgery, or trauma may require an increase in methylprednisolone dosage.
• Stress to the patient/family that follow-up visits and laboratory tests are a necessary part of treatment and that children must be assessed for growth retardation.
• Tell the patient/family to inform the patient's dentist or other physicians of methylprednisolone therapy now or within past 12 mos.
• Explain that steroids often cause mood swings, ranging from euphoria to depression.

Prednisolone

pred-**niss**-oh-lone
(AK-Pred, AK-Tate [CAN], Econopred, Inflamase, Minims-Prednisolone [CAN], Novo-Prednisolone [CAN], Pediapred, Pred Mild, Prelone)

CATEGORY AND SCHEDULE

Pregnancy Risk Category: C (D if used in first trimester)

MECHANISM OF ACTION

An adrenal corticosteroid that inhibits accumulation of inflammatory cells at inflammation sites, phagocytosis, lysosomal enzyme release and synthesis, and release of mediators of inflammation. ***Therapeutic Effect:*** Prevents or suppresses cell-mediated immune reactions. Decreases or prevents tissue response to the inflammatory process.

AVAILABILITY

Ophthalmic Suspension: 0.12%, 0.125%, 1%.
Ophthalmic Solution: 0.125%, 1%.
Oral Solution: 5 mg/5 mL, 15 mg/5 mL.
Oral Suspension: 5 mg/5 mL
Tablets: 5 mg, 20 mg.

INDICATIONS AND DOSAGES

▸ Acute asthma
PO
Adolescents and children. 1–2 mg/kg/day in divided doses.
IV
Adolescents and children. 2–4 mg/kg/day in 3–4 divided doses.

▸ Anti-inflammation or immunosuppression
PO/IV
Adolescents and children. 0.1–2 mg/kg/day in divided doses.

▸ Nephrotic syndrome
PO
Adolescents and children. Initially give 2 mg/kg/day in 3–4 divided doses until the urine is free from protein for 5 days. Maximum: 80 mg/day. If proteinuria persists, give a 4 mg/kg/dose every other day for 28 additional days. Maximum: 120 mg/day. Normal maintenance dose is 2 mg/kg/dose every other day for 28 days tapered off over 4–6 wks.
OPHTHALMIC SOLUTION
Children. 1–2 drops q1h during the day; q2h during the night; after response, decrease dosage to 1 drop q4h, then 1 drop 3–4 times/day.

CONTRAINDICATIONS

Hypersensitivity to prednisolone or any related component. Acute superficial herpes simplex keratitis, systemic fungal infections, varicella.

INTERACTIONS

Drug

Amphotericin: May increase hypokalemia.
Digoxin: May increase the risk of toxicity of this drug caused by hypokalemia.
Diuretics, insulin, oral hypoglycemics, potassium supplements: May decrease the effects of diuretics, insulin, oral hypoglycemics, and potassium supplements.
Liver enzyme inducers: May decrease the effects of prednisolone.
Live virus vaccines: May decrease the patient's antibody response to vaccine, increase vaccine side effects, and potentiate virus replication.

Herbal

None known.

Food

None known.

DIAGNOSTIC TEST EFFECTS

May decrease serum calcium, potassium, and thyroxine levels. May increase blood glucose, serum lipid, amylase, and sodium levels.

SIDE EFFECTS

Frequent
Insomnia, heartburn, nervousness, abdominal distention, increased sweating, acne, mood swings, increased appetite, facial flushing, delayed wound healing, increased susceptibility to infection, diarrhea or constipation
Occasional
Headache, edema, change in skin color, frequent urination
Rare
Tachycardia, allergic reaction, such as rash and hives, psychic changes, hallucinations, depression
Ophthalmic: stinging or burning, posterior subcapsular cataracts

SERIOUS REACTIONS

! The serious effects of long-term therapy are hypocalcemia, hypokalemia, muscle wasting, especially in the arms and legs, osteoporosis, spontaneous fractures, amenorrhea, cataracts, glaucoma, peptic ulcer disease, and CHF.
! Abruptly withdrawing the drug after long-term therapy may cause anorexia, nausea, fever, headache, severe or sudden joint pain, rebound inflammation, fatigue, weakness, lethargy, dizziness, and orthostatic hypotension.
! Sudden discontinuance may be fatal.

PEDIATRIC CONSIDERATIONS

Baseline Assessment

- Determine whether the patient has a hypersensitivity to any corticosteroids.
- Obtain the patient's baseline blood pressure, blood glucose and serum electrolyte levels, height, and weight.
- Evaluate the results of initial tests, such as a tuberculosis skin test, radiographs, and EKG.
- Determine whether the patient has diabetes mellitus, and anticipate an increase in his or her antidiabetic drug regimen because of raised blood glucose levels.
- Find out whether your patient takes digoxin, and if so plan to draw blood for measurement of serum digoxin levels.
- Remember never to give this patient population a live virus vaccine, such as smallpox.

Precautions

- Use cautiously in pts with cirrhosis, CHF, diabetes mellitus, hypertension, hypothyroidism, myasthenia gravis, ocular herpes simplex, osteoporosis, peptic ulcer disease, thromboembolic disorders, and ulcerative colitis.

Intervention and Evaluation

- Be alert to signs and symptoms of infection such as fever, sore throat, or vague symptoms.
- Assess the patient's mouth daily for signs of *Candida* infection, such as white patches and painful mucous membranes and tongue.

Patient/Family Teaching

- Warn the patient/family to notify the physician if the patient experiences fever, muscle aches, sore throat, and sudden weight gain, or swelling.
- Urge the patient/family to avoid alcohol and to limit the patient's caffeine intake during prednisolone therapy.
- Caution the patient/family against abruptly discontinuing the drug without the physician's approval.
- Tell the patient/family to avoid exposure to chickenpox or measles.
- Explain that steroids often cause mood swings, ranging from euphoria to depression.

Prednisone

pred-nih-sewn

(Apo-Prednisone [CAN], Deltasone, Meticorten, Panafcort [AUS], Sone [AUS], Winpred [CAN])

Do not confuse with prednisolone or Primidone.

CATEGORY AND SCHEDULE

Pregnancy Risk Category: C (D if used in first trimester)

MECHANISM OF ACTION

An adrenal corticosteroid that inhibits accumulation of inflammatory cells at inflammation sites, phagocytosis, lysosomal enzyme release and synthesis, and release of mediators of inflammation. ***Therapeutic Effect:*** Prevents or suppresses cell-mediated immune reactions. Decreases or prevents tissue response to inflammatory process.

PHARMACOKINETICS

Well absorbed from the GI tract. Protein binding: 70%–90%. Widely distributed. Metabolized in liver and converted to prednisolone. Primarily excreted in urine. Not removed by hemodialysis. ***Half-Life:*** 3.4–3.8 hrs.

AVAILABILITY

Tablets: 1 mg, 2.5 mg, 5 mg, 10 mg, 20 mg, 50 mg.

Oral Solution: 5 mg/5 mL, 5 mg/mL.

INDICATIONS AND DOSAGES

▸ **Acute asthma**

PO

Adolescents and children. 0.5–2 mg/kg/day in divided doses. Maximum: 20–40 mg/day.

▸ **Anti-inflammation and immunosuppression**

PO

Adolescents and children. 0.05–2 mg/kg/day in divided doses.

▸ **Nephrotic syndrome**

PO

Adolescents and children. Initially give 2 mg/kg/day in 3–4 divided doses until the urine is free from protein for 5 days. Maximum: 80 mg/day. If proteinuria persists, give 4 mg/kg/dose every other day for 28 additional days. Maximum: 120 mg/day. Normal maintenance dose is 2 mg/kg/dose every other day for 28 days tapered off over 4–6 wks.

▸ **Physiologic replacement**
PO
Adolescents and children. 4–5 mg/m²/dose in 2 divided doses.

CONTRAINDICATIONS

Hypersensitivity to prednisone or any related component. Acute superficial herpes simplex keratitis, systemic fungal infections, varicella.

INTERACTIONS

Drug

Amphotericin: May increase hypokalemia.
Digoxin: May increase the risk of toxicity of this drug caused by hypokalemia
Diuretics, insulin, oral hypoglycemics, potassium supplements: May decrease the effects of diuretics, insulin, oral hypoglycemics, and potassium supplements.
Salicylates, NSAIDs, caffeine, alcohol: May increase the risk for GI bleeding.
Liver enzyme inducers: May decrease the effects of prednisone.
Live virus vaccines: May decrease the patient's antibody response to vaccine, increase vaccine side effects, and potentiate virus replication.

Herbal

None known.

Food

None known.

DIAGNOSTIC TEST EFFECTS

May decrease serum calcium, potassium, and thyroxine levels. May increase blood glucose, serum lipid, amylase, and sodium levels.

SIDE EFFECTS

Frequent
Insomnia, heartburn, nervousness, abdominal distention, increased sweating, acne, mood swings, increased appetite, facial flushing, delayed wound healing, increased susceptibility to infection, diarrhea or constipation
Occasional
Headache, edema, change in skin color, frequent urination
Rare
Tachycardia, allergic reaction, including rash and hives, psychic changes, hallucinations, depression

SERIOUS REACTIONS

! The serious reactions of long-term therapy are muscle wasting in the arms and legs, osteoporosis, spontaneous fractures, amenorrhea, cataracts, glaucoma, peptic ulcer disease, and CHF.
! Abruptly withdrawing the drug after long-term therapy may cause anorexia, nausea, fever, headache, sudden or severe joint pain, rebound inflammation, fatigue, weakness, lethargy, dizziness, and orthostatic hypotension.
! Sudden discontinuance of the drug may be fatal.

PEDIATRIC CONSIDERATIONS

Baseline Assessment

- Determine whether the patient has a hypersensitivity to any corticosteroids.
- Obtain the patient's baseline blood pressure (B/P), blood glucose and serum electrolyte levels, height, and weight.
- Determine whether the patient has diabetes mellitus, and anticipate an increase in his or her antidiabetic drug regimen because of raised blood glucose levels.
- Find out whether your patient takes digoxin, and if so plan to draw blood for measurement of serum digoxin levels.

• Check the results of initial patient tests, such as a tuberculosis skin test, radiographs, and EKG.
• Remember never to give this patient population live virus vaccine, such as smallpox.
• Be aware that prednisone crosses the placenta and is distributed in breast milk.
• Be aware that chronic prednisone use in the first trimester of pregnancy causes cleft palate in the neonate.
• Be aware that prolonged treatment or high dosages may decrease cortisol secretion and short-term growth rate of children.
• Be aware that this medication has a bitter taste. Interventions need to be conducted to help decrease this taste in pediatric pts.
• Be sure not to confuse this medication with prednisolone.

Precautions

• Use cautiously in pts with cirrhosis, CHF, hypertension, hyperthyroidism, myasthenia gravis, ocular herpes simplex, osteoporosis, peptic ulcer disease, thromboembolic disorders, and ulcerative colitis.

Administration and Handling

PO

• Give prednisone without regard to meals; give with food if GI upset occurs.
• Give single doses before 9 A.M.; give multiple doses at evenly spaced intervals.

Intervention and Evaluation

• Monitor the patient's B/P, blood glucose and electrolyte levels, and height. In pediatric pts also monitor weight.
• Be alert to signs and symptoms of infection such as fever, sore throat, or vague symptoms.
• Assess the patient's mouth daily for signs of *Candida* infection, such as white patches and painful mucous membranes and tongue.

Patient/Family Teaching

• Warn the patient/family to notify the physician if the patient experiences fever, muscle aches, sore throat, or sudden weight gain or swelling.
• Urge the patient/family to avoid alcohol and limit the patient's caffeine intake during prednisone therapy.
• Caution the patient/family against abruptly discontinuing prednisone without the physician's approval.
• Warn the patient/family to avoid exposure to chickenpox or measles.
• Explain that steroids often cause mood swings, ranging from euphoria to depression.

Triamcinolone 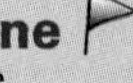

try-am-**sin**-oh-lone
(Aristocort)

Triamcinolone Acetonide

(Aristocort, Azmacort, Kenalog, Nasacort AQ, Triaderm [CAN])

Triamcinolone Diacetate

(Amcort, Aristocort Intralesional)

Triamcinolone Hexacetonide

(Aristospan)
Do not confuse with Triaminicin or Triaminicol.

CATEGORY AND SCHEDULE

Pregnancy Risk Category: C (D if used in first trimester)

MECHANISM OF ACTION
An adrenocortical steroid that inhibits accumulation of inflammatory cells at inflammation sites, phagocytosis, lysosomal enzyme release, and synthesis and release of mediators of inflammation. ***Therapeutic Effect:*** Prevents or suppresses cell-mediated immune reactions. Decreases or prevents tissue response to the inflammatory process.

AVAILABILITY
Tablets: 4 mg, 8 mg.
Syrup: 4 mg/ 5 mL.
Aerosol: 0.1% (acetonide).
Injection: 10 mg/mL, 40 mg/mL.
Oral paste: 0.1%.
Ointment: 0.025%, 0.1%, 0.5%.
Lotion: 0.025%, 0.1%.
Cream: 0.025%, 0.1%, 0.5%.
Aerosol (nasal spray): 55 mcg/inhalation.
Oral Inhalation (Azmacort): 100 mcg/actuation.
Diacetate
Injection: 25 mg/mL, 40 mg/mL.
Hexacetone
Injection: 5 mg/mL, 20 mg/mL.

INDICATIONS AND DOSAGES
▸ Adrenal insufficiency
PO
Children older than 12 yrs: 4–100 mg/day in 1–4 divided doses.
▸ Control of bronchial asthma
INHALATION
Children 6–12 yrs. 1–2 puffs acetonide 3–4 times/day. Maximum: 12 inhalations/day.
▸ Rhinitis
INTRANASAL
Children older than 6 yrs. 2 sprays each nostril daily.
▸ Topical anti-inflammatory
TOPICAL (AS TRIAMCINOLONE)
Children. Apply acetonide, 0.025% cream, ointment, or lotion as a thin film 2–3 times/day or 0.015% aerosol spray daily.
▸ Anti-inflammatory
IM (AS ACETONIDE OR HEXACETONIDE)
Children 6–12 yrs: 0.03–0.2 mg/kg at 1–7 day intervals.
INTRA-ARTICULAR, INTRASYNOVIAL (AS ACETONIDE OR HEXACETONIDE)
Children 6–12 yrs: 2.5–15 mg as needed.
Children older than 12 yrs: 2–20 mg q3–4wks (hexacetonide).
Children older than 12 yrs: 2.5–40 mg as needed (as diacetate or acetonide).

CONTRAINDICATIONS
Hypersensitivity to triamcinolone or any related component. Avoid immunizations, especially smallpox vaccination; hypersensitivity to any corticosteroid or tartrazine, IM injection, oral inhalation not for children younger than 6 yrs of age, peptic ulcers (except life-threatening situations), systemic fungal infection.
Topical: Marked circulation impairment.

INTERACTIONS
Drug
Amphotericin: May increase hypokalemia.
Digoxin: May increase the risk of toxicity of this drug caused by hypokalemia.
Diuretics, insulin, oral hypoglycemics, potassium supplements: May decrease the effects of diuretics, insulin, oral hypoglycemics, and potassium supplements.
Liver enzyme inducers: May decrease the effects of triamcinolone.

Live virus vaccines: May decrease the patient's antibody response to vaccine, increase vaccine side effects, and potentiate virus replication.
Salicylates, NSAIDs, caffeine, alcohol: May increase the risk of GI ulcer.

Herbal
None known.

Food
None known.

DIAGNOSTIC TEST EFFECTS

May decrease serum calcium, potassium, and thyroxine levels. May increase blood glucose, serum lipid, amylase, and sodium levels.

SIDE EFFECTS

Frequent
Insomnia, dry mouth, heartburn, nervousness, abdominal distention, diaphoresis, acne, mood swings, increased appetite, facial flushing, delayed wound healing, increased susceptibility to infection, diarrhea or constipation

Occasional
Headache, edema, change in skin color, frequent urination

Rare
Tachycardia, allergic reaction, including rash and hives, mental changes, hallucinations, depression
Topical: Allergic contact dermatitis.

SERIOUS REACTIONS

! The serious reactions of long-term therapy are muscle wasting in the arms or legs, osteoporosis, spontaneous fractures, amenorrhea, cataracts, glaucoma, peptic ulcer disease, and CHF.
! Abruptly withdrawing the drug after long-term therapy may cause anorexia, nausea, fever, headache, joint pain, rebound inflammation, fatigue, weakness, lethargy, dizziness, and orthostatic hypotension.
! Anaphylaxis with parenteral administration occurs rarely.
! Sudden discontinuance of the drug may be fatal.
! Blindness has occurred rarely after intralesional injection around the face and head.

PEDIATRIC CONSIDERATIONS

Baseline Assessment

- Determine whether the patient is hypersensitive to any corticosteroids or tartrazine (Kenacort).
- Obtain the patient's baseline blood pressure (B/P), blood glucose and serum electrolyte levels, height, and weight.
- Determine whether the patient has diabetes mellitus, and anticipate an increase in his or her antidiabetic drug regimen because of raised blood glucose levels.
- Find out whether your patient takes digoxin, and if so plan to draw blood for measurement of serum digoxin levels.
- Check the results of initial patient tests, such as a tuberculosis skin test, radiographs, and EKG.
- Remember never to give this patient population a live virus vaccine, such as smallpox.
- It is important to limit topical application in children to the least amount that is effective.

Precautions

- Use cautiously in pts with cirrhosis, CHF, a history of tuberculosis (because it may reactivate the disease), hypertension, hypothyroidism, nonspecific ulcerative colitis, psychosis, and renal insufficiency.
- Discontinue prolonged therapy slowly.

Administration and Handling

PO

• Give triamcinolone with food or milk.

• Give single doses before 9 A.M.; give multiple doses at evenly spaced intervals.

IM

• Do not give IV.

• Give IM injection deeply in the gluteus maximus.

INHALATION

• Shake container well; instruct the patient to exhale as completely as possible.

• Place the mouthpiece fully into the patient's mouth and while holding the inhaler upright, have the patient inhale deeply and slowly while pressing the top of the canister. Instruct the patient to hold his or her breath as long as possible before slowly exhaling.

• Wait 1 min between inhalations when multiple inhalations are ordered to allow for deeper bronchial penetration.

• Rinse the patient's mouth with water immediately after inhalation to prevent thrush.

TOPICAL

• Gently cleanse the area before application.

• Use occlusive dressings only as ordered.

• Apply sparingly and rub into the area thoroughly.

Intervention and Evaluation

• Monitor the patient's blood glucose level, B/P, and intake and output. Record the patient's daily weight.

• Assess the patient for edema.

• Check the patient's vital signs at least 2 times/day.

• Be alert to signs and symptoms of infection such as fever, sore throat, or vague symptoms.

• Evaluate the patient for signs and symptoms of hypocalcemia, such as cramps, muscle twitching, or a positive Chvostek or Trousseau sign, or hypokalemia, such as EKG changes, irritability, muscle cramps and weakness, nausea and vomiting, or numbness and tingling in the lower extremities.

• Assess the patient's ability to sleep and emotional status.

• Check the mucous membranes for signs of fungal infection in pts taking triamcinolone for oral inhalation.

• Monitor the growth rate in pediatric pts.

• Check the patient's laboratory results for blood coagulability and clinical evidence of thromboembolism.

• Assist the patient with ambulation.

Patient/Family Teaching

• Tell the patient/family taking oral triamcinolone to notify the physician if the patient experiences difficulty breathing, muscle weakness, sudden weight gain, or swelling of the face.

• Instruct the patient/family taking oral triamcinolone to take the drug with food or after meals.

• Warn the patient/family to notify the physician if the patient's condition worsens.

• Caution the patient/family against abruptly discontinuing oral triamcinolone without physician approval.

• Explain to the patient/family that oral triamcinolone may cause dry mouth.

• Urge the patient/family to avoid alcohol during oral triamcinolone therapy.

• Instruct the patient/family taking inhaled triamcinolone not to take the drug for acute asthma attacks.
• Tell the patient/family taking inhaled triamcinolone to rinse the patient's mouth after drug administration to decrease the risk of mouth soreness.
• Warn the patient/family taking inhaled triamcinolone to notify the physician if the patient experiences mouth lesions or soreness.
• Warn the patient/family taking nasal triamcinolone to notify the physician if the patient experiences persistent nasal bleeding, burning or infection, or unusual cough or spasm.
• Explain that steroids often cause mood swings, ranging from euphoria to depression.

REFERENCES

Miller, S. & Fioravanti, J. (1997). Pediatric medications: a handbook for nurses. St. Louis: Mosby.
Taketomo, C. K., Hodding, J. H. & Kraus, D. M. (2003–2004). Pediatric dosage handbook (10th ed.). Hudson, OH: Lexi-Comp.

61 Antidiabetic Agents

Insulin
Metformin Hydrochloride

Uses: All antidiabetic agents are used to treat diabetes. *Insulin* is used to manage insulin-dependent diabetes mellitus (type 1) and non–insulin-dependent diabetes mellitus (type 2). It is also used in acute situations, such as ketoacidosis, severe infections, and major surgery in otherwise non–insulin-dependent diabetes mellitus. It is administered to pts receiving parenteral nutrition and is the drug of choice during pregnancy.

Biguanides, such as metformin, are used along with diet to lower the blood glucose level in pts with type 2 diabetes mellitus whose hyperglycemia cannot be managed by diet alone.

Action: Antidiabetic agents act in different ways to control diabetes. *Insulin* is a hormone synthesized and secreted by beta-cells in the islets of Langerhans in the pancreas. It controls the storage and use of glucose, amino acids, and fatty acids by activated transport systems and enzymes. It also inhibits the breakdown of glycogen, fat, and protein. Insulin lowers the blood glucose level by inhibiting glycogenolysis and gluconeogenesis in the liver and by stimulating glucose uptake by muscle and adipose tissue. Insulin activity is initiated by binding to cell surface receptors.

Biguanides decrease hepatic glucose output and enhance peripheral glucose uptake.

COMBINATION PRODUCTS

AVANDAMET: metformin/rosiglitazone (an antidiabetic) 500 mg/1 mg; 500 mg/2 mg; 500 mg/4 mg; 1 g/2 mg; 1 g/4 mg.

GLUCOVANCE: glyburide/metformin (an antidiabetic) 1.25 mg/250 mg; 2.5 mg/500 mg; 5 mg/500 mg.

METAGLIP: glipizide/metformin (an antidiabetic) 2.5 mg/250 mg; 2.5 mg/500 mg; 5 mg/500 mg.

Insulin

in-sull-in

Rapid acting: Insulin lispro (Humalog), Insulin aspart (NovoLog, Novorapid [AUS]), Regular Insulin (Actrapid [AUS], Humulin R, Novolin R, Regular Iletin II)
Intermediate acting: NPH (Humulin N, Novolin N, pork), lente: (Humulin L, Lente Iletin II, Monotard [AUS], Novolin L)
NPH/regular mixture (70%/30%): Humulin 70/30, Novolin 70/30
NPH/regular mixture (50%/50%): Humulin 50/50
NPH/lispro mixture (75%/25%): Humalog Mix 75/25, NovoLog Mix 70/30
Long acting: Insulin glargine (Lantus)

CATEGORY AND SCHEDULE

Pregnancy Risk Category: B

MECHANISM OF ACTION

An exogenous insulin that facilitates passage of glucose, potassium, and magnesium across cellular membranes of skeletal and cardiac muscle, adipose tissue; controls storage and metabolism of carbohydrates, protein, and fats. Promotes conversion of glucose to glycogen in liver. ***Therapeutic Effect:*** Controls glucose levels in diabetic pts.

PHARMACOKINETICS

Drug Form	Onset (hrs)	Peak (hrs)	Duration (hrs)
Lispro	¼	½–1½	4–5
Insulin aspart	⅙	1–3	3–5
Regular	¼–1	2–4	5–7
NPH	1–2	6–14	24+
Lente	1–3	6–14	24+
Insulin glargine	N/A	N/A	24

AVAILABILITY

Fast-acting:
NovoLog (human)
Lispro (human)
Short-acting:
Humulin R (human)
Novolin R (human)
Iletin II Regular (purified pork)
Intermediate-acting:
Humulin L (human)
Novolin L (human)
Lente (pork)
Iletin II (pork)
Humulin N (human)
Novolin N (human)
NPH Iletin (pork)
Long-acting:
Lantus (human)
Humulin U Ultralente (human)
Combination, intermediate-acting:
Novolog Mix 70/30
Humalog Mix 75/25
Humulin 50/50
Humulin 70/30
Novolin 70/30

INDICATIONS AND DOSAGES

▸ **Treatment of insulin-dependent type 1 diabetes mellitus, non–insulin-dependent type 2 diabetes mellitus when diet or weight control therapy has failed to maintain satisfactory blood glucose levels or in event of fever, infection, pregnancy, severe endocrine, liver or renal dysfunction, surgery, or trauma, regular insulin used in emergency treatment of ketoacidosis, to promote passage of glucose across cell membrane in**

hyperalimentation, to facilitate intracellular shift of potassium in hyperkalemia
SC (DOSES MUST BE INDIVIDUALIZED FOR THE PATIENT)
Children. 0.5–1 unit/kg/day in divided doses.
Adolescents (during growth spurt). 0.8–1.2 units/kg/day in divided doses.

CONTRAINDICATIONS

Hypersensitivity or insulin resistance may require change of type or species source of insulin.

INTERACTIONS

Drug

These drugs may increase the hypoglycemic effects of insulin: ACE inhibitors, alcohol (acute use), alpha-blockers, anabolic steroids, beta-blockers, calcium, chloroquine, clofibrate, disopyramide, fluoxetine, guanethidine, lithium, MAO inhibitors, mebendazole, octreotide, oral hypoglycemic drugs, pentamidine, phenylbutazone, propoxyphene, pyridoxine, salicylates, sulfinpyrazones, sulfonamides, tetracyclines.
These drugs may decrease the hypoglycemic effects of insulin: acetazolamide, alcohol (chronic use), antiretrovirals, asparaginase, calcitonin, oral contraceptives, corticosteroids, cyclophosphamide, danazol, diazoxide, diltiazem, dobutamine, epinephrine, estrogens, ethacrynic acid, isoniazid, lithium, morphine, niacin, nicotine, phenothiazine, phenytoin, somatropin, terbutaline, thiazide diuretics, thyroid hormones.

Herbal

None known.

Food

None known.

DIAGNOSTIC TEST EFFECTS

May decrease serum magnesium, phosphate, and potassium concentrations.

IV INCOMPATIBILITIES

Digoxin (Lanoxin), diltiazem (Cardizem), dopamine (Intropin), nafcillin (Nafcil)

IV COMPATIBILITIES

Amiodarone (Cordarone), ampicillin/sulbactam (Unasyn), cefazolin (Ancef), cimetidine (Tagamet), digoxin (Lanoxin), dobutamine (Dobutrex), famotidine (Pepcid), gentamicin, heparin, magnesium sulfate, metoclopramide (Reglan), midazolam (Versed), milrinone (Primacor), morphine, nitroglycerin, potassium chloride, propofol (Diprivan), vancomycin (Vancocin)

SIDE EFFECTS

Occasional
Local redness, swelling, itching, caused by improper injection technique or allergy to cleansing solution or insulin
Infrequent
Somogyi effect, including rebound hyperglycemia with chronically excessive insulin doses, systemic allergic reaction, marked by rash, angioedema, and anaphylaxis, lipodystrophy or depression at injection site due to breakdown of adipose tissue, lipohypertrophy or accumulation of subcutaneous tissue at injection site due to lack of adequate site rotation
Rare
Insulin resistance

SERIOUS REACTIONS

! Severe hypoglycemia caused by hyperinsulinism may occur as a result of overdose of insulin, a decrease or delay of food intake, and excessive exercise or in those with brittle diabetes.

! Diabetic ketoacidosis may result from stress, illness, omission of insulin dose, or long-term poor insulin control.

PEDIATRIC CONSIDERATIONS

Baseline Assessment

- Check the patient's blood glucose level.
- Discuss the patient's lifestyle to determine the extent of his or her emotional and learning needs.
- Be aware that insulin is the drug of choice for treating diabetes mellitus during pregnancy, but close medical supervision is needed. After delivery, the patient's insulin needs may drop for 24–72 hrs, then rise to prepregnancy levels.
- Be aware that insulin is not secreted in breast milk and that lactation may decrease insulin requirements.
- Be aware that there are no age-related precautions noted in children.

Administration and Handling

◂ALERT▸ Know that insulin dosages are individualized and monitored. Adjust dosage, as prescribed, to achieve premeal and bedtime glucose level of 80–140 mg/dL in adults, and 100–200 mg/dL in children younger than 5 yrs.

SC

- Store currently used insulin at room temperature, avoiding extreme temperatures and direct sunlight. Store extra vials in refrigerator.
- Discard unused vials if not used for several weeks. No insulin should have a precipitate or discoloration.
- Give SC only. Regular insulin is the only insulin that may be given IV or IM for ketoacidosis or other specific situations.
- Warm the drug to room temperature; do not give cold insulin.
- Roll the drug vial gently between the hands; do not shake. Regular insulin normally appears clear. No insulin should have a precipitate or discoloration.
- Administer insulin approximately 30 min before a meal. Insulin lispro may be given up to 15 min before meals. Check the patient's blood glucose concentration before administration. Insulin dosages are highly individualized.
- Always draw regular insulin first when insulin is mixed. Mixtures must be administered at once because binding can occur within 5 min. Humalog may be mixed with Humulin N and Humulin L.
- Give SC injections in the abdomen, buttocks, thigh, upper arm, or upper back if there is adequate adipose tissue.
- Maintain a careful record of rotated injection sites.
- For home situations, prefilled syringes are stable for 1 wk under refrigeration, including stabilized mixtures, 15 min for NPH/regular and 24 hrs for lente/regular. Prefilled syringes should be stored in the vertical or oblique position to avoid plugging; the plunger should be pulled back slightly and the syringe rocked to remix the solution before injection.

IV (regular)

- Use only if solution is clear.
- May give undiluted.

Intervention and Evaluation

• Monitor the sleeping patient for diaphoresis and restlessness.
• Assess the patient for hypoglycemia, including anxiety, cool, wet skin, diplopia, dizziness, headache, hunger, numbness in the mouth, tachycardia, and tremors, or hyperglycemia, including deep, rapid breathing, dim vision, fatigue, nausea, polydipsia, polyphagia, polyuria, and vomiting.
• Be alert to conditions that alter blood glucose requirements, such as fever, increased activity, stress, or a surgical procedure.

Patient/Family Teaching

• Make sure that the patient/family is adept at drawing up the prescribed dose of insulin, and knows the proper injection technique. Also ensure that the patient can perform self blood glucose testing at the prescribed intervals.
• Stress to the patient/family that exercise, hygiene, including foot care, the prescribed diet, and weight control are integral parts of treatment. Warn the patient/family to avoid smoking and not to skip or delay meals.
• Ensure that the patient/family knows the signs and symptoms of hypo- and hyperglycemia. Tell the patient to carry candy, sugar packets, or other sugar supplements for immediate response to hypoglycemia.
• Urge the patient/family to have the patient wear medical alert identification.
• Instruct the patient/family to notify the physician when the patient's glucose demands are altered, such as by fever, heavy physical activity, infection, stress, and trauma.
• Tell the patient/family to inform the patient's dentist, other physicians, or surgeons of insulin therapy before any treatment is given.
• Encourage the patient not to drink alcohol while taking insulin.

Metformin Hydrochloride

met-**for**-min
(Diabex [AUS], Diaformin [AUS], Glucohexal [AUS], Glucomet [AUS], Glucophage, Glucophage XL, Glycon [CAN], Novo-Metformin [CAN], Riomet)

CATEGORY AND SCHEDULE

Pregnancy Risk Category: B

MECHANISM OF ACTION

An antihyperglycemic that decreases liver production of glucose, decreases absorption of glucose, and improves insulin sensitivity. ***Therapeutic Effect:*** Provides improvement in glycemic control, stabilizes or decreases body weight, and improves lipid profile.

PHARMACOKINETICS

Slowly, incompletely absorbed after PO administration or food delays or decrease extent of absorption. Protein binding: Negligible. Primarily distributed to intestinal mucosa, salivary glands. Primarily excreted unchanged in urine. Removed by hemodialysis. ***Half-Life:*** 3–6 hrs.

AVAILABILITY

Tablets: 500 mg, 850 mg, 1,000 mg.
Tablets (extended release): 500 mg, 750 mg, 1,000 mg.
Oral Solution: 100 mg/mL. (not available in the United States)

INDICATIONS AND DOSAGES

Diabetes mellitus (500-mg, 1,000-mg tablet)

PO

Children 17 yrs or older. Initially, 500 mg twice daily, with morning and evening meals. May increase dosage in 500-mg increments every week, in divided doses. Can be given 2 times/day up to 2,000 mg/day, for example, 1,000 mg 2 times/day with morning and evening meals. If a 2,500 mg/day dose is required, give 3 times/day with meals. Maximum per day: 2,500 mg.

Children 10–16 yrs. Initially, 500 mg 2 times/day. May increase by 500 mg/day at weekly intervals. Maximum: 2,000 mg/day.

▸ **Diabetes mellitus (850-mg tablet)**

PO

Children 17 yrs or older. Initially, 850 mg/day, with morning meal. May increase dosage in 850-mg increments every other week, in divided doses. Maintenance: 850 mg 2 times/day, with morning and evening meals. Maximum per day: 2,550 mg (850 mg 3 times/day).

▸ **Diabetes mellitus (extended-release tablets)**

PO

Children 17 yrs or older. Initially, 500 mg once daily. May increase by 500 mg/day at weekly intervals. Maximum: 2,000 mg/day once daily.

▸ **Adjunct to insulin therapy**

PO

Children 17 yrs or older. Initially, 500 mg/day. May increase by 500 mg at 7-day intervals. Maximum: 2,500 mg (2,000 mg for extended release).

UNLABELED USES

Treatment of metabolic complications of AIDS, prediabetes, weight reduction.

CONTRAINDICATIONS

Hypersensitivity to metformin or any related component. Acute myocardial infarction (MI), acute CHF, cardiovascular collapse, renal disease or dysfunction, respiratory failure, septicemia.

INTERACTIONS

Drug

Alcohol, amiloride, cimetidine, digoxin, furosemide, morphine, nifedipine, procainamide, quinidine, quinine, ranitidine, triamterene, trimethoprim, vancomycin: Increase metformin blood concentration.

Furosemide, hypoglycemia-causing medications: May decrease the dosage of metformin needed.

Iodinated contrast studies: May produce acute renal failure, increases risk of lactic acidosis.

Herbal

None known.

Food

Food may decrease the absorption of metformin.

DIAGNOSTIC TEST EFFECTS

None known.

SIDE EFFECTS

Occasional (greater than 3%)

GI disturbances are transient and resolve spontaneously during therapy, including diarrhea, nausea, vomiting, abdominal bloating, flatulence, and anorexia

Rare (3%–1%)

Unpleasant or metallic taste that resolves spontaneously during therapy

SERIOUS REACTIONS

! Lactic acidosis occurs rarely (0.03 cases/1,000 pts) but is a serious, often fatal (50%) complication. Lactic acidosis is characterized by an increase in blood lactate levels (greater than 5 mmol/L), a decrease in blood pH, and electrolyte disturbances. Symptoms include unexplained hyperventilation, myalgia, malaise, and somnolence. Lactic acidosis may advance to cardiovascular collapse (shock), acute CHF, acute MI, and prerenal azotemia.

PEDIATRIC CONSIDERATIONS

Baseline Assessment

- Inform the patient of the potential advantages and risks of metformin therapy and of alternative modes of therapy.
- Assess the patient's blood Hgb and Hct concentrations, RBC count, and serum creatinine levels before beginning metformin therapy and annually thereafter.
- Be aware that insulin is the drug of choice during pregnancy.
- Be aware that metformin is distributed in breast milk in animals.
- Be aware that the safety and efficacy of metformin have not been established in children.

Precautions

- Use cautiously in pts with conditions that cause hyperglycemia or hypoglycemia or delay food absorption, such as diarrhea, high fever, malnutrition, gastroparesis, and vomiting.
- Use cautiously in cardiovascular pts, in debilitated, liver-impaired, or malnourished pts with renal impairment, and in pts concurrently taking drugs that affect renal function.
- Use cautiously in pts with CHF, chronic respiratory difficulty, and uncontrolled hyperthyroidism or hypothyroidism.
- Use cautiously in pts who consume excessive amounts of alcohol.

Administration and Handling

◀ **ALERT** ▶ Plan to decrease the insulin dosage if blood glucose levels fall below 120 mg/dL.

◀ **ALERT** ▶ Be aware that lactic acidosis, is a rare but potentially severe consequence of metformin therapy. Withhold metformin in pts with conditions that may predispose them to lactic acidosis, such as dehydration, hypoperfusion, hypoxemia, and sepsis.

PO

- Do not crush film-coated tablets.
- Give metformin with meals.

Intervention and Evaluation

- Monitor the patient's fasting blood glucose, Hgb A, and folic acid levels and renal function.
- Assess the patient concurrently taking oral sulfonylureas for signs and symptoms of hypoglycemia, including anxiety, cool, wet skin, diplopia, dizziness, headache, hunger, numbness in the mouth, tachycardia, and tremors.
- Be alert to conditions that alter blood glucose requirements, such as fever, increased activity, stress, or a surgical procedure.

Patient/Family Teaching

- Warn the patient/family to notify the physician and discontinue metformin therapy, as prescribed, if the patient experiences signs or symptoms of lactic acidosis, such as extreme tiredness, muscle aches, unexplained hyperventilation, and unusual sleepiness.
- Stress to the patient/family that the prescribed diet is a principal part of treatment. Warn the patient/family not to skip or delay meals.
- Tell the patient/family that diabetes mellitus requires lifelong control.
- Urge the patient/family to avoid consuming alcohol.

• Instruct the patient/family to notify the physician if the patient experiences diarrhea, easy bleeding or bruising, change in the color of stool or urine, headache, nausea, persistent skin rash, and vomiting.

REFERENCES

Miller, S. & Fioravanti, J. (1997). Pediatric medications: a handbook for nurses. St. Louis: Mosby.

Taketomo, C. K., Hodding, J. H. & Kraus, D. M. (2003–2004). Pediatric dosage handbook (10th ed.). Hudson, OH: Lexi-Comp.

62 Estrogens and Progestins

Estradiol, Estradiol Cypionate, Estradiol Transdermal, Estradiol Valerate
Medroxyprogesterone Acetate

Uses: Estrogens and progestins are commonly used for contraception. They are also used to treat dysfunctional uterine bleeding and female hypogonadism.

Action: As ovarian sex hormones, estrogens and progestins provide different actions.

Estrogens, such as estradiol, mainly promote proliferation and growth of specific cells in the body and are responsible for the development of most secondary sex characteristics, such as the breasts and milk-producing apparatus. These agents primarily cause the cellular proliferation and growth of female reproductive organs, including the ovaries, fallopian tubes, uterus, and vagina.

Progestins, stimulate secretion by the uterine endometrium during the latter half of the female sexual cycle, preparing the uterus for implantation of the fertilized ovum. These hormones decrease the frequency of uterine contractions, which helps prevent expulsion of the implanted ovum. Progesterone also promotes breast development.

Estradiol

ess-tra-**dye**-ole
(Estrace, Estraderm MX [AUS], Sandrena Gel [AUS], Zumenon [AUS])

Estradiol Cypionate

(Depo Estradiol, Depogen)

Estradiol Transdermal

(Alora, Climara, Esclim, Estraderm, Vivelle, Vivelle Dot)

Estradiol Valerate

(Delestrogen, Valergen)
Do not confuse with Testoderm.

CATEGORY AND SCHEDULE

Pregnancy Risk Category: X

MECHANISM OF ACTION

An estrogen that increases synthesis of DNA, RNA, and proteins in target tissues; reduces release of gonadotropin-releasing hormone from the hypothalamus; and reduces follicle-stimulating hormone and luteinizing hormone (LH) release from the pituitary. ***Therapeutic Effect:*** Promotes normal growth and development of female sex organs, maintaining GU function and vasomotor stability. Prevents accelerated bone loss by inhibiting bone resorption, restoring the balance of bone resorption and formation. Inhibits LH and decreases the serum concentration of testosterone.

PHARMACOKINETICS

Well absorbed from the GI tract. Widely distributed. Protein binding: 50%–80%. Metabolized in liver. Primarily excreted in urine. ***Half-Life:*** Unknown.

AVAILABILITY

Tablets: 0.5 mg (Estrace), 1 mg (Estrace), 2 mg (Estrace).
Injection: 5 mg/mL (Cypionate), 10 mg/mL (Valerate), 20 mg/mL (Valerate), 40 mg/mL (Valerate).
Transdermal: 0.025 mg, 0.0375 mg, 0.05 mg, 0.075 mg, 0.1 mg.
Vaginal Cream: 100 mcg/g.
Vaginal Ring: 0.05 mg, 0.1 mg, 2 mg.

INDICATIONS AND DOSAGES

▸ Female hypogonadism

IM
Adolescents. 1.5–2 mg/mo (Cypionate), 10–20 mg/mo (Valerate).
PO
Adolescents. 0.5–2 mg/day cyclically (3 wks on, 1 wk off).
TRANSDERMAL
Adolescents. 0.025–0.05 mg/day patch put on once weekly (Climara), 0.05 mg 2 times/wk cyclically (3 wks using the patch and 1 wk off) in pts with an intact uterus, or continuous in pts without a uterus (other transdermal patches).

▸ Vaginal or vulvae atrophy

INTRAVAGINAL
Adolescents. Initially, 200–400 mcg/day (2–4 g of cream) estradiol daily for 1–2 wks; then 100–200 mcg (1–2 g) daily for 1–2 wks. Maintenance: After vaginal mucosa is restored: 100 mcg 1–3 times/wk for 3 wks, off 1 wk per cycle.

UNLABELED USES

Treatment of Turner syndrome.

CONTRAINDICATIONS

Hypersensitivity to estradiol or any related component. Abnormal vaginal bleeding, active arterial thrombosis, blood dyscrasias, estrogen-dependent cancer, known or suspected breast cancer, pregnancy, thrombophlebitis or thromboembolic disorders, thyroid dysfunction.

INTERACTIONS

Drug

Bromocriptine: May interfere with the effects of bromocriptine.
Cyclosporine: May increase the blood concentration and risk of liver toxicity and nephrotoxicity of cyclosporine.
Liver toxic medications: May increase the risk of liver toxicity.
Rifampin, phenobarbital, carbamazepine: May decrease the effects of estrogens.
Erythromycin, ketoconazole, clarithromycin itraconazole, ritonavir: May increase concentration and effects of estrogens.

Herbal

Saw palmetto: Increases the effects of saw palmetto.
St. John's wort: May decrease the effects of estrogens.

Food

Vitamin C: Large doses of vitamin C may increase the adverse effects of estradiol.
Grapefruit juice: May increase concentrations and effects of estradiol.

DIAGNOSTIC TEST EFFECTS

May affect metapyrone testing and thyroid function tests. May decrease serum cholesterol and lactate dehydrogenase levels. May increase blood glucose, high-density lipoprotein, serum calcium, and triglyceride levels.

SIDE EFFECTS

Frequent

Anorexia, nausea, swelling of breasts, peripheral edema, evidenced by swollen ankles, feet

Transdermal route: Skin irritation, redness

Occasional

Vomiting, especially with high dosages, headache that may be severe, intolerance to contact lenses, increased blood pressure (B/P), glucose intolerance, brown spots on exposed skin

Vaginal route: Local irritation, vaginal discharge, changes in vaginal bleeding, including spotting, breakthrough or prolonged bleeding

Rare

Chorea or involuntary movements, hirsutism or abnormal hairiness, loss of scalp hair, depression

SERIOUS REACTIONS

! Prolonged administration increases risk of gallbladder disease, thromboembolic disease, and breast, cervical, vaginal, endometrial, and liver carcinoma.

! Cholestatic jaundice occurs rarely.

PEDIATRIC CONSIDERATIONS

Baseline Assessment

• Determine whether the patient is hypersensitive to estrogen and whether she has had previous jaundice or thromboembolic disorders associated with pregnancy or estrogen therapy.

• Determine whether the patient is pregnant.

• Be aware that estradiol is distributed in breast milk and may be harmful to offspring. Estradiol should not be used during breast-feeding.

• Be aware that estradiol should be used cautiously in children whose bone growth is not complete as the drug may accelerate epiphyseal closure.

Precautions

• Use cautiously in pediatric pts whose bone growth is incomplete.

• Use cautiously in pts with diseases exacerbated by fluid retention and liver or renal insufficiency.

Administration and Handling

PO

• Administer estradiol at the same time each day.

IM

• Rotate the vial to disperse the drug in solution.

• Give IM injection deeply into the gluteus maximus.

VAGINAL

• Apply estradiol cream at bedtime for best absorption.

• Insert the end of the filled applicator into the patient's vagina, directed slightly toward the sacrum; push the plunger down completely.

• Avoid skin contact with cream to prevent skin absorption of the drug.

TRANSDERMAL

◂ **ALERT** ▸ Transdermal Climara is administered once weekly; others are administered twice weekly.

• Remove the old patch and select a new site. Consider using the buttocks as an alternative application site.

• Peel off the protective strip on the patch to expose the adhesive surface.

• Apply to clean, dry, intact skin on the trunk of the patient's body in an area with as little hair as possible.

• Press in place for at least 10 sec. Do not apply the patch to the patient's breasts or waistline.

Intervention and Evaluation

• Monitor the patient's B/P, blood glucose, hepatic enzyme, and serum calcium levels and weight.

Patient/Family Teaching

• Urge the patient/family to limit the patient's alcohol and caffeine intake.
• Encourage the patient/family to stop smoking tobacco.
• Warn the patient/family to notify the physician if the patient experiences calf or chest pain, mental depression, numbness or weakness of an extremity, severe abdominal pain, shortness of breath, speech or vision disturbance, sudden headache, unusual bleeding, and vomiting.

Medroxyprogesterone Acetate

meh-drocks-ee-pro-**jes**-ter-own
(Depo-Provera, Novo-Medrone [CAN], Provera, Ralovera [AUS])
Do not confuse with Ambien, hydroxyprogesterone, methylprednisolone, or methyltestosterone.

CATEGORY AND SCHEDULE

Pregnancy Risk Category: X

MECHANISM OF ACTION

A hormone that transforms endometrium from proliferative to secretory in an estrogen-primed endometrium; inhibits secretion of pituitary gonadotropins. ***Therapeutic Effect:*** Prevents follicular maturation and ovulation. Stimulates growth of mammary alveolar tissue; relaxes uterine smooth muscle. Restores hormonal imbalance.

PHARMACOKINETICS

Slow absorption after IM administration. Protein binding: 90%. Metabolized in liver. Primarily excreted in urine. ***Half-Life:*** 30 days.

AVAILABILITY

Tablets: 2.5 mg, 5 mg, 10 mg.
Injection: 150 mg/mL, 400 mg/mL.

INDICATIONS AND DOSAGES

▸ **Secondary amenorrhea**

PO

Adolescents. 5–10 mg/day for 5–10 days to begin at any time during the menstrual cycle or 2.5 mg/day.

▸ **Abnormal uterine bleeding**

PO

Adolescents. 5–10 mg/day for 5–10 days to begin on calculated day 16 or day 21 of the menstrual cycle.

▸ **Pregnancy prevention**

IM

Adolescents. 150 mg q3mos.

UNLABELED USES

Hormonal replacement therapy in estrogen-treated menopausal women, treatment of endometriosis.

CONTRAINDICATIONS

Hypersensitivity to medroxyprogesterone or any related component. Carcinoma of breast, estrogen-dependent neoplasm, history of or active thrombotic disorders, such as cerebral apoplexy, thrombophlebitis, or thromboembolic disorders, hypersensitivity to progestins, known or suspected pregnancy, missed abortion, severe liver dysfunction, undiagnosed abnormal genital bleeding, undiagnosed vaginal bleeding, use as pregnancy test.

INTERACTIONS

Drug

Bromocriptine: May interfere with the effects of bromocriptine.

Herbal

None known.

Food

None known.

DIAGNOSTIC TEST EFFECTS

Altered thyroid and liver function tests, prothrombin time, and metapyrone test results.

SIDE EFFECTS

Frequent

Transient menstrual abnormalities, including spotting, a change in menstrual flow or cervical secretions, and amenorrhea, at initiation of therapy

Occasional

Edema, weight change, breast tenderness, nervousness, insomnia, fatigue, dizziness

Rare

Alopecia, mental depression, dermatologic changes, headache, fever, nausea

SERIOUS REACTIONS

! Thrombophlebitis, pulmonary or cerebral embolism, and retinal thrombosis occur rarely.

PEDIATRIC CONSIDERATIONS

Baseline Assessment

• Determine whether the patient is hypersensitive to progestins or pregnant before beginning medroxyprogesterone therapy.
• Plan to obtain the patient's baseline blood glucose level, blood pressure (B/P), and weight.
• Be aware that medroxyprogesterone use should be avoided during pregnancy, especially in the first 4 mos as the drug may cause congenital heart and limb reduction defects in the neonate.
• Be aware that medroxyprogesterone is distributed in breast milk.
• Be aware that the safety and efficacy of this drug have not been established in children.

Precautions

• Use cautiously in pts with conditions aggravated by fluid retention, including asthma, seizures, migraine, and cardiac or renal dysfunction, diabetes mellitus, and a history of mental depression.

Administration and Handling

PO

• Give medroxyprogesterone without regard to meals.

IM

• Shake vial immediately before administering to ensure complete suspension.
• Inject IM only in upper arm or upper outer aspect of buttock. Rarely, a residual lump, change in skin color, or sterile abscess occurs at injection site.
• For first dose IM, administer only during the first 5 days of the normal menstrual period, only within 5 days postpartum if the patient is not breast-feeding, or only at the 6th postpartum week if the patient is breast-feeding.

Intervention and Evaluation

• Monitor the patient's weight daily and report weekly gain of 5 lbs or more.
• Monitor the patient's B/P periodically.
• Assess the patient's skin for rash and urticaria.
• Immediately report pain, redness, swelling, or warmth in the calf, chest pain, migraine headache, numbness of an arm or leg, a

sudden decrease in vision, and sudden shortness of breath.

Patient/Family Teaching

• Warn the patient/family to notify the physician if she experiences chest pain, hemoptysis, numbness in the arm or leg, severe headache, severe pain or swelling in the calf, severe pain or tenderness in the abdominal area, sudden loss of vision, or unusually heavy vaginal bleeding.

• Encourage the patient/family to stop smoking tobacco.

REFERENCES

Taketomo, C. K., Hodding, J. H. & Kraus, D. M. (2003–2004). Pediatric dosage handbook (10th ed.). Hudson, OH: Lexi-Comp.

63 Oxytocics

Methylergonovine
Mifepristone
Oxytocin

Uses: Oxytocic agents are used to induce or augment labor when maternal or fetal need exists. They are also used to control postpartum hemorrhage, to cause uterine contractions after cesarean delivery or during other uterine surgery, and to induce therapeutic abortion. In addition, oxytocin is used to promote breast milk ejection.

Action: Oxytocics stimulate the frequency and force of contractions of uterine smooth muscle. They increase the responsiveness of the uterus closer to term. Some agents, such as oxytocin, stimulate the breasts to release milk by causing myoepithelial cells around the mammary glands to contract.

Methylergonovine

meth-ill-er-go-**noe**-veen
(Methergine)

CATEGORY AND SCHEDULE

Pregnancy Risk Category: C

MECHANISM OF ACTION

An ergot alkaloid that stimulates alpha-adrenergic and serotonin receptors, producing arterial vasoconstriction. Causes vasospasm of coronary arteries. Directly stimulates uterine muscle. ***Therapeutic Effect:*** Increases strength and frequency of contractions; decreases uterine bleeding.

PHARMACOKINETICS

Route	Onset	Peak	Duration
PO	5–10 min	N/A	N/A
IM	2–5 min	N/A	N/A
IV	Immediate	N/A	3 hrs

Rapidly absorbed from the GI tract and after IM administration. Distributed rapidly to plasma, extracellular fluid, and tissues. Metabolized in liver and undergoes a first-pass effect. Primarily excreted in urine.

AVAILABILITY

Tablets: 0.2 mg.
Injection: 0.2 mg/ml.

INDICATIONS AND DOSAGES

▸ **Prevents and treats postpartum and postabortion hemorrhage due to atony or involution; not for induction or augmentation of labor.**

PO

Adolescents. 0.2 mg 3–4 times/day. Continue for up to 7 days.

IM/IV

Adolescents. Initially, 0.2 mg after delivery of anterior shoulder, after delivery of placenta, or during puerperium. May repeat no more often than q2–4h for no more than 5 doses total.

UNLABELED USES

Treatment of incomplete abortion.

CONTRAINDICATIONS

Hypersensitivity to methylergonovine or any related component, hypertension, pregnancy, toxemia, untreated hypocalcemia.

INTERACTIONS

Drug

Vasoconstrictors, vasopressors: May increase the effects of methylergonovine.
Protease inhibitors: May increase risk of toxicity of methylergonovine
Erythromycin, clarithromycin, ketoconazole, itraconazole, voriconazole: May increase risk of vasospasm
MAO inhibitors, SSRIs, sumatriptan, trazodone: May increase risk for development of serotonin syndrome
Metoclopramide: May decrease effects of methylergonovine

Herbal

None known.

Food

Grapefruit juice: May increase risk of vasospasm

DIAGNOSTIC TEST EFFECTS

May decrease prolactin concentration.

IV INCOMPATIBILITIES

No information available for Y-site administration.

IV COMPATIBILITIES

Heparin, potassium

SIDE EFFECTS

Frequent
Nausea, uterine cramping, vomiting
Occasional
Abdominal or stomach pain, diarrhea, dizziness, diaphoresis, tinnitus, bradycardia, chest pain
Rare
Allergic reaction, such as rash and itching, dyspnea, severe or sudden hypertension

SERIOUS REACTIONS

! Severe hypertensive episodes may result in a cerebrovascular accident, serious arrhythmias, and seizures. Hypertensive effects are more frequent with patient susceptibility, rapid IV administration, and concurrent use of regional anesthesia or vasoconstrictors.
! Peripheral ischemia may lead to gangrene.

PEDIATRIC CONSIDERATIONS

Baseline Assessment

- Determine the patient's baseline blood pressure (B/P), pulse, and serum calcium level.
- Assess the patient's bleeding before administration.
- Be aware that methylergonovine use is contraindicated during pregnancy and that small amounts of the drug are found in breast milk.
- No information on methylergonovine use in young children is available.

Precautions

- Use cautiously in pts with coronary artery disease, liver or renal impairment, occlusive peripheral vascular disease, and sepsis.

Administration and Handling

- May give PO, IM, or IV.
- Refrigerate ampoules.
- Initial dose may be given parenterally, followed by oral regimen.
- Use IV in life-threatening emergencies only, as prescribed.
- Dilute to volume of 5 mL with 0.9% NaCl.
- Give over at least 1 min, carefully monitoring the patient's B/P.

Intervention and Evaluation

- Monitor the patient's bleeding, B/P, pulse, and uterine tone every 15 min until stable for 1–2 hrs.
- Assess the patient's extremities for color, movement, pain, and warmth.

• Report any chest pain the patient experiences promptly.
• Assist the patient with ambulation if she experiences dizziness.

Patient/Family Teaching

• Urge the patient/family to avoid smoking because of the added effects of vasoconstriction.
• Warn the patient/family to notify the physician if she experiences increased bleeding, cold or pale feet or hands, cramping, or foul-smelling lochia.

Mifepristone

my-fih-**priss**-tone
(Mifeprex)
Do not confuse with Mirapex.

CATEGORY AND SCHEDULE

Pregnancy Risk Category: X

MECHANISM OF ACTION

An abortifacient that has antiprogestational activity resulting from competitive interaction with progesterone. Inhibits the activity of endogenous or exogenous progesterone. Also has antiglucocorticoid and weak antiandrogenic activity. ***Therapeutic Effect:*** Terminates pregnancy.

AVAILABILITY

Tablets: 200 mg.

INDICATIONS AND DOSAGES

▸ **Termination of pregnancy**

PO

Adolescents. (Must be used under the direct supervision of a physician)
Day 1: 600 mg as single dose. Day 3: 400 mcg misoprostol. Day 14: Post-treatment examination for confirmation of pregnancy termination.

UNLABELED USES

Cushing syndrome, endometriosis, intrauterine fetal death or nonviable early pregnancy, postcoital contraception or contragestation, unresectable meningioma.

CONTRAINDICATIONS

Hypersensitivity to mifepristone, misoprostol or other related prostaglandins. Chronic adrenal failure, concurrent long-term steroid or anticoagulant therapy, confirmed or suspected ectopic pregnancy, intrauterine device (IUD) in place, hemorrhagic disorders, inherited porphyries. Inadequate or lack of access to emergency medical services or inability to comply or understand effects of the treatment.

INTERACTIONS

Drug

Carbamazepine, phenobarbital, phenytoin, rifampin: May increase the metabolism of mifepristone.
Erythromycin, itraconazole, ketoconazole: May inhibit the metabolism of mifepristone.

Herbal

St. John's wort: May increase the metabolism of mifepristone.

Food

Grapefruit: May inhibit the metabolism of mifepristone.

DIAGNOSTIC TEST EFFECTS

May decrease blood Hgb and Hct and RBC count. hCG levels will not be useful to confirm pregnancy termination until 10 days after mifepristone treatment.

SIDE EFFECTS

Frequent (greater than 10%)
Headache, dizziness, abdominal pain, nausea, vomiting, diarrhea, fatigue

Occasional (10%–3%)
Uterine hemorrhage, back pain, insomnia, vaginitis, dyspepsia, back pain, fever, viral infections, rigors (chills or shaking)
Rare (2%–1%)
Anxiety, syncope, anemia, asthenia, leg pain, sinusitis, leukorrhea, septic shock

SERIOUS REACTIONS

! Postmarketing reports of adverse events exist, including bacterial infection following use, prolonged vaginal bleeding and ectopic pregnancy.
! In rare cases, septic shock has been a complication of the bacterial infections. Infections may be severe and sometimes fatal. Sustained fever, abdominal pain, or pelvic tenderness should be promptly evaluated. Most women will experience vaginal bleeding for 9–16 days. Up to 8% of women will experience bleeding or spotting for as long as 30 days or more. In some cases, bleeding may be prolonged and heavy and could potentially lead to life-threatening hypovolemic shock.
! Pts should seek medical attention in cases of syncope or excessive bleeding (soaking through two thick sanitary pads per hr for 2 consecutive hrs). Ultrasound may not identify all cases of ectopic pregnancy and health care providers should be alert for signs and symptoms that may be related to undiagnosed ectopic pregnancy in any patient who receives mifepristone.

PEDIATRIC CONSIDERATIONS

Baseline Assessment

• Determine whether the patient is taking anticonvulsants, erythromycin, itraconazole, ketoconazole, or rifampin as these drugs may inhibit the metabolism of mifepristone.
• Ask the patient if she has an IUD in place, and do not give the drug until it is removed.
• Make sure that an ectopic pregnancy has been ruled out.
• Patient must be instructed of the treatment procedure and expected effects. A signed agreement form must be kept in the patient's file (forms are available from Danco Laboratories at 1-877-432-7596). Adverse effects must be reported in writing to the medication distributor.
• Medication can only be distributed directly to physicians who have completed and filed a signed agreement with the distributor. Mifepristone is not available at pharmacies.
• Medication can only be administered by physicians who can date pregnancy, diagnose ectopic pregnancy, provide access to surgical abortion (if needed), and provide access to emergency care.
• Safety and efficacy in pediatric pts has not been established.

Precautions

• Use cautiously in pts with cardiovascular disease, diabetes, hypertension, liver or renal impairment, and severe anemia.

Administration and Handling

◂ **ALERT** ▸ Be aware that treatment with mifepristone and misoprostol requires three office visits.

Intervention and Evaluation

• Monitor the patient's blood Hgb and Hct levels.

Patient/Family Teaching

• Explain to the patient/family the treatment procedure, its effects, and the need for a follow-up visits.

• Tell the patient/family that she may experience uterine cramping and vaginal bleeding that is heavier than a normal menstrual period. She should report to her physician immediately if the bleeding is prolonged or severe (soaking two thick sanitary pads within 2 hrs).

• Explain to the patient that she may experience nausea, vomiting and diarrhea.

• Tell the patient that it is possible to get pregnant before her next period. Once the pregnancy has been proved to be ended, she should start contraception before having sexual intercourse.

Oxytocin

ox-ih-**toe**-sin

(Pitocin, Syntocinon INJ [AUS])

Do not confuse with Pitressin.

CATEGORY AND SCHEDULE

Pregnancy Risk Category: X

MECHANISM OF ACTION

An oxytocic that acts on uterine myofibril activity. Stimulates mammary smooth muscle. ***Therapeutic Effect:*** Contracts uterine smooth muscle. Enhances milk ejection from breasts.

PHARMACOKINETICS

Route	Onset	Peak	Duration
IM	3–5 min	N/A	2–3 hrs
IV	Immediate	N/A	1 hr
Intra nasal	Few minutes	N/A	20 min

Rapidly absorbed through nasal mucous membranes. Protein binding: 30%. Distributed in extracellular fluid. Metabolized in liver, kidney. Primarily excreted in urine. ***Half-Life:*** 1–6 min.

AVAILABILITY

Injection: 10 units/mL.

INDICATIONS AND DOSAGES

▸ Induction or stimulation of labor

IV INFUSION

Adolescents. Initially, 0.001–0.002 units/min. May increase by 0.001–0.002 units q15–30min until a contraction pattern has been established.

▸ Incomplete or inevitable abortion

IV INFUSION

Adolescents. 10 units in 500 mL (20 munits/mL) D_5W or 0.9% NaCl infused at 20–40 munits/min.

▸ Control of postpartum bleeding

IV INFUSION

Adolescents. 10–40 units (maximum: 40 units/1,000 mL) infused at rate of 20–40 munits/min after delivery of infant.

IM

Adolescents. 10 units after delivery of placenta.

▸ Postabortion hemorrhage

IV INFUSION

Adolescents. 10 units infused at rate of 20–100 munits/min.

CONTRAINDICATIONS

Hypersensitivity to oxytocin or any related component. Adequate uterine activity that fails to progress, cephalopelvic disproportion, fetal distress without imminent delivery, grand multiparity, hyperactive or hypertonic uterus, nasal spray during pregnancy, obstetric emergencies that favor surgical intervention, prematurity, unengaged fetal head, unfavorable fetal position or presentation, when vaginal delivery is contraindicated, such as with active genital herpes infection, placenta previa, and cord presentation.

INTERACTIONS

Drug

Caudal block anesthetics, vasopressors: May increase pressor effects.
Other oxytocics: May cause cervical lacerations, uterine hypertonus, or uterine rupture.

Herbal

None known.

Food

None known.

DIAGNOSTIC TEST EFFECTS

None known.

IV INCOMPATIBILITIES

No known incompatibilities via Y-site administration.

IV COMPATIBILITIES

Heparin, insulin, multivitamins, potassium chloride, sodium bicarbonate, thiopental, verapamil

SIDE EFFECTS

Occasional

Tachycardia, premature ventricular contractions, hypotension, nausea, vomiting

Rare

Nasal: Lacrimation or tearing, nasal irritation, rhinorrhea, unexpected uterine bleeding or contractions

SERIOUS REACTIONS

! Hypertonicity with tearing of uterus, increased bleeding, abruptio placenta, and cervical and vaginal lacerations may occur.
! In the fetus, bradycardia, CNS or brain damage, trauma due to rapid propulsion, low Apgar score at 5 min, and retinal hemorrhage occur rarely.
! Prolonged IV infusion of oxytocin with excessive fluid volume has caused severe water intoxication with seizures, coma, and death.

PEDIATRIC CONSIDERATIONS

Baseline Assessment

• Assess the patient's baseline blood pressure (B/P), pulse, and fetal heart rate.
• Determine the duration, frequency, and strength of patient contractions.
• Be aware that oxytocin should be used as indicated and is not expected to present a risk of fetal abnormalities.
• Be aware that oxytocin is present in small amounts in breast milk. Breast-feeding is not recommended in this patient population.
• Be aware that oxytocin should not be used in young children.

Precautions

• Induction should be for medical, not elective, reasons.

Administration and Handling

IV

• Store at room temperature.
• Dilute 10–40 units (1–4 mL) in 1,000 mL of 0.9% NaCl, lactated Ringer's solution, or D_5W to provide a concentration of 10–40 munits/mL solution.
• Give by IV infusion and use an infusion device to carefully control rate of flow as ordered by physician.

Intervention and Evaluation

• Monitor the patient's B/P, contractions, including duration, frequency, and strength, fetal heart rate, intrauterine pressure, pulse, respirations, fetal heart rate, and intrauterine pressure every 15 min.
• Notify the physician of any patient contractions that last

longer than 1 min, occur more frequently than every 2 min, or stop.

• Maintain careful intake and output records for the patient.

• Be alert to potential water intoxication of the patient.

• Check the patient for blood loss.

Patient/Family Teaching

• Explain the labor progress to the patient and family.

• Teach the patient/family the proper use of the oxytocin nasal spray.

• Explain to the patient/family that the drug will be present in the breast milk, so breast-feeding is not recommended.

REFERENCES

Taketomo, C. K., Hodding, J. H. & Kraus, D. M. (2003–2004). Pediatric dosage handbook (10th ed.). Hudson, OH: Lexi-Comp.

64 Pituitary Hormones

Desmopressin
Somatrem
Somatropin
Vasopressin

Uses: Pituitary hormones have various uses. *Antidiuretic hormones,* such as desmopressin and vasopressin, are used to treat diabetes insipidus, postoperative abdominal distention, nocturnal enuresis, hemophilia A, and von Willebrand disease. *Growth hormones,* such as somatrem and somatropin, are used to treat pediatric growth hormone (GH) deficiency, chronic renal insufficiency, Turner syndrome, and cachexia or wasting in pts with AIDS.

Action: The actions of pituitary hormones also vary greatly. *Antidiuretic hormones* act on the collecting ducts of the kidneys to increase their permeability to water, resulting in increased water reabsorption. In higher concentrations, these agents constrict arterioles throughout the body, which increases blood pressure. *Growth hormones* cause growth in almost all body tissues: a childhood deficiency of GH results in dwarfism; an excess results in acromegaly. Metabolic effects of these agents include an increased rate of protein synthesis, mobilization of fatty acids from adipose tissue, and a decreased rate of glucose use.

Desmopressin

des-moe-**press**-in
(DDAVP, Minirin [AUS], Octostim [CAN], Stimate)

CATEGORY AND SCHEDULE

Pregnancy Risk Category: B

MECHANISM OF ACTION

A synthetic pituitary hormone that increases reabsorption of water by increasing permeability of collecting ducts of the kidneys. Plasminogen activator. ***Therapeutic Effect:*** Decreases urinary output. Increases plasma factor VIII (antihemophilic factor).

PHARMACOKINETICS

Route	Onset	Peak	Duration
PO	1 hr	2–7 hrs	6–8 hrs
Intranasal	15 min –1 hr	1–5 hrs	5–21 hrs
IV	15–30 min	1.5–3 hrs	N/A

Poorly absorbed after PO/nasal administration. Metabolism: unknown. ***Half-Life:*** Oral: 1.5–2.5 hrs. Nasal: 3.3–3.5 hrs. IV: 0.4–4 hrs.

AVAILABILITY

Tablets (DDAVP): 0.1 mg, 0.2 mg.
Injection (DDAVP): 4 mcg/mL (DDAVP).
Nasal Solution (DDAVP): 100 mcg/mL (DDAVP).

Nasal Spray: 1.5 mg/mL (150 mcg/spray) (Stimate), 100 mcg/mL (10 mcg/spray) (DDAVP).

INDICATIONS AND DOSAGES

▸ Primary nocturnal enuresis

INTRANASAL

Children 6 yrs and older. Initially, 20 mcg (0.2 mL) at bedtime; use one-half dose each nostril. Adjust up to 40 mcg.

PO

Children older than 6 yrs. 0.2–0.6 mg once before bedtime.

▸ Central cranial diabetes insipidus

PO

Children 12 yrs and older. Initially, 0.05 mg 2 times/day. Titrate to response. Range: 0.1–1.2 mg/day in 2–3 divided doses.

Children younger than 12 yrs. Initially 0.05 mg, 2 times/day. Titrate to response. Range: 0.1–0.8 mg daily.

INTRANASAL

Children older than 12 yrs. 5–40 mcg (0.05–0.4 mL) in 1–3 doses/day.

Children 3 mos–12 yrs. Initially, 5 mcg (0.05 mL)/day, divided 1–2 times/day. Range: 5–30 mcg (0.05–0.3 mL)/day.

SC/IV

Children older than 12 yrs. 2–4 mcg/day in 2 divided doses or ¹⁄₁₀ of maintenance intranasal dose.

▸ Hemophilia A, von Willebrand disease (type I)

IV INFUSION

Children weighing 10 kg or more. 0.3 mcg/kg diluted in 50 mL 0.9% NaCl.

Children weighing less than 10 kg. 0.3 mcg/kg diluted in 10 mL 0.9% NaCl.

INTRANASAL

Children 12 yrs and older weighing more than 50 kg. 300 mcg; use 1 spray each nostril.

Children 12 yrs and older weighing less than 50 kg. 150 mcg as single spray.

CONTRAINDICATIONS

Hypersensitivity to desmopressin or any related component. Hemophilia A with factor VIII levels less than 5% or hemophilia B, severe type I, type IIB, or platelet-type von Willebrand disease

INTERACTIONS

Drug

Carbamazepine, chlorpropamide, clofibrate: May increase the effects of desmopressin.

Demeclocycline, lithium, norepinephrine: May decrease effects of desmopressin.

Herbal

None known.

Food

None known.

DIAGNOSTIC TEST EFFECTS

None known.

IV INCOMPATIBILITIES

Information not available.

SIDE EFFECTS

Occasional

IV: Pain, redness, or swelling at injection site, headache, abdominal cramps, vulval pain, flushed skin, mild elevation of blood pressure (B/P), nausea with high dosages

Nasal: Rhinorrhea, nasal congestion, slight elevation of B/P

SERIOUS REACTIONS

! Water intoxication or hyponatremia, marked by headache, drowsiness, confusion, decreased urination, rapid weight gain, seizures, and coma, may occur in overhydration. Children and infants are especially at risk.

PEDIATRIC CONSIDERATIONS

Baseline Assessment

• Establish the patient's baseline B/P, electrolytes, pulse, urine specific gravity, and weight.
• Plan to check the patient's laboratory values for factor VIII coagulant concentration for hemophilia A and von Willebrand disease and bleeding times.
• Use cautiously in neonates younger than 3 mos as this age group is at an increased risk of fluid balance problems.
• Be aware that careful fluid restrictions are recommended in infants.

Precautions

• Use cautiously in pts with conditions that affect fluid or electrolyte imbalance, coronary artery disease, hypertensive cardiovascular disease, and a predisposition to thrombus formation.

Administration and Handling

INTRANASAL

• Refrigerate DDAVP nasal solution and Stimate nasal spray. Nasal solution and Stimate nasal spray are stable for 3 wks at room temperature if unopened.
• Remember that DDAVP nasal spray is stable at room temperature.
• Draw up a measured quantity of desmopressin with a calibrated catheter (rhinyle). Insert one end in the patient's nose and have the patient blow on the other end to deposit the solution deep in the nasal cavity. For infants, young children, and obtunded pts, an air-filled syringe may be attached to the catheter to deposit the solution.

SC

• Estimate therapeutic response by adequacy of sleep duration.
• Plan to adjust morning and evening doses separately.

IV

• Refrigerate. Know that the drug is stable for 2 wks at room temperature.
• For IV infusion, dilute in 10–50 mL 0.9% NaCl.
• Prepare to infuse over 15–30 min.
• For preoperative use, administer 30 min before procedure, as prescribed.
• Monitor the patient's B/P and pulse during IV infusion.
• Remember that the IV dose is $\frac{1}{10}$ the intranasal dose.

Intervention and Evaluation

• Check the patient's B/P and pulse with IV infusion.
• Monitor for signs of diabetes insipidus, as well as the patient's serum electrolyte levels, fluid intake, serum osmolality, urine volume, urine specific gravity, and body weight.
• Assess the patient's factor VIII antigen levels, activated partial thromboplastin time and factor VIII activity level for hemophilia.

Patient/Family Teaching

• Caution the patient/family to avoid overhydration.
• Teach the patient/family the proper technique for intranasal administration.
• Warn the patient/family to notify the physician if the patient experiences abdominal cramps, headache, heartburn, nausea, or shortness of breath.
• Tell the parent of a child treated for nocturnal enuresis to carefully monitor the child's sleeping pattern.

Somatrem

soe-ma-trem
(Protropin)
Do not confuse with Proloprim, protamine, Protopam, or somatropin.

CATEGORY AND SCHEDULE
Pregnancy Risk Category: C

MECHANISM OF ACTION
A polypeptide hormone that increases the number and size of muscle cells and RBC mass. Affects carbohydrate metabolism by antagonizing action of insulin, increasing the mobilization of fats, and increasing cellular protein synthesis. ***Therapeutic Effect:*** Stimulates linear growth.

AVAILABILITY
Powder for Injection: 5 mg, 10 mg.

INDICATIONS AND DOSAGES
▸ **Long-term treatment of children who have growth failure due to endogenous growth hormone deficiency**
IM/SC
Children. Up to 0.1 mg/kg (0.26 international units/kg) 3 times/wk. Maximum: 0.3 mg/kg/wk.

CONTRAINDICATIONS
Hypersensitivity to growth hormone or any related component. Children with closed epiphyses, evidence of active malignancy, intracranial tumors.

INTERACTIONS
Drug
Corticosteroids: May inhibit growth response.
Herbal
None known.
Food
None known.

DIAGNOSTIC TEST EFFECTS
May increase serum parathyroid hormone, serum alkaline phosphatase, and inorganic phosphorus levels.

SIDE EFFECTS
Frequent (30%)
Persistent antibodies to growth hormone, but generally does not cause failure to respond to somatrem
Occasional
Headache, muscle pain, weakness, mild hyperglycemia, allergic reaction, including rash and itching, pain and swelling at injection site, pain in hip or knee

PEDIATRIC CONSIDERATIONS
Baseline Assessment
- Establish the patient's baseline blood glucose levels and thyroid function studies.
- Use with caution in children who have diabetes or a treated neoplasm.
- Monitor children's growth and development and thyroid function during treatment.
- Be aware that the diluent contains benzyl alcohol, which in large amounts can lead to neonatal toxicity.

Precautions
- Use cautiously in pts with diabetes mellitus, malignancy, and untreated hypothyroidism.

Intervention and Evaluation
- Monitor the patient's blood glucose, parathyroid hormone, phosphorus, and serum calcium levels, bone age, growth rate, renal function, and thyroid function studies.

Patient/Family Teaching

- Instruct the patient/family in the correct reconstitution procedure for IM/SC administration.
- Teach the patient/family the safe handling and disposal of needles.
- Stress to the patient/family the importance of regular follow-up appointments with the physician.

Somatropin

soe-mah-**troe**-pin

(Humatrope, Norditropin, Nutropin, Nutropin AQ, Nutropin Depot)

Do not confuse with somatrem or sumatriptan.

CATEGORY AND SCHEDULE

Pregnancy Risk Category: C

MECHANISM OF ACTION

A polypeptide hormone that increases the number and size of muscle cells; increases RBC mass. Affects carbohydrate metabolism by antagonizing the action of insulin, increasing the mobilization of fats, and increasing cellular protein synthesis. ***Therapeutic Effect:*** Stimulates linear growth.

AVAILABILITY

Injection:

Genotropin: 1.5 mg (preservative free), 5.8 mg

Genotropin Miniquick (preservative free): 0.2 mg, 0.4 mg, 0.6 mg, 0.8 mg, 1 mg, 1.2 mg, 1.4 mg, 1.6 mg, 1.8 mg, 2 mg

Humatrope: 5 mg, 6 mg, 12 mg, 24 mg

Norditropin: 4 mg

Nutropin: 5 mg

Nutropin AQ: 5 mg/mL

Nutropin (depot): 13.5 mg, 18 mg, 22.5 mg.

INDICATIONS AND DOSAGES

▸ **Growth hormone deficiency (doses should be individualized)**

IM/SC

Children. Genotropin: 0.16-0.24 mg/kg/weekly divided into 7 daily doses

Humatrope: 0.18 mg/kg weekly divided into equal doses given on alternate days or 6 times weekly. Maximum weekly dose: 0.3 mg/kg

Norditropin: 0.024-0.034 mg/kg/dose 6–7 times weekly

Nutropin: 0.3 mg/kg weekly divided into 7 daily doses. Maximum dose: 0.7 mg/kg weekly.

SC

Children. Nutropin Depot: 1.5 mg/kg 1 time/mo on the same day of the month OR 0.75 mg/kg 2 times/mo on the same days of the month.

▸ **Chronic renal insufficiency**

SC

Children. 0.35 mg/kg/wk (Nutropin).

▸ **Turner syndrome**

SC

Children. Humatrope: 0.375 mg/kg/wk divided into 3–7 equal daily doses or on 3 alternate days.

CONTRAINDICATIONS

Hypersensitivity to human growth hormone or any related component. Children with closed epiphyses, evidence of active malignancy, intracranial tumors.

INTERACTIONS

Drug

Corticosteroids: May inhibit growth response.

Herbal

None known.

Food

None known.

DIAGNOSTIC TEST EFFECTS

May increase serum parathyroid hormone, serum alkaline phosphatase, and inorganic phosphorus levels.

SIDE EFFECTS

Frequent

Development of persistent antibodies to growth hormone, generally does not cause failure to respond to somatropin; hypercalciuria during first 2–3 mos of therapy

Occasional

Headache, muscle pain, weakness, mild hyperglycemia, allergic reaction, including rash and itching, pain or swelling at injection site, pain in hip or knee

PEDIATRIC CONSIDERATIONS

Baseline Assessment

- Establish the patient's baseline blood glucose levels and thyroid function studies.
- Use with caution in children who have diabetes or treated neoplasm.
- Monitor children's growth and development and thyroid function during treatment.

Precautions

- Use cautiously in pts with diabetes mellitus, malignancy, and untreated hypothyroidism.

Intervention and Evaluation

- Monitor the patient's blood glucose, parathyroid hormone, phosphorus, and serum calcium levels, bone age, growth rate, renal function, and thyroid function studies.
- Observe the HIV-positive patient for decreased wasting.

Patient/Family Teaching

- Instruct the patient/family in the correct reconstitution procedure and injection technique for IM or SC administration.
- Teach the patient/family the safe handling and disposal of needles.
- Stress to the patient/family the importance of regular follow-up appointments with the physician.

Vasopressin

vay-sew-**press**-in

(Pitressin, Pressyn [CAN])

CATEGORY AND SCHEDULE

Pregnancy Risk Category: B

MECHANISM OF ACTION

A posterior pituitary hormone that increases reabsorption of water by the renal tubules. Directly stimulates smooth muscle in the GI tract. Directly stimulates receptors in the pituitary gland resulting in increased ACTH production. ***Therapeutic Effect:*** Increases water permeability at the distal tubule and collecting duct decreasing urine volume. Causes peristalsis. Causes vasoconstriction.

PHARMACOKINETICS

Route	Onset	Peak	Duration
IM/SC	1–2 hrs	N/A	2–8 hrs
IV	N/A	N/A	0.5–1 hr

Distributed throughout extracellular fluid. Metabolized in liver and kidney. Primarily excreted in urine. ***Half-Life:*** 10–20 min.

AVAILABILITY

Injection: 20 units/mL.

INDICATIONS AND DOSAGES

▸ **Diabetes insipidus (dose should be individualized to effect)**

IM/SC

Children. 2.5–10 units, 2–4 times/day.

IV INFUSION
Children. 0.005 units/kg/hr. May double dose q30min as needed. Maximum: 10 milliunits/kg/hr.

▸ **GI hemorrhage**
IV INFUSION
Children. 0.002–0.005 units/kg/min. Titrate as needed. Maximum: 0.01 units/kg/min.

UNLABELED USES

Adjunct in treatment of acute, massive hemorrhage.

CONTRAINDICATIONS

Hypersensitivity to vasopressin or any related component.

INTERACTIONS

Drug

Carbamazepine, chlorpropamide, clofibrate: May increase the effects of vasopressin.
Demeclocycline, lithium, norepinephrine: May decrease the effects of vasopressin.

Herbal

None known.

Food

None known.

DIAGNOSTIC TEST EFFECTS

None known.

IV INCOMPATIBILITIES

Amphotericin B complex (Abelcet, AmBisome, Amphotec), diazepam (Valium), etomidate (Amidate), furosemide (Lasix), thiopental

IV COMPATIBILITIES

Dobutamine (Dobutrex), dopamine (Intropin), heparin, lorazepam (Ativan), midazolam (Versed), milrinone (Primacor), verapamil (Calan, Isoptin)

SIDE EFFECTS

Frequent

Pain at injection site with vasopressin tannate

Occasional

Stomach cramps, nausea, vomiting, diarrhea, dizziness, diaphoresis, paleness, circumoral pallor, trembling, headache, eructation, flatulence

Rare

Chest pain, confusion
Allergic reaction: Rash or hives, pruritus, wheezing or difficulty breathing, swelling of face and extremities. Sterile abscess with vasopressin tannate

SERIOUS REACTIONS

! Anaphylaxis, myocardial infarction, and water intoxication have occurred.

! The very young are at higher risk for water intoxication.

PEDIATRIC CONSIDERATIONS

Baseline Assessment

• Establish the patient's baselines for blood pressure (B/P), serum electrolyte levels, pulse, urine specific gravity, and weight.
• Be aware that vasopressin should be used cautiously in breast-feeding women.
• Be aware that vasopressin should be used cautiously in children because of the risk of water intoxication and hyponatremia.
• Monitor and assess weight and urine osmolality in pediatric pts.

Precautions

• Use cautiously in pts with arteriosclerosis, asthma, cardiac disease, goiter with cardiac complications, migraine, nephritis, renal disease, seizures, and vascular disease.

Administration and Handling

◂ **ALERT** ▸ May administer intranasally on cotton pledgets or by nasal spray; individualize dosage.

SC/IM

• Give with 1–2 glasses of water to reduce side effects.

IV

• Store at room temperature.
• Dilute with D_5W or 0.9% NaCl to a concentration of 0.1–1 unit/mL.
• Give as IV infusion.

Intervention and Evaluation

• Monitor the patient's fluid intake and output closely, and restrict the patient's intake as ordered to prevent water intoxication.
• Weigh the patient daily, if indicated.
• Check the patient's B/P and pulse 2 times/day.
• Monitor the patient's serum electrolyte levels and urine specific gravity.
• Evaluate the patient's injection site for abscess, erythema, and pain.
• Report side effects experienced by the patient to the physician for dose reduction.
• Be alert for early signs of water intoxication, such as drowsiness, headache, and listlessness.
• Withhold the medication, as prescribed, and report immediately if the patient experiences any allergic symptoms or chest pain.

Patient/Family Teaching

• Warn the patient/family to notify the physician if the patient experiences any chest pain, headache, shortness of breath, or other symptoms.
• Stress to the patient/family the importance of monitoring the patient's fluid intake and output.
• Urge the patient/family to avoid alcohol during vasopressin therapy.

REFERENCES

Miller, S. & Fioravanti, J. (1997). Pediatric medications: a handbook for nurses. St. Louis: Mosby.

Taketomo, C. K., Hodding, J. H. & Kraus, D. M. (2003–2004). Pediatric dosage handbook (10th ed.). Hudson, OH: Lexi-Comp.

65 Thyroid Agents

Levothyroxine
Liothyronine
Methimazole
Propylthiouracil

Uses: Two *thyroid hormones*—levothyroxine and liothyronine—are used to treat primary or secondary hypothyroidism, myxedema, cretinism, or simple goiter. Levothyroxine is also used in thyroid cancer management. Levothyroxine and liothyronine are used in thyroid suppression tests.

Propylthiouracil and *methimazole* are used to treat hyperthyroidism, especially before thyroid surgery or radioactive iodine therapy.

Action: *Thyroid hormones* are essential for normal growth, development, and energy metabolism. They promote growth and development by controlling DNA transcription and protein synthesis, which are required for nervous system development. These agents stimulate energy use by increasing the basal metabolic rate, which increases oxygen consumption and heat production. They also act as cardiac stimulants by increasing the heart rate, force of cardiac contractions, and cardiac output.

Propylthiouracil blocks the oxidation of iodine in the thyroid gland, thereby preventing the synthesis of thyroid hormones.

COMBINATION PRODUCTS

THYROLAR: levothyroxine/liothyronine 12.5 mcg/3.1 mcg; 25 mcg/6.25 mcg; 50 mcg/12.5 mcg; 100 mcg/25 mcg; 150 mcg/37.5 mcg.

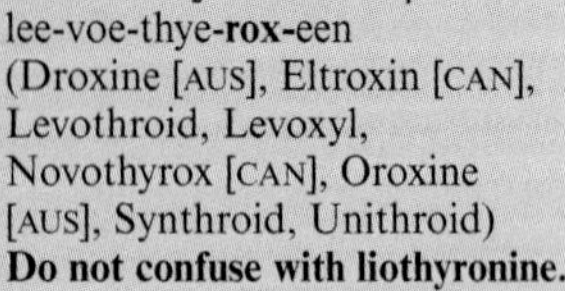

Levothyroxine

lee-voe-thye-**rox**-een
(Droxine [AUS], Eltroxin [CAN], Levothroid, Levoxyl, Novothyrox [CAN], Oroxine [AUS], Synthroid, Unithroid)
Do not confuse with liothyronine.

CATEGORY AND SCHEDULE

Pregnancy Risk Category: A

MECHANISM OF ACTION

A synthetic isomer of thyroxine involved in normal metabolism, growth, and development, especially for the CNS of infants. Possesses catabolic and anabolic effects. ***Therapeutic Effect:*** Increases basal metabolic rate, enhances gluconeogenesis, and stimulates protein synthesis.

PHARMACOKINETICS

Variable, incomplete absorption from the GI tract. Protein binding: greater than 99%. Widely distributed. Deiodinated in peripheral tissues, minimal metabolism in liver. Eliminated by urinary and biliary excretion. ***Half-Life:*** 6–7 days.

AVAILABILITY

Tablets: 0.025 mg, 0.05 mg, 0.075 mg, 0.088 mg, 0.1 mg, 0.112 mg, 0.125 mg, 0.137 mg, 0.15 mg, 0.175 mg, 0.2 mg, 0.3 mg.
Injection: 200 mcg, 500 mcg.

INDICATIONS AND DOSAGES

▸ Hypothyroidism

PO

Children older than 12 yrs. 150 mcg/day.
Children 6–12 yrs. 100–125 mcg/day.
Children older than 1–5 yrs. 75–100 mcg/day.
Children older than 6–12 mos. 50–75 mcg/day.
Children older than 3–6 mos. 25–50 mcg/day.
Children 3 mos and younger. 10–15 mcg/kg/day.

IV

IV doses are 50–75% of the PO dosages.

CONTRAINDICATIONS

Hypersensitivity to any component of tablets, such as tartrazine, allergy to aspirin, myocardial infarction, and thyrotoxicosis uncomplicated by hypothyroidism or treatment of obesity

INTERACTIONS

Drug

Antacids, cholestyramine, colestipol, iron salts, sucralfate: May decrease the absorption of levothyroxine.
Oral anticoagulants: May alter the effects of oral anticoagulants.
Sympathomimetics, tricyclic antidepressants, SSRIs: May increase the effects and coronary insufficiency of levothyroxine.
Phenytoin, Phenobarbital, carbamazepine, rifampin, amiodarone, beta-adrenergic antagonists: May decrease levothyroxine levels

Herbal

None known.

Food

Soybeans, walnuts, dietary fiber: May decrease absorption of levothyroxine

DIAGNOSTIC TEST EFFECTS

None known.

IV INCOMPATIBILITIES

Do not use or mix with other IV solutions.

SIDE EFFECTS

Occasional

Children may have reversible hair loss upon initiation.

Rare

Dry skin, GI intolerance, skin rash, hives, pseudotumor cerebri or severe headache in children

SERIOUS REACTIONS

! Excessive dosage produces signs and symptoms of hyperthyroidism including weight loss, palpitations, increased appetite, tremors, nervousness, tachycardia, hypertension, headache, insomnia, and menstrual irregularities.
! Cardiac arrhythmias occur rarely.

PEDIATRIC CONSIDERATIONS

Baseline Assessment

• Determine whether the patient is hypersensitive to aspirin, lactose, and tartrazine.
• Obtain the patient's baseline weight and vital signs.
• Know that the signs and symptoms of adrenal insufficiency, diabetes insipidus, diabetes mellitus, and hypopituitarism may become intensified.

• Treat the patient with adrenocortical steroids, as prescribed, before thyroid therapy in coexisting hypoadrenalism and hypothyroidism.
• Be aware that levothyroxine does not cross the placenta and is minimally excreted in breast milk.
• There are no age-related precautions noted in children.
• Be aware that levothyroxine should be used cautiously in neonates in interpreting thyroid function tests.
• Monitor growth and development (bone age and head circumference) in infants.

Precautions

• Use cautiously in pts with angina pectoris, hypertension, or other cardiovascular disease.

Administration and Handling

◂ **ALERT** ▸ Do not interchange brands because there have been problems with bioequivalence between manufacturers.

◂ **ALERT** ▸ Begin therapy with small doses and increase the dosage gradually, as prescribed.

PO

• Give at same time each day to maintain hormone levels.
• Administer before breakfast to prevent insomnia.
• Crush tablets as needed.

IV

• Store vials at room temperature.
• Reconstitute 200-mcg or 500-mcg vial with 5 mL 0.9% NaCl to provide a concentration of 40 or 100 mcg/mL, respectively; shake until clear.
• Use immediately, and discard unused portions.
• Give each 100 mcg or less over 1 min.

Intervention and Evaluation

• Monitor the patient's pulse for rate and rhythm. Report a marked increase in pulse rate or one that exceeds of 100 beats/min.
• Assess the patient for nervousness and tremors.
• Evaluate the patient's appetite and sleep pattern.

Patient/Family Teaching

• Caution the patient/family against discontinuing the drug. Explain to the patient that replacement therapy for hypothyroidism is life-long.
• Stress to the patient/family that follow-up office visits and thyroid function tests are essential.
• Instruct the patient/family to take the drug at the same time each day, preferably in the morning.
• Teach the patient/family to monitor the patient's pulse, and advise the patient to notify the physician if there is a change in rhythm, a marked increase in rate, or a pulse of 100 beats or more.
• Instruct the patient/family not to change brands of the drug.
• Warn the patient/family to notify the physician promptly if the patient experiences chest pain, insomnia, nervousness, tremors, or weight loss.
• Tell the pediatric patient and his or her caregiver that children may have reversible hair loss or increased aggressiveness during the first few months of therapy.
• Warn the patient/family that the full therapeutic effect of the drug may take 1–3 weeks to appear.

Liothyronine 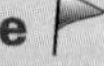

lye-oh-**thigh**-roe-neen
(Cytomel, Tertroxin [AUS], Triostat)
Do not confuse with levothyroxine.

CATEGORY AND SCHEDULE

Pregnancy Risk Category: A

MECHANISM OF ACTION

A synthetic form of thyroid hormone involved in normal metabolism, growth, and development, especially for the CNS of infants. Possesses catabolic and anabolic effects. ***Therapeutic Effect:*** Increases basal metabolic rate, enhances gluconeogenesis, and stimulates protein synthesis.

AVAILABILITY

Tablets: 5 mcg, 25 mcg, 50 mcg.
Injection: 10 mcg/mL.

INDICATIONS AND DOSAGES

▸ **Nontoxic goiter**

PO

Children. 5 mcg/day. May increase by 5 mcg q1–2wks. Maintenance: 15–20 mcg/day.

▸ **Congenital hypothyroidism**

PO

Children. Maintenance: *Infants.* 20 mcg/day. Initially, 5 mcg/day. Increase by 5 mcg/day q3–4days. *Children 1–3 yrs.* 50 mcg/day. *Children older than 3 yrs.* 25 mcg/day increase by 12.5–25 mcg/day q1–2wks. Maximum: 100 mcg/day.

CONTRAINDICATIONS

Hypersensitivity to liothyronine or any related component. Adrenal insufficiency. Myocardial infarction and thyrotoxicosis uncomplicated by hypothyroidism, treatment of obesity.

INTERACTIONS

Drug

Antacids, cholestyramine, colestipol, sucralfate iron salts: May decrease the absorption of liothyronine.
Antidepressants: May increase risk of toxicity of these drugs.
Oral anticoagulants, digoxin: May alter the effects of these drugs.
Sympathomimetics: May increase the effects and coronary insufficiency of liothyronine.
Theophylline, caffeine: May decrease clearance of these drugs. Monitor for toxicity.

Herbal

None known.

Food

None known.

DIAGNOSTIC TEST EFFECTS

None known.

SIDE EFFECTS

Occasional

Children may have reversible hair loss upon initiation

Rare

Dry skin, GI intolerance, skin rash, hives, pseudotumor cerebri or severe headache in children

SERIOUS REACTIONS

! Excessive dosage produces signs and symptoms of hyperthyroidism including weight loss, palpitations, increased appetite, tremors, nervousness, tachycardia, increased blood pressure, headache, insomnia, and menstrual irregularities.
! Cardiac arrhythmias occur rarely.

PEDIATRIC CONSIDERATIONS

Baseline Assessment

- Determine whether the patient is hypersensitive to aspirin and tartrazine.
- Obtain the patient's baseline weight and vital signs.
- Know that the signs and symptoms of adrenal insufficiency, diabetes insipidus, diabetes mellitus, and hypopituitarism may become intensified.

PRECAUTIONS

• Use cautiously in pts with adrenal insufficiency, cardiovascular disease, coronary artery disease, diabetes insipidus, and diabetes mellitus.

Administration and Handling

◀ **ALERT** ▶ Initial and subsequent dosage based on patient's clinical status and response. Administer IV dose over 4 hrs but no longer than 12 hrs apart.

Intervention and Evaluation

• Monitor the patient's pulse for rate and rhythm (report pulse of 100 beats or a marked increase).
• Assess the patient for nervousness and tremors.
• Evaluate the patient's appetite and sleep pattern.

Patient/Family Teaching

• Caution the patient/family against discontinuing the drug. Explain to the patient that replacement for hypothyroidism is lifelong.
• Stress to the patient/family that follow-up office visits and thyroid function tests are essential.
• Instruct the patient/family to take the drug at the same time each day, preferably in the morning.
• Teach the patient/family to monitor the patient's pulse and advise the patient to notify the physician if there is a change in rhythm, a marked increase in rate, or a pulse of 100 beats or more.
• Tell the patient/family not to change brands of the drug.
• Warn the patient/family to notify the physician promptly if the patient experiences chest pain, insomnia, nervousness, tremors, or weight loss.
• Explain to the pediatric patient and his or her caregiver that children may have reversible hair loss or increased aggressiveness during the first few months of therapy.

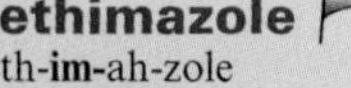

Methimazole

meth-**im**-ah-zole
(Tapazole)

CATEGORY AND SCHEDULE

Pregnancy Risk Category: D

MECHANISM OF ACTION

A thioimidazole derivative that inhibits synthesis of thyroid hormone by interfering with incorporation of iodine into tyrosyl residues. ***Therapeutic Effect:*** Effective in the treatment of hyperthyroidism.

AVAILABILITY

Tablets: 5 mg, 10 mg.

INDICATIONS AND DOSAGES

▸ **Hyperthyroidism**

PO

Children. Initially, 0.4 mg/kg/day in 3 divided doses. Maintenance: 0.2 mg/kg/day in 3 divided doses.

CONTRAINDICATIONS

Hypersensitivity to methimazole or any related component.

INTERACTIONS

Drug

Amiodarone, iodinated glycerol, iodine, potassium iodide: May decrease response.
Digoxin: May increase the blood concentration of digoxin as patient becomes euthyroid.
Iodine-131: May decrease thyroid uptake of iodine-131.
Oral anticoagulants: May decrease the effects of oral anticoagulants.

Herbal
None known.
Food
None known.

DIAGNOSTIC TEST EFFECTS

May increase prothrombin time and lactate dehydrogenase, serum alkaline phosphatase, bilirubin, SGOT (AST), and SGPT (ALT) levels. May decrease prothrombin level and WBC count.

SIDE EFFECTS

Frequent (5%–4%)
Fever, rash, pruritus
Occasional (3%–1%)
Dizziness, loss of taste, nausea, vomiting, stomach pain, peripheral neuropathy, or numbness in fingers, toes, face
Rare (less than 1%)
Swollen lymph nodes or salivary glands

SERIOUS REACTIONS

! Agranulocytosis, which may occur for as long as 4 mos after therapy, pancytopenia, and hepatitis have occurred.

PEDIATRIC CONSIDERATIONS

Baseline Assessment
- Obtain the patient's baseline pulse and weight.
- Expect to perform baseline thyroid function studies.

Precautions
- Use cautiously in pts older than 40 yrs of age, in pts taking methimazole in combination with other agranulocytosis-inducing drugs, and in pts with impaired liver function.

Intervention and Evaluation
- Monitor the patient's pulse and weight daily.
- Assess the patient's skin for rash, pruritus, and swollen lymph glands.
- Monitor the patient's complete blood count, prothrombin time, and serum hepatic enzymes.
- Evaluate the patient for signs and symptoms of bleeding and infection.

Patient/Family Teaching
- Caution the patient/family against exceeding the ordered dose.
- Instruct the patient/family to space drug doses evenly around the clock.
- Teach the patient/family to take the patient's resting pulse daily to monitor therapeutic results.
- Urge the patient/family to restrict the patient's consumption of iodine products and seafood.
- Warn the patient/family to notify the physician immediately if the patient experiences illness, fever, sore throat, rash, yellowing of skin or unusual bleeding or bruising.

Propylthiouracil

pro-pill-thye-oh-**your**-ah-sill
(Propylthiouracil, Propyl-Thyracil [CAN])

CATEGORY AND SCHEDULE

Pregnancy Risk Category: D

MECHANISM OF ACTION

A thiourea derivative that blocks oxidation of iodine in the thyroid gland and blocks synthesis of thyroxine and triiodothyronine. ***Therapeutic Effect:*** Inhibits synthesis of thyroid hormone.

AVAILABILITY

Tablets: 50 mg.

INDICATIONS AND DOSAGES

▸ Hyperthyroidism

PO

Children. Initially: 5–7 mg/kg/day in divided doses q8h.
Maintenance: one-third to two-thirds of initial dose in divided doses q8–12h.
Neonates. 5–10 mg/kg/day in divided doses q8h.

CONTRAINDICATIONS

Hypersensitivity to propylthiouracil or any related component.

INTERACTIONS

Drug

Amiodarone, iodinated glycerol, iodine, potassium iodide: May decrease response.
Digoxin: May increase the blood concentration of this drug as patient becomes euthyroid.
Iodine-131: May decrease thyroid uptake of iodine-131.
Oral anticoagulants: May decrease the effects of oral anticoagulants.

Herbal

None known.

Food

None known.

DIAGNOSTIC TEST EFFECTS

May increase prothrombin time and lactate dehydrogenase (LDH), serum alkaline phosphatase, bilirubin, SGOT (AST), and SGPT (ALT) levels.

SIDE EFFECTS

Frequent

Urticaria, rash, pruritus, nausea, skin pigmentation, hair loss, headache, paresthesia

Occasional

Drowsiness, lymphadenopathy, vertigo

Rare

Drug fever, lupus-like syndrome

SERIOUS REACTIONS

! Agranulocytosis may occur as long as 4 mos after therapy; pancytopenia and fatal hepatitis have occurred.

PEDIATRIC CONSIDERATIONS

Baseline Assessment

- Obtain the patient's baseline pulse and weight.
- Expect to obtain baseline laboratory tests, including prothrombin time and LDH, serum alkaline phosphatase, bilirubin, SGOT (AST), and SGPT (ALT) levels.
- Assess for signs of bone marrow suppression (sore throat, fatigue, and/or fever).

Precautions

- Use cautiously in pts older than 40 yrs of age and in pts taking methimazole in combination with other agranulocytosis-inducing drugs.

Intervention and Evaluation

- Monitor the patient's pulse and weight daily.
- Assess the patient's skin for eruptions, itching, and swollen lymph glands.
- Monitor the patient's hematology results for bone marrow suppression.
- Be alert to signs and symptoms of hepatitis including drowsiness, jaundice, nausea, and vomiting.
- Evaluate the patient for signs and symptoms of bleeding and infection.

Patient/Family Teaching

- Instruct the patient/family to space drug doses evenly around the clock.

• Teach the patient/family to take the patient's resting pulse daily to monitor therapeutic results.
• Urge the patient/family to restrict the patient's consumption of iodine-containing products and seafood.
• Warn the patient/family to notify the physician immediately if the patient experiences cold intolerance, depression, or weight gain.

REFERENCES

Miller, S. & Fioravanti, J. (1997). Pediatric medications: a handbook for nurses. St. Louis: Mosby.
Taketomo, C. K., Hodding, J. H. & Kraus, D. M. (2003–2004). Pediatric dosage handbook (10th ed.). Hudson, OH: Lexi-Comp.

66 Miscellaneous Hormonal Agents

Glucagon Hydrochloride
Imiglucerase
Octreotide Acetate
Testosterone, Testosterone Cypionate, Testosterone Enanthate, Testosterone Propionate, Testosterone Transdermal

Uses: Miscellaneous hormonal agents have a wide variety of indications. *Glucagon* is used for treatment of severe hypoglycemia in diabetic pts and as an aid in radiographs of the GI tract. *Imiglucerase* is helpful in managing Gaucher disease. *Octreotide* is prescribed to control the symptoms of metastatic carcinoid tumors, vasoactive intestinal peptide-secreting tumors, and secretory diarrhea. *Testosterone* is used to treat male hypogonadism and delayed male puberty.

Action: Because miscellaneous hormonal agents belong to different subclasses, their actions vary widely. *Glucagon* promotes hepatic glycogenolysis and gluconeogenesis. *Imiglucerase* catalyzes the hydrolysis of glycolipid glucocerebrosidase to glucose and ceramide. *Octreotide* suppresses the secretion of serotonin and gastroenteropancreatic peptides, which enhances fluid and electrolyte absorption from the GI tract. *Testosterone* mimics the endogenous androgen, promoting the development of male sex organs and maintaining secondary sex characteristics in androgen-deficient men.

Glucagon Hydrochloride

glue-ka-gon
(Glucagen [AUS], Glucagon Emergency Kit)
Do not confuse with Glaucon.

CATEGORY AND SCHEDULE

Pregnancy Risk Category: B

MECHANISM OF ACTION

A glucose–elevating agent that promotes hepatic glycogenolysis and gluconeogenesis. Stimulates enzyme to increase production of cyclic adenosine monophosphate. ***Therapeutic Effect:*** Increases plasma glucose concentration and the relaxant effect on smooth muscle and exerts an inotropic myocardial effect.

AVAILABILITY

Powder for Injection: 1 mg.

INDICATIONS AND DOSAGES

▸ **Hypoglycemia**

SC/IM/IV

Children weighing greater than 20 kg. 0.5–1 mg. May repeat 1–2 additional doses every 20 min as needed.

Children weighing 20 kg or less. 0.02–0.03 mg/kg or 0.5 mg. May repeat 1–2 additional doses every 20 min as needed.

UNLABELED USES

Esophageal obstruction due to foreign bodies, treatment of toxicity associated with beta-blockers and calcium channel blockers.

CONTRAINDICATIONS

Hypersensitivity to glucagon protein or any related component and pheochromocytoma.

INTERACTIONS

Drug

Anticoagulants: May increase the effects of these drugs.
Phenytoin, propranolol: May decrease the clinical effects of glucagon

Herbal

None known.

Food

None known.

DIAGNOSTIC TEST EFFECTS

May decrease serum potassium levels.

IV INCOMPATIBILITIES

Do not mix with any other medications.

SIDE EFFECTS

Occasional
Nausea, vomiting
Rare
Allergic reaction, such as urticaria, respiratory distress, and hypotension

SERIOUS REACTIONS

! Overdose may produce persistent nausea or vomiting and hypokalemia, marked by severe weakness, decreased appetite, irregular heartbeat, and muscle cramps.

PEDIATRIC CONSIDERATIONS

Baseline Assessment

- Obtain an immediate assessment of the patient, including clinical signs and symptoms and history.
- Give glucagon immediately, as prescribed, if hypoglycemic coma is established.
- It is important to turn the unconscious child on his or her side to decrease the risk of aspiration with vomiting.

Precautions

- Use cautiously in pts with history of insulinoma or pheochromocytoma.

Administration and Handling

◂ALERT▸ Place the patient on his or her side to avoid potential aspiration because glucagon, as well as hypoglycemia, may produce nausea and vomiting.
◂ALERT▸ Administer IV dextrose if the patient fails to respond to glucagon.
SC/IM/IV
- Store vial at room temperature.
- Remember that after reconstitution, the solution is stable for 48 hrs if refrigerated. If reconstituted with Sterile Water for Injection, use immediately. Do not use glucagon solution unless clear.
- Reconstitute powder with manufacturer's diluent when preparing doses of 2 mg or less. For doses greater than 2 mg, dilute with Sterile Water for Injection.
- To provide 1 mg glucagon/mL, use 1 mL diluent for 1-mg vial of glucagon.
- Patient will usually awaken in 5–20 min. Although 1–2 additional doses may be administered, the concern for the effects of continuing cerebral hypoglycemia requires consideration of parenteral glucose.
- When the patient awakens, give supplemental carbohydrate to restore hepatic glycogen stores and prevent secondary hypoglycemia. If the patient fails to respond to glucagon, give IV glucose as prescribed.

Intervention and Evaluation

- Monitor the patient's response time carefully.
- Have IV dextrose readily available if the patient does not awaken within 5–20 min.
- Assess the patient for a possible allergic reaction, including hypotension, respiratory difficulty, and urticaria.
- Give oral carbohydrates when the patient is conscious.

Patient/Family Teaching

- Teach the patient/family to recognize the significance of identifying the symptoms of hypoglycemia, including anxiety, diaphoresis, difficulty concentrating, headache, hunger, nausea, nervousness, pale and cool skin, shakiness, unconsciousness, unusual tiredness, and weakness.
- Instruct the patient, family, or friends to give a sugar form first, such as hard candy, honey, orange juice, sugar cubes, or table sugar dissolved in water or juice, followed by a protein source, such as cheese and crackers or half a sandwich or glass of milk, if symptoms of hypoglycemia develop.
- Recommend to the patient/family that the patient wear a medical identification bracelet.

Imiglucerase

im-ih-**gloo**-sir-ace
(Cerezyme)
Do not confuse with Cerebyx or Ceredase.

CATEGORY AND SCHEDULE

Pregnancy Risk Category: C

MECHANISM OF ACTION

An enzyme analogue of the enzyme β-glucocerebrosidase, which catalyzes hydrolysis of glycolipid glucocerebroside to glucose and ceramide. ***Therapeutic Effect:*** Minimizes conditions associated with Gaucher disease, such as anemia and bone disease.

AVAILABILITY

Powder for Injection: 200 units, 424 units.

INDICATIONS AND DOSAGES

▸ Gaucher disease (dose is dependent on severity of disease symptoms)

IV INFUSION (OVER 1–2 HRS)
Children. Initially, 2.5 units/kg 3 times/wk up to 60 units/kg/wk. Maintenance: Progressive reduction in dosage every 3–6 mos while monitoring patient response.

CONTRAINDICATIONS

Hypersensitivity to imiglucerase or any related component.

INTERACTIONS

Drug
None known.
Herbal
None known.
Food
None known.

DIAGNOSTIC TEST EFFECTS

None known.

IV INCOMPATIBILITIES

Do not mix with any other medication.

SIDE EFFECTS

Frequent (3%)
Headache
Occasional (less than 3%–1%)
Nausea, abdominal discomfort, dizziness, pruritus, rash, small decrease in blood pressure, or urinary frequency

PEDIATRIC CONSIDERATIONS

Baseline Assessment

- Expect to perform baseline laboratory tests, including a complete blood count (CBC), serum hepatic enzyme levels, and platelets.
- Be sure to use the preservative-free form with children.
- In clinical trials 16% of pts developed IgG antibodies and less than 1% experienced anaphylactic reactions.

Administration and Handling

IV

- Refrigerate.
- Once reconstituted, the solution is stable for 24 hrs if refrigerated.
- Reconstitute with 5.1 mL sterile water to provide concentration of 40 units/mL.
- Further dilute with 100–200 mL 0.9% NaCl.
- Infuse over 1–2 hrs.

Intervention and Evaluation

- Monitor the patient's CBC, hepatic enzyme levels, and platelets.
- If the patient experiences anaphylactoid reactions, you may need to reduce the infusion rate and/or pretreat with an antihistamine or corticosteroid.

Patient/Family Teaching

- Let the patient/family know about any required follow-up tests.
- Instruct the patient/family to tell you about any side effects, such as headache.

Octreotide Acetate

ock-**tree**-oh-tide
(Sandostatin, Sandostatin LAR)
Do not confuse with OctreoScan, Sandimmune, or Sandoglobulin.

CATEGORY AND SCHEDULE

Pregnancy Risk Category: B

MECHANISM OF ACTION

A secretory inhibitory, growth hormone suppressant that suppresses secretion of serotonin and gastroenteropancreatic peptides. Enhances fluid and electrolyte absorption from the GI tract. ***Therapeutic Effect:*** Prolongs intestinal transit time.

PHARMACOKINETICS

Route	Onset	Peak	Duration
SC	N/A	N/A	Up to 12 hrs

Rapidly, completely absorbed from injection site. Metabolized extensively by the liver. Excreted in urine. Removed by hemodialysis. ***Half-Life:*** 1.5 hrs.

AVAILABILITY

Injection (Sandostatin): 0.05 mg/mL, 0.1 mg/mL, 0.2 mg/mL, 0.5 mg/mL, 1 mg/mL.
Suspension for Injection (Sandostatin-LAR; Depot formulation): 10-mg, 20-mg, 30-mg vials.

INDICATIONS AND DOSAGES

▸ **Diarrhea (Sandostatin)**

IV/SC

Children. 1–10 mcg/kg q12h have been used in clinical trials.

▸ **Chylothorax**

IV/SC

Children. 1-4 mcg/kg/hr continuous infusion has been used. Titrate to response

▸ **GI Bleeding**

IV/SC

Children. 1 mcg/kg bolus, followed by 1 mcg/kg/hr continuous infusion. Titrate to effect. Taper dose by 50% every 12 hrs after active bleeding has been stopped for

24 hrs. Discontinue when dose is 25% of initial dose.

UNLABELED USES

AIDS-associated secretory diarrhea, chemotherapy-induced diarrhea, control of bleeding of esophageal varices, insulinomas, small bowel fistulas

CONTRAINDICATIONS

Hypersensitivity to octreotide or any related component.

INTERACTIONS

Drug

Glucagon, growth hormone, insulin, oral hypoglycemics: May alter glucose concentrations with glucagon, growth hormone, insulin, and oral hypoglycemics.
Cyclosporin: May decrease cyclosporine serum concentrations.

Herbal

None known.

Food

Dietary Fats: May decrease absorption of dietary fats.

DIAGNOSTIC TEST EFFECTS

May decrease thyroxine concentration.

SIDE EFFECTS

Frequent (10%–6%, 58%–30% in pts with acromegaly)
Diarrhea, nausea, abdominal discomfort, headache, pain at injection site
Occasional (5%–1%)
Vomiting, flatulence, constipation, alopecia, flushing, itching, dizziness, fatigue, arrhythmias, bruising, blurred vision
Rare (less than 1%)
Depression, decreased libido, vertigo, palpitations, shortness of breath

SERIOUS REACTIONS

! There is an increased risk of cholelithiasis.
! There is a potential for hypothyroidism with prolonged high therapy.
! GI bleeding, hepatitis, and seizures occur rarely.

PEDIATRIC CONSIDERATIONS

Baseline Assessment

- Establish the patient's baseline blood glucose and electrolyte levels, blood pressure (B/P), and weight.
- Be aware that it is unknown whether octreotide is excreted in breast milk.
- Be aware that the dosage is not established in children.

Precautions

- Use cautiously in pts with insulin-dependent diabetes and renal failure.

Administration and Handling

◂ALERT▸ Sandostatin may be given IV, IM, and SC.

SC

- Do not use if particulates or discoloration is noted.
- Avoid multiple injections at the same site within short periods of time.

IM

- Give immediately after mixing.
- Administer intragluteally at 4-wk intervals.
- Avoid deltoid injections.

Intervention and Evaluation

- Monitor the patient's blood glucose levels, fecal fat, fluid and electrolyte balance, and thyroid function tests.
- Monitor growth hormone levels in acromegaly pts.
- Weigh the patient every 2–3 days and report more than a 5-lb weight gain in a week.

• Monitor the patient's B/P, pulse, and respirations periodically during treatment.
• Be alert for decreased urinary output and edema of the ankles and fingers in the patient.
• Assess the patient's pattern of daily bowel frequency and stool consistency.

Patient/Family Teaching

• Therapy should provide significant improvement of symptoms.
• Tell the patient/family to weigh the patient daily and to report a weight gain of greater than 5 lbs/wk.

Testosterone

tess-**toss**-ter-own
(Andronaq, Delatestryl [CAN], Histerone, Striant)

Testosterone Cypionate

(Depotest, Depo-Testosterone)

Testosterone Enanthate

(Delatest)

Testosterone Propionate

(Testex)

Testosterone Transdermal

(Androderm, Testim, Testoderm, Testoderm TTS)
Do not confuse with testolactone.

CATEGORY AND SCHEDULE

Pregnancy Risk Category: X

MECHANISM OF ACTION

A primary endogenous androgen that promotes growth and development of male sex organs and maintains secondary sex characteristics in androgen-deficient males.

PHARMACOKINETICS

Well absorbed after IM administration. Protein binding: 98%. Metabolized in liver (undergoes first-pass metabolism). Primarily excreted in urine. Unknown whether removed by hemodialysis. ***Half-Life:*** 10–20 min.

AVAILABILITY

Injection: 100 mg/mL (aqueous suspension, Cypionate, Propionate), 200 mg/mL (Cypionate and Enanthate).
*Pellets for Subcutaneous Implanta*tion: 75 mg.
Transdermal Gel: 25 mg (2.5 g gel/pack), 50 mg (5 g gel/pack).
Transdermal System: 2.5 mg/day, 4 mg/day, 5 mg/day, 6 mg/day.
Buccal System: 30 mg.

INDICATIONS AND DOSAGES

▸ Male hypogonadism

IM

Children. 40–50 mg/m²/dose every mo (Cypionate or enanthate, initial pubertal growth), 100 mg/m²/dose every mo (terminal growth phase). Maintenance virilizing dose: 100 mg/m²/dose 2 times/mo.

▸ Delayed puberty

IM

Children. 40–50 mg/m²/dose every mo for 6 mos.

▸ Postpubertal cryptorchism

IM

Children. 10–25 mg 2–3 times/wk (testosterone or testosterone propionate).

CONTRAINDICATIONS

Hypersensitivity to testosterone or any related component, including testosterone that is derived from soy. Cardiac impairment, hypercalcemia, pregnancy, prostatic or breast cancer in males, severe liver or renal disease.

INTERACTIONS

Drug

Liver toxic medications: May increase liver toxicity.
Oral anticoagulants: May increase the effects of oral anticoagulants.

Herbal

None known.

Food

None known.

DIAGNOSTIC TEST EFFECTS

May increase blood Hgb and Hct, low-density lipoprotein, serum alkaline phosphatase, bilirubin, calcium, potassium, SGOT (AST), and sodium levels. May decrease high-density lipoprotein concentrations.

SIDE EFFECTS

Frequent

Gynecomastia, acne, amenorrhea or other menstrual irregularities Females: Hirsutism, deepening of voice, clitoral enlargement that may not be reversible when drug is discontinued

Occasional

Edema, nausea, insomnia, oligospermia, priapism, male pattern of baldness, bladder irritability, hypercalcemia in immobilized pts or those with breast cancer, hypercholesterolemia, inflammation and pain at IM injection site

Rare

Polycythemia with high dosage, hypersensitivity

SERIOUS REACTIONS

! Peliosis hepatitis or liver, spleen replaced with blood-filled cysts, hepatic neoplasms, and hepatocellular carcinoma have been associated with prolonged high-dosage, anaphylactic reactions.

PEDIATRIC CONSIDERATIONS

Baseline Assessment

- Establish the patient's baseline blood Hgb and Hct, blood pressure (B/P), and weight.
- Check the patient's serum cholesterol and electrolyte levels and hepatic enzyme test results, if ordered.
- Know that wrist radiographs may be ordered to determine bone maturation in children.
- Assess and monitor for growth rate, pubertal status, and bone age in children.

Precautions

- Use cautiously in pts with diabetes and liver or renal impairment.
- Be aware that testosterone use is contraindicated during lactation.
- Be aware that the safety and efficacy of testosterone have not been established in children, so use with caution.

Administration and Handling

IM

- Give deep in gluteal muscle.
- Do not give IV.
- Warming and shaking redissolves crystals that may form in long-acting preparations.
- A wet needle may cause the solution to become cloudy; this does not affect potency.

Intervention and Evaluation

- Weigh the patient daily and report weekly gains of more than 5 lbs.
- Evaluate the patient for edema.

• Monitor the patient's intake and output and sleep patterns.
• Check the patient's B/P at least 2 times/day.
• Assess the patient's blood Hgb and Hct periodically when giving high dosages, as ordered. Also plan to check serum cholesterol and electrolyte levels, as well as liver function test results.
• Expect to perform a radiologic examination of the hand or wrist when using in prepubertal children.
• Monitor pts with breast cancer or immobility for hypercalcemia, confusion, irritability, lethargy, and muscle weakness.
• Ensure that the patient consumes adequate calories and protein.
• Assess the patient for signs of virilization, such as deepening of the voice.
• Examine the patient's injection site for pain, redness, or swelling.

Patient/Family Teaching

• Stress to the patient/family the importance of monitoring tests and regular visits to the physician.
• Warn the patient/family not to take any other medications, including OTC drugs, without first consulting the physician.
• Teach the patient/family to consume a diet high in calories and protein. Tell the patient that food may be better tolerated if he or she consumes small, frequent meals.
• Instruct the patient/family to weigh the patient each day and to report to the physician weight gains of 5 lbs or more per week.
• Warn the patient/family to notify the physician if the patient experiences acne, nausea, pedal edema, or vomiting. Tell female pts to also promptly report deepening of voice, hoarseness, and menstrual irregularities. Tell male pts to report difficulty urinating, frequent erections, and gynecomastia.

REFERENCES

Taketomo, C. K., Hodding, J. H. & Kraus, D. M. (2003–2004). Pediatric dosage handbook (10th ed.). Hudson, OH: Lexi-Comp.

67 Antirheumatic Agents

Auranofin, Aurothioglucose
Gold Sodium Thiomalate
Methotrexate Sodium
Sulfasalazine

Uses: Antirheumatic agents are used to relieve symptoms of rheumatoid arthritis, especially in pts with an insufficient therapeutic response to NSAIDs. Specific antirheumatic agents may be used to treat malaria (hydroxychloroquine), trophoblastic neoplasms and other cancers (methotrexate), and ulcerative colitis and inflammatory bowel disease (sulfasalazine).

Action: Disease-modifying antirheumatic drugs include gold compounds and immunosuppressive and antimalarial agents. *Gold compounds,* such as auranofin, aurothioglucose, and gold sodium thiomalate, depress leukocyte migration and suppress prostaglandin activity. They may also inhibit the destructive lysosomal enzymes in leukocytes, which are released at joints. Some *immunosuppressive agents,* such as methotrexate, suppress the inflammatory process of rheumatoid arthritis. *Antimalarial agents,* such as hydroxychloroquine, act by an unknown mechanism in rheumatoid arthritis.

Auranofin
aur-an-**oh**-fin
(Ridaura)
Do not confuse with Cardura.

Aurothioglucose
ah-row-thigh-oh-**glue**-cose
(Gold-50 [AUS], Solganal)

CATEGORY AND SCHEDULE
Pregnancy Risk Category: C

MECHANISM OF ACTION
A gold compound that alters cellular mechanisms, collagen biosynthesis, enzyme systems, and immune responses. ***Therapeutic Effect:*** Suppresses synovitis of the active stage of rheumatoid arthritis.

PHARMACOKINETICS
Auranofin (29% gold): Moderately absorbed from the GI tract. Protein binding: 60%. Rapidly metabolized. Primarily excreted in urine. ***Half-Life:*** 21–31 days. Aurothioglucose (50% gold): Slow, erratic absorption after IM administration. Protein binding: 95%–99%. Primarily excreted in urine. ***Half-Life:*** 3–27 days (half-life increased with increased number of doses).

AVAILABILITY
Capsules: 3 mg.
Injection: 50 mg/mL suspension.

INDICATIONS AND DOSAGES
▸ **Rheumatoid arthritis**

IM

Children. 0.25 mg/kg/dose once weekly, may increase by 0.25

mg/kg each week. Maintenance: 0.75–1 mg/kg/dose. Maximum: 25 mg/dose for a total of 20 doses, then q2–4wks.
PO
Children. 0.1 mg/kg/day in 1–2 divided doses. Maintenance: 0.15 mg/kg/day. Maximum: 0.2 mg/kg/day.

UNLABELED USES
Treatment of pemphigus, psoriatic arthritis.

CONTRAINDICATIONS
Hypersensitivity to auranofin or any related component. Bone marrow aplasia, history of gold-induced pathologic conditions, including blood dyscrasias, exfoliative dermatitis, necrotizing enterocolitis, and pulmonary fibrosis, serious adverse effects with previous gold therapy, severe blood dyscrasias.

INTERACTIONS
Drug
Bone marrow depressants; hepatotoxic, nephrotoxic medications: May increase the risk of aurothioglucose toxicity.
Penicillamine: May increase risk of hematologic or renal adverse effects of aurothioglucose.
Antimalarials, hydroxychloroquine, cytotoxic agents, immunosuppressive agents: May increase toxicity of auranofin.
Herbal
None known.
Food
None known.

DIAGNOSTIC TEST EFFECTS
May decrease Hgb and Hct levels and platelet and WBC count. May alter liver function tests. May increase urine protein level.

SIDE EFFECTS
Frequent
Auranofin: Diarrhea (50%), pruritic rash (26%), abdominal pain (14%), stomatitis (13%), nausea (10%)
Aurothioglucose: Rash (39%), stomatitis (19%), diarrhea (13%)
Occasional
Nausea, vomiting, anorexia, abdominal cramps

SERIOUS REACTIONS
! Gold toxicity is the primary serious reaction. Signs and symptoms of gold toxicity include decreased Hgb level, leukopenia (WBC count less than 4,000/mm^3), reduced granulocyte counts (less than 150,000/mm^3), proteinuria, hematuria, stomatitis (sores, ulcers, and white spots in the mouth and throat), blood dyscrasias (anemia, leukopenia, thrombocytopenia, and eosinophilia), glomerulonephritis, nephritic syndrome, and cholestatic jaundice.

PEDIATRIC CONSIDERATIONS
Baseline Assessment
- Determine whether the patient is pregnant before beginning treatment.
- Check the results of the patient's complete blood count (CBC), particularly platelet count, blood urea nitrogen, Hct, Hgb, serum alkaline phosphatase, creatinine, SGOT (AST), and SGPT (ALT) levels to assess renal and liver function and urinalysis, before therapy begins.
- Be aware that aurothioglucose crosses the placenta and is distributed in breast milk. Use only when the drug's benefits outweigh the possible hazard to the fetus.
- There are no age-related precautions noted in children.

Precautions

• Use cautiously in pts with blood dyscrasias, compromised cerebral or cardiovascular circulation, eczema, a history of sensitivity to gold compounds, marked by hypertension, renal or liver impairment, severe debilitation, Sjögren syndrome in rheumatoid arthritis, and systemic lupus erythematosus.

Administration and Handling

PO

• Give without regard to food.

IM

◂ **ALERT** ▸ Give as weekly injections.

• Give in upper outer quadrant of gluteus maximus.

Intervention and Evaluation

• Assess the patient's pattern of daily bowel activity and stool consistency.

• Test the patient's urine for hematuria and proteinuria.

• Monitor the results of the patient's blood chemistry analysis, CBC, and renal and liver function studies.

• Assess the patient for pruritus, which may be the first sign of an impending rash.

• Assess the patient's skin daily for ecchymoses, purpura, and rash.

• Examine the patient's oral mucous membranes, palate, pharynx, and tongue borders for ulceration. Investigate any patient complaints of a metallic taste in the mouth as this is a sign of stomatitis.

• Evaluate the patient for the expected therapeutic response, including improved grip strength, increased joint mobility, reduced joint tenderness, and relief of pain, stiffness, and swelling.

Patient/Family Teaching

• Advise the patient/family that the therapeutic response of the drug may be expected in 3–6 mos.

• Warn the patient/family to avoid exposure to sunlight. Explain that sun exposure may cause a gray to blue pigment to appear on the skin.

• Urge the patient/family to notify the physician if indigestion, metallic taste, pruritus, rash, or sore mouth occurs.

• Stress to the patient/family that the patient maintain diligent oral hygiene to help prevent stomatitis.

Gold Sodium Thiomalate

gold sodium thigh-oh-**mal**-ate
(Myochrysine, Myocrisin [AUS])

CATEGORY AND SCHEDULE

Pregnancy Risk Category: C

MECHANISM OF ACTION

A gold compound whose mechanism of action is unknown. May decrease prostaglandin synthesis or alter cellular mechanisms by inhibiting sulfhydryl systems. ***Therapeutic Effect:*** Decreases synovial inflammation, retards cartilage and bone destruction, suppresses or prevents but does not cure, arthritis and synovitis.

AVAILABILITY

Injection: 50 mg/mL.

INDICATIONS AND DOSAGES

▸ **Rheumatoid arthritis**

IM

Children. Initially, 10 mg test dose, then 1 mg/kg/wk for 20 wks. Maximum single dose: 50 mg. Maintenance: 1 mg/kg/dose at 2- to 4-wk intervals.

▸ **Dosage in renal impairment**

Creatinine Clearance	Dosage
50–80 mL/min	50% of usual dosage
Less than 50 mL/min	not recommended

UNLABELED USES

Treatment of psoriatic arthritis.

CONTRAINDICATIONS

Hypersensitivity to gold compounds or related components and heavy metals. Colitis, concurrent use of antimalarials, immunosuppressive agents, penicillamine, or phenylbutazone, congestive heart failure, exfoliative dermatitis, history of blood dyscrasias, severe liver or renal impairment, systemic lupus erythematosus.

INTERACTIONS

Drug

Bone marrow depressants, liver toxic, nephrotoxic medications: May increase the risk of toxicity.
Penicillamine: May increase the risk of adverse hematologic or renal effects.
Antimalarial agents, immunosuppressive agents, cytoxic agents: Use not recommended due to increased risk of toxicity.

Herbal

None known.

Food

None known.

DIAGNOSTIC TEST EFFECTS

May decrease blood Hgb and Hct and platelet and WBC counts. May alter liver function tests. May increase urine protein.

SIDE EFFECTS

Frequent
Pruritic dermatitis, stomatitis, marked by erythema, redness, shallow ulcers of oral mucous membranes, sore throat, and difficulty swallowing, diarrhea or loose stools, abdominal pain, nausea
Occasional
Vomiting, anorexia, flatulence, dyspepsia, conjunctivitis, photosensitivity
Rare
Constipation, urticaria, rash

SERIOUS REACTIONS

! Signs of gold toxicity including decreased Hgb, leukopenia (WBC less than 4,000 mm^3), reduced granulocyte counts (less than 150,000/mm^3), proteinuria, hematuria, blood dyscrasias, including anemia, leukopenia, thrombocytopenia, and eosinophilia, glomerulonephritis, nephrotic syndrome, and cholestatic jaundice may occur.

PEDIATRIC CONSIDERATIONS

Baseline Assessment

- Determine whether the patient is pregnant before beginning treatment.
- Plan to perform a complete blood count (CBC), particularly blood urea nitrogen, Hct, Hgb, platelet and WBC count, and serum alkaline phosphatase, creatinine, SGOT (AST), and SGPT (ALT) levels to assess liver and renal function and a urinalysis of the patient before beginning therapy.

Administration and Handling

◂ **ALERT** ▸ Give gold sodium thiomalate as weekly injections, as prescribed.

Intervention and Evaluation

- Assess the patient's pattern of daily bowel activity and stool consistency.
- Assess the patient's urine tests for hematuria or proteinuria.
- Monitor the patient's CBC and liver and renal function studies.
- Assess the patient's skin daily for ecchymoses, purpura, and rash.
- Assess the patient's borders of tongue, oral mucous membranes, palate, and pharynx for ulceration.
- Evaluate any patient complaints of metallic taste sensation or sign of stomatitis.
- Evaluate the patient for a therapeutic response, improved grip strength, increased joint mobility, reduced joint tenderness, and relief of pain, stiffness, and swelling.

Patient/Family Teaching

- Tell the patient/family that the drug's therapeutic response may take 6 mos or more to appear.
- Warn the patient/family to avoid exposure to sunlight. Explain that a gray to blue skin pigment may appear.
- Stress to the patient/family that the patient must maintain diligent oral hygiene during gold sodium thiomalate therapy.

Methotrexate Sodium

See antimetabolites

Sulfasalazine

See miscellaneous anti-infective agents

REFERENCES

Taketomo, C. K., Hodding, J. H. & Kraus, D. M. (2003–2004). Pediatric dosage handbook (10th ed.). Hudson, OH: Lexi-Comp.

68 Immune Globulins

Hepatitis B Immune Globulin (Human)
Immune Globulin IV (IGIV)
Lymphocyte Immune Globulin N
Respiratory Syncytial Immune Globulin
Rh_0 (D) Immune Globulin

Uses: Immune globulins are primarily used to immunize pts against infectious diseases, such as hepatitis B virus and respiratory syncytial virus infections. In addition, *antithymocyte globulin* is used to prevent and treat allograft rejection, to treat aplastic anemia, and to prevent graft-vs-host disease after bone marrow transplantation. *Immune globulin IV* is used to treat primary immunodeficiency syndromes, Kawasaki disease, and idiopathic thrombocytopenic purpura; to prevent bacterial infections in pts with hypogammaglobulinemia; and as an adjunct in bone marrow transplantation. *Rh_0 (D) immune globulin* is used to prevent isoimmunization in Rh-negative pts exposed to Rh-positive blood.

Action: These immune globulins provide passive immunization, which involves administration of preformed antibodies. Passive immunity is not permanent and does not last as long as active immunity, which results from immunization with an antigen to develop defenses against a future exposure.

Hepatitis B Immune Globulin (Human)

(BayHep B, Nabi-HB)

CATEGORY AND SCHEDULE
Pregnancy Risk Category: C

MECHANISM OF ACTION

An immune globulin of inactivated hepatitis B virus that provides passive immunization against hepatitis B virus.

AVAILABILITY

Injection: 5-mL vial.

INDICATIONS AND DOSAGES

▸ **Acute exposure**

IM

Children. 0.06 mL/kg usual dose; 3–5 mL for postexposure prophylaxis. Repeat at 28–30 days after exposure.

Neonates born to hepatitis B surface antigen–positive mothers. 0.5 mL within 12 hr of birth. Repeat at 3 and 6 mos if hepatitis B vaccine is refused.

CONTRAINDICATIONS

Hypersensitivity to hepatitis immune globulin, blood products, or any related component. Allergies to gamma globulin or thimerosal, immunoglobulin (Ig) A deficiency, IM injections in pts with coagulation disorders or thrombocytopenia.

INTERACTIONS

Drug
None known.

Herbal
None known.

Food
None known.

DIAGNOSTIC TEST EFFECTS
None known.

SIDE EFFECTS
Frequent
Headache (26%), local pain (12%)
Occasional (5%)
Malaise, nausea, myalgia

SERIOUS REACTIONS
! None significant.

PEDIATRIC CONSIDERATIONS
Baseline Assessment
• Ask the patient whether he or she has a known allergy to thimerosal, eggs, or chicken products before administering.
• Expect to obtain baseline hepatic enzyme levels and hepatitis B antibodies.
Precautions
• Use cautiously in pts with coagulation disorders and thrombocytopenia.
• Know that the drug is contraindicated in pts with allergies to gamma globulin or thimerosal and IgA deficiency.
Administration and Handling
◂ **ALERT** ▸ Avoid giving IM injections in pts with coagulation disorders or thrombocytopenia.
IM
• Refrigerate, do not freeze.
• Give via IM injection only in gluteal or deltoid area.
Intervention and Evaluation
◂ **ALERT** ▸ This drug is for IM injection only.
• Use care when administering to pts with bleeding disorders and thrombocytopenia.
• Plan to obtain periodic liver function studies and hepatitis B antibody levels.
Patient/Family Teaching
• Advise the patient/family to complete the full course of immunization.
• Tell the patient/family to report any side effects, as soon as possible, including headache or injection site pain.
• Teach the patient/family how hepatitis B is transmitted, such as by blood and body fluid.

Immune Globulin IV (IGIV)
(BayGam, Gamimune N, Gammagard, Gammar-IV, ***Gammunex, Polygam, Sandoglobulin, Venoglobulin-I)
Do not confuse with Sandimmune or Sandostatin.

CATEGORY AND SCHEDULE
Pregnancy Risk Category: C

MECHANISM OF ACTION
An immune serum that increases antibody titer and antigen-antibody reaction. ***Therapeutic Effect:*** Provides passive immunity against infection. Induces rapid increase in platelet counts. Produces an anti-inflammatory effect.

PHARMACOKINETICS
Evenly distributed between intravascular and extravascular space. ***Half-Life:*** 21–29 days.

AVAILABILITY
Injection (powder for reconstitution):
Carimune: 1 g, 3 g, 6 g, 10 g.
Gammar-P IV: 1 g, 2.5 g, 5 g, 10 g.
Iveegam EN: 0.5 g, 1 g, 2.5 g, 5 g.
Panglobulin: 1 g, 3 g, 6 g, 12 g.
Gammagard S/D: 2.5 g, 5 g, 10 g (solvent/detergent treated).

Polygam S/D: 2.5 g, 5 g, 10 g (solvent/detergent treated).
Solution for injection:
Gamimune N: 10%
Venoglobulin S: 5%, 10%.

INDICATIONS AND DOSAGES

▸ Primary immunodeficiency syndrome

IV INFUSION

Children. 300–400 mg/kg/dose q1mo to maintain trough immunoglobulin (Ig) G concentration of 500 mg/dL.

▸ Idiopathic thrombocytopenia purpura (ITP)

IV INFUSION

Children. 400–1,000 mg/kg/day for 2–5 days.

▸ Kawasaki disease

IV INFUSION

Children. 2 g/kg as a single dose given over 10–12 hrs.

▸ Chronic lymphocytic leukemia

IV INFUSION

Children. 400 mg/kg q3–4wks.

▸ Congenital and acquired AIDS

IV INFUSION

Children. 100–400 mg/kg/dose q3–4wks.

▸ Bone marrow transplant

IV INFUSION

Children. 400–500 mg/kg/dose every wk for 3 mo, then once/mo.

UNLABELED USES

Control and prevention of infections in infants and children immunosuppressed in association with AIDS or AIDS-related complex, prevention of acute infections in immunosuppressed pts, prophylaxis and treatment of infections in high-risk, preterm, low-birth-weight neonates, treatment of chronic inflammatory demyelinating polyneuropathies, multiple sclerosis

CONTRAINDICATIONS

Hypersensitivity to immune globulin, blood products, or any related component. Allergic response to thimerosal, any coagulation disorder for IM administration, a history of allergic response to gamma globulin or anti-IgA antibodies, isolated IgA deficiency (may use Gammagard S/D or Polygam S/D), severe thrombocytopenia for IM administration.

INTERACTIONS

Drug

Live virus vaccines: May decrease the patient's antibody response to the vaccine, increase vaccine side effects, and potentiate virus replication. Example: measles, mumps, rubella.

Herbal

None known.

Food

None known.

DIAGNOSTIC TEST EFFECTS

None known.

IV INCOMPATIBILITIES

Do not mix with any other medications.

SIDE EFFECTS

Frequent

Tachycardia, backache, headache, joint or muscle pain

Occasional

Fatigue, wheezing, rash or pain at injection site, leg cramps, hives, bluish color of lips and nailbeds, lightheadedness

SERIOUS REACTIONS

! Anaphylactic reactions occur rarely, but there is increased incidence when repeated injections of immune globulin are given.

Epinephrine should be readily available.
! Overdose may produce chest tightness, chills, diaphoresis, dizziness, flushed face, nausea, vomiting, fever, and hypotension.

PEDIATRIC CONSIDERATIONS

Baseline Assessment

- Determine the patient's history and patient's family history of exposure to the disease.
- Have epinephrine readily available in case of an anaphylactic reaction.
- Make sure the patient is well hydrated before giving immune globulin IV.
- Be aware that it is unknown whether immune globulin IV crosses the placenta or is distributed in breast milk.
- There are no age-related precautions noted in children.

Precautions

- Use cautiously in pts with cardiovascular disease, diabetes mellitus, a history of thrombosis, impaired renal function, sepsis, and volume depletion.
- Use cautiously in pts who concomitantly use nephrotoxic drugs.

Administration and Handling

IV

- Refer to individual IV preparations for storage requirements and stability after reconstitution.
- Reconstitute only with diluent provided by manufacturer.
- Discard partially used or turbid preparations.
- Give by infusion only.
- After reconstituted, administer through separate tubing.
- Avoid mixing with other medication or IV infusion fluids.
- Remember that the rate of infusion varies among products.
- Monitor the patient's blood pressure (B/P) and vital signs diligently during and immediately after IV administration. Be aware that a precipitous fall in B/P may indicate anaphylactic reaction.
- Stop patient infusion immediately if anaphylactic reaction is suspected. Epinephrine should be readily available.

Intervention and Evaluation

- Control the rate of IV infusion carefully. Too rapid infusion increases the risk of a precipitous fall in B/P and signs of anaphylaxis such as chest tightness, chills, diaphoresis, facial flushing, fever, nausea, and vomiting. Stop the infusion temporarily if the aforementioned signs are noted.
- Assess the patient closely during infusion, especially in the first hour.
- Monitor the patient's vital signs continuously.
- Monitor the patient's platelets for treatment of ITP.

Patient/Family Teaching

- Explain to the patient/family the rationale for therapy.
- Explain to the patient/family that the patient should have a rapid response to therapy, lasting 1–3 mo.
- Warn the patient/family to notify the physician if the patient experiences decreased urine output, edema, fluid retention, shortness of breath, or sudden weight gain.

Lymphocyte Immune Globulin N

lym-phow-site
(Atgam)
Do not confuse with Ativan.

CATEGORY AND SCHEDULE

Pregnancy Risk Category: C

MECHANISM OF ACTION
A biologic response modifier that acts as a lymphocyte selective immunosuppressant, reducing the number of circulating thymus-dependent lymphocytes (T-lymphocytes) and altering the function of T-lymphocytes, which are responsible for cell-mediated and humoral immunity. Antithymocyte globulin (ATG) also stimulates the release of hematopoietic growth factors. ***Therapeutic Effect:*** Prevents allograft rejection and treats aplastic anemia.

AVAILABILITY
Injection: 50 mg/mL.

INDICATIONS AND DOSAGES
▸ Prevent or treat renal allograft rejection
IV INFUSION
Children. Usual dosage: 5–25 mg/kg/day.
▸ Delay of onset of rejection
IV INFUSION
Children. 15 mg/kg/day for 14 days, then 15 mg/kg/day every other day for 14 days. Give first dose within 24 hrs before or after transplant.
▸ Treatment of rejection
IV INFUSION
Children. 10–15 mg/kg/day for 14 days. May continue with alternate-day therapy for up to 21 doses.
▸ Aplastic anemia protocol
IV INFUSION
Children. 10–20 mg/kg/day for 8–14 days, then 10–30 mg/kg/dose every other day for 7 more doses.

UNLABELED USES
Immunosuppressant in bone marrow, heart, and liver transplants, treatment of pure red cell aplasia, multiple sclerosis, myasthenia gravis, and scleroderma.

CONTRAINDICATIONS
Hypersensitivity to ATG thimerosal, or other equine gamma globulins. Systemic hypersensitivity reaction to previous injection of ATG. Severe leucopenia or thrombocytopenia.

INTERACTIONS
Drug
None known.
Herbal
None known.
Food
None known.

DIAGNOSTIC TEST EFFECTS
May alter renal function tests.

IV INCOMPATIBILITIES
No information is available for Y-site administration.

SIDE EFFECTS
Frequent
Fever (51%), thrombocytopenia (30%), rash (2%), chills (16%), leukopenia (14%), systemic infection (13%).
Occasional (10%–5%)
Serum sickness-like symptoms, dyspnea, apnea, arthralgia, chest pain, back pain, flank pain, nausea, vomiting, diarrhea, phlebitis.

SERIOUS REACTIONS
! Thrombocytopenia occurs but is generally transient.
! Severe hypersensitivity reaction, including anaphylaxis, occurs rarely.

PEDIATRIC CONSIDERATIONS
Baseline Assessment
• To prevent chemical phlebitis, avoid using a peripheral vein for IV infusion. Instead, expect to use a central venous catheter,

Groshong catheter, or peripherally inserted central catheter.

• An intradermal test dose is recommended before the first dose of ATG. Use 0.1 mL of a 1:1,000 dilution of ATG in 0.9% NaCl. Observe closely every 15 min for 1 hr. A wheal or local reaction greater than 10 mm in diameter should be considered a positive skin test.

• Pts may need to be pretreated before the infusion with an antipyretic, antihistamine and/or corticosteroid to prevent chills, fever, itching, and erythema.

Precautions

• Use cautiously in pts receiving concurrent immunosuppressive therapy.

Administration and Handling

IV

• Keep refrigerated before and after dilution.

• Discard diluted solution after 24 hrs.

• Further dilute the total daily dose with 0.9% NaCl, as prescribed, to a final concentration that doesn't exceed 4 mg/mL.

• Gently rotate diluted solution; avoid shaking solution.

• Use a 0.2- to 1-micron filter. Give the total daily dose over a minimum of 4 hrs.

Intervention and Evaluation

• Expect to monitor the patient frequently for chills, erythema, fever, and itching. Obtain an order for prophylactic antihistamines or corticosteroids to treat these possible side effects.

Patient/Family Teaching

• Stress the importance of avoiding exposure to colds or infections and to notify the physician as soon as signs or symptoms develop.

• Explain that during the IV infusion, the patient/family should immediately report chest pain, rapid or irregular heartbeats, shortness of breath or wheezing, or swelling of the face or throat.

Respiratory Syncytial Immune Globulin

(RespiGam)

CATEGORY AND SCHEDULE

Pregnancy Risk Category: C

MECHANISM OF ACTION

An immune serum with a high concentration of neutralizing and protective antibodies specific for respiratory syncytial virus (RSV).

AVAILABILITY

Injection: 2,500 mcg RSV immune globulin (50 mg/mL).

INDICATIONS AND DOSAGES

▸ Prevents RSV in children with bronchopulmonary dysplasia and history of premature birth

IV INFUSION

Children younger than 24 mos. 750 mg/kg (15 mL/kg). Initially, 1.5 mL/kg/hr for the first 15 min, then 3.6 mL/kg/hr for the remainder of the infusion. Administer monthly for a total of 5 doses beginning in September or October or during the RSV season.

CONTRAINDICATIONS

Hypersensitivity to RSV-immune globulin or any related component and immunoglobulin A deficiency.

INTERACTIONS

Drug

Live virus vaccines: May reduce antibody response and may not replicate successfully. Examples include measles, mumps, rubella, diphtheria-pertussis-tetanus (DPT), *Haemophilus influenza.*

Herbal

None known.

Food

None known.

DIAGNOSTIC TEST EFFECTS

None known.

SIDE EFFECTS

Occasional (6%–2%)

Fever, vomiting, wheezing.

Rare (less than 1%)

Diarrhea, rash, tachycardia, hypertension, hypoxia, injection site inflammation

PEDIATRIC CONSIDERATIONS

Baseline Assessment

- Assess the patient's routine arterial blood gas values, blood chemistry, electrolyte levels, osmolality, and total protein level.
- Determine the patient's cardiopulmonary status and vital signs before giving the drug, before each dosage or rate increase, and at 30-min intervals during the infusion and ending 30 min after the infusion is completed.
- Record the child's body weight in kilograms.
- Perform a baseline pulmonary assessment, including lung sounds, the presence of intercostal retraction, and respiratory rate.

Precautions

- Use cautiously in pts with pulmonary disease.

Administration and Handling

IV

- Refrigerate vials. Do not freeze.
- Do not shake.
- Start infusion within 6 hrs and complete within 12 hrs of vial entry.
- Use an initial infusion rate of 1.5 mL/kg/hr for the first 15 min, then increase to 3 mL/kg/hr for the next 15 min. Use an infusion rate of 6 mL/kg/hr 30 min to the end of the infusion. Maximum infusion rate is 6 mL/kg/hr.

Intervention and Evaluation

- Monitor the patient's arterial blood gas values, blood pressure, heart rate, respiratory rates, RSV antibody titers, and temperature.
- Observe the patient for rales, intercostals or supraventricular retractions, and wheezing.

Patient/Family Teaching

- Advise the patient/family to notify the physician if the patient has any heart disease or lung impairment.
- Warn the patient/family to notify the physician if the patient experiences any allergic reactions (e.g., chest tightness, facial swelling, itching, or tingling in the mouth or throat), drowsiness, fever, muscle stiffness, nausea, or vomiting.
- Teach parents how to minimize their child's exposure to infected individuals.
- Encourage the parents to have their child immunized, as recommended.
- Teach the parents to monitor the child for signs of infection, including fever.

Rh_o (D) Immune Globulin

(BayRho-D full dose, BayRho Minidose, MICRhoGAM, RhoGAM, WinRho SDF)

CATEGORY AND SCHEDULE

Pregnancy Risk Category: C

MECHANISM OF ACTION

An immune globulin that is responsible for most cases of Rh sensitization (occurs when Rh-positive fetal RBCs enter the maternal circulation of an Rh-negative woman). Injection of anti-D globulin results in opsonization of the fetal RBCs, which are then phagocytized in the spleen, preventing immunization of the mother. Injection of anti-D into an Rh-positive patient with idiopathic thrombocytopenic purpura (ITP) coats the patient's own D-positive RBCs with antibody and, as they are cleared by the spleen, they saturate the capacity of the spleen to clear antibody-coated cells, sparing antibody-coated platelets.

AVAILABILITY

Injection, Powder for Reconstitution (WinRho SDF): 120 mcg, 300 mcg, 1,000 mcg.
Injection Solution (BayRho-D): 50 mcg, 300 mcg.

INDICATIONS AND DOSAGES

▸ ITP

IV

Children. WinRho SDF: Initially, 50 mcg/kg as a single dose (reduce to 25–40 mcg/kg if Hgb level less than 10 g/dL). Maintenance: 25–60 mcg/kg based on platelet and Hgb levels.

▸ Abortion, miscarriage, termination of ectopic pregnancy

IM (BayRho-D, RhoGAM)

Adolescents. 300 mcg if older than 13 wks' gestation at time of administration, 50 mcg if younger than 13 wks' gestation at time of adminstration.

IM/IV (WinRho SDF)

Adolescents. 120 mcg after 34 wks' gestation given immediately or within 72 hrs of procedure or miscarriage.

CONTRAINDICATIONS

Hypersensitivity to any component, immunoglobulin A deficiency, Rh_o (D)-positive mother or pregnant woman, transfusion of Rh_o (D)-positive blood in previous 3 mos, prior sensitization to Rh_o (D), mothers whose Rh group or immune status is uncertain.

INTERACTIONS

Drug

Live virus vaccines: May interfere with immune response to live virus vaccines.

Herbal

None known.

Food

None known.

DIAGNOSTIC TEST EFFECTS

None known.

SIDE EFFECTS

Hypotension, pallor, vasodilation (IV formulation), fever, headache, chills, dizziness, somnolence, lethargy, rash, pruritus, abdominal pain, diarrhea, discomfort and swelling at injection site, back pain, myalgia, arthralgia, weakness

SERIOUS REACTIONS

None known.

PEDIATRIC CONSIDERATIONS

Baseline Assessment

- Assess the patient for bleeding disorders.
- Assess the patient's Hgb levels. Administer this drug cautiously in pts with an Hgb level less than 8 g/dL.

Precautions

- Use cautiously in pts with bleeding disorders, particularly thrombocytopenia, and blood Hgb level less than 8 g/dl.

Administration and Handling

◂**ALERT**▸ Must give this drug within 72 hrs after exposure to an incompatible blood transfusion or a massive fetal hemorrhage.

IV

- Refrigerate vials (do not freeze).
- Once reconstituted, solution is stable for 12 hrs at room temperature.
- Reconstitute 120 and 300 mcg with 2.5 mL 0.9% NaCl (8.5 mL for 1,000-mcg vial).
- Gently swirl; do not shake.
- Infuse over 3–5 min.

IM

- Reconstitute 120 and 300 mcg with 2.5 mL 0.9% NaCl (8.5 mL for 1,000-mcg vial).
- Administer into the deltoid muscle of the upper arm or the anterolateral aspect of the upper thigh.

Intervention and Evaluation

- Monitor the patient's complete blood count, especially blood urea nitrogen, Hgb level, platelet count, serum creatinine level, reticulocyte count, and urinalysis.
- Assess the patient for signs and symptoms of hemolysis.

Patient/Family Teaching

- Teach the patient/family that this drug is given only by injection. Advise the patient that he or she may experience pain at the injection site.
- Warn the patient/family to notify the physician if the patient experiences chills, dizziness, fever, headache, or rash.

REFERENCES

Miller, S. & Fioravanti, J. (1997). Pediatric medications: a handbook for nurses. St. Louis: Mosby.

Taketomo, C. K., Hodding, J. H. & Kraus, D. M. (2003–2004). Pediatric dosage handbook (10th ed.). Hudson, OH: Lexi-Comp.

69 Immunologic Agents

Azathioprine
Basiliximab
Cyclosporine
Daclizumab
Etanercept
Interferon γ-1b
Muromonab-CD3
Sirolimus
Tacrolimus

Uses: Immunologic agents can stimulate or suppress immune function. *Immunostimulants,* such as interferons and peginterferons, are used to treat infection, immunodeficiency disorders, and cancer. *Immunosuppressants,* such as basiliximab and tacrolimus, are used to inhibit the immune response in autoimmune diseases and to improve short-term and long-term allograft survival. For additional uses, see the specific entries in this chapter.

Action: *Immunostimulants* enhance immune activity, including increased phagocytosis by macrophages and augmentation of specific cytotoxicity by T-lymphocytes. *Immunosuppressants* dampen the immune response; most of them do this by affecting interleukin-2, others by affecting inosine monophosphate dehydrogenase. For additional actions, see the specific entries in this chapter.

Azathioprine

asia-**thigh**-oh-preen
(Alti-Azathioprine [CAN], Azasan, Imuran, Thioprine [AUS])
Do not confuse with Azulfidine, Elmiron, or Imferon.

CATEGORY AND SCHEDULE

Pregnancy Risk Category: D

MECHANISM OF ACTION

An immunologic agent that antagonizes purine metabolism and inhibits DNA, protein, and RNA synthesis. ***Therapeutic Effect:*** Suppresses cell-mediated hypersensitivities; alters antibody production and immune response in transplant recipients. Reduces arthritis severity.

AVAILABILITY

Tablets: 25 mg, 50 mg, 75 mg, 100 mg.
Injection: 100-mg vial.

INDICATIONS AND DOSAGES

▸ **Kidney transplantation**

IV/PO

Children. Initially, 2–5 mg/kg/day on the day of the transplant, then 1–3 mg/kg/day as a maintenance dose.

▸ **Dosage in renal impairment**

Creatinine Clearance	Dose
10–50 mL/min	75%
Less than 10 mL/min	50%

UNLABELED USES

Treatment of biliary cirrhosis, chronic active hepatitis, glomerulonephritis, inflammatory bowel disease, inflammatory myopathy, multiple sclerosis, myasthenia gravis, nephrotic syndrome, pemphigoid, pemphigus, polymyositis, systemic lupus erythematosus.

CONTRAINDICATIONS

Hypersensitivity to azathioprine or any related component.

Pregnant rheumatoid arthritis pts.
Lactating pts.

INTERACTIONS

Drug

Allopurinol: May increase the activity of azathioprine and the risk for azathioprine toxicity.
Bone marrow depressants: May increase the bone marrow depression of these drugs.
Live virus vaccines: May potentiate virus replication, increase the vaccine's side effects, and decrease the patient's antibody response to the vaccine.
Other immunosuppressants: May increase the risk of infection or development of neoplasms.
Captopril, enalapril: May result in severe anemia.

Herbal

None known.

Food

None known.

DIAGNOSTIC TEST EFFECTS

May decrease serum albumin, Hgb, and serum uric acid levels. May increase serum alkaline phosphatase, serum amylase, serum bilirubin, SGOT (AST), and SGPT (ALT) levels.

IV INCOMPATIBILITIES

Methyl and propyl parabens, phenol

SIDE EFFECTS

Frequent
Nausea, vomiting, anorexia, particularly during early treatment and with large doses
Occasional
Rash
Rare
Severe nausea, vomiting with diarrhea, stomach pain, hypersensitivity reaction

SERIOUS REACTIONS

! There is an increased risk of neoplasia and new, abnormal growth tumors.
! Significant leukopenia and thrombocytopenia may occur, particularly in those undergoing kidney rejection.
! Hepatotoxicity occurs rarely.

PEDIATRIC CONSIDERATIONS

Baseline Assessment

- If azathioprine is being given for arthritis, assess the duration, location, onset, and type of fever, inflammation, or pain. Inspect the appearance of affected joints for deformities, immobility, and skin condition.

Precautions

- Use cautiously in immunosuppressed pts.
- Use cautiously in pts previously treated for rheumatoid arthritis with alkylating agents such as chlorambucil, cyclophosphamide, and melphalan.
- Use cautiously in pts with chickenpox currently or who have recovered recently, and those with decreased liver or renal function, gout, herpes zoster, or infection.

Administration and Handling

PO

- Give during or after meals to reduce the potential for GI disturbances.
- Store the oral form at room temperature.

IV

- Store the parenteral form at room temperature.
- After reconstitution, the IV solution is stable for 24 hrs.
- Reconstitute 100-mg vial with 10 mL Sterile Water for Injection to provide a concentration of 10 mg/mL.

• Swirl the vial gently to dissolve the solution.
• May further dilute solution in 50 mL D_5W or 0.9% NaCl.
• Infuse the solution over 30–60 min. Range: 5 min–8 hrs.

Intervention and Evaluation

• Perform and monitor complete blood count, especially platelet count and serum hepatic enzyme levels weekly during the first month of therapy, twice monthly during the second and third months of treatment, then monthly thereafter.
• Expect to reduce or discontinue the drug dose if a rapid fall in the WBC count occurs.
• Assess the patient for delayed bone marrow suppression. Routinely watch for any change from normal.
• In pts receiving azathioprine to treat arthritis, evaluate for signs of a therapeutic response including improved grip strength, increased joint mobility, reduced joint tenderness, and relief of pain, stiffness, and swelling.

Patient/Family Teaching

• Warn the patient/family to notify the physician if abdominal pain, fever, mouth sores, sore throat, or unusual bleeding occurs.
• Explain to the rheumatoid arthritis patient/family that the drug's therapeutic response may take up to 12 wks to manifest.
• Caution women of childbearing age to avoid pregnancy.

Basiliximab

bay-zul-**ix**-ah-mab
(Simulect)

CATEGORY AND SCHEDULE

Pregnancy Risk Category: B

MECHANISM OF ACTION

This monoclonal antibody binds to interleukin–2 (IL-2) receptor complex and inhibits IL–2 binding. ***Therapeutic Effect:*** Prevents lymphocytic activity and impairs the response of the immune system to antigens.

PHARMACOKINETICS

Half-Life: Adults 4–10 days. Children 5–17 days.

AVAILABILITY

Powder for Injection: 20 mg.

INDICATIONS AND DOSAGES

▸ Prophylaxis of organ rejection

IV

Children weighing 35 kg or more. Two doses of 20 mg each in reconstituted volume of 50 mL given as an IV infusion over 20–30 min. Give the first dose of 20 mg within 2 hrs before transplant surgery and the second dose of 20 mg 4 days after transplant.

Children weighing less than 35 kg. 10 mg dose as above.

CONTRAINDICATIONS

Hypersensitivity to basiliximab or any related component.

INTERACTIONS

Drug

None known.

Herbal

None known.

Food

None known.

DIAGNOSTIC TEST EFFECTS

Alters serum calcium and potassium, blood glucose, Hgb, and Hct levels. Increases BUN, serum cholesterol, creatinine, and uric acid levels. Decreases serum magnesium and serum phosphate levels and platelet count.

IV INCOMPATIBILITIES

Specific information not available. Other medications should not be added simultaneously through same IV line.

SIDE EFFECTS

Frequent (greater than 10%)
GI disturbances, as evidenced by constipation, diarrhea, and dyspepsia, CNS effects, manifested as dizziness, headache, insomnia, and tremor, respiratory infection, dysuria, acne, leg or back pain, peripheral edema, hypertension
Occasional (10%–3%)
Angina, neuropathy, abdominal distention, tachycardia, rash, hypotension, urinary disturbances as evidenced by frequent micturition, genital edema, and hematuria, joint pain, increased hair growth, muscle pain

SERIOUS REACTIONS

None known.

PEDIATRIC CONSIDERATIONS

Baseline Assessment

- Expect to obtain the patient's baseline BUN, blood glucose, and serum calcium, creatinine, phosphatase, potassium, and uric acid levels.
- Obtain the patient's vital signs, particularly blood pressure (B/P) and pulse rate before beginning therapy.
- Breast-feeding is not recommended in female pts receiving basiliximab.
- Be aware that it is unknown whether basiliximab crosses the placenta or is distributed in breast milk.
- Be aware that there are no well-controlled studies of this medication in pediatric pts.
- There are no age-related precautions noted in children.

Precautions

- Use cautiously in pts with a history of malignancy or who have an infection.

Administration and Handling

IV

- Refrigerate the drug. After reconstitution, use within 4 hrs (24 hrs if refrigerated).
- Discard the solution if a precipitate forms.
- Reconstitute with 5 mL Sterile Water for Injection.
- Shake gently to dissolve.
- Further dilute with 50 mL 0.9% NaCl or D_5W. Gently invert to avoid foaming.
- Infuse over 20–30 min.

Intervention and Evaluation

- Diligently monitor all of the patient's laboratory test results, especially the patient's complete blood count.
- Assess the patient's B/P for signs of hypertension or hypotension.
- Assess the patient's pulse for evidence of tachycardia.
- Determine whether the patient is experiencing adverse CNS effects, GI disturbances, and urinary changes.
- Monitor the patient for signs or symptoms of a wound infection or systemic infection, including fever, sore throat, and unusual bleeding or bruising.

Patient/Family Teaching

- Warn the patient/family to report difficulty in breathing or swallowing, itching, rapid heartbeat, rash, swelling of the lower extremities, or weakness to the physician.

• Caution women of childbearing age to avoid pregnancy while taking basiliximab.

Cyclosporine

sigh-klo-**spore**-in
(Neoral, Restasis, Sandimmune Neoral [AUS], Sandimmune)
Do not confuse with cycloserine or Cyklokapron.
(See Color Plate)

CATEGORY AND SCHEDULE

Pregnancy Risk Category: C

MECHANISM OF ACTION

A cyclic polypeptide that inhibits interleukin-2, a proliferative factor needed for T-cell activity. ***Therapeutic Effect:*** Inhibits both cellular and humoral immune responses.

PHARMACOKINETICS

Variably absorbed from the GI tract. Widely distributed. Protein binding: 90%. Metabolized in liver. Eliminated primarily by biliary or fecal excretion. Not removed by hemodialysis. ***Half-Life:*** Adults 10–27 hrs. Children 7–19 hrs.

AVAILABILITY

Capsules: 25 mg, 100 mg.
Oral Solution: 100 mg/mL in a 50-mL calibrated liquid measuring device.
IV Solution: 50 mg/mL (5-mL ampules).
Ophthalmic Emulsion: 0.05%.

INDICATIONS AND DOSAGES

▸ Prevention of allograft rejection
PO
Children. Initially, 15 mg/kg as a single dose 4–12 hrs before transplantation, continue daily dose of 10–14 mg/kg/day for 1–2 wks. Taper dose by 5%/wk over 6–8 wks. Maintenance: 5–10 mg/kg/day.
IV
Children. Give one-third of oral dose (5–6 mg/kg) as single dose 4–12 hrs before transplantation, continue this daily single dose until the patient is able to take oral medication. Maintenance: 2–10 mg/kg/day in divided doses every 8–24 hrs.

UNLABELED USES

Treatment of alopecia areata, aplastic anemia, atopic dermatitis, Behçet disease, biliary cirrhosis, corneal transplantation.

CONTRAINDICATIONS

History of hypersensitivity to cyclosporine or polyoxyethylated castor oil or other related component.

INTERACTIONS

Drug

Angiotensin-converting enzyme inhibitors, potassium-sparing diuretics, potassium supplements: May cause hyperkalemia.
Cimetidine, danazol, diltiazem, erythromycin, ketoconazole: May increase blood concentration and risk of liver toxicity and nephrotoxicity.
Immunosuppressants: May increase the risk of infection and lymphoproliferative disorders.
Live virus vaccines: May decrease the patient's antibody response to the vaccine, increase vaccine side effects, and potentiate virus replication.
Lovastatin: May increase the risk of acute renal failure and rhabdomyolysis.

Herbal
St. John's wort: May alter the absorption of cyclosporine.
Food
Grapefruit and grapefruit juice: May increase the absorption and risk of toxicity of cyclosporine.

DIAGNOSTIC TEST EFFECTS

May increase blood BUN, serum alkaline phosphatase, amylase, bilirubin, creatinine, potassium, uric acid, SGOT (AST), and SGPT (ALT) levels. May decrease magnesium levels. Therapeutic blood peak serum level is 50–300 ng/mL; toxic blood serum level is greater than 400 ng/mL. Therapeutic serum concentrations may vary depending on assay used and type of transplant performed.

IV INCOMPATIBILITIES

Amphotericin B complex (AmBisome, Amphotec, Abelcet), magnesium

IV COMPATIBILITIES

Propofol (Diprivan)

SIDE EFFECTS

Frequent
Mild to moderate hypertension (26%), increased hair growth or hirsutism (21%), tremor (12%)
Occasional (4%–2%)
Acne, cramping, gingival hyperplasia, marked by red, bleeding, and tender gums, paresthesia, diarrhea, nausea, vomiting, headache
Rare (less than 1%)
Hypersensitivity reaction, abdominal discomfort, gynecomastia, sinusitis

SERIOUS REACTIONS

! Mild nephrotoxicity occurs in 25% of renal transplants after transplantation, 38% of cardiac transplants, and 37% of liver transplants.
! Liver toxicity occurs in 4% of renal, 7% of cardiac, and 4% of liver transplant pts. Both toxicities are usually responsive to dosage reduction.
! Severe hyperkalemia and hyperuricemia occur occasionally.

PEDIATRIC CONSIDERATIONS

Baseline Assessment
• Note that if nephrotoxicity occurs, mild toxicity is generally noted 2–3 mos after transplantation, and more severe toxicity is generally noted early after transplantation.
• Know that liver toxicity may be noted during first month after transplantation.
• Be aware that cyclosporine readily crosses the placenta and is distributed in breast milk. Breast-feeding should be avoided in this patient population.
• There are no age-related precautions noted in pediatric transplant pts.
• Absorption rates of cyclosporine can be erratic; therefore, it is important to monitor levels in pediatric pts regularly.
Precautions
• Use cautiously in pregnant pts and pts with cardiac impairment, chickenpox, herpes zoster infection, hypokalemia, liver impairment, malabsorption syndrome, and renal impairment.
• Use cautiously in ophthalmic pts with active eye infection.
Administration and Handling
◀ **ALERT** ▶ Remember that the oral solution is available in bottle form with a calibrated liquid measuring device. Expect to begin therapy with the oral form as soon as possible.

◀ **ALERT** ▶ Expect to give with adrenal corticosteroids. Know that administering other immunosuppressive agents with cyclosporine increases the susceptibility to infection and the development of lymphoma.

PO

• Oral solution may be mixed in glass container with chocolate milk, milk, or orange juice, preferably at room temperature. Stir well. Drink immediately. Avoid using Styrofoam containers, because the liquid form of the drug can adhere to the wall of the container.
• Add more diluent to a glass container and mix with remaining solution to ensure that the total amount is given.
• Dry the outside of the calibrated liquid measuring device before replacing the cover. Do not rinse with water.
• Avoid refrigeration of oral solution because separation of solution may occur. Discard oral solution after 2 mos once bottle is opened.

IV

• Store parenteral form at room temperature.
• Protect IV solution from light.
• After diluted, solution is stable for 24 hrs.
• Dilute each 1 mL concentrate with 20–100 mL 0.9% NaCl or D_5W.
• Infuse over 2–6 hrs.
• Monitor the patient continuously for the first 30 min after instituting the infusion and frequently thereafter for a hypersensitivity reaction, including facial flushing and dyspnea.

Intervention and Evaluation

• Diligently monitor the patient's BUN, lactate dehydrogenase, serum bilirubin, creatinine, SGOT (AST), and SGPT (ALT) levels for liver toxicity or nephrotoxicity. Mild toxicity is noted by a slow rise in serum levels; more overt toxicity noted by a rapid rise in levels. Hematuria is also noted in nephrotoxicity.
• Monitor the patient's serum potassium level for hyperkalemia.
• Encourage the patient to maintain diligent oral hygiene to prevent gum hyperplasia.
• Monitor the patient's blood pressure for hypertension.
• Know that the peak therapeutic serum level of cyclosporine is 50–300 ng/mL and that the toxic serum level of cyclosporine is greater than 400 ng/mL.

Patient/Family Teaching

• Instruct the patient/family to take the drug at the same times each day and to notify the physician for further instructions if the patient forgets to take a dose.
• Tell the patient/family to take the drug after a trough blood level has been measured.
• Stress to the patient/family that routine blood testing while receiving cyclosporine is essential to therapy.
• Tell the patient/family that the patient may experience headache and tremor as a response to the medication.
• Warn the patient/family to avoid consuming grapefruit and grapefruit juice as these foods increase the blood concentration and side effects of cyclosporine.
• Tell the patient/family to maintain good oral hygiene to prevent gingivitis caused by gingival hyperplasia.
• Tell the patient/family to keep the gel caps in a dry, cool environment, away from direct light. Keep the gel caps in their original foil

wrapping. Keep the liquid form in the amber-colored glass container.
• Instruct the patient/family to avoid prolonged exposure to the sun, and to wear sunscreen.

Daclizumab

day-**cly**-zu-mab
(Zenapax)

CATEGORY AND SCHEDULE

Pregnancy Risk Category: C

MECHANISM OF ACTION

A monoclonal antibody that binds to and inhibits interleukin-2–mediated lymphocyte activation, a critical pathway in the cellular immune response involved in allograft rejection. ***Therapeutic Effect:*** Prevents organ rejection.

PHARMACOKINETICS

Half-Life: Adults 20 days. Children 13 days.

AVAILABILITY

Injection: 5 mg/mL.

INDICATIONS AND DOSAGES

▸ Prophylaxis of acute organ rejection in pts receiving renal transplants, in combination with an immunosuppressive regimen

IV

Children. 1 mg/kg over 15 min. First dose no more than 24 hrs before transplantation, then q14days for a total of 5 doses. Maximum: 100 mg.

UNLABELED USES

Graft-vs-host disease.

CONTRAINDICATIONS

Hypersensitivity to daclizumab or any related component.

INTERACTIONS

Drug

None known.

Herbal

None known.

Food

None known.

DIAGNOSTIC TEST EFFECTS

None known.

IV INCOMPATIBILITIES

Do not mix with any other medication.

SIDE EFFECTS

Occasional (greater than 2%)

Constipation, nausea, diarrhea, vomiting, abdominal pain, edema, headache, dizziness, fever, pain, fatigue, insomnia, weakness, arthralgia, myalgia, increased sweating

SERIOUS REACTIONS

None known.

PEDIATRIC CONSIDERATIONS

Baseline Assessment

• Expect to obtain the patient's baseline laboratory values, including a complete blood count (CBC), and vital signs, particularly blood pressure (B/P) and pulse rate.
• Be aware that it is unknown whether daclizumab crosses the placenta or is distributed in breast milk.
• There are no age-related precautions noted in children.
• Adolescents of childbearing age should avoid becoming pregnant while taking daclizumab. Use an effective form of birth control before beginning therapy, during therapy, and for 4 mos after discontinuation of daclizumab.

Precautions
• Use cautiously in pts with a history of malignancy and infection.

Administration and Handling

IV
• Protect from light; refrigerate vials.
• Once reconstituted, solution is stable for 4 hrs at room temperature, 24 hrs if refrigerated.
• Dilute in 50 mL 0.9% NaCl.
• Invert gently. Avoid shaking.
• Infuse over 15 min.

Intervention and Evaluation
• Diligently monitor all blood serum levels and CBC.
• Assess the patient's B/P for hypertension and hypotension and pulse for evidence of tachycardia.
• Determine whether the patient is experiencing GI disturbances and urinary changes.
• Monitor the patient for signs and symptoms of systemic infection such as fever or sore throat, unusual bleeding or bruising, and wound infection.

Patient/Family Teaching
• Warn the patient/family to notify the physician if the patient experiences difficulty in breathing or swallowing, itching or swelling of the lower extremities, rash, tachycardia, and weakness.
• Caution the patient/family to avoid pregnancy during daclizumab therapy.
• Tell the patient/family to avoid circumstances that place the patient at risk for infection, such as crowded areas.

Etanercept

ee-**tan**-er-cept
(Enbrel)

CATEGORY AND SCHEDULE
Pregnancy Risk Category: B

MECHANISM OF ACTION
A protein that binds to tumor necrosis factor (TNF), blocking its interaction with cell surface receptors. TNF is involved in inflammatory and immune responses; elevated TNF is found in synovial fluid of rheumatoid arthritis pts. ***Therapeutic Effect:*** Reduces rheumatoid arthritis effects.

PHARMACOKINETICS
Slowly but well absorbed after subcutaneous administration. Blocks interactions with cell surface TNF receptors. ***Half-Life:*** Adults: 115 hrs.

AVAILABILITY
Powder for Injection: 25 mg.

INDICATIONS AND DOSAGES
▸ **Rheumatoid arthritis**
SC
Children 4–17 yrs. 0.4 mg/kg/dose (maximum: 25 mg dose) twice weekly given 72–96 hrs apart.

UNLABELED USES
Crohn disease.

CONTRAINDICATIONS
Hypersensitivity to etanercept or any related component (mannitol, sucrose, tromethamine, or benzyl alcohol). Serious active infection or sepsis.

INTERACTIONS
Drug
Live vaccines: Secondary transmission of the infection may occur.
Herbal
None known.
Food
None known.

DIAGNOSTIC TEST EFFECTS
None known.

SIDE EFFECTS

Frequent (37%)
Injection site reaction, including erythema, itching, pain, and swelling, incidence of abdominal pain, and vomiting (more common in children than in adults)
Occasional (16%–4%)
Headache, rhinitis, dizziness, pharyngitis, cough, asthenia, abdominal pain, dyspepsia
Rare (less than 3%)
Sinusitis, allergic reaction

SERIOUS REACTIONS

! Infection, including pyelonephritis, cellulitis, osteomyelitis, wound infection, leg ulcer, septic arthritis, and diarrhea, and upper respiratory tract infection, including bronchitis and pneumonia, occur frequently (29%–38%).
! Formation of autoimmune antibodies may occur.
! Serious adverse effects, such as heart failure, hypertension, hypotension, pancreatitis, gastrointestinal (GI) hemorrhage, and dyspnea, occur rarely.

PEDIATRIC CONSIDERATIONS

Baseline Assessment
- Assess the duration, location, onset, and type of inflammation or pain the patient is experiencing.
- Temporarily discontinue therapy and expect to treat the patient with varicella-zoster immune globulin, as prescribed, if the patient experiences significant exposure to varicella virus during treatment.
- Be aware that it is unknown whether etanercept is excreted in breast milk.
- There are no age-related precautions noted in children older than 4 yrs of age.
- Be aware that etanercept contains benzyl alcohol, which may cause allergic reactions in certain pts. Large amounts of benzyl alcohol have been associated with a fatal toxicity in neonates.

Precautions
- Use cautiously in pts with a history of recurrent infections or illnesses that predispose to infection, such as diabetes mellitus.

Administration and Handling
◀ALERT▶ Do not add other medications to solution. Do not use a filter during reconstitution or administration.
SC
- Refrigerate.
- Once reconstituted, may be stored under refrigeration for up to 6 hrs.
- Reconstitute with 1 mL of Sterile Bacteriostatic Water for Injection (0.9% benzyl alcohol). Do not reconstitute with other diluents.
- Slowly inject the diluent into the vial. Some foaming will occur. To avoid excessive foaming, slowly swirl the contents until the powder is dissolved over less than 5 min.
- Inspect the solution for particles or discoloration. Reconstituted solution normally appears clear and colorless. If solution is discolored or cloudy or if particles remain, discard the solution; do not use.
- Withdraw all the solution into syringe. The final volume should be approximately 1 mL.
- Inject into the patient's abdomen, thigh, or upper arm. Rotate injection sites.
- Give a new injection at least 1 inch from an old site and never into area when the skin is tender, bruised, hard, or red.

Intervention and Evaluation

• Assess the patient for joint swelling, pain, and tenderness.
• Obtain the patient's complete blood count and erythrocyte sedimentation rate or C-reactive protein level.

Patient/Family Teaching

• Instruct the patient/family in SC injection technique, including areas of the body acceptable as injection sites.
• Explain to the patient/family that an injection site reaction generally occurs in the first month of treatment and decreases in frequency during continued etanercept therapy.
• Caution the patient/family against receiving live vaccines during treatment.
• Warn the patient/family to notify the physician if the patient experiences bleeding, bruising, pallor, or persistent fever.

Interferon γ-1b

inn-ter-**fear**-on
(Actimmune, Imukin [AUS])

CATEGORY AND SCHEDULE

Pregnancy Risk Category: C

MECHANISM OF ACTION

A biologic response modifier that induces activation of macrophages in blood monocytes to phagocytes, which is necessary in cellular immune response to intracellular and extracellular pathogens. ***Therapeutic Effect:*** Enhances phagocytic function and antimicrobial activity of monocytes.

PHARMACOKINETICS

Slowly absorbed after SC administration.

AVAILABILITY

Injection: 100 mcg (3 million units).

INDICATIONS AND DOSAGES

▸ **Chronic granulomatous disease, severe, malignant osteopetrosis**

SC

Children older than 1 yr. 50 mcg/m^2 (1 million units/m^2) in pts with body surface area (BSA) greater than 0.5 m^2; 1.5 mcg/kg/dose in pts with BSA 0.5 m^2 or less. Give 3 times/wk.

CONTRAINDICATIONS

Hypersensitivity to *Escherichia coli* products.

INTERACTIONS

Drug

Bone marrow depressants: May increase bone marrow depression.

Herbal

None known.

Food

None known.

DIAGNOSTIC TEST EFFECTS

None known.

SIDE EFFECTS

Frequent

Fever (52%); headache (33%); rash (17%); chills, fatigue, diarrhea (14%)

Occasional (13%–10%)

Vomiting, nausea

Rare (6%–3%)

Weight loss, myalgia, anorexia

SERIOUS REACTIONS

! May exacerbate preexisting CNS disturbances, including decreased mental status, gait disturbance, and dizziness, as well as cardiac disorders.

PEDIATRIC CONSIDERATIONS

Baseline Assessment

• Plan to perform blood chemistry analysis, including BUN, serum alkaline phosphatase, creatinine, SGOT (AST), and SGPT (ALT) levels, to assess hepatic and renal function, complete blood count, and urinalysis before beginning drug therapy and at 3-mo intervals during the course of treatment.
• Be aware that it is unknown whether interferon γ-1b crosses the placenta or is distributed in breast milk.
• Be aware that the safety and efficacy of interferon γ-1b have not been established in children younger than 1 year of age.
• Be aware that children experience flu-like symptoms more frequently.

Precautions

• Use cautiously in pts with compromised CNS function, myelosuppression, preexisting cardiac diseases, including arrhythmias, congestive heart failure, and myocardial ischemia, and seizure disorders.

Administration and Handling

◂ALERT▸ Avoid excessive agitation of vial; do not shake.

SC

• Refrigerate vials. Do not freeze.
• Do not keep at room temperature for longer than 12 hrs; discard after 12 hrs.
• Vials are single dose; discard the unused portion.
• Do not use if discolored or precipitate forms; solution normally appears clear, colorless.
• When given 3 times/wk, administer in left deltoid, right deltoid, or anterior thigh muscle.

Intervention and Evaluation

• Monitor the patient for flu-like symptoms, including chills, fatigue, fever, and muscle aches.
• Assess the patient's skin for rash.
• Acetaminophen may be administered to the patient to prevent or partially alleviate fever and headache after injection.

Patient/Family Teaching

• Tell the patient/family that flu-like symptoms, such as chills, fatigue, fever, and muscle aches, are generally mild and tend to disappear as treatment continues. Explain to the patient that symptoms may be minimized with bedtime administration.
• Warn the patient/family to avoid performing tasks that require mental alertness or motor skills until the patient's response to the drug is established.
• Instruct the patient/family the proper technique of administration and disposal of needles and syringes.
• Teach the patient/family that vials should remain refrigerated.

Muromonab-CD3 

meur-oh-mon-ab
(Orthoclone, OKT3)

CATEGORY AND SCHEDULE

Pregnancy Risk Category: C

MECHANISM OF ACTION

An antibody derived from purified immunoglobulin G_2 immune globulin that reacts with T3 (CD3) antigen of human T-cell membranes. Blocks function of T cells, which has a major role in acute renal rejection. ***Therapeutic Effect:*** Reverses graft rejection.

AVAILABILITY

Injection: 1 mg/mL.

INDICATIONS AND DOSAGES

▸ Treat acute allograft rejection

IV

Children older than 12 yrs. 5 mg/day for 10–14 days. Begin when acute renal rejection is diagnosed.
Children younger than 12 yrs. 0.1 mg/kg/day for 10–14 days.

CONTRAINDICATIONS

History of hypersensitivity to muromonab-CD3 or any product of murine origin, pts with fluid overload evidenced by chest radiograph or a greater than 3% weight gain within the week before initial treatment.

INTERACTIONS

Drug

Live virus vaccines: May decrease the patient's response to the vaccine, increase the vaccine's side effects, and potentiate virus replication.
Other immunosuppressants: May increase the risk of infection or development of lymphoproliferative disorders.

Herbal

Echinacea: May decrease the effects of muromonab.

Food

None known.

DIAGNOSTIC TEST EFFECTS

None known.

IV INCOMPATIBILITIES

Do not mix with any other medications.

SIDE EFFECTS

Frequent

First-dose reaction: Fever, chills, dyspnea, or malaise occurs 30 min–6 hrs after the first dose and will markedly diminish with subsequent dosing after the first 2 days of treatment.

Occasional

Chest pain, nausea, vomiting, diarrhea, tremor

SERIOUS REACTIONS

! Cytokine release syndrome may range from flu-like illness to a life-threatening shock-like reaction.
! Occasionally fatal hypersensitivity reactions occur.
! Severe pulmonary edema occurs in less than 2% of those treated with muromonab-CD3.
! Infection, caused by immunosuppression, generally occurs within 45 days after initial treatment, cytomegalovirus infection occurs in 19% of pts, and herpes simplex occurs in 27% of pts.
! Severe and life-threatening infection occurs in less than 4.8% of pts.

PEDIATRIC CONSIDERATIONS

Baseline Assessment

- Plan to obtain a chest radiograph within 24 hrs of beginning muromonab therapy to ensure that the patient's lungs are clear of fluid.
- Know that the patient's weight should be 3% or less above minimum weight the week before beginning treatment; pulmonary edema occurs when fluid overload is present before muromonab treatment.
- Have resuscitative drugs and equipment immediately available.
- It is strongly recommended that methylprednisolone sodium succinate 1 mg/kg IV be administered 2–6 hrs before the first dose of muromonab-CD3 and that hydro-

cortisone sodium succinate 50–100 mg IV be given 30 min after administration to prevent serious reactions with the first dose. Patient temperature should not exceed 100°F at the time of administration.

Precautions

• Use cautiously in pts with impaired cardiac, liver, or renal function.

Administration and Handling

IV

• Refrigerate ampoule. If left out of refrigerator for longer than 4 hrs, do not use.
• Do not shake ampoule before using.
• Fine translucent particles may develop but does not affect potency.
• Draw solution into syringe through 0.22-micron filter. Discard filter; use needle for IV administration.
• Administer IV push over less than 1 min.
• Give methylprednisolone 1 mg/kg before and 100 mg hydrocortisone 30 min after the drug dose, as prescribed, to decrease adverse reactions to the first dose.

Intervention and Evaluation

• Monitor the patient's immunologic tests, including plasma levels and quantitative T-lymphocyte surface phenotyping, liver and renal function tests, and WBC count, before beginning and during therapy.
• Give antipyretics to pts experiencing fevers exceeding 100°F.
• Expect to monitor the patient for fluid overload by chest radiograph, and monitor the patient's weight. Observe the patient for any weight gain of more than 3% over his or her pretherapy weight.
• Assess the patient's lung sounds for fluid overload.
• Monitor the patient's intake and output.
• Assess the patient's daily pattern of bowel activity and stool consistency.

Patient/Family Teaching

• Tell the patient/family that the patient may experience a first-dose reaction, including chest tightness, chills, diarrhea, fever, nausea, vomiting, and wheezing.
• Warn the patient/family to avoid receiving immunizations during therapy.
• Caution the patient/family to avoid crowds and those with known infections during muromonab therapy.

Sirolimus

sigh-row-**lie**-mus
(Rapamune)

CATEGORY AND SCHEDULE

Pregnancy Risk Category: C

MECHANISM OF ACTION

An immunosuppressant that inhibits T-lymphocyte proliferation induced by stimulation of cell surface receptors, mitogens, alloantigens, and lymphokines. Prevents activation of an enzyme called target of rapamycin, a key regulatory kinase in cell cycle progression. ***Therapeutic Effect:*** Inhibits T- and B-cell proliferation, essential components of the immune response.

AVAILABILITY

Oral Solution: 1 mg/mL.
Tablets: 1 mg, 2 mg.

INDICATIONS AND DOSAGES

▸ Prophylaxis of organ rejection
PO
Children 13 yrs and older weighing less than 40 kg. 3 mg/m^2 loading dose; then, 1 mg/m^2/day.

CONTRAINDICATIONS

Current malignancy, hypersensitivity to sirolimus, current malignancy.

INTERACTIONS

Drug

Cyclosporine, diltiazem, ketoconazole: May increase blood concentration and risk of toxicity of sirolimus.
Rifampin: May decrease the blood concentration and effects of sirolimus.

Herbal

None known.

Food

Grapefruit juice: May decrease the metabolism of sirolimus.

DIAGNOSTIC TEST EFFECTS

May decrease blood Hgb and Hct levels and platelet count. May increase serum cholesterol, creatinine, and triglyceride levels.

SIDE EFFECTS

Occasional
Hypercholesterolemia, hyperlipidemia, hypertension, rash
High dose (5 mg/day): Anemia, arthralgia, diarrhea, hypokalemia, thrombocytopenia

SERIOUS REACTIONS

! None known.

PEDIATRIC CONSIDERATIONS

Baseline Assessment

- Determine whether the female patient is pregnant or breast-feeding.
- Determine whether the patient is taking other medications, especially cyclosporine, diltiazem, ketoconazole, and rifampin.
- Determine whether the patient has chickenpox, herpes zoster, infection, or a malignancy.
- Expect to perform baseline laboratory tests, including a complete blood count and lipid profile.

Precautions

- Use cautiously in pts with chickenpox, herpes zoster, impaired liver function, and infection.

Intervention and Evaluation

- Monitor the patient's serum hepatic enzyme levels function periodically.

Patient/Family Teaching

- Tell the patient/family to avoid consuming grapefruit or grapefruit juice.
- Caution the patient/family against contact with those with colds or other infections.
- Stress to the patient/family that close monitoring by the physician is an important part of sirolimus therapy.
- Tell the patient/family to take the drug at the same time each day and to notify the physician if the patient misses a dose.

Tacrolimus

tack-row-**lee**-mus
(Prograf, Protopic)

CATEGORY AND SCHEDULE

Pregnancy Risk Category: C

MECHANISM OF ACTION

An immunologic agent that binds to intracellular protein, forming a complex, inhibiting phosphatase activity. Inhibits T-lymphocyte activation. ***Therapeutic Effect:***

Suppresses the immunologically mediated inflammatory response. Assists in preventing organ transplant rejection.

PHARMACOKINETICS

Variably absorbed after PO administration (food reduces absorption). Protein binding: 75%–97%. Extensively metabolized in the liver. Excreted in urine. Not removed by hemodialysis. ***Half-Life:*** 11.7 hrs.

AVAILABILITY

Capsules: 0.5 mg, 1 mg, 5 mg.
Injection: 5 mg/mL.
Ointment: 0.03%, 0.1%.

INDICATIONS AND DOSAGES

▸ Prophylaxis of transplant rejection

IV INFUSION

Children. 0.03–0.15 mg/kg/day.

PO

Children. 0.15–0.4 mg/kg/day in 2 divided doses 12 hrs apart.

IV INFUSION

Children (without preexisting liver or renal dysfunction). 0.03–0.15 mg/kg/day.

PO

Children (without preexisting liver or renal dysfunction). 0.3 mg/kg/day.

▸ Atopic dermatitis

TOPICAL

Children 2 yrs and older. 0.03% ointment to affected area 2 times/day. Continue for 1 wk after symptoms have cleared.

UNLABELED USES

Prophylaxis of organ rejection in pts receiving allogeneic bone marrow, cardiac, pancreas, pancreatic island cell, and small bowel transplantation, treatment of autoimmune disease, severe recalcitrant psoriasis.

CONTRAINDICATIONS

Concurrent use with cyclosporine increases the risk of ototoxicity, hypersensitivity to HCO-60 (polyoxyl 60 hydrogenated castor oil) used in solution for injection, hypersensitivity to tacrolimus.

INTERACTIONS

Drug

Aminoglycosides, amphotericin B, cisplatin: Increases the risk of renal dysfunction.
Antacids: Decrease the absorption of the drug.
Antifungals, bromocriptine, calcium channel blockers, cimetidine, clarithromycin, cyclosporine, danazol, diltiazem, erythromycin, methylprednisolone, metoclopramide: Increase tacrolimus blood concentration.
Carbamazepine, phenobarbital, phenytoin, rifamycin: Decrease tacrolimus blood concentrations.
Cyclosporine: Increases the risk of nephrotoxicity.
Live virus vaccines: May decrease the patient's antibody response to the vaccine, increase the patient's antibody response to the vaccine, and potentiate virus replication.
Other immunosuppressants: May increase the risk of infection or development of lymphomas.

Herbal

Echinacea: May decrease the effects of tacrolimus.

Food

Grapefruit, grapefruit juice: May alter the effects of the drug.

DIAGNOSTIC TEST EFFECTS

May increase blood glucose, BUN, and serum creatinine levels and WBC count. May decrease serum magnesium and RBC and thrombocyte counts. Alters serum potassium level.

IV INCOMPATIBILITIES

No known specific drug incompatibilities. Do not mix with other medications if possible.

IV COMPATIBILITIES

Calcium gluconate, dexamethasone (Decadron), diphenhydramine (Benadryl), dobutamine (Dobutrex), dopamine (Intropin), furosemide (Lasix), heparin, hydromorphone (Dilaudid), insulin, leucovorin, lorazepam (Ativan), morphine, nitroglycerin, potassium chloride

SIDE EFFECTS

Frequent (greater than 30%)
Headache, tremor, insomnia, paresthesia, diarrhea, nausea, constipation, vomiting, abdominal pain, hypertension

Occasional (29%–10%)
Rash, pruritus, anorexia, asthenia, peripheral edema, photosensitivity

SERIOUS REACTIONS

! Nephrotoxicity and pleural effusion occur frequently.
! Overt nephrotoxicity is characterized by increasing serum creatinine levels and a decrease in urine output.
! Thrombocytopenia, leukocytosis, anemia, and atelectasis occur occasionally.
! Neurotoxicity, including tremor, headache, and mental status changes, occurs commonly.
! Sepsis and infection occur occasionally.
! Significant anemia, thrombocytopenia, and leukocytosis may occur.

PEDIATRIC CONSIDERATIONS

Baseline Assessment

- Assess the patient's drug history, especially for other immunosuppressants, and medical history, especially renal function.
- Prepare an aqueous solution of epinephrine 1:1,000 to have available at the bedside as well as O_2 before beginning IV infusion.
- Assess the patient continuously for the first 30 min after the start of infusion and at frequent intervals thereafter.
- Plan to obtain baseline laboratory tests, including a complete blood count and BUN, hepatic enzyme, serum creatinine, and serum electrolyte levels.
- Be aware that tacrolimus crosses the placenta and is distributed in breast milk. Breast-feeding should be avoided in this patient population.
- Be aware that hyperkalemia and renal dysfunction are noted in neonates.
- Be aware that children may require higher drug dosages due to decreased bioavailability and increased clearance.
- Be aware that post-transplant lymphoproliferative disorder is more common in children, especially children younger than 3 yrs of age.

Precautions

- Use cautiously in pts with immunosuppression and liver and renal function impairment.

Administration and Handling

◂ **ALERT** ▸ In pts unable to take capsules, initiate therapy with an IV infusion. Give an oral dose 8–12 hrs after discontinuing the IV infusion. Titrate dosing based on clinical assessments of rejection and patient tolerance. In pts with liver or renal function impairment, give the lowest IV and oral dosing range, as prescribed. Plan to delay dosing up to 48 hrs or longer in pts with postoperative oliguria.

PO
• Administer tacrolimus on an empty stomach.
• Use a polyethylene oral syringe or glass container when giving the oral solution; avoid plastic or Styrofoam.
• Do not give with grapefruit or grapefruit juice or within 2 hrs of antacids.
TOPICAL
• For external use only.
• Do not cover with an occlusive dressing.
• Rub in gently and completely onto clean, dry skin.
IV
• Store diluted infusion solution in glass or polyethylene containers and discard after 24 hrs.
• Do not store in a container made from PVC because the drug is less stable, and there is a risk of drug absorption into the container.
• Dilute with an appropriate amount, 250 to 1,000 mL 0.9% NaCl or D_5W, to provide a concentration between 0.004 and 0.02 mg/mL, depending on desired dose.
• Give tacrolimus as continuous IV infusion.
• Continuously monitor the patient for anaphylaxis for at least 30 min after starting the infusion.
• Stop the infusion immediately at the first sign of a hypersensitivity reaction.

Intervention and Evaluation
• Closely monitor pts with impaired renal function.
• Monitor the patient's laboratory values, especially complete blood count (CBC) and hepatic enzyme and serum creatinine and potassium levels.
• Monitor the patient's intake and output closely.
• Perform a CBC weekly during the first month of therapy, twice monthly during second and third months of treatment, and then monthly throughout the first year.
• Report any major change in the assessment of the patient.

PATIENT/FAMILY TEACHING
• Instruct the patient/family to take the drug dose at the same time each day. Tell the patient/family to notify the physician if the patient misses a dose.
• Caution the patient/family to avoid crowds and those with an infection.
• Warn the patient/family to notify the physician if the patient experiences chest pain, dizziness, headache, decreased urination, rash, respiratory infection, or unusual bleeding or bruising.
• Urge the patient/family to avoid exposure to sunlight and artificial light as this may cause a photosensitivity reaction.
• Instruct the patient/family on the proper administration of the drug. Instruct the patient to avoid grapefruit and to take the oral solution in the oral syringe or glass container on an empty stomach.

REFERENCES
Taketomo, C. K., Hodding, J. H. & Kraus, D. M. (2003–2004). Pediatric dosage handbook (10th ed.). Hudson, OH: Lexi-Comp.

70 Minerals and Electrolytes

Aluminum Hydroxide
Calcium Acetate, Calcium Carbonate, Calcium Chloride, Calcium Citrate, Calcium Glubionate, Calcium Gluconate
Citrates: Potassium Citrate, Potassium Citrate and Citric Acid, Sodium Citrate and Citric Acid, Tricitrates
Fluoride
Magnesium, Magnesium Chloride, Magnesium Citrate, Magnesium Hydroxide, Magnesium Oxide, Magnesium Protein Complex, Magnesium Sulfate
Phosphates
Potassium Acetate, Potassium Bicarbonate/Citrate, Potassium Chloride, Potassium Gluconate

Uses: Minerals and electrolytes are used as replacements to correct specific electrolyte imbalances, such as hypokalemia, hyponatremia, and hypermagnesemia. Additional uses vary greatly. *Aluminum* is used to treat hyperacidity and gastroesophageal reflux disease (GERD) and to prevent GI bleeding and phosphate calculi formation. *Calcium* is also prescribed to treat hyperacidity. *Citrates* treat metabolic acidosis. *Fluoride* prevents dental caries in children. *Magnesium* is also used to treat hypertension, torsades de pointes, encephalopathy, constipation, hyperacidity, and seizures from acute nephritis. *Phosphates* are used to prevent and treat hypophosphatemia, to treat constipation, to evacuate the colon for examination, and to acidify the urine and reduce calcium calculi formation. *Sodium bicarbonate* is used to manage metabolic acidosis and hyperacidity, alkalinize urine, stabilize acid-base balance, and treat cardiac arrest. *Sodium chloride* is also used to promote hydration, assess renal function, and manage hyperosmolar diabetes; in addition, it has nasal and ophthalmic uses. *Zinc oxide* is used to protect the skin from mild irritation and abrasions and to promote the healing of chapped skin and diaper rash. *Zinc sulfate* helps prevent zinc deficiency and is used to promote wound healing.

Action: Minerals are needed for normal body function. Electrolytes are substances that carry a positive or negative charge. Their functions include transmission of nerve impulses to contract skeletal and smooth muscles. Additional specific actions vary with the agent. *Aluminum* reduces gastric acid, binds with phosphate, and may increase calcium absorption. (See illustration, *Sites of Action: Drugs Used to Treat GERD,* page 601.) *Calcium* neutralizes or reduces gastric acid. *Citrates* increase urinary pH and citrate, decrease calcium activity, increase plasma bicarbonate, and buffer excess hydrogen ions. *Fluoride* increases tooth resistance to acid dissolution. *Magnesium* neutralizes gastric acid, produces osmotic effects on the small

Sodium Bicarbonate
Sodium Chloride
Zinc Oxide, Zinc Sulfate

intestine, and blocks neuromuscular transmission. *Phosphates* participate in bone deposition, calcium metabolism, B-complex vitamin use, and acid-base buffering. *Sodium bicarbonate* dissociates to provide bicarbonate ions, which raise blood and urine pH. *Sodium chloride* controls water distribution and fluid and electrolyte balance; it also helps maintain acid-base balance. As an astringent, *zinc oxide* forms a protective coating for the skin. As a cofactor for enzymes important to protein and carbohydrate metabolism, *zinc sulfate* maintains normal growth and tissue repair as well as skin hydration.

COMBINATION PRODUCTS

GAVISCON: (oral suspension) aluminum hydroxide/magnesium carbonate (an antacid) 31.7 mg/119.3 mg.
GAVISCON: (tablets) aluminum hydroxide/magnesium trisilicate (an antacid) 80 mg/20 mg.
GELUSIL: aluminum hydroxide/magnesium hydroxide (an antacid)/simethicone (an antiflatulent) 200 mg/200 mg/25 mg.
HALEY'S M-O: magnesium/mineral oil (a laxative) 300 mg/1.25 mL.
MAALOX: aluminum hydroxide/magnesium hydroxide (an antacid) 200 mg/200 mg (oral suspension); 225 mg/200 mg (tablets).
MAALOX PLUS: aluminum hydroxide/magnesium hydroxide (an antacid)/simethicone (an antiflatulent) 200 mg/200 mg/25 mg.
MYLANTA: aluminum hydroxide/magnesium hydroxide (an antacid)/simethicone (an antiflatulent) 200 mg/200 mg/20 mg; 400 mg/400 mg/40 mg.
PEPCID COMPLETE: calcium chloride/magnesium hydroxide (an antacid)/famotidine (a histamine [H_2] antagonist) 800 mg/165 mg/10 mg.
SILAIN-GEL: aluminum hydroxide/magnesium hydroxide (an antacid)/simethicone (an antiflatulent).

Aluminum Hydroxide

(ALternaGEL, Alu-Cap, Alu-Tab, Amphojel, Basaljel [CAN])

CATEGORY AND SCHEDULE

Pregnancy Risk Category: C
(Considered safe unless chronic, high-dose usage)
OTC

MECHANISM OF ACTION

An antacid that reduces gastric acid by binding with phosphate in the intestine and then is excreted as aluminum carbonate in feces. Aluminum carbonate may increase the absorption of calcium due to decreased serum phosphate levels. The drug also has astringent and adsorbent properties. ***Therapeutic Effect:*** Neutralizes or increases gastric pH; reduces phosphates in urine, preventing formation of phosphate urinary stones; reduces serum phosphate levels; decreases fluidity of stools.

AVAILABILITY

Capsules: 400 mg, 500 mg.
Tablets: 500 mg, 600 mg.
Suspension: 320 mg/5 mL, 600 mg/5 mL.
Suspension (concentrate): 450 mg/5 mL, 675 mg/5 mL.

INDICATIONS AND DOSAGES

▸ **Peptic ulcer disease**
PO
Children. 5–15 mL every 3–6 hrs or 1–3 hrs after meals and at bedtime.

▸ **GI bleeding prevention**
PO
Children. 5–15 mL q1–2h.

▸ **Hyperphosphatemia**
PO
Children. 50–150 mg/kg in divided doses q4–6h.

CONTRAINDICATIONS

Children 6 yrs or younger: intestinal obstruction

INTERACTIONS

Drug

Anticholinergics, quinidine: May decrease excretion of aluminum hydroxide.
Iron preparations, digoxin, isoniazid, ketoconazole, quinolones, tetracyclines: May decrease absorption of aluminum hydroxide.
Methenamine: May decrease effects of methenamine.
Salicylate: May increase salicylate excretion.

Herbal

None known.

Food

None known.

DIAGNOSTIC TEST EFFECTS

May increase serum gastrin levels and systemic and urinary pH. May decrease serum phosphate levels.

SIDE EFFECTS

Frequent

Chalky taste, mild constipation, stomach cramps

Occasional

Nausea, vomiting, speckling or whitish discoloration of stools

SERIOUS REACTIONS

! Prolonged constipation may result in intestinal obstruction.
! Excessive or chronic use may produce hypophosphatemia manifested as anorexia, malaise, muscle weakness or bone pain and resulting in osteomalacia and osteoporosis.
! Prolonged use may produce urinary calculi.

PEDIATRIC CONSIDERATIONS

Baseline Assessment

- Do not give other oral medications within 1–2 hrs of antacid administration.

Precautions

- Use cautiously in pts with Alzheimer's disease, chronic diarrhea, constipation, dehydration, fecal impaction, fluid restrictions, gastric outlet obstruction, GI or rectal bleeding, impaired renal function, or symptoms of appendicitis and in elderly pts.

Administration and Handling

PO

◂ **ALERT** ▸ Administer 1–3 hrs after meals.

- Expect the dosage to be individualized based on the neutralizing capacity of the antacid.
- For chewable tablets, instruct the patient to thoroughly chew tablets

before swallowing and then to drink a glass of water or milk.
• If administering a suspension, shake well before use.

Intervention and Evaluation
• Assess the patient's pattern of daily bowel activity and stool consistency.
• Expect to monitor the patient's serum aluminum, serum calcium, serum phosphate, and uric acid levels.
• Evaluate and document the patient's relief from gastric distress.

Patient/Family Teaching
• Instruct the patient/family to chew tablets thoroughly before swallowing and to then drink a glass of water or milk.
• Explain to the patient/family that the tablets may discolor the patient's stool and provide reassurance that this is expected and will resolve when the medication is discontinued.
• Stress to the patient/family that the patient should maintain adequate fluid intake.

Calcium Acetate
(PhosLo)

Calcium Carbonate
(Apo-Cal [CAN], Calsan [CAN], Caltrate [CAN], Dicarbosil, Os-Cal, Titralac, Tums)

Calcium Chloride
(Calcijex [CAN])

Calcium Citrate
(Citracal, Calcitrate)

Calcium Glubionate
(Calcione, Calciquid)

Calcium Gluconate
Do not confuse with Asacol, Citrucel, or PhosChol.

CATEGORY AND SCHEDULE
Pregnancy Risk Category: C
OTC (acetate, carbonate, citrate, glubionate, gluconate [tablets only])

MECHANISM OF ACTION
An electrolyte replenisher that is essential for the function and integrity of nervous, muscular, and skeletal systems. These agents play an important role in normal cardiac and renal function, respiration, blood coagulation, and cell membrane and capillary permeability. Assists in regulating release and storage of neurotransmitters and hormones. Neutralizes or reduces gastric acid (increases pH). Calcium acetate: Combines with dietary phosphate, forming insoluble calcium phosphate. ***Therapeutic Effect:*** Replaces calcium in deficiency states; controls hyperphosphatemia in end-stage renal disease.

PHARMACOKINETICS
Moderately absorbed from small intestine (dependent on presence of vitamin D metabolites and pH). Primarily eliminated in feces.

AVAILABILITY
Calcium Acetate
Tablets: 667 mg (equivalent to 169 mg elemental calcium).

Capsules: 667 mg (equivalent to 169 mg elemental calcium).

Calcium Carbonate

Tablets: 500 mg (equivalent to 200 mg elemental calcium), 650 mg (equivalent to 260 mg elemental calcium), 1,250 mg (equivalent to 500 mg elemental calcium), 1,500 mg (equivalent to 600 mg elemental calcium).

Tablets (chewable): 350 mg (equivalent to 140 mg elemental calcium), 500 mg (equivalent to 200 mg elemental calcium), 750 mg (equivalent to 300 mg elemental calcium), 1,000 mg (equivalent to 400 mg elemental calcium).

Capsules: 1,250 mg (equivalent to 500 mg elemental calcium).

Calcium Chloride

Injection: 10%.

Calcium Citrate

Tablets: 250 mg (equivalent to 53 mg elemental calcium), 950 mg (equivalent to 200 mg elemental calcium).

Calcium Glubionate

Syrup: 1.8 g/5 mL (equivalent to 115 mg elemental calcium/5 mL).

Calcium Gluconate

Tablets: 500 mg (equivalent to 45 mg elemental calcium), 650 mg (equivalent to 58.5 mg elemental calcium), 975 mg (equivalent to 87.75 mg elemental calcium).

Injection: 10%.

INDICATIONS AND DOSAGES

▸ **Hypocalcemia (dose expressed in mg of elemental calcium)**

PO

Children. 45–65 mg/kg/day in 3–4 divided doses.

▸ **Antihypocalcemic (calcium glubionate)**

PO

Children 1–4 yrs. 10 mL calcium glubionate 3 times/day.

Children younger than 1 yr. 5 mL calcium glubionate 5 times/day.

▸ **Cardiac arrest (calcium chloride)**

IV

Children. 20 mg/kg calcium chloride. May repeat in 10 min.

▸ **Hypocalcemia (calcium chloride)**

IV

Children. 2.5–5 mg/kg/dose of calcium chloride q4–6h.

▸ **Hypocalcemia tetany (calcium chloride)**

IV

Children. 10 mg/kg of calcium chloride over 5–10 min. May repeat in 6–8 hrs.

▸ **Hypocalcemia (calcium gluconate)**

IV

Children. 200–500 mg/kg/day of calcium gluconate as continuous infusion or in 4 divided doses.

▸ **Hypocalcemia tetany (calcium gluconate)**

IV

Children. 100–200 mg/kg/dose of calcium gluconate q6–8h.

UNLABELED USES

Calcium carbonate: Treatment of hyperphosphatemia.

CONTRAINDICATIONS

Hypersensitivity to calcium dose formulation. Calcium renal calculi, hypercalcemia, hypercalciuria, sarcoidosis, digoxin toxicity, sarcoidosis, ventricular fibrillation.

Calcium acetate: Hypoparathyroidism, decreased renal function.

INTERACTIONS

Drug

Digoxin: May increase the risk of arrhythmias.

Etidronate, gallium: May antagonize the effects of these drugs.

Ketoconazole, fluoroquinolones, phenytoin, tetracyclines: May decrease the absorption of these drugs.
Methenamine, parenteral magnesium: May decrease the effects of these drugs.

Herbal

None known.

Food

None known.

DIAGNOSTIC TEST EFFECTS

May increase blood gastrin, blood pH, and serum calcium. May decrease serum phosphate and potassium.

IV INCOMPATIBILITIES

Calcium chloride: amphotericin B complex (AmBisome, Abelcet), propofol (Diprivan), sodium bicarbonate
Calcium gluconate: amphotericin c complex (AmBisome, Abelcet), fluconazole (Diflucan)

IV COMPATIBILITIES

Calcium chloride: Amikacin (Amikin), dobutamine (Dobutrex), lidocaine, milrinone (Primacor), morphine, norepinephrine (Levophed)
Calcium gluconate: Ampicillin, aztreonam (Azactam), cefazolin (Ancef), cefepime (Maxipime), ciprofloxacin (Cipro), dobutamine (Dobutrex), enalapril (Vasotec), famotidine (Pepcid), furosemide (Lasix), heparin, lidocaine, magnesium sulfate, meropenem (Merrem IV), midazolam (Versed), milrinone (Primacor), norepinephrine (Levophed), piperacillin tazobactam (Zosyn), potassium chloride, propofol (Diprivan)

SIDE EFFECTS

Frequent

Parenteral: Hypotension, flushing, feeling of warmth, nausea, vomiting; pain, rash, redness, burning at injection site; sweating, decreased blood pressure (B/P)
PO: Chalky taste

Occasional

PO: Mild constipation, fecal impaction, swelling of hands and feet, metabolic alkalosis (muscle pain, restlessness, slow breathing, poor taste)
Calcium carbonate: Milk-alkali syndrome (headache, decreased appetite, nausea, vomiting, unusual tiredness)

Rare

Difficult or painful urination

SERIOUS REACTIONS

! Hypercalcemia is a serious reaction from calcium acetate use. The early signs of hypercalcemia are constipation, headache, dry mouth, increased thirst, irritability, decreased appetite, metallic taste, fatigue, weakness, and depression. Later signs of hypercalcemia are confusion, drowsiness, increased B/P, increased light sensitivity, irregular heartbeat, nausea, vomiting, and increased urination.

PEDIATRIC CONSIDERATIONS

Baseline Assessment

- Assess the patient's B/P, EKG, serum magnesium, potassium, and phosphate levels, as well as BUN and serum creatinine levels to assess renal function tests.
- Be aware that calcium acetate is distributed in breast milk and that it is unknown whether calcium chloride or gluconate is distributed in breast milk.

• Be aware that children experience extreme irritation and possible tissue necrosis or sloughing with the IV form. Restrict IV use in children because of their small vasculature.

Precautions

• Use cautiously in pts with chronic renal impairment, decreased cardiac function, dehydration, a history of renal calculi, and ventricular fibrillation during cardiac resuscitation.

Administration and Handling

PO

• Give tablets with a full glass of water 0.5–1 hr after meals.
• Give syrup, diluted in juice or water, before meals to increase absorption.
• Chewable tablets must be well chewed before swallowing.

IV

• Store at room temperature.
• May give calcium chloride undiluted or may dilute with equal amount of 0.9% NaCl or Sterile Water for Injection.
• May give calcium gluconate undiluted or may dilute in up to 1,000 mL NaCl.
• Give calcium chloride by slow IV push: 0.5–1 mL/min. Rapid administration may produce bradycardia, chalky or metallic taste, a drop in B/P, peripheral vasodilation, and a sensation of heat.
• Give calcium gluconate by IV push: 0.5–1 mL/min. Rapid administration may produce arrhythmias, a drop in B/P, myocardial infarction, and vasodilation.
• The maximum rate for intermittent IV calcium gluconate infusion is 200 mg/min (e.g., 10 mL/min when 1 g diluted with 50 mL diluent).

Intervention and Evaluation

• Monitor the patient's B/P, EKG, and serum magnesium, phosphate, and potassium levels as well as renal function tests and urine calcium concentrations.
• Monitor the patient for signs and symptoms of hypercalcemia.

Patient/Family Teaching

• Stress to the patient/family the importance of diet.
• Instruct the patient/family to take tablets with a full glass of water, ½–1 hr after meals.
• Teach the patient/family to consume liquid before meals.
• Advise the patient/family not to take the vitamin within 1–2 hrs of other fiber-containing foods and oral medications.
• Urge the patient/family to avoid consuming excessive amounts of alcohol, caffeine, and tobacco.

Citrates (Potassium Citrate, Potassium Citrate and Citric Acid, Sodium Citrate and Citric Acid, Tricitrates)

(Bicitra, Oracit, Polycitra, Urocit-K)

CATEGORY AND SCHEDULE

Pregnancy Risk Category: C (potassium citrate) (Other forms not expected to cause fetal harm)

MECHANISM OF ACTION

This alkalinizer increases urinary pH and increases the solubility of cystine in urine and the ionization of uric acid to urate ion. Increasing urinary pH and urinary citrate concentration decreases calcium ion activity and decreases saturation of calcium oxalate. Increases plasma bicarbonate and buffers excess hydrogen ion concentration. ***Therapeutic Effect:*** Increases blood pH and reverses acidosis.

AVAILABILITY

Tablets (Urocit-K as potassium citrate): 5 mEq, 10 mEq.
Syrup.
Cytra-3: Potassium citrate 550 mg and sodium citrate 500 mg/5 mL (equivalent to 1 mEq/mL sodium, 1 mEq/mL potassium and 2 mEq/mL bicarbonate)
Polycitra: Potassium citrate 550 mg and sodium citrate 500 mg and citric acid 334 mg/5mL (equivalent to 1 mEq/mL sodium, 1 mEq/mL potassium and 2 mEq/mL bicarbonate)
Polycitra-LC: Potassium citrate 550 mg and sodium citrate 500 mg and citric acid 334 mg/5mL (equivalent to 1 mEq/mL sodium, 1 mEq/mL potassium and 2 mEq/mL bicarbonate)
Oral Solution.
Bicitra, Cytra-2: sodium citrate 500 mg and citric acid 334 mg/5mL (equivalent to 1 mEq/mL sodium and 1 mEq/mL bicarbonate)
Cytra-K: Potassium citrate 1,100 mg and citric acid 334 mg/5mL (equivalent to 2 mEq/mL potassium and 2 mEq/mL bicarbonate)
Oracit: Sodium citrate 490 mg and citric acid 640 mg/5mL (equivalent to 1 mEq/mL sodium and 1 mEq/mL bicarbonate)

INDICATIONS AND DOSAGES

▸ Treatment of metabolic acidosis
PO
Children. 5–15 mL after meals and at bedtime or 2–3 mEq/kg/day in 3–4 divided doses.

CONTRAINDICATIONS

Acute dehydration, anuria, azotemia, heat cramps, hypersensitivity to citrate, pts with sodium-restricted diet, severe myocardial damage, severe renal impairment, or untreated Addison' disease
Urocit K: anticholinergics, intestinal obstruction or stricture, pts with delayed gastric emptying or severe peptic ulcer disease.

INTERACTIONS

Drug
Angiotensin-converting enzyme inhibitors, NSAIDs, potassium-containing medication, potassium-sparing diuretics: May increase the risk of hyperkalemia.
Antacids: May increase the risk of systemic alkalosis.
Methenamine: May decrease the effects of methenamine.
Quinidine: May increase the excretion of quinidine.
Herbal
None known.
Food
None known.

DIAGNOSTIC TEST EFFECTS

None known.

SIDE EFFECTS

Occasional
Diarrhea, mild abdominal pain, nausea, vomiting

SERIOUS REACTIONS

! Metabolic alkalosis, bowel obstruction or perforation, hyperkalemia, and hypernatremia occur rarely.

PEDIATRIC CONSIDERATIONS

Precautions

• Use cautiously in pts with CHF, hypertension, and pulmonary edema.

• Use cautiously because citrate use may increase the risk of urolithiasis.

Intervention and Evaluation

• Assess the EKG and urinary pH in pts with cardiac disease.

• Assess the patient's complete blood count, particularly blood Hct and Hgb levels, serum acid-base balance, and serum creatinine levels.

Patient/Family Teaching

• Instruct the patient/family to take citrates after meals.

• Teach the patient/family to mix citrates in juice or water and to follow citrate consumption with additional liquid.

Fluoride

flur-eyd

(Fluor-A-Day, Fluoritab, Fluotic [CAN], Luride)

CATEGORY AND SCHEDULE

Pregnancy Risk Category: C

MECHANISM OF ACTION

A trace element that increases tooth resistance to acid dissolution. ***Therapeutic Effect:*** Promotes remineralization of decalcified enamel, inhibits dental plaque bacteria, increases resistance to development of caries. Maintains bone strength.

AVAILABILITY

Topical Cream: 1.1%.
Gel-Drops: 1.1%.
Topical Gel: 0.4%, 1.1%.
Lozenge: 2.2 mg.
Oral Solution Drops: 1.1 mg/mL.
Oral Solution Rinse: 0.05%, 0.2%, 0.44%.
Tablets (chewable): 0.58 mg, 1.1 mg, 2.2 mg.

INDICATIONS AND DOSAGES

▸ Dietary supplement for the prevention of dental caries in children

Water Fluoride	Age	mg/day
Less than 0.3 ppm	younger than 2 yrs	0.25 mg/day
	2–3 yrs	0.5 mg/day
	3–13 yrs	1 mg/day
0.3–0.7 ppm	less than 2 yrs	None
	2–3 yrs	0.25 mg/day
	3–13 yrs	0.5 mg/day
Greater than 0.7 ppm	None	None

CONTRAINDICATIONS

Hypersensitivity to fluoride or any related component. Arthralgia, GI ulceration, severe renal insufficiency.

INTERACTIONS

Drug

Aluminum hydroxide, calcium: May decrease the absorption of fluoride.

Herbal

None known.

Food

None known.

DIAGNOSTIC TEST EFFECTS

May increase serum alkaline phosphatase and SGOT (AST) levels.

SIDE EFFECTS

Rare

Oral mucous membrane ulceration

SERIOUS REACTIONS

! Hypocalcemia, tetany, bone pain (especially of the ankles and feet), electrolyte disturbances, and arrhythmias occur rarely.
! Fluoride use may cause skeletal fluorosis, osteomalacia, and osteosclerosis.

PEDIATRIC CONSIDERATIONS

Patient/Family Teaching

- Instruct the patient/family not to take fluoride with dairy products as these foods decrease absorption.
- Teach the patient/family to apply gels and rinses at bedtime after brushing or flossing. Stress to the patient that he or she should expectorate excess fluoride, not swallow it.
- Advise the patient/family not to drink, eat, or rinse the mouth after application.

Magnesium

See laxatives

Phosphates

(Fleet enema, Fleet Phosphosoda, K-Phosphate, Neutra-Phos K, Uro KP)

CATEGORY AND SCHEDULE

Pregnancy Risk Category: C

MECHANISM OF ACTION

An electrolyte that participates in bone deposition, calcium metabolism, utilization of B complex vitamins, buffer in acid-base equilibrium.
Laxative: Exerts osmotic effect in small intestine. ***Therapeutic Effect:*** Produces distention; promotes peristalsis and evacuation of bowel.

PHARMACOKINETICS

Poorly absorbed after PO administration. PO form excreted in feces, IV forms excreted in urine.

AVAILABILITY

Injection: 3 mM/mL (available as sodium phosphate or potassium phosphate).
Tablets.
K-Phos M.F.: phosphorus 4 mM, potassium 1.1 mEq and sodium 2.9 mEq/tablet
K-Phos Neutral: phosphorus 8 mM, potassium 1.1 mEq and sodium 13 mEq/tablet
K-Phos No. 2: phosphorus 8 mM, potassium 2.3 mEq and sodium 5.8 mEq/tablet
K-Phos Original: phosphorus 3.7 mM and potassium 3.7 mEq/tablet
Uro-KP-Neutral: phosphorus 8 mM, potassium 1.27 mEq and sodium 10.9 mEq/tablet
Oral Solution.
Fleet Phospho-Soda: phosphate 4 mM and sodium 4.82 mEq/mL
Enema.
Fleet Enema: monobasic sodium phosphate 19 g and dibasic sodium phosphate 3.5 g/118 mL
Fleet Enema for Children: monobasic sodium phosphate 9.5 g and dibasic sodium phosphate 3.5 g/59 mL
Powder.
Neutra-Phos: phosphorus 8 mM, potassium 7.125 mEq and sodium 7.125 mEq/packet
Neutra-Phos-K: phosphorus 8 mM and potassium 14.25 mEq/packet

INDICATIONS AND DOSAGES

▸ Hypophosphatemia

IV

Children. 0.5–1.5 mM/kg/day.

PO

Children. 2–3 mM/kg/day in divided doses.

▸ Laxative

PO

Children older than 4 yrs. 1–2 capsules/packets (8–16 mM) 4 times/day.

Children 4 yrs and younger. 1 capsule/packet (8 mM) 4 times/day.

RECTAL

Children 12 yrs and older. 4.5-oz enema as single dose. May repeat.

Children younger than 12 yrs. 2.25-oz enema as single dose. May repeat.

UNLABELED USES

Prevention of calcium renal calculi.

CONTRAINDICATIONS

Abdominal pain (from rectal dosage form) CHF, fecal impaction, hypocalcemia, hyperkalemia, hypomagnesemia, hypernatremia, hyperphosphatemia, phosphate kidney stones, severe renal function impairment.

INTERACTIONS

Drug

Angiotensin-converting enzyme inhibitors, NSAIDs, potassium-containing medications, potassium-sparing diuretics, salt substitutes with potassium phosphate: May increase potassium blood concentration.

Antacids: May decrease the absorption of phosphate.

Calcium-containing medications: May increase the risk of calcium deposition in soft tissues and decrease phosphate absorption.

Digoxin, potassium phosphate: May increase the risk of heart block caused by hyperkalemia.

Glucocorticoids: May cause edema with sodium phosphate.

Phosphate-containing medications: May increase the risk of hyperphosphatemia.

Sodium-containing medication with sodium phosphate: May increase the risk of edema.

Herbal

None known.

Food

None known.

DIAGNOSTIC TEST EFFECTS

None known.

IV INCOMPATIBILITIES

Dobutamine (Dobutrex)

IV COMPATIBILITIES

Diltiazem (Cardizem), enalapril (Vasotec), famotidine (Pepcid), magnesium sulfate, metoclopramide (Reglan)

SIDE EFFECTS

Frequent

Mild laxative effect first few days of therapy

Occasional

GI upset, including diarrhea, nausea, abdominal pain, and vomiting

Rare

Headache, dizziness, mental confusion, heaviness of legs, fatigue, muscle cramps, numbness or tingling of hands or feet or around lips, peripheral edema, irregular heartbeat, weight gain, thirst

SERIOUS REACTIONS

! High phosphate levels may produce extraskeletal calcification.

PEDIATRIC CONSIDERATIONS

Baseline Assessment

- Assess for the presence of GI pain. Note its pattern, duration, quality, intensity, location, and areas of radiation, as well as factors that relieve or worsen the pain.
- Assess the amount, color, and consistency of the stool of the patient taking phosphates as a laxative.
- Assess the pattern of daily bowel activity and evaluate the bowel sounds for peristalsis of the patient taking phosphates as a laxative.
- Assess the patient for a history of recent abdominal surgery, nausea, vomiting, and weight loss.
- Assess baseline phosphate levels and urine pH.
- Be aware that it is unknown whether phosphates cross the placenta or are distributed in breast milk.
- There are no age-related precautions noted in children.

Precautions

- Use cautiously in pts with adrenal insufficiency, cirrhosis, and renal impairment.
- Use cautiously in pts concurrently receiving potassium-sparing drugs.

Administration and Handling

PO

- Dissolve tablets/contents of packets in water.
- Give after meals or with food to decrease GI upset.
- Maintain high fluid intake to prevent kidney stones.

IV

- Store at room temperature.
- Dilute before using.
- Infuse at a maximum rate of 0.06 mM phosphate/kg/hr, as prescribed.

Intervention and Evaluation

- Monitor the patient's serum alkaline phosphatase, bilirubin, calcium, phosphorus, potassium, sodium, SGOT (AST), and SGPT (ALT) levels routinely.

Patient/Family Teaching

- Warn the patient/family to notify the physician if the patient experiences diarrhea, nausea, or vomiting.

Potassium Acetate

(Potassium acetate)

Potassium bicarbonate/citrate

(K-Lyte)

Potassium Chloride

(Apo-K [CAN], Kaochlor, K-Dur, K-Lor, K-Lor-Con M 15, Klotrix, K-Lyte-Cl, Micro-K, Slow-K)

Potassium Gluconate

(Kaon)

Do not confuse with Cardura or Slow-FE.

CATEGORY AND SCHEDULE

Pregnancy Risk Category: C (A for potassium chloride)

MECHANISM OF ACTION

An electrolyte that is necessary for multiple cellular metabolic processes. Its primary action is intracellular. ***Therapeutic Effect:*** Necessary for nerve impulse conduction, contraction of cardiac, skeletal, and smooth muscle; maintains normal renal function and acid-base balance.

PHARMACOKINETICS

Well absorbed from the GI tract. Enters cells via active transport from extracellular fluid. Primarily excreted in urine.

AVAILABILITY

Acetate
Injection: 2 mEq/mL, 4 mEq/mL.
Bicarbonate and Citrate
Effervescent Tablets: 25 mEq, 50 mEq.
Chloride
Tablets: 6.7 mEq, 8 mEq, 10 mEq, 20 mEq.
Liquid: 20 mEq/15 mL, 40 mEq/15 mL.
Oral Powder: 20 mEq, 25 mEq.
Injection: 2 mEq/mL.
Gluconate
Liquid: 20 mEq/15 mL.

INDICATIONS AND DOSAGES

▸ **Prevention of hypokalemia (on diuretic therapy)**
PO
Children. 1–2 mEq/kg in 1–2 divided doses.
▸ **Treatment of hypokalemia**
IV
Children. 1 mEq/kg over 1–2 hrs.
PO
Children. 1–2 mEq/day, further doses based on laboratory values.

CONTRAINDICATIONS

Digitalis toxicity, heat cramps, hyperkalemia, pts receiving potassium-sparing diuretics, postoperative oliguria, severe burns, severe renal impairment, shock with dehydration or hemolytic reaction, untreated Addison' disease.

INTERACTIONS

Drug
Anticholinergics: May increase the risk of GI lesions.
Angiotensin-converting enzyme inhibitors, beta-adrenergic blockers, heparin, NSAIDs, potassium-containing medications, potassium-sparing diuretics, salt substitutes: May increase potassium blood concentration.
Herbal
None known.
Food
None known.

DIAGNOSTIC TEST EFFECTS

None known.

IV INCOMPATIBILITIES

Amphotericin B complex (Abelcet, AmBisome, Amphotec), methylprednisolone (Solu-Medrol), phenytoin (Dilantin)

IV COMPATIBILITIES

Aminophylline, amiodarone (Cordarone), atropine, aztreonam (Azactam), calcium gluconate, cefepime (Maxipime), ciprofloxacin (Cipro), clindamycin (Cleocin), dexamethasone (Decadron), digoxin (Lanoxin), diltiazem (Cardizem), diphenhydramine (Benadryl), dobutamine (Dobutrex), dopamine (Intropin), enalapril (Vasotec), famotidine (Pepcid), fluconazole (Diflucan), furosemide (Lasix), granisetron (Kytril), heparin, hydrocortisone (Solu-Cortef), insulin, lidocaine, lorazepam (Ativan), magnesium sulfate, methylprednisolone (Solu-Medrol), midazolam (Versed), milrinone (Primacor), metoclopramide

(Reglan), morphine, norepinephrine (Levophed), ondansetron (Zofran), oxytocin (Pitocin), piperacillin/tazobactam (Zosyn), procainamide (Pronestyl), propofol (Diprivan), propranolol (Inderal)

SIDE EFFECTS

Occasional

Nausea, vomiting, diarrhea, flatulence, abdominal discomfort with distention, phlebitis with IV administration (particularly when potassium concentration of greater than 40 mEq/L is infused).

Rare

Rash

SERIOUS REACTIONS

! Hyperkalemia (observed particularly in pts with impaired renal function) manifested as paresthesia of extremities, heaviness of legs, cold skin, grayish pallor, hypotension, mental confusion, irritability, flaccid paralysis, and cardiac arrhythmias may occur.

PEDIATRIC CONSIDERATIONS

Baseline Assessment

- Give the patient oral doses after meals or with food with a full glass of fruit juice or water to minimize GI irritation.
- Be aware that it is unknown whether potassium crosses the placenta and is distributed in breast milk.
- There are no age-related precautions noted in children.

Precautions

- Use cautiously in pts with cardiac disease and tartrazine sensitivity, which is most common in those with aspirin hypersensitivity.

Administration and Handling

◂ **ALERT** ▸ Know that potassium dosage is individualized.

PO

Give with or after meals and with full glass of water to decrease GI upset.

- Mix or dissolve effervescent tablets, liquids, and powder with juice or water before administering.
- Instruct the patient to swallow the tablets whole and avoid chewing or crushing the tablets.

IV

Store at room temperature.

- For IV infusion only, must dilute before administration; mix well.
- Avoid adding potassium to hanging the IV infusion.
- Infuse slowly; the rate should not exceed 1 mEq/kg/hr. Maximum concentration for a peripheral line: 80 mEq/L. Maximum concentration for a central line: 150 mEq/L or 15 mEq/100 mL.
- Check the patient's IV site closely during infusion for phlebitis as evidenced by hardness of the vein, heat, pain, and red streaking of skin over the vein, and extravasation manifested as cool skin, little or no blood return, pain, and swelling.

Intervention and Evaluation

- Monitor the patient's serum potassium level, particularly in those with renal function impairment.
- Dilute the preparation further or give with meals if the patient experiences GI disturbance.
- Be alert to a decrease in the patient's urinary output, which may be an indication of renal insufficiency.
- Assess the patient's pattern of daily bowel activity and stool consistency.
- Monitor the patient's intake and output diligently for diuresis and

IV site for extravasation and phlebitis.
• Be alert to signs and symptoms of hyperkalemia, including cold skin, a feeling of heaviness of the legs, paresthesia of the extremities and tongue, and skin pallor.

Patient/Family Teaching

• Give the patient/family a list of foods rich in potassium including apricots, avocados, bananas, beans, beef, broccoli, Brussels sprouts, cantaloupe, chicken, dates, fish, ham, lentils, milk, molasses, potatoes, prunes, raisins, spinach, turkey, watermelon, veal, and yams.
• Warn the patient/family to notify the physician if the patient experiences a feeling of heaviness in the legs or numbness of the extremities or tongue.

Sodium Bicarbonate

CATEGORY AND SCHEDULE

Pregnancy Risk Category: C
OTC

MECHANISM OF ACTION

An alkalinizing agent that dissociates to provide bicarbonate ion. ***Therapeutic Effect:*** Neutralizes hydrogen ion concentration, raises blood and urinary pH.

PHARMACOKINETICS

Route	Onset	Peak	Duration
PO	15 min	N/A	1–3 hrs
IV	Immediate	N/A	8–10 min

After administration, sodium bicarbonate dissociates to sodium and bicarbonate ions. Forms or excretes carbon dioxide (CO_2). With increased hydrogen ions, combines to form carbonic acid and then dissociates to CO_2, which is excreted by the lungs. Plasma concentration regulated by the kidneys, which have the ability to excrete or make bicarbonate.

AVAILABILITY

Tablets: 325 mg, 650 mg.
Injection: 0.5 mEq/mL (4.2%), 0.6 mEq/mL (5%), 0.9 mEq/mL (7.5%), 1 mEq/mL (8.4%).

INDICATIONS AND DOSAGES

▸ Cardiac arrest

IV

Children and infants. Initially, 1 mEq/kg slow IV push.

▸ Metabolic acidosis (less severe)

IV INFUSION

Children. 2–5 mEq/kg over 4–8 hrs. May repeat based on laboratory values.

▸ Renal tubular acidosis (distal)

PO

Children. 2–3 mEq/kg/day in divided doses.

▸ Renal tubular acidosis (proximal)

PO

Children. 5–10 mEq/kg/day in divided doses.

▸ Alkalinization of urine

PO

Children. 84–840 mg/kg/day in divided doses.

CONTRAINDICATIONS

Excessive chloride loss due to diarrhea or GI suction or vomiting, hypocalcemia, metabolic or respiratory alkalosis

INTERACTIONS

Drug

Calcium-containing products: May result in milk-alkali syndrome.

Lithium, salicylates: May increase the excretion of these drugs.
Methenamine: May decrease the effects of methenamine.
Quinidine, ketoconazole, tetracyclines: May decrease the excretion of these drugs.
Herbal
None known.
Food
Milk, milk products: May result in milk-alkali syndrome.

DIAGNOSTIC TEST EFFECTS

May increase serum or urinary pH.

IV INCOMPATIBILITIES

Ascorbic acid, diltiazem (Cardizem), dobutamine (Dobutrex), dopamine (Intropin), hydromorphone (Dilaudid), magnesium sulfate, midazolam (Versed), morphine, norepinephrine (Levophed)

IV COMPATIBILITIES

Aminophylline, calcium chloride, furosemide (Lasix), heparin, insulin, lidocaine, mannitol, milrinone (Primacor), morphine, phenylephrine (Neo-Synephrine), phenytoin (Dilantin), potassium chloride, propofol (Diprivan), vancomycin (Vancocin)

SIDE EFFECTS

Frequent
Abdominal distention, flatulence, belching

SERIOUS REACTIONS

! Excessive or chronic use may produce metabolic alkalosis (irritability, twitching, numbness or tingling of extremities, cyanosis, slow or shallow respirations, headache, thirst, nausea).
! Fluid overload results in headache, weakness, blurred vision, behavioral changes, incoordination, muscle twitching, a rise in blood pressure, a decrease in pulse rate, rapid respirations, wheezing, coughing, and distended neck veins.
! Extravasation may occur at the IV site, resulting in necrosis and ulceration.

PEDIATRIC CONSIDERATIONS

Baseline Assessment
- Do not give other oral medication within 1–2 hrs of antacid administration.
- Be aware that sodium bicarbonate use may produce hypernatremia and increase tendon reflexes in the neonate or fetus whose mother is a chronic, high-dose user.
- Be aware that sodium bicarbonate may be distributed in breast milk.
- There are no age-related precautions noted in children.
- Be aware that sodium bicarbonate should not be used as an antacid in children younger than 6 yrs of age.

Precautions
- Use cautiously in pts with CHF, receiving corticosteroid therapy, in edematous states, and with renal insufficiency.

Administration and Handling
◂ **ALERT** ▸ May give by IV push, IV infusion, or orally. Drug doses are individualized and are based on laboratory values, patient age, clinical conditions, weight, and severity of acidosis. Know that metabolic alkalosis may result if the bicarbonate deficit is fully corrected during the first 24 hrs.

PO
Give 1–3 hrs after meals.

IV

◂ALERT▸ If sodium bicarbonate is being given for acidosis, give when plasma bicarbonate is less than 15 mEq/L.

• Store at room temperature.
• May give undiluted.

◂ALERT▸ For direct IV administration in neonates and infants, use 0.5 mEq/mL concentration.

• For IV push, give up to 1 mEq/kg over 1–3 min for myocardial infarction.
• For IV infusion, do not exceed rate of infusion of 50 mEq/hr. For children younger than 2 yrs of age, premature infants, or neonates, administer by slow infusion, up to 8 mEq/min.

Intervention and Evaluation

• Monitor the patient's blood and urine pH partial pressure of carbon dioxide in arterial blood, CO_2 level, plasma bicarbonate, and serum electrolyte levels.
• Observe the patient for signs and symptoms of fluid overload and metabolic alkalosis.
• Assess the patient for clinical improvement of metabolic acidosis, including relief from disorientation, hyperventilation, and weakness.
• Assess the patient's pattern of daily bowel activity and stool consistency.
• Monitor the patient's serum calcium, phosphate, and uric acid levels.
• Assess the patient for relief of gastric distress.

Patient/Family Teaching

• Advise the patient/family that the patient who is considering breast-feeding should consult with her physician before taking sodium bicarbonate.
• Encourage the patient/family to check with the physician before taking any OTC medications, which may contain sodium.

Sodium Chloride

(Ocean Mist, Salinex, Sodium chloride [CAN])

CATEGORY AND SCHEDULE

Pregnancy Risk Category: C
OTC (tablets, nasal solution, ophthalmic solution, ophthalmic ointment)

MECHANISM OF ACTION

Sodium is a major cation of extracellular fluid that controls water distribution, fluid and electrolyte balance, and osmotic pressure of body fluids and maintains acid-base balance.

PHARMACOKINETICS

Well absorbed from the GI tract. Widely distributed. Primarily excreted in urine.

AVAILABILITY

Tablets: 1 g.
Nasal Solution (OTC): 0.4%, 0.6%, 0.75%.
Ophthalmic Solution (OTC): 2%, 5%.
Ophthalmic Ointment (OTC): 5%.
Injection (concentrate): 14.6%, 23.4%.
Injection (infusion): 0.45%, 0.9%, 3%, 5%.
Irrigation: 0.45%, 0.9%.

INDICATIONS AND DOSAGES

▸ Prevention and treatment of sodium and chloride deficiencies; source of hydration

IV INFUSION
Premature infants: 2-8 mEq/kd/day

Term neonates: 1-4 mEq/kg/day
Infants and children: 3-4 mEq/kg/day; Max 100-150 mEq/day

▸ Prevention of heat prostration and muscle cramps from excessive perspiration
PO
Adolescents: 0.5-1 G up to 5-10 times/day; Max 5 g/day.
Relieves dry and inflamed nasal membranes, restores moisture
INTRANASAL
Use as often as needed.
Diagnostic aid in ophthalmoscopic exam, therapy in reduction of corneal edema
OPHTHALMIC SOLUTION
Apply once daily or more often as needed.
OPHTHALMIC OINTMENT
Apply once daily or more often as needed.

CONTRAINDICATIONS

Hypersensitivity to sodium chloride or any related component; fluid retention, hypernatremia.

INTERACTIONS

Drug

Hypertonic saline and oxytocics: May cause uterine hypertonus, possible uterine ruptures or lacerations.

Herbal

None known.

Food

None known.

DIAGNOSTIC TEST EFFECTS

None known.

SIDE EFFECTS

Frequent

Facial flushing

Occasional

Fever, irritation, phlebitis, or extravasation at injection site
Ophthalmic: Temporary burning or irritation

SERIOUS REACTIONS

! Too rapid administration may produce peripheral edema, CHF, and pulmonary edema.
! Excessive dosage produces hypokalemia, hypervolemia, and hypernatremia.

PEDIATRIC CONSIDERATIONS

Baseline Assessment

- Assess the patient's fluid balance, including daily weight, edema, intake and output, and lung sounds.
- There are no age-related precautions noted in children.

Precautions

- Use cautiously in pts with cirrhosis, CHF, hypertension, and renal impairment.
- Do not use sodium chloride preserved with benzyl alcohol in neonates.

Administration and Handling

◂ ALERT ▸ Drug dosage is based on the patient's acid-base status, age, clinical condition, fluid and electrolyte status, and weight.
PO
Do not crush or break enteric-coated or extended-release tablets.
- Administer with a full glass of water.

NASAL
- Instruct the patient to begin inhaling slowly just before releasing medication into the nose.
- Teach the patient to inhale slowly, then release air gently through the mouth.
- Continue this technique for 20–30 sec.

OPHTHALMIC
- Place a gloved finger on the patient's lower eyelid and pull it

out until a pocket is formed between the patient's eye and lower lid.
• Hold the dropper above the pocket and place the prescribed number of drops (or apply a thin strip of ointment) into pocket.
• Instruct the patient to close the eyes gently so that medication will not be squeezed out of sac.
• When the lower lid is released, have the patient keep the affected eye open without blinking for at least 30 sec for solution; for ointment, have patient close the affected eye and roll the eyeball around to distribute the medication.
• When using drops, apply gentle finger pressure to the lacrimal sac (bridge of the nose, inside corner of the eye) for 1–2 min after administration of solution to reduce systemic absorption.

IV

Hypertonic solutions (3%–5%) are administered via a large vein; avoid infiltration, and do not exceed 100 mL/hr.
• Vials containing 2.5–4 mEq/mL (concentrated sodium chloride) must be diluted with D_5W or $D_{10}W$ before administration.

Intervention and Evaluation

• Monitor the patient's fluid balance and IV site for extravasation.
• Monitor the patient's acid-base balance, blood pressure (B/P), and serum electrolyte levels.
• Assess the patient for hypernatremia associated with edema, elevated B/P, and weight gain and hyponatremia associated with dry mucous membranes, muscle cramps, nausea, and vomiting.

Patient/Family Teaching

• Advise the patient/family that the patient may experience temporary burning or irritation upon instillation of ophthalmic medication.
• Instruct the patient/family to discontinue ophthalmic medication and notify the physician if the patient experiences acute redness of eyes, double vision, headache, pain on exposure to light, a rapid change in vision (side and straight ahead), severe pain, or the sudden appearance of floating spots.

Zinc Oxide

(Balmex, Desitin)
zinc sulfate
(Orazinc)

CATEGORY AND SCHEDULE

Pregnancy Risk Category: C

MECHANISM OF ACTION

A mineral that acts as an enzyme cofactor and skin protectant.
Oxide: Mild astringent, protector. ***Therapeutic Effect:*** Protective coating for skin.
Sulfate: Cofactor for enzymes important for protein and carbohydrate metabolism. ***Therapeutic Effect:*** Maintains normal growth and tissue repair, as well as skin hydration.

AVAILABILITY

Oxide

Ointment: 10%, 20%, 40%.

Sulfate

Capsules: 110 mg, 220 mg.
Tablets: 110 mg.
Injection: 1 mg/mL.

INDICATIONS AND DOSAGES

▸ **Oxide: Protective for mild skin irritation and abrasions. Promotes healing of chapped skin, diaper rash**

TOPICAL

Children. Apply as needed.

CONTRAINDICATIONS
Hypersensitivity to zinc oxide or any related component.

INTERACTIONS
Drug
Histamine H_2 blockers, such as famotidine: May decrease zinc absorption.
Quinolones, such as ciprofloxacin, tetracycline: May decrease the absorption of quinolones and tetracycline.
Herbal
None known.
Food
Coffee, dairy products: May decrease zinc absorption.

DIAGNOSTIC TEST EFFECTS
None known.

SIDE EFFECTS
Indigestion, nausea, vomiting (rare).

SERIOUS REACTIONS
None available.

PEDIATRIC CONSIDERATIONS

Baseline Assessment
- Assess the skin for signs of infection before application of topical zinc.
- Avoid using during pregnancy, unless prescribed.

Administration and Handling
TOPICAL
- For external use only.
- Avoid use in the eyes.

Patient/Family Teaching
- Explain that coffee and dairy products may decrease the absorption of zinc oxide.
- Instruct the patient/family to notify the physician if the skin condition does not improve after using zinc oxide for 7 days.

71 Vitamins

Ascorbic Acid (Vitamin C)
Cyanocobalamin (Vitamin B_{12})
Folic Acid (Vitamin B_9), Sodium Folate
Leucovorin Calcium (Folinic Acid, Citrovorum Factor)
Niacin, Nicotinic Acid (Vitamin B_3)
Pyridoxine Hydrochloride (Vitamin B_6)
Thiamine Hydrochloride (Vitamin B_1)
Vitamin A
Vitamin D, Calcitriol, Dihydrotachysterol, Ergocalciferol, Paricalcitol
Vitamin E
Vitamin K, Phytonadione

Uses: Vitamins are primarily used to supplement the diet to meet the body's need for the organic substances required for growth, reproduction, and maintenance of health. The need for vitamin supplementation may result from inadequate dietary intake, increased physiologic need (such as during pregnancy), or certain disorders or conditions, such as Crohn disease, renal disease, and gastrectomy. Some vitamins have additional uses. *Vitamin C* is used to prevent and treat scurvy. *Leucovorin* is used to prevent and treat methotrexate, pyrimethamine, and trimethoprim toxicity. As an adjunct, *niacin* is used to treat hyperlipidemias and peripheral vascular disease. *Pyridoxine* is used to treat isoniazid poisoning, seizures in neonates that do not respond to conventional therapy, and sideroblastic anemia caused by increased serum iron concentrations. *Thiamine* is helpful in treating alcoholic pts with altered sensorium. *Vitamin K* is used to prevent and treat hemorrhagic states in neonates and to act as the antidote for hemorrhage caused by oral anticoagulants.

Action: Vitamins are essential for energy transformation and regulation of metabolic processes. There are catalysts for all reactions using proteins, fats, and carbohydrates for energy, growth, and cell maintenance.

Water-soluble vitamins, such as folic acid and vitamins C, B_1, B_2, B_3, B_6, and B_{12}, act as coenzymes for almost every cellular reaction in the body. B-complex vitamins differ from one another in structure and function but are grouped together because they were first isolated from the same source (yeast and liver).

Fat-soluble vitamins, such as vitamins A, D, E, and K, are soluble in lipids, are stored in body tissue when excessive quantities are consumed, and may be toxic when taken in large quantities. Vitamin A is needed for normal retinal function, night vision, bone growth, gonadal function, embryonic development, and epithelial cell integrity. Vitamin D is essential for calcium absorption and use and for normal calcification of bone.

Vitamin E prevents oxidation and protects fatty acids from free radicals. Vitamin K is required for hepatic formation of coagulation factors II, VII, IX, and X.

Ascorbic Acid (Vitamin C)

(Apo-C [CAN], Cecon, Cenolate, Pro-C [AUS], Redoxon [CAN])

CATEGORY AND SCHEDULE

Pregnancy Risk Category: A (C if used in doses exceeding the recommended daily allowance [RDA])
OTC

MECHANISM OF ACTION

This vitamin assists in collagen formation and tissue repair and is involved in oxidation-reduction reactions and other metabolic reactions. ***Therapeutic Effect:*** Involved in carbohydrate utilization, metabolism, and synthesis of carnitine, lipids, and proteins. Preserves blood vessel integrity.

PHARMACOKINETICS

Readily absorbed from the GI tract. Protein binding: 25%. Metabolized in liver. Excreted in urine. Removed by hemodialysis.

AVAILABILITY

Tablets: 100 mg, 250 mg, 500 mg, 1 g.
Tablets (chewable): 60 mg, 100 mg, 250 mg, 500 mg.
Tablets (controlled release): 500 mg, 1 g, 1,500 mg.
Capsules (controlled release): 500 mg.
Liquid: 500 mg/5 mL.
Solution: 500 mg/mL.
Injection: 250 mg/mL, 500 mg/mL.

INDICATIONS AND DOSAGES

▸ Dietary supplement

PO

Children older than 4 yrs. 35–100 mg/day.

▸ Scurvy

PO

Children. 100–300 mg/day in divided doses

▸ RDA

PO/IM/IV/SC

Adolescents 14–18 yrs. Males 75 mg; females 65 mg.
Children 9–13 yrs. 45 mg.
Children 4–8 yrs. 25 mg.
Children 1–3 yrs. 15 mg.

UNLABELED USES

Prevention of the common cold, control of idiopathic methemoglobinemia, urinary acidifier.

CONTRAINDICATIONS

Hypersensitivity to ascorbic acid or any related component. Large doses in pregnancy.

INTERACTIONS

Drug

Deferoxamine: May increase iron toxicity.
Aspirin: May increase aspirin toxicity.
Iron: May increase the absorption of iron at high doses.
Oral contraceptives: Increases estrogen levels.
Warfarin: Decreases the anticoagulant effects of warfarin.

Herbal
None known.

Food
None known.

DIAGNOSTIC TEST EFFECTS

May decrease serum bilirubin level and urinary pH. May increase uric acid and urine oxalate levels. May give a false-negative amine-dependent stool occult blood test.

IV INCOMPATIBILITIES

No information available via Y-site administration.

IV COMPATIBILITIES

Calcium gluconate, heparin

SIDE EFFECTS

Rare
Abdominal cramps, nausea, vomiting, diarrhea, increased urination with doses exceeding 1 g
Parenteral: Flushing, headache, dizziness, sleepiness or insomnia, soreness at injection site

SERIOUS REACTIONS

! Ascorbic acid may produce urine acidification, leading to crystalluria.
! Prolonged use of large doses of ascorbic acid may result in scurvy when dosage is reduced to normal.

PEDIATRIC CONSIDERATIONS

Baseline Assessment
- Be aware that ascorbic acid crosses the placenta and is excreted in breast milk.
- Be aware that large doses of ascorbic acid during pregnancy may produce scurvy in neonates.
- There are no age-related precautions noted in children.
- Some products may contain aspartame, which should be avoided or used with caution in pts with phenylketonuria.

Precautions
- Use cautiously in pts who receive daily doses of a salicylate, those with diabetes mellitus, a history of renal stones, and sodium restrictions, and those who are receiving warfarin therapy.

Administration and Handling
PO
- May give without regard to food.

IV
Refrigerate and protect from freezing and sunlight.
- May give undiluted or dilute in D_5W, 0.9% NaCl, or lactated Ringer's solution.
- For IV push, dilute with equal volume of D_5W or 0.9% NaCl and infuse over 10 min. For IV solution, infuse over 4–12 hrs.

Intervention and Evaluation
- Assess the patient for signs of clinical improvement, such as an improved sense of well-being and improved sleep patterns.
- Monitor for signs and symptoms of the recurrence of vitamin C deficiency, including bleeding gums, digestive difficulties, gingivitis, poor wound healing, and joint pain.

Patient/Family Teaching
- Alert the patient/family that abrupt vitamin C withdrawal may produce rebound deficiency. Instruct the patient/family to reduce ascorbic acid dosage gradually, as prescribed.
- Inform the patient/family to eat foods rich in vitamin C, including black currant jelly, Brussels sprouts, citrus fruits, guava, green peppers, rose hips, spinach, strawberries, and watercress.

Cyanocobalamin (Vitamin B_{12})

sye-ah-no-koe-**bal**-a-min
(LA-12, Nascobal, Bedoz [CAN], Cytamen [AUS])

CATEGORY AND SCHEDULE

Pregnancy Risk Category: A (C if used at dosages exceeding the RDA)

MECHANISM OF ACTION

A coenzyme for metabolic functions, including fat and carbohydrate metabolism and protein synthesis. ***Therapeutic Effect:*** Necessary for growth, cell replication, hematopoiesis, and myelin synthesis.

PHARMACOKINETICS

Absorbed in the lower half of ileum in the presence of calcium. Initially, bound to intrinsic factor; this complex passes down intestine, binding to receptor sites on the ileal mucosa. In presence of calcium, absorbed systemically. Protein binding: High. Metabolized in liver. Primarily eliminated in urine unchanged. ***Half-Life:*** 6 days.

AVAILABILITY

Tablets: 50 mcg, 100 mcg, 250 mcg, 500 mcg, 660 mcg, 1 mg, 2 mg, 2.5 mg, 5 mg.
Tablet (controlled release): 1,000 mcg, 1,500 mcg.
Lozenges: 50 mcg, 100 mcg, 250 mcg, 500 mcg.
Injection: 1,000 mcg/mL.
Intranasal Gel: 500 mcg per actuation of 0.1 mL.

INDICATIONS AND DOSAGES

▸ RDA
PO
Children. 0.3–2 mcg.

▸ Vitamin B_{12} deficiency
IM/SC
Children. 0.2 mcg/kg for 2 days, then 1,000 mcg/day for 2–7 days followed by 100 mcg/wk for 1 mo.

▸ Supplement
PO
Children. 0.3–2 mcg/day.

CONTRAINDICATIONS

Folate-deficient anemia, hereditary optic nerve atrophy, a history of allergy to cobalamin.

INTERACTIONS

Drug

Alcohol, colchicines: May decrease the absorption of cyanocobalamin.
Ascorbic acid: May destroy vitamin B_{12} if used in large doses.
Folic acid (large doses): May decrease cyanocobalamin blood concentration.
Aminoglycosides, extended-release potassium, phenytoin, phenobarbital: May decrease the absorption of cyanocobalamin.

Herbal

None known.

Food

None known.

DIAGNOSTIC TEST EFFECTS

None known.

SIDE EFFECTS

Occasional
Diarrhea, itching

SERIOUS REACTIONS

! A rare allergic reaction, generally due to impurities in preparation, may occur.

! May produce peripheral vascular thrombosis, pulmonary edema, hypokalemia, and CHF.

PEDIATRIC CONSIDERATIONS

Baseline Assessment

- Be aware that cyanocobalamin crosses the placenta and is excreted in breast milk.
- There are no age-related precautions noted in children.

Administration and Handling

PO

- Give cyanocobalamin with meals to increase absorption.

IM/SC

- Avoid IV administration.
- Administer IM or deep SC.

INTRANASAL

- Administer 1 hr before or after ingestion of hot foods or liquids to avoid loss of drug from increased nasal secretions.

Intervention and Evaluation

- Assess the patient for signs and symptoms of CHF and hypokalemia, especially in pts receiving cyanocobalamin by the SC or IM route, and pulmonary edema.
- Monitor the patient's serum potassium levels, which normally ranges between 3.5 and 5 mEq/L, and serum B_{12} levels, which normally range between 200 and 800 mcg/mL. Also monitor the patient for a rise in the blood reticulocyte count, which peaks in 5–8 days.
- Evaluate the patient for reversal of deficiency symptoms including anorexia, ataxia, fatigue, hyporeflexia, insomnia, irritability, loss of positional sense, pallor, and palpitations on exertion.
- Know that the patient's therapeutic response to treatment is usually dramatic and occurs within 48 hrs.

Patient/Family Teaching

- Stress to the pernicious anemia patient that lifetime treatment may be necessary.
- Warn the patient/family to notify the physician if the patient experiences symptoms of an infection.
- Suggest to the patient/family that the patient eat foods rich in vitamin B_{12} including clams, dairy products, egg yolks, fermented cheese, herring, muscle meats, organ meats, oysters, and red snapper.

Folic Acid (Vitamin B_9)

foe-lick

(Apo-Folic [CAN], Folvite, Megafol [AUS])

Do not confuse with Florvite.

Sodium Folate

(Folvite-parenteral)

CATEGORY AND SCHEDULE

Pregnancy Risk Category: A (C if used at dosages exceeding the RDA)

OTC (0.4 mg and 0.8 mg tablets only)

MECHANISM OF ACTION

A coenzyme that stimulates production of platelets, RBCs, and WBCs. ***Therapeutic Effect:*** Essential for nucleoprotein synthesis and maintenance of normal erythropoiesis.

PHARMACOKINETICS

The oral form is almost completely absorbed from the GI tract (upper duodenum). Protein binding: High. Metabolized in liver and plasma to the active form.

Excreted in urine. Removed by hemodialysis.

AVAILABILITY

Tablets: 0.4 mg, 0.8 mg, 1 mg.
Injection: 5 mg/mL.

INDICATIONS AND DOSAGES

▸ **Vitamin B_9 deficiency**
IV/IM/SC/PO
Children older than 10 yrs. Initially, 1 mg/day. Maintenance: 0.5 mg/day.
Children 1–10 yrs. Initially 1 mg/day. Maintenance: 0.1–0.4 mg/day.
Infants. 50 mcg/day or 15 mcg/kg/dose.

▸ **Supplement**
PO/IM/IV/SC
Children older than 4 yrs. 0.4 mg/day.
Children 1–4 yrs. 0.3 mg/day.
Children younger than 1 yr. 0.1 mg/day.

UNLABELED USES

Decreases risk of colon cancer.

CONTRAINDICATIONS

Hypersensitivity to folic acid or any related component. Anemias (aplastic, normocytic, pernicious, and refractory).

INTERACTIONS

Drug

Analgesics, anticonvulsants, carbamazepine, estrogens: May increase folic acid requirements.
Antacids, cholestyramine: May decrease the absorption of folic acid.
Hydantoin anticonvulsants: May decrease the effects of these drugs.
Methotrexate, triamterene, trimethoprim: May antagonize the effects of folic acid.

Herbal

None known.

Food

None known.

DIAGNOSTIC TEST EFFECTS

May decrease vitamin B_{12} concentration.

SIDE EFFECTS

None known.

SERIOUS REACTIONS

! Allergic hypersensitivity occurs rarely with the parenteral form. Oral folic acid is nontoxic.

PEDIATRIC CONSIDERATIONS

Baseline Assessment

- Know that the physician will rule out pernicious anemia with a Schilling test and vitamin B_{12} blood level before beginning folic acid therapy because the signs of pernicious anemia may be masked while irreversible neurologic damage progresses.
- Know that resistance to treatment may occur if alcoholism, use of antimetabolic drugs, decreased hematopoiesis, or deficiency of vitamin B_6, B_{12}, C, or E is evident.
- Be aware that folic acid is distributed in breast milk.
- There are no age-related precautions noted in children.
- Be aware that the injectable form of folic acid contains benzyl alcohol, which may cause toxicity in neonates when given in large doses.

Administration and Handling

◂ **ALERT** ▸ Know that the parenteral form is used in acutely ill pts, pts receiving enteral or parenteral alimentation, and pts unresponsive to the oral route in GI malabsorption syndrome and that folic acid dosages greater than 0.1 mg/day may conceal signs of pernicious anemia.

Intervention and Evaluation

• Assess the patient for therapeutic improvement, an improved sense of well-being, and relief from iron deficiency symptoms, which include fatigue, headache, pallor, shortness of breath, and sore tongue.

Patient/Family Teaching

• Encourage the patient/family to eat foods rich in folic acid including fruits, organ meats, and vegetables.

Leucovorin Calcium (Folinic Acid, Citrovorum Factor)

lou-**koe**-vor-in

(Calcium Leucovorin [AUS], Lederle, Leucovorin, Wellcovorin)

Do not confuse with Wellbutrin or Wellferon.

CATEGORY AND SCHEDULE

Pregnancy Risk Category: C

MECHANISM OF ACTION

A folic acid antagonist that competes with methotrexate for the same transport processes into cells; limits methotrexate action on normal cells. ***Therapeutic Effect:*** Allows purine, DNA, RNA, and protein synthesis.

PHARMACOKINETICS

Readily absorbed from the GI tract. Widely distributed. Primarily concentrated in liver. Metabolized in liver and intestinal mucosa to the active metabolite. Primarily excreted in urine. ***Half-Life:*** 15 min (metabolite: 30–35 min).

AVAILABILITY

Tablets: 5 mg, 10 mg, 15 mg, 25 mg.
Injection: 10 mg/mL.
Powder for Injection: 50 mg, 100 mg, 200 mg, 350 mg, 500 mg.

INDICATIONS AND DOSAGES

▸ **Conventional rescue dosage**

IV

Children. 10 mg/m^2 parenterally one time then q6h orally until serum methotrexate level is less than 10^{-8} M. If 24-hr serum creatinine level is increased by 50% or more over baseline or methotrexate level is greater than 5×10^{-6} M or 48-hr level is greater than 9×10^{-7} M, increase to 100 mg/m^2 IV q3h until methotrexate level is less than 1×10^{-8} M.

▸ **Folic acid antagonist overdosage**

PO

Children. 2–15 mg/day for 3 days or 5 mg q3days.

▸ **Folate-deficient megaloblastic anemia**

IM

Children. 1 mg/day.

▸ **Megaloblastic anemia**

IM

Children. 3–6 mg/day.

▸ **Prevention of hematologic toxicity (for toxoplasmosis)**

IV/PO

Children. 5–10 mg/day, repeat q3days.

▸ **Prevention of hematologic toxicity, *Pneumocystis carnii* pneumonia**

IV/PO

Children. 25 mg once weekly.

UNLABELED USES

Ewing sarcoma, gestational trophoblastic neoplasms, non-Hodgkin lymphoma, treatment adjunct for head and neck carcinoma.

CONTRAINDICATIONS

Hypersensitivity to leucovorin or any related component. Pernicious anemia or other megaloblastic anemias secondary to vitamin B_{12} deficiency.

INTERACTIONS

Drug

5-Fluorouracil: May increase the effects and toxicity of 5-fluorouracil.
Anticonvulsants: May decrease the effects of anticonvulsants.

Herbal

None known.

Food

None known.

DIAGNOSTIC TEST EFFECTS

None known.

IV INCOMPATIBILITIES

Amphotericin B complex (Abelcet, AmBisome, Amphotec), droperidol (Inapsine), foscarnet (Foscavir)

IV COMPATIBILITIES

Cisplatin (Platinol AQ), cyclophosphamide (Cytoxan), doxorubicin (Adriamycin), etoposide (VePesid), filgrastim(Neupogen), fluorouracil, gemcitabine (Gemzar), granisetron (Kytril), heparin, methotrexate, metoclopramide (Reglan), mitomycin (Mutamycin), piperacillin-tazobactam (Zosyn), vinblastine (Velban), vincristine (Oncovin)

SIDE EFFECTS

Frequent
With 5-fluorouracil: Diarrhea, stomatitis, nausea, vomiting, lethargy or malaise or fatigue, alopecia, anorexia

Occasional
Urticaria, dermatitis

SERIOUS REACTIONS

! Excessive dosage may negate the chemotherapeutic effect of folic acid antagonists.
! Anaphylaxis occurs rarely.
! Diarrhea may cause rapid clinical deterioration and death.

PEDIATRIC CONSIDERATIONS

Baseline Assessment

- Give leucovorin, as prescribed, as soon as possible, preferably within 1 hr, for treatment of accidental overdosage of folic acid antagonists.
- Be aware that it is unknown whether leucovorin crosses the placenta or is distributed in breast milk.
- Be aware that leucovorin use in children may increase the risk of seizures by counteracting the anticonvulsant effects of barbiturate and hydantoins.

Precautions

- Use cautiously in pts with bronchial asthma and a history of allergies.
- Use leucovorin with 5-fluorouracil cautiously in pts with GI toxicities.
- Administer promptly. When time between doses is increased, the risk of significant loss of effectiveness increases.

Administration and Handling

◀ **ALERT** ▶ For rescue therapy in cancer chemotherapy, refer to the specific protocol being used for optimal dosage and sequence of leucovorin administration.

PO
- Scored tablets may be crushed.

IV
- Store vials for parenteral use at room temperature.

• Injection normally appears as clear, yellowish solution.
• Use immediately if reconstituted with Sterile Water for Injection; is stable for 7 days if reconstituted with Bacteriostatic Water for Injection.
• Reconstitute each 50-mg vial with 5 mL Sterile Water for Injection or Bacteriostatic Water for Injection containing benzyl alcohol to provide a concentration of 10 mg/mL.
• Because of benzyl alcohol in 1-mg ampule and in Bacteriostatic Water for Injection, reconstitute doses greater than 10 mg/m^2 with Sterile Water for Injection.
• Further dilute with D_5W or 0.9% NaCl.
• Do not exceed 160 mg/min if given by IV infusion (because of calcium content).
• Do not administer leucovorin intrathecally or intraventricularly.

Intervention and Evaluation

• Monitor the patient for vomiting, which may require a change from oral to parenteral therapy.
• Observe debilitated pts closely because of the risk of severe toxicities.
• Assess the patient's BUN, complete blood count, and serum creatinine level to assess renal function (important in leucovorin rescue).
• Assess electrolyte levels and liver function tests of pts also taking 5-fluorouracil in combination with leucovorin.

Patient/Family Teaching

• Explain to the patient/family the purpose of medication in the treatment of cancer.
• Warn the patient/family to notify the physician if the patient experiences an allergic reaction or vomiting.

Niacin, Nicotinic Acid

See antihyperlipidemics

Pyridoxine Hydrochloride (Vitamin B_6)

pie-rih-**docks**-in
(Hexa-Betalin [CAN], Pyridoxine, Pyroxin [AUS])
Do not confuse with paroxetine, pralidoxime, or Pyridium.

CATEGORY AND SCHEDULE

Pregnancy Risk Category: A (C if used as dose exceeding the RDA)
OTC

MECHANISM OF ACTION

A coenzyme for various metabolic functions that maintains metabolism of proteins, carbohydrates, and fats. Aids in release of liver and muscle glycogen and in the synthesis of γ-aminobutyric acid in the CNS.

PHARMACOKINETICS

Readily absorbed, primarily in jejunum. Stored in liver, muscle, and brain. Metabolized in liver. Primarily excreted in urine. Removed by hemodialysis. ***Half-Life:*** 15–20 days.

AVAILABILITY

Injection: 100 mg/mL.
Tablets: 25 mg, 50 mg, 100 mg, 250 mg, 500 mg.
Tablets (enteric coated): 20 mg.

INDICATIONS AND DOSAGES

▸ **Pyridoxine deficiency**

PO

Children. 5–25 mg/day for 3 wks, then 1.5–2.5 mg/day.

▸ **Seizures in neonates**

IM/IV

Neonates. 10–100 mg/day; then oral therapy of 50–100 mg/day for life.

▸ **Drug-induced neuritis**

PO

Children. 50–100 mg/day as treatment, then 1–2 mg/kg/day as prophylaxis.

▸ **RDA**

PO

Adolescents 14–19 yrs.
Males 1.3 mg; females 1.2 mg.
Children 9–13 yrs. 1 mg.
Children 4–8 yrs. 0.6 mg.
Children 1–3 yrs. 0.5 mg.

CONTRAINDICATIONS

Hypersensitivity to pyridoxine or any related component.

INTERACTIONS

Drug

Immunosuppressants, isoniazid, penicillamine: May antagonize pyridoxine (may cause anemia or peripheral neuritis).

Levodopa: Reverses the effects of levodopa.

Phenobarbital, phenytoin: May decrease the serum concentrations of these drugs.

Herbal

None known.

Food

None known.

DIAGNOSTIC TEST EFFECTS

False-positive urobilinogen spot test.

IV INCOMPATIBILITIES

Do not mix with any other medications.

SIDE EFFECTS

Occasional

Stinging at IM injection site

Rare

Headache, nausea, somnolence, High dosages cause sensory neuropathy (paresthesia, unstable gait, and clumsiness of hands).

SERIOUS REACTIONS

! Long-term megadoses (2–6 g over longer than 2 mos) may produce sensory neuropathy (reduced deep tendon reflex, profound impairment of sense of position in distal limbs, and gradual sensory ataxia). Toxic symptoms reverse with drug discontinuance.

! Seizures have occurred after IV megadoses.

PEDIATRIC CONSIDERATIONS

Baseline Assessment

• Be aware that pyridoxine crosses the placenta and is excreted in breast milk.

• Be aware that high dosages of pyridoxine in utero may produce seizures in neonates.

• There are no age-related precautions noted in children.

Administration and Handling

◂ **ALERT** ▸ Give orally unless malabsorption, nausea, or vomiting occurs. Avoid IV use in cardiac pts.

IV

• Give undiluted or may be added to IV solutions and given as infusion.

• Watch heart rate, blood pressure, and respiratory rate when administering large IV doses.

Intervention and Evaluation

• Observe the patient for improvement of deficiency symptoms, including nervous system abnormalities (anxiety, depression, insomnia, motor difficulty, peripheral numbness, and tremors), and skin lesions (glossitis and seborrhea-like lesions around the eyes, mouth, and nose).

- Evaluate the patient for nutritional adequacy.

Patient/Family Teaching

- Advise the patient/family that the patient may experience discomfort with IM injection.
- Encourage the patient/family to eat foods rich in pyridoxine, including avocados, bananas, bran, carrots, eggs, hazelnuts, legumes, organ meats, shrimp, soybeans, sunflower seeds, tuna, and wheat germ.

Thiamine Hydrochloride (Vitamin B_1)

thigh-ah-min
(Betalin, Betaxin [CAN])

CATEGORY AND SCHEDULE

Pregnancy Risk Category: A (C if used in dosages exceeding the RDA)
OTC (tablets)

MECHANISM OF ACTION

A water-soluble vitamin that combines with adenosine triphosphate in liver, kidney, and leukocytes to form thiamine diphosphate.
Therapeutic Effect: Necessary for carbohydrate metabolism.

PHARMACOKINETICS

Readily absorbed after IM administration. Poor oral absorption. Widely distributed. Metabolized in liver. Primarily excreted in urine.

AVAILABILITY

Tablets: 50 mg, 100 mg, 250 mg.
Tablets (enteric coated): 20 mg.
Injection: 100 mg/mL.

INDICATIONS AND DOSAGES

▸ **Dietary supplement**
PO
Children. 0.5–1 mg/day.
Infants. 0.3–0.5 mg/day.

▸ **Thiamine deficiency**
PO
Children. 10–50 mg/day in 3 divided doses.

▸ **Critically ill or malabsorption syndrome**
IM/IV
Children. 10–25 mg/day.

▸ **Metabolic disorders**
PO
Children. 10–20 mg/day; up to 4 g in divided doses/day.

▸ **RDA**
Adolescents 14–19 yrs. Male 1.2 mg; Female 1.1 mg.
Children 9–13 yrs. 0.9 mg.
Children 4–8 yrs. 0.6 mg.
Children 1–3 yrs. 0.5 mg.

CONTRAINDICATIONS

Hypersensitivity to thiamine or any related component.

INTERACTIONS

Drug

Neuromuscular blocking agents: Thiamine may increase the effects of these drugs.

Herbal

None known.

Food

None known.

DIAGNOSTIC TEST EFFECTS

False-positive for uric acid and urobilinogen. Large doses may alter the determination of theophylline concentrations.

IV COMPATIBILITIES

Famotidine (Pepcid), multivitamins

SIDE EFFECTS

Frequent

Pain, induration, tenderness at IM injection site

SERIOUS REACTIONS

! Rare, severe hypersensitivity reaction with IV administration may result in feeling of warmth, pruritus, urticaria, weakness, diaphoresis, nausea, restlessness, tightness in the throat, angioedema (swelling of the face or lips), cyanosis, pulmonary edema, GI tract bleeding, and cardiovascular collapse.

PEDIATRIC CONSIDERATIONS

Baseline Assessment

- Be aware that thiamine crosses the placenta and that it is unknown whether thiamine is excreted in breast milk.
- There are no age-related precautions noted in children.

Administration and Handling

◂ALERT▸ Know that the IM and IV routes of administration are used only in acutely ill pts or in those who are unresponsive to the PO route, such as pts with GI malabsorption syndrome. Be aware that the IM route is preferred to the IV route. Give by IV push, or add to most IV solutions and give as an infusion.

Intervention and Evaluation

- Monitor the patient's EKG and laboratory values for erythrocyte count.
- Assess the patient for signs and symptoms of improvement, including an improved sense of well-being and weight gain.
- Observe the patient for reversal of deficiency symptoms. For neurologic signs and symptoms, expect a decrease in peripheral neuropathy, ataxia, hyporeflexia, muscle weakness, nystagmus, ophthalmoplegia, and peripheral neuropathy. For cardiac signs and symptoms, assess for a decrease in peripheral edema, a bounding arterial pulse, tachycardia, and venous hypertension. Also assess for a decreased confused state.

Patient/Family Teaching

- Advise the patient/family that the patient may experience discomfort with IM injection.
- Encourage the patient/family to consume foods rich in thiamine including legumes, nuts, organ meats, pork, rice, bran, seeds, wheat germ, whole grain and enriched cereals, and yeast.
- Advise the patient/family that the patient's urine may appear bright yellow during thiamine therapy.

Vitamin A

(Aquasol A)

Do not confuse with Anusol.

CATEGORY AND SCHEDULE

Pregnancy Risk Category: A (X if used in dosages exceeding the RDA)

MECHANISM OF ACTION

A fat-soluble vitamin that may be a cofactor in biochemical reactions. ***Therapeutic Effect:*** Is essential for normal function of retina. Necessary for visual adaptation to darkness, bone growth, testicular and ovarian function, embryonic development; preserves integrity of epithelial cells.

PHARMACOKINETICS

Absorption is dependent on bile salts, pancreatic lipase, and dietary fat. Transported in blood to liver, stored in parenchymal liver cells, and then transported in plasma as retinol, as needed. Metabolized in liver. Excreted in bile and, to a lesser amount, in urine.

AVAILABILITY

Capsules: 8,000 units, 10,000 units, 15,000 units, 25,000 units.
Injection: 50,000 units/mL.
Tablets: 5,000 units, 10,000 units, 15,000 units.

INDICATIONS AND DOSAGES

▸ **Severe deficiency with xerophthalmia**

IM

Children older than 8 yrs. 50,000–100,000 units/day for 3 days, then 50,000 units/day for 14 days.
Children 1–8 yrs. 17,500–35,000 units/day for 10 days.

PO

Children older than 8 yrs. 500,000 units/day for 3 days, then 50,000 units/day for 14 days, then 10,000–20,000 units/day for 2 mo.
Children 1–8 yrs. 5,000 units/kg/day for 5 days or until recovery occurs.

▸ **Malabsorption syndrome**

PO

Children older than 8 yrs. 10,000–50,000 units/day.

▸ **Dietary supplement**

PO

Children 7–10 yrs. 3,300–3,500 units/day.
Children 4–6 yrs. 2,500 units/day.
Children 6 mos–3 yrs. 1,500–2,000 units/day.
Neonates younger than 6 mos. 1,500 units/day.

▸ **RDA**

Adolescents. Male 1,000 mcg (3,330 units); female 800 mcg (2,670 units).
Children 7–10 yrs. 2,330 units.
Children 4–6 yrs. 1,670 units.
Children 1–3 yrs. 1,330 units.
Infants younger than 1 yr. 1,250 units.

CONTRAINDICATIONS

Hypersensitivity to vitamin A or any related component; hypervitaminosis A, oral use in malabsorption syndrome.

INTERACTIONS

Drug

Cholestyramine, colestipol, mineral oil: May decrease the absorption of vitamin A.
Isotretinoin: May increase the risk of toxicity.
Warfarin: Increases the effects of warfarin.

Herbal

None known.

Food

None known.

DIAGNOSTIC TEST EFFECTS

May increase BUN, serum cholesterol, serum calcium, and serum triglyceride levels. May decrease blood erythrocyte and leukocyte counts.

SIDE EFFECTS

None known.

SERIOUS REACTIONS

! Chronic overdosage produces malaise, nausea, vomiting, drying or cracking of skin or lips, inflammation of tongue or gums, irritability, loss of hair, and night sweats.
! Bulging fontanelles in infants have been noted.

PEDIATRIC CONSIDERATIONS

Baseline Assessment

- Be aware that vitamin A crosses the placenta and is distributed in breast milk.
- Use vitamin A with caution at higher doses in children.

Precautions

- Use cautiously in pts with renal impairment.

Administration and Handling

◂ **ALERT** ▸ Know that the IM route of administration is used only in acutely ill pts or pts unresponsive to the oral route, such as those with GI malabsorption syndrome.

PO

- Do not crush, open, or break capsule form.
- Give vitamin A without regard to food.

IM

- For IM injection in adults, if dosage is 1 mL (50,000 units), may give in deltoid muscle; if dosage is greater than 1 mL, give in gluteus maximus muscle. Know that the anterolateral thigh is the site of choice for infants and children younger than 7 mos.

Intervention and Evaluation

- Closely assess the patient for overdosage symptoms during prolonged daily administration greater than 25,000 units.
- Monitor the patient for therapeutic serum vitamin A levels, 180–300 units/mL.

Patient/Family Teaching

- Encourage the patient/family to consume foods rich in vitamin A, including cod, halibut, tuna, and shark. Explain to the patient/family that naturally occurring vitamin A is found only in animal sources.
- Warn the patient/family to avoid taking cholestyramine (Questran) and mineral oil during vitamin A therapy.

Vitamin D

calcitriol
(Calcijex [AUS], Rocaltrol)

Dihydrotachysterol

(DHT, Hytakerol)

Ergocalciferol

(Calciferol, Deltalin, Drisdol, Ostelin [AUS])

Paricalcitol

(Zemplar)

CATEGORY AND SCHEDULE

Pregnancy Risk Category: A (D if used in dosages exceeding the RDA)

MECHANISM OF ACTION

A fat-soluble vitamin that is essential for absorption, utilization of calcium phosphate, and normal calcification of bone. ***Therapeutic Effect:*** Stimulates calcium and phosphate absorption from the small intestine, promotes secretion of calcium from bone to blood, promotes renal tubule phosphate resorption, and acts on bone cells to stimulate skeletal growth and on parathyroid gland to suppress hormone synthesis and secretion.

PHARMACOKINETICS

Readily absorbed from the small intestine with the presence of bile. Concentrated primarily in liver and fat deposits. Activated in liver and kidney. Eliminated via the

biliary system; excreted in urine.
Half-Life: Calcifediol: 10–22 days.
Calcitriol: 3–6 hrs.
Ergocalciferol: 19–48 hrs.

AVAILABILITY

Calcitriol (Calcijex, Rocaltrol)
Capsule: 0.25 mcg, 0.5 mcg.
Injection: 1 mcg/mL, 2 mcg/mL.
Oral Solution: 1 mcg/mL.
Dihydrotachysterol (DHT)
Oral Solution: 0.2 mg/mL.
Tablets: 0.125 mg, 0.2 mg, 0.4 mg.
Ergocalciferol (Calciferol, Drisdol)
Capsules: 50,000 units.
Liquid Drops: 8,000 units/mL.
Paricalcitol (Zemplar)
Injection: 2 mcg/mL, 5 mcg/mL.

INDICATIONS AND DOSAGES

▸ **Dietary supplement**
PO
Children. 10 mcg (400 units)/day.
Neonates. 10–20 mcg (400–800 units)/day.
▸ **Renal failure**
PO
Children. 0.1–1 mg/day.
▸ **Hypoparathyroidism**
PO
Children. 1.25–5 mg/day (with calcium supplements).
▸ **Vitamin D-dependent rickets**
PO
Children. 75–125 mcg/day.
Maximum: 1,500 mcg/day.
▸ **Nutritional rickets and osteomalacia**
PO
Children. 25–125 mcg/day for 8–12 wks.
Children (malabsorption). 250–625 mcg/day.
▸ **Vitamin D-resistant rickets**
PO
Children. Initially 1,000–2,000 mcg/day (with phosphate supplements). May increase at 3- to 4-mo intervals in 250- to 500-mcg increments.

CONTRAINDICATIONS

Hypercalcemia, malabsorption syndrome, vitamin D toxicity.

INTERACTIONS

Drug
Aluminum-containing antacid (long-term use): May increase aluminum concentration and aluminum bone toxicity.
Calcium-containing preparations, thiazide diuretics: May increase the risk of hypercalcemia.
Magnesium-containing antacids: May increase magnesium concentration.
Herbal
None known.
Food
None known.

DIAGNOSTIC TEST EFFECTS

May increase serum cholesterol, calcium, magnesium, and phosphate levels. May decrease serum alkaline phosphatase level.

SIDE EFFECTS

Nausea, vomiting, loss of appetite, constipation, metallic taste

SERIOUS REACTIONS

! Early signs of overdosage are manifested as weakness, headache, somnolence, nausea, vomiting, dry mouth, constipation, muscle and bone pain, and metallic taste sensation.
! Later signs of overdosage are evidenced by polyuria, polydipsia, anorexia, weight loss, nocturia, photophobia, rhinorrhea, pruritus, disorientation, hallucinations, hyperthermia, hypertension, and cardiac arrhythmias.

PEDIATRIC CONSIDERATIONS

Baseline Assessment

• Know that vitamin D therapy should begin at the lowest possible dosage.
• Be aware that it is unknown whether vitamin D crosses the placenta or is distributed in breast milk.
• Be aware that children may be more sensitive to the effects of vitamin D.
• Assess for and monitor weight and development.

Precautions

• Use cautiously in pts with coronary artery disease, kidney stones, and renal impairment.

Administration and Handling

◂ **ALERT** ▸ 1 mcg = 40 units.

PO

Give vitamin D without regard to food.
• Have the patient swallow the vitamin whole and avoid crushing, chewing, or opening the capsules.

Intervention and Evaluation

• Monitor the patient's BUN, serum alkaline phosphatase, serum calcium, serum creatinine, serum magnesium, serum phosphate, and urinary calcium levels. Know that the therapeutic serum calcium level is 9–10 mg/dL.
• Estimate the patient's daily dietary calcium intake.
• Encourage the patient to maintain adequate fluid intake.

Patient/Family Teaching

• Encourage the patient/family to consume foods rich in vitamin D including eggs, leafy vegetables, margarine, meats, milk, vegetable oils, and vegetable shortening.
• Warn the patient/family not to take mineral oil during vitamin D therapy.
• Advise the patient/family receiving chronic renal dialysis not to take magnesium-containing antacids during vitamin D therapy.
• Encourage the patient/family to drink plenty of liquids.

Vitamin E

(Aquasol E)

Do not confuse with Anusol.

CATEGORY AND SCHEDULE

Pregnancy Risk Category: A (C if used in dosages exceeding the RDA)

OTC

MECHANISM OF ACTION

An antioxidant that prevents oxidation of vitamins A and C, protects fatty acids from attack by free radicals, and protects RBCs from hemolysis by oxidizing agents.

PHARMACOKINETICS

Variably absorbed from the GI tract (requires bile salts, dietary fat, normal pancreatic function). Primarily concentrated in adipose tissue. Metabolized in liver. Primarily eliminated via the biliary system.

AVAILABILITY

Capsules: 100 units, 200 units, 400 units, 600 units, 800 units, 1,000 units.

Tablets: 100 units, 200 units, 400 units, 500 units, 800 units.

Oral Drops: 15 units/0.3 mL.

INDICATIONS AND DOSAGES

▸ **Vitamin E deficiency**

PO

Children. 1 unit/kg/day.
Neonates. 25–50 unit/day until 6–19 wks of age or 7 unit/L of formula.

▸ **Cholestasis, biliary atresia, fat malabsorption**

PO

Children. Water-soluble form: 15–25 units/kg/day, decreased as levels reach normal.

▸ **Cystic fibrosis**

PO

Children. 100–400 units/day.

▸ **β-Thalassemia**

PO

Children. 750 units/day.

▸ **Sickle cell anemia**

PO

Children. 450 units/day.

UNLABELED USES

Decreases severity of tardive dyskinesia.

CONTRAINDICATIONS

Hypersensitivity to vitamin E or any related component.

INTERACTIONS

Drug

Cholestyramine, colestipol, mineral oil: May decrease the absorption of vitamin E.
Iron (large doses): May increase vitamin E requirements.
Warfarin: May increase the effects of warfarin.

Herbal

None known.

Food

None known.

DIAGNOSTIC TEST EFFECTS

None known.

SIDE EFFECTS

Mild nausea, diarrhea, intestinal cramps, headache

SERIOUS REACTIONS

! Chronic overdosage produces fatigue, weakness, nausea, headache, blurred vision, flatulence, and diarrhea.

PEDIATRIC CONSIDERATIONS

Baseline Assessment

- Be aware that it is unknown whether vitamin E crosses the placenta or is distributed in breast milk.
- There are no age-related precautions noted for normal dosages in children.
- Necrotizing enterocolitis has been associated with large oral doses of vitamin E (greater than 200 units/day) in low-birth-weight infants.

Precautions

- Vitamin E use may impair the hematologic response in pts with iron deficiency anemia.

Administration and Handling

PO

- Do not crush, open, or break capsules or tablets.
- Give vitamin E without regard to food.

Patient/Family Teaching

- Instruct the patient/family to swallow capsules whole and not to chew, open, or crush them.
- Warn the patient/family to notify the physician if the patient experiences signs and symptoms of toxicity including blurred vision, diarrhea, dizziness, flu-like symptoms, headache, and nausea.
- Encourage the patient/family to consume foods rich in vitamin E, including eggs, leafy vegetables,

margarine, meats, milk, vegetable oils, and vegetable shortening.

Vitamin K
(vitamin K_1)

Phytonadione
fy-toe-na-**dye**-own
(AquaMEPHYTON, Mephyton)
Do not confuse with melphalan or mephenytoin.

CATEGORY AND SCHEDULE
Pregnancy Risk Category: C

MECHANISM OF ACTION
A fat-soluble vitamin that is necessary for hepatic formation of coagulation factors II, VII, IX, and X. ***Therapeutic Effect:*** Essential for normal clotting of blood.

PHARMACOKINETICS
Readily absorbed from the GI tract (duodenum) in the presence of bile, after IM or SC administration. Metabolized in liver. Excreted in urine, eliminated via the biliary system. Parenteral: Controls hemorrhage within 3–6 hrs and normal prothrombin time in 12–14 hrs. PO: Effect in 6–10 hrs.

AVAILABILITY
Tablets: 5 mg.
Injection: 2 mg/mL, 10 mg/mL.

INDICATIONS AND DOSAGES
▸ **Oral anticoagulant overdose**
IV/SC/PO
Children. 0.5–5 mg, depending on the need for further anticoagulation and severity of bleeding.
▸ **Vitamin K deficiency**
IV/IM/SC
Children. 1–2 mg/dose as a single dose.
PO
Children. 2.5–5 mg/24 hrs.
▸ **Hemorrhagic disease in newborn**
IM/SC
Neonate. Treatment: 1–2 mg/day. Prophylaxis: 0.5–1 mg within 1 hr of birth. May repeat in 6–8 hrs if necessary.

CONTRAINDICATIONS
Hypersensitivity to phytonadione or any related component.

INTERACTIONS
Drug
Broad-spectrum antibiotics, high-dose salicylates: May increase vitamin K requirements.
Cholestyramine, colestipol, mineral oil, sucralfate: May decrease the absorption of vitamin K.
Oral anticoagulants: May decrease the effects of these drugs.
Herbal
None known.
Food
None known.

DIAGNOSTIC TEST EFFECTS
None known.

IV INCOMPATIBILITIES
No known incompatibility noted via Y-site administration.

IV COMPATIBILITIES
Heparin, potassium chloride

SIDE EFFECTS
Occasional
Pain; soreness; swelling at IM injection site; with repeated injections, pruritic erythema, flushed face, unusual taste

SERIOUS REACTIONS

! Vitamin K may produce hyperbilirubinemia in newborns (especially premature infants).

! Rarely, severe reaction occurs immediately after IV administration (cramplike pain, chest pain, dyspnea, facial flushing, dizziness, rapid or weak pulse, rash, diaphoresis, hypotension that may progress to shock, and cardiac arrest).

PEDIATRIC CONSIDERATIONS

Baseline Assessment

- Be aware that vitamin K crosses the placenta and is distributed in breast milk.
- There are no age-related precautions noted in children.

Administration and Handling

◂ALERT▸ The SC route is preferred. IV/IM routes are restricted to emergency situations.

◂ALERT▸ Know that the PO or SC route of administration is less likely to produce side effects than the IM or IV route.

PO

- Scored tablets may be crushed.

SC/IM

- Inject into the anterolateral aspect of the thigh or deltoid region.

IV

- Store at room temperature.
- May dilute with preservative-free 0.9% NaCl or D_5W immediately before use. Do not use other diluents. Discard unused portions.
- Administer IV infusion slowly at a rate of 1 mg/min.
- Monitor the patient continuously for signs and symptoms of hypersensitivity.
- Monitor the patient for an anaphylactic reaction during and immediately after IV administration.

Intervention and Evaluation

- Monitor the international normalized ratio and prothrombin time routinely in pts taking anticoagulants.
- Examine the patient's skin for bruises and petechiae.
- Assess the patient's gums for erythema and gingival bleeding.
- Test the patient's urine for hematuria.
- Assess the patient's blood Hct level, platelet count, and stool and urine samples for occult blood.
- Monitor the patient for abdominal or back pain, a decrease in blood pressure, an increase in pulse rate, and severe headache, which may indicate hemorrhage.
- Determine whether the patient has an increase in the amount of discharge during menses.
- Assess the patient's peripheral pulses.
- Examine the patient for excessive bleeding from minor cuts and scratches.

Patient/Family Teaching

- Advise the patient/family that the patient may experience discomfort with parenteral administration.
- Warn the patient/family to notify the physician if the patient experiences black or red stool, coffee-ground vomitus, red or dark urine, or red-speckled mucus from cough.
- Caution the patient/family against taking any other medications, including OTC preparations, without physician approval because they may interfere with platelet aggregation.
- Encourage the patient/family to consume foods rich in vitamin K, including cow's milk, egg yolks, leafy green vegetables, meat, tomatoes, and vegetable oil.

REFERENCES

Miller, S. & Fioravanti, J. (1997). Pediatric medications: a handbook for nurses. St. Louis: Mosby.

Taketomo, C. K., Hodding, J. H. & Kraus, D. M. (2003–2004). Pediatric dosage handbook (10th ed.). Hudson, OH: Lexi-Comp.

72 Cholinergics

Bethanechol Chloride
Neostigmine
Physostigmine
Pyridostigmine Bromide

Uses: Cholinergics are primarily used to treat urine retention and myasthenia gravis and to reverse nondepolarizing neuromuscular blockade. Neostigmine is used to prevent postoperative urine retention and to diagnose myasthenia gravis. Physostigmine and pilocarpine are used to treat glaucoma. Physostigmine is also used to reverse anticholinergic and tricyclic antidepressant toxicity.

Action: Some cholinergics, such as bethanechol and pilocarpine, directly bind to cholinergic (muscarinic) receptors and activate them, mimicking the action of acetylcholine. Others, such as neostigmine and physostigmine, inhibit the enzyme acetylcholinesterase, preventing the destruction of acetylcholine. Cholinergic agents mainly affect the heart, exocrine glands, and smooth muscle. In the heart, they can lead to bradycardia. In the exocrine glands, they may increase sweating, salivation, and bronchial secretions. In smooth muscle, they promote contraction. Several also stimulate ciliary muscles, leading to miosis.

Bethanechol Chloride

be-**than**-eh-coal
(Duvoid [CAN], Myotonachol [CAN], Urecholine)
Do not confuse with betaxolol.

CATEGORY AND SCHEDULE

Pregnancy Risk Category: C

MECHANISM OF ACTION

A cholinergic that acts directly at cholinergic receptors of smooth muscle of urinary bladder and the GI tract. Increases tone of the detrusor muscle. ***Therapeutic Effect:*** May initiate micturition and bladder emptying. Stimulates gastric and intestinal motility.

AVAILABILITY

Tablets: 5 mg, 10 mg, 25 mg, 50 mg.

INDICATIONS AND DOSAGES

▸ **Postoperative and postpartum urinary retention, atony of bladder**

PO

Children. 0.6 mg/kg/day in 3–4 divided doses.

SC

Children. 0.1–0.2 mg/kg/dose given 0.5–1 hr before meals. Maximum: 4 doses/day.

UNLABELED USES

Treatment of congenital megacolon, gastroesophageal reflux, postoperative gastric atony.

CONTRAINDICATIONS

Hypersensitivity to bethanechol or any related component. Active or latent bronchial asthma, acute inflammatory GI tract conditions, anastomosis, bladder wall instability, cardiac disease, coronary artery disease, epilepsy, hypertension, hyperthyroidism, hypotension, mechanical GI and urinary obstruction or recent GI resection, parkinsonism, peptic ulcer, pronounced bradycardia, vasomotor instability.

INTERACTIONS

Drug

Cholinesterase inhibitors: May increase the effects and risk of toxicity of bethanechol.
Procainamide, quinidine: May decrease the effects of bethanechol.
Anticholinergic agents: May decrease the effects of bethanechol.

Herbal

None known.

Food

None known.

DIAGNOSTIC TEST EFFECTS

May increase serum amylase, lipase, and SGOT (AST) levels.

SIDE EFFECTS

Occasional

Belching, change in vision, blurred vision, diarrhea, frequent urinary urgency

Rare

SC: Shortness of breath, chest tightness, bronchospasm

SERIOUS REACTIONS

! Overdosage produces CNS stimulation, including insomnia, nervousness, and orthostatic hypotension, and cholinergic stimulation, such as headache, increased salivation and sweating, nausea, vomiting, flushed skin, stomach pain, and seizures.

PEDIATRIC CONSIDERATIONS

Baseline Assessment

- Avoid giving IM or IV because it will precipitate a violent cholinergic reaction, including bloody diarrhea, circulatory collapse, myocardial infarction, severe hypotension, and shock. The antidote is 0.6–1.2 mg atropine sulfate.

Administration and Handling

◀ **ALERT** ▶ Realize that the side effects are more noticeable with SC administration.

Intervention and Evaluation

- Assess the patient for a cholinergic reaction manifested as blurred vision, excessive salivation and sweating, a feeling of facial warmth, GI cramping or discomfort, lacrimation, pallor, and urinary urgency.
- Observe the patient for difficulty chewing or swallowing and progressive muscle weakness.
- Measure and record fluid intake and output.

Patient/Family Teaching

- Tell the patient/family to notify the physician if the patient experiences diarrhea, difficulty breathing, increased salivary secretions, irregular heartbeat, muscle weakness, nausea, severe abdominal pain, sweating, and vomiting.

Neostigmine

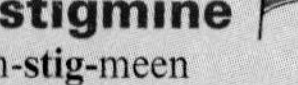

nee-oh-**stig**-meen
(Prostigmin)
Do not confuse with physostigmine.

CATEGORY AND SCHEDULE

Pregnancy Risk Category: C

MECHANISM OF ACTION

A cholinergic that prevents destruction of acetylcholine by attaching to the enzyme, anticholinesterase. ***Therapeutic Effect:*** Improves intestinal and skeletal muscle tone; increases secretions and salivation.

AVAILABILITY

Injection: 0.5 mg/mL, 1 mg/mL.
Tablets: 15 mg.

INDICATIONS AND DOSAGES

▸ Myasthenia gravis

PO

Children. 2 mg/kg/day or 60 mg/m²/day every 3–4 hrs. Maximum: 375 mg/day.

SC/IM/IV

Children. 0.01–0.04 mg/kg q2–4h.

▸ Diagnosis of myasthenia gravis

IM

Children. 0.025–0.04 mg/kg IM preceded by atropine sulfate 0.011 mg/kg SC.

▸ Reversal of neuromuscular blockade

IV

Children. 0.025–0.08 mg/kg/dose with atropine or glycopyrrolate.
Infants. 0.025–0.1 mg/kg/dose with atropine or glycopyrrolate.

CONTRAINDICATIONS

Hypersensitivity to neostigmine, bromides, or any related component. GI and GU obstruction, peritonitis.

INTERACTIONS

Drug

Anticholinergics: Reverse or prevent the effects of neostigmine.
Cholinesterase inhibitors: May increase the risk of toxicity.
Neuromuscular blocking agents: Antagonizes neuromuscular blocking agents.
Procainamide, quinidine: May antagonize the action of neostigmine.

Herbal

None known.

Food

None known.

DIAGNOSTIC TEST EFFECTS

None known.

IV INCOMPATIBILITIES

None known.

IV COMPATIBILITIES

Glycopyrrolate (Robinul), heparin, ondansetron (Zofran), potassium chloride, thiopental (Pentothal)

SIDE EFFECTS

Frequent

Muscarinic effects, including diarrhea, increased sweating or watering of mouth, nausea, vomiting, and stomach cramps or pain

Occasional

Muscarinic effects, including increased frequency or urge to urinate, increased bronchial secretions, and unusually small pupils or watering of eyes

SERIOUS REACTIONS

! Overdose produces a cholinergic reaction manifested as abdominal discomfort or cramping, nausea, vomiting, diarrhea, flushing, a feeling of warmth or heat about the face, excessive salivation and sweating, lacrimation, pallor, bradycardia or tachycardia, hypotension, urinary urgency, blurred vision, bronchospasm, pupillary contraction, and involuntary muscular contraction visible under the skin.

PEDIATRIC CONSIDERATIONS

Baseline Assessment

• Expect to give larger doses at the time of the patient's greatest fatigue.

• Avoid giving large doses to pts with megacolon or reduced GI motility.

Precautions

• Use cautiously in pts with arrhythmias, asthma, bradycardia, epilepsy, hyperthyroidism, peptic ulcer disease, and a recent coronary artery occlusion.

Administration and Handling

◀ **ALERT** ▶ Discontinue all anticholinesterase therapy at least 8 hrs before testing, as prescribed. Plan to give 0.011 mg/kg atropine sulfate IV simultaneously with neostigmine or IM 30 min before administering neostigmine to prevent adverse effects.

Intervention and Evaluation

• Monitor the patient's muscle strength and vital signs.

• Monitor the patient for a therapeutic response to the drug, decreased fatigue, improved chewing and swallowing, and increased muscle strength.

• Monitor the patient's fluid intake and output.

• Palpate the patient's bladder for signs of distension.

Patient/Family Teaching

• Warn the patient/family to notify the physician if the patient experiences diarrhea, difficulty breathing, increased salivary secretions, irregular heartbeat, muscle weakness, nausea, severe abdominal pain, sweating, and vomiting.

• Tell the patient/family to keep a log of the patient's energy levels and muscle strength to get a better idea of drug dosing.

Physostigmine

(Antilirium)

Do not confuse with Prostigmin or pyridostigmine.

CATEGORY AND SCHEDULE

Pregnancy Risk Category: C

MECHANISM OF ACTION

A parasympathomimetic (cholinergic) that inhibits destruction of acetylcholine by the enzyme acetylcholinesterase. ***Therapeutic Effect:*** Improves skeletal muscle tone; stimulates salivary and sweat gland secretion.

AVAILABILITY

Injection: 1 mg/mL.

INDICATIONS AND DOSAGES

▸ **Antidote**

IM/IV

Children. 0.01–0.03 mg/kg/dose. May give additional doses at 5- to 10-min intervals until response occurs, adverse cholinergic effects occur, or a total dose of 2 mg is given.

UNLABELED USES

Systemic: Treatment of hereditary ataxia.

CONTRAINDICATIONS

Active uveal inflammation, angle-closure (narrow-angle) glaucoma before iridectomy, asthma, cardiovascular disease, diabetes, gangrene, glaucoma associated with iridocyclitis, hypersensitivity to cholinesterase inhibitors or any component of the preparation, mechanical obstruction of the intestinal and urogenital tract, pts receiving ganglionic blocking agents, vagotonic state.

INTERACTIONS

Drug

Cholinesterase agents, including bethanechol and carbachol: May increase the effects of cholinesterase agents.
Succinylcholine: May prolong the action of succinylcholine.

Herbal

None known.

Food

None known.

DIAGNOSTIC TEST EFFECTS

None known.

SIDE EFFECTS

Expected

Miosis, increased GI and skeletal muscle tone, reduced pulse rate

Occasional

Hypertensive pts may react with a marked fall in blood pressure.

Rare

Allergic reaction

SERIOUS REACTIONS

! Parenteral overdosage produces a cholinergic reaction manifested as abdominal discomfort or cramping, nausea, vomiting, diarrhea, flushing, a feeling of warmth or heat about the face, excessive salivation, diaphoresis, urinary urgency, and blurred vision. This requires a withdrawal of all anticholinergic drugs and immediate use of 0.6–1.2 mg atropine sulfate IM/IV for adults or 0.01 mg/kg for infants and children younger than 12 yrs of age.

PEDIATRIC CONSIDERATIONS

Baseline Assessment

- Have tissues readily available at the patient's bedside.
- Plan to discontinue ophthalmic physostigmine at least 3 wks before ophthalmic surgery.
- Be aware that injectable solutions may contain benzyl alcohol, which has been associated with fatal gasping syndrome in neonates.

Precautions

- Use cautiously in pts with bradycardia, bronchial asthma, disorders that may respond adversely to vagotonic effects, epilepsy, GI disturbances, hypotension, parkinsonism, peptic ulcer disease, and recent myocardial infarction.
- Expect to use ophthalmic physostigmine only when shorter-acting miotics are not adequate, except in aphakic pts.

Intervention and Evaluation

- Assess the patient's vital signs immediately before and every 15–30 min after parenteral physostigmine administration.
- Monitor the patient for a cholinergic reaction, such as abdominal pain, dyspnea, hypotension, irregular heartbeat, muscle weakness, and sweating, after parenteral physostigmine administration.

Patient/Family Teaching

- Tell the patient/family that the adverse effects of the drug often subside after the first few days of therapy.
- Warn the patient/family to avoid night driving and activities requiring visual acuity in dim light during physostigmine therapy.

Pyridostigmine Bromide

pier-id-oh-**stig**-meen
(Mestinon, Regonol)
Do not confuse with mesantoin, Metatensin, physostigmine, Renagel, Reglan, or Regroton.

CATEGORY AND SCHEDULE

Pregnancy Risk Category: C

MECHANISM OF ACTION

An anticholinesterase that prevents destruction of acetylcholine by the enzyme anticholinesterase.
Therapeutic Effect: Produces miosis; increases tone of intestinal and skeletal muscles; stimulates salivary and sweat gland secretions.

AVAILABILITY

Tablets: 60 mg.
Tablets (sustained release): 180 mg.
Syrup: 60 mg/5 mL.
Injection: 5 mg/mL.

INDICATIONS AND DOSAGES

▸ Myasthenia gravis

PO

Children. Initially, 7 mg/kg/day in 5–6 divided doses.
Neonates. 5 mg q4–6h.

IM

Children and neonates. 0.05–0.15 mg/kg q4–6h. Maximum single dose: 10 mg.

▸ Reversal of nondepolarizing muscle relaxants

IM/IV

Children. 0.1–0.25 mg/kg/dose preceded by atropine or glycopyrrolate.

CONTRAINDICATIONS

Hypersensitivity to pyridostigmine, bromides, or any related component. Mechanical GI and urinary obstruction.

INTERACTIONS

Drug

Anticholinergics: Prevents or reverses the effects of pyridostigmine.
Cholinesterase inhibitors: May increase the risk of toxicity.
Neuromuscular blocking agents: Antagonizes neuromuscular blocking agents.
Procainamide, quinidine: May antagonize the action of pyridostigmine.

Herbal

None known.

Food

None known.

DIAGNOSTIC TEST EFFECTS

None known.

IV INCOMPATIBILITIES

Do not mix with any other medications.

SIDE EFFECTS

Frequent
Miosis, increased GI and skeletal muscle tone, reduced pulse rate, constriction of bronchi and ureters, salivary and sweat gland secretion

Occasional
Headache, rash, a slight temporary decrease in diastolic blood pressure (B/P) with mild reflex tachycardia, short periods of atrial fibrillation in hyperthyroid pts, a marked fall in B/P with hypertensive pts

SERIOUS REACTIONS

! Overdosage may produce a cholinergic crisis, manifested by increasingly severe muscle weakness that appears first in muscles involving chewing and swallowing, followed by muscular weakness of the shoulder girdle and upper extremities and respiratory muscle paralysis followed by pelvis girdle and leg muscle paralysis. This requires withdrawal of all cholinergic drugs and immediate use of 1–4 mg atropine sulfate IV for adults or 0.01 mg/kg for infants and children younger than 12 yrs of age.

PEDIATRIC CONSIDERATIONS

Baseline Assessment

• Give larger doses at the time of the patient's greatest fatigue.
• Assess the patient's muscle strength before testing for diagnosis of myasthenia gravis and after drug administration.
• Avoid giving large doses in pts with megacolon or reduced GI motility.
• Use caution with children who have asthma or experience seizures.
• The injection contains benzyl alcohol, which may cause allergic reactions in those pts who are sensitive. Large doses of benzyl alcohol have been associated with serious and/or fatal toxicity in neonates.

Precautions

• Use cautiously in pts with bradycardia, bronchial asthma, cardiac arrhythmias, epilepsy, hyperthyroidism, peptic ulcer disease, a recent coronary artery occlusion, and vagotonia.

Administration and Handling

◂ **ALERT** ▸ Remember that drug dosage and frequency of administration depend on the daily clinical patient response, including exacerbations, physical and emotional stress, and remissions.

PO

• Give pyridostigmine with food or milk.
• Crush tablets as needed. Instruct pts that extended-release tablets may be broken but not to chew or crush them.
• Give larger doses at times of increased fatigue, for example, for pts who have difficulty chewing, give 30–45 min before meals.

IM/IV

• Give large parenteral doses concurrently with 0.6–1.2 mg atropine sulfate IV, as prescribed, to minimize side effects.

Intervention and Evaluation

• Monitor the patient's respirations closely during myasthenia gravis testing or if dosage is increased.
• Assess the patient diligently for a cholinergic reaction, as well as bradycardia in the myasthenic patient in crisis.
• Coordinate dosage time versus periods of patient fatigue and increased or decreased muscle strength.
• Monitor the patient for a therapeutic response to the medication, including decreased fatigue, improved chewing and swallowing, and increased muscle strength.
• Have tissues available at the patient's bedside.

Patient/Family Teaching

• Warn the patient/family to notify the physician if the patient experiences diarrhea, difficulty breathing, increased salivary secretions, irregular heartbeat, muscle weakness, nausea, severe abdominal pain, sweating, or vomiting.
• Tell the patient/family to keep a log of the patient's energy levels and muscle strength to get a better idea of drug dosing.

REFERENCES

Miller, S. & Fioravanti, J. (1997). Pediatric medications: a handbook for nurses. St. Louis: Mosby.
Taketomo, C. K., Hodding, J. H. & Kraus, D. M. (2003–2004). Pediatric dosage handbook (10th ed.). Hudson, OH: Lexi-Comp.

73 Diuretics

Amiloride Hydrochloride
Bumetanide
Furosemide
Hydrochlorothiazide
Mannitol
Metolazone
Spironolactone
Triamterene

Uses: Several subclasses of diuretics have slightly different indications. *Thiazide diuretics,* such as hydrochlorothiazide and metolazone, are used to manage edema caused by various disorders, including CHF and hepatic cirrhosis. They are also used alone or with other antihypertensives to control hypertension. *Loop diuretics,* such as bumetanide and furosemide, are prescribed to manage edema caused by CHF, hepatic cirrhosis, and renal disease. Whether used alone or with other antihypertensives, furosemide is also administered to treat hypertension. *Potassium-sparing diuretics,* such as amiloride and spironolactone, are used as adjuncts to thiazide or loop diuretics in treating CHF and hypertension. *Osmotic diuretics,* such as mannitol, are used to prevent and treat the oliguric phase of acute renal failure, to reduce increased intracranial pressure, and to promote the urinary excretion of certain toxic substances.

Action: Diuretics act to increase the excretion of water, sodium, and other electrolytes by the kidneys. Although their exact mechanism in hypertension is unknown, these agents may act by reducing plasma volume or decreasing peripheral vascular resistance. They are subclassified based on their mechanism and site of action. *Thiazide diuretics* act at the cortical diluting segment of the nephron, blocking sodium, chloride, and water reabsorption and promoting the excretion of sodium, chloride, potassium, and water. *Loop diuretics* act primarily at the thick ascending limb of the loop of Henle to inhibit sodium, chloride, and water absorption. Among the *potassium-sparing diuretics,* amiloride and triamterene act on the distal nephron, decreasing sodium reuptake and reducing potassium excretion, and spironolactone blocks aldosterone from acting on the distal nephron, which causes potassium retention and sodium excretion. *Osmotic diuretics* work in the proximal convoluted tubule by increasing the osmotic pressure of the glomerular filtrate and inhibiting the passive reabsorption of water, sodium, and chloride. (See illustration, *Sites of Action: Diuretics,* page 827.)

COMBINATION PRODUCTS

ACCURETIC: hydrochlorothiazide/quinapril (an angiotensin-converting enzyme [ACE] inhibitor) 12.5 mg/10 mg; 12.5 mg/20 mg; 25 mg/20 mg.

ALDACTAZIDE: hydrochlorothiazide/spironolactone (a potassium-sparing diuretic) 25 mg/25 mg; 50 mg/50 mg.

ALDORIL: hydrochlorothiazide/methyldopa (an antihypertensive) 15 mg/250 mg; 25 mg/250 mg; 30 mg/500 mg; 50 mg/500 mg.

APRESAZIDE: hydrochlorothiazide/hydralazine (a vasodilator) 25 mg/25 mg; 50 mg/50 mg; 50 mg/100 mg.

ATACAND HCT: hydrochlorothiazide/candesartan (an angiotensin II receptor antagonist) 12.5 mg/16 mg; 12.5 mg/32 mg.

AVALIDE: hydrochlorothiazide/irbesartan (an angiotensin II receptor antagonist) 12.5 mg/150 mg; 12.5 mg/300 mg.

BENICAR HCT: hydrochlorothiazide/olmesartan (an angiotensin II receptor antagonist) 12.5 mg/20 mg; 12.5 mg/40 mg; 25 mg/40 mg.

CAPOZIDE: hydrochlorothiazide/captopril (an ACE inhibitor) 15 mg/25 mg; 15 mg/50 mg; 25 mg/25 mg; 25 mg/50 mg.

DIOVAN HCT: hydrochlorothiazide/valsartan (an angiotensin II receptor antagonist) 12.5 mg/80 mg; 12.5 mg/160 mg.

DYAZIDE: hydrochlorothiazide/triamterene (a potassium-sparing diuretic) 25 mg/37.5 mg; 25 mg/50 mg; 50 mg/75 mg.

HYZAAR: hydrochlorothiazide/losartan (an angiotensin II receptor antagonist) 12.5 mg/50 mg; 25 mg/100 mg.

INDERIDE: hydrochlorothiazide/propranolol (a beta-blocker) 25 mg/40 mg; 25 mg/80 mg; 50 mg/80 mg; 50 mg/120 mg; 50 mg/160 mg.

INDERIDE LA: hydrochlorothiazide/propranolol (a beta-blocker) 50 mg/80 mg; 50 mg/120 mg; 50 mg/160 mg.

LOPRESSOR HCT: hydrochlorothiazide/metoprolol (a beta-blocker) 25 mg/50 mg; 25 mg/100 mg; 50 mg/100 mg.

LOTENSIN HCT: hydrochlorothiazide/benazepril (an ACE inhibitor) 6.25 mg/5 mg; 12.5 mg/10 mg; 12.5 mg/20 mg; 25 mg/20 mg.

MAXZIDE: hydrochlorothiazide/triamterene (a potassium-sparing diuretic) 25 mg/37.5 mg; 25 mg/50 mg; 50 mg/75 mg.

MICARDIS HCT: hydrochlorothiazide/telmisartan (an angiotensin II receptor antagonist) 12.5 mg/40 mg; 12.5 mg/80 mg.

MODURETIC: hydrochlorothiazide/amiloride (a potassium-sparing diuretic) 50 mg/5 mg.

NORMOZIDE: hydrochlorothiazide/labetalol (a beta-blocker) 25 mg/100 mg; 25 mg/300 mg.

PRINZIDE: hydrochlorothiazide/lisinopril (an ACE inhibitor) 12.5 mg/10 mg; 12.5 mg/20 mg; 25 mg/20 mg.

TEVETEN HCT: hydrochlorothiazide/eprosartan (an angiotensin II receptor antagonist) 12.5 mg/600 mg; 25 mg/600 mg.

TIMOLIDE: hydrochlorothiazide/timolol (a beta-blocker) 25 mg/10 mg.

UNIRETIC: hydrochlorothiazide/moexipril (an ACE inhibitor) 12.5 mg/7.5 mg; 25 mg/15 mg.

VASERETIC: hydrochlorothiazide/enalapril (an ACE inhibitor) 12.5 mg/5 mg; 25 mg/10 mg.

ZESTORETIC: hydrochlorothiazide/lisinopril (an ACE inhibitor)

12.5 mg/10 mg; 12.5 mg/20 mg; 25 mg/20 mg.

ZIAC: hydrochlorothiazide/bisoprolol (a beta-blocker) 6.25 mg/5 mg; 6.25 mg/10 mg.

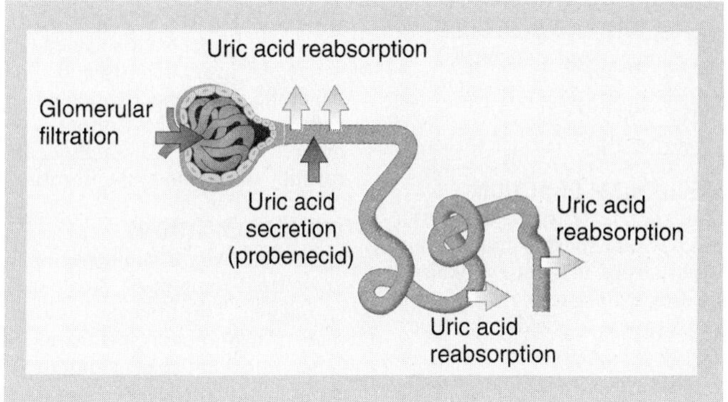

Sites of Action: Diuretics

Diuretics act primarily to increase water and sodium excretion by the kidneys, thereby increasing urine output. In the process, chloride, potassium, and other electrolytes may also be excreted. Generally, most diuretics act by blocking sodium, water, and chloride reabsorption by peritubular capillaries in the nephrons. As a result, water and electrolytes remain in the convoluted tubules to be excreted as urine. The increased water and electrolyte excretion reduces blood volume and ultimately blood pressure.

Diuretics belong to four major subclasses: thiazide, loop, potassium-sparing, and osmotic. Although similar in action, drugs in each subclass act at different sites along the nephron. Also, because the solute concentration decreases as the filtrate passes through the nephron's tubules, drugs that act earlier in the process can block more water and electrolytes, promoting greater diuresis.

Thiazide diuretics, such as hydrochlorothiazide, act in the early portion of the distal convoluted tubule, called the cortical diluting segment. These drugs block sodium, chloride, and water reabsorption and promote their excretion along with potassium.

Loop diuretics, such as furosemide, act primarily in the thick ascending limb of the loop of Henle, blocking sodium, water, and chloride reabsorption. Then these substances are excreted along with potassium.

Potassium-sparing diuretics, such as spironolactone, act in the late portion of the distal convoluted tubule and collecting tubule. Here, they inhibit the action of aldosterone, leading to sodium excretion and potassium retention. Although triamterene and amiloride, two other potassium-sparing diuretics, act at the same site, they do not affect aldosterone. Instead, these drugs directly block the exchange of sodium and potassium, leading to decreased sodium reabsorption and decreased potassium excretion.

Osmotic diuretics, such as mannitol, work in the proximal convoluted tubule. As their name implies, these diuretics increase the osmotic pressure of the glomerular filtrate, inhibiting the passive reabsorption of water, sodium, and chloride.

Amiloride Hydrochloride

ah-**mill**-or-ride
(Kaluril [AUS], Midamor)
Do not confuse with amiodarone or amlodipine.

CATEGORY AND SCHEDULE

Pregnancy Risk Category: B
(D if used in pregnancy-induced hypertension)

MECHANISM OF ACTION

A guanidine derivative that acts as a potassium-sparing diuretic, antihypertensive, and antihypokalemic by directly interfering with sodium reabsorption in the distal tubule. ***Therapeutic Effect:*** Increases sodium and water excretion and decreases potassium excretion.

PHARMACOKINETICS

Route	Onset	Peak	Duration
PO	2 hrs	6–10 hrs	24 hrs

Incompletely absorbed from the GI tract. Protein binding: Minimal. Primarily excreted in urine; partially eliminated in feces. ***Half-Life:*** Adults: 6–9 hrs.

AVAILABILITY

Tablets: 5 mg.

INDICATIONS AND DOSAGES

▸ To counteract potassium loss induced by other diuretics

PO

Children weighing more than 20 kg. 5–10 mg/day. Maximum: 20 mg.
Children weighing 6–20 kg. 0.625 mg/kg/day. Maximum: 10 mg/day.

▸ Dosage in renal impairment

Creatinine Clearance	Dosage
10–50 mL/min	50% of normal
Less than 10 mL/min	avoid use

UNLABELED USES

Treatment of edema associated with CHF, liver cirrhosis, and nephrotic syndrome, treatment of hypertension, reduces lithium-induced polyuria, slows pulmonary function decline in cystic fibrosis

CONTRAINDICATIONS

Hypersensitivity to amiloride or any related component. Acute or chronic renal insufficiency, anuria, diabetic nephropathy, pts taking other potassium-sparing diuretics, serum potassium level greater than 5.5 mEq/L.

INTERACTIONS

Drug

ACE inhibitors, including captopril, and potassium-containing diuretics: May increase potassium levels.
Anticoagulants, including heparin: May decrease effect of anticoagulants, including heparin.
Lithium: May decrease lithium clearance and increase risk of amiloride toxicity.
NSAIDs: May decrease antihypertensive effect.
Cyclosporin and tacrolimus: May increase potassium levels.
Digoxin: May increase risk for toxicity with digoxin.

Herbal

None known.

Food

Licorice: May lead to sodium and water retention and potassium loss.

DIAGNOSTIC TEST EFFECTS

May increase calcium excretion, and BUN, glucose, serum creatinine, serum magnesium, serum potassium, and uric acid levels. May decrease serum sodium levels.

SIDE EFFECTS

Frequent (8%–3%)
Headache, nausea, diarrhea, vomiting, decreased appetite
Occasional (3%–1%)
Dizziness, constipation, abdominal pain, weakness, fatigue, cough, impotence
Rare (less than 1%)
Tremors, vertigo, confusion, nervousness, insomnia, thirst, dry mouth, heartburn, shortness of breath, increased urination, hypotension, rash

SERIOUS REACTIONS

! Severe hyperkalemia may produce irritability, anxiety, a feeling of heaviness in the legs, paresthesia of the hands, face, and lips, hypotension, bradycardia, tented T waves, widening of the QRS complex, and ST segment depression.

PEDIATRIC CONSIDERATIONS

Baseline Assessment
- As appropriate, assess the patient's serum electrolyte levels, especially for low potassium.
- Monitor the patient's renal function test results and serum hepatic enzyme levels.
- Determine the location and extent of edema and assess the patient's skin turgor. Note the skin temperature and moisture level.
- Check the patient's mucous membranes to determine his or her hydration status.
- Assess the patient's muscle strength and mental status.
- Determine the patient's baseline weight.
- Initiate strict intake and output procedures and document.
- Obtain a baseline 12-lead EKG.
- Assess the patient's pulse rate and rhythm.
- Be aware that it is unknown whether amiloride crosses the placenta or is distributed in breast milk.
- There are no age-related precautions noted in children.

Precautions
- Use cautiously in pts with a BUN level greater than 30 mg/dL or serum creatinine level greater than 1.5 mg/dL.
- Use cautiously in debilitated pts.
- Use cautiously in pts with cardiopulmonary disease, diabetes mellitus, or liver insufficiency.

Administration and Handling
PO
- Give with food or milk to avoid GI distress.

Intervention and Evaluation
- Expect to monitor the patient's blood pressure, vital signs, electrolyte levels, intake and output, and weight. Note the extent of diuresis.
- Watch for changes from the initial assessment. Hyperkalemia may result in cardiac arrhythmias, a change in mental status, muscle cramps, muscle strength changes, or tremor.
- Monitor the patient's serum potassium level, particularly during initial therapy.
- Weigh the patient each day.
- Assess lung sounds for rales, rhonchi, or wheezing.

Patient/Family Teaching
- Advise the patient/family to expect an increase in the volume and frequency of urination.

• Explain to the patient/family that the therapeutic effect of the drug takes several days to begin and can last for several days after the drug is discontinued.
• Warn the patient/family that a high-potassium diet and potassium supplements can be dangerous, especially if the patient has liver or kidney problems. Caution the patient to avoid foods high in potassium such as apricots, bananas, legumes, meat, orange juice, raisins, whole grains, including cereals, and white and sweet potatoes.
• Instruct the patient/family to notify the physician if the patient experiences the signs and symptoms of hyperkalemia, including confusion, difficulty breathing, irregular heartbeat, nervousness, numbness of the hands, feet, or lips, unusual tiredness, and weakness in the legs.

Bumetanide

byew-**met**-ah-nide
(Bumex, Burinex [CAN])

CATEGORY AND SCHEDULE

Pregnancy Risk Category: C (D if used in pregnancy-induced hypertension)

MECHANISM OF ACTION

A loop diuretic that enhances excretion of sodium, chloride, and to lesser degree, potassium, by direct action at the ascending limb of the loop of Henle and in the proximal tubule. ***Therapeutic Effect:*** Produces diuresis.

PHARMACOKINETICS

Route	Onset	Peak	Duration
PO	30–60 min	60–120 min	4–6 hrs
IM	40 min	60–120 min	4–6 hrs
IV	rapid	15–30 min	2–3 hrs

Completely absorbed from the GI tract (absorption is decreased in CHF and nephrotic syndrome). Protein binding: 94%–96%. Partially metabolized in liver. Primarily excreted in urine. Not removed by hemodialysis. ***Half-Life:*** 1–1.5 hrs.

AVAILABILITY

Tablets: 0.5 mg, 1 mg, 2 mg.
Injection: 0.25 mg/mL.

INDICATIONS AND DOSAGES

▸ Edema

Children older than 18 yrs. 0.5–2 mg given as a single dose in morning. May repeat at 4- to 5-hr intervals. Maximum: 10 mg/day.
IV/IM/PO
Children. 0.15–0.1 mg/kg/dose q6–24h. Maximum: 10 mg/day.

▸ Hypertension

IV/IM/PO
Children. 0.015–0.1 mg/kg/dose q6–24h. Maximum: 10 mg/day.

UNLABELED USES

Treatment of hypercalcemia and hypertension.

CONTRAINDICATIONS

Hypersensitivity to bumetanide or any related component. Anuria, hepatic coma, severe electrolyte depletion.

INTERACTIONS

Drug

Amphotericin, nephrotoxic agents, ototoxic agents: May increase the risk of toxicity.
Anticoagulants, heparin: May decrease the effects of anticoagulants and heparin.
Hypokalemia-causing agents: May increase the risk of hypokalemia.
Lithium: May increase the risk of toxicity of lithium.

Herbal

None known.

Food

None known.

DIAGNOSTIC TEST EFFECTS

May increase blood glucose, BUN, uric acid, and urinary phosphate levels. May decrease serum calcium, chloride, magnesium, potassium, and sodium levels.

IV INCOMPATIBILITIES

Midazolam (Versed)

IV COMPATIBILITIES

Aztreonam (Azactam), cefepime (Maxipime), diltiazem (Cardizem), dobutamine (Dobutrex), furosemide (Lasix), lorazepam (Ativan), milrinone (Primacor), morphine, piperacillin, propofol (Diprivan), tazobactam (Zosyn)

SIDE EFFECTS

Expected

Increase in urine frequency and volume

Frequent

Orthostatic hypotension, dizziness

Occasional

Blurred vision, diarrhea, headache, anorexia, premature ejaculation, impotence, GI upset

Rare

Rash, urticaria, pruritus, weakness, muscle cramps, nipple tenderness

SERIOUS REACTIONS

! Vigorous diuresis may lead to profound water and electrolyte depletion, resulting in hypokalemia, hyponatremia, dehydration, coma, and circulatory collapse.
! Acute hypotensive episodes may occur.
! Ototoxicity manifested as deafness, vertigo, and tinnitus or ringing in ears may occur, especially in pts with severe renal impairment or who are taking other ototoxic drugs.
! Blood dyscrasias have been reported.

PEDIATRIC CONSIDERATIONS

Baseline Assessment

- Check the patient's vital signs, especially blood pressure (B/P) for hypotension before administration.
- Assess the patient's baseline electrolyte levels, particularly for low potassium.
- Evaluate the patient for edema.
- Determine the patient's hydration status.
- Measure and record the patient's fluid intake and output.
- Be aware that it is unknown whether bumetanide is distributed in breast milk.
- Be aware that the safety and efficacy of bumetanide have not been established in children.
- Be aware that the injectable form of bumetanide contains benzyl alcohol, which has been associated with allergic reactions in certain pts and with toxicity when used in large doses in neonates. Use with caution in neonates.

Precautions
• Use cautiously in pts with diabetes mellitus, hypersensitivity to sulfonamides, and impaired liver or renal function.

Administration and Handling
PO
• Give bumetanide with food to avoid GI upset, preferably with breakfast to help prevent nocturia.

IV
• Store at room temperature.
• Drug is stable for 24 hrs if diluted.
• May give undiluted but is compatible with D_5W, 0.9% NaCl, or lactated Ringer's solution.
• Administer IV push over 1–2 min.
• May give as continuous infusion.

Intervention and Evaluation
• Continue to monitor the patient's B/P, electrolyte levels, intake and output, vital signs, and weight.
• Note the extent of patient diuresis.
• Observe the patient for changes from his or her initial assessment. Hypokalemia may result in cardiac arrhythmias, a change in mental status, muscle cramps, muscle strength changes, and tremor. Hyponatremia may result in clammy or cold skin, confusion, and thirst.

Patient/Family Teaching
• Tell the patient/family to expect the patient to have hearing abnormalities, such as a sense of fullness or ringing in the ears, and increased frequency and volume of urination.
• Encourage the patient/family to consume foods high in potassium such as apricots, bananas, legumes, meat, orange juice, white and sweet potatoes, raisins, and whole grains, including cereals.
• Instruct the patient/family to rise slowly from a sitting or lying position.
• Tell the patient/family to take the drug with food to avoid GI distress.

Furosemide

feur-**oh**-sah-mide
(Apo-Furosemide [CAN], Lasix, Uremide [AUS], Urex-M [AUS])
Do not confuse with torsemide.

CATEGORY AND SCHEDULE

Pregnancy Risk Category: C (D if used in pregnancy-induced hypertension)

MECHANISM OF ACTION

A loop diuretic that enhances excretion of sodium, chloride, and potassium by direct action at the ascending limb of the loop of Henle. ***Therapeutic Effect:*** Produces a diuretic effect.

PHARMACOKINETICS

Route	Onset	Peak	Duration
PO	30–60 min	1–2 hrs	6–8 hrs
IM	30 min	N/A	N/A
IV	5 min	20–60 min	2 hrs

Well absorbed from the GI tract. Protein binding: 91%–97%. Partially metabolized in liver. Primarily excreted in urine in severe renal impairment; nonrenal clearance increases. Not removed by hemodialysis. ***Half-Life:*** Adults: 30–90 min. Half-life is increased in pts with impaired renal or liver function and in neonates.

AVAILABILITY

Tablets: 20 mg, 40 mg, 80 mg.
Oral Solution: 10 mg/mL, 40 mg/5 mL.
Injection: 10 mg/mL.

INDICATIONS AND DOSAGES

▸ **Edema and hypertension**
PO
Children. 1–6 mg/kg/day in divided doses q6–12h.
IM/IV
Children. 1–2 mg/kg/dose q6–12h.
Neonates. 1–2 mg/kg/dose q12–24h.
▸ **IV continuous infusion**
Children. 0.05 mg/kg/hr; titrate to desired effect.

UNLABELED USES

Treatment of hypercalcemia

CONTRAINDICATIONS

Hypersensitivity to furosemide or any related component. Anuria, liver coma, severe electrolyte depletion.

INTERACTIONS

Drug

Amphotericin, nephrotoxic and ototoxic agents: May increase the risk of toxicity.
Anticoagulants, heparin: May decrease the effects of anticoagulants and heparin.
Hypokalemia-causing agents: May increase the risk of hypokalemia.
Lithium: May increase the risk of toxicity of lithium.
Probenecid: May increase furosemide blood concentration.
Indomethacin: May decrease the diuretic effect of furosemide.

Herbal

None known.

Food

Licorice: May lead to increased potassium excretion, sodium retention, and edema.

DIAGNOSTIC TEST EFFECTS

May increase blood glucose, BUN, and serum uric acid levels. May decrease serum calcium, chloride, magnesium, potassium, and sodium levels.

IV INCOMPATIBILITIES

Ciprofloxacin (Cipro), diltiazem (Cardizem), dobutamine (Dobutrex), dopamine (Intropin), doxorubicin (Adriamycin), droperidol (Inapsine), esmolol (Brevibloc), famotidine (Pepcid), filgrastim (Neupogen), fluconazole (Diflucan), gemcitabine (Gemzar), gentamicin (Garamycin), idarubicin (Idamycin), labetalol (Trandate), meperidine (Demerol), metoclopramide (Reglan), midazolam (Versed), milrinone (Primacor), nicardipine (Cardene), ondansetron (Zofran), quinidine, thiopental (Pentothal), vecuronium (Norcuron), vinblastine (Velban), vincristine (Oncovin), vinorelbine (Navelbine)

IV COMPATIBILITIES

Aminophylline, amiodarone (Cordarone), bumetanide (Bumex), calcium gluconate, cimetidine (Tagamet), heparin, hydromorphone (Dilaudid), lidocaine, morphine, nitroglycerin, norepinephrine (Levophed), potassium chloride, propofol (Diprivan)

SIDE EFFECTS

Expected
Increase in urinary frequency and volume

Frequent
Nausea, gastric upset with cramping, diarrhea, or constipation, electrolyte disturbances
Occasional
Dizziness, lightheadedness, headache, blurred vision, paresthesia, photosensitivity, rash, weakness, urinary frequency or bladder spasm, restlessness, diaphoresis
Rare
Flank pain, loin pain

SERIOUS REACTIONS

! Vigorous diuresis may lead to profound water loss and electrolyte depletion, resulting in hypokalemia, hyponatremia, and dehydration.
! Sudden volume depletion may result in an increased risk of thrombosis, circulatory collapse, and sudden death.
! Acute hypotensive episodes may also occur, sometimes several days after the beginning of therapy.
! Ototoxicity manifested as deafness, vertigo, and tinnitus or ringing and roaring in ears may occur, especially in pts with severe renal impairment.
! Furosemide use can exacerbate diabetes mellitus, systemic lupus erythematosus, gout, and pancreatitis.
! Blood dyscrasias have been reported.

PEDIATRIC CONSIDERATIONS

Baseline Assessment

• Monitor the patient's vital signs, especially blood pressure (B/P), for hypotension before giving furosemide.
• Assess the patient's baseline electrolyte levels, particularly for low potassium.
• Evaluate the patient's edema, mucous membranes, and skin turgor for hydration status.
• Evaluate the patient's mental status and muscle strength.
• Record the patient's skin moisture and temperature.
• Obtain the patient's baseline weight.
• Begin monitoring the patient's fluid intake and output.
• Be aware that furosemide crosses the placenta and is distributed in breast milk.
• Be aware that the half-life of the drug is increased in neonates and may require an increased dosage interval.
• Use caution when administering furosemide to neonates because of the extended half-life of the medication.
• Be aware that neonates have poor oral absorption of furosemide.

Precautions

• Use cautiously in pts with liver cirrhosis.

Administration and Handling

PO
• Give furosemide with food to avoid GI upset, preferably with breakfast to help prevent nocturia.
IM
• Monitor the patient for temporary pain at the injection site.
IV
• Solution normally appears clear, colorless.
• Discard yellow solutions.
• May give undiluted but is compatible with D_5W, 0.9% NaCl, or lactated Ringer's solution.
• Administer each 40 mg or fraction by IV push over 1–2 min. Do not exceed administration rate of 4 mg/min in pts with renal impairment.

Intervention and Evaluation

• Monitor the patient's B/P, electrolyte levels, fluid intake and output, vital signs, and weight.
• Note the extent of patient diuresis.
• Observe the patient for changes from the initial assessment. Hypokalemia may result in cardiac arrhythmias, changes in mental status and muscle strength, muscle cramps, and tremor. Hyponatremia may result in clammy and cold skin, confusion, and thirst.

Patient/Family Teaching

• Tell the patient/family to expect an increase in the frequency and volume of urination.
• Warn the patient/family to notify the physician if the patient experiences hearing abnormalities, such as ringing or roaring in the ears, or a sense of fullness in the ears, irregular heartbeat, or signs of electrolyte imbalances.
• Encourage the patient/family to eat foods high in potassium such as apricots, bananas, legumes, meat, orange juice, white or sweet potatoes, raisins, and whole grains, such as cereals.
• Urge the patient/family to avoid overexposure to artificial lights, such as sun lamps, and sunlight.

Hydrochlorothiazide

high-drow-chlor-oh-**thigh**-ah-zide
(Apo-Hydro [CAN], Dichlotride [AUS], Esidrix, HydroDIURIL, Microzide, Oretic)

CATEGORY AND SCHEDULE

Pregnancy Risk Category: B (D if used in pregnancy-induced hypertension)

MECHANISM OF ACTION

A sulfonamide derivative that acts as a thiazide diuretic and antihypertensive. As a diuretic blocks reabsorption of water and the electrolytes sodium and potassium at the cortical diluting segment of distal tubule. As an antihypertensive reduces plasma and extracellular fluid volume and decreases peripheral vascular resistance by a direct effect on blood vessels. ***Therapeutic Effect:*** Promotes diuresis; reduces blood pressure (B/P).

PHARMACOKINETICS

Route	Onset	Peak	Duration
PO (diuretic)	2 hrs	4–6 hrs	6–12 hrs

Variably absorbed from the GI tract. Primarily excreted unchanged in urine. Not removed by hemodialysis. ***Half-Life:*** Adults: 5.6–14.8 hrs.

AVAILABILITY

Capsules: 12.5 mg.
Tablets: 25 mg, 50 mg, 100 mg.
Oral Solution: 50 mg/5 mL.

INDICATIONS AND DOSAGES

▸ **Edema, hypertension**

PO

Children 6 mos–12 yrs.
2 mg/kg/day divided q12h.
Maximum: 200 mg/day.
Children younger than 6 mos. 2–4 mg/kg/day divided q12h.
Maximum: 37.5 mg/day.

UNLABELED USES

Treatment of diabetes insipidus, prevention of calcium-containing renal stones.

CONTRAINDICATIONS

Anuria, a history of hypersensitivity to sulfonamides or thiazide diuretics, renal decompensation.

INTERACTIONS

Drug

Cholestyramine, colestipol: May decrease the absorption and effects of hydrochlorothiazide.
Digoxin: May increase the risk of toxicity of digoxin caused by hypokalemia.
Lithium: May increase the risk of toxicity of lithium.
NSAIDs: May decrease the antihypertensive effects of hydrochlorothiazide.

Herbal

None known.

Food

Licorice: May lead to increased potassium excretion, edema, and sodium retention.

DIAGNOSTIC TEST EFFECTS

May increase blood glucose levels, serum cholesterol, low-density lipoprotein, bilirubin, calcium, creatinine, uric acid, and triglyceride levels. May decrease urinary calcium and serum magnesium, potassium, and sodium levels.

SIDE EFFECTS

Expected
Increase in urine frequency and volume
Frequent
Potassium depletion
Occasional
Postural hypotension, headache, GI disturbances, photosensitivity reaction

SERIOUS REACTIONS

! Vigorous diuresis may lead to profound water loss and electrolyte depletion, resulting in hypokalemia, hyponatremia, and dehydration.
! Acute hypotensive episodes may occur.
! Hyperglycemia may be noted during prolonged therapy.
! GI upset, pancreatitis, dizziness, paresthesias, headache, blood dyscrasias, pulmonary edema, allergic pneumonitis, and dermatologic reactions occur rarely.
! Overdosage can lead to lethargy and coma without changes in electrolytes or hydration.

PEDIATRIC CONSIDERATIONS

Baseline Assessment

- Monitor the patient's vital signs, especially B/P for hypotension before giving hydrochlorothiazide.
- Plan to assess the patient's baseline electrolyte levels, particularly for hypokalemia.
- Evaluate the patient's mucous membranes, peripheral edema, and skin turgor for hydration status.
- Evaluate the patient's mental status and muscle strength.
- Record the patient's skin moisture and temperature.
- Obtain and record the patient's baseline weight.
- Begin monitoring the patient's fluid intake and output.
- Be aware that hydrochlorothiazide crosses the placenta and a small amount is distributed in breast milk. Breast-feeding is not recommended in this patient population.
- Be aware that the injectable product contains a benzyl alcohol derivative. Use in neonates in large amounts may lead to a fatal toxicity. Avoid use of injection in neonates.
- There are no age-related precautions noted in children, except that

jaundiced infants may be at risk for hyperbilirubinemia.

Precautions

• Use cautiously in debilitated pts.
• Use cautiously in pts with diabetes mellitus, impaired liver function, severe renal disease, and thyroid disorders.

Administration and Handling

PO

• May give hydrochlorothiazide with food or milk if GI upset occurs, preferably with breakfast to help prevent nocturia.

Intervention and Evaluation

• Continue to monitor the patient's B/P, electrolyte levels, intake and output, vital signs, and weight daily.
• Record the extent of patient diuresis.
• Observe the patient for changes from the initial assessment. Hypokalemia may result in a change in mental status, muscle cramps, nausea, tachycardia, tremor, vomiting, and weakness. Hyponatremia may result in clammy and cold skin, confusion, and thirst.
• Be especially alert for signs of potassium depletion in pts taking digoxin, such as cardiac arrhythmias.
• Give the patient potassium supplements, if ordered.
• Assess the patient for constipation, which may occur with exercise diuresis.

Patient/Family Teaching

• Tell the patient/family to expect an increase in the frequency and volume of urination.
• Instruct the patient/family to rise slowly from a lying to a sitting position and to permit the legs to dangle momentarily before standing to reduce the hypotensive effect of the drug.
• Encourage the patient/family to eat foods high in potassium such as apricots, bananas, legumes, meat, orange juice, white and sweet potatoes, raisins, and whole grains, such as cereals.
• Urge the patient/family to protect the patient's skin from sunlight and ultraviolet rays as a photosensitivity reaction may occur.

Mannitol

man-ih-toll
(Osmitrol)

CATEGORY AND SCHEDULE

Pregnancy Risk Category: C

MECHANISM OF ACTION

An osmotic diuretic, antiglaucoma, and antihemolytic agent that elevates osmotic pressure of the glomerular filtrate; increases the flow of water into interstitial fluid and plasma, inhibiting renal tubular reabsorption of sodium and chloride. Enhances flow of water from eye into plasma. ***Therapeutic Effect:*** Produces diuresis, reduces intraocular pressure (IOP).

PHARMACOKINETICS

Indication	Onset	Peak	Duration
Diuresis	1–3 hrs	N/A	N/A
Reduced IOP	15 min	N/A	3–6 hrs

Remains in extracellular fluid. Primarily excreted in urine. Removed by hemodialysis. ***Half-Life:*** 100 min. Onset of diuresis occurs in 1–3 hrs; decreases IOP in 0.5–1 hr, duration 4–6 hrs. Decreases cerebrospinal fluid pressure in 15 min, duration 3–8 hrs.

AVAILABILITY

Injection: 5%, 10%, 15%, 20%, 25%.

INDICATIONS AND DOSAGES

▸ **Prevention and treatment of oliguric phase of acute renal failure, before evidence of permanent renal failure, promotes urinary excretion of toxic substances, such as aspirin, barbiturates, bromides, and imipramine, reduces increased intracranial pressure because of cerebral edema, edema of injured spinal cord, IOP due to acute glaucoma**

IV

Children. Test dose 200 mg/kg over 3–5 min to start urine flow of 1 mL/kg/hr for 1–3 hrs. Maximum: 12.5 g. Initial dose: 0.5–1 g/kg. Maintenance dose: 0.25–0.5 g/kg q4–6 h.

CONTRAINDICATIONS

Hypersensitivity to mannitol or any related component. Dehydration, intracranial bleeding, severe pulmonary edema and congestion, severe renal disease.

INTERACTIONS

Drug

Digoxin: May increase the risk of toxicity of digoxin caused by hypokalemia.

Herbal

None known.

Food

None known.

DIAGNOSTIC TEST EFFECTS

May decrease serum phosphate, potassium, and sodium levels.

IV INCOMPATIBILITIES

Cefepime (Maxipime), doxorubicin liposome (Doxil), filgrastim (Neupogen)

IV COMPATIBILITIES

Cisplatin (Platinol), ondansetron (Zofran), propofol (Diprivan)

SIDE EFFECTS

Frequent

Dry mouth, thirst

Occasional

Blurred vision, increased urination, headache, arm pain, backache, nausea, vomiting, urticaria or hives, dizziness, hypotension or hypertension, tachycardia, fever, angina-like chest pain

SERIOUS REACTIONS

! Fluid and electrolyte imbalance may occur because of the rapid administration of large doses or inadequate urinary output resulting in overexpansion of extracellular fluid.

! Circulatory overload may produce pulmonary edema and CHF.

! Excessive diuresis may produce hypokalemia and hyponatremia.

! Fluid loss in excess of electrolyte excretion may produce hypernatremia and hyperkalemia.

PEDIATRIC CONSIDERATIONS

Baseline Assessment

- Monitor the patient's vital signs, especially blood pressure, for hypotension before giving mannitol.
- Evaluate the patient's mucous membranes, peripheral edema, and skin turgor for hydration status.
- Obtain and record the patient's baseline weight.
- Begin monitoring the patient's fluid intake and output.

• Be aware that it is unknown whether mannitol crosses the placenta or is distributed in breast milk.
• Be aware that the safety and efficacy of mannitol have not been established in children younger than 12 yrs of age.

Administration and Handling

◀ **ALERT** ▶ Assess the patient's IV site for patency before each dose. Pain and thrombosis are noted with extravasation.

◀ **ALERT** ▶ Test a dose of 12.5 g for adults (200 mg/kg for children) over 3–5 min to produce a urine flow of at least 30–50 mL/hr over 2–3 hrs (1 mL/kg/hr for children).

IV

• Store at room temperature.
• If crystals are noted in solution, warm the bottle in hot water and shake vigorously at intervals. Do not use if crystals remain after the warming procedure.
• Cool to body temperature before administration.
• Use an in-line filter (less than 5 microns) for drug concentrations greater than 20%.
• The test dose for oliguria is IV push over 3–5 min. The test dose for cerebral edema or elevated intracranial pressure is IV infusion over 20–30 min. Maximum concentration: 25%.
• Do not add potassium chloride (KCl) or sodium chloride (NaCl) to mannitol 20% or greater.
• Do not add to whole blood for transfusion.

Intervention and Evaluation

• Monitor the patient's urine output to ascertain a therapeutic response.
• Monitor the results of the patient's BUN, electrolyte, and serum hepatic enzyme level tests.
• Weigh the patient daily.
• Observe the patient for changes from the initial assessment. Know that hypokalemia may result in cardiac arrhythmias, a change in mental status, muscle cramps, nausea, tachycardia, tremor, vomiting, and weakness; hyperkalemia may result in arrhythmias, colic, diarrhea, and muscle twitching followed by paralysis or weakness; hyponatremia may result in clammy and cold skin, confusion, drowsiness, and thirst.

Patient/Family Teaching

• Tell the patient/family to expect an increase in the frequency and volume of urination.
• Explain to the patient/family that mannitol may cause dry mouth.
• Tell the patient/family to weigh the patient daily.

Metolazone

me-**toh**-lah-zone
(Mykrox, Zaroxolyn)
Do not confuse with methazolamide, metoprolol, or Zarontin.

CATEGORY AND SCHEDULE

Pregnancy Risk Category: B (D if used in pregnancy-induced hypertension)

MECHANISM OF ACTION

A thiazide-like diuretic and antihypertensive. As a diuretic, blocks reabsorption of sodium, potassium, and chloride at the distal convoluted tubule, promoting delivery of sodium to the potassium side, increasing potassium excretion and (Na-K) exchange. ***Therapeutic Effect:*** Produces renal excretion of sodium and water. As an antihypertensive, reduces plasma and extracellular fluid volume. ***Therapeutic Effect:***

Decreases peripheral vascular resistance; reduces blood pressure (B/P) by a direct effect on blood vessels.

PHARMACOKINETICS

Route	Onset	Peak	Duration
PO (diuretic)	1 hr	2 hrs	12–24 hrs

Incompletely absorbed from the GI tract. Protein binding: 95%. Primarily excreted unchanged in urine. Not removed by hemodialysis. ***Half-Life:*** 14 hrs.

AVAILABILITY

Tablets: 2.5 mg, 5 mg, 10 mg.
Tablets (Mykrox): 0.5 mg.

INDICATIONS AND DOSAGES

▸ Usual pediatric dosage

PO

Children. 0.2–0.4 mg/kg/day in divided doses q12–24h.

CONTRAINDICATIONS

Hypersensitivity to metolazone or any related component. Anuria, a history of hypersensitivity to sulfonamides or thiazide diuretics, liver coma or precoma, renal decompensation.

INTERACTIONS

Drug

Cholestyramine, colestipol: May decrease the absorption and effects of metolazone.
Digoxin: May increase the risk of toxicity of digoxin caused by hypokalemia.
Allopurinol: Use with metolazone may increase the risk of hypersensitivity reactions.
Lithium: May increase the risk of toxicity of lithium.

Herbal

None known.

Food

Licorice: May increase the risk for hypokalemia; increases edema and sodium retention.

DIAGNOSTIC TEST EFFECTS

May increase blood glucose, serum cholesterol, low-density lipoprotein, bilirubin, calcium, creatinine, uric acid, and triglyceride levels. May decrease urinary calcium, and serum magnesium, potassium, and sodium levels.

SIDE EFFECTS

Expected
Increase in urine frequency and volume
Frequent (10%–9%)
Dizziness, lightheadedness, headache
Occasional (6%–4%)
Muscle cramps and spasm, fatigue, lethargy
Rare (less than 2%)
Weakness, palpitations, depression, nausea, vomiting, abdominal bloating, constipation, diarrhea, urticaria

SERIOUS REACTIONS

! Vigorous diuresis may lead to profound water loss and electrolyte depletion, resulting in hypokalemia, hyponatremia, and dehydration.
! Acute hypotensive episodes may occur.
! Hyperglycemia may be noted during prolonged therapy.
! GI upset, pancreatitis, dizziness, paresthesias, headache, blood dyscrasias, pulmonary edema, allergic pneumonitis, and dermatologic reactions occur rarely.
! Overdosage can lead to lethargy and coma without changes in electrolytes or hydration.

PEDIATRIC CONSIDERATIONS

Baseline Assessment

- Monitor the patient's B/P for hypotension before giving metolazone.
- Assess the patient's baseline electrolyte levels, particularly for hypokalemia.
- Evaluate the patient's mucous membranes, peripheral edema, and skin turgor for hydration status.
- Evaluate the patient's mental status and muscle strength.
- Assess the patient's skin moisture and temperature.
- Obtain and record the patient's baseline weight.
- Begin monitoring the patient's fluid intake and output.
- Be aware that metolazone crosses the placenta and a small amount is distributed in breast milk. Breast-feeding is not recommended in this patient population.
- There are no age-related precautions noted in children.

Precautions

- Use cautiously in pts with diabetes, elevated cholesterol and triglyceride levels, gout, impaired liver function, lupus erythematosus, and severe renal disease.

Administration and Handling

PO

- May give metolazone with food or milk if GI upset occurs, preferably with breakfast to help prevent nocturia.

Intervention and Evaluation

- Continue to monitor the patient's B/P, electrolyte levels, intake and output, vital signs, and weight.
- Record the extent of patient diuresis.
- Observe the patient for changes from the initial assessment. Hypokalemia may result in a change in mental status, muscle cramps, nausea, tachycardia, tremor, vomiting, and weakness. Hyponatremia may result in clammy and cold skin, confusion, and thirst.

Patient/Family Teaching

- Tell the patient/family to expect an increase in the frequency and volume of urination.
- Instruct the patient/family to rise slowly from a lying to a sitting position and to permit the legs to dangle momentarily before standing to reduce the hypotensive effect of the drug.
- Encourage the patient/family to eat foods high in potassium such as apricots, bananas, legumes, meat, orange juice, white and sweet potatoes, raisins, and whole grains, such as cereals.

Spironolactone 

spear-own-oh-**lak**-tone
(Aldactone, Novospiroton [CAN], Spiractin [AUS])

CATEGORY AND SCHEDULE

Pregnancy Risk Category: C
(D if used in pregnancy-induced hypertension)

MECHANISM OF ACTION

An aldosterone antagonist that competitively inhibits the action of aldosterone. Interferes with sodium reabsorption in distal tubule. ***Therapeutic Effect:*** Increases potassium retention while promoting sodium and water excretion.

PHARMACOKINETICS

Route	Onset	Peak	Duration
PO	24–48 hrs	48–72 hrs	48–72 hrs

Well absorbed from the GI tract (increased with food). Protein binding: 91%–98%. Metabolized in liver to the active metabolite. Primarily excreted in urine. Unknown whether removed by hemodialysis. ***Half-Life:*** 1–1.5 hrs. Metabolite: 13–24 hrs.

AVAILABILITY

Tablets: 25 mg, 50 mg, 100 mg.

INDICATIONS AND DOSAGES

▸ Diuretic, hypertension

PO

Children. 1.5–3.3 mg/kg/day in divided doses q6–24h.
Neonates. 1–3 mg/kg/day q12–24h.

▸ Diagnosis of primary aldosteronism

PO

Children. 100–400 mg/m²/day in 1–2 divided doses.

▸ Dosage in renal impairment

Creatinine Clearance	Interval
10–50 mL/min	12–24 hrs
Less than 10 mL/min	avoid use

UNLABELED USES

Treatment of female hirsutism, polycystic ovary syndrome.

CONTRAINDICATIONS

Hypersensitivity to spironolactone or any related component. Acute renal insufficiency and impairment, anuria, hyperkalemia, BUN and serum creatinine levels over twice normal values.

INTERACTIONS

Drug

Angiotensin-converting enzyme inhibitors, such as captopril, potassium-containing medications, potassium supplements: May increase serum potassium levels.
Anticoagulants, heparin: May decrease the effects of anticoagulants and heparin.
Digoxin: May increase the half-life of digoxin.
Lithium: May decrease the clearance and increase the risk of toxicity of lithium.
NSAIDs: May decrease the antihypertensive effect.

Herbal

None known.

Food

Licorice: May increase the risk for hypokalemia and increases edema and sodium retention.

DIAGNOSTIC TEST EFFECTS

May increase blood glucose, BUN, serum creatinine, magnesium, and potassium, and uric acid levels, and calcium excretion. May decrease serum sodium levels.

SIDE EFFECTS

Frequent

Hyperkalemia for pts taking potassium supplements or with renal insufficiency, dehydration, hyponatremia, lethargy

Occasional

Nausea, vomiting, anorexia, cramping, diarrhea, headache, ataxia, drowsiness, confusion, fever
Male: Gynecomastia, impotence, decreased libido
Female: Menstrual irregularities or amenorrhea, postmenopausal bleeding, breast tenderness

Rare

Rash, urticaria, hirsutism

SERIOUS REACTIONS

! Severe hyperkalemia may produce arrhythmias, bradycardia, EKG changes (tented T waves, widening QRS complex), and depression. These may proceed to a cardiac standstill or ventricular fibrillation.

! Cirrhosis pts are at risk for hepatic decompensation if dehydration or hyponatremia occurs.

! Pts with primary aldosteronism may experience rapid weight loss and severe fatigue during high-dose therapy.

PEDIATRIC CONSIDERATIONS

Baseline Assessment

- Monitor the patient's baseline vital signs and note the patient's pulse rate and quality.
- Assess the patient's baseline BUN, serum creatinine, serum electrolyte, and serum hepatic enzyme levels to evaluate renal function and urinalysis results. Also expect to perform a baseline EKG.
- Evaluate the patient's mucous membranes and skin turgor for hydration status.
- Evaluate the patient for edema and note its extent and location.
- Obtain and record the patient's baseline weight.
- Begin monitoring the patient's fluid intake and output.
- Be aware that an active metabolite of spironolactone is excreted in breast milk. Breast-feeding is not recommended in this patient population.
- There are no age-related precautions noted in children.

Precautions

- Use cautiously in pts who concurrently take supplemental potassium and who are dehydrated.
- Use cautiously in pts with hyponatremia and impaired liver or renal function.

Administration and Handling

PO

- Oral suspension containing crushed tablets in cherry syrup is stable for up to 30 days if refrigerated.
- Drug absorption is enhanced if spironolactone is taken with food.
- Crush scored tablets as needed.

Intervention and Evaluation

- Monitor the patient's blood pressure and electrolyte values, particularly for hyperkalemia. Hyperkalemia may result in arrhythmias, colic, diarrhea, and muscle twitching followed by paralysis and weakness.
- Obtain an EKG, as ordered, if hyperkalemia is severe.
- Observe the patient for hyponatremia. Hyponatremia may result in clammy and cold skin, confusion, drowsiness, dry mouth, and thirst.
- Obtain and record the patient's daily weight.
- Record changes in the patient's edema and skin turgor.

Patient/Family Teaching

- Tell the patient/family to expect an increase in the frequency and volume of urination.
- Caution the patient/family to avoid consuming foods high in potassium such as apricots, bananas, legumes, meat, orange juice, white and sweet potatoes, raisins, and whole grains, such as cereals.
- Warn the patient/family that the therapeutic effect of spironolactone takes several days to begin and can last for several days once the drug is discontinued. Explain that this time frame may not apply if the patient is taking a potassium-losing drug concomitantly. Expect the physician to help establish the patient's diet and use of supplements.
- Warn the patient/family to notify the physician if the patient

experiences electrolyte imbalance or an irregular or slow pulse.
• Inform the patient/family that spironolactone may cause drowsiness. Warn the patient to avoid performing tasks that require mental alertness or motor skills until his or her response to the drug is established.

Triamterene

try-**am**-tur-een
(Dyrenium)
Do not confuse with diazoxide, Maxidex, and trimipramine.

CATEGORY AND SCHEDULE

Pregnancy Risk Category: B (D if used in pregnancy-induced hypertension)

MECHANISM OF ACTION

A potassium-sparing diuretic that inhibits sodium, potassium adenosine triphosphatase. Interferes with sodium and potassium exchange in the distal tubule, cortical collecting tubule, and collecting duct. ***Therapeutic Effect:*** Increases sodium excretion and decreases potassium excretion. Also increases magnesium level and decreases calcium loss.

PHARMACOKINETICS

Route	Onset	Peak	Duration
PO	2–4 hrs	N/A	7–9 hrs

Incompletely absorbed from the GI tract. Widely distributed. Metabolized in liver. Primarily eliminated in feces via biliary route. ***Half-Life:*** 1.5–2.5 hrs. Half-life is increased in pts with impaired renal function.

AVAILABILITY

Capsules: 50 mg, 100 mg.

INDICATIONS AND DOSAGES

▸ **Edema, hypertension**
PO
Children. 2–4 mg/kg/day in 1 or 2 divided doses. Maximum: 6 mg/kg/day or 300 mg/day.

UNLABELED USES

Treatment adjunct for hypertension, prophylaxis, and treatment of hypokalemia.

CONTRAINDICATIONS

Hypersensitivity to triamterene or any related component. Drug-induced or preexisting hyperkalemia, progressive or severe renal disease, severe liver disease.

INTERACTIONS

Drug
Angiotensin-converting enzyme inhibitors, such as captopril, potassium-containing medications, potassium supplements: May increase serum potassium levels.
Anticoagulants, heparin: May decrease the effects of anticoagulants and heparin.
Lithium: May decrease the clearance and increase the risk of toxicity of lithium.
NSAIDs: May decrease the antihypertensive effect.
Herbal
None known.
Food
None known.

DIAGNOSTIC TEST EFFECTS

May increase blood glucose, BUN, calcium, serum creatinine, potassium, and uric acid levels. May decrease serum magnesium and sodium levels.

SIDE EFFECTS

Occasional

Fatigue, nausea, diarrhea, abdominal distress, leg aches, headache

Rare

Anorexia, weakness, rash, dizziness

SERIOUS REACTIONS

! May produce hyponatremia (drowsiness, dry mouth, increased thirst, and lack of energy) or severe hyperkalemia (irritability, anxiety, heaviness of the legs, paresthesia, hypotension, bradycardia, and EKG changes [tented T waves, a widening QRS complex, and ST segment depression]).

! Agranulocytosis, nephrolithiasis, and thrombocytopenia occur rarely.

PEDIATRIC CONSIDERATIONS

Baseline Assessment

• Assess the patient's baseline electrolyte levels, particularly for low serum potassium levels.

• Assess the patient's BUN, serum creatinine, and serum hepatic enzyme levels to assess renal function.

• Examine the patient for edema and note its extent and location.

• Evaluate the patient's mucous membranes and skin turgor for hydration status.

• Evaluate the patient's mental status and muscle strength.

• Assess the patient's skin moisture and temperature.

• Obtain and record the patient's baseline weight.

• Begin monitoring the patient's fluid intake and output.

• Assess the patient's pulse rate and rhythm.

• Be aware that triamterene crosses the placenta and is distributed in breast milk. Breast-feeding is not recommended in this patient population.

• Be aware that the safety and efficacy of this drug have not been established in children.

Precautions

• Use cautiously in pts with diabetes mellitus, a history of renal calculi, and impaired liver and renal functions.

• Use cautiously in pts receiving other potassium-sparing diuretics or potassium supplements.

Administration and Handling

PO

• Give triamterene with food if GI disturbances occur.

• Do not crush or break capsules.

Intervention and Evaluation

• Monitor the patient's blood pressure, electrolyte levels, particularly potassium levels, fluid intake and output, vital signs, and daily weight.

• Record the amount of patient diuresis.

• Observe the patient for changes from the initial assessment. Hypokalemia may result in a change in mental status, muscle cramps, nausea, tachycardia, tremor, vomiting, and weakness.

• Assess the patient's lung sounds for rhonchi and wheezing.

Patient/Family Teaching

• Tell the patient/family to expect an increase in the frequency and volume of urination.

• Instruct the patient/family to take triamterene in the morning to help prevent nocturia.

• Inform the patient/family that the therapeutic effect of the drug takes several days to begin and can last for several days after the drug is discontinued.

• Warn the patient/family to notify the physician if the patient experiences dry mouth, fever, headache, nausea, persistent or severe weakness, sore throat, unusual bleeding or bruising, and vomiting.

- Encourage the patient/family to avoid excessive intake of foods high in potassium and to avoid salt substitutes.

REFERENCES

Miller, S. & Fioravanti, J. (1997). Pediatric medications: a handbook for nurses. St. Louis: Mosby.

Taketomo, C. K., Hodding, J. H. & Kraus, D. M. (2003–2004). Pediatric dosage handbook (10th ed.). Hudson, OH: Lexi-Comp.

Flavoxate
Oxybutynin
Phenazopyridine Hydrochloride

Uses: Spasmolytic agents are used to treat urinary frequency and urgency or urge incontinence. Flavoxate also relieves other symptoms of cystitis, prostatitis, urethritis, and related disorders. Oxybutynin also minimizes other symptoms of neurogenic bladder. Phenazopyridine also relieves other symptoms of urinary mucosal irritation, which may be caused by infection, trauma, or surgery.

Action: Most spasmolytics competitively block the actions of acetylcholine at muscarinic receptors. Because of this cholinergic blockade, flavoxate and oxybutynin relax detrusor and other smooth muscle, counteracting muscle spasms in the urinary tract. Phenazopyridine exerts a topical analgesic effect on the urinary mucosa.

COMBINATION PRODUCTS

ZOTRIM: phenazopyridine/ trimethoprim (an anti-infective)/ sulfamethoxazole (a sulfonamide) 200 mg/160 mg/800 mg.

Flavoxate

flay-**vocks**-ate
(Urispas)
Do not confuse with Urised.

CATEGORY AND SCHEDULE

Pregnancy Risk Category: B

MECHANISM OF ACTION

An anticholinergic that relaxes detrusor and other smooth muscle by cholinergic blockade, counteracting muscle spasms of the urinary tract. ***Therapeutic Effect:*** Produces anticholinergic, local anesthetic, and analgesic effects, relieving urinary symptoms.

AVAILABILITY

Tablets: 100 mg.

INDICATIONS AND DOSAGES

▸ **Urinary antispasmodic**

PO
Adolescents.
100–200 mg 3–4 times/day.

CONTRAINDICATIONS

Duodenal or pyloric obstruction, GI hemorrhage, GI obstruction, ileus, obstructions of the lower urinary tract.

INTERACTIONS

Drug
None known.

Herbal
None known.

Food
None known.

DIAGNOSTIC TEST EFFECTS

None known.

SIDE EFFECTS

Generally well tolerated. Side effects are usually mild and transient.

Frequent
Drowsiness, dry mouth, throat

Occasional
Constipation, difficult urination, blurred vision, dizziness, headache, increased light sensitivity, nausea, vomiting, stomach pain
Rare
Confusion, hypersensitivity, increased intraocular pressure, leukopenia

SERIOUS REACTIONS

! An anticholinergic effect may occur with overdose, including unsteadiness, severe dizziness, drowsiness, fever, flushed face, shortness of breath, nervousness, and irritability.

PEDIATRIC CONSIDERATIONS

Baseline Assessment
- Assess the patient's dysuria, urinary frequency, incontinence, suprapubic pain, and urinary urgency.
- Plan to obtain a urine sample for culture and sensitivity testing and urinalysis.
- Be aware that this product contains castor oil.

Precautions
- Use cautiously in pts with glaucoma.

Intervention and Evaluation
- Monitor the patient for symptomatic relief.

Patient/Family Teaching
- Warn the patient/family to avoid performing tasks that require mental alertness or motor skills until the patient's response to the drug is established.
- Teach the patient/family about the adverse side effects of the drug, which are related to overdose, including unsteadiness, severe dizziness, drowsiness, fever, flushed face, shortness of breath, nervousness, and irritability.

Oxybutynin

ox-ee-**byoo**-tih-nin
(Ditropan, Ditropan XL, Oxytrol)
Do not confuse with diazepam or Oxycontin.

CATEGORY AND SCHEDULE

Pregnancy Risk Category: B

MECHANISM OF ACTION

An anticholinergic that exerts antispasmodic (papaverine-like) and antimuscarinic or atropine-like action on the detrusor smooth muscle of the bladder. ***Therapeutic Effect:*** Increases bladder capacity, diminishes frequency of uninhibited detrusor muscle contraction, and delays desire to void.

PHARMACOKINETICS

Route	Onset	Peak	Duration
PO	0.5–1 hr	3–6 hrs	6–10 hrs

Rapid absorption from the GI tract. Metabolized in liver. Primarily excreted in urine. Unknown whether removed by hemodialysis. ***Half-Life:*** Adults: 1–2.3 hrs.

AVAILABILITY

Tablets: 5 mg.
Syrup: 5 mg/5 mL.
Tablets (extended release): 5 mg, 10 mg, 15 mg.
Transdermal: 3.9 mg/day.

INDICATIONS AND DOSAGES

▸ **Neurogenic bladder**
PO
Children older than 5 yrs. 5 mg 2 times/day up to 5 mg 4 times/day.

Children 1–5 yrs. 0.2 mg/kg/dose 2–4 times/day.

CONTRAINDICATIONS

Hypersensitivity to oxybutynin or any related component. GI obstruction, GU obstruction, glaucoma, myasthenia gravis, partial or complete GU obstruction, toxic megacolon, ulcerative colitis.

INTERACTIONS

Drug

Medications with anticholinergic effects, such as antihistamines: May increase the effects of oxybutynin.
Digoxin: May increase serum concentrations of digoxin, leading to an increased risk for toxicity.
Haloperidol: May decrease serum concentrations of haloperidol, leading to decreased antipsychotic effects.

Herbal

None known.

Food

None known.

DIAGNOSTIC TEST EFFECTS

None known.

SIDE EFFECTS

Frequent
Constipation, dry mouth, drowsiness, decreased sweating
Occasional
Decreased lacrimation, salivary or sweat gland secretion, and sexual ability, urinary hesitancy and retention, suppressed lactation, blurred vision, mydriasis, nausea or vomiting, insomnia

SERIOUS REACTIONS

! Overdosage produces CNS excitation, including nervousness, restlessness, hallucinations, and irritability, hypotension or hypertension, confusion, fast heartbeat or tachycardia, flushed or red face, and respiratory depression, such as shortness of breath or troubled breathing.

PEDIATRIC CONSIDERATIONS

Baseline Assessment

• Assess the patient's dysuria, urinary frequency, incontinence, and urinary urgency.
• Be aware that it is unknown whether oxybutynin crosses the placenta or is distributed in breast milk.
• There are no age-related precautions noted in children older than 5 yrs of age.

Precautions

• Use cautiously in pts with cardiovascular disease, hypertension, hyperthyroidism, liver or renal impairment, neuropathy, prostatic hypertrophy, and reflux esophagitis.

Administration and Handling

PO
• Give oxybutynin without regard to meals.

Intervention and Evaluation

• Monitor the patient for symptomatic relief.
• Monitor the patient's intake and output and palpate the patient's bladder for signs of urinary retention.
• Assess the patient's pattern of daily bowel activity and stool consistency.

Patient/Family Teaching

• Urge the patient/family to avoid alcohol during oxybutynin therapy.
• Warn the patient/family to avoid performing tasks requiring mental alertness or motor skills until the patient's response to the drug is established.

• Alert the patient that the tablet shell may be seen in the stool.
• Tell the patient/family that oxybutynin may cause drowsiness and dry mouth.

Phenazopyridine Hydrochloride

feen-ah-zoe-**peer**-ih-deen
(Azo-Gesic, Azo-Standard, Phenazo [CAN], Prodium, Pyridium, Pyronium [CAN], Uristat)
Do not confuse with pyridoxine.

CATEGORY AND SCHEDULE

Pregnancy Risk Category: B

MECHANISM OF ACTION

An interstitial cystitis agent that exerts a topical analgesic effect on the urinary tract mucosa. ***Therapeutic Effect:*** Provides relief of urinary pain, burning, urgency, and frequency.

PHARMACOKINETICS

Well absorbed from the GI tract. Partially metabolized in liver. Primarily excreted in urine.

AVAILABILITY

Tablets: 95 mg, 97.2 mg, 100 mg, 150 mg, 200 mg.

INDICATIONS AND DOSAGES

▸ **Analgesic**

PO

Children older than 6 yrs. 12 mg/kg/day in 3 divided doses for 2 days.

▸ **Dose interval in renal impairment**

Creatinine Clearance	Interval
50–80 mL/min	q8–16h
Less than 50 mL/min	avoid use

CONTRAINDICATIONS

Hypersensitivity to phenazopyridine or any related component. Liver and renal insufficiency.

INTERACTIONS

Drug

None known.

Herbal

None known.

Food

None known.

DIAGNOSTIC TEST EFFECTS

May interfere with urinalysis color reactions, such as urinary glucose and ketone tests, urinary protein, or determination of urinary steroids.

SIDE EFFECTS

Occasional

Headache, GI disturbance, rash, pruritus

SERIOUS REACTIONS

! Overdosage levels or pts with impaired renal function or severe hypersensitivity may develop renal toxicity, hemolytic anemia, and liver toxicity.
! Methemoglobinemia generally occurs as a result of massive and acute overdosage.

PEDIATRIC CONSIDERATIONS

Baseline Assessment

• Be aware that it is unknown whether phenazopyridine crosses the placenta or is distributed in breast milk.
• There are no age-related precautions noted in children older than 6 yrs of age.

Administration and Handling

PO

• Give phenazopyridine with meals.

Intervention and Evaluation

• Assess the patient for a therapeutic response, including relief of pain or burning and decreased frequency of urination and urgency.

Patient/Family Teaching

• Tell the patient/family that the patient's urine will turn a reddish orange color during phenazopyridine therapy.

• Explain to the patient/family that this drug may stain fabric.

• Explain to the patient/family that this drug may stain soft contact lenses.

• Instruct the patient/family to take phenazopyridine with meals to reduce the possibility of GI upset.

REFERENCES

Miller, S. & Fioravanti, J. (1997). Pediatric medications: a handbook for nurses. St. Louis: Mosby.

Taketomo, C. K., Hodding, J. H. & Kraus, D. M. (2003–2004). Pediatric dosage handbook (10th ed.). Hudson, OH: Lexi-Comp.

75 Antihistamines

Azelastine
Cetirizine
Clemastine Fumarate
Desloratidine
Diphenhydramine Hydrochloride
Fexofenadine Hydrochloride
Hydroxyzine
Loratadine
Promethazine Hydrochloride

Uses: Antihistamines are chiefly used to relieve symptoms of upper respiratory allergic disorders. They are also used to manage allergic reactions to other drugs as well as blood transfusion reactions. These agents are used as a second choice in treating angioneurotic edema. Some can be used to provide preoperative and postoperative sedation, to manage insomnia, to relieve anxiety and tension, and to control muscle spasms. They also may be used to treat acute urticaria, other dermatologic conditions, motion sickness, and Parkinson disease.

Action: As histamine (H_1) antagonists, antihistamines cause vasoconstriction, which helps decrease edema, bronchodilation, and mucus secretion. These agents also block the increased capillary permeability and formation of edema and wheals caused by histamine. Many antihistamines can bind to receptors in the CNS, causing primarily depression (with decreased alertness, slowed reaction times, and somnolence) but also stimulation (with restlessness, nervousness, and an inability to sleep). Some may counter motion sickness. (See illustration, *Sites of Action: Respiratory Agents,* page 853.)

COMBINATION PRODUCTS

ALLEGRA-D: fexofenadine/-pseudoephedrine (a nasal decongestant) 60 mg/120 mg.
CALADRYL: diphenhydramine/calamine (an astringent)/camphor (a counterirritant).
CLARITIN-D: loratadine/pseudo-ephedrine (a nasal decongestant) 5 mg/120 mg; 10 mg/240 mg.
PHENERGAN WITH CODEINE: promethazine/codeine (a cough suppressant) 6.25 mg/10 mg per 5 mL.
PHENERGAN VC: promethazine/phenylephrine (a vasopressor) 6.25 mg/5 mg per 5 mL.
PHENERGAN VC WITH CODEINE: promethazine/phenylephrine (a vasopressor)/codeine (a cough suppressant) 6.25 mg/5 mg/10 mg per 5 mL.
ZYRTEC D-12 HOUR TABLETS: cetirizine/pseudoephedrine (a nasal decongestant) 5 mg/120 mg.

Azelastine

aye-zeh-**las**-teen
(Astelin, Optivar)

CATEGORY AND SCHEDULE

Pregnancy Risk Category: C

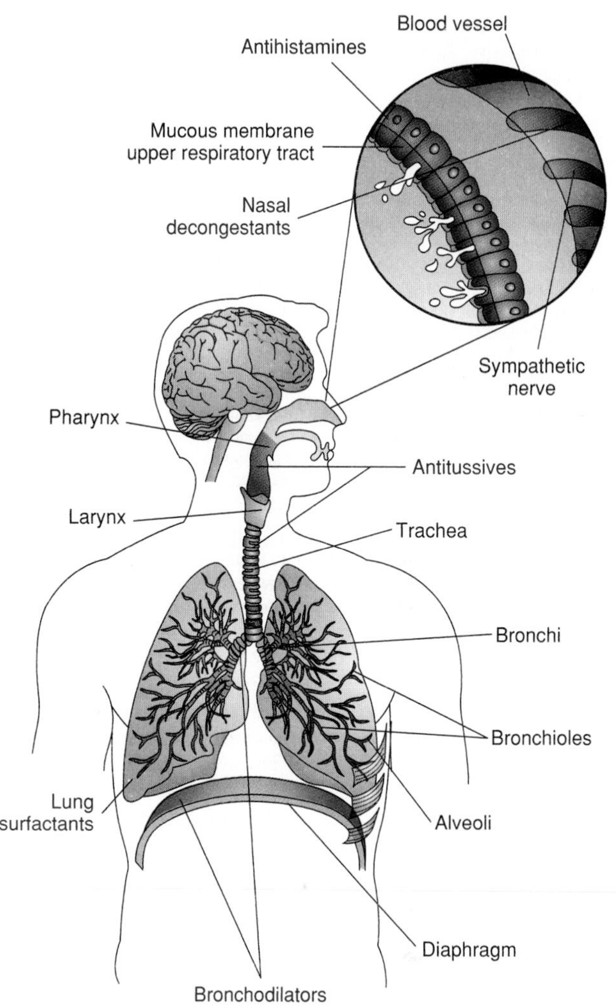

Sites of Action: Respiratory Agents

Drugs from several classes are used to manage respiratory disorders. Each class of drugs and individual drugs within each class can act at different sites in the respiratory tract. Antihistamines, such as diphenhydramine, help relieve symptoms of upper respiratory allergic disorders by blocking the stimulation of histamine$_1$ (H_1)-receptors primarily in the mucous membranes of the upper respiratory tract. Normally, H_1-receptor stimulation

(continued)

Sites of Action: Respiratory Agents—cont'd

results in vasodilation, increased capillary permeability and mucous secretion, and bronchoconstriction. When antihistamines block H_1-receptors, vasoconstriction occurs, which decreases edema, capillary permeability, and mucous secretion. The drugs also cause bronchodilation, improving airflow to and from the lungs. Unlike first-generation antihistamines, such as diphenhydramine, which cross the blood-brain barrier and cause sedation, second-generation antihistamines, such as loratadine, do not cross the blood-brain barrier and produce little or no sedation.

Non-narcotic antitussives, such as benzonatate, act on the stretch and cough receptors in the respiratory tract, including the pharynx, larynx, and tracheobronchial tree. Because benzonatate also has local anesthetic properties, it anesthetizes irritated tissues and suppresses cough. Another antitussive, guaifenesin, has an expectorant action that alters respiratory tract secretions, making mucus more viscous and less adhesive and making the cough more productive.

All bronchodilators open the bronchioles to improve airflow. However, subclasses of bronchodilators work in different ways. $Beta_2$-adrenergic agonists may be short-acting, such as albuterol, and long-acting, such as salmeterol. Both types stimulate $beta_2$-receptors in the lungs, resulting in relaxation of bronchial smooth muscle, increased vital capacity, and decreased airway resistance. These agents also block histamine release from mast cells, decreasing capillary permeability and mucous secretion.

Anticholinergics, such as ipratropium, block muscarinic cholinergic receptors in the bronchi, leading to bronchodilation. These drugs exert more action on larger airways, whereas $beta_2$-adrenergic agonists act primarily on smaller airways, Methylxanthines, such as aminophylline, work by inhibiting phosphodiesterase and adenosine, relaxing bronchial smooth muscle and promoting bronchodilation. These drugs also increase the contractility of the diaphragm and may enhance mucus clearance.

Lung surfactants, such as beractant, restore pulmonary surfactant in infants who have a deficiency of it. They work by lowering the surface tension on alveoli. As a result, the alveoli become more stable and less likely to collapse. These actions lead to improved lung compliance and respiratory gas exchange.

Nasal decongestants, such as pseudoephedrine, constrict blood vessels in the nose by mimicking the actions of the sympathetic nervous system. They directly stimulate $alpha_1$-adrenergic receptors in the smooth muscle of nasal blood vessels, which shrinks swollen mucous membranes and decreases mucus production by reducing fluid exudation.

MECHANISM OF ACTION

An antihistamine that competes with histamine for histamine receptor sites on cells in the blood vessels, GI tract, and respiratory tract. ***Therapeutic Effect:*** Inhibits symptoms associated with seasonal allergic rhinitis such as increased mucus production and sneezing.

PHARMACOKINETICS

Route	Onset	Peak	Duration
Nasal spray	0.5–1 hr	2–3 hrs	12 hrs
Ophthalmic	N/A	3 min	8 hrs

Well absorbed through nasal mucosa. Primarily excreted in feces. ***Half-Life:*** 22 hrs.

AVAILABILITY

Nasal Spray: 137 mcg/spray.
Ophthalmic Solution: 0.05%.

INDICATIONS AND DOSAGES

Allergic rhinitis

NASAL

Children 12 yrs or older. 2 sprays to each nostril 2 times/day.
Children 5–11 yrs. 1 spray to each nostril 2 times/day.

Vasomotor rhinitis
NASAL
Children 12 yrs or older: 2 sprays to each nostril twice daily.
Allergic conjunctivitis Ophthalmic
Children 3 yrs or older: 1 drop into affected eye twice daily.

CONTRAINDICATIONS

A history of hypersensitivity to antihistamines, newborn or premature infants, nursing mothers, third trimester of pregnancy.

INTERACTIONS

Drug

Alcohol, CNS depressants: May increase CNS depression.
Cimetidine: May increase azelastine blood concentration.

Herbal

None known.

Food

None known.

DIAGNOSTIC TEST EFFECTS

May suppress flare and wheal reaction to antigen skin testing unless drug is discontinued 4 days before testing. May increase SGPT (AST) levels.

SIDE EFFECTS

Frequent (20%–15%)
Headache, bitter taste
Rare
Nasal burning, paroxysmal sneezing
Ophthalmic: Transient eye burning or stinging, bitter taste, headache

SERIOUS REACTIONS

! Epistaxis or nosebleed occurs rarely.

PEDIATRIC CONSIDERATIONS

Baseline Assessment

• Determine whether the patient has a hypersensitivity to antihistamines.
• Be aware that it is unknown whether azelastine crosses the placenta or is distributed in breast milk.
• Do not use azelastine in pts during the third trimester of pregnancy.
• Be aware that the safety and efficacy of azelastine have not been established in children younger than 12 yrs of age.

Precautions

• Use cautiously in pts with renal function impairment.

Administration and Handling

NASAL
• Clear the patient's nasal passages as much as possible before use.
• Tilt the patient's head slightly forward.
• Insert the spray tip into one of the patient's nostrils, pointing the spray toward the nasal passage, away from nasal septum.
• Spray into the patient's nostril while holding the patient's other nostril closed and instruct the patient to inhale at the same time through his or her nose to deliver the medication as high into the nasal passages as possible.
OPHTHALMIC
• Tilt the patient's head back; place solution in conjunctival sac.
• Have the patient close his or her eyes, then press gently on the lacrimal sac for 1 min.

Intervention and Evaluation

• Assess the patient's therapeutic response to the medication.

Patient/Family Teaching

• Advise the patient/family to clear the patient's nasal passages before using azelastine.
• Teach the patient/family that before using the medication the first time, the patient should prime the pump with 4 sprays or until a fine mist appears. After the first

use and if the pump has not been used for 3 or more days, tell the patient to prime the pump with 2 sprays or until a fine mist appears.
• Teach the patient/family to wipe the tip of the applicator with a clean, damp tissue and to replace the cap immediately after use.
• Warn the patient/family to avoid spraying the medication in the eyes.

Cetirizine

sih-**tier**-eh-zeen
(Reactine [CAN], Zyrtec)
Do not confuse with Zyprexa.

CATEGORY AND SCHEDULE

Pregnancy Risk Category: B

MECHANISM OF ACTION

A second-generation piperazine that competes with histamine for H_1-receptor sites on effector cells in the GI tract, blood vessels, and respiratory tract. ***Therapeutic Effect:*** Prevents allergic response, produces mild bronchodilation, and blocks histamine-induced bronchitis.

PHARMACOKINETICS

Route	Onset	Peak	Duration
PO	less than 1 hr	4–8 hrs	less than 24 hrs

Rapidly, almost completely absorbed from the GI tract. Protein binding: 93%. Food has no effect on absorption. Undergoes low first-pass metabolism; not extensively metabolized. Primarily excreted in urine (greater than 80% as unchanged drug). Minimally removed by dialysis. ***Half-Life:*** 6.5–10 hrs.

AVAILABILITY

Tablets: 5 mg, 10 mg.
Syrup: 5 mg/5 mL.

INDICATIONS AND DOSAGES

Allergic rhinitis, hives
PO
Children 6–11 yrs. 5–10 mg once daily.
Children 2–5 yrs. Initially, 2.5 mg once daily. Maximum: 5 mg once daily or 2.5 mg q12h.
Children 6 mos–2 yrs. Initially 2.5 mg once daily. May increase dose to maximum of 2.5 mg q12h.

UNLABELED USES

Treatment of bronchial asthma.

CONTRAINDICATIONS

Hypersensitivity to cetirizine, hydroxyzine.

INTERACTIONS

Drug
Alcohol, CNS depressants: May increase CNS depression.
Theophylline: May decrease clearance of cetirizine.
Herbal
None known.
Food
None known.

DIAGNOSTIC TEST EFFECTS

May suppress wheal and flare reactions to antigen skin testing, unless antihistamines are discontinued 4 days before testing.

SIDE EFFECTS

Minimal anticholinergic effects
Occasional (10%–2%)
Pharyngitis, dry mouth, nose, throat, nausea, vomiting, abdominal pain, headache, dizziness,

fatigue, thickening mucus, drowsiness, increased sensitivity of skin to sun

SERIOUS REACTIONS

! Children may experience a dominant paradoxical reaction, including restlessness, insomnia, euphoria, nervousness, and tremors.

PEDIATRIC CONSIDERATIONS

Baseline Assessment

• Assess the patient's lung sounds.
• Assess the severity of the patient's rhinitis, urticaria, or other symptoms.
• Expect to obtain the patient's baseline serum hepatic enzyme levels to assess liver function.
• Be aware that cetirizine use is not recommended during the early months of pregnancy.
• Be aware that it is unknown whether cetirizine is excreted in breast milk. Breast-feeding is not recommended in this patient population.
• Be aware that cetirizine is less likely to cause anticholinergic effects in children.

Precautions

• Use cautiously in pts with impaired liver or renal function.
• Remember that cetirizine may cause drowsiness at dosages greater than 10 mg/day.

Administration and Handling

PO

• Give cetirizine without regard to meals.

Intervention and Evaluation

• Ensure that the patient with upper respiratory allergies increases fluid intake to maintain thin secretions and offset thirst.
• Monitor the patient's symptoms for a therapeutic response.

Patient/Family Teaching

• Warn the patient/family to avoid performing tasks that require motor skills if the patient experiences drowsiness during cetirizine therapy.
• Tell the patient/family to avoid alcohol during cetirizine therapy.
• Urge the patient/family to avoid prolonged exposure to sunlight.

Clemastine Fumarate

kleh-**mass**-teen
(Dayhistol, Tavist, Tavist-1)

CATEGORY AND SCHEDULE

Pregnancy Risk Category: B

MECHANISM OF ACTION

An ethanolamine that competes with histamine on effector cells in the GI tract, blood vessels, and respiratory tract. ***Therapeutic Effect:*** Relieves allergic conditions, including urticaria and pruritus. Anticholinergic effects cause drying of nasal mucosa.

PHARMACOKINETICS

Route	Onset	Peak	Duration
PO	15–60 min	5–7 hrs	10–12 hrs

Well absorbed from GI tract. Metabolized in liver. Excreted primarily in urine.

AVAILABILITY

Tablets: 1.34 mg, 2.68 mg.
Syrup: 0.67 mg/5 mL, 0.5 mg/5 mL.

INDICATIONS AND DOSAGES

Allergic rhinitis
PO
Children older than 12 yrs. 1.34–2.68 mg 3 times/day. Maximum: 8.04 mg/day.
Children 6–12 yrs. 0.67–1.34 mg 2 times/day. Maximum: 4.02 mg/day.
Children younger than 6 yrs. 0.335–0.67 mg/day in 2–3 divided doses. Maximum: 1.34 mg (1 mg base).

Allergic urticaria, angioedema
PO
Children older than 12 yrs. 2.68 mg 1–3 times/day. Do not exceed 8.04 mg/day.
Children 6–12 yrs. 1.34 mg 2 times/day. Do not exceed 4.02 mg/day.

CONTRAINDICATIONS

Hypersensitivity to clemastine, narrow-angle glaucoma, pts receiving MAOIs.

INTERACTIONS

Drug

Alcohol, CNS depressants: May increase CNS depressant effects.
MAOIs: May increase anticholinergic and CNS depressant effects.

Herbal

None known.

Food

None known.

DIAGNOSTIC TEST EFFECTS

May suppress wheal and flare reactions to antigen skin testing, unless antihistamines are discontinued 4 days before testing.

SIDE EFFECTS

Frequent
Drowsiness, dizziness, dry mouth, nose, or throat, urinary retention, thickening of bronchial secretions

SERIOUS REACTIONS

! Children may experience a dominant paradoxical reaction, including restlessness, insomnia, euphoria, nervousness, and tremors.
! Overdosage in children may result in hallucinations, convulsions, and death.
! A hypersensitivity reaction, marked by eczema, pruritus, rash, cardiac disturbances, angioedema, and photosensitivity, may occur.
! Overdosage may vary from CNS depression, including sedation, apnea, cardiovascular collapse, or death to a severe paradoxical reaction, such as hallucinations, tremor, and seizures.

PEDIATRIC CONSIDERATIONS

Baseline Assessment

- Obtain the history of recently ingested drugs and foods, environmental exposure, and emotional stress of the patient undergoing allergic reaction.
- Monitor the depth, quality, rate, and rhythm of the patient's pulse.
- Monitor the patient's respirations. Assess the patient's lung sounds for crackles, rhonchi, and wheezing.
- Be aware that clemastine is excreted in breast milk.
- Be aware that the safety and efficacy of clemastine have not been established in children younger than 6 yrs of age.

Precautions

- Use cautiously in pts with asthma, GI or GU obstruction, peptic ulcer disease, and prostatic hypertrophy.

Administration and Handling

◂ALERT▸ Be aware that the fixed-combination form (Tavist-D) may produce mild CNS stimulation.

PO
Give clemastine without regard to meals.

• Crush scored tablets as needed. Do not crush extended-release or film-coated forms.

Intervention and Evaluation

• Monitor blood pressure in pts who are at an increased risk of developing hypotension.
• Monitor pediatric pts closely for a paradoxical reaction.

Patient/Family Teaching

• Tell the patient/family that the patient will develop tolerance to the antihistaminic effect of the drug.
• Explain to the patient/family that the patient may develop tolerance to the sedative effect of the drug.
• Warn the patient/family to avoid performing tasks that require mental alertness or motor skills until the patient's response to the drug is established.
• Inform the patient/family that dizziness, drowsiness, and dry mouth are expected side effects of clemastine. Explain to the patient/family that consuming coffee and tea may help reduce the patient's drowsiness.
• Urge the patient/family to avoid alcohol during antihistamine therapy.

Desloratidine

des-low-**rah**-tah-deen
(Clarinex, Aerius [CAN])

CATEGORY AND SCHEDULE

Pregnancy Risk Category: C

MECHANISM OF ACTION

A nonsedating antihistamine that exhibits selective peripheral histamine H_1-receptor blocking action. Competes with histamine at receptor sites. Desloratidine has 2.5–4 times greater potency than its parent compound, loratadine. ***Therapeutic Effect:*** Prevents the allergic response mediated by histamine, such as rhinitis and urticaria.

PHARMACOKINETICS

Rapidly, almost completely absorbed from the GI tract. Distributed mainly in liver, lungs, GI tract, and bile. Metabolized in liver to the active metabolite and undergoes extensive first-pass metabolism. Excreted in urine and eliminated in feces. ***Half-Life:*** 27 hrs. Half-life is increased in the pts with liver or renal disease.

AVAILABILITY

Tablets: 5 mg.
Reditabs: 5 mg.

INDICATIONS AND DOSAGES

Allergic rhinitis, hives
PO
Children older than 12 yrs. 5 mg once daily.

Liver or renal impairment
Children older than 12 yrs. 5 mg every other day.

CONTRAINDICATIONS

Hypersensitivity to desloratidine or any related component.

INTERACTIONS

Drug

Erythromycin, ketoconazole: May increase desloratidine blood concentrations.

Herbal

None known.

Food

None known.

DIAGNOSTIC TEST EFFECTS

May suppress wheal and flare reactions to antigen skin testing, unless antihistamines are discontinued 4 days before testing.

SIDE EFFECTS

Frequent (12%)
Headache
Occasional (3%)
Dry mouth, somnolence
Rare (less than 3%)
Fatigue, dizziness, diarrhea, nausea

SERIOUS REACTIONS

None known.

PEDIATRIC CONSIDERATIONS

Baseline Assessment

- Assess the patient's lung sounds for wheezing and skin for urticaria.
- Plan to discontinue the drug 4 days before antigen skin testing.
- Be aware that desloratidine is excreted in breast milk.
- Be aware that children are more sensitive to anticholinergic effects, such as dry mouth, nose, and throat.

Precautions

- Use cautiously in pts with liver impairment.
- Be aware that the safety of desloratidine in children younger than 6 yrs of age is unknown.
- Be aware that the oral-disintegrating tablet contains aspartame.

Administration and Handling

PO

- Do not crush or break film-coated tablets.

Intervention and Evaluation

- Increase the fluid intake in pts with upper respiratory allergies to decrease the viscosity of secretions, offset thirst, and replace lost fluids from diaphoresis.
- Monitor the patient for therapeutic response.

Patient/Family Teaching

- Tell the patient/family that desloratidine does not cause drowsiness.
- Warn the patient/family to avoid driving and performing tasks that require visual acuity if the patient experiences blurred vision or eye pain.
- Urge the patient/family to avoid consuming alcohol during desloratidine therapy.

Diphenhydramine Hydrochloride

dye-phen-**high**-dra-meen
(Allerdryl [CAN], Benadryl, Nytol [CAN], Unisom Sleepgels [AUS])
Do not confuse with benazepril, Bentyl, Benylin, calamine, or dimenhydrinate.

CATEGORY AND SCHEDULE

Pregnancy Risk Category: B
OTC (capsules, tablets, chewable tablets, syrup, elixir, cream, spray)

MECHANISM OF ACTION

An ethanolamine that competes with histamine at histaminic receptor sites. Inhibits central acetylcholine. ***Therapeutic Effect:*** Results in anticholinergic, antipruritic, antitussive, and antiemetic effects. Produces antidyskinetic and sedative effects.

PHARMACOKINETICS

Route	Onset	Peak	Duration
PO	15–30 min	1–4 hrs	4–6 hrs
IM/IV	less than 15 min	1–4 hrs	4–6 hrs

Well absorbed after PO and parenteral administration. Widely distributed. Protein binding: 98%–99%. Metabolized in liver. Primarily excreted in urine. ***Half-Life:*** 1–4 hrs.

AVAILABILITY

Capsules: 25 mg, 50 mg.
Tablets: 25 mg, 50 mg.
Tablets (chewable): 12.5 mg.
Syrup: 12.5 mg/5 mL.
Injection: 10 mg/mL, 50 mg/mL.
Cream: 1%, 2%.
Spray: 1%, 2%.

INDICATIONS AND DOSAGES

Moderate to severe allergic reaction, dystonic reaction
PO/IM/IV
Children. 5 mg/kg/day in divided doses q6–8h. Maximum: 300 mg/day.
Motion sickness, minor allergic rhinitis
PO/IM/IV
Children 12 yrs. 25–50 mg q4–6 hrs. Maximum: 300 mg/day.
Children 6–11 yrs. 12.5–25 mg q4–6h. Maximum: 150 mg/day.
Children 2–6 yrs. 6.25 mg q4–6h. Maximum: 37.5 mg/day.
Antitussive
PO
Children 12 yrs and older. 25 mg q4h. Maximum: 150 mg/day.
Children 6–11 yrs. 12.5 mg q4h. Maximum: 75 mg/day.
Children 2–5 yrs. 6.25 mg q4h. Maximum: 37.5 mg/day.
Nighttime sleep aid
PO
Children 12 yrs and older. 50 mg qhs 30 min before bedtime.
Children 2–11 yrs. 1 mg/kg/dose 30 min before bedtime. Maximum: 50 mg.
Pruritus relief
TOPICAL
Children 12 yrs and older. 1% or 2% strength: Apply 3–4 times/day.
Children 2–11 yrs. 1% strength: Apply 3–4 times/day.

CONTRAINDICATIONS

Hypersensitivity to diphenhydramine or any related component. Acute asthmatic attack, pts receiving MAOIs.

INTERACTIONS

Drug

Alcohol, CNS depressants: May increase CNS depressant effects.
Anticholinergics: May increase anticholinergic effects.
MAOIs: May increase anticholinergic and CNS depressant effects.

Herbal

None known.

Food

None known.

DIAGNOSTIC TEST EFFECTS

May suppress wheal and flare reactions to antigen skin testing unless antihistamines are discontinued 4 days before testing.

IV INCOMPATIBILITIES

Allopurinol (Aloprim), amphotericin B complex (Abelcet, AmBisome, Amphotec), cefepime (Maxipime), dexamethasone (Decadron), foscarnet (Foscavir)

IV COMPATIBILITIES

Atropine, cisplatin (Platinol), cyclophosphamide (Cytoxan), cytarabine (ARA-C), droperidol (Inapsine), fentanyl, glycopyrrolate (Robinul), heparin, hydrocortisone (Solu-Cortef), hydromorphone (Dilaudid), hydroxyzine (Vistaril), lidocaine, metoclopramide (Reglan), ondansetron (Zofran), promethazine (Phenergan), potassium chloride, propofol (Diprivan)

SIDE EFFECTS

Frequent

Drowsiness, dizziness, muscular weakness, hypotension, dry mouth, nose, throat, and lips, urinary retention, thickening of bronchial secretions

SERIOUS REACTIONS

! Children may experience dominant paradoxical reactions, including restlessness, insomnia, euphoria, nervousness, and tremors.

! Overdosage in children may result in hallucinations, seizures, and death.

! Hypersensitivity reaction, such as eczema, pruritus, rash, cardiac disturbances, and photosensitivity, may occur.

! Overdosage may vary from CNS depression, including sedation, apnea, hypotension, cardiovascular collapse, or death to severe paradoxical reaction, such as hallucinations, tremor, and seizures.

PEDIATRIC CONSIDERATIONS

Baseline Assessment

- Obtain the history of recently ingested drugs and food, emotional stress, and environmental exposure in pts having acute allergic reaction.
- Monitor the depth, rate, rhythm, and type of patient respirations and the quality and rate of the patient's pulse.
- Assess the patient's lung sounds for crackles, rhonchi, and wheezing.
- Plan to discontinue drug 4 days before antigen skin testing.
- Be aware that diphenhydramine crosses the placenta and is detected in breast milk. Also know that diphenhydramine use may inhibit lactation and that diphenhydramine use in breast-feeding women may produce irritability in their infants.
- Be aware that there is an increased risk of seizures in neonates and premature infants if the drug is used during the third trimester of pregnancy.
- Be aware that diphenhydramine use is not recommended in newborns or premature infants as these groups are at an increased risk of experiencing a paradoxical reaction.

Precautions

- Use cautiously in pts with asthma, cardiovascular disease, chronic obstructive pulmonary disease, hypertension, hyperthyroidism, narrow-angle glaucoma, increased intraocular pressure, peptic ulcer disease, prostatic hypertrophy, pyloroduodenal or bladder neck obstruction, and seizure disorders.

Administration and Handling

PO

- Give diphenhydramine without regard to meals.
- Crush scored tablets as needed.
- Do not crush, break, or open capsules or film-coated tablets.

IM

- Give IM injection deeply into a large muscle mass.

IV

- May be given undiluted.
- Give IV injection over at least 1 min.

Intervention and Evaluation

- Monitor the patient's blood pressure, because of increased risk of hypotension.

• Monitor pediatric pts closely for paradoxical reaction.

Patient/Family Teaching

• Explain to the patient/family that the patient will not develop a tolerance to the antihistaminic effects of the drug but may develop tolerance to its sedative effects.
• Warn the patient/family to avoid performing tasks that require mental alertness or motor skills until the patient's response to the drug is established.
• Warn the patient/family that expected responses to the drug include dizziness, drowsiness, and dry mouth.
• Urge the patient/family to avoid consuming alcohol during diphenhydramine therapy.

Fexofenadine Hydrochloride

fecks-**oh**-fen-ah-deen
(Allegra, Telfast [AUS])

CATEGORY AND SCHEDULE

Pregnancy Risk Category: C

MECHANISM OF ACTION

A piperidine that prevents and antagonizes most histamine effects, such as urticaria and pruritus. ***Therapeutic Effect:*** Relieves allergic rhinitis symptoms.

PHARMACOKINETICS

Rapidly absorbed after PO administration. Does not cross the blood-brain barrier. Protein binding: 60%–70%. Minimally metabolized. Eliminated in feces and excreted in urine. Not removed by hemodialysis. ***Half-Life:*** 14.4 hrs. Half-life is increased in pts with impaired renal function.

AVAILABILITY

Capsules: 60 mg.
Tablets: 30 mg, 60 mg, 180 mg.

INDICATIONS AND DOSAGES

Allergic rhinitis

PO

Children 12 yrs and older. 60 mg 2 times/day or 180 mg once daily.
Children 6–11 yrs. 30 mg 2 times/day.

Dosage in renal impairment

PO

Children 12 yrs and older. 60 mg once daily.
Children 6–11 yrs. 30 mg once daily.

CONTRAINDICATIONS

Hypersensitivity to fexofenadine or any related component.

INTERACTIONS

Drug

Ketoconazole, erythromycin: May increase fexofenadine blood concentrations.

Herbal

St. John's wort: May decrease absorption of fexofenadine.

Food

None known.

DIAGNOSTIC TEST EFFECTS

May suppress wheal and flare reactions to antigen skin testing. Discontinue at least 4 days before testing.

SIDE EFFECTS

Rare (less than 2%)

Drowsiness, headache, fatigue, nausea, vomiting, abdominal distress, dysmenorrhea

SERIOUS REACTIONS

None known.

PEDIATRIC CONSIDERATIONS

Baseline Assessment

- Obtain the history of recently ingested drugs and foods, emotional stress, and environmental exposure in pts undergoing an allergic reaction.
- Monitor depth, rate, rhythm, and type of patient respirations and the quality and rate of the patient's pulse.
- Assess the patient's lung sounds for crackles, rhonchi, and wheezing.
- Plan to discontinue the drug 4 days before antigen skin testing.
- Be aware that it is unknown whether fexofenadine crosses the placenta or is distributed in breast milk.
- Be aware that the safety and efficacy of fexofenadine have not been established in children younger than 12 yrs of age.

Precautions

- Use cautiously in pts with severe renal impairment.

Administration and Handling

PO

- Give fexofenadine without regard to food.

Intervention and Evaluation

- Assess the patient for therapeutic response relief from allergy symptoms including itching, red, watery eyes, rhinorrhea, and sneezing.

Patient/Family Teaching

- Warn the patient/family to avoid performing tasks that require mental alertness or motor skills until the patient's response to the drug is established.
- Urge the patient/family to avoid alcohol during antihistamine therapy.
- Tell the patient/family that drinking coffee or tea may help reduce drowsiness.

Hydroxyzine

See antianxiety agents

Loratadine

low-**rah**-tah-deen
(Claratyne [AUS], Claritin, Claritin Reditabs)

CATEGORY AND SCHEDULE

Pregnancy Risk Category: B

MECHANISM OF ACTION

An antihistamine that is long acting with selective peripheral histamine H_1-receptor antagonist action. Competes with histamine for receptor site. ***Therapeutic Effect:*** Prevents allergic responses mediated by histamine, such as urticaria and pruritus.

PHARMACOKINETICS

Route	Onset	Peak	Duration
PO	1–3 hrs	8–12 hrs	longer than 24 hrs

Rapidly, almost completely absorbed from the GI tract. Protein binding: 97% (metabolite: 73%–77%). Distributed mainly in liver, lungs, GI tract, and bile. Metabolized in liver to the active metabolite and undergoes extensive first-pass metabolism. Excreted in urine and eliminated in feces. Not removed by hemodialysis. ***Half-Life:*** 8.4 hrs. Metabolite: 28 hrs. Half-life increased in pts with liver disease.

AVAILABILITY

Tablets: 10 mg.
Rapid Dissolution Tablet: 10 mg.
Syrup: 10 mg/10 mL.

INDICATIONS AND DOSAGES

▸ **Allergic rhinitis, hives**

PO

Children 6 yrs and older. 10 mg once daily.

Children 2–5 yrs. 5 mg once daily.

▸ **Dosage in hepatic impairment**

Children. 10 mg every other day.

UNLABELED USES

Adjunct treatment of bronchial asthma.

CONTRAINDICATIONS

Hypersensitivity to loratadine or any ingredient.

INTERACTIONS

Drug

Clarithromycin, erythromycin, fluconazole, ketoconazole: May increase loratadine blood concentrations.

Herbal

None known.

Food

Delays the absorption of loratadine.

DIAGNOSTIC TEST EFFECTS

May suppress wheal and flare reactions to antigen skin testing, unless antihistamines are discontinued 4 days before testing.

SIDE EFFECTS

Frequent (12%–8%)

Headache, fatigue, drowsiness

Occasional (3%)

Dry mouth, nose, throat

Rare

Photosensitivity

SERIOUS REACTIONS

! None known.

PEDIATRIC CONSIDERATIONS

Baseline Assessment

- Assess the patient for allergy symptoms.
- Assess the patient's lung sounds for crackles, rhonchi, and wheezing and skin for urticaria.
- Expect to discontinue the drug 4 days before antigen skin testing.
- Be aware that loratadine is excreted in breast milk.
- Be aware that children are more sensitive to the anticholinergic effects of the drug, such as dry mouth, nose, and throat.

Precautions

- Use cautiously in breast-feeding women, children, and pts with liver impairment.

Administration and Handling

PO

- Give on an empty stomach as food delays drug absorption.

Intervention and Evaluation

- Increase the fluid intake to maintain thin secretions and offset thirst and loss of fluids from increased sweating in pts with upper respiratory allergies.
- Monitor the patient for therapeutic response.

Patient/Family Teaching

- Instruct the patient/family to drink plenty of water to help prevent dry mouth.
- Urge the patient/family to avoid consuming alcohol during antihistamine therapy.
- Explain to the patient/family that loratadine use may cause drowsiness.
- Warn the patient/family to avoid tasks requiring mental alertness or motor skills until the patient's response to the drug is established.
- Tell the patient/family that loratadine use may cause photosensitivity reactions. Stress to the

patient that he or she should avoid direct exposure to sunlight and should wear sunscreen.

Promethazine Hydrochloride

pro-**meth**-ah-zeen
(Histantil [CAN], Insomn-Eze [AUS], Phenergan)
Do not confuse with promazine.

CATEGORY AND SCHEDULE

Pregnancy Risk Category: C

MECHANISM OF ACTION

A phenothiazine that acts as an antiemetic, antihistamine, and sedative-hypnotic. As an antihistamine, inhibits histamine at histamine receptor sites. ***Therapeutic Effect:*** Prevents and antagonizes most allergic effects, such as urticaria and pruritus. As an antiemetic, diminishes vestibular stimulation, depresses labyrinthine function, and acts on the chemoreceptor trigger zone.
Therapeutic Effect: Produces an antiemetic effect. As a sedative-hypnotic, decreases stimulation to the brainstem reticular formation.
Therapeutic Effect: Produces CNS depression.

PHARMACOKINETICS

Route	Onset	Peak	Duration
PO	20 min	N/A	2–8 hrs
IM	20 min	N/A	2–8 hrs
Rectal	20 min	N/A	2–8 hrs
IV	3–5 min	N/A	2–8 hrs

Well absorbed from the GI tract and after IM administration. Widely distributed. Metabolized in liver. Primarily excreted in urine. Not removed by hemodialysis.
Half-Life: 16–19 hrs.

AVAILABILITY

Tablets: 25 mg, 50 mg.
Syrup: 6.25 mg/5 mL.
Suppository: 12.5 mg, 25 mg, 50 mg.
Injection: 25 mg/mL, 50 mg/mL.

INDICATIONS AND DOSAGES

Promethazine should not be used in pts younger than 2 yrs because of the potential for fatal respiratory depression.

▸ **Allergic symptoms**
PO
Children. 0.1 mg/kg/dose (maximum: 12.5 mg) 3 times/day plus 0.5 mg/kg/dose (maximum: 25 mg) at bedtime.

▸ **Motion sickness**
PO/RECTAL
Children. 0.5 mg/kg (maximum: 25 mg) 30 min–1 hr before leaving, then may administer q12h as needed.

▸ **Prevention of nausea, vomiting**
PO/IM/IV/RECTAL
Children. 0.25–1 mg/kg (maximum: 25 mg) q4–6h as needed.

▸ **Preoperative and postoperative sedation; adjunct to analgesics**
IM/IV
Children. 0.5–1 mg/kg/dose. Maximum: 50 mg.

CONTRAINDICATIONS

Hypersensitivity to promethazine or any related component. Cross-sensitivity with phenothiazines may occur. GI or GU obstruction, narrow-angle glaucoma, severe CNS depression or coma. Age younger than 2 yrs.

INTERACTIONS

Drug

Alcohol, CNS depressants: May increase CNS depressant effects.
Anticholinergics: May increase anticholinergic effects.
MAOIs: May intensify and prolong anticholinergic and CNS depressant effects.

Herbal

None known.

Food

None known.

DIAGNOSTIC TEST EFFECTS

May suppress wheal and flare reactions to antigen skin testing unless discontinued 4 days before testing.

IV INCOMPATIBILITIES

Allopurinol (Aloprim), amphotericin B complex (Abelcet, AmBisome, Amphotec), heparin, ketorolac (Toradol), nalbuphine (Nubain), piperacillin tazobactam (Zosyn)

IV COMPATIBILITIES

Atropine, diphenhydramine (Benadryl), glycopyrrolate (Robinul), hydromorphone (Dilaudid), hydroxyzine (Vistaril), midazolam (Versed), morphine

SIDE EFFECTS

Expected
Drowsiness, disorientation
Frequent
Dry mouth, urinary retention, thickening of bronchial secretions
Occasional
Epigastric distress, flushing, visual disturbances, hearing disturbances, wheezing, paresthesia, sweating, chills
Rare
Dizziness, urticaria, photosensitivity, nightmares
Fixed-combination form with pseudoephedrine: mild CNS stimulation

SERIOUS REACTIONS

! Paradoxical reaction, particularly in children, manifested as excitation, nervousness, tremor, hyperactive reflexes, and convulsions.
! CNS depression has occurred in infants and young children, such as respiratory depression, sleep apnea, and sudden infant death syndrome.
! Long-term therapy may produce extrapyramidal symptoms noted as dystonia or abnormal movements or pronounced motor restlessness, which occurs most frequently in children.
! Blood dyscrasias, particularly agranulocytosis, have occurred.

PEDIATRIC CONSIDERATIONS

Baseline Assessment

- Assess the patient's blood pressure (B/P) and pulse rate if the patient is given the parenteral form of promethazine.
- Assess the patient for dehydration, including dry mucous membranes, longitudinal furrows in the tongue, and poor skin turgor, if promethazine is used as an antiemetic.
- Expect to discontinue the drug 4 days before antigen skin testing.
- Be aware that promethazine readily crosses the placenta, and it is unknown whether the drug is excreted in breast milk.
- Be aware that promethazine use may inhibit platelet aggregation in neonates if taken within 2 wks of birth.
- Be aware that promethazine use may produce extrapyramidal

symptoms and jaundice in neonates if taken during pregnancy.
• Be aware that children may experience increased excitement.
• Be aware that promethazine use is not recommended for children younger than 2 yrs of age.
• Be aware that the FDA issued a Black Box warning for promethazine due to cases of respiratory depression including fatalities in pediatric pts younger than 2 yrs. A wide range of weight-based doses of promethazine have resulted in respiratory depression in these pts.
• Exercise caution when administering promethazine to pediatric pts 2 yrs of age and older. It is recommended that the lowest effective dose be used and that concomitant administration of other drugs with respiratory depressant effects be avoided.

Precautions

• Use cautiously in pts with asthma, a history of seizures, impaired cardiovascular disease, liver function impairment, pts suspected of having Reye syndrome, peptic ulcer disease, and sleep apnea.

Administration and Handling

PO
• Give promethazine without regard to meals.
• Crush scored tablets as needed.

IM
◀ **ALERT** ▶ Avoid giving SC because significant tissue necrosis may occur. Inject carefully because inadvertent intra-arterial injection may produce severe arteriospasm, resulting in severe circulation impairment.
• Give IM injection deeply.

IV
• Store at room temperature.
• May be given undiluted or dilute with 0.9% NaCl; final dilution should not exceed 25 mg/mL.
• Administer at a 25 mg/min rate through the IV infusion tube, as prescribed.
• Inject slowly because a too rapid rate of infusion may result in a transient fall in B/P, producing orthostatic hypotension and reflex tachycardia.
• If the patient complains of pain at the IV site, stop the injection immediately because of the possibility of intra-arterial needle placement and perivascular extravasation.

RECTAL
• Refrigerate suppository.
• Moisten suppository with cold water before inserting well into the rectum.

Intervention and Evaluation

• Monitor serum electrolyte levels in pts with severe vomiting.
• Assist the patient with ambulation if he or she experiences drowsiness and lightheadedness.

Patient/Family Teaching

• Instruct the patient/family that drowsiness and dry mouth are expected responses to the drug.
• Suggest to the patient/family that sips of tepid water and sugarless gum may relieve dry mouth.
• Tell the patient/family that drinking coffee or tea may help reduce drowsiness.
• Warn the patient/family to notify the physician if the patient experiences visual disturbances.
• Warn the patient/family to avoid performing tasks that require mental alertness or motor skills until the patient's response to the drug is established.
• Urge the patient/family to avoid alcohol and other CNS depressants during promethazine therapy.

REFERENCES

Miller, S. & Fioravanti, J. (1997). Pediatric medications: a handbook for nurses. St. Louis: Mosby.

Taketomo, C. K., Hodding, J. H. & Kraus, D. M. (2003–2004). Pediatric dosage handbook (10th ed.). Hudson, OH: Lexi-Comp.

76 Antitussives (Non-Narcotic)

Benzonatate
Guaifenesin (Glyceryl Guaiacolate)

Uses: Antitussives are used to suppress cough. Specifically, *benzonatate* is used to relieve nonproductive cough, including acute cough caused by minor throat and bronchial irritation. *Guaifenesin* is used to relieve cough when mucus is present in the respiratory tract.

Action: Antitussives act in different ways to relieve cough. *Benzonatate* decreases the sensitivity of stretch receptors in the respiratory tract, which reduces cough production. *Guaifenesin* stimulates respiratory tract secretions by decreasing the adhesiveness and viscosity or phlegm, which promotes the removal of viscous mucus. (See illustration, *Sites of Action: Respiratory Agents,* page 853.)

COMBINATION PRODUCTS

ROBITUSSIN AC: guaifenesin/codeine (a narcotic analgesic) 100 mg/10 mg; 75 mg/2.5 mg per 5 mL.
ROBITUSSIN DM: guaifenesin/dextromethorphan (a cough suppressant) 100 mg/10 mg per 5 mL.

Benzonatate

ben-**zow**-nah-tate
(Tessalon Perles)

CATEGORY AND SCHEDULE

Pregnancy Risk Category: C

MECHANISM OF ACTION

A non-narcotic antitussive that anesthetizes stretch receptors in respiratory passages, lungs, and pleura. ***Therapeutic Effect:*** Reduces cough production.

AVAILABILITY

Capsules: 100 mg, 200 mg.

INDICATIONS AND DOSAGES

▸ **Antitussive**
PO
Children older than 10 yrs. 100–200 mg 3 times/day, up to 600 mg/day.

CONTRAINDICATIONS

Hypersensitivity to benzonatate or any related component.

INTERACTIONS

Drug
CNS depressants: May increase the effects of benzonatate.
Herbal
None known.
Food
None known.

DIAGNOSTIC TEST EFFECTS

None known.

SIDE EFFECTS

Occasional
Mild drowsiness, mild dizziness, constipation, GI upset, skin eruptions, nasal congestion

SERIOUS REACTIONS

! Paradoxical reaction, including restlessness, insomnia, euphoria, nervousness, and tremors, has been noted.

PEDIATRIC CONSIDERATIONS

Baseline Assessment

- Assess the frequency, severity, and type of patient cough.
- Monitor the amount, color, and consistency of the patient's sputum.
- Be aware that this product has not been studied in children younger than 10 yrs of age.

Precautions

- Use cautiously in pts with productive cough.
- Be aware that hallucinations and behavioral changes have occurred in pts taking benzonatate.

Administration and Handling

PO

- Give benzonatate without regard to meals.
- Swallow whole; do not chew pills or dissolve in the mouth because benzonatate may produce temporary local anesthesia or choking.

Intervention and Evaluation

- Have the patient begin deep breathing and coughing exercises, particularly in pts with impaired pulmonary function.
- Monitor the patient for a paradoxical reaction.
- Increase the patient's environmental humidity and fluid intake to lower the viscosity of his or her lung secretions.
- Assess the patient for clinical improvement and record onset of relief of the patient's cough.

Patient/Family Teaching

- Tell the patient/family to avoid tasks that require mental alertness or motor skills until the patient's response to the drug is established.
- Explain to the patient/family that dizziness, drowsiness, and dry mouth occur often.
- Instruct the patient/family to swallow the pill whole, not to chew it or allow it to dissolve in the mouth.

Guaifenesin (Glyceryl Guaiacolate)

guay-**fen**-ah-sin
(Balminil [CAN], Benylin E [CAN], Humibid, Mucinex, Robitussin)

CATEGORY AND SCHEDULE

Pregnancy Risk Category: C
OTC

MECHANISM OF ACTION

An expectorant that stimulates respiratory tract secretion by decreasing phlegm adhesiveness, viscosity, and fluid volume. ***Therapeutic Effect:*** Promotes removal of viscous mucus.

PHARMACOKINETICS

Well absorbed from the GI tract. Metabolized in liver. Excreted in urine.

AVAILABILITY

Tablets: 100 mg, 200 mg, 400 mg.
Tablets (sustained release): 600 mg.
Capsules: 200 mg.
Capsules (sustained release): 300 mg.
Syrup: 100 mg/5 mL.
Liquid: 200 mg/5 mL, 100 mg/5 mL.

INDICATIONS AND DOSAGES

▸ **Expectorant**

PO

Children older than 12 yrs. 200–400 mg q4h. Maximum: 2.4 g/day.
Children 6–12 yrs. 100–200 mg q4h. Maximum: 1.2 g/day.
Children 2–5 yrs. 50–100 mg q4h. Maximum: 600 mg/day.
Children younger than 2 yrs. 12 mg/kg/day in 6 divided doses.

CONTRAINDICATIONS

Hypersensitivity to guaifenesin or any related component.

INTERACTIONS

Drug
None known.
Herbal
None known.
Food
None known.

DIAGNOSTIC TEST EFFECTS

None known.

SIDE EFFECTS

Rare
Dizziness, headache, rash, diarrhea, nausea, vomiting, stomach pain

SERIOUS REACTIONS

! Excessive dosage may produce nausea and vomiting.

PEDIATRIC CONSIDERATIONS

Baseline Assessment

- Assess the frequency, severity, and type of patient cough.
- Increase the patient's environmental humidity and fluid intake to lower the viscosity of the patient's lung secretions.
- Ask about a history of cigarette smoking, asthma, and chronic bronchitis because the drug is not recommended for use with coughs caused by these conditions.
- Be aware that it is unknown whether guaifenesin crosses the placenta or is distributed in breast milk.
- There are no age-related precautions noted in children.
- Be aware that guaifenesin should be used cautiously in pts younger than 2 yrs of age with persistent cough.

Administration and Handling

◂ **ALERT** ▸ Give extended-release capsules at 12-hr intervals, as prescribed.

PO

- Store syrup, liquid, or capsules at room temperature.
- Give guaifenesin without regard to meals.
- Do not crush or break sustained-release capsules. May sprinkle contents on soft food, then swallow without chewing or crushing.

Intervention and Evaluation

- Have the patient begin deep breathing and coughing exercises, particularly in pts with impaired pulmonary function.
- Assess the patient for clinical improvement and record the onset of relief of the patient's cough.

Patient/Family Teaching

- Caution the patient/family to avoid performing tasks that require mental alertness or motor skills until the patient's response to the drug is established.
- Tell the patient/family not to take guaifenesin for chronic cough.
- Urge the patient/family to maintain adequate hydration by drinking plenty of fluids.
- Warn the patient/family to notify the physician if the patient's cough persists or if fever, rash, headache, or sore throat is present with cough.

REFERENCES

Miller, S. & Fioravanti, J. (1997). Pediatric medications: a handbook for nurses. St. Louis: Mosby.

Taketomo, C. K., Hodding, J. H. & Kraus, D. M. (2003–2004). Pediatric dosage handbook (10th ed.). Hudson, OH: Lexi-Comp.

77 Bronchodilators

Albuterol
Aminophylline (Theophylline Ethylenediamine), Theophylline
Formoterol Fumarate
Ipratropium Bromide
Levalbuterol
Metaproterenol Sulfate
Salmeterol
Terbutaline Sulfate

Uses: Bronchodilators are used to relieve bronchospasm that occurs during anesthesia and in bronchial asthma, bronchitis, emphysema, and chronic obstructive pulmonary disease. Some may also be prescribed to prevent bronchospasm. Terbutaline is also used to delay premature labor.

Action: Each bronchodilator subclass works by a different mechanism of action. *Beta$_2$-adrenergic agonists,* such as albuterol and formoterol, stimulate beta–receptors in the lungs, resulting in relaxed bronchial smooth muscle, increased vital capacity, and decreased airway resistance. Terbutaline also relaxes uterine muscle, inhibiting labor contractions. *Anticholinergics,* such as ipratropium, inhibit cholinergic receptors on bronchial smooth muscle, blocking the action of acetylcholine. This causes bronchodilation and inhibits secretions from glands in the nasal mucosa. *Methylxanthines,* such as aminophylline, directly relax smooth muscle in the bronchial airways and pulmonary blood vessels, relieving bronchospasm and increasing vital capacity. They also produce cardiac and skeletal muscle stimulation. (See illustration, *Sites of Action: Respiratory Agents,* page 000.)

COMBINATION PRODUCTS

ADVAIR: salmeterol/fluticasone (a corticosteroid) 50 mcg/100 mcg; 50 mcg/250 mcg; 50 mcg/500 mcg.
COMBIVENT: ipratropium/albuterol (a bronchodilator) 18 mcg/103 mcg per actuation from the mouthpiece.
DUONEB: ipratropium/albuterol base (a bronchodilator) 0.5 mg/2.5 mL per 3 mL.

Albuterol

ale-**beut**-er-all
(Airomir [AUS], Asmol CFC-Free [AUS], Epaq Inhaler [AUS], Novosalmol [CAN], Proventil, Respax [AUS], Ventolin, Ventolin CFC-Free [AUS], Volmax, Vospire ER)
Do not confuse with atenolol or Prinivil.

CATEGORY AND SCHEDULE

Pregnancy Risk Category: C

MECHANISM OF ACTION

A sympathomimetic (adrenergic agonist) that stimulates $beta_2$-adrenergic receptors in the lungs, resulting in relaxation of bronchial smooth muscle. ***Therapeutic Effect:*** Relieves bronchospasm, reduces airway resistance.

PHARMACOKINETICS

Route	Onset	Peak	Duration
PO	15–30 min	2–3 hrs	4–6 hrs
PO extended release	30 min	2–4 hrs	12 hrs
Inhalation	5–15 min	0.5–2 hrs	2–5 hrs

Rapidly, well absorbed from the GI tract; gradual absorption from bronchi after inhalation. Metabolized in liver. Primarily excreted in urine. ***Half-Life:*** Oral: 2.7–5 hrs; Inhalation: 3.8 hrs.

AVAILABILITY

Tablets: 2 mg, 4 mg.
Tablets (extended release): 4 mg, 8 mg.
Syrup: 2 mg/5 mL.
Aerosol: Metered dose inhaler (90 mcg/spray).
Solution for Inhalation: 0.083% (0.83 mg/mL), 0.5% (5 mg/mL).

INDICATIONS AND DOSAGES

▸ Bronchospasm

PO

Children 7–12 yrs. 2 mg 3–4 times/day. Repetabs: 4 mg 2 times/day.

Children 2–6 yrs. 0.1–0.2 mg/kg 3–4 times/day. Maximum: 4 mg 3 times/day.

INHALATION

Children 12 yrs and older. Metered dose inhaler: 1–2 inhalations q4–6h. Maximum: 12 inhalations/day.

Children younger than 12 yrs. 1–2 inhalations 4 times/day.

NEBULIZATION

Children. 0.15 mg/kg (minimum: 2.5 mg) every 20 min for 3 doses followed by 0.15–0.3 mg/kg (maximum: 10 mg) q1–4h as needed or continuous nebulization of 0.5 mg/kg/hr.

▸ Exercise-induced bronchospasm

INHALATION

Children older than 12 yrs. 2 inhalations 30 min before exercise.

CONTRAINDICATIONS

History of hypersensitivity to sympathomimetics.

INTERACTIONS

Drug

Beta-adrenergic blocking agents (beta-blockers): Antagonizes effects of albuterol.
Digoxin: May increase risk of arrhythmias with digoxin.
MAOIs, tricyclic antidepressants: May potentiate cardiovascular effects.

Herbal

None known.

Food

None known.

DIAGNOSTIC TEST EFFECTS

May increase blood glucose levels. May decrease serum potassium levels.

SIDE EFFECTS

Frequent

Headache (27%); nausea (15%); restlessness, nervousness, trembling (20%); dizziness (less than 7%); throat dryness and irritation, pharyngitis (less than 6%); blood pressure (B/P) changes including hypertension (5%–3%); heartburn, transient wheezing (less than 5%)

Occasional (3%–2%)

Insomnia, weakness, unusual or bad taste or taste or smell change. Inhalation: Dry, irritated mouth or throat; coughing; bronchial irritation.

Rare

Drowsiness, diarrhea, dry mouth, flushing, sweating, anorexia

SERIOUS REACTIONS

! Excessive sympathomimetic stimulation may produce palpitations, extrasystoles, tachycardia, chest pain, a slight increase in B/P followed by a substantial decrease, chills, sweating, and blanching of skin.

! Too frequent or excessive use may lead to loss of bronchodilating effectiveness and severe, paradoxical bronchoconstriction.

PEDIATRIC CONSIDERATIONS

Baseline Assessment

- Offer emotional support. Pts receiving this drug may become anxious because of their difficulty in breathing and also from the sympathomimetic response to the drug.
- Be aware that albuterol appears to cross the placenta, and it is unknown whether albuterol is distributed in breast milk.
- Albuterol may inhibit uterine contractility.
- Be aware that safety and efficacy have not been established in children younger than 2 years of age (syrup) or younger than 6 years of age (tablets).

Precautions

- Use cautiously in pts with cardiovascular disease, diabetes mellitus, hypertension, or hyperthyroidism.

Administration and Handling

PO

- Do not crush or break extended-release tablets.
- May give without regard to food.

INHALATION

- Shake container well and have the patient exhale completely through the mouth. Have the patient place the mouthpiece into the mouth and close the lips while holding the inhaler upright.
- Ask the patient to inhale deeply through the mouth while fully depressing the top of the canister, and to hold his or her breath as long as possible before exhaling slowly.
- Have the patient wait 2 min before inhaling the second dose because this allows for deeper bronchial penetration.
- Have the patient rinse his or her mouth with water immediately after inhalation to prevent mouth and throat dryness.
- For best results, use a spacer in conjunction with the metered dose inhaler.

NEBULIZATION

- Dilute 0.5 mL 0.5% solution to a final volume of 3 mL with 0.9% NaCl to provide 2.5 mg.
- Administer over 5–15 min.
- The nebulizer should be used with compressed air or O_2 at a rate of 6–10 L/min.

Intervention and Evaluation

- Monitor the 12-lead EKG, arterial blood gas determinations, quality and rate of the pulse the rate, depth, rhythm, and type of respirations, and serum potassium levels.
- Assess the patient's lung sounds for signs of bronchoconstriction, such as wheezing, and for rales.

Patient/Family Teaching

- Instruct the patient/family on the proper use of an inhaler.
- Encourage the patient/family to increase fluid intake to decrease the viscosity of the patient's pulmonary secretions.
- Inform the patient/family not to take more than 2 inhalations at any one time (excessive use may produce paradoxical bronchoconstriction or a decreased bronchodilating effect).
- Advise the patient/family that rinsing the mouth with water immediately after inhalation may prevent mouth and throat dryness.
- Urge the patient/family to avoid excessive use of caffeine derivatives, such as chocolate, cocoa, coffee, cola, and tea.

Aminophylline (Theophylline Ethylenediamine)

am-in-**ah**-phil-lin
(Aminophylline)
Do not confuse with amitriptyline or ampicillin.

Theophylline

(Slo-Bid, Theo-Dur, Theolair, Uniphyl)
Immediate-release: Aerolate, Theolair. Extended-release: Theo-24, Uniphyl.
Do not confuse with Dolobid.

CATEGORY AND SCHEDULE

Pregnancy Risk Category: C

MECHANISM OF ACTION

A xanthine derivative that acts as a bronchodilator by directly relaxing smooth muscle of the bronchial airway and pulmonary blood vessels. ***Therapeutic Effect:*** Relieves bronchospasm, increases vital capacity. Produces cardiac and skeletal muscle stimulation.

AVAILABILITY

Theophylline
Capsules: 100 mg, 200 mg.
Capsules (sustained release): 100 mg, 125 mg, 200 mg, 300 mg.
Capsules (sustained release 24 hrs): 100 mg, 200 mg, 300 mg.
Elixir: 80 mg/15 mL.
Injection: 25 mg/mL, 800 mg/500 mL.
Syrup: 150 mg/15 mL.
Tablet: 100 mg, 125 mg, 200 mg, 300 mg.
Tablet (controlled release): 100 mg, 200 mg, 300 mg, 400 mg, 600 mg.
Tablet (controlled release 12 hrs): 100 mg, 200 mg, 300 mg, 450 mg.
Aminophylline
Tablets: 100 mg (equivalent to 79 mg theophylline), 200 mg (equivalent to 158 mg theophylline).
Liquid: 105 mg/5 mL (equivalent to 90 mg theophylline/5 mL).
Injection: 250 mg/10 mL (equivalent to 197 mg theophylline/10 mL).
Suppository: 250 mg, 500 mg.

INDICATIONS AND DOSAGES

▸ **Acute bronchospasm**
PO LOADING DOSE FOR THEOPHYLLINE
Infants and children who have not received theophylline in the previous 24 hrs. 5 mg/kg.
Infants and children who have received theophylline in the previous 24 hrs. 2.5 mg/kg.
▸ **Chronic bronchospasm**
PO MAINTENANCE DOSE FOR THEOPHYLLINE
Infants 6 wks–6 mos. 10 mg/kg/day.

Infants 6 mos–1 yr. 12–18 mg/kg/day.
Children 1–9 yrs. 20–24 mg/kg/day.
Children 9–12 yrs. 16 mg/kg/day.
Adolescents (nonsmokers). 13 mg/kg/day.
Adolescents (smokers). 16 mg/kg/day.

▸ **Acute bronchospasm**

IV LOADING DOSE FOR AMINOPHYLLINE
Infants and children. 6 mg/kg over 20–30 min.
IV MAINTENANCE DOSE FOR AMINOPHYLLINE
Infants 6 wks–6 mos. 0.5 mg/kg/hr.
Infants 6 mos–1 yr. 0.6–0.7 mg/kg/hr.
Children 1–9 yrs. 1–1.2 mg/kg/hr.
Children 9–12 yrs. 0.9 mg/kg/hr.
Adolescents (nonsmokers). 0.7 mg/kg/hr.
Adolescents (smokers). 0.9 mg/kg/hr.

UNLABELED USES
Treatment of apnea in neonates.

CONTRAINDICATIONS
History of hypersensitivity to caffeine or xanthines. Uncontrolled arrhythmias.

INTERACTIONS
Drug
Beta-blockers: May decrease effects of aminophylline.
Cimetidine, ciprofloxacin, erythromycin, norfloxacin: May increase aminophylline blood concentration and risk of aminophylline toxicity.
Glucocorticoids: May produce hypernatremia.
Phenytoin, primidone, rifampin: May increase aminophylline metabolism.
Smoking: May decrease aminophylline blood concentration.

Herbal
None known.

Food
None known.

DIAGNOSTIC TEST EFFECTS
None known.

IV INCOMPATIBILITIES
Amiodarone (Cordarone), ciprofloxacin (Cipro), dobutamine (Dobutrex), ondansetron (Zofran)

IV COMPATIBILITIES
Aztreonam (Azactam), ceftazidime (Fortaz), fluconazole (Diflucan), heparin, morphine, potassium chloride

SIDE EFFECTS
Frequent
Momentary change in sense of smell during IV administration, shakiness, restlessness, tachycardia, trembling
Occasional
Heartburn, vomiting, headache, mild diuresis, insomnia, nausea

SERIOUS REACTIONS
! Too rapid a rate of IV administration may produce a marked fall in blood pressure with accompanying faintness and lightheadedness, palpitations, tachycardia, hyperventilation, nausea, vomiting, angina-like pain, seizures, ventricular fibrillation, and cardiac standstill.

PEDIATRIC CONSIDERATIONS
Baseline Assessment
- Offer the patient emotional support. Anxiety may occur because of difficulty in breathing and from the sympathomimetic response to the drug.
- As ordered, obtain the peak serum concentration 1 hr after IV dose, 1–2 hrs after immediate-

release dose, and 3–8 hours after extended-release dose. Obtain the serum trough level just before next dose.

- This medication is not indicated for infants younger than 16 mos of age.
- Be aware that aminophylline is a salt form of theophylline.

Precautions

- Use cautiously in pts with diabetes mellitus, glaucoma, hypertension, hyperthyroidism, impaired cardiac, renal or liver function, peptic ulcer disease, or a seizure disorder.

Administration and Handling

PO

- Give with food to avoid GI distress.
- Do not crush or break extended-release forms.

IV

- Store at room temperature.
- Discard if solution contains a precipitate.
- Give loading dose diluted in 100–200 mL of D_5W or 0.9% NaCl. Prepare maintenance dose in a larger volume parenteral infusion.
- Do not exceed flow rate of 1 mL/min (25 mg/min) for either piggyback or infusion.
- Administer loading dose over 20–30 min.
- Use infusion pump or microdrip to regulate IV administration.

Intervention and Evaluation

◂ **ALERT** ▸ Aminophylline dosage is calculated based on lean body weight. The dosage is also based on peak serum theophylline concentrations, the patient's clinical condition, and the absence of theophylline toxicity.

- Expect to monitor the rate, depth, rhythm, and type of breathing as well as to assess lung sounds for rhonchi, wheezing, or rales.
- Expect to monitor the patient's arterial blood gases and the quality and rate of the pulse.
- Examine the patient's lips and fingernails for evidence of oxygen depletion such as blue or gray lips, blue or dusky colored fingernails in light-skinned pts; and gray fingernails in dark-skinned pts.
- Assess the patient for clavicular retractions and hand tremor.
- Evaluate the patient for signs of clinical improvement such as cessation of clavicular retractions, quieter and slower respirations, and a relaxed facial expression.
- Monitor serum theophylline levels. The therapeutic serum level range is 10–20 mcg/mL.

Patient/Family Teaching

- Encourage the patient/family to increase the patient's fluid intake to decrease the thickness of lung secretions.
- Urge the patient/family to avoid excessive use of caffeine derivatives such as chocolate, coffee, cola, cocoa, and tea.
- Explain to the patient/family that smoking and consumption of charcoal-broiled food or a high-protein, low-carbohydrate diet may decrease theophylline level.

Formoterol Fumarate

four-**moh**-tur-all
(Foradil Aerolizer, Foradile [AUS], Oxis [AUS])

CATEGORY AND SCHEDULE

Pregnancy Risk Category: C

MECHANISM OF ACTION

A long-acting bronchodilator that stimulates $beta_2$-adrenergic receptors in the lungs, resulting in relaxation of bronchial smooth muscle. Also inhibits release of mediators from various cells in the lungs, including mast cells, with little effect on heart rate. ***Therapeutic Effect:*** Relieves bronchospasm, reduces airway resistance. Produces improved bronchodilation, nighttime improved asthma control, and improved peak flow rates.

PHARMACOKINETICS

Route	Onset	Peak	Duration
Inhalation	1–3 min	0.5–1 hr	12 hrs

Absorbed from bronchi after inhalation. Metabolized in liver. Primarily excreted in urine. Unknown whether removed by hemodialysis. ***Half-Life:*** 10 hrs.

AVAILABILITY

Inhalation Powder in Capsules: 12 mcg.

INDICATIONS AND DOSAGES

▸ Maintenance treatment of asthma

INHALATION

Children older than 5 yrs. Inhale aerosolized contents of 1 capsule every 12 hrs.

▸ Exercise-induced asthma

INHALATION

Children older than 12 yrs. Inhale aerosolized contents of 1 capsule at least 15 min before exercise.

CONTRAINDICATIONS

Hypersensitivity to formoterol, adrenergic amines, or any related component.

INTERACTIONS

Drug

Beta-adrenergic blocking agents: May antagonize bronchodilating effects.

Diuretics, steroids, xanthine derivatives: May increase the risk of hypokalemia.

Drugs that can prolong QT interval, including erythromycin, quinidine, and thioridazine, MAOIs, tricyclic antidepressants: May potentiate cardiovascular effects with drugs that can prolong QT interval.

Herbal

None known.

Food

None known.

DIAGNOSTIC TEST EFFECTS

May decrease serum potassium levels. May increase blood glucose levels.

SIDE EFFECTS

Occasional

Tremor, cramps, tachycardia, insomnia, headache, irritability, irritation of mouth or throat

SERIOUS REACTIONS

! Excessive sympathomimetic stimulation may produce palpitations, extrasystoles, and chest pain.

PEDIATRIC CONSIDERATIONS

Baseline Assessment

- Ask the patient about a history of cardiovascular disease, convulsive disorder, hypertension, and thyrotoxicosis.
- Check the patient's baseline EKG, and measure the QT interval.
- Check the patient's baseline peak flow readings.
- Be aware that it is unknown whether formoterol crosses the

placenta or is distributed in breast milk.

• Be aware that the safety and efficacy of formoterol have not been established in children younger than 5 yrs of age.

Precautions

• Use cautiously in pts with cardiovascular disease, convulsive disorder, hypertension, and thyrotoxicosis.

Administration and Handling

• Maintain capsules in individual blister pack until immediately before use. Do not swallow capsules. Do not use with a spacer.

INHALATION

• Pull off Aerolizer inhaler cover, twisting mouthpiece in direction of the arrow to open.

• Place capsule in chamber. Capsule is pierced by pressing and releasing buttons on the side of the Aerolizer, once only.

• Have the patient exhale completely; place mouthpiece into the patient's mouth and have the patient close his or her lips.

• Instruct the patient to inhale quickly and deeply through mouth because this causes the capsule to spin and dispense the drug. Next tell the patient to hold his or her breath as long as possible before exhaling slowly.

• Check capsule to make sure all the powder is gone. If not, instruct the patient to inhale again to receive the rest of the dose.

• Have the patient rinse his or her mouth with water immediately after inhalation to prevent mouth and throat dryness.

Intervention and Evaluation

• Monitor the depth, rate, rhythm, and type of patient respirations.

• Monitor the quality and rate of the patient's pulse.

• Monitor the patient's arterial blood gases, EKG, and serum potassium levels.

• Assess the patient's lung sounds for rhonchi and wheezing, signs of bronchoconstriction.

Patient/Family Teaching

• Instruct the patient/family on the proper use of the inhaler.

• Teach the patient/family to increase the patient's fluid intake to decrease lung secretion viscosity.

• Tell the patient/family that rinsing the mouth with water immediately after inhalation may prevent mouth and throat irritation.

• Urge the patient/family to avoid excessive use of caffeine derivatives such as chocolate, coffee, cola, and tea.

• Teach the patient/family how to measure peak flow readings and keep a log of measurements.

Ipratropium Bromide

ih-prah-**trow**-pea-um

(Aproven [AUS], Atrovent)

Do not confuse with Alupent.

CATEGORY AND SCHEDULE

Pregnancy Risk Category: B

MECHANISM OF ACTION

An anticholinergic that blocks the action of acetylcholine at parasympathetic sites in bronchial smooth muscle. ***Therapeutic Effect:*** Causes bronchodilation and inhibits secretions from the glands lining the nasal mucosa.

PHARMACOKINETICS

Route	Onset	Peak	Duration
Inhalation	1–3 min	1–2 hrs	4–6 hrs

Minimal systemic absorption. Metabolized in liver (systemic absorption). Primarily eliminated in feces. ***Half-Life:*** 1.5–4 hrs.

AVAILABILITY

Oral Inhalation: 18 mcg/actuation.
Aerosol Solution for Inhalation: 0.02% (500-mcg vial).
Nasal Spray: 0.03%, 0.06%.

INDICATIONS AND DOSAGES

▸ **Bronchospasm**

INHALATION

Children 3–12 yrs. 1–2 inhalations 3 times/day. Maximum: 6 inhalations/24 hrs.

NEBULIZATION

Children. 125–250 mcg 3 times/day.
Neonates. 25 mcg/kg/dose 3 times/day.

▸ **Rhinorrhea**

INTRANASAL

Children 6–12 yrs (0.03%). 2 sprays each nostril 2–3 times/day.
Children older than 12 yrs (0.06%). 2 sprays each nostril 3–4 times/day.

CONTRAINDICATIONS

History of hypersensitivity to atropine or ipratropium.

INTERACTIONS

Drug

Cromolyn inhalation solution: Avoid mixing these drugs because they form a precipitate.

Herbal

None known.

Food

None known.

DIAGNOSTIC TEST EFFECTS

None known.

SIDE EFFECTS

Frequent

Inhalation (6%–3%): Cough, dry mouth, headache, nausea
Nasal: Dry nose and mouth, headache, nasal irritation

Occasional

Inhalation (2%): Dizziness, transient increased bronchospasm

Rare (less than 1%)

Hypotension, insomnia, metallic and unpleasant taste, palpitations, urinary retention
Nasal: Diarrhea or constipation, dry throat, stomach pain, stuffy nose

SERIOUS REACTIONS

! Worsening of narrow-angle glaucoma, acute eye pain, and hypotension occur rarely.

PEDIATRIC CONSIDERATIONS

Baseline Assessment

- Offer the patient emotional support because of the high incidence of anxiety caused by breathing difficulty and the sympathomimetic response to the drug.
- Be aware that it is unknown whether ipratropium is distributed in breast milk.
- There are no age-related precautions noted in children.

Precautions

- Use cautiously in pts with bladder neck obstruction, narrow-angle glaucoma, and prostatic hypertrophy.

Administration and Handling

INHALATION

- Shake container well, have the patient exhale completely through his or her mouth; place mouthpiece into the patient's mouth and have the patient close his or her lips, holding the inhaler upright.
- Instruct the patient to inhale deeply through the mouth while fully depressing the top of the canister. Tell the patient to hold

his or her breath as long as possible before exhaling slowly.
• Wait 2 min before inhaling the second dose to allow for deeper bronchial penetration.
• Have the patient rinse his or her mouth with water immediately after inhalation to prevent mouth and throat dryness.

Intervention and Evaluation

• Monitor the depth, rate, rhythm, and type of patient respirations.
• Monitor the quality and rate of the patient's pulse.
• Assess the patient's lung sounds for crackles, rhonchi, and wheezing.
• Monitor the patient's arterial blood gases.
• Observe the patient's fingernails and lips for blue or dusky color in light-skinned pts or gray in dark-skinned pts.
• Observe the patient for clavicular, intercostal, and sternal retractions, and hand tremor.
• Evaluate the patient for clinical improvement, such as cessation of retractions, quieter and slower respirations, and a relaxed facial expression.

Patient/Family Teaching

• Instruct the patient/family to increase the patient's fluid intake to decrease the viscosity of his or her lung secretions.
• Teach the patient/family not to take more than 2 inhalations at any one time. Explain to the patient that excessive use may produce paradoxical bronchoconstriction or a decreased bronchodilating effect.
• Suggest to the patient/family that rinsing the mouth with water immediately after inhalation may prevent mouth and throat dryness.
• Urge the patient/family to avoid excessive use of caffeine derivatives such as chocolate, cocoa, coffee, and tea.

Levalbuterol

lee-val-**bwet**-err-all
(Xopenex)
Do not confuse with Xanax.

CATEGORY AND SCHEDULE

Pregnancy Risk Category: C

MECHANISM OF ACTION

A sympathomimetic that stimulates beta$_2$-adrenergic receptors in the lungs, resulting in relaxation of bronchial smooth muscle.
Therapeutic Effect: Relieves bronchospasm, reduces airway resistance.

PHARMACOKINETICS

Route	Onset	Peak	Duration
Inhalation	10–17 min	1.5 hrs	5–6 hrs

Metabolized in the liver to inactive metabolite. ***Half-Life:*** 3.3–4 hrs.

AVAILABILITY

Solution for Nebulization: 0.31 in 3-mL vials, 0.63 mg in 3-mL vials; 1.25 mg in 3-mL vials.

INDICATIONS AND DOSAGES

▸ Treatment and prevention of bronchospasm

NEBULIZATION

Children 12 yrs and older. Initially, 0.63 mg 3 times/day 6–8 hrs apart. May increase to 1.25 mg 3 times/day with dose monitoring.
Children 6–11 yrs. Initially 0.31 mg 3 times/day. Maximum: 0.63 mg 3 times/day.

CONTRAINDICATIONS

History hypersensitivity to sympathomimetics.

INTERACTIONS

Drug

Beta-adrenergic blocking agents (beta-blockers): Antagonize the effects of levalbuterol.
Digoxin: May increase the risk of arrhythmias with digoxin.
MAOIs, tricyclic antidepressants: May potentiate cardiovascular effects.

Herbal

None known.

Food

None known.

DIAGNOSTIC TEST EFFECTS

May increase serum potassium levels.

SIDE EFFECTS

Frequent
Tremor, nervousness, headache, throat dryness and irritation
Occasional
Dry, irritated mouth or throat, coughing, bronchial irritation
Rare
Drowsiness, diarrhea, dry mouth, flushing, diaphoresis, anorexia

SERIOUS REACTIONS

! Excessive sympathomimetic stimulation may produce palpitations, extrasystoles, tachycardia, chest pain, and a slight increase in blood pressure followed by a substantial decrease, chills, diaphoresis, and blanching of skin.
! Too frequent or excessive use may lead to loss of bronchodilating effectiveness and severe, paradoxical bronchoconstriction.

PEDIATRIC CONSIDERATIONS

Baseline Assessment

- Offer the patient emotional support because of a high incidence of anxiety resulting from difficulty in breathing and a sympathomimetic response to drug.
- Be aware that levalbuterol crosses the placenta, and it is unknown whether the drug is distributed in breast milk.
- Be aware that the safety and efficacy of levalbuterol have not been established in pts younger than 12 years of age.

Precautions

- Use cautiously in pts with cardiovascular disorders, such as cardiac arrhythmias, diabetes mellitus, hypertension, and seizures.

Administration and Handling

NEBULIZATION

- Do not dilute.
- Protect from light and excessive heat. Store at room temperature.
- Once foil is opened, use within 2 wks.
- Discard if solution is not colorless.
- Do not mix with other medications.
- Give over 5–15 min.

Intervention and Evaluation

- Monitor the depth, rate, rhythm, and type of patient respirations.
- Monitor the patient's arterial blood gases, EKG, quality and rate of the pulse, and serum potassium levels.
- Assess the patient's lung sounds for crackles and wheezing, signs of bronchoconstriction.

Patient/Family Teaching

- Instruct the patient/family to increase the patient's fluid intake to decrease the viscosity of his or her lung secretions.

• Tell the patient/family that rinsing the mouth with water immediately after inhalation may prevent mouth and throat dryness.
• Urge the patient/family to avoid excessive use of caffeine derivatives such as chocolate, coffee, cola, and tea.
• Warn the patient/family to notify the physician if the patient experiences chest pain, dizziness, headache, palpitations, tachycardia, or tremors.

Metaproterenol Sulfate

met-ah-pro-**tair**-in-all
(Alupent)
Do not confuse with Atrovent, metipranolol, or metoprolol.

CATEGORY AND SCHEDULE

Pregnancy Risk Category: C

MECHANISM OF ACTION

A sympathomimetic or adrenergic agonist that stimulates $beta_2$-adrenergic receptors, resulting in relaxation of bronchial smooth muscle. ***Therapeutic Effect:*** Relieves bronchospasm; reduces airway resistance.

AVAILABILITY

Solution for Oral Inhalation: 0.4%, 0.6%, 5%.
Aerosol for Oral Inhalation: 0.65 mg/inhalation.
Syrup: 10 mg/5 mL.
Tablets: 10 mg, 20 mg.

INDICATIONS AND DOSAGES

▸ Treatment of bronchospasm

PO
Children older than 9 yrs. 20 mg 3–4 times/day.
Children 6–9 yrs. 10 mg 3–4 times/day.
Children 2–5 yrs. 1.3–2.6 mg/kg/day in 3–4 divided doses.
Children younger than 2 yrs. 0.4 mg/kg 3–4 times/day.
INHALATION
Children older than 12 yrs. 2–3 inhalations q3–4h. Maximum: 12 inhalations/24 hrs.
NEBULIZATION
Children 12 yrs and older. 10–15 mg (0.2–0.3 mL) of 5% q4–6h.
Children younger than 12 yrs and infants. 0.5–1 mg/kg (0.01–0.02 mL/kg) of 5% q4–6h.

CONTRAINDICATIONS

Hypersensitivity to metaproterenol or any related component. Narrow-angle glaucoma, preexisting cardiac arrhythmias associated with tachycardia.

INTERACTIONS

Drug

Beta-blockers: May decrease the effects of beta-blockers.
Digoxin, other sympathomimetics: May increase the risk of arrhythmias.
MAOIs: May increase the risk of hypertensive crises.
Tricyclic antidepressants: May increase cardiovascular effects.

Herbal

None known.

Food

None known.

DIAGNOSTIC TEST EFFECTS

May decrease serum potassium levels.

SIDE EFFECTS

Frequent (10% or greater)

Shakiness, nervousness, nausea, dry mouth

Occasional (9%–1%)
Dizziness, vertigo, weakness, headache, GI distress, vomiting, cough, dry throat
Rare (less than 1%)
Drowsiness, diarrhea, unusual taste

SERIOUS REACTIONS

! Excessive sympathomimetic stimulation may cause palpitations, extrasystoles, tachycardia, chest pain, and a slight increase in blood pressure followed by a substantial decrease, chills, diaphoresis, and blanching of skin.
! Too frequent or excessive use may lead to loss of bronchodilating effectiveness and severe, paradoxical bronchoconstriction.

PEDIATRIC CONSIDERATIONS

Baseline Assessment
• Offer the patient emotional support because of the high incidence of anxiety caused by breathing difficulty and the sympathomimetic response to drug.
Precautions
• Use cautiously in pts with arrhythmias, congestive heart failure, diabetes mellitus, hypertension, hyperthyroidism, ischemic heart disease, and seizure disorder.
Intervention and Evaluation
• Monitor the depth, rate, rhythm, and type of patient respirations.
• Monitor the patient's arterial blood gases and pulmonary function tests.
• Assess the patient's lung sounds for rhonchi and wheezing and signs of bronchoconstriction.
• Observe the patient's fingernails and lips for a blue or dusky color in light-skinned pts or gray in dark-skinned pts and signs of hypoxemia.
• Evaluate the patient for clinical improvement, cessation of clavicular, intercostal, and sternal retractions, quieter and slower respirations, and a relaxed facial expression.
Patient/Family Teaching
• Instruct the patient/family to increase the patient's fluid intake to decrease the viscosity of his or her lung secretions.
• Teach the patient/family not to exceed the recommended dosage.
• Tell the patient/family that metaproterenol may cause inability to sleep, nervousness, and restlessness.
• Warn the patient/family to notify the physician if the patient experiences chest pain, difficulty breathing, dizziness, flushing, headache, palpitations, tachycardia, and tremors.
• Urge the patient/family to avoid excessive use of caffeine derivatives such as chocolate, cocoa, coffee, cola, and tea.

Salmeterol

sal-**met**-er-all
(Serevent Diskus)
Do not confuse with Serentil.

CATEGORY AND SCHEDULE

Pregnancy Risk Category: C

MECHANISM OF ACTION

An adrenergic agonist that stimulates beta$_2$-adrenergic receptors in the lungs, resulting in relaxation of bronchial smooth muscle.
Therapeutic Effect: Relieves bronchospasm, reducing airway resistance.

PHARMACOKINETICS

Route	Onset	Peak	Duration
Inhalation	10–20 min	3 hrs	12 hrs

Primarily acts in lung; low systemic absorption. Protein binding: 95%. Metabolized by hydroxylation. Primarily eliminated in feces. ***Half-life:*** 3–4 hrs.

AVAILABILITY

Aerosol Powder: 50 mcg.

INDICATIONS AND DOSAGES

▸ **Maintenance and prevention of asthma**

INHALATION

Children older than 4 yrs. Diskus: 1 activation (50 mcg) q12h.

Prevention of exercise-induced bronchospasm.

INHALATION

Children older than 4 yrs. 1 inhalation at least 30 min before exercise.

CONTRAINDICATIONS

Hypersensitivity to salmeterol or any related component. History of hypersensitivity to sympathomimetics.

INTERACTIONS

Drug

Beta-adrenergic blockers: May decrease the effects of beta-adrenergic blockers.

Herbal

None known.

Food

None known.

DIAGNOSTIC TEST EFFECTS

May decrease serum potassium levels.

SIDE EFFECTS

Frequent (28%)

Headache

Occasional (7%–3%)

Cough, tremor, dizziness, vertigo, throat dryness or irritation, pharyngitis

Rare (less than 3%)

Palpitations, tachycardia, shakiness, nausea, heartburn, GI distress, diarrhea

SERIOUS REACTIONS

! May prolong QT interval, which may lead to ventricular arrhythmias.

! Black pts may be at a higher risk for asthma-related death and serious reactions with the use of salmeterol.

! May cause hypokalemia and hyperglycemia.

PEDIATRIC CONSIDERATIONS

Baseline Assessment

- Ask the patient about a history of sensitivity to sympathomimetics.
- Assess a baseline EKG, and measure the QT interval.
- Check the patient's baseline peak flow readings.
- Be aware that it is unknown whether salmeterol is excreted in breast milk.
- There are no age-related precautions noted in children older than 4 years of age.

Precautions

- Use cautiously in pts with cardiovascular disorders, such as coronary insufficiency, arrhythmias, hypertension, seizure disorder, and thyrotoxicosis.
- Salmeterol use is not for acute symptoms and may cause paradoxical bronchospasm.

Administration and Handling

INHALATION

- Shake container well. Instruct the patient to exhale completely through the mouth. Place mouth-

piece into the patient's mouth and have the patient close his or her lips, holding the inhaler upright.
• Have the patient inhale deeply through the mouth while fully depressing the top of canister. Instruct the patient to hold his or her breath as long as possible before exhaling slowly.
• Teach the patient to wait 2 min before inhaling a second dose to allow for deeper bronchial penetration.
• Instruct the patient to rinse his or her mouth with water immediately after inhalation to prevent mouth and throat dryness.

Intervention and Evaluation

• Monitor the depth, rate, rhythm, and type of patient respirations.
• Monitor the patient's blood pressure and the quality and rate of the patient's pulse.
• Assess the patient's lungs for crackles, rhonchi, and wheezing.
• Periodically evaluate the patient's serum potassium levels.

Patient/Family Teaching

• Explain to the patient/family that salmeterol use is not for relief of acute episodes.
• Teach the patient/family to keep the drug canister at room temperature. Inform the patient that cold decreases the drug's effects.
• Caution the patient/family against abruptly discontinuing the drug or exceeding the recommended dosage.
• Warn the patient/family to notify the physician if the patient experiences chest pain or dizziness.
• Instruct the patient/family to wait at least 1 full min before the second inhalation.
• Teach the patient/family to administer the dose 30–60 min before exercising when the drug is used to prevent exercise-induced bronchospasm.
• Urge the patient/family to avoid excessive consumption of caffeine derivatives such as chocolate, coffee, colas, and tea.
• Teach the patient/family how to measure peak flow readings, and keep a log of measurements.

Terbutaline Sulfate

tur-**byew**-ta-leen
(Brethine)
Do not confuse with Brethaire, terbinafine, or tolbutamide.

CATEGORY AND SCHEDULE

Pregnancy Risk Category: B

MECHANISM OF ACTION

A sympathomimetic or adrenergic agonist that stimulates $beta_2$-adrenergic receptors. ***Therapeutic Effect:*** Bronchospasm: Relaxes bronchial smooth muscle, relieves bronchospasm, reduces airway resistance.
Labor: Relaxes uterine muscle, inhibiting uterine contractions.

AVAILABILITY

Tablets: 2.5 mg, 5 mg.
Injection: 1 mg/mL.

INDICATIONS AND DOSAGES

▸ Bronchospasm

PO

Children older than 15 yrs. Initially, 2.5 mg 3–4 times/day. Maintenance: 2.5–5 mg 3 times/day q6h while awake. Maximum: 15 mg/day.
Children 12–15 yrs. 2.5 mg 3 times/day. Maximum: 7.5 mg/day.
Children younger than 12 yrs. Initially, 0.05 mg/kg/dose q8h.

May increase up to 0.15 mg/kg/dose. Maximum: 5 mg.
SC
Children 12 yrs and older. Initially, 0.25 mg. Repeat in 15–30 min if substantial improvement does not occur. Maximum: No more than 0.75 mg/4 hrs.
Children younger than 12 yrs. 0.005–0.01 mg/kg/dose to a maximum of 0.4 mg/dose q15–20min for 3 doses.

CONTRAINDICATIONS

History of hypersensitivity to sympathomimetics.

INTERACTIONS

Drug

Beta-blockers: May decrease the effects of beta-blockers.
Digoxin, sympathomimetics: May increase the risk of arrhythmias.
MAOIs: May increase the risk of hypertensive crises.
Tricyclic antidepressants: May increase cardiovascular effects.

Herbal

None known.

Food

None known.

DIAGNOSTIC TEST EFFECTS

May decrease serum potassium levels.

SIDE EFFECTS

Frequent (23%–18%)
Tremor, shakiness, nervousness
Occasional (11%–10%)
Drowsiness, headache, nausea, heartburn, dizziness
Rare (3%–1%)
Flushing, weakness, drying or irritation of oropharynx noted with inhalation therapy

SERIOUS REACTIONS

! Too frequent or excessive use may lead to loss of bronchodilating effectiveness and severe, paradoxical bronchoconstriction.
! Excessive sympathomimetic stimulation may cause palpitations, extrasystoles, tachycardia, chest pain, and a slight increase in blood pressure followed by a substantial decrease, chills, sweating, and blanching of skin.

PEDIATRIC CONSIDERATIONS

Baseline Assessment

- Offer emotional support to the patient taking terbutaline for bronchospasm because these pts have a high incidence of anxiety because of difficulty in breathing and sympathomimetic response to drug.
- Safety and effectiveness of this medication in children has not been established.

Precautions

- Use cautiously in pts with diabetes mellitus, a history of seizures, hypertension, hyperthyroidism, and impaired cardiac function.

Administration and Handling

PO
- Give terbutaline without regard to food. May give terbutaline with food if the patient experiences GI upset.
- Crush tablets as needed.

SC
- Do not use if solution appears discolored.
- Inject SC into lateral deltoid region.

Intervention and Evaluation

- Monitor the depth, rate, rhythm, and type of patient respirations.
- Monitor the quality and rate of the patient's pulse.
- Assess the patient's lungs for rhonchi and wheezing.
- Periodically evaluate the patient's serum potassium levels.

• Monitor the patient's arterial blood gases.
• Observe the patient's fingernails and lips for a blue or dusky color in light-skinned pts or gray in dark-skinned pts and signs of hypoxemia.
• Observe the patient for clavicular retractions and hand tremor.
• Evaluate the patient for clinical improvement, cessation of clavicular retractions, quieter and slower respirations, and a relaxed facial expression.
• Monitor the duration and frequency of the patient's contractions when the drug is used for preterm labor.
• Diligently monitor the pregnant patient's fetal heart rate.

Patient/Family Teaching

• Warn the patient/family to notify the physician if the patient experiences chest pain, difficulty breathing, dizziness, flushing, headache, muscle tremors, or palpitations.
• Tell the patient/family that terbutaline may cause nervousness and shakiness.
• Urge the patient/family to avoid excessive consumption of caffeine derivatives such as chocolate, coffee, colas, and tea.

REFERENCES

Miller, S. & Fioravanti, J. (1997). Pediatric medications: a handbook for nurses. St. Louis: Mosby.

Taketomo, C. K., Hodding, J. H. & Kraus, D. M. (2003–2004). Pediatric dosage handbook (10th ed.). Hudson, OH: Lexi-Comp.

78 Lung Surfactants

Beractant
Calfactant
Poractant Alfa

Uses: Lung surfactants are used to prevent and treat respiratory distress syndrome (RDS) in premature neonates, often improving oxygenation within minutes of administration.

Action: By replenishing pulmonary surfactant, which is deficient in premature neonates, lung surfactants lower the surface tension on alveolar surfaces during respiration. These agents also stabilize the alveoli to prevent the collapse that may occur with resting transpulmonary pressures. Their actions improve lung compliance and respiratory gas exchange. (See illustration, *Sites of Action: Respiratory Agents,* page 853.)

Beractant

burr-**act**-ant
(Survanta)
Do not confuse with Sufenta.

CATEGORY AND SCHEDULE

Pregnancy Risk Category: This drug is not indicated for use in pregnant women.

MECHANISM OF ACTION

A natural bovine lung extract that lowers surface tension on alveolar surfaces during respiration, stabilizes alveoli, inhibiting alveolar collapse that may occur at resting transpulmonary pressures. ***Therapeutic Effect:*** Replenishes surfactant, restores surface activity to lungs.

PHARMACOKINETICS

Not absorbed systemically.

AVAILABILITY

Suspension: 25 mg/mL vial.

INDICATIONS AND DOSAGES

▸ **Prevention and rescue treatment of RDS or hyaline membrane disease in premature infants**

INTRATRACHEAL

Infants. 100 mg of phospholipids/kg birth weight (4 mL/kg). Give within 15 min of birth if infant weighs less than 1,250 g with evidence of surfactant deficiency; give within 8 hrs when RDS is confirmed by x-ray and infant requires mechanical ventilation. May repeat 6 hrs or longer after preceding dose. As many as 4 doses may be given during the first 48 hrs of life.

CONTRAINDICATIONS

None known.

INTERACTIONS

Drug

None known.

Herbal

None known.

Food

None known.

DIAGNOSTIC TEST EFFECTS
None known.

SIDE EFFECTS
Frequent
Transient bradycardia, O_2 desaturation; increased CO_2 retention
Occasional
Endotracheal tube reflux
Rare
Apnea, endotracheal tube blockage, hypotension/hypertension, pallor, vasoconstriction

SERIOUS REACTIONS
! Nosocomial sepsis may occur and is associated with increased mortality.

PEDIATRIC CONSIDERATIONS

Baseline Assessment
- Administer the drug in a highly supervised setting. Clinicians in care of the neonate must be experienced with intubation and ventilator management.
- Offer emotional support to the patient's parents.
- There are no age-related precautions noted for neonates.

Precautions
- Use cautiously in pts at risk for circulatory overload.

Administration and Handling
INTRATRACHEAL
- Refrigerate vials.
- Warm by standing vial at room temperature for 20 min or warm in hand 8 min.
- If settling occurs, gently swirl vial—do not shake—to disperse.
- After warming, may return to refrigerator within 8 hrs one time only.
- Each vial should be injected with a needle only one time; discard unused portions.
- Color normally appears off-white to light brown.
- Instill through catheter inserted into the infant's endotracheal tube. Do not instill into the main stem of the bronchus.
- Monitor for bradycardia and decreased O_2 saturation during administration. Stop the dosing procedure, as prescribed, if the patient experiences these effects and then begin appropriate measures before reinstituting therapy.

Intervention and Evaluation
- Monitor the infant with arterial or transcutaneous measurement of systemic O_2 and CO_2.
- Assess the patient's lung sounds for crackles, rales, and rhonchi.

Patient/Family Teaching
- Tell parents the purpose of treatment and the expected outcome.
- Limit visitors during treatment, and monitor for handwashing and other infection control measures to minimize the risk of nosocomial infections.

Calfactant
cal-**fak**-tant
(Infasurf)

CATEGORY AND SCHEDULE
Pregnancy Risk Category: This drug is not indicated for use in pregnant women.

MECHANISM OF ACTION
A natural lung extract that modifies alveolar surface tension, stabilizing the alveoli. ***Therapeutic Effect:*** Restores surface activity to infant lungs; improves lung compliance and respiratory gas exchange.

AVAILABILITY
Intratracheal Suspension: 35 mg/mL vial.

INDICATIONS AND DOSAGES

▸ **RDS**

INTRATRACHEAL

Neonates. Instill 3 mL/kg of birth weight as soon as possible after birth, administered as 2 doses of 1.5 mL/kg. Repeat doses of 3 mL/kg of birth weight, up to a total of 3 doses, 12 hrs apart.

CONTRAINDICATIONS

None known.

INTERACTIONS

Drug

None known.

Herbal

None known.

Food

None known.

DIAGNOSTIC TEST EFFECTS

None known.

SIDE EFFECTS

Frequent

Cyanosis (65%), airway obstruction (39%), bradycardia (34%), reflux of surfactant into endotracheal tube (21%), requirement of manual ventilation (16%)

Occasional (3%)

Reintubation

SERIOUS REACTIONS

! Complications may occur as apnea, patent ductus arteriosus, intracranial hemorrhage, sepsis, pulmonary air leaks, pulmonary hemorrhage, and necrotizing enterocolitis.

PEDIATRIC CONSIDERATIONS

Baseline Assessment

- Administer drug in a highly supervised setting. Clinicians in care of the neonate must be experienced with intubation and ventilator management.
- Offer emotional support to the patient's parents.
- There are no age-related precautions noted in neonates.
- This drug is only for use in neonates.

Precautions

- Use cautiously in pts with a hypersensitivity to calfactant.

Administration and Handling

INTRATRACHEAL

- Refrigerate.
- Unopened, unused vials may be returned to refrigerator only once after having been warmed to room temperature.
- Do not shake.
- Enter only once, discard unused suspension.

Intervention and Evaluation

- Monitor the neonate with arterial or transcutaneous measurement of systemic O_2 and CO_2.
- Assess the patient's lung sounds for crackles, rales, and rhonchi.

Patient/Family Teaching

- Tell parents the purpose of treatment and the expected outcome.
- Limit visitors during treatment, and monitor for hand washing and other infection control measures to minimize the risk of nosocomial infections.

Poractant Alfa

pour-**act**-tant

(Curosurf, Curosurg [CAN])

CATEGORY AND SCHEDULE

Pregnancy Risk Category: This drug is not indicated for use in pregnant women.

MECHANISM OF ACTION

A pulmonary surfactant that reduces surface tension of alveoli during ventilation; stabilizes alveoli against collapse that may occur at resting transpulmonary pressures. ***Therapeutic Effect:*** Prevents alveoli from collapsing during expiration by lowering surface tension between air and alveolar surfaces.

AVAILABILITY

Intratracheal Suspension: 1.5 mL (120 mg), 3 mL (240 mg).

INDICATIONS AND DOSAGES

▸ RDS

ENDOTRACHEAL

Infants. Initially, 2.5 mL/kg birth weight (BW). Up to 2 subsequent doses of 1.25 mL/kg BW at 12-hr intervals. Maximum total dose: 5 mL/kg.

UNLABELED USES

Adult RDS due to viral pneumonia, HIV-infected infants with *Pneumocystis carinii* pneumonia, prophylaxis for RDS, treatment in adult RDS after near-drowning

CONTRAINDICATIONS

None known.

INTERACTIONS

Drug

None known.

Herbal

None known.

Food

None known.

DIAGNOSTIC TEST EFFECTS

None known.

SIDE EFFECTS

Frequent

Transient bradycardia, O_2 desaturation, increased CO_2 tension

Occasional

Endotracheal tube reflux

Rare

Apnea, endotracheal tube blockage, hypotension/hypertension, pallor, vasoconstriction

SERIOUS REACTIONS

! Pneumonia (17%), septicemia (14%), bronchopulmonary dysplasia (18%), intracranial hemorrhage (51%), patent ductus arteriosus (60%), pneumothorax (21%), and pulmonary interstitial emphysema (21%) may occur.

PEDIATRIC CONSIDERATIONS

Baseline Assessment

- Plan to correct acidosis, anemia, hypoglycemia, hypotension, and hypothermia before beginning poractant alfa administration.
- Change ventilator settings, as prescribed, to 40–60 breaths/min, inspiratory time 0.5 sec, and supplemental O_2 sufficient to maintain SaO_2 greater than 92% immediately before poractant alfa administration.
- Administer the drug in a highly supervised setting. Clinicians in care of the neonate must be experienced with intubation and ventilator management.
- Offer emotional support to the neonate patient's parents.
- There are no age-related precautions noted for the neonate.

Precautions

- Use cautiously in pts at risk for circulatory overload.

Administration and Handling

INTRATRACHEAL

- Refrigerate vials.
- Warm by standing the vial at room temperature for 20 min or warm in hand for 8 min.
- To obtain uniform suspension, turn upside down gently and swirl the vial, but do not shake.

• After warming, may return to refrigerator one time only.
• Withdraw entire contents of vial into a 3- or 5-mL plastic syringe through a large-gauge needle (20 gauge or larger).
• Attach syringe to a catheter and instill through the catheter inserted into the infant's endotracheal tube.
• Monitor the infant for bradycardia and decreased O_2 saturation during administration. Stop the dosing procedure if the infant experiences these effects, then begin appropriate measures before reinstituting therapy.

Intervention and Evaluation

• Monitor the infant with arterial or transcutaneous measurement of systemic O_2 and CO_2.
• Assess the patient's lung sounds for crackles, rales, and rhonchi.
• Monitor the patient's heart rate.

Patient/Family Teaching

• Tell parents the purpose of treatment and the expected outcome.
• Limit visitors during treatment, and monitor for hand washing and other infection control measures to minimize the risk of nosocomial infections.

REFERENCES

Taketomo, C. K., Hodding, J. H. & Kraus, D. M. (2003–2004). Pediatric dosage handbook (10th ed.). Hudson, OH: Lexi-Comp.

79 Nasal Decongestants

Naphazoline
Phenylephrine Hydrochloride
Pseudoephedrine Hydrochloride, Pseudoephedrine Sulfate
Sodium Chloride

Uses: Nasal decongestants are used to relieve stuffiness caused by conditions such as the common cold, acute or chronic rhinitis, hay fever, and other allergies. Sodium chloride is administered nasally to restore moisture and relieve dry, inflamed nasal membranes.

Action: Most nasal decongestants stimulate alpha$_1$-adrenergic receptors on nasal blood vessels, causing vasoconstriction that shrinks swollen membranes and allows nasal drainage. As a major extracellular cation, sodium chloride soothes the nasal passages. (See illustration, *Sites of Action: Respiratory Agents,* page 853.)

COMBINATION PRODUCTS

ALLEGRA-D: pseudoephedrine/fexofenadine (an antihistamine) 120 mg/60 mg.
CHILDREN'S ADVIL COLD: pseudoephedrine/ibuprofen (an NSAID) 15 mg/100 mg per 5 mL.
CLARITIN-D: pseudoephedrine/loratadine (an antihistamine) 120 mg/5 mg; 240 mg/10 mg.
NAPHCON-A: naphazoline/pheniramine (an antihistamine) 0.25%/0.3%.
PHENERGAN VC: phenylephrine/promethazine (an antihistamine) 5 mg/6.25 mg per 5 mL.
PHENERGAN VC WITH CODEINE: phenylephrine/promethazine (an antihistamine)/codeine (a narcotic analgesic) 5 mg/6.25 mg/10 mg per 5 mL.
ZYRTEC D-12 HOUR TABLETS: pseudoephedrine/cetirizine (an antihistamine) 120 mg/5 mg.

Naphazoline

na-**faz**-oh-leen
(Albalon Liquifilm [AUS], AK-Con, Clear Eyes [AUS], Naphcon, Privine, Vasocon)

CATEGORY AND SCHEDULE
Pregnancy Risk Category: C

MECHANISM OF ACTION
A sympathomimetic that directly acts on alpha-adrenergic receptors in arterioles of conjunctiva. ***Therapeutic Effect:*** Causes vasoconstriction, with subsequent decreased congestion to area.

AVAILABILITY
Ophthalmic Solution: 0.012%, 0.02%, 0.1%.
Nasal Drops: 0.05%.
Nasal Spray: 0.05%.

INDICATIONS AND DOSAGES

▸ **Relief of nasal congestion due to acute or chronic rhinitis, common cold, hay fever or other allergies**

INTRANASAL

Children older than 12 yrs. 1–2 drops/sprays (0.05%) in each nostril q3–6h.

Children 6–12 yrs. 1 spray (0.05%)/drop q6h as needed.

▸ **Control of hyperemia in pts with superficial corneal vascularity, relief of congestion, itching, and minor irritation, may be used during some ocular diagnostic procedures**

OPHTHALMIC

Children older than 6 yrs. 1–2 drops q3–4h for 3–4 days.

CONTRAINDICATIONS

Hypersensitivity to naphazoline or any related component. Before peripheral iridectomy, eyes capable of angle closure, narrow-angle glaucoma, or pts with a narrow angle who do not have glaucoma.

INTERACTIONS

Drug

Maprotiline, tricyclic antidepressants: May increase the hypertensive effects of naphazoline.

Anesthetics (cyclopropane, halothane): May sensitize the myocardium.

Herbal

None known.

Food

None known.

DIAGNOSTIC TEST EFFECTS

None known.

SIDE EFFECTS

Occasional

Nasal: Burning, stinging, drying nasal mucosa, sneezing, rebound congestion

Ophthalmic: Blurred vision, large pupils, increased eye irritation

SERIOUS REACTIONS

! Large doses may produce tachycardia, palpitations, lightheadedness, nausea, and vomiting.

! Overdosage in pts older than 60 yrs of age may produce hallucinations, CNS depression, and seizures.

PEDIATRIC CONSIDERATIONS

Baseline Assessment

• Ask the patient if he or she takes tricyclic antidepressants before administering drug.

Precautions

• Use cautiously in pts with cerebral arteriosclerosis, coronary artery disease, diabetes, heart disease, hypertension, hypertensive cardiovascular disease, hyperthyroidism, and long-standing bronchial asthma.

Administration and Handling

◂ **ALERT** ▸ Be aware that if naphazoline is systemically absorbed, the patient may experience a fast, irregular, and pounding heartbeat, headache, insomnia, lightheadedness, nausea, nervousness, and trembling.

Patient/Family Teaching

• Caution the patient/family not to use naphazoline for longer than 72 hrs without consulting a physician.

• Warn the patient/family to use caution when performing tasks that require visual acuity during naphazoline therapy.

• Tell the patient/family to discontinue the drug and contact the physician if the patient experiences acute eye redness, dizziness, eye pain, floating spots, headache, insomnia, irregular heartbeat, pain

with light exposure, tremor, vision changes, or weakness.
• Explain to the patient/family that if naphazoline is used too frequently the patient may experience rebound effects.

Phenylephrine Hydrochloride

See vasopressors

Pseudoephedrine Hydrochloride

su-do-eh-**fed**-rin
(Dimetapp sinus liquid caps [AUS], Eltor [CAN], Sudafed)

Pseudoephedrine Sulfate

(Afrinol Repetabs)

CATEGORY AND SCHEDULE

Pregnancy Risk Category: C
OTC

MECHANISM OF ACTION

A sympathomimetic that directly stimulates alpha-adrenergic and beta-adrenergic receptors. ***Therapeutic Effect:*** Produces vasoconstriction of respiratory tract mucosa; shrinks nasal mucous membranes; reduces edema and nasal congestion.

PHARMACOKINETICS

Route	Onset	Peak	Duration
PO tablets, syrup	15–30 min	N/A	4–6 hrs
PO extended release	N/A	N/A	8–12 hrs

Well absorbed from the GI tract. Partially metabolized in liver. Primarily excreted in urine. Not removed by hemodialysis. ***Half-Life:*** 9–16 hrs. Children 3.1 hrs.

AVAILABILITY

Gelcaps: 30 mg.
Liquid: 15 mg/5 mL.
Oral Drops: 7.5 mg/0.8 mL.
Syrup: 30 mg/5 mL.
Tablets: 30 mg, 60 mg.
Tablets (chewable): 15 mg.
Tablets (extended-release): 120 mg, 240 mg.

INDICATIONS AND DOSAGES

▸ **Decongestant**

PO
Children older than 12 yrs. 60 mg q4–6h. Maximum: 240 mg/day.
Children 6–12 yrs. 30 mg q6h. Maximum: 120 mg/day.
Children 2–5 yrs. 15 mg q6h. Maximum: 60 mg/day.
Children younger than 2 yrs. 4 mg/kg/day in divided doses q6h.
PO (EXTENDED RELEASE)
Children older than 12 yrs. 120 mg q12h.

CONTRAINDICATIONS

Hypersensitivity to pseudoephedrine or any related component. Coronary artery disease, lactating women, MAOI therapy, severe hypertension.

INTERACTIONS

Drug

Antihypertensives, beta-adrenergic blockers, diuretics: May decrease the effects of antihypertensives, beta-adrenergic blockers, and diuretics.
MAOIs: May increase cardiac stimulant and vasopressor effects.

Herbal
None known.
Food
None known.

DIAGNOSTIC TEST EFFECTS
None known.

SIDE EFFECTS
Occasional (10%–5%)
Nervousness, restlessness, insomnia, trembling, headache
Rare (4%–1%)
Increased sweating, weakness

SERIOUS REACTIONS
! Large doses may produce tachycardia and palpitations, particularly in those with cardiac disease, lightheadedness, nausea, and vomiting.

PEDIATRIC CONSIDERATIONS

Baseline Assessment
- Ask the patient if he or she takes antihypertensives, beta-adrenergic blockers, diuretics, or MAOIs before administering the drug.
- Be aware that pseudoephedrine crosses the placenta and is distributed in breast milk.
- Be aware that the safety and efficacy of pseudoephedrine have not been established in children younger than 2 yrs of age.

Precautions
- Use cautiously in pts with diabetes, heart disease, and hyperthyroidism.

Administration and Handling
PO
- Do not chew or crush extended-release tablets; swallow whole.

Patient/Family Teaching
- Tell the patient/family to discontinue the drug if the patient experiences adverse reactions.
- Warn the patient/family to notify the physician if the patient experiences dizziness, insomnia, irregular or rapid heartbeat, or tremors.

Sodium Chloride 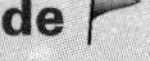
See minerals/electrolytes

REFERENCES
Taketomo, C. K., Hodding, J. H. & Kraus, D. M. (2003–2004). Pediatric dosage handbook (10th ed.). Hudson, OH: Lexi-Comp.

80 Respiratory Inhalants and Intranasal Steroids

Acetylcysteine (*N*-Acetylcysteine)
Beclomethasone Dipropionate
Budesonide
Cromolyn Sodium
Flunisolide
Fluticasone Propionate
Mometasone Furoate Monohydrate
Nedocromil Sodium
Triamcinolone, Triamcinolone Acetonide, Triamcinolone Diacetate, Triamcinolone Hexacetonide

Uses: Most respiratory inhalants and intranasal steroids are used to treat seasonal and perennial rhinitis, to prevent all major symptoms of rhinitis, and to manage bronchial asthma. Acetylcysteine is prescribed as an adjunct to treat bronchopulmonary disease and pulmonary complications of cystic fibrosis. It' is also used in tracheostomy care and in the treatment of acetaminophen overdose. Beclomethasone is also used to prevent nasal polyp recurrence after surgery.

Action: Several mechanisms of action account for the effects of respiratory inhalants and intranasal steroids. *Acetylcysteine* splits the disulfide linkages between mucoproteins, reducing the viscosity of pulmonary secretions. *Intranasal steroids,* such as beclomethasone and fluticasone, prevent the inflammatory response to allergens. *Cromolyn* and *nedocromil* prevent the release of inflammatory mediators from mast cells.

COMBINATION PRODUCTS

ADVAIR: fluticasone/salmeterol (a bronchodilator) 100 mcg/50 mcg; 250 mcg/50 mcg; 500 mcg/50 mcg.
MYCO-II: triamcinolone/nystatin (an antifungal) 0.1%/100,000 units/g.
MYCOLOG II: triamcinolone/nystatin (an antifungal) 0.1%/100,000 units/g.
MYCO-TRIACET: triamcinolone/nystatin (an antifungal) 0.1%/100,000 units/g.

Acetylcysteine (*N*-Acetylcysteine)

ah-sea-tyl-**sis**-teen
(Mucomyst, Parvolex [CAN])
Do not confuse with acetylcholine.

CATEGORY AND SCHEDULE

Pregnancy Risk Category: B

MECHANISM OF ACTION

An intratracheal respiratory inhalant that splits the linkage of mucoproteins. ***Therapeutic Effect:*** Reduces the viscosity of pulmonary secretions, facilitates removal by coughing, postural drainage, and mechanical means. Protects against acetaminophen overdose–induced liver toxicity.

AVAILABILITY

Solution: 10%, 20%.

INDICATIONS AND DOSAGES

▸ Adjunctive treatment for viscid mucus secretions from chronic bronchopulmonary disease and for pulmonary complications of cystic fibrosis.

NEBULIZATION

Children (20% solution). 3–5 mL 3–4 times/day. Range: 1–10 mL q2–6h.

Children (10% solution). 6–10 mL 3–4 times/day. Range: 2–20 mL q2–6h.

Infants. 1–2 mL (20%) or 2–4 mL (10%) 3–4 times/day.

▸ To treat viscid mucus secretions in pts with a tracheostomy

INTRATRACHEAL INSTILLATION

Children. 1–2 mL of 10%–20% solution instilled into tracheostomy q1–4h.

▸ Acetaminophen overdose

ORAL SOLUTION (5%)

Children. Loading dose of 140 mg/kg, followed in 4 hrs by maintenance dose of 70 mg/kg q4h for 17 additional doses (unless acetaminophen assay reveals nontoxic level).

UNLABELED USES

Prevention of renal damage from dyes given during certain diagnostic tests (e.g., computed tomography scans).

CONTRAINDICATIONS

Hypersensitivity to acetylcysteine or any related component.

INTERACTIONS

Drug

None known.

Herbal

None known.

Food

None known.

DIAGNOSTIC TEST EFFECTS

None known.

SIDE EFFECTS

Frequent

Inhalation: Stickiness on face, transient unpleasant odor

Occasional

Inhalation: Increased bronchial secretions, irritated throat, nausea, vomiting, rhinorrhea

Rare

Inhalation: Skin rash

Oral: Facial edema, bronchospasm, wheezing

SERIOUS REACTIONS

! Large dosage may produce severe nausea and vomiting.

PEDIATRIC CONSIDERATIONS

Baseline Assessment

- Assess pretreatment respirations for their rate, depth, and rhythm when this drug is used as a mucolytic.

Precautions

- Use cautiously in pts with bronchial asthma or who are debilitated with severe respiratory insufficiency.
- Be aware that acetylcysteine is foul smelling and may induce bronchospasm.

Intervention and Evaluation

- Discontinue treatment and notify the physician if bronchospasm occurs. Expect to administer a bronchodilator as needed.

• Monitor the rate, depth, rhythm, and type of respirations, such as abdominal or thoracic.
• Check the sputum for its color, consistency, and amount.

Patient/Family Teaching

• Explain to the patient/family that a slight, disagreeable odor from the solution may be noticed during initial administration but that the odor disappears quickly.
• Stress to the patient/family the importance of drinking plenty of fluids to maintain adequate hydration.
• Teach the patient/family proper coughing and deep breathing activities.

Beclomethasone Dipropionate

beck-low-**meth**-ah-sewn
(Aqueous Nasal Spray [AUS], Beclodisk [CAN], Becloforte inhaler [CAN], Beconase AQ, Becotide [AUS], Qvar)
Do not confuse with baclofen.

CATEGORY AND SCHEDULE

Pregnancy Risk Category: C

MECHANISM OF ACTION

An adrenocorticosteroid that controls the rate of protein synthesis, depresses migration of polymorphonuclear leukocytes and fibroblasts, prevents or controls inflammation, and reverses capillary permeability. ***Therapeutic Effect:*** Inhalation: Inhibits bronchoconstriction, produces smooth muscle relaxation, and decreases mucus secretion. Intranasal: Decreases response to seasonal and perennial rhinitis.

PHARMACOKINETICS

Rapidly absorbed from pulmonary, nasal, and GI tissue. Protein binding: 87%. Metabolized in liver and undergoes an extensive first-pass effect. Primarily eliminated in feces. ***Half-Life:*** 15 hrs.

AVAILABILITY

Aerosol for Inhalation: 40 mcg/actuation, 80 mcg/actuation.
Intranasal Suspension: 42 mcg/actuation.

INDICATIONS AND DOSAGES

▸ **Control of bronchial asthma in pts requiring chronic steroid therapy**

ORAL INHALATION

Children older than 12 yrs. 2 puffs 3–4 times a day. Maximum: 20 puffs/day.
Children 6–12 yrs. 1–2 puffs 3–4 times/day. Maximum: 10 puffs/day.

▸ **Relief of seasonal or perennial rhinitis, prevention of nasal polyps from recurring after surgical removal, treatment of nonallergic rhinitis**

NASAL INHALATION

Children 12 yrs and older. 1–2 sprays in each nostril 2 times/day.
Children 6–11 yrs. 1 spray in each nostril 2 times/day. May increase up to 2 sprays 2 times/day into each nostril.

UNLABELED USES

Nasal: Prophylaxis of seasonal rhinitis.

CONTRAINDICATIONS

Hypersensitivity to beclomethasone. Status asthmaticus.

INTERACTIONS

Drug

None known.

Herbal

None known.

Food
None known.

DIAGNOSTIC TEST EFFECTS
None known.

SIDE EFFECTS
Frequent
Inhalation (14%–4%): Throat irritation, dry mouth, hoarseness, cough
Intranasal: Burning, dryness inside nose
Occasional
Inhalation (3%–2%): Localized fungal infection (thrush)
Intranasal: Nasal-crusting nosebleed, sore throat, ulceration of nasal mucosa
Rare
Inhalation: Transient bronchospasm, esophageal candidiasis
Intranasal: Nasal and pharyngeal candidiasis, eye pain

SERIOUS REACTIONS
! Acute hypersensitivity reaction as evidenced by urticaria, angioedema, and severe bronchospasm occurs rarely.
! Any transfer from systemic to local steroid therapy may unmask previously suppressed bronchial asthma condition.

PEDIATRIC CONSIDERATIONS

Baseline Assessment
- Determine whether the patient has any hypersensitivity to corticosteroids.
- Be aware that it is unknown whether beclomethasone crosses the placenta or is distributed in breast milk.
- In children, prolonged treatment and high dosages may decrease the patient's short-term growth rate and cortisol secretion.

Precautions
- Use cautiously in pts with cirrhosis, glaucoma, hypothyroidism, osteoporosis, tuberculosis, and untreated systemic infections.

Administration and Handling
INHALATION
- Shake the container well, instruct the patient to exhale completely, and place the mouthpiece between the patient's lips. Have the patient inhale and hold his or her breath as long as possible before exhaling.
- Allow at least 1 min between inhalations.
- Have the patient rinse his or her mouth after each use to decrease dry mouth and hoarseness.

INTRANASAL
- Have the patient clear his or her nasal passages as much as possible.
- Insert the spray tip into the patient's nostril, pointing toward the nasal passages, away from the nasal septum.
- Spray beclomethasone into the nostril while holding the patient's other nostril closed and at the same time, have the patient inhale through the nose to deliver the medication as high into the nasal passages as possible.

Intervention and Evaluation
- In those pts receiving bronchodilators by inhalation concomitantly with inhalation of steroid therapy, advise the patient to use a bronchodilator several minutes before taking the corticosteroid aerosol to enhance the penetration of the steroid into the bronchial tree.

Patient/Family Teaching
- Advise the patient/family not to change the dose schedule or stop taking beclomethasone. Explain to the patient/family that the patient must stop beclomethasone use gradually under medical supervision.

- Encourage the patient/family receiving beclomethasone by inhalation to maintain careful mouth hygiene. Instruct the patient/family to rinse the patient's mouth with water immediately after inhalation to prevent mouth or throat dryness and fungal infection of the mouth. Urge the patient to notify the physician or nurse if he or she develops a sore throat or mouth.
- In pts receiving beclomethasone intranasally, warn the patient/family to notify the physician if nasal irritation occurs or there is no improvement in symptoms, such as sneezing.
- Teach the patient/family to clear the patient's nasal passages before intranasal beclomethasone use.
- Advise the patient/family that the patient should notice symptom improvement in several days.

Budesonide

byew-**des**-oh-nyd
(Entocort, Pulmicort, Rhinocort, Rhinocort Aqua, Rhinocort Aqueous [AUS], Rhinocort Hayfever [AUS])

CATEGORY AND SCHEDULE

Pregnancy Risk Category: B

MECHANISM OF ACTION

A glucocorticosteroid that decreases and prevents tissue response to an inflammatory process. ***Therapeutic Effect:*** Inhibits accumulation of inflammatory cells.

PHARMACOKINETICS

Minimally absorbed from nasal tissue; moderately absorbed from inhalation. Protein binding: 88%. Primarily metabolized in liver. ***Half-Life:*** 2–3 hrs.

AVAILABILITY

Capsule: 3 mg (Entocort EC).
Powder for Oral Inhalation: 200 mcg (Pulmicort Turbuhaler).
Suspensions for Oral Inhalation: 0.25 mg/2 mL; 0.5 mg/2 mg (Pulmicort Respules).
Nasal Spray Suspension: 32 mcg/spray (Rhinocort Aqua).

INDICATIONS AND DOSAGES

▸ Allergic rhinitis

INTRANASAL

Children 6 yrs and older. Rhinocort: 2 sprays to each nostril 2 times/day or 4 sprays to each nostril in morning.
Rhinocort Aqua: 1 spray to each nostril once daily. Maximum: Adults and children older than 12 yrs: 8 sprays/day. Children younger than 12 yrs: 4 sprays/day.

NEBULIZATION

Children 6 mos–8 yrs. 0.25–1 mg/day titrated to the lowest effective dosage.

INHALATION

Children 6 yrs and older. Initially, 200–400 mcg 2 times/day. Maximum: Adults: 800 mcg 2 times/day. Children: 400 mcg 2 times/day.

UNLABELED USES

Treatment of vasomotor rhinitis.

CONTRAINDICATIONS

Hypersensitivity to any corticosteroid or components, persistently positive sputum cultures for *Candida albicans*, primary treatment of status asthmaticus, systemic fungal infections, untreated localized infection involving nasal mucosa.

INTERACTIONS

Drug

None known.

Herbal

None known.

Food

None known.

DIAGNOSTIC TEST EFFECTS

None known.

SIDE EFFECTS

Frequent (greater than 3%)

Nasal: Mild nasopharyngeal irritation, burning, stinging, dryness, headache, cough
Inhalation: Flu-like syndrome, headache, pharyngitis

Occasional (3%–1%)

Nasal: Dry mouth, dyspepsia, rebound congestion, rhinorrhea, loss of sense of taste
Inhalation: Back pain, vomiting, altered taste and voice, abdominal pain, nausea, dyspepsia

SERIOUS REACTIONS

! Acute hypersensitivity reaction, including urticaria, angioedema, and severe bronchospasm, occurs rarely.

PEDIATRIC CONSIDERATIONS

Baseline Assessment

• Determine whether the patient is hypersensitive to any corticosteroids or components of the drug.
• Be aware that it is unknown whether budesonide crosses the placenta or is distributed in breast milk.
• Be aware that prolonged treatment and high dosages may decrease the cortisol secretion and short-term growth rates in children.

Precautions

• Use cautiously in pts with adrenal insufficiency, cirrhosis, glaucoma, hypothyroidism, osteoporosis, tuberculosis, and untreated infection.

Administration and Handling

INHALATION

• Shake the container well. Instruct the patient to exhale completely, then place the mouthpiece between the patient's lips, have the patient inhale, and instruct the patient to hold his or her breath as long as possible before exhaling.
• Allow at least 1 min between inhalations.
• Have the patient rinse his or her mouth after each use to decrease dry mouth and hoarseness.

INTRANASAL

• Have the patient clear his or her nasal passages before using budesonide.
• Tilt the patient's head slightly forward.
• Insert the spray tip into the patient's nostril, pointing toward the nasal passages and away from nasal septum.
• Spray into 1 nostril while holding the patient's other nostril closed. Concurrently have the patient inspire through the nostril to allow medication as high into nasal passages as possible.

Intervention and Evaluation

• Monitor the patient for relief of symptoms.

Patient/Family Teaching

• Tell the patient/family that the patient may experiences symptomatic improvement in 24 hrs, but the drug's full effect may take 3–7 days to appear.
• Warn the patient/family to notify the physician if the patient

experiences nasal irritation, no symptomatic improvement, or sneezing.

Cromolyn Sodium

krom-oh-lin
(Apo-Cromolyn [CAN], Crolom, Gastrocom, Intal, Nasalcrom, Opticrom, Rynacrom [AUS])

CATEGORY AND SCHEDULE

Pregnancy Risk Category: B

MECHANISM OF ACTION

An antiasthmatic and antiallergic agent that prevents mast cell release of histamine, leukotrienes, and slow-reacting substances of anaphylaxis by inhibiting degranulation after contact with antigens. ***Therapeutic Effect:*** Prevents release of histamine from mast cells after exposure to allergens.

PHARMACOKINETICS

Minimal absorption after PO, inhalation, or nasal administration. Absorbed portion excreted in urine or via biliary elimination. ***Half-Life:*** 80–90 min.

AVAILABILITY

Aerosol: 800 mcg/inhalation.
Oral Solution: 100 mg/5 mL.
Nasal Spray: 40 mg/mL.
Nebulization: 20 mg/2 mL.
Ophthalmic Drops: 4%.

INDICATIONS AND DOSAGES

▸ **Asthma**
INHALATION (NEBULIZATION)
Children older than 2 yrs. 20 mg 3–4 times/day.
AEROSOL SPRAY
Children 12 yrs and older. Initially, 2 inhalations 4 times/day. Maintenance: 2–4 sprays 3–4 times/day.
Children 5–11 yrs. Initially, 2 inhalations 4 times/day, then 1–2 sprays 3–4 times/day.

▸ **Prevention of bronchospasm**
INHALATION (NEBULIZATION)
Children older than 2 yrs. 20 mg not longer than 1 hr before exercise or allergic exposure.
AEROSOL SPRAY
Children older than 5 yrs. 2 inhalations not longer than 1 hr before exercise or allergic exposure.

▸ **Food allergy, inflammatory bowel disease**
PO
Children older than 12 yrs. 200–400 mg 4 times/day.
Children 2–12 yrs. 100–200 mg 4 times/day. Maximum: 40 mg/kg/day.

▸ **Allergic rhinitis**
INTRANASAL
Children older than 6 yrs. 1 inhalation each nostril 3–4 times/day. May increase up to 6 times/day.

▸ **Systemic mastocytosis**
PO
200 mg 4 times/day.
Children 2–12 yrs. 100 mg 4 times/day. Maximum: 40 mg/kg/day.
Children younger than 2 yrs. 20 mg/kg/day in 4 divided doses. Maximum (children 6 mos–2 yrs): 30 mg/kg/day.

▸ **Conjunctivitis**
OPHTHALMIC
Children older than 4 yrs. 1–2 drops in both eyes 4–6 times/day.

CONTRAINDICATIONS

Hypersensitivity to cromolyn or any related component. Status asthmaticus.

INTERACTIONS

Drug
None known.
Herbal
None known.
Food
None known.

DIAGNOSTIC TEST EFFECTS

None known.

SIDE EFFECTS

Frequent
Inhalation: Cough, dry mouth and throat, stuffy nose, throat irritation, unpleasant taste
Nasal: Burning, stinging, irritation of nose, increased sneezing
Ophthalmic: Burning, stinging of eye
PO: Headache, diarrhea
Occasional
Inhalation: Bronchospasm, hoarseness, watering eyes
Nasal: Cough, headache, unpleasant taste, postnasal drip
Ophthalmic: Increased watering and itching of eye
PO: Skin rash, abdominal pain, joint pain, nausea, insomnia
Rare
Inhalation: Dizziness, painful urination, muscle and joint pain, skin rash
Nasal: Nosebleeds, skin rash
Ophthalmic: Chemosis or edema of conjunctiva, eye irritation

SERIOUS REACTIONS

! Anaphylaxis occurs rarely when cromolyn is given via inhalation, nasal, and PO.

PEDIATRIC CONSIDERATIONS

Baseline Assessment
- Perform baseline assessment of lung sounds, auscultating for adventitious sounds.
- Determine the patient's baseline exercise and activity tolerance.
- Measure baseline peak flow readings, and if ordered, pulmonary function testing.
- Be aware that it is unknown whether cromolyn crosses the placenta or is distributed in breast milk.
- There are no age-related precautions noted in children.

Precautions
- Use cautiously in pts with arrhythmias and coronary artery disease.
- Discontinue and taper doses cautiously as symptoms may recur.

Administration and Handling
INHALATION
- Shake container well. Instruct the patient to exhale completely. Place the mouthpiece fully into the patient's mouth and have the patient inhale deeply and slowly while depressing the canister. Instruct the patient to hold his or her breath as long as possible before exhaling.
- Wait 1–10 min before inhaling the second dose to allow for deeper bronchial penetration.
- Have the patient rinse his or her mouth with water immediately after inhalation to prevent mouth and throat dryness.
- Instruct the patient on the use of a Spinhaler if he or she is to receive cromolyn by nebulization or inhalation capsules.

OPHTHALMIC
- Place a gloved finger on the patient's lower eyelid and pull it down until a pocket is formed between the patient's eye and lower lid.
- Hold the dropper above the pocket and place the prescribed number of drops in the patient's pocket.

• Instruct the patient to close his or her eyes gently so that medication will not be squeezed out of the lacrimal sac.
• Apply gentle finger pressure to the patient's lacrimal sac at the inner canthus for 1 min after installation to lessen the risk of systemic absorption.

PO

Give cromolyn at least 30 min before meals.
• Pour contents of capsule in hot water, stirring until completely dissolved; add an equal amount of cold water while stirring.
• Do not mix with food, fruit juice, or milk.

NASAL

• Nasal passages should be clear, which may require nasal decongestant.
• Inhale through the nose.

Intervention and Evaluation

• Monitor the depth, rate, rhythm, and type of patient respirations.
• Monitor the quality and rate of the patient's pulse.
• Assess the patient's lung sounds for crackles, rhonchi, and wheezing.
• Observe the patient's fingernails and lips for a blue or dusky color in light-skinned pts or gray color in dark-skinned pts (signs of hypoxemia).

Patient/Family Teaching

• Instruct the patient/family to increase the patient's fluid intake to decrease the viscosity of his or her lung secretions.
• Teach the patient/family to rinse the patient's mouth with water immediately after inhalation to prevent mouth and throat dryness.
• Tell the patient/family that the effects of therapy are dependent on administering the drug at regular intervals.
• Instruct the patient/family on the use of a Spinhaler if the patient is to receive cromolyn by nebulization or inhalation capsules.

Flunisolide

flew-**nis**-oh-lide
(AeroBid, Nasalide, Nasarel, Rhinalar [CAN])
Do not confuse with fluocinonide or Nasalcrom.

CATEGORY AND SCHEDULE

Pregnancy Risk Category: C

MECHANISM OF ACTION

An adrenocorticosteroid that controls the rate of protein synthesis, depresses migration of polymorphonuclear leukocytes, reverses capillary permeability, and stabilizes lysosomal membranes. ***Therapeutic Effect:*** Prevents or controls inflammation.

AVAILABILITY

Aerosol: 250 mcg/activation.
Nasal Spray: 25 mcg/activation.

INDICATIONS AND DOSAGES

▸ Control of bronchial asthma in those requiring chronic steroid therapy

INHALATION

Children 6–15 yrs. 2 inhalations 2 times/day.

▸ Relief of symptoms of perennial and seasonal rhinitis

INTRANASAL

Children 6–14 yrs. Initially, 1 spray to each nostril 3 times/day or 2 sprays 2 times/day. Maximum: 4 sprays each nostril/day.
Maintenance: Smallest amount to control symptoms.

UNLABELED USES

Prevents recurrence of postsurgical nasal polyps.

CONTRAINDICATIONS

Hypersensitivity to any corticosteroid. Persistently positive sputum cultures for *Candida albicans,* primary treatment of status asthmaticus, systemic fungal infections.

INTERACTIONS

Drug

None known.

Herbal

None known.

Food

None known.

DIAGNOSTIC TEST EFFECTS

None known.

SIDE EFFECTS

Frequent

Inhalation (25%–10%): Unpleasant taste, nausea, vomiting, sore throat, diarrhea, upset stomach, cold symptoms, nasal congestion

Occasional

Inhalation (9%–3%): Dizziness, irritability, nervousness, shakiness, abdominal pain, heartburn, fungal infection in mouth, pharynx, and larynx, edema

Intranasal: Mild nasopharyngeal irritation, dryness, rebound congestion, bronchial asthma, rhinorrhea, loss of sense of taste

SERIOUS REACTIONS

! Acute hypersensitivity reaction, including urticaria, angioedema, and severe bronchospasm, occurs rarely.

! A transfer from systemic to local steroid therapy may unmask previously suppressed bronchial asthma condition.

PEDIATRIC CONSIDERATIONS

Baseline Assessment

• Establish whether the patient has a history of asthma and rhinitis.

Precautions

• Use cautiously in pts with adrenal insufficiency.

Administration and Handling

◂ALERT▸ Expect to see improvement of the patient's symptoms within a few days or relief of symptoms within 3 wks. Prepare to discontinue the drug beyond 3 wks if the patient does not experience any significant improvement.

INHALANT

• Shake container well. Have the patient exhale as completely as possible.

• Place the mouthpiece fully into the patient's mouth, then while holding the inhaler upright, have the patient inhale deeply and slowly while pressing the top of the canister. Instruct the patient to hold his or her breath as long as possible before exhaling and then to exhale slowly.

• Wait 1 min between inhalations when multiple inhalations are ordered to allow for deeper bronchial penetration.

• Have the patient rinse his or her mouth with water immediately after inhalation to prevent mouth and throat dryness and oral candidiasis.

INTRANASAL

• Ensure that the patient clears his or her nasal passages before using flunisolide. The patient may need topical nasal decongestants 5–15 min before flunisolide use.

• Tilt the patient's head slightly forward.

• Insert the spray tip up in one patient nostril, pointing toward the

inflamed nasal turbinates and away from nasal septum.
- Pump medication into one of the patient's nostrils while holding his or her other nostril closed. Instruct the patient to concurrently inspire through the nose.
- Discard opened nasal solution after 3 mos.

Intervention and Evaluation
- Tell pts receiving bronchodilators by inhalation concomitantly with steroid inhalation therapy to use the bronchodilator several minutes before corticosteroid aerosol to enhance penetration of the steroid into the bronchial tree.
- Monitor the depth, rate, rhythm, and type of patient's respirations.
- Monitor the patient's arterial blood gas values and the quality and rate of the patient's pulse.
- Assess the patient's lung sounds for rales, rhonchi, and wheezing.

Patient/Family Teaching
- Caution the patient/family against abruptly discontinuing the drug or changing the drug's dose schedule. Explain to the patient/family that the patient must taper off drug doses gradually under medical supervision.
- Urge the patient/family to maintain careful oral hygiene.
- Instruct the patient/family to rinse the patient's mouth with water immediately after inhalation to prevent mouth and throat dryness and oral candidiasis.
- Instruct the patient/family to increase the patient's fluid intake to decrease the viscosity of his or her lung secretions.
- Teach pts taking flunisolide intranasally the proper use of nasal spray. Instruct the patient to clear his or her nasal passages before use.
- Warn the patient/family to notify the physician if the patient experiences nasal irritation, no improvement in symptoms, or sneezing.
- Explain to the patient/family that the patient should notice symptomatic improvement in several days.

Fluticasone Propionate

flew-**tih**-cah-sewn
(Cutivate, Flixotide Disks [AUS], Flixotide Inhaler AUS], Flonase, Flovent)

CATEGORY AND SCHEDULE

Pregnancy Risk Category: C

MECHANISM OF ACTION

A corticosteroid that controls the rate of protein synthesis, depresses migration of polymorphonuclear leukocytes, reverses capillary permeability, and stabilizes lysosomal membranes. ***Therapeutic Effect:*** Prevents or controls inflammation.

PHARMACOKINETICS

Inhalation/intranasal: Protein binding: 91%. Undergoes extensive first-pass metabolism in liver. Excreted in urine. ***Half-Life:*** 3–7.8 hrs. Topical: Amount absorbed depends on the drug, area, and skin condition. Absorption is increased with elevated skin temperature, hydration, and inflamed or denuded skin.

AVAILABILITY

Aerosol for Oral Inhalation (Flovent): 44 mcg/inhalation, 110 mcg/inhalation, 220 mcg/inhalation.
Topical Cream (Cutivate): 0.05%.

Topical Ointment (Cutivate): 0.005%.
Powder for Oral Inhalation (Flovent Diskus, Flovent Rotadisk): 50 mcg, 100 mcg, 250 mcg.
Intranasal Spray (Flonase): 50 mcg/inhalation.

INDICATIONS AND DOSAGES

▸ Allergic rhinitis

INTRANASAL

Children older than 4 yrs. Initially, 100 mcg (1 spray each nostril once daily). Maximum: 200 mcg/day.

▸ Relief of inflammation and pruritus associated with steroid-responsive disorders, such as contact dermatitis and eczema

TOPICAL

Children older than 3 mos. Apply sparingly to affected area 1–2 times/day.

▸ Maintenance treatment of asthma for those requiring oral corticosteroid therapy using dry powder formulation

INHALATION

Children 4–11 yrs. 50–100 mcg twice daily.

▸ Previous treatment: bronchodilators

INHALATION

Children older than 12 yrs. Initially, 100 mcg q12h. Maximum: 500 mcg/day.

▸ Previous treatment: inhaled steroids

INHALATION

Children older than 12 yrs. Initially, 100–250 mcg q12h. Maximum: 500 mcg q12h.

▸ Previous treatment with oral steroids

INHALATION

Children older than 12 yrs. Diskus: 500–1,000 mcg 2 times/day. Rotadisk: 1,000 mcg 2 times/day.

CONTRAINDICATIONS

Hypersensitivity to fluticasone or any related component. Untreated localized infection of nasal mucosa.
Inhalation: Primary treatment of status asthmaticus or other acute asthma episodes.

INTERACTIONS

Drug

None known.

Herbal

None known.

Food

None known.

DIAGNOSTIC TEST EFFECTS

None known.

SIDE EFFECTS

Frequent

Inhalation: Throat irritation, hoarseness, dry mouth, coughing, temporary wheezing, localized fungal infection in mouth, pharynx, and larynx, particularly if mouth is not rinsed with water after each administration
Intranasal: Mild nasopharyngeal irritation; nasal irritation, burning, stinging, dryness, rebound congestion, rhinorrhea, loss of sense of taste

Occasional

Intranasal: Nasal and pharyngeal candidiasis, headache
Inhalation: Oral candidiasis
Topical: Burning and itching of skin

SERIOUS REACTIONS

None known.

PEDIATRIC CONSIDERATIONS

Baseline Assessment

- Establish the patient's baseline history of asthma, rhinitis, and skin disorder.

• Be aware that it is unknown whether fluticasone crosses the placenta or is distributed in breast milk.
• Be aware that the safety and efficacy of fluticasone have not been established in children younger than 4 yrs of age.
• Be aware that children older than 4 yrs of age may experience growth suppression with prolonged or high doses.

Precautions

• Use cautiously in pts with active or quiescent tuberculosis and untreated fungal, bacterial, or systemic ocular herpes simplex and viral infections.

Administration and Handling

INHALATION

• Shake container well. Have the patient exhale as completely as possible.
• Place the mouthpiece fully into the patient's mouth; then while holding the inhaler upright, have the patient inhale deeply and slowly while pressing the top of the canister. Instruct the patient to hold his or her breath as long as possible before exhaling and then to exhale slowly.
• Wait 1 min between inhalations when multiple inhalations are ordered to allow for deeper bronchial penetration.
• Have the patient rinse his or her mouth with water immediately after inhalation to prevent mouth and throat dryness.

INTRANASAL

• Ensure that the patient clears his or her nasal passages before using fluticasone. The patient may need topical nasal decongestants 5–15 min before fluticasone use.
• Tilt the patient's head slightly forward.
• Insert spray tip up in one patient nostril, pointing toward inflamed nasal turbinates, away from the nasal septum.
• Pump medication into one of the patient's nostrils while holding his or her other nostril closed. Instruct the patient to concurrently inspire through the nose.

Intervention and Evaluation

• Monitor the depth, rate, rhythm, and type of patient respirations.
• Monitor the patient's arterial blood gas values and the quality and rate of the patient's pulse.
• Assess the patient's lung sounds for rales, rhonchi, and wheezing.
• Evaluate the patient's oral mucous membranes for evidence of candidiasis.
• Monitor growth in pediatric pts.
• Examine the involved area for a therapeutic response to irritation in pts using topical fluticasone.

Patient/Family Teaching

• Tell pts/families receiving bronchodilators by inhalation concomitantly with steroid inhalation therapy to use the bronchodilator several minutes before corticosteroid aerosol to enhance penetration of the steroid into the bronchial tree.
• Caution the patient/family against abruptly discontinuing the drug or changing the dose schedule of the drug. Explain to the patient/family that the patient must taper off drug doses gradually under medical supervision.
• Urge the patient/family to maintain careful oral hygiene.
• Instruct the patient/family to rinse the patient's mouth with water immediately after inhalation to prevent mouth and throat dryness and oral candidiasis.
• Instruct the patient/family to increase the patient's fluid intake

to decrease the viscosity of his or her lung secretions.
• Teach pts taking fluticasone intranasally the proper use of nasal spray. Instruct the patient/family to clear his or her nasal passages before use.
• Warn the patient/family to notify the physician if the patient experiences nasal irritation, no improvement in symptoms, or sneezing.
• Tell the patient/family that the patient should notice symptomatic improvement in several days.
• Instruct the patient/family using topical fluticasone to rub a thin film gently onto the affected area.
• Teach pts/families to use topical fluticasone only for the prescribed area and not longer than prescribed. Warn the patient to avoid topical fluticasone contact with eyes.

Mometasone Furoate Monohydrate

(Nasonex)

CATEGORY AND SCHEDULE

Pregnancy Risk Category: C

MECHANISM OF ACTION

An adrenocorticosteroid that acts as an anti-inflammatory agent. Inhibits early activation of allergic reaction and release of inflammatory cells into nasal tissue.
Therapeutic Effect: Decreases response to seasonal and perennial rhinitis.

PHARMACOKINETICS

Undetectable in plasma. Protein binding: 98%–99%. The portion of the dose that is swallowed undergoes extensive metabolism. Excreted into bile and, to a lesser extent, into the urine.

AVAILABILITY

Nasal Spray. 50 mcg/spray.

INDICATIONS AND DOSAGES

▸ Allergic rhinitis

NASAL SPRAY

Children older than 12 yrs. 2 sprays in each nostril once daily.
Children 2–12 yrs. 1 spray in each nostril once daily. Improvement occurs within 11 hrs–2 days after the first dose. Maximum benefit is achieved within 1–2 wks.

CONTRAINDICATIONS

Hypersensitivity to any corticosteroid. Persistently positive sputum cultures for *Candida albicans*, systemic fungal infections, untreated localized infection involving nasal mucosa.

INTERACTIONS

Drug

None known.

Herbal

None known.

Food

None known.

DIAGNOSTIC TEST EFFECTS

None known.

SIDE EFFECTS

Occasional

Nasal irritation, stinging

Rare

Nasal or pharyngeal candidiasis

SERIOUS REACTIONS

! Acute hypersensitivity reaction, including urticaria, angioedema, and severe bronchospasm, occurs rarely.

! A transfer from systemic to local steroid therapy may unmask a previously suppressed bronchial asthma condition.

PEDIATRIC CONSIDERATIONS

Baseline Assessment

• Determine whether the patient is hypersensitive to any corticosteroids.
• Be aware that it is unknown whether mometasone crosses the placenta or is distributed in breast milk.
• Be aware that high dosages and prolonged treatment may decrease cortisol secretion and short-term growth rate in children.

Precautions

• Use cautiously in pts with adrenal insufficiency, cirrhosis, glaucoma, hypothyroidism, osteoporosis, tuberculosis, and untreated infection.

Administration and Handling

INTRANASAL

• Shake well before each use. Ensure that the patient clears his or her nasal passages before using mometasone.
• Insert the spray tip up in one patient nostril, pointing toward the inflamed nasal turbinates, away from the nasal septum.
• Pump medication into one of the patient's nostrils while holding his or her other nostril closed. Instruct the patient to concurrently inspire through the nose to permit the medication as high into nasal passages as possible.

Patient/Family Teaching

• Teach the patient/family the proper use of mometasone nasal spray.
• Instruct the patient/family to clear the patient's nasal passages before using mometasone.
• Caution the patient/family against abruptly discontinuing the drug or changing the dose schedule of the drug. Explain to the patient/family that the patient must taper off drug doses gradually under medical supervision.
• Warn the patient/family to notify the physician if the patient experiences nasal irritation, no improvement in symptoms, or sneezing.

Nedocromil Sodium

ned-oh-**crow**-mul
(Alocril, Mireze [CAN], Tilade)

CATEGORY AND SCHEDULE

Pregnancy Risk Category: B

MECHANISM OF ACTION

A mast cell stabilizer that prevents activation and release of mediators of inflammation, such as histamine, leukotrienes, mast cells, eosinophils, and monocytes. ***Therapeutic Effect:*** Prevents both early and late asthmatic responses.

AVAILABILITY

Aerosol for Inhalation: 1.75 mg/activation.
Ophthalmic Solution: 2%.

INDICATIONS AND DOSAGES

▸ **Mild to moderate asthma**

ORAL INHALATION

Children 6 yrs and older. 2 inhalations 4 times/day. May decrease to 3 times/day then 2 times/day as control of asthma occurs.

▸ **Allergic conjunctivitis**

OPHTHALMIC

Children 3 yrs and older. 1–2 drops in each eye 2 times/day.

UNLABELED USES

Prevention of bronchospasm in pts with reversible obstructive airway disease.

CONTRAINDICATIONS

Hypersensitivity to nedocromil or any related component.

INTERACTIONS

Drug

None known.

Herbal

None known.

Food

None known.

DIAGNOSTIC TEST EFFECTS

None known.

SIDE EFFECTS

Frequent (10%–6%)

Cough, pharyngitis, bronchospasm, headache, unpleasant taste

Occasional (5%–1%)

Rhinitis, upper respiratory tract infection, abdominal pain, fatigue

Rare (less than 1%)

Diarrhea, dizziness

SERIOUS REACTIONS

None known.

PEDIATRIC CONSIDERATIONS

Baseline Assessment

• Perform baseline assessment of lung sounds, auscultating for adventitious sounds.

• Determine the patient's baseline exercise and activity tolerance.

• Measure baseline peak flow readings, and, if ordered, pulmonary function testing.

Precautions

• Remember that nedocromil is not used for reversing acute bronchospasm.

Intervention and Evaluation

• Evaluate the patient for therapeutic response, less frequent or severe asthmatic attacks, and reduced dependence on antihistamines.

Patient/Family Teaching

• Instruct the patient/family to increase the patient's fluid intake to decrease the viscosity of his or her lung secretions.

• Explain to the patient/family that the drug must be administered at regular intervals, even when the patient is symptom-free, to achieve optimal results of therapy.

• Tell the patient/family that the unpleasant taste the patient experiences after nedocromil inhalation may be relieved by rinsing his or her mouth with water immediately after inhalation.

• Teach the patient/family how to use a peak flow meter and to record the values in a log.

Triamcinolone

See adrenocortical steroids

REFERENCES

Miller, S. & Fioravanti, J. (1997). Pediatric medications: a handbook for nurses. St. Louis: Mosby.

Taketomo, C. K., Hodding, J. H. & Kraus, D. M. (2003–2004). Pediatric dosage handbook (10th ed.). Hudson, OH: Lexi-Comp.

81 Miscellaneous Respiratory Agents

Dornase Alfa
Montelukast
Omalizumab
Zafirlukast

Uses: Because they belong to separate subclasses, miscellaneous respiratory agents have different indications. Along with standard therapy, *dornase alfa* is used to reduce the frequency of respiratory infections and improve pulmonary function in pts with advanced cystic fibrosis. *Montelukast* and *zafirlukast* are used for prophylaxis and long-term treatment of asthma. *Omalizumab* is prescribed to treat moderate to severe persistent asthma triggered by year-round allergens.

Action: Miscellaneous respiratory agents act by various mechanisms. *Dornase alfa* selectively splits and hydrolyzes DNA in sputum, reducing sputum viscidity and elasticity. *Montelukast* and *zafirlukast* act on leukotriene receptors. This decreases the effects of leukotrienes, which increase eosinophil migration, producing mucus and edema of the airway wall and causing bronchoconstriction. *Omalizumab* works by blocking immunoglobulin E, an underlying cause of allergic asthma.

Dornase Alfa

door-naze al-fah
(Pulmozyme)

CATEGORY AND SCHEDULE

Pregnancy Risk Category: B

MECHANISM OF ACTION

A respiratory inhalant enzyme that selectively splits and hydrolyzes DNA in sputum. ***Therapeutic Effect:*** Reduces sputum viscid elasticity.

AVAILABILITY

Inhalation: 2.5 mg ampules for nebulization (1 mg/mL).

INDICATIONS AND DOSAGES

▸ **Management of pulmonary function in cystic fibrosis**

NEBULIZATION

Children older than 5 yrs. 2.5 mg (1 ampule) once daily via a recommended nebulizer. May increase to twice daily dosing.

CONTRAINDICATIONS

Sensitivity to dornase alfa, epoetin alfa (Chinese hamster ovary cell products), or any related component.

INTERACTIONS

Drug
None known.
Herbal
None known.
Food
None known.

DIAGNOSTIC TEST EFFECTS

None known.

SIDE EFFECTS

Frequent (greater than 10%)
Pharyngitis, chest pain or discomfort, sore throat, changes in voice

Occasional (10%–3%)
Conjunctivitis, hoarseness, skin rash

SERIOUS REACTIONS

None significant.

PEDIATRIC CONSIDERATIONS

Baseline Assessment

- Assess the patient's arterial blood gas values, dyspnea, fatigue, lung sounds, and pulmonary secretions for amount, color, and viscosity.
- Use of this product has not been established in children younger than 5 yrs of age or in pts with forced vital capacity less than 40% of normal.
- Safety of this product during breast-feeding has not been established.

Administration and Handling

NEBULIZATION

- Refrigerate and protect from light.
- Do not expose to room temperature for longer than 24 hrs.
- Discard solution if cloudy or discolored.
- Do not mix with other medications in the nebulizer.

Intervention and Evaluation

- Provide emotional support to the patient and his or her family.
- Assess the patient for relief of dyspnea and fatigue.
- Examine the patient for decreased viscosity of pulmonary secretions.
- Encourage the patient to increase his or her fluid intake.

Patient/Family Teaching

- Instruct the patient/family not to dilute or mix dornase alfa with other medications. Teach the patient to refrigerate the drug.
- Explain to the patient/family that the patient may have hoarseness or other upper airway irritation during dornase alfa therapy.
- Teach the patient/family how to use and clean the nebulizer.

Montelukast

mon-**tee**-leu-cast
(Singulair)

CATEGORY AND SCHEDULE

Pregnancy Risk Category: B

MECHANISM OF ACTION

An antiasthmatic that inhibits cysteinyl leukotriene receptors, producing inhibition of the effects on bronchial smooth muscle. ***Therapeutic Effect:*** Attenuates bronchoconstriction and decreases vascular permeability, mucosal edema, and mucus production.

PHARMACOKINETICS

Route	Onset	Peak	Duration
PO	N/A	N/A	24 hrs
PO, chewable	N/A	N/A	24 hrs

Rapidly absorbed from the GI tract. Protein binding: 99%. Extensively metabolized in the liver. Excreted almost exclusively in the feces via the biliary system. ***Half-Life:*** 2.7–5.5 hrs.

AVAILABILITY

Tablets: 10 mg.
Tablets (chewable): 4 mg, 5 mg.
Oral Granules: 4 mg/packet.

INDICATIONS AND DOSAGES

▸ Bronchial asthma

PO

Adolescents older than 14 yrs. One 10-mg tablet daily, taken in the evening.
Children 6–14 yrs. One 5-mg chewable tablet daily, taken in the evening.
Children 1–5 yrs. One 4-mg chewable tablet daily, taken in the evening.

CONTRAINDICATIONS

Hypersensitivity to montelukast or any related component.

INTERACTIONS

Drug

Phenobarbital, rifampin: May reduce the duration of action of montelukast.

Herbal

None known.

Food

None known.

DIAGNOSTIC TEST EFFECTS

May increase SGOT (AST) and SGPT (ALT) levels.

SIDE EFFECTS

Adults and adolescents older than 14 yrs

Frequent (18%)

Headache

Occasional (4%)

Influenza

Rare (3%–2%)

Abdominal pain, cough, dyspepsia, dizziness, fatigue, dental pain

Children 6–14 yrs

Rare (less than 2%)

Diarrhea, laryngitis, pharyngitis, nausea, otitis media, sinusitis, viral infection

SERIOUS REACTIONS

None known.

PEDIATRIC CONSIDERATIONS

Baseline Assessment

- Inform parents of phenylketonuric pts that the montelukast chewable tablet contains phenylalanine, a component of aspartame.
- Do not abruptly substitute montelukast for inhaled or oral corticosteroids.
- Be aware that it is unknown whether montelukast is excreted in breast milk. Use montelukast during pregnancy only if necessary.
- There are no age-related precautions noted in children older than 6 yrs of age.

Precautions

- Use cautiously in pts with impaired liver function and those whose systemic corticosteroid treatment is being reduced during montelukast therapy.
- Be aware that the chewable tablets contain aspartame.

Administration and Handling

PO

- Administer montelukast in the evening without regard to food ingestion.

Intervention and Evaluation

- Monitor the depth, rate, rhythm, and type of patient respirations.
- Monitor the quality and rate of the patient's pulse.
- Assess the patient's lung sounds for crackles, rhonchi, and wheezing.

• Observe the patient's fingernails and lips for a blue or dusky color in light-skinned pts and gray color in dark-skinned pts (signs of hypoxemia).

Patient/Family Teaching

• Instruct the patient/family to increase the patient's fluid intake to decrease the viscosity of his or her lung secretions.
• Teach the patient/family to take the drug as prescribed, even during symptom-free periods as well as during exacerbations of asthma.
• Caution the patient/family not to alter the dosage or abruptly discontinue the patient's other asthma medications.
• Explain to the patient/family that montelukast is not for the treatment of acute asthma attacks.
• Tell pts/families with aspirin sensitivity to avoid aspirin and NSAIDs while taking montelukast.

Omalizumab

oh-mah-**liz**-uw-mab
(Xolair)

CATEGORY AND SCHEDULE

Pregnancy Risk Category: B

MECHANISM OF ACTION

A monoclonal antibody that selectively binds to human immunoglobulin E (IgE). Inhibits the binding of IgE on the surface of mast cells and basophiles. ***Therapeutic Effect:*** Reduction of surface-bound IgE limits the degree of release of mediators of the allergic response, reducing or preventing asthmatic attacks.

PHARMACOKINETICS

After SC administration, absorbed slowly, with peak concentration in 7–8 days. Excreted in the liver reticuloendothelial system and endothelial cells. ***Half-Life:*** 26 days.

AVAILABILITY

Powder for Injection: 129.6 mg (75 mg/0.6 mL after reconstitution), 202.5 mg (150 mg/1.2 mL after reconstitution).

INDICATIONS AND DOSAGES

▸ **Treatment of moderate to severe persistent asthma in those reactive to a perennial allergen and inadequately controlled asthma symptoms with inhaled corticosteroids**

SC

Children older than 12 yrs. 150–375 mg every 2–4 wks, with dosing and frequency depending on immunoglobulin E (IgE) level and body weight.

▸ **SC dosage given every 4 wks**

UNLABELED USES

Treatment of seasonal allergic rhinitis.

CONTRAINDICATIONS

Severe hypersensitivity to omalizumab.

INTERACTIONS

Drug

None known.

Herbal

None known.

Food

None known.

DIAGNOSTIC TEST EFFECTS

Total IgE levels do not return to pretreatment levels for up to 1 yr after discontinuation of omalizumab.

SIDE EFFECTS

Frequent (45%–11%)
Injection site reaction, including bruising, redness, warmth, stinging, hive formation, viral infections, sinusitis, headache, pharyngitis

Occasional (8%–3%)
Arthralgia, leg pain, fatigue, dizziness

Rare (2%)
Arm pain, earache, dermatitis, pruritus

SERIOUS REACTIONS

! Anaphylaxis, starting within 2 hrs of the first or subsequent administration, occurs in 0.1% of pts.

! Malignant neoplasms occur in 0.5% of pts.

PEDIATRIC CONSIDERATIONS

Baseline Assessment

- Obtain the patient's baseline serum total IgE levels before beginning omalizumab therapy because the omalizumab dosage is based on these pretreatment levels.
- Remember that omalizumab is not for the treatment of acute exacerbations of asthma, acute bronchospasm, or status asthmaticus.
- Be aware that since IgE is present in breast milk, it is assumed that omalizumab is present in breast milk. Use omalizumab only if clearly needed.
- Be aware that the safety and efficacy of omalizumab have not been established in children younger than 12 yrs of age.

Precautions

- Be aware that omalizumab is not for use in reversing acute bronchospasm or status asthmaticus.

Administration and Handling

◀ **ALERT** ▶ Remember that testing of IgE levels during omalizumab treatment cannot be used as a guide for omalizumab dose determination because IgE levels remain elevated for up to 1 yr after discontinuation of omalizumab treatment. Expect to base omalizumab dosage on IgE levels obtained before beginning omalizumab treatment.

- Use only clear or slightly opalescent solution; solution is slightly viscous.
- Store in refrigerator.
- Reconstituted solution is stable for 8 hrs if refrigerated or for 4 hrs after reconstitution when stored at room temperature.
- Use only Sterile Water for Injection to prepare for SC administration.
- Medication takes 15–20 min to dissolve.
- Draw 1.4 mL Sterile Water for Injection into a 3-mL syringe with a 1-inch, 18-gauge needle and inject contents into powdered vial.
- Swirl vial for approximately 1 min but do not shake. Then swirl the vial again for 5–10 sec every 5 min until no gel-like particles appear in the solution. Do not use if contents do not dissolve completely by 40 min.
- Invert the vial for 15 sec to allow the solution to drain toward the stopper.
- Using a new 3-mL syringe with a 1-inch 18-gauge needle, withdraw the required 1.2 mL dose and replace 18-gauge needle with a 25-gauge needle for SC administration.

• SC administration may take 5–10 sec because of the viscosity of omalizumab.

Intervention and Evaluation

• Monitor the depth, rate, rhythm, and type of patient respirations and the quality and rate of the patient's pulse.
• Assess the patient's lung sounds for rales, rhonchi, and wheezing.
• Observe the patient's fingernails and lips for a blue or dusky color in light-skinned pts or gray color in dark-skinned pts (signs of hypoxemia).

Patient/Family Teaching

• Instruct the patient/family to increase the patient's fluid intake to decrease lung secretion viscosity.
• Warn the patient/family not to alter the dosage of omalizumab or discontinue other asthma medications.

Zafirlukast

zay-**fur**-leu-cast
(Accolate)
Do not confuse with Accupril or Aclovate.

CATEGORY AND SCHEDULE

Pregnancy Risk Category: B

MECHANISM OF ACTION

An antiasthma agent that binds to leukotriene receptors. Inhibits bronchoconstriction due to sulfur dioxide, cold air, specific antigens, such as grass, cat dander, and ragweed. ***Therapeutic Effect:*** Reduces airway edema and smooth muscle constriction; alters cellular activity associated with inflammatory process.

PHARMACOKINETICS

Rapidly absorbed after PO administration (food reduces absorption). Protein binding: 99%. Extensively metabolized in liver. Primarily excreted in feces. Unknown if removed by hemodialysis. ***Half-Life:*** 10 hrs.

AVAILABILITY

Tablets: 10 mg, 20 mg.

INDICATIONS AND DOSAGES

▸ Bronchial asthma

PO

Children older than 12 yrs. 20 mg twice daily.
Children 5–12 yrs. 10 mg twice daily.

CONTRAINDICATIONS

Hypersensitivity to zafirlukast or any related component.

INTERACTIONS

Drug

Aspirin: Increases zafirlukast blood concentration.
Erythromycin, theophylline: Decreases zafirlukast blood concentration.
Warfarin: Coadministration of warfarin increases prothrombin time.

Herbal

None known.

Food

Food reduces absorption of zafirlukast.

DIAGNOSTIC TEST EFFECTS

May increase SGPT (ALT) levels.

SIDE EFFECTS

Frequent (13%)
Headache
Occasional (3%)
Nausea, diarrhea

Rare (less than 3%)
Generalized pain, asthenia, myalgia, fever, dyspepsia, vomiting, dizziness

SERIOUS REACTIONS

! Coadministration of inhaled corticosteroids increases the risk of upper respiratory infection.

PEDIATRIC CONSIDERATIONS

Baseline Assessment

- Obtain the patient's medication history.
- Assess the patient's hepatic enzyme levels.
- Be aware that zafirlukast is distributed in breast milk. Zafirlukast use is not recommended in breast-feeding women.
- Be aware that the safety and efficacy of this drug have not been established in children younger than 5 yrs of age.

Precautions

- Use cautiously in pts with impaired liver function.

Administration and Handling

PO

- Give zafirlukast 1 hr before or 2 hrs after meals.
- Do not crush or break tablets.

Intervention and Evaluation

- Monitor the depth, rate, rhythm, and type of patient respirations.
- Monitor the quality and rate of the patient's pulse.
- Monitor the patient's liver function test results.
- Assess the patient's lung sounds for crackles, rhonchi, and wheezing.
- Observe the patient's fingernails and lips for a blue or dusky color in light-skinned pts or gray in dark-skinned pts (signs of cyanosis).

Patient/Family Teaching

- Instruct the patient/family to increase the patient's fluid intake to decrease the viscosity of his or her lung secretions.
- Teach the patient/family to take the drug as prescribed, even during symptom-free periods.
- Caution the patient/family not to alter the dosage or abruptly discontinue the patient's other asthma medications.
- Explain to the patient/family that zafirlukast is not for the treatment of acute asthma episodes.
- Warn breast-feeding mothers not to breast-feed during zafirlukast therapy.
- Warn the patient/family to notify the physician if the patient experiences abdominal pain, flu-like symptoms, jaundice, nausea, or worsening of asthma.

REFERENCES

Miller, S. & Fioravanti, J. (1997). Pediatric medications: a handbook for nurses. St. Louis: Mosby.
Taketomo, C. K., Hodding, J. H. & Kraus, D. M. (2003–2004). Pediatric dosage handbook (10th ed.). Hudson, OH: Lexi-Comp.

Appendix A

CALCULATION OF BODY SURFACE AREA

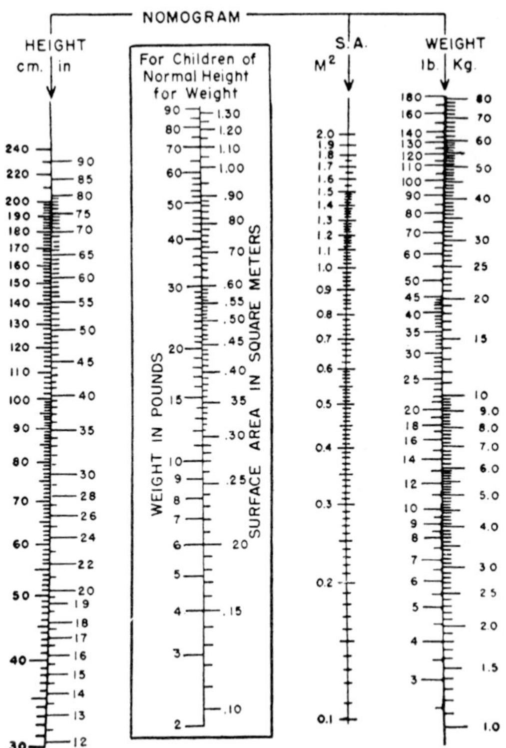

Place a straight edge from the patient's height in the left column to the patient's weight in the right column. The point of intersection on the body surface area column indicates the body surface area (BSA). (Reproduced in Behrman RE, Kliegman RM, Jenson HB: *Nelson textbook of pediatrics*, ed 17, Philadelphia, 2004, WB Saunders: Nomogram modified from data of E. Boyd by CD West.)

$$\text{BSA (m}^2\text{)} = \frac{\sqrt{\text{height (cm) x weight (kg)}}}{3600}$$

Appendix B
CONTROLLED SUBSTANCES CLASSIFICATION

Drugs	United States	Canada
Heroin, LSD, peyote, marijuana, mescaline	Schedule I • High abuse potential • No currently accepted medical use	Schedule H
Opium (morphine), meperidine, amphetamines, cocaine, short-acting barbiturates (secobarbital)	Schedule II • High abuse potential; potentially severe psychologic or physical dependence • Currently accepted medical use but may be severely restricted • Telephone orders only in emergencies if written Rx follows promptly • No refills	Schedule G
Glutethimide, paregoric, phendimetrazine	Schedule III • Abuse potential less than the drugs/substances in Schedules I and II; potentially moderate or low physical dependence or high psychologic dependence • Currently accepted medical use • Telephone orders permitted • Prescriber may authorize limited refills	Schedule F
Chloral hydrate, chlordiazepoxide, diazepam, mazindol, meprobamate, phenobarbital (Canada–G)	Schedule IV • Low abuse potential relative to drugs/substances in Schedule III; potentially limited physical or psychologic dependence • Currently accepted medical use • Telephone orders permitted • Prescriber may authorize limited refills	Schedule F

(continued)

Drugs	United States	Canada
Antidiarrheals with opium (Canada–G), antitussives	Schedule V • Lowest abuse potential; potentially very limited physical or psychologic dependence • Currently accepted medical use • Prescriber determines refills • Some products containing limited amounts of Schedule V substances (e.g., cough suppressants) available OTC to pts >18 yr	Schedule F

Appendix C
WEIGHTS AND EQUIVALENTS

METRIC SYSTEM

Weight

kilogram = kg = 1000 grams
gram = g = 1 gram
milligram = mg = 0.001 gram
microgram = mcg = 0.001 milligram

Volume

liter = L = 1 L
milliliter = ml = 0.001 L

AVOIRDUPOIS WEIGHT

1 ounce (oz) = 437.5 grains
1 pound (lb) = 16 ounces = 7000 grains

METRIC AND APOTHECARY EQUIVALENTS

Exact weight equivalents

Metric	Apothecary
1 mg	1/64.8 grain
64.8 mg	1 grain
324 mg	5 grains
1 g	15.432 grains
31.103 g	1 ounce = 480 grains

Exact volume equivalents

Metric	Apothecary
1.00 ml	16.23 minims
3.69 ml	1 fluidram = 60 minims
29.57 ml	1 fluid ounce = 480 minims
473.16 ml	1 pint = 7,680 minims
946.33 ml	1 quart = 15,360 minims

Appendix D

FORMULAS FOR DRUG CALCULATIONS

SURFACE AREA RULE:

$$\text{Child dose} = \frac{\text{Surface area (m}^2\text{)}}{1.73\ \text{m}^2} \times \text{Adult dose}$$

CALCULATING STRENGTH OF A SOLUTION:

Solution Strength: *Desired Solution:*

$$\frac{\times}{100} = \frac{\text{Amount of drug desired}}{\text{Amount of finished solution}}$$

CALCULATING FLOW RATE FOR IV:

$$\text{Rate of flow} = \frac{\text{Amount of fluid} \times \text{Administration set calibration}}{\text{Running time}}$$

$$\frac{x}{1} = \frac{\text{(ml) (gtt m/min)}}{\text{min}}$$

CALCULATION OF MEDICATION DOSAGES:

Formula method:

$$\frac{\text{Amount ordered}}{\text{Amount on hand}} \times \text{Vehicle} = \text{Number of tablets, capsules, or amount of liquid}$$

Vehicle is the drug form or amount of liquid containing the dosage. Amounts used in calculation by formula must be in same system.

Ratio–proportion method:

1 tablet:tablet in mg on hand::*x* tablet order in mg

Know or have::Want to know or order

Multiply means and extremes, divide both sides by known amount to get *x*. Amounts used in equation must be in same system.

Dimensional analysis method:

$$\text{Order in mg} \times \frac{\text{1 tablet or capsule}}{\text{What 1 tablet or capsule is in mg}} = \text{Tablets or capsules to be given}$$

If amounts are in different systems:

$$\text{Order in mg} \times \frac{\text{1 tablet or capsule}}{\text{What 1 tablet or capsule is in g}} \times \frac{1}{\text{1000 mg}} = \text{Tablets or capusles to be given}$$

Appendix E
HERBAL PRODUCTS

Herb	Uses
acidophilus	Diarrhea, vaginal and other candida infections, urinary tract infections, atopic dermatitis (eczema), atopic disease, irritable bowel syndrome, respiratory infections
alfalfa	*External:* Boils and insect bites *Internal:* Constipation, arthritis, increase blood clotting, diuretic, relieve inflammation of the prostate, treat acute or chronic cystitis, nutrient source
aloe (aloe vera gel)	Minor burns, skin irritations, minor wounds, frostbite, radiation-caused injuries
angelica	Poor blood flow to the extremities, headaches, backaches, osteoporosis, asthma, allergies, skin disorders, diuretic, antispasmodic, cholagogue, stomach cancer, mild antiseptic, expectorant, bronchitis, ease rheumatic pains, stomach cramps, muscle spasms
anise	*External:* Treat catarrhs of respiratory system (Inhalent), lice, neuralgia, rash, scabies; *Internal:* expectorant, bronchitis, cancer, cholera, colic, dysmenorrheal, emphysema, epilepsy, indigestion, insomnia, migraine, nausea, whooping cough, given to children to reduce gas, colic and respiratory symptoms; antibacterial, antispasmodic, abortifacient (large quantities), diaphoretic, diuretic, stimulant, tonic, flavoring in food
astragalus	Bronchitis, chronic obstructive pulmonary disease, colds, flu, GI conditions, weakness, fatigue, chronic hepatitis, ulcers, hypertension and viral myocarditis, immune stimulant, aphrodisiac and improve sperm motility
bilberry	Improve night vision, prevent cataracts, macular degeneration, glaucoma, varicose veins, hemorrhoids, diabetic retinopathy, myopia, mild diarrhea, dyspepsia in adults or children, controlling insulin levels, diuretic, urinary antiseptic
black cohosh	Smooth-muscle relaxant, antispasmodic, antitussive, astringent, diuretic, antidiarrheal, antiarthritic, hormone balancer in perimenopausal women, decrease uterine spasms in first trimester of pregnancy, antiabortion agent, dysmenorrheal
buckthorn	Powerful laxative

Herb	Uses
capsicum peppers	*External:* diabetic neuropathy, psoriasis, postmastectomy pain, Raynaud's syndrome, herpes zoster, arthritic, mascular pain, poor peripheral circulation *Internal:* cardiovascular health, CAD, reduce cholesterol and blood clotting, peptic ulcer disease, cold, flu
cascara	Laxative
chamomile	*External:* an antiseptic and soothing agent for inflamed skin and minor wounds. *Internal:* an antispasmodic, antianxiety, gas-relieving, and anti-inflammatory agent for the treatment of digestive problems; light sleep aid and sedative
chondroitin	Alone or in combination with glucosamine for joint conditions, as an antithrombotic, extravasation therapy agent, for ischemic heart disease, hyperlipidemia
chromium	Essential trace mineral required for proper metabolic functioning, decreases glucose tolerance, arteriosclerosis, elevated cholesterol, glaucoma, hypoglycemia, diabetes, obesity
coenzyme Q10	Ischemic heart disease, CHF, angina pectoris, hypertension, arrhythmias, diabetes mellitus, deafness, Bell's palsy, decreased immunity, mitral valve prolapse, periodontal disease, infertility
dong quai	Menopausal symptoms, menstrual irregularities, headache neuralgia, herpes infections, malaria, vitiligo, anemia
echinacea	*External:* Wound healing, bruises, burns, scratches, leg ulcers *Internal:* Immune stimulant, prophylaxis for colds, influenza, other infections
eyebright	Internally and externally to relieve eye fatigue, redness, sty and eye infections, nasal catarrh in sinusitis and hay fever
feverfew	Menstrual irregularities, threatened spontaneous abortion, arthritis, fever
flax	*External:* Inflammatory *Internal:* Laxative anticholesteremic
garlic	Antilipidemic, antimicrobial, antiasthmatic, anti-inflammatory, possible antihypertensive, treatment for some heavy metal poisonings

(continued)

Herb	Uses
ginger	Antioxidant, nausea, motion sickness, vomiting, sore throat, migraine headaches
ginkgo	Poor circulation, age-related decline in cognition, memory; vascular disease, antioxidant, depressive mood disorders, sexual dysfunction, asthma, glaucoma, menopausal symptoms, multiple sclerosis, headaches, tinnitus, dizziness, arthritis, altitude sickness, intermittent claudication
ginseng	Physical and mental exhaustion, stress, sluggishness, fatigue, weak immunity, as a tonic
goldenseal	Gastritis, GI ulceration, peptic ulcer disease, mouth ulcer, bladder infection, sore throat, postpartum hemorrhage, skin disorders, cancer, tuberculosis, wound healing, antiinflammatory, in combination with echinacea for cold and flu
green tea	Antioxidant, anticancer agent, diuretic, stimulant, antibacterial, antilipidemic, antiatherosclerotic
hops	Analgesic, hyperactivity, anthelmintic, mild sedative, insomnia, menopausal symptoms
kava	Anxiolytic, antiepileptic, antidepressant, antipsychotic, nervous anxiety, hyperactivity, restlessness, sleep disturbances, headache, muscle relaxant, wound healing
khat	Fatigue, obesity, gastric ulcers, depression
lemon balm	*External:* Cold sores *Internal:* Insomnia, anxiety, gastric conditions, psychiatric conditions, Grave's disease, attention deficit disorder (ADD)
licorice	Allergies, arthritis, asthma, constipation, esophagitis, gastritis, hepatitis, inflammatory conditions, peptic ulcers, poor adrenal function, poor appetite
lysine	Cold sores, herpes infections, Bell's palsy, rheumatoid arthritis, detoxify opiates
maitake	Diabetes, hypertension, high cholesterol, obesity, cancer
melatonin	Insomnia, inhibit cataract formation, increase longevity, epilepsy, hypertension, various cancers, jet lag, cancer protection, oral contraceptive
panax ginseng	Increase stamina and well being, fatigue, hypercholesterolemia, diabetes, COPD

Herb	Uses
papain	Anti-inflammatory, digestive aid
papaya	*External:* Debridement of worms. *Internal:* Intestinal worms, GI disorders, injection in a herniated lumbar intervetebral disk
SAM-e	Depression, Alzheimer's disease, migraine headache, hypersensitivity, chronic liver disease, fibromyalgia pain, inflammation in osteoarthritis
St. John's wort	*External:* Anti-inflammatory, relieve hemorrhoids, treat vitiligo, burns. *Internal:* Depression, anxiety
saw palmetto	Benign prostatic hypertrophy, mild diuretic, chronic and subacute cystitis, increase breast size, sperm count, sexual potency
senna	Laxative
siberian ginseng	Increase immunity, energy and performance, decrease inflammation and insomnia
turmeric	Menstrual disorders, colic, inflammation, bruising, dyspepsia, hematuria, flatulence
valerian	Sedative
wintergreen	*External:* Sore, inflamed muscles and joints *Internal:* Bladder inflammation, urinary tract diseases, diseases of prostate and kidney
yohimbe	Aphrodisiac, hallucinogenic

From Skidmore-Roth L: *Mosby's handbook of herbs and natural supplements*, ed 3, St. Louis, 2006, Mosby.

Appendix F

FDA PREGNANCY GUIDELINES

Alert: Medications should be used during pregnancy only if clearly needed.

A: Adequate and well-controlled studies have failed to show a risk to the fetus in the first trimester of pregnancy (also, no evidence of risk has been seen in later trimesters). Possibility of fetal harm appears remote.

B: Animal reproduction studies have failed to show a risk to the fetus and there are no adequate/well-controlled studies in pregnant women.

C: Animal reproduction studies have shown an adverse effect on the fetus and there are no adequate/well-controlled studies in humans. However, the benefits may warrant use of the drug in pregnant women despite potential risks.

D: There is positive evidence of human fetal risk based on data from investigational or marketing experience or from studies in humans, but the potential benefits may warrant use of the drug despite potential risks (e.g., use in life-threatening situations in which other medications cannot be used or are ineffective).

X: Animal or human studies have shown fetal abnormalities and/or there is evidence of human fetal risk based on adverse reaction data from investigational or marketing experience where the risks in using the medication clearly outweigh potential benefits.

Appendix G

RECOMMENDED CHILDHOOD IMMUNIZATION SCHEDULE

Recommended Childhood and Adolescent Immunization Schedule UNITED STATES • 2005

Vaccine ▼ / Age ▶	Birth	1 month	2 months	4 months	6 months	12 months	15 months	18 months	24 months	4–6 years	11–12 years	13–18 years
Hepatitis B[1]	HepB #1		HepB #2			HepB #3					HepB Series	
Diphtheria, Tetanus, Pertussis[2]			DTaP	DTaP	DTaP		DTaP			DTaP	Td	Td
Haemophilus influenzae type b[3]			Hib	Hib	Hib	Hib						
Inactivated Poliovirus			IPV	IPV		IPV				IPV		
Measles, Mumps, Rubella[4]						MMR #1				MMR #2	MMR #2	
Varicella[5]							Varicella				Varicella	
Pneumococcal Conjugate[6]			PCV	PCV	PCV	PCV			PCV	PPV		
Influenza[7]						Influenza (Yearly)				Influenza (Yearly)		
Vaccines below red line are for selected populations												
Hepatitis A[8]										Hepatitis A Series		

This schedule indicates the recommended ages for routine administration of currently licensed childhood vaccines, as of December 1, 2004, for children through age 18 years. Any dose not administered at the recommended age should be administered at any subsequent visit when indicated and feasible.

Indicates age groups that warrant special effort to administer those vaccines not previously administered. Additional vaccines may be licensed and recommended during the year. Licensed combination vaccines may be used whenever any components of the combination are indicated and other components of the vaccine are not contraindicated. Providers should consult the manufacturers' package inserts for detailed recommendations. Clinically significant adverse events that follow immunization should be reported to the Vaccine Adverse Event Reporting System (VAERS). Guidance about how to obtain and complete a VAERS form is available at www.vaers.org or by telephone, 800-822-7967.

Range of recommended ages

Preadolescent assessment

Only if mother HBsAg(–)

Catch-up immunization

DEPARTMENT OF HEALTH AND HUMAN SERVICES
CENTERS FOR DISEASE CONTROL AND PREVENTION

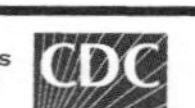

The Childhood and Adolescent Immunization Schedule is approved by:
Advisory Committee on Immunization Practices www.cdc.gov/nip/acip
American Academy of Pediatrics www.aap.org
American Academy of Family Physicians www.aafp.org

Footnotes

Recommended Childhood and Adolescent Immunization Schedule

UNITED STATES 2005

1. **Hepatitis B (HepB) vaccine.** All infants should receive the first dose of HepB vaccine soon after birth and before hospital discharge; the first dose may also be administered by age 2 months if the mother is hepatitis B surface antigen (HBsAg) negative. Only monovalent HepB may be used for the birth dose. Monovalent or combination vaccine containing HepB may be used to complete the series. Four doses of vaccine may be administered when a birth dose is given. The second dose should be administered at least 4 weeks after the first dose, except for combination vaccines which cannot be administered before age 6 weeks. The third dose should be given at least 16 weeks after the first dose and at least 8 weeks after the second dose. The last dose in the vaccination series (third or fourth dose) should not be administered before age 24 weeks.

   Infants born to HBsAg-positive mothers should receive HepB and 0.5 mL of hepatitis B immune globulin (HBIG) at separate sites within 12 hours of birth. The second dose is recommended at age 1–2 months. The final dose in the immunization series should not be administered before age 24 weeks. These infants should be tested for HBsAg and antibody to HBsAg (anti-HBs) at age 9–15 months.

   Infants born to mothers whose HBsAg status is unknown should receive the first dose of the HepB series within 12 hours of birth. Maternal blood should be drawn as soon as possible to determine the mother's HBsAg status; if the HBsAg test is positive, the infant should receive HBIG as soon as possible (no later than age 1 week). The second dose is recommended at age 1–2 months. The last dose in the immunization series should not be administered before age 24 weeks.

2. **Diphtheria and tetanus toxoids and acellular pertussis (DTaP) vaccine.** The fourth dose of DTaP may be administered as early as age 12 months, provided 6 months have elapsed since the third dose and the child is unlikely to return at age 15–18 months. The final dose in the series should be given at age ≥4 years. **Tetanus and diphtheria toxoids (Td)** is recommended at age 11–12 years if at least 5 years have elapsed since the last dose of tetanus and diphtheria toxoid-containing vaccine. Subsequent routine Td boosters are recommended every 10 years.

3. ***Haemophilus influenzae* type b (Hib) conjugate vaccine.** Three Hib conjugate vaccines are licensed for infant use. If PRP-OMP (PedvaxHIB® or ComVax® [Merck]) is administered at ages 2 and 4 months, a dose at age 6 months is not required. DTaP/Hib combination products should not be used for primary immunization in infants at ages 2, 4 or 6 months but can be used as boosters after any Hib vaccine. The final dose in the series should be administered at age ≥12 months.

4. **Measles, mumps, and rubella vaccine (MMR).** The second dose of MMR is recommended routinely at age 4–6 years but may be administered during any visit, provided at least 4 weeks have elapsed since the first dose and both doses are administered beginning at or after age 12 months. Those who have not previously received the second dose should complete the schedule by age 11–12 years.

5. **Varicella vaccine.** Varicella vaccine is recommended at any visit at or after age 12 months for susceptible children (i.e., those who lack a reliable history of chickenpox). Susceptible persons aged ≥13 years should receive 2 doses administered at least 4 weeks apart.

6. **Pneumococcal vaccine.** The heptavalent **pneumococcal conjugate vaccine (PCV)** is recommended for all children aged 2–23 months and for certain children aged 24–59 months. The final dose in the series should be given at age ≥12 months. **Pneumococcal polysaccharide vaccine (PPV)** is recommended in addition to PCV for certain high-risk groups. See ***MMWR*** 2000;49(RR-9):1-35.

7. **Influenza vaccine.** Influenza vaccine is recommended annually for children aged ≥6 months with certain risk factors (including, but not limited to, asthma, cardiac disease, sickle cell disease, human immunodeficiency virus [HIV], and diabetes), healthcare workers, and other persons (including household members) in close contact with persons in groups at high risk (see ***MMWR*** 2004;53[RR-6]:1-40). In addition, healthy children aged 6–23 months and close contacts of healthy children aged 0–23 months are recommended to receive influenza vaccine because children in this age group are at substantially increased risk for influenza-related hospitalizations. For healthy persons aged 5–49 years, the intranasally administered, live, attenuated influenza vaccine (LAIV) is an acceptable alternative to the intramuscular trivalent inactivated influenza vaccine (TIV). See ***MMWR*** 2004;53(RR-6):1-40. Children receiving TIV should be administered a dosage appropriate for their age (0.25 mL if aged 6–35 months or 0.5 mL if aged ≥3 years). Children aged ≤8 years who are receiving influenza vaccine for the first time should receive 2 doses (separated by at least 4 weeks for TIV and at least 6 weeks for LAIV).

8. **Hepatitis A vaccine.** Hepatitis A vaccine is recommended for children and adolescents in selected states and regions and for certain high-risk groups; consult your local public health authority. Children and adolescents in these states, regions, and high-risk groups who have not been immunized against hepatitis A can begin the hepatitis A immunization series during any visit. The 2 doses in the series should be administered at least 6 months apart. See ***MMWR*** 1999;48(RR-12):1-37.

Recommended Immunization Schedule
for Children and Adolescents Who Start Late or Who Are More Than 1 Month Behind
UNITED STATES 2005

The tables below give catch-up schedules and minimum intervals between doses for children who have delayed immunizations. There is no need to restart a vaccine series regardless of the time that has elapsed between doses. Use the chart appropriate for the child's age.

CATCH-UP SCHEDULE FOR CHILDREN AGED 4 MONTHS THROUGH 6 YEARS

Vaccine	Minimum Age for Dose 1	Minimum Interval Between Doses			
		Dose 1 to Dose 2	Dose 2 to Dose 3	Dose 3 to Dose 4	Dose 4 to Dose 5
Diphtheria, Tetanus, Pertussis	6 wks	4 weeks	4 weeks	6 months	6 months[1]
Inactivated Poliovirus	6 wks	4 weeks	4 weeks	4 weeks[2]	
Hepatitis B[3]	Birth	4 weeks	8 weeks (and 16 weeks after first dose)		
Measles, Mumps, Rubella	12 mo	4 weeks[4]			
Varicella	12 mo				
Haemophilus influenzae type b[5]	6 wks	**4 weeks** if first dose given at age <12 months **8 weeks (as final dose)** if first dose given at age 12-14 months **No further doses needed** if first dose given at age ≥15 months	**4 weeks**[6] if current age <12 months **8 weeks (as final dose)**[6] if current age ≥12 months and second dose given at age <15 months **No further doses needed** if previous dose given at age ≥15 mo	**8 weeks (as final dose)** This dose only necessary for children aged 12 months–5 years who received 3 doses before age 12 months	
Pneumococcal Conjugate[7]	6 wks	**4 weeks** if first dose given at age <12 months and current age <24 months **8 weeks (as final dose)** if first dose given at age ≥12 months or current age 24–59 months **No further doses needed** for healthy children if first dose given at age ≥24 months	**4 weeks** if current age <12 months **8 weeks (as final dose)** if current age ≥12 months **No further doses needed** for healthy children if previous dose given at age ≥24 months	**8 weeks (as final dose)** This dose only necessary for children aged 12 months–5 years who received 3 doses before age 12 months	

CATCH-UP SCHEDULE FOR CHILDREN AGED 7 YEARS THROUGH 18 YEARS

Vaccine	Minimum Interval Between Doses		
	Dose 1 to Dose 2	Dose 2 to Dose 3	Dose 3 to Booster Dose
Tetanus, Diphtheria	4 weeks	6 months	6 months[8] if first dose given at age <12 months and current age <11 years 5 years[8] if first dose given at age ≥12 months and third dose given at age <7 years and current age ≥11 years 10 years[8] if third dose given at age ≥7 years
Inactivated Poliovirus[9]	4 weeks	4 weeks	IPV[2,9]
Hepatitis B	4 weeks	8 weeks (and 16 weeks after first dose)	
Measles, Mumps, Rubella	4 weeks		
Varicella[10]	4 weeks		

Footnotes

Children and Adolescents Catch-up Schedules UNITED STATES • 2005

1. **DTaP.** The fifth dose is not necessary if the fourth dose was administered after the fourth birthday.
2. **IPV.** For children who received an all-IPV or all-oral poliovirus (OPV) series, a fourth dose is not necessary if third dose was administered at age ≥4 years. If both OPV and IPV were administered as part of a series, a total of 4 doses should be given, regardless of the child's current age.
3. **HepB.** All children and adolescents who have not been immunized against hepatitis B should begin the HepB immunization series during any visit. Providers should make special efforts to immunize children who were born in, or whose parents were born in, areas of the world where hepatitis B virus infection is moderately or highly endemic.
4. **MMR.** The second dose of MMR is recommended routinely at age 4–6 years but may be administered earlier if desired.
5. **Hib.** Vaccine is not generally recommended for children aged ≥5 years.
6. **Hib.** If current age <12 months and the first 2 doses were PRP-OMP (PedvaxHIB® or ComVax® [Merck]), the third (and final) dose should be administered at age 12–15 months and at least 8 weeks after the second dose.
7. **PCV.** Vaccine is not generally recommended for children aged ≥5 years.
8. **Td.** For children aged 7–10 years, the interval between the third and booster dose is determined by the age when the first dose was administered. For adolescents aged 11–18 years, the interval is determined by the age when the third dose was given.
9. **IPV.** Vaccine is not generally recommended for persons aged ≥18 years.
10. **Varicella.** Administer the 2-dose series to all susceptible adolescents aged ≥13 years.

Report adverse reactions to vaccines through the federal Vaccine Adverse Event Reporting System. For information on reporting reactions following immunization, please visit **www.vaers.org** or call the 24-hour national toll-free information line **800-822-7967**. Report suspected cases of vaccine-preventable diseases to your state or local health department.

For additional information about vaccines, including precautions and contraindications for immunization and vaccine shortages, please visit the National Immunization Program Web site at **www.cdc.gov/nip** or call **800-CDC-INFO / 800-232-4636** (English or Spanish)

Appendix H

EQUIANALGESIA (SELECTED ANALGESICS)

Drug*	Equal to IM/IV Morphine (mg)	Equal to Oral Morphine (mg)
Hydromorphone (Dilaudid), 1 mg	4	1.3
Codeine, 30 mg	4.5	1.5
Meperidine (Demerol), 50 mg	4.8	1.6
Codeine, 30 mg + acetaminophen, 300 mg (Tylenol No. 3)	7.2	2.4
Oxycodone, 5 mg + acetaminophen, 325 mg (Percocet)	7.2	2.4
Oxycodone, 5 mg + aspirin, 325 mg (Percodan)	7.2	2.4
Hydrocodone, 5 mg + acetaminophen, 500 mg (Vicodin, Lortab)	9	3
Oxycodone, 5 mg + acetaminophen, 500 mg (Tylox)	9	3
Dolophine (Methadone), 10 mg	15	7.5
Acetaminophen (Tylenol), 325 mg	2.7	0.9
Aspirin, 325 mg	2.7	0.9
Acetaminophen (Tylenol Extra Strength), 500 mg	4	1.3
Codeine, 60 mg + acetaminophen, 300 mg (Tylenol No. 4)	11.7	3.9
Transdermal fentanyl patch (Duragesic) (based on 25 μg/hr patch applied every 3 days = 50 mg oral morphine every 24 hours or divided into six doses = 8.3 mg) or use:	2.77	

From Hockenberry MJ: *Wong's essentials of pediatric nursing*, ed 7, St. Louis, 2005, Mosby. Courtesy of Betty R. Ferrell, PhD, FAAN, 1999. Used with permission.)

NOTE: When converting to oral oxycodone from oral morphine, an appropriate conservative estimate is 15–20 mg of oxycodone per 30 mg of morphine; however, when converting to oral morphine from oral oxycodone, an appropriate conservative estimate is 30 mg of morphine per 30 mg of oxycodone. (McCaffery M, Pasero C: Pain: a clinical manual, ed 2, St. Louis, 1999, Mosby, p 198.)

*Oral medication with exception of fentanyl.

Recommended Initial Duragesic Dose Based on Daily Oral Morphine Dose*

Oral 24-hour Morphine (mg/day)	Duragesic Dose (mg/hr)
45–134	25
135–224	50
225–314	75
315–404	100
405–494	125
495–584	150
585–674	175
675–764	200
765–854	225
855–944	250
945–1034	275
1035–1124	300

From *Mosby's Nursing Drug Reference 2004,* St. Louis: Mosby.
*Data from Duragesic package insert, Janssen, Pharmaceutical Products, Titusville, NJ, 2001.

Appendix I

PATIENT/FAMILY TEACHING

Each drug monograph contains a Patient/Family Teaching section, which offers key points that should be discussed with the pts and family about a medication. Also included are several more general topics that should be included when teaching pts and families about any medication use. Each topic is not listed in every monograph because the information would be repetitive and the length of the book would be prohibitive. The following teaching topics, nonetheless, should be included in patient care management.

- Explain the rationale for using the medication and the anticipated patient response to the medication.
- Teach the proper administration technique for the medication being prescribed. Information should include whether or not the oral tablet can be crushed, how to accurately measure liquid medications, how to use inhalers and nebulizers, and how to administer medications such as ear and eye drops and rectal and vaginal suppositories.
- Discuss how to prepare the patient for medication administration. Strategies include using concrete terms appropriate to the child's level of understanding, being honest with the child about unpleasant aspects of the medication, using distractions (such as tape recordings), and using relaxation techniques.
- Provide information about how often the medication should be taken and for what length of time it should be used. Discourage overusage and underusage of medications. Explain which signs and symptoms the patient or parent should use to determine when prn medications should be used.
- Instruct family members to keep all medications out of the reach of children. This is particularly important with medications requiring refrigeration; children may assume that they are food.
- Discourage parents from referring to medications as candy, particularly medications such as pleasant-tasting chewable tablets or oral liquids. Children may believe that these medications are to be eaten as snacks or treats.
- Teach pts or parents to discard any unused medications; advise pts or parents never to use expired or outdated medications.
- Discuss the possible side effects and symptoms of hypersensitivity for each medication. Tell the parents which side effects are of particular concern and warrant notifying the care provider.
- Discuss specific activities to be monitored or restricted as related to specific medications. (For example, activities such as biking, skating, or skateboarding might need to be restricted if the child is experiencing drowsiness as a side effect from antihistamines, anticonvulsants, or psychotropic drugs.) Insulin doses may need to be modified as activity levels change. Certain drugs may cause drowsiness upon arising.
- Determine whether the family can afford to purchase the medication, both on an immediate basis and a long-term basis. A referral to the

social work department of the health care agency when needed may be helpful.

- Provide information to the patient or parent about whom they can contact with questions about medications. This may be the primary care provider, a specialist, a pharmacist, or a hospital clinic.
- Stress the importance of compliance with any follow-up or ongoing care. Be sure the patient or parent knows when and with whom to seek follow-up care.

From Miller S, Fioravanti J: *Pediatric medications: a handbook for nurses*, St. Louis, 1997, Mosby-Year Book, Inc.

Appendix J

CULTURAL ASPECTS OF DRUG THERAPY

The term *ethnopharmacology* was first used to describe the study of medicinal plants used by indigenous cultures. More recently, it is being used as a reference to the action and effects of drugs in people from diverse racial, ethnic, and cultural backgrounds. Although there are insufficient data from investigations involving people from diverse backgrounds that would provide reliable information on ethnic-specific responses to all medications, there is growing evidence that modifications in dosages are needed for some members of racial and ethnic groups. There are wide variations in the perception of side effects by pts from diverse cultural backgrounds. These differences may be related to metabolic differences that result in higher or lower levels of the drug, individual differences in the amount of body fat, or cultural differences in the way individuals perceive the meaning of side effects and toxicity. Nurses and other health care providers need to be aware that variations can occur with side effects, adverse reactions, and toxicity so that pts from diverse cultural backgrounds can be monitored.

Some cultural differences in response to medications include the following:

African Americans: Generally, African Americans are less responsive to beta-blockers (e.g., propranolol [Inderal]) and angiotensin-converting enzyme (ACE) inhibitors (e.g., enalapril [Vasotec]).

Asian Americans: On average, Asian Americans have a lower percentage of body fat, so dosage adjustments must be made for fat-soluble vitamins and other drugs (e.g., vitamin K used to reverse the anticoagulant effect of warfarin).

Hispanic Americans: Hispanic Americans may require lower dosages and may experience a higher incidence of side effects with the tricyclic antidepressants (e.g., amitryptyline).

Native Americans: Alaskan Eskimos may suffer prolonged muscle paralysis with the use of succinylcholine when administered during surgery.

There has been a desire to exert more responsibility over one's health and, as a result, a resurgence of self-care practices. These practices are often influenced by folk remedies and the use of medicinal plants. In the United States, there are several major ethnic population subgroups (European, African, Hispanic, Asian, and Native Americans). Each of these ethnic groups has a wide range of practices that influence beliefs and interventions related to health and illness. At any given time, in any group, treatment may consist of the use of traditional herbal therapy, a combination of ritual and prayer with medicinal plants, customary dietary and environmental practices, or the use of Western medical practices.

AFRICAN AMERICANS

Many African Americans carry the traditional health beliefs of their African heritage. Health denotes harmony with nature of the body, mind, and spirit, whereas illness is seen as disharmony that results from natural causes or divine punishment. Common practices to the art of healing include treatments with herbals and rituals known empirically to restore health. Specific forms of healing include using home remedies, obtaining medical advice from a physician, and seeking spiritual healing.
Examples of healing practices include the use of hot baths and warm compresses for rheumatism, the use of herbal teas for respiratory illnesses, and the use of kitchen condiments in folk remedies. Lemon, vinegar, honey, saltpeter, alum, salt, baking soda, and Epsom salt are common kitchen ingredients used. Goldenrod, peppermint, sassafras, parsley, yarrow, and rabbit tobacco are a few of the herbals used.

HISPANIC AMERICANS

The use of folk healers, medicinal herbs, magic, and religious rituals and ceremonies are included in the rich and varied customs of Hispanic Americans. This ethnic group believes that God is responsible for allowing health or illness to occur. Wellness may be viewed as good luck, a reward for good behavior, or a blessing from God. Praying, using herbals and spices, wearing religious objects such as medals, and maintaining a balance in diet and physical activity are methods considered appropriate in preventing evil or poor health.
Hispanic ethnopharmacology is more complementary to Western medical practices. After the illness is identified, appropriate treatment may consist of home remedies (e.g., use of vegetables and herbs), use of over-the-counter patent medicines, and use of physician-prescribed medications.

ASIAN AMERICANS

For Asian Americans, harmony with nature is essential for physical and spiritual well-being. Universal balance depends on harmony between the elemental forces: fire, water, wood, earth, and metal. Regulating these universal elements are two forces that maintain physical and spiritual harmony in the body: the *yin* and the *yang.* Practices shared by most Asian cultures include meditation, special nutritional programs, herbology, and martial arts.
Therapeutic options available to the traditional Chinese physicians include prescribing herbs, meditation, exercise, nutritional changes, or acupuncture.

NATIVE AMERICANS

The theme of total harmony with nature is fundamental to traditional Native American beliefs about health. It is dependent on maintaining a state of equilibrium among the physical body, the mind, and the environment. Health practices reflect this holistic approach. The method of healing is determined traditionally by the medicine man, who diagnoses the ailment and recommends the appropriate intervention. Treatment may include heat, herbs, sweat baths, massage, exercise, diet changes, or other interventions performed in a curing ceremony.

EUROPEAN AMERICANS

Europeans often use home treatments as the front-line interventions. Traditional remedies practiced are based on the magical or empirically validated experience of ancestors. These cures are often practiced in combination with religious rituals or spiritual ceremonies.
Household products, herbal teas, and patent medicines are familiar preparations used in home treatments (e.g., salt water gargle for sore throat).

Appendix K

ENGLISH TO SPANISH DRUG PHRASES AND TERMS

TAKING THE MEDICATION HISTORY

Are you allergic to any medications? (If yes:)
Es alérgico a algún medicamento? (sí:)
(Ehs ah-lehr-hee-koh ah ahl-goon meh-dee-kah-mehn-toh) (see:)

—Which medications are you allergic to?
¿A cuál medicamento es alérgico?
(ah koo-ahl meh-dee-kah-mehn-toh ehs ah-lehr-hee-koh)

—What happens when you develop an allergic reaction?
¿Qué le pasa cuando desarrolla una reacción alérgica?
(Keh leh pah-sah koo-ahn-doh deh-sah-roh-yah oo-nah reh-ahk-see-ohn ah-lehr-hee-kah)

—What did you do to relieve or stop the allergic reaction?
¿Qué hizo para aliviar o detener la reacción alérgica?
(Keh ee-soh pah-rah ah-lee-bee-ahr oh deh-teh-nehr lah reh-ahk-see-ohn ah-lehr-hee-kah)

Do you take any over-the-counter, prescription, or herbal medications? (If yes:)
¿Toma medicamentos sin receta, con receta, o naturistas (hierbas medicinales)? (sí:)
(Toh-mah meh-dee-kah-mehn-tohs seen reh-seh-tah, kohn reh-seh-tah, oh nah-too-rees-tahs [ee-ehr-bahs meh-dee-see-nah-lehs]) (see:)

—Why do you take each medication?
¿Porqué toma cada medicamento?
(Pohr-keh toh-mah kah-dah meh-dee-kah-mehn-toh)

—What is the dosage for each medication?
¿Cuál es la dosis de cada medicamento?
(Koo-ahl ehs lah doh-sees deh kah-dah meh-dee-kah-mehn-toh)

—How often do you take each medication?
¿Con qué frequencia toma cada medicamento?
(Kohn keh freh-koo-ehn-see-ah toh-mah kah-dah meh-dee-kah-mehn-toh)

Once a day?	¿Una vez por día; diariamente? (Oo-nah behs pohr dee-ah; dee-ah-ree-ah-mehn-teh)
Twice a day?	¿Dos veces por día? (dohs beh-sehs pohr dee-ah)

Three times a day?	¿Tres veces por día? (Trehs beh-sehs pohr dee-ah)
Four times a day?	¿Cuatro veces por día? (Koo-ah-troh beh-sehs pohr-dee-ah)
Every other day?	¿Cada tercer día? (Kah-dah tehr-sehr dee-ah)
Once a week?	¿Una vez por semana? (Oo-nah behs pohr seh-mah-nah)

How does each medication make you feel?
¿Como le hace sentir cada medicamento?
(Koh-moh leh ah-seh sehn-teer kah-dah meh-dee-kah-mehn-toh)

—Does the medication make you feel better?
¿Le hace sentir mejor el medicamento?
(Heh ah-seh sehn-teer meh-hohr ehl meh-dee-kah-mehn-toh)

—Does the medication make you feel the same or unchanged?
¿Le hace sentir igual o sin cambio el medicamento?
(Leh ah-seh sehn-teer ee-goo-ahl oh seen kam-bee-oh ehl meh-dee-kah-mehn-toh)

—Does the medication make you feel worse? (If yes:)
¿Se siente peor con el medicamento? (si:)
(Seh see-ehn teh peh-ohr kohn ehl meh-dee-kah-mehn-toh) (see:)

—What do you do to make yourself feel better?
¿Qué hace para sentirse mejor?
(Keh ah-seh pah-rah sehn-teer-seh meh-hohr)

PREPARING FOR TREATMENT TO MEDICATION THERAPY

Medication Purpose

This medication will help relieve:
Este medicamento le ayudará a aliviar:
(Ehs-teh meh-dee-kah-mehn-toh leh ah-yoo-dah-rah ah ah-lee-bee-ahr)

English	Spanish	Pronunciation
Abdominal gas	Gases intestinales	(Gah-sehs een-tehs-tee-nah-lehs)
Abdominal pain	Dolor intestinal; dolor en el abdomen	(Doh-lohr een-tehs-tee-nahl; doh-lohr ehn ehl ahb-doh-mehn)
Chest congestion	Congestión del pecho	(Kohn-hehs-tee-ohn dehl peh-choh)
Chest pain	Dolor del pecho	(Doh-lohr dehl peh-choh)
Constipation	Constipación; estreñimiento	(Kohns-tee-pah-see-ohn; ehs-treh-nyee-mee-ehn-toh)

English	Spanish	Pronunciation
Cough	Tos	(Tohs)
Headache	Dolor de cabeza	(Doh-lohr-deh kah-beh-sah)
Muscle aches and pains	Achaques musculares y dolores	(Ah-chah-kehs moos-koo-lah-rehs ee doh-loh-rehs)
Pain	Dolor	(Doh-lohr)

This medication will prevent:
Este medicamento prevendrá:
(Ehs-teh meh-dee-kah-mehn-toh preh-behn-drah)

English	Spanish	Pronunciation
Blood clots	Coágulos de sangre	(Koh-ah-goo-lohs deh sahn-greh)
Constipation	Constipación; estreñimiento	(Kohns-tee-pah-see-ohn; ehs-treh-nyee-mee-ehn-toh)
Contraception	Contracepción; embarazo	(Kohn-trah-sehp-see-ohn; ehm-bah-rah-soh)
Diarrhea	Diarrea	(Dee-ah-reh-ah)
Infection	Infección	(Een-fehk-see-ohn)
Seizures	Convulciónes; ataque epiléptico	(Kohn-bool-see-ohn-ehs; ah-tah-keh eh-pee-lehp-tee-koh)
Shortness of breath	Respiración corta; falta de aliento	(Rehs-pee-rah-see-ohn kohr-tah; fahl-tah deh ah-lee-ehn-toh)
Wheezing	El resollar; la respiración ruidosa, sibilante	(Ehl reh-soh-yahr; lah rehs-pee-rah-see-ohn roo-ee-doh-sah, see-bee-lahn-teh)

This medication will increase your:
Este medicamento aumentará su:
(Ehs-teh meh-dee-kah-mehn-toh ah-oo-mehn-tah-rah soo:)

English	Spanish	Pronunciation
Ability to fight Infections	Habilidad a combatir infecciones	(Ah-bee-lee-dahd ah kohm-bah-teer een-fehk-see-oh-nehs)
Appetite	Apetito	(Ah-peh-tee-toh)
Blood iron levels	Nivel de hierro en la sargre	(Nee-behl deh ee-eh-roh ehn lah sahn-greh)
Blood sugar	Azúcar en la sangre	(Ah-soo-kahr ehn lah sahn-greh)
Heart rate	Pulso; latido	(Pool-soh; lah-tee-doh)

English	Spanish	Pronunciation
Red blood cell Count	Cuenta de células Rojas	(Koo-ehn-tah deh seh-loo-lahs roh-hahs)
Thyroid Hormone levels	Niveles de Hormona tiroide	(Nee-beh-lehs deh ohr-moh- nah tee-roh-ee-deh)
Urine volume	Volumen de orina	(Boh-loo-mehn deh oh-ree-nah)

This medication will decrease your:
Este medicamento reducirá su:
(Ehs-teh meh-dee-kah-mehn-toh reh-doo-see-rah soo:)

English	Spanish	Pronunciation
Anxiety	Ansiedad	(Ahn-see-eh-dahd)
Blood Cholesterol level	Nivel de colesterol En la sangre	(Nee-behl deh koh-lehs-teh- rohl ehn lah sahn-greh)
Blood lipid level	Nivel de lípido en la sangre	(Nee-behl deh lee-pee-doh ehn lah sahn-greh)
Blood pressure	Presión arterial; de sangre	(Preh-see-ohn ahr teh-ree-ahl; deh sahn-greh)
Blood sugar Level	Nivel de azúcar En la sangre	(Nee-behl deh ah-soo-kahr ehn lah sahn-greh)
Heart rate	Pulso; latido	(Pool-soh; lah-tee-doh)
Stomach acid	Ácido en el estómago	(Ah-see-doh ehn ehl ehs-toh-mah-goh)
Thyroid Hormone levels	Niveles de Hormona tiroide	(Nee-beh-lehs deh ohr-moh- nah tee-roh-ee-deh)
Weight	Peso	(Peh-soh)

This medication will treat:
Este medicamento sirve para:
(Ehs-teh meh-dee-kah-mehn-toh seer-beh pah-rah)

English	Spanish	Pronunciation
Cancer of your	Cancer de su	(Kahn-sehr deh soo)
Depression	Depresión	(Deh-preh-see-ohn)
HIV infection	Infección de VIH	(Een-fehk-see-ohn deh beh ee ah-cheh)
Inflammation	Infamación	(Een-flah-mah-see-ohn)
Swelling	Hinchazón	(Een-chah-sohn)
the infection in your	La infección en su	(lah een-fehk-see-ohn ehn soo)
Your abnormal Heart rhythm	Su ritmo anormal De corazón	(Soo reet-moh ah-nohr-mahl deh koh-rah-sohn)
Your allergy to	Su alergia a	(Soo eh-lehr-hee-ah ah)
Your rash	Su erupción; Sarpullido	(Soo eh-roop-see-ohn; sahr-poo-yee-doh)

ADMINISTERING MEDICATION

Swallow this medication with water or juice.
Tragüe este medicamento con agua o jugo
(Trah-geh ehs-teh meh dee-kah-mehn-toh kohn ah-goo-ah oh hoo-goh)

If you cannot swallow the medication whole, I can crush it and put it in food.
Si no puede tragar el medicamento entero puedo aplastarlo (triturarlo) y ponerlo en el alimento.
(See noh poo-eh-deh trah-gahr ehl meh-dee-kah-mehn-toh ehn-teh-roh poo-eh-doh ah-plahs-tahr-loh [tree-too-rahr-loh] ee poh-nehr-loh ehn ehl ah lee-mehn-toh)

I need to mix this medication with water or juice before you drink it.
Necesito mezclar este medicamento en agua o jugo antes de que lo tome.
(Neh-seh-see-toh mehs-klahr ehs-teh meh-dee-kah-mehn-toh ehn ah-goo-ah oh hoo-goh ahn-tehs deh keh loh toh-meh)

Do not chew this medication. Swallow it whole.
No mastique este medicamento. Tragüelo entero.
(Noh mahs-tee-keh ehs-teh meh-dee-kah-mehn-toh. Trah-geh-loh ehn-teh-roh)

Gargle with this medication and then swallow it.
Haga gargaras con este medicamento y luego tragüelo.
(Ah-gah gahr-gah-rahs koh ehs-teh meh-dee-kah-mehn-toh ee loo-eh-goh trah-geh-loh)

Place this medication under your tongue and let it dissolve.
Ponga este medicamento bajo la lengua y deje que se disuelva
(Pohn-gah ehs-teh meh-dee-kah-mehn-toh bah-hoh lah lehn-goo-ah ee deh-heh keh seh dee-soo-ehl-bah)

I would like to give this injection in your:
Quiero aplicar esta injección en su:
(Kee-eh-roh ah-plee-kahr ehs-tah een-yehk-see-ohn ehn soo:)

—abdomen
abdomen
(ahb-doh-mehn)

—arm
brazo
(brah-soh)

—buttocks
nalga
(nahl-gah)

—hip
cadera
(kah-deh-rah)

—thigh
muslo
(moos-loh)

I will give you this medication through your intravenous line.
Le daré este medicamento por el tubo de suero intravenoso.
(Leh dah-reh ehs-teh meh-dee-kah-mehn-toh pohr ehl too-boh deh soo-eh-roh een-trah-beh-noh-soh)

Let me know if you feel burning or pain at the intravenous site.
Digame si siente ardor o dolor en el sitio del suero intravenoso.
(Dee-gah-meh see see-ehn-teh ahr-dohr oh doh-lohr ehn ehl see-tee-oh dehl soo-eh-roh een-trah-beh-noh-soh)

I need to insert this suppository into your rectum (or vagina).
Necesito meter este supositorio en el recto (o vagina).
(Neh-seh-see-toh meh-tehr ehs-teh soo-poh-see-toh-ree-oh ehn ehl rehk-toh [oh bah-hee-nah])

I need to put this medication into each ear; left ear; right ear.
Necesito poner este medicamento en cada oreja; oreja izquierda; oreja derecha.
(Neh-seh-see-toh poh-nehr ehs-teh meh-dee-kah-mehn-toh ehn kah-dah oh-reh-hah; oh-reh-hah ees-kee-ehr-dah; -oh-reh-hah deh-reh-chah)

I need to put this medication into each eye; left eye; right eye.
Necesito poner este medicamento en cada ojo; ojo izquierdo; ojo derecho.
(Neh-seh-see-toh poh-nehr ehs-teh meh-dee-kah-mehn-toh ehn kah-dah oh-hoh; oh-hoh ees-kee-ehr-doh; oh-hoh deh-reh-choh)

PREPARING FOR DISCHARGE

The generic name for this medication is.
El nombre genérico (sin marca) de este medicamento es.
(Ehl nohn-breh heh-neh-ree-koh ?seen mahr-kah] deh ehs-teh meh-dee-kah-mehn-toh ehs)

The trade name for this medication is.
El nombre comercial de este medicamento es.
(Ehs nohm-breh koh-mehr-see-ahl deh ehs-teh meh-dee-kah-mehn-toh ehs)

Take the medication exactly as prescribed.
Tome el medicamento exactamente como se receta.
(Toh-meh ehl meh-dee-kah-mehn-toh ehx-ahk-tah-mehn-teh koh-moh seh reh-seh-tah)

You can safely break a scored tablet in half.
Puede partir por la mitad la tableta que tiene una muesca (marca).
(Poo-eh-deh pahr-teer pohr lah mee-tahd lah tah-bleh-tah keh tee-eh-neh oo-nah moo-ehs-kah [mahr-kah])

Do not crush or chew enteric-coated, extended-release, or sustained-release tablets or capsules.
No aplaste (triture) o mastique una tableta con capa entérica, de acción prolongada o de mantenimiento.
(Noh ah-plahs-teh [tree-too-reh] oh mahs-tee-keh oo-nah tah-bleh-tah kohn-kah-pah ehn-teh-ree-kah, deh ahk-see-ohn proh-lohn-gah-dah oh deh mahn-teh-nee-mee-ehn-toh)

If you miss a dose:
Si pierde una dosis:
(See pee-ehr-deh oo-nah doh-sees:)

—take it as soon as you remember it.
tómela tan pronto se acuerde.
(toh-meh-lah tahn prohn-toh seh ah-koo-ehr-deh)

—wait until the next dose.
espere hasta la siguiente dosis.
(ehs-peh-reh ahs-tah lah see-ghee-ehn-teh doh-sees)

—do not double the next dose.
No doble la siguiente dosis.
(noh doh-bleh lah see-ghee-ehn-teh doh-sees)

—contact your physician.
llame a su médico.
(yah-meh ah soo meh-dee-koh)

Do not stop taking your medication without first speaking with your physician.
No deje de tomar su medicamento sin hablar primero con su médico.
(Noh deh-heh deh toh-mahr soo meh-dee-kah-ehn-toh seen ah-blahr pree-meh-roh kohn soo meh-dee-koh)

Do not drink alcohol while taking this medication.
No tome alcohol cuando tome este medicamento.
(Noh toh-meh ahl-kohl koo-ahn-doh toh-meh ehs-teh meh-dee-kah-mehn-toh)

Do not drive or operate machinery while taking this medication.
No maneje o use maquinaria cuando toma este medicamento.
(Noh mah-neh-heh oh oo-seh mah-kee-nah-ree-ah koo-ahn-doh toh-mah ehs-teh meh-dee-kah-mehn-toh)

Notify your physician right away if you experience a dangerous side effect.
Llame a su médico inmediatamente si tiene efectos secundarios peligrosos.
(Llah-meh ah soo meh-dee-koh een-meh-dee-ah-tah-mehn-teh see tee-eh-neh eh-fehk-tohs seh-koon-dah-ree-ohs peh-lee-groh-sohs)

Check with your physician before taking any over-the-counter medications.
Cheque con su médico antes de tomar medicamentos sin receta.
(Cheh-keh kohn soo meh-dee-koh ahn-tehs deh toh-mahr meh-dee-kah-mehn-tohs seen reh-seh-tah)

Notify your physician if you are pregnant or are planning to become pregnant while taking this medication.
Dígale a su médico si está embarazada o planea el embarazo cuando toma este medicamento.
(Dee-gah-leh ah soo meh-dee-koh see ehs-tah ehm-bah-rah-sah-dah oh plah-neh-ah ehl ehm-bah-rah-soh koo-ahn-doh toh-mah ehs-teh meh-dee-kah-mehn-toh)

Notify your physician if you are breast-feeding while taking this medication.
Dígale a su médico si está amamantando (dando de pecho) cuando toma este medicamento.
(Dee-gah-leh ah soo meh-dee-koh see ehs-tah ah-mah-mahn-tahn-doh [dahn-doh deh peh-choh] koo-ahn-doh toh-mah ehs-teh meh-dee-kah-mehn-toh)

Refill your prescription right away, unless you don't need it anymore.
Rellene su receta inmediatamente, a menos que no la necesite.
(Reh-yeh-neh soo reh-seh-tah een-meh-dee-ah-tah-mehn-teh, ah meh-nohs keh noh lah neh-seh-see-teh)

PROPER MEDICATION STORAGE

Discard expired medications because they may become dangerous or ineffective.
Tire los medicamentos con fecha vencida (caducados) porque pueden ser peligrosos o inefectivos.
(Tee-reh lohs meh-dee-kah-mehn-tohs kohn feh-chah behn-see-dah [kah-doo-kah-dohs] pohr-keh poo-eh-dehn sehr peh-lee-groh-sohs oh een-eh-fehk-tee-bohs)

Keep all medications out of the reach of children at all times.
Guarde todos los medicamentos fuera del alcance de los niños todo el tiempo.
(Goo-ahr-deh toh-dohs lohs meh-dee-kah-mehn-tohs foo-eh-rah dehl ahl-kahn-seh deh lohs nee-nyohs toh-doh ehl tee-ehm-poh)

Store the medication:
Almacene (guarde) el medicamento:
(Ahl-mah-seh-neh [goo-ahr-deh] ehl meh-dee-kah-mehn-toh:)

—in its original container.
en su empaque original.
(ehn-soo ehm-pah-keh oh-ree-hee-nahl)

—in a cool, dry place.
en un lugar fresco y seco.
(ehn oon loo-gahr frehs-koh ee seh-koh)

—away from heat.
lejos del calor.
(leh-hohs dehl kah-lohr)

—at room temperature.
a temperatura ambiente
(ah tehm-peh-rah-too-rah ahm-bee-ehn-teh)

—out of direct sunlight.
fuera de la luz directa del sol.
(foo-eh-rah deh lah loos dee-rehk-tah dehl sohl)

—in the refrigerator.
en el refrigerador.
(ehn ehl reh-free-heh-rah-dohr)

Selected Drug Classes
Clasificación de Drogas Selectas (Medicamentos Selectos)
(Klah see-fee-kah-see-ohn deh droh-gahs seh-lehk-tahs [Meh-dee-kah-mehn-tohs Seh-lehk-tohs])

English	Spanish	Pronunciation
Analgesic (narcotic, nonnarcotic)	Analgésico (narcótico, no narcótico)	(Ah-nahl-heh-see-koh [nahr-koh-tee-koh, noh nahr-koh-tee-koh])
Antacid	Antiácido	(Ahn-tee-ah-see-doh)
Antianginal	Antianginoso	(Ahn-tee-ahn-hee-noh-soh)
Antianxiety	Ansiolítico	(Ahn-see-oh-lee-tee-koh)
Antiarrhythmic	Antiarritmico	(Ahn-tee-ah-reet-mee-koh)
Antibiotic	Antibiótico	(Ahn-tee-bee-oh-tee-koh)
Anticoagulant	Anticoagulante	(Ahn-tee-koh-ah-goo-lahn-teh)
Anticonvulsant	Anticonvulsivo	(Ahn-tee-kohn-bool-see-boh)
Antidepressant	Antidepresivo	(Ahn-tee-deh-preh-see-boh)
Antidiarrheal	Antidiarréicos	(Ahn-tee-dee-ah-reh-ee-kohs)
Antifungal	Antimicótico	(Ahn-tee-mee-koh-tee-koh)
Antihistamine	Antihistamínico	(Ahn-tee-ees-tah-mee-nee-koh)
Antihyperlipemic	Antihiperlipémico	(Ahn-tee-ee-pehr-lee-peh-mee-koh)
Antihypertensive	Antihipertensivo	(Ahn-tee-ee-pehr-tehn-see-boh)
Anti-inflamatory	Antiinflamatorio; Contra la inflamación	(Ahn-tee-een-flah-mah-toh-ree-oh; kohn-trah lah een-flah-mah-see-ohn)
Antimigraine	Antimigrañoso	(Ahn-tee-mee-grah-nyoh-soh)
Antiparkinsonian	Contra el Parkinson	(Kohn-trah ehl Pahr-keen-sohn)
Antipsychotic	Medicamentos sicóticos	(Meh-dee-kah-mehn-tohs see-koh-tee-kohs)
Antipyretic	Antitérmicos	(Ahn-tee-tehr-mee-kohs)
Antiseptic	Antiséptico	(Ahn-tee-sehp-tee-koh)
Antispasmodic	Antiespasmódico	(Ahn-tee-ehs-pahs-moh-dee-koh)
Antithyroid	Antitiroideos	(Ahn-tee-tee-roh-ee-deh-ohs)
Antituberculosis	Antifímicos	(Ahn-tee-fee-mee-kohs)

English	Spanish	Pronunciation
Antitussive	Antitusígenos	(Ahn-tee-too-see-heh-nohs)
Antiviral	Antivirales	(Ahn-tee-bee-rah-lehs)
Appetite suppressant	Antisupresivos del apetito	(Ahn-tee-soo-preh-see-bohs dehl ah-peh-tee-toh)
Appetite stimulant	Estimulantes del apetito	(Ehs-tee-moo-lahn-tehs dehl ah-peh-tee-toh)
Bronchodilator	Bronquiolíticos	(Brohn-kee-oh-lee-tee-kohs)
Cancer chemotherapy	Quimioterapia de cancer	(Kee-mee-oh teh-rah-pee-ah deh kahn-sehr)
Decongestant	Anticongestivo	(Ahn-tee-kohn-hehs-tee-boh)
Digestant	Digestible	(Dee-hehs-tee-bleh)
Diuretic	Diurético	(Dee-oo-reh-tee-koh)
Emetic	Emético	(Eh-meh-tee-koh)
Fertility	Inductor de la ovulación	(Een-doohk-tohr deh lah oh-boo-lah-see-ohn)
Herbal	Medicamentos naturales; hierbas medicinales	(Meh-dee-kah-mehn-tohs nah-too-rah-lehs, ee-ehr-bhas meh-dee-see-nah-lehs)
Hypnotic	Hipnótico	(Eep-noh-tee-koh)
Insulin	Insulina	(Een-soo-lee-nah)
Laxative	Laxante	(Lahx-ahn-teh)
Mineral	Mineral	(Mee-neh-rahl)
Muscle relaxant	Relajante muscular	(Reh-lah-hahn-teh moos-koo-lahr)
Oral contraceptive	Anticonceptivos orales	(Ahn-tee-kohn-sehp-tee-bohs oh-rah-lehs)
Oral hypoglycemic	Hipoglicémico oral	(Ee-poh-glee-seh-mee-koh oh-rahl)
Sedative	Sedantes	(Seh-dahn-tehs)
Steroid	Esteroide	(Ehs-teh-roh-ee-deh)
Thyroid hormone	Tiroideos, hormona tiroide	(Tee-roh-ee-deh-ohs, ohr-moh-nah tee-roh-ee-deh)
Vaccine	Vacuna	(Bah-koo-nah)

(continued)

Administration Routes
Modo de Uso
(Moh-doh deh Oo-soh)

English	Spanish	Pronunciation
By mouth	Oral	(Oh-rahl)
Intradermal	Intradermica	(Een-trah-dehr-mee-kah)
Intramuscular	Intramuscular	(Een-trah-moos-koo-lahr)
Intravenous	Intravenosa	(Een-trah-beh-noh-sah)
Nasal	Nasal	(Nah-sahl)
Oral	Oral	(Oh-rahl)
Otic	Ótica	(Oh-tee-kah)
Patch	Parche	(Pahr-cheh)
Rectal	Rectal	(Rehk-tahl)
Subcutaneous	Subcutanea	(Soob-koo-tah-neh-ah)
Sublingual	Sublingual	(Soob-leen-goo-ahl)
Topical	Topical, local	(Toh-pee-kahl, loh-kahl)
Vaginal	Vaginal	(Bah-hee-nahl)

Drug Preparations
Presentación del Medicamento
(Preh-sehn-tah-see-ohn dehl Meh-dee-kah-mehn-toh)

English	Spanish	Pronunciation
Capsule	Cápsula	(Kahp-soo-lah)
Cream	Crema	(Kreh-máh)
Drops	Gotas	(Goh-tahs)
Elixir	Elixir, jarabe	(Eh-leex-eer, hah-rah-beh)
Fluid	Líquido	(Lee-kee-doh)
Gel	Gel, jalea	(Hehl, hah-leh-ah)
Inhaler	Inhalador*	(Een-ah-lah-dohr)
Injection	Inyección	(Een-yehk-see-ohn)
Liquid	Líquido	(Lee-kee-doh)
Lotion	Loción	(Loh-see-ohn)
Lozenge	Trocisco, pastilla	(Troh-sees-koh, pahs-tee-yah)
Ointment	Ungüento	(Oon-goo-ehn-toh)
Pill	Píldora, pastilla	(Peel-doh-rah, pahs-tee-yah)
Powder	Polvo	(Pohl-boh)

English	Spanish	Pronunciation
Spray	Spray	(Sp-rah-ee)
Suppository	Supositorio	(Soo-poh-see-toh-ree-oh)
Syrup	Jarabe	(Hah-rah-beh)
Tablet	Tableta	(Tah-bleh-tah)

*The h is silent.

Administration Frequency
Frecuencia de la Administración
(Freh-koo-ehn-see-ah deh lah Ahd-mee-nees-trah-see-ohn)

English	Spanish	Pronunciation
Once a day	Una vez por día; diariamente	(Oo-nah behs pohr dee-ah; dee-ah-ree-ah-mehn-teh)
Twice a day	Dos veces por día	(Dohs beh-sehs pohr dee-ah)
Three times a day	Tres veces por día	(Trehs beh-sehs pohr dee-ah)
Four times a day	Cuatro veces por día	(Koo-ah-troh beh-sehs pohr dee-ah)
Every other day	Cada tercer día	(Kah-dah tehr-sehr dee-ah)
Once a week	Una vez por semana	(Oo-nah behs pohr seh-mah-nah)
Every 4 hours	Cada cuatro horas	(Kah-dah koo-ah-troh oh-rahs)
Every 6 hours	Cada seis horas	(Kah-dah seh-ees oh-rahs)
Every 8 hours	Cada ocho horas	(Kah-dah oh-choh oh-rahs)
Every 12 hours	Cada doce horas	(Kah-dah doh-seh oh-rahs)
In the morning	En la mañana	(Ehn lah mah-nyah-nah)
In the afternoon	En la tarde	(Ehn lah tahr-deh)

English	Spanish	Pronunciation
In the evening	En la noche	(Ehn lah noh-cheh)
Before bedtime	Antes de acostarse	(Ahn-tehs deh ah-kohs-tahr-seh)
Before meals	Antes de la comida; antes del alimento	(Ahn-tehs deh lah koh-mee-dah; ahn-tehs dehl ah-lee-mehn-toh)
With meals	Con los alimentos; Con la comida	(Kohn lohs ah-lee-mehn-tohs; kohn lah koh-mee-dah)

(continued)

English	Spanish	Pronunciation
After meals	Después de los alimentos; después de la comida	(Dehs-poo-ehs deh lohs ah-lee-mehn-tohs; dehs-poo-ehs deh lah koh-mee-dah)
Only when you need it	Solo cuando la necesite	(Soh-loh koo-ahn-doh lah neh-seh-see-teh)
When you have	Cuando tiene	(Koo-ahn-doh tee-eh-neh)
(pain)	(dolor)	(doh-lohr)

50 Common Side Effects
Cincuenta Efectos Secundarios Comúnes
(Seen-koo-ehn-tah Eh-fehk-tohs Seh-koon-dah-ree-ohs Koh-moo-nehs)

English	Spanish	Pronunciation
Abdominal cramps	Retorcijón abdominal	(Reh-tohr-see-hohn ahb-doh-mee-nahl)
Abdominal pain	Dolor abdominal	(Doh-lohr ahb-doh-mee-nahl)
Abdominal swelling	Inflamación abdominal	(Een-flah-mah-see-ohn ahb-doh-mee-nahl)
Anxiety	Ansiedad	(Ahn-see-eh-dahd)
Blood in the stool	Sangre en el excremento	(Sahn-greh ehn ehl ehx-kreh-mehn-toh)
Blood in the urine	Sangre en la orina	(Sahn-greh ehn la oh-ree-nah)
Bone pain	Dolor de hueso*	(Doh-lohr deh oo-eh-soh)
Chest pain	Dolor de pecho	(Doh-lohr deh peh-choh)
Chest pounding	Palpitación; latidos fuertes en el pecho	(Pahl-pee-tah-see-ohn; lah-tee-dohs foo-ehr-tehs ehn ehl peh-choh)
Chills	Escalofrío	(Ehs-kah-loh-free-oh)
Confusion	Confusión	(Kohn-foo-see-ohn)
Constipation	Constipación, estreñimiento	(Kohns-tee-pah-see-ohn, ehs-treh-nyee-mee-ehn-toh)
Cough	Tos	(Tohs)
Mental depression	Depresión mental	(Deh-preh-see-ohn mehn-tahl)
Diarrhea	Diarrea	(Dee-ah-reh-ah)
Difficult urination	Dificultad al orinar	(Dee-fee-kool-tahd ahl oh-ree-nahr)

English	Spanish	Pronunciation
Difficulty breathing	Dificultad al respirar	(Dee-fee-kool-tahd ahl rehs-pee-rahr)
Difficulty sleeping	Dificultad al dormir	(Dee-fee-kool-tahd ahl dohr-meer)
Dizziness	Mareos; vahídos	(Mah-reh-ohs; bah-ee-dohs)
Dry mouth	Boca seca	(Boh-kah seh-kah)
Easy bruising	Fragilidad capilar; le salen moretones con facilidad	(Frah-hee-lee-dahd kah-pee-lahr; leh sah-lehn moh-reh-toh-nehs kohn fah-see-lee-dahd)
Faintness	Desvanecimiento; sintió un vahído	(Dehs-bah-neh-see-mee-ehn-toh; seen-tee-oh oon bah-ee-doh)
Fatigue	Fatiga, cansancio	(Fah-tee-gah, kahn-sahn-see-oh)
Fever	Fiebre	(Fee-eh-breh)
Frequent urination	Orina frecuente	(Oh-ree-nah freh-koo-ehn-teh)
Headache	Dolor de cabeza	(Doh-lohr deh kah-beh-sah)
Impotence	Impotencia	(Eem-poh-tehn-see-ah)
Increased appetite	Aumento en el apetito	(Ah-oo-mehn-toh ehn ehl ah-peh-tee-toh)
Increased gas	Flatulencia	(Flah-too-lehn-see-ah)
Increased perspiration	Aumento en el sudor	(Ah-oo-mehn-toh ehn ehl soo-dohr)
Indigestion	Indigestión	(Een-dee-hehs-tee-ohn)
Itching	Comezón	(Koh-meh-sohn)
Loss of appetite	Pérdida en el apetito	(Pehr-dee-dah ehn ehl ah-peh-tee-toh)
Menstrual changes	Cambios en la menstruación; cambio en el ciclo menstrual	(Kahm-bee-ohs ehn la mehns-truh-ah-see-ohn; kahm-bee-oh ehn ehl see-kloh mehns-truh-ahl)
Mood changes	Cambio en el humor; cambio en la disposición	(Kahm-bee-oh ehn ehl oo-mohr, kahm-bee-oh ehn lah dees-poh-see-see-ohn)
Muscle pain	Dolores musculares	(Doh-loh-rehs moos-koo-lah-rehs)

(continued)

English	Spanish	Pronunciation
Muscle aches	Achaques musculares	(Ah-chah-kehs moos-koo-lah-rehs)
Muscle cramps	Calambre muscular	(Kah-lahm-breh moos-koo-lahr)
Nasal congestion	Congestión nasal	(Kohn-hehs-tee-ohn nah-sahl)
Nausea	Nausea	(Nah-oo-seh-ah)
Ringing in the ears	Zumbido en los oidos	(Soom-bee-doh ehn lohs oh-ee-dohs)
Skin rash	Erupción en la piel	(Eh-roop-see-ohn ehn lah pee-ehl)
Swelling on the hands, legs, or feet	Hinchazón en las manos, piernas, o pies	(Een-chah-sohn ehn lahs mah-nohs, pee-ehr-nahs, oh pee-ehs)
Vaginal bleeding	Sangrado vaginal	(Sahn-grah-doh bah-hee-nahl)
Vision changes	Cambios en la visión; cambios en la vista	(Kahm-bee-ohs ehn lah bee-see-ohn; cahm-bee-ohs ehn lah bees-tah)
Vomiting	Vomitando	(Boh-mee-tahn-doh)
Weakness	Debilidad	(Deh-bee-lee-dahd)
Weight gain	Aumento de peso	(Ah-oo-mehn-toh deh peh-soh)
Weight loss	Pérdida de peso	(Pehr-dee-day deh peh-soh)
Wheezing	Resollar; respiración sibilante	(Reh-soh-yahr; rehs-pee-rah-see-ohn see-bee-lahn-teh)

*The h is silent.

Appendix L

TECHNIQUES OF MEDICATION ADMINISTRATION

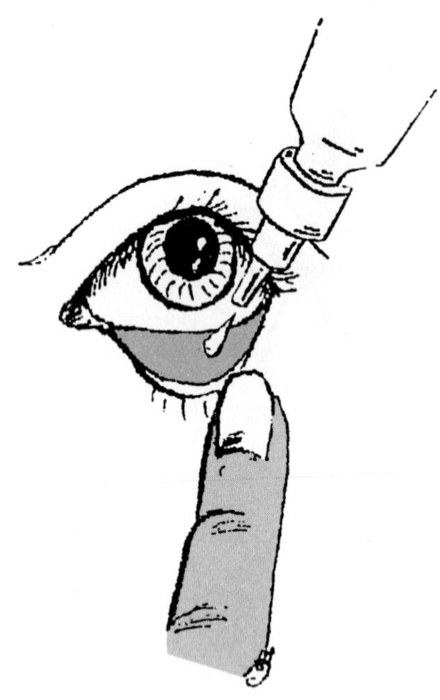

OPHTHALMIC

Eye Drops

1. Wash hands.
2. Instruct patient to lie down or tilt head backward and look up.
3. Gently pull lower eyelid down until a pocket (pouch) is formed between eye and lower lid (conjunctival sac).
4. Hold dropper above pocket. Without touching tip of eye dropper to eyelid or conjunctival sac, place prescribed number of drops into the center pocket (placing drops directly onto eye may cause a sudden squeezing of eyelid, with subsequent loss of solution). Continue to hold the eyelid for a moment after the drops are applied (allows medication to distribute along entire conjunctival sac).
5. Instruct patient to close eyes gently so that medication will not be squeezed out of the sac.
6. Apply gentle finger pressure to the lacrimal sac at the inner canthus (bridge of the nose, inside corner of the eye) for 1–2 min (promotes

absorption, minimizes drainage into nose and throat, lessens risk of systemic absorption).

7. Remove excess solution around eye with a tissue.
8. Wash hands immediately to remove medication on hands. Never rinse eye dropper.

Eye Ointment

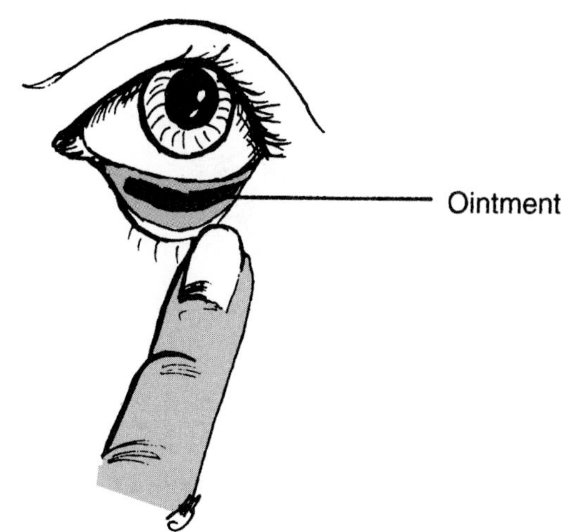

1. Wash hands.
2. Instruct patient to lie down or tilt head backward and look up.
3. Gently pull lower eyelid down until a pocket (pouch) is formed between eye and lower lid (conjunctival sac).
4. Hold applicator tube above pocket. Without touching the applicator tip to eyelid or conjunctival sac, place prescribed amount of ointment (¼–½ inch) into the center pocket (placing ointment directly onto eye may cause discomfort).
5. Instruct patient to close eye for 1–2 min, rolling eyeball in all directions (increases contact area of drug to eye).
6. Inform patient of temporary blurring of vision. If possible, apply ointment just before bedtime.
7. Wash hands immediately to remove medication on hands. Never rinse tube applicator.

OTIC

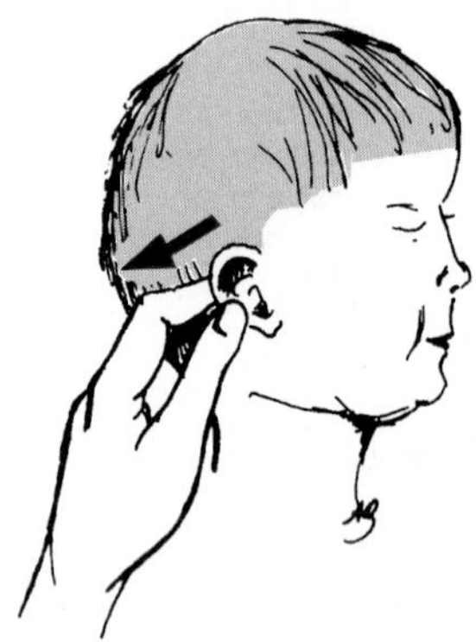

1. Ear drops should be at body temperature (wrap hand around bottle to warm contents). Body temperature instillation prevents startling of patient.
2. Instruct patient to lie down with head turned so affected ear is upright (allows medication to drip into ear).
3. Instill prescribed number of drops toward the canal wall, not directly on eardrum.
4. To promote correct placement of ear drops in children, pull the auricle down and posterior.

NASAL

Nose Drops and Sprays

1. Instruct patient to blow nose to clear nasal passages as much as possible.
2. Tilt head slightly forward if instilling nasal spray, slightly backward if instilling nasal drops.
3. Insert spray tip into one nostril, pointing toward inflamed nasal passages, away from nasal septum.
4. Spray or drop medication into one nostril while holding other nostril closed and concurrently inspire through nose to permit medication as high into nasal passages as possible.
5. Discard unused nasal solution after 3 mos.

INHALATION

Aerosol (Multidose Inhalers)

1. Shake container well before each use.
2. Exhale slowly and as completely as possible through the mouth.
3. Place mouthpiece fully into mouth, holding inhaler upright, and close lips fully around mouthpiece.
4. Inhale deeply and slowly through the mouth while depressing the top of the canister with the middle finger.
5. Hold breath as long as possible before exhaling slowly and gently.
6. When 2 puffs are prescribed, wait 2 min and shake container again before inhaling a second puff (allows for deeper bronchial penetration).
7. Rinse mouth with water immediately after inhalation (prevents mouth and throat dryness).

SUBLINGUAL

1. Administer while seated.
2. Dissolve sublingual tablet under tongue (do not chew or swallow tablet).
3. Do not swallow saliva until tablet is dissolved.

TOPICAL

1. Gently cleanse area prior to application.
2. Use occlusive dressings only as ordered.
3. Without touching applicator tip to skin, apply sparingly; gently rub into area thoroughly unless ordered otherwise.
4. When using aerosol, spray area for 3 sec from a 15-cm distance; avoid inhalation.

TRANSDERMAL

1. Apply transdermal patch to clean, dry, hairless skin on upper arm or body (not below knee or elbow).
2. Rotate sites (prevents skin irritation).
3. Do not trim patch to adjust dose.

RECTAL

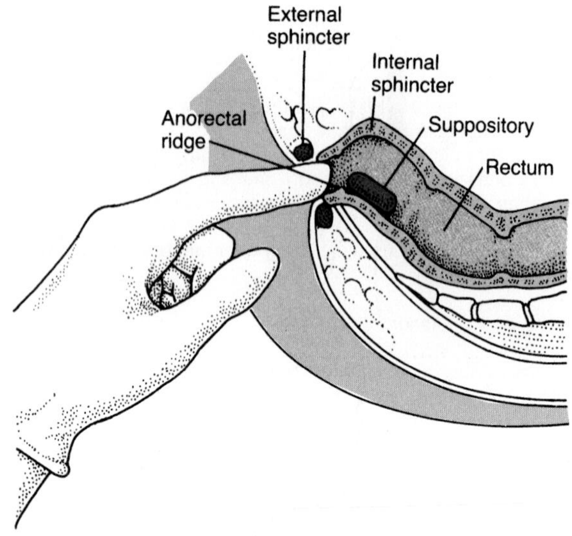

1. Instruct patient to lie in left lateral Sims position.
2. Moisten suppository with cold water or water-soluble lubricant.
3. Instruct patient to slowly exhale (relaxes anal sphincter) while inserting suppository well up into rectum.
4. Inform patient as to length of time (20–30 min) before desire for defecation occurs or the length of time (<60 min) for systemic absorption to occur, depending on purpose for suppository.

SUBCUTANEOUS

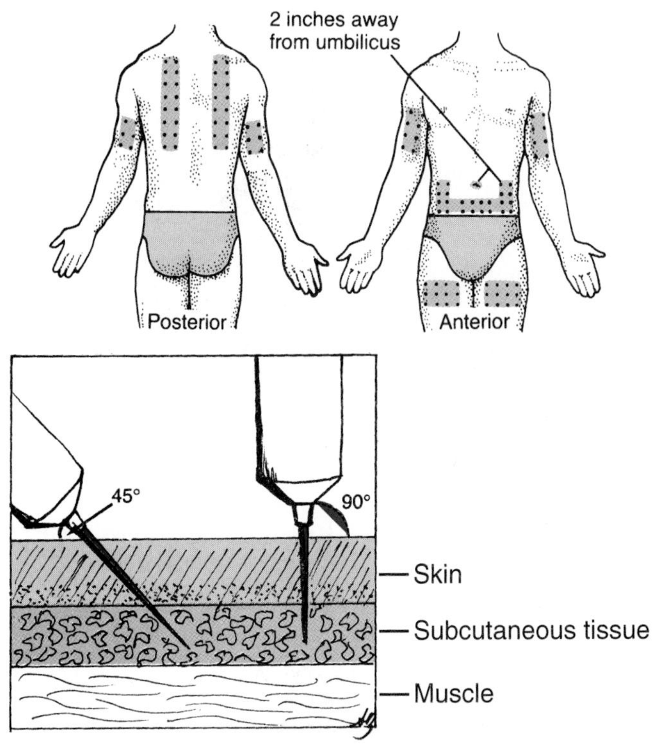

1. Use 25- to 27-gauge, 1/2 - to 5/8 -inch needle; 1-3 ml. Angle of insertion depends on body size: 90° if patient is obese. If patient is very thin, gather the skin at the area of needle insertion and administer also at a 90° angle. A 45° angle may be used in a patient with average weight.
2. Cleanse area to be injected with circular motion.
3. Avoid areas of bony prominence, major nerves, blood vessels.
4. Aspirate syringe before injecting (to avoid intra-arterial administration), except insulin, heparin.
5. Inject slowly; remove needle quickly.

IM
Injection Sites

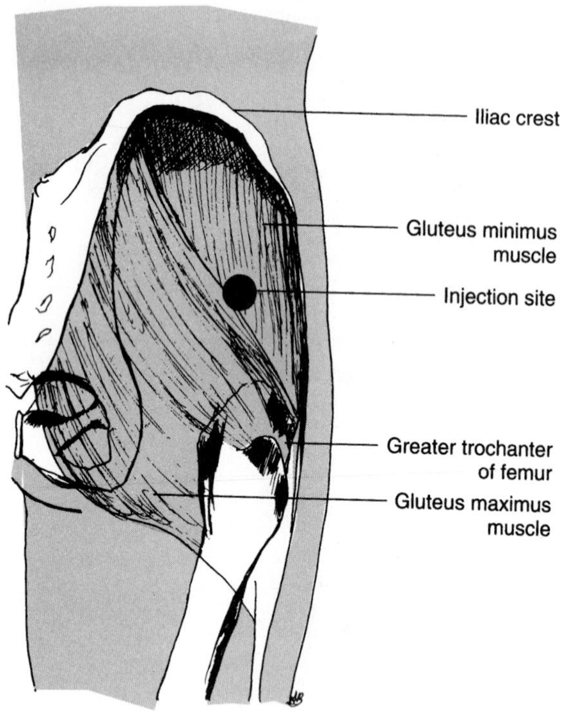

1. Use this site if volume to be injected is 1-3 ml. Use 18- to 23-gauge, 1.25- to 3-inch needle. Needle should be long enough to reach the middle of the muscle.
2. Do not use this site in children <2 yrs or in those who are emaciated. Patient should be in prone position.
3. Using 90° angle, flatten the skin area using the middle and index fingers and inject between them.

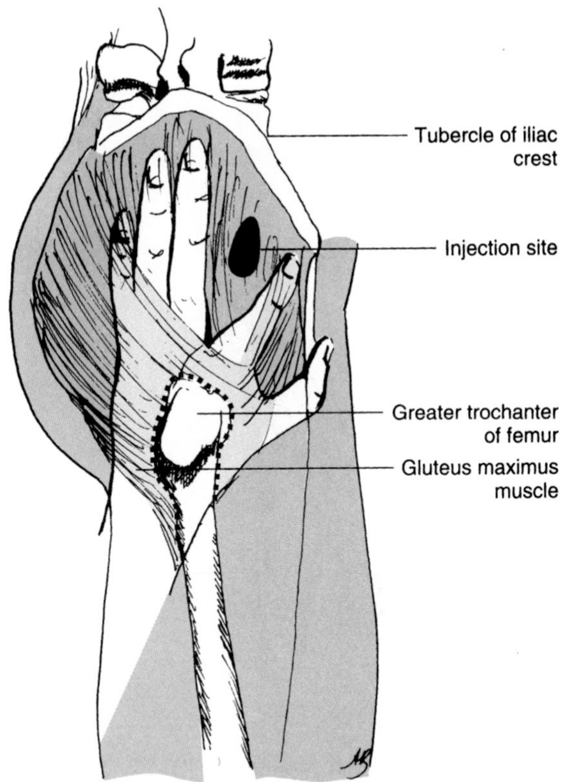

1. Use this site if volume to be injected is 1 to 5 ml. Use 20- to 23-gauge, 1.25- to 2.5-inch needle. Needle should be long enough to reach the middle of the muscle.
2. Preferred site for children younger than 7 mos. Patient should be in supine lateral position.
3. Using 90° angle, flatten the skin area using the middle and index fingers and inject between them.

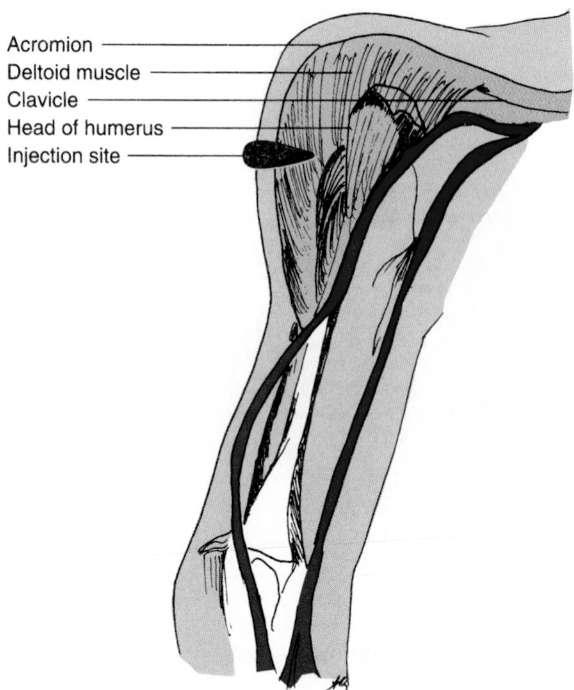

1. Use this site if volume to be injected is 0.5 to 1 ml. Use 23- to 25-gauge, 1/8- to 1/2-inch needle. Needle should be long enough to reach the middle of the muscle.
2. Patient may be in prone, sitting, supine, or standing position.
3. Using 90° angle or angled slightly toward acromion, flatten the skin area using the thumb and index finger and inject between them.

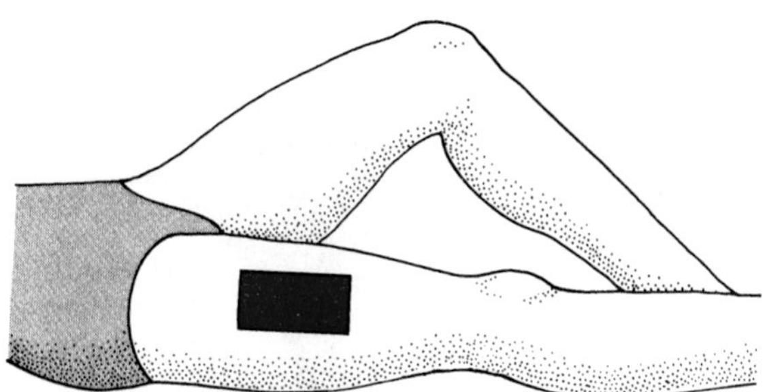

1. Anterolateral thigh is site of choice for infants and children younger than 7 mos. Use 22- to 25-gauge, 5/8- to 1-inch needle.
2. Patient may be in supine or sitting position.
3. Using 90° angle, flatten the skin area using the thumb and index finger and inject between them.

Z-TRACK TECHNIQUE

1. Draw up medication with one needle, and use new needle for injection (minimizes skin staining).
2. Administer deep IM in upper outer quadrant of buttock only (dorsogluteal site).
3. Displace the skin lateral to the injection site before inserting the needle.
4. Withdraw the needle before releasing the skin.

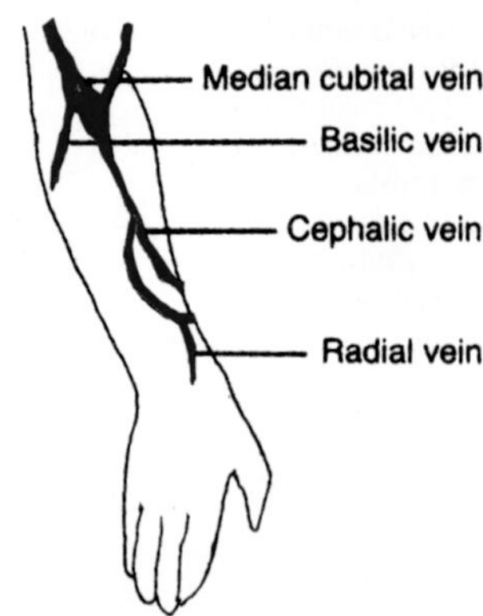

1. Medication may be given as direct IV, intermittent (piggyback), or continuous infusion.
2. Ensure that medication is compatible with solution being infused (see IV compatibility chart in this drug handbook).
3. Do not use if precipitate is present or discoloration occurs.
4. Check IV site frequently for correct infusion rate, evidence of infiltration, extravasation.

Intravenous medications are administered by the following:

1. Continuous infusing solution.
2. Piggyback (intermittent infusion).
3. Volume control setup (medication contained in a chamber between the IV solution bag and the patient).
4. Bolus dose (a single dose of medication given through an infusion line or heparin lock). Sometimes this is referred to as an IV push.

Adding medication to a newly prescribed IV bag:

1. Remove the plastic cover from the IV bag.
2. Cleanse rubber port with an alcohol swab.
3. Insert the needle into the center of the rubber port.
4. Inject the medication.
5. Withdraw the syringe from the port.
6. Gently rotate the container to mix the solution.
7. Label the IV including the date, time, medication, and dosage. It should be placed so it is easily read when hanging.
8. Spike the IV tubing and prime the tubing.

Hanging an IV piggyback (IVPB):

1. When using the piggyback method, lower the primary bag at least 6 inches below the piggyback bag.
2. Set the pump as a secondary infusion when entering the rate of infusion and volume to be infused.

3. Most piggyback medications contain 50 to 100 cc and usually infuse in 20 to 60 min, although larger-volume bags will take longer.

Administering IV medications through a volume control setup (Buretrol):

1. Insert the spike of the volume control set (Buretrol, Soluset, Pediatrol) into the primary solution container.
2. Open the upper clamp on the volume control set and allow sufficient fluid into volume control chamber.
3. Fill the volume control device with 30 cc of fluid by opening the clamp between the primary solution and the volume control device.

Administering an IV bolus dose:

1. If an existing IV is infusing, stop the infusion by pinching the tubing above the port.
2. Insert the needle into the port and aspirate to observe for a blood return.
3. If the IV is infusing properly with no signs of infiltration or inflammation, it should be patent.
4. Blood indicates that the intravenous line is in the vein.
5. Inject the medication at the prescribed rate.
6. Remove the needle and regulate the IV as prescribed.

General Index

Entries can be identified as follows: **bold** = main drug entry; *italics* = classification name

E

G

O